Management
of Urologic Malignancies

Commissioning Editor: Sue Hodgson
Project Manager: Rory MacDonald
Design Direction: Andy Chapman
Illustration Manager: Mick Ruddy
Illustrations: Lynda Payre

Management of Urologic Malignancies

Edited by

Freddie C Hamdy MD FRCSEd (Urol)
Professor and Head of Urology, School of Medicine and Biomedical Sciences,
University of Sheffield, Sheffield, UK

Joseph W Basler PhD MD
Associate Professor of Urologic Surgery, Division of Urology, University of Texas
Health Sciences Center, San Antonio, Texas, USA

David E Neal MS FRCS
Professor of Surgery, School of Surgical and Reproductive Sciences, University of
Newcastle, Newcastle upon Tyne, UK

William J Catalona MD
Professor of Urologic Surgery, Division of Urology, Washington University at St Louis,
St Louis, Missouri, USA

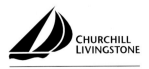

CHURCHILL
LIVINGSTONE

London • Edinburgh • New York • Philadelphia • St Louis • Sydney • Toronto 2002

Churchill Livingstone
An imprint of Elsevier Science Limited

First published 2002

ISBN 0 443 05478 9

British Library Cataloguing in Publication Data
A catalogue record for this book is available from the British Library

Library of Congress Cataloging in Publication Data
A catalog record for this book is available from the Library of Congress

Note
Medical knowledge is constantly changing. As new information becomes available, changes in treatment, procedures, equipment and the use of drugs become necessary. The editors and the publishers have taken care to ensure that the information given in this text is accurate and up to date. However, readers are strongly advised to confirm that the information, especially with regard to drug usage, complies with the latest legislation and standards of practice.

The
publisher's
policy is to use
**paper manufactured
from sustainable forests**

Printed in China by RDC Group Limited

Contents

Contributors *ix*

Preface *xv*

Part One **Bladder Cancer** 1

1   Incidence, etiology, epidemiology and genetics
     M A Knowles 3

2   Natural history
     D E Neal and T R L Griffiths 11

3   Pathology
     M C Robinson 17

4   Bladder carcinoma presentation, diagnosis and staging
     J W Basler and C Magee 37

5   Treatment of superficial transitional cell carcinoma

5.1 Surgical treatment of superficial transitional cell carcinoma
     J Carbone, C Magee and J W Basler 42

5.2 Intravesical treatment of superficial transitional cell carcinoma
     M F Sarosdy 45

5.3 The follow up of superficial bladder cancer
     R R Hall 52

6   Treatment of carcinoma in situ
     K H Kurth 57

7   Treatment of invasive transitional cell carcinoma

7.1 Surgical ablation of invasive transitional cell carcinoma of the bladder
     J P Stein and D G Skinner 67

7.2 Urinary diversion and bladder replacement
     D E Neal 76

7.3 Bladder preserving treatment for muscle invasive bladder cancer
     R R Hall 85

7.4 Systemic chemotherapy for transitional cell carcinoma of the urinary tract
     J T Roberts 88

7.5 Radiotherapy in the management of bladder cancer
     J T Roberts 94

8   Adenocarcinoma of the bladder
     J Catto and F C Hamdy 97

9.1 Squamous tumors of the urinary bladder
     M A Ghoneim 103

Part Two **Prostate Cancer** 109

10   Epidemiology and etiology
     D W Keetch 111

11   Natural history
     P Stattin and J Damber 117

12   Pathology
     D G Bostwick 127

13   Presentation and diagnosis
     M M Ahmed and J E Oesterling 139

14   Staging
     S D Graham Jr and W H Sanders 151

15   Treatment of early organ-confined disease

15.1 Issues and options: patient and tumor factors
     J W Basler 162

15.2 Watchful-waiting
     J S Palmer and G W Chodak 164

15.3 Prostate cancer treatment: radical prostatectomy for early organ-confined disease
     C E Bermejo Jr, D Shepherd and J W Basler 167

15.4 Radiotherapy for organ-confined prostate cancer
     J T Roberts 176

16   Treatment of locally advanced disease

16.1 Hormonal downstaging: myth or reality?
     M Perrotti, B R Kava, N Stroumbakis and W R Fair 180

16.2 Surgery: Is there a rationale?
     D van den Ouden and F H Schröder 186

16.3 Radiation Therapy
     C A Perez 190

16.4 Locally advanced prostate cancer – hormonal treatment
     T H Lynch and J M Fitzpatrick 203

17   Treatment of metastatic prostate cancer

17.1 Endocrine therapy
     F Rabbani and M E Gleave 210

17.2   Immediate versus deferred hormonal treatment
   D Kirk 226

17.3   Radiation therapy
   C A Perez 233

17.4   Strontium^{89} in metastatic disease
   J Bolger 242

17.5   The use of bisphosphonates in prostate carcinoma metastatic to the skeleton
   N A T Hamdy 244

17.6   The role of monoclonal antibody imaging in the management of prostate cancer
   D Khan, J C Austin and R D Williams 248

17.7   Chemotherapy in patients with androgen independent prostate cancer
   P M Swanson, E M O'Reilly and W K Kelly 254

18   Management of sequelae, voiding dysfunction and renal failure
   J W Basler and J Herschman 259

Part Three **Upper Urinary Tract, Adrenal and Retroperitoneal Tumors** *271*

19   Renal cell carcinoma: Incidence, etiology, epidemiology and genetics
   R B Nadler and J M Kozlowski 273

20   Pathology of renal tumors
   D J M DiMaio 277

21   Renal cell carcinoma: Presentation, diagnosis and staging
   D K Ornstein and G L Andriole 285

22   Surgical treatment of renal cell carcinoma

22.1   Radical nephrectomy
   R J Krane 296

22.2   Surgery for neoplastic involvement of the renal vein and inferior vena cava
   T J Polascik and F F Marshall 300

22.3   Partial radical nephrectomy
   T J Polascik and F F Marshall 304

22.4   Von Hippel-Lindau disease
   E R Maher 306

23   Minimally invasive therapy

23.1   Focused ultrasound ablation
   K U Köhrmann and P Alken 311

23.2   Focused microwave ablation and cryotherapy
   E Keahey and J W Basler 316

23.3   Laparoscopic surgery
   R V Clayman, D Hoenig and E M McDougall 316

24   Metastatic renal cancer

24.1   The role of surgery and tumor embolization
   A P Patel and J B deKernion 325

24.2   The role of immunotherapy
   C A Kim and R K Babayan 329

24.3   The role of chemotherapy
   G Veilkova and P J Selby 337

25   Transitional cell carcinoma of the upper urinary tract: Incidence, etiology, epidemiology and genetics
   S E Robbins and M J Droller 349

26   Transitional cell carcinoma of the upper urinary tract: Presentation, diagnosis and staging
   S J Savage and M J Droller 355

27   Transitional cell carcinoma of the upper urinary tract: Pathology
   D Ansell 361

28   Transitional cell carcinoma of the upper urinary tract: Surgical treatment

28.1   Nephro-ureterectomy and partial ureterectomy
   C R J Woodhouse 368

28.2   Percutaneous, ureteroscopic resection and novel approaches
   E R Goldfischer and G S Gerber 372

29   Chemotherapy and immunotherapy for upper urinary tract transitional cell carcinoma
   F S Freiha and M F Sarosdy 379

30   Rare renal tumors
   W P Tongco, T Hodges, A Szmit and J W Basler 383

31   Adrenal tumors
   C K Naughton and G L Andriole 389

32   Retroperitoneal malignancies and processes
   S B Bhayani, K Rockers, C K Naughton and J W Basler 397

33   Pathology of adrenal and retroperitoneal tumors
   D J M DiMaio 407

Part Four **Testicular Cancer** *413*

34   Incidence, etiology, epidemiology and genetics
   A Heidenreich and J W Moul 415

35   Pathology
      P Harnden and M C Parkinson 423

36   Presentation, diagnosis and staging
      M I Johnson and F C Hamdy 431

37   Carcinoma in situ
      S Fosså and E H Wanderås 435

38   Non-seminomatous germ-cell tumors

38.1 Germ cell tumors: surveillance and adjuvant
      chemotherapy
      M Cullen 440

38.2 Surgical treatment
      R S Foster and J P Donohue 445

38.3 Practical approaches to the use of
      chemotherapy
      R T D Oliver 452

39   Seminomatious germ cell tumor

39.1 Treatment of seminomas
      R S Foster and J P Donohue 462

39.2 Radiotherapy
      W G Jones 463

39.3 Background, rationale and results from use
      of chemotherapy in metastatic and localized
      seminoma
      R T D Oliver 467

40   Non-germ cell testicular tumors
      C E Bermejo and J W Basler 475

Part Five **Spermatic Cord and Scrotal
         Cancer** *479*

41   Tumors of the spermatic cord

41.1 Epidemiology and etiology
      J Petros and P D LaFontaine 482

41.2 Presentation, staging and diagnosis
      J Petros and P D LaFontaine 482

41.3 Pathology of malignant tumors of the
      spermatic cord
      P A Humphrey 483

41.4 Paratesticular sarcomas
      J Petros and P D LaFontaine 486

41.5 Radiotherapy
      J Michalski 487

41.6 Systemic chemotherapy
      A Tolcher 488

42   Tumors of the scrotum

42.1 Epidemiology and etiology
      J Petros and P D LaFontaine 489

42.2 Presentation, diagnosis & staging of
      squamous cell carcinoma
      J Petros and P D LaFontaine 490

42.3 Pathology of malignant tumors of the scrotum
      P A Humphrey 491

42.4 Surgical management of scrotal carcinoma
      J Petros 493

42.5 Radiotherapy for scrotal carcinoma
      J Michalski 494

42.6 Chemotherapy for scrotal carcinoma
      J W Basler 495

Part Six **Carcinoma of the Penis** *497*

43   Incidence, etiology and epidemiology
      S D Graham Jr and W H Sanders 499

44   Presentation, diagnosis and staging
      J Nelson and J W Basler 503

45   Pathology of carcinoma of the penis
      P A Humphrey 507

46   Surgical Management

46.1 Surgical Management
      J Petros and P D LaFontaine 515

46.2 The role of radiotherapy in the management
      of squamous carcinoma
      J T Roberts 519

46.3 Chemotherapy
      A Tolcher 521

Part Seven **Carcinoma of the Urethra** *523*

47   Carcinoma of the urethra
      C E Bermejo Jr and J W Basler 525

48   Pathology of urethral carcinoma
      P A Humphrey 529

49   Treatment *535*

49.1 Surgery
      V J Gnanapragasam and H Y Leung 538

49.2 Radiotherapy for urethral cancer
      P Grigsby 541

49.3 Chemotherapy
      J W Basler 546

Part Eight **Urological Aspects of
           Gynecologic Malignancies** *547*

50   Overview of gynecologic malignancies

50.1 Epithelial ovarian cancer
      K O Easley and D G Mutch 549

50.2   Cervical cancer
       K O Easley and D G Mutch 553

50.3   Uterine cancer
       K O Easley and D G Mutch 558

51   The role of exenteration and urinary
       diversion in gynecological malignancies
       A R Mundy and S Venn 563

52   Management of urogynecologic fistulae
       L D Kowalski and D G Mutch 571

**Part Nine Common Pediatric Urologic
             Malignancies 577**

53   Neuroblastoma
       D C S Gough and N Wright 579

54   Wilms' tumor
       H M Landa 585

55   Urologic manifestations of pediatric
       rhabdomyosarcoma
       O Lesani, E Espinosa and J W Basler 591

**Part Ten Patient Support and Palliative
            Care 595**

56   Palliative care
       P McNamara and C Regnard 597

       Index *617*

Contributors

Muzammil Ahmed
Clinical Instructor of Urology
Oakwood Healthcare System
Westland, MI, USA

Peter Alken
Professor of Urology
University Hospital
Mannheim, Germany

Gerald L Andriole
Chief and Professor of Urologic
Surgery
Washington University School of
Medicine
St Louis, MO, USA

David Ansell
Consultant Histopathologist
Nottingham City Hospital
Nottingham, UK

J C Austin
c/o D Khan
Groote Schuur Hospital
Cape Town, South Africa

Richard Babayan
Professor of Urology
Boston University School of
Medicine
Boston, MA, USA

Joseph W Basler
Associate Professor of Urologic
Surgery
Division of Urology
University of Texas Health
Sciences Center
San Antonio, TX, USA

C E Bermejo
University of Texas Health
Sciences Center
San Antonio, TX, USA

Sam B Bhayani
Assistant (House Staff)
Department of Urology
Washington University School of
Medicine
St Louis, MO, USA

Jonathan Bolger (deceased)
Formerly Consultant Clinical
Oncologist
Weston Park Hospital
Sheffield, UK

David Bostwick
Medical Director
Bostwick Laboratories
Richmond, VA, USA

Joseph M Carbone
Danville Urologic Clinic
Danville, VA, USA

James W S Catto
Research Fellow in Urology
Academic Urology Unit
University of Sheffield
Sheffield, UK

Gerald W Chodak
Clinical Instructor
Department of Urology
University of Chicago Medical
School
Chicago, IL, USA

Ralph Clayman
Professor of Urology &
Radiology
Washington University School of
Medicine
St Louis, MO, USA

Michael Cullen
Consultant Medical Oncologist
Cancer Centre at the Queen
Elizabeth Hospital
Birmingham, UK

Jan-Erik Damber
Professor of Urology
Sahlgrenska University Hospital
Gothemburg, Sweden

Dominick J DiMaio
Assistant Professor
Department of Pathology
University of Nebraska Medical
Center

Omaha, NE, USA

John P Donohue
Professor of Urology
Indiana University Hospital
Indianapolis, IN, USA

Michael J Droller
Professor of Urology
Mount Sinai Medical Center
New York, NY, USA

Kevin O Easley
Chief, Division of Gynecologic
Oncology
St John's Mercy Medical
Center
St Louis, MO, USA

Eric Espinosa
Resident Physician
Department of Urology
University of Cincinatti College
of Medicine
Cincinatti, OH, USA

William R Fair (deceased)
Formerly Chief of Urologic
Surgery
Memorial Sloan Kettering
Cancer Center
New York, NY, USA

John M Fitzpatrick
Professor of Surgery
Department of Urology
Mater Misericordiae Hospital
Dublin, Ireland

Sophie D Fosså
Professor of Medical Oncology
and Radiology
The Norwegien Radium
Hospital
Oslo, Norway

Richard S Foster
Professor of Urology
Indiana University Hospital
Indianapolis, IN, USA

Gus S Freiha
Department of Urology
McKenna Memorial Hospital
New Braunfels, TX, USA

Glenn S Gerber
Associate Professor of Surgery
University of Chicago
Chicago, IL, USA

Mohamed Ghoneim
Director
Al-Mansoura University
Hospital
Mansoura, Egypt

Martin E Gleave
Professor of Surgery
University of British Columbia
Vancouver, BC, Canada

Vincent J Gnanapragasam
CRC Clinical Research Fellow
Department of Surgery
University of Newcastle Medical
School
Newcastle upon Tyne, UK

Evan R Goldfischer
Hudson Valley Urology
Poughkeepsie, NY, USA

David C S Gough
Consultant Paediatric Urologist
Royal Manchester Children's
Hospital
Manchester, UK

Sam D Graham Jr
Urologist
Virginia Urology Center
Richmond, VA, USA

T R L Griffiths
Registrar in Urology
University of Newcastle Medical
School
Newcastle upon Tyne, UK

Perry Grigsby
Professor of Radiation
Oncology
Washington University School of
Medicine
St Louis, MO, USA

Reginald R Hall
Director, Northern Cancer
Network
Freeman Hospital
Newcastle upon Tyne, UK

Freddie C Hamdy
Professor and Head of Urology
School of Medicine and
Biomedical Sciences
University of Sheffield
Sheffield, UK

Neveen A T Hamdy
Consultant Physician and Head
of Clinical Section
Department of Endocrinology &
Metabolic Diseases
Leiden University Medical
Centre
Leiden, Netherlands

Patricia Harnden
Consultant Urological
Pathologist
ICRF Cancer Medicine Research
Unit
St James's University Hospital
Leeds, UK

Axel Heidenreich
Department of Urology
Hospital of the Phillipps-
University
Marburg, Germany

J Herschman
Division of Urology
Washington University School of
Medicine
St Louis, MO, USA

T Hodges
University of Texas Health
Sciences Center
San Antonio, TX, USA

David M Hoenig
Assistant Professor of Urology
Montefiore Medical Center
New York, NY, USA

Peter A Humphrey
Associate Professor of Pathology
and Urology

Washington University School of
Medicine
St Louis, MO, USA

Mark I Johnson
Specialist Registrar
Department of Urology
Freeman Hospital
Newcastle upon Tyne, UK

William G Jones
Consultant in Radiotherapy &
Oncology
Leeds Teaching Hospitals NHS
Trust
Leeds, UK

Bruce R Kava
Assistant Professor
Department of Urology
University of Miami
Miami, FL, USA

Eric Keahey
University of Texas Health
Science Center
San Antonio, TX, USA

David W Keetch
Urologist and Surgeon
Urology Consultants Ltd
St Louis, MO, USA

Wm Kevin Kelly
Assistant Attending Physician
Department of Medical
Oncology
Memorial Sloan-Kettering
Cancer Center
New York, NY, USA

Jean deKernion
Chair, Department of Urology
UCLA
Los Angeles, CA, USA

D Khan
Senior Specialist & Lecturer
Department of Surgery
Groote Schuur Hospital
Cape Town, South Africa

Cadence Kim
Boston University Medical Center
Boston, MA, USA

David Kirk
Consultant Urologist
Gartnavel General Hospital
Glasgow, UK

Margaret A Knowles
Professor of Experimental
Cancer Research
St James's University Hospital
Leeds, UK

Kai U Kohrmann
Associate Professor
Department of Urology
Ruprecht-Karls University
Heidelberg, Germany

Lynn D Kowalski
Women's Cancer Center of
Southern Nevada
Las Vegas, NV, USA

James M Kozlowski
Associate Professor of Urology
and Surgery
Northwestern University
Medical School
Chicago, IL, USA

Robert J Krane (deceased)
Formerly Professor of Urology
Boston University School of
Medicine
Boston, MA, USA

Karlheinz H Kurth
Professor of Urology
University of Amsterdam
Medical Center
Amsterdam
Netherlands

P D LaFontaine
c/o John Petros
Emory Clinic
Atlanta, GA, USA

Howard M Landa
Associate Professor of Surgery
Loma Linda University Urology
Medical Group
Loma Linda, CA, USA

O Lesani
University of Texas Health
Sciences Center
San Antonio, TX, USA

Hing Y Leung
Senior Lecturer in Urological
Surgery
University of Newcastle
Newcastle upon Tyne, UK

Thomas H Lynch
Consultant Urologist
Royal Victoria Hospital
Belfast, Northern Ireland

C Magee
University of Texas Health
Sciences Center
San Antonio, TX, USA

Eamonn Maher
Professor of Medical Genetics
University of Birmingham
Birmingham, UK

Fray Marshall
Professor and Chairman of
Urology
Emory University
Atlanta, GA, USA

Elspeth McDougall
Professor of Urologic Surgery
Vanderbilt University Medical
Centre
Nashville, TN, USA

Paul J G McNamara
Medical Director & Consultant
in Palliative Medicine
St Oswald's Hospice
Newcastle upon Tyne, UK

Jeff M Mickalski
Assistant Professor of Radiology
Washington University School of
Medicine
St Louis, MO, USA

Judd Moul
Professor of Surgery
Uniformed Services University
of the Health Sciences
Bethesda, MD, USA

Anthony R Mundy
Professor of Urology
University College London
Medical School
London, UK

David G Mutch
Professor of Obstetrics and
Gynecology
Washington University School of
Medicine
St Louis, MO, USA

Robert B Nadler
Assistant Professor of
Urology
Northwestern University
Medical School
Chicago, IL, USA

Cathy K Naughton
Assistant Professor Urologic
Surgery
Washington University School of
Medicine
St Louis, MO, USA

David E Neal
Professor of Surgery
& Honorary Consultant
Urologist
University of Newcastle
Newcastle upon Tyne, UK

J Nelson
University of Texas Health
Sciences Center
San Antonio, TX, USA

Joseph Oesterling
Michigan, USA

RTD Oliver
Sir Maxwell Joseph Professor in
Medical Oncology
Medical Oncology Department
St Bartholomew's Hospital
London, UK

Eileen M O'Reilly
Assistant Attending
Department of Medicine
Memorial Sloan-Kettering
Cancer Center
New York, NY, USA

David K Ornstein
Assistant Professor of Surgery
and Urology
University of North Carolina
Chapel Hill, NC, USA

Dies van den Ouden
Department of Urology
St Clara Hospital
Rotterdam, Netherlands

Jeffrey Palmer
c/o Gerald W Chodak
University of Chicago Medical
School
Chicago, IL, USA

M Constance Parkinson
Consultant Histopathologist
University College London
London, UK

Anup Patel
Consultant Urological Surgeon
St Mary's Hospital at ICSM
London, UK

Carlos Perez
Professor and Chairman
Radiation Oncology Center
Washington University Medical
Center
St Louis, MO, USA

Michael Perrotti
Assistant Professor of Surgery
Division of Urology
Robert Wood Johnson Medical
School
New Brunswick, NJ, USA

John Petros
Associate Professor of Urology
Emory Clinic
Atlanta, GA, USA

Thomas J Polascik
Assistant Professor of Urologic
Surgery
Duke University Medical
Center
Durham, NC, USA

Farhang Rabbani
Clinical Assistant Attending
Department of Urology
Memorial Sloan-Kettering
Cancer Center
New York, NY, USA

Claud F B Regnard
Consultant in Palliative
Medicine
St Oswald's Hospice
Newcastle upon Tyne, UK

S Robbins
c/o Michael J Droller
Mount Sinai Medical Center
New York, NY, USA

J Trevor Roberts
Consultant Clinical Oncologist &
Clinical Director
Northern Centre for Cancer
Treatment
Newcastle Upon Tyne, UK

Mary C Robinson
Consultant Pathologist
Freeman Hospital
Newcastle upon Tyne, UK

K Rockers
University of Texas Health
Sciences Center
San Antonio, TX, USA

William H Sanders
Emory University School of
Medicine
Atlanta, GA, USA

Michael Sarosdy
South Texas Urology and
Urologic Oncology
San Antonio, TX, USA

Stephen J Savage
Assistant Professor of
Urology
Mount Sinai Medical Center
New York, NY, USA

Fritz H Schröder
Professor of Urology
Erasmus University
Rotterdam, Netherlands

P Selby
Professor of Cancer Medicine
ICRF Cancer Medicine Research
Unit
St James's University Hospital
Leeds, UK

D Shepherd
University of Texas Health
Sciences Center
San Antonio, TX, USA

Donald Skinner
Professor and Chairman
Department of Urology
Keck School of Medicine
Los Angeles, CA, USA

Par Stattin
Associate Professor of Urology
Umea University Hospital
Umea, Sweden

John Stein
Fellow in Genitourinary Oncology
USC
Los Angeles, CA, USA

Nicholas Stroumbakis
Fellow in Urological Oncology
Memorial Sloan Kettering
Cancer Center
New York, NY, USA

Paul Swanson
Memorial Sloan Kettering
Cancer Center
New York, NY, USA

A Szmit
Erasmus University
Rotterdam, Netherlands

Anthony Tolcher
Associate Director Clinical
Research
Institute for Drug Development
University of Texas Health
Science Center
San Antonio, TX, USA

W P Tongco
Chief Resident
Division of Urology
University of Texas Health
Science Center
San Antonio, TX, USA

Galina Velikova
Senior Clinical Research Fellow
ICRF Medical Oncology Unit
St James's University Hospital
Leeds, UK

Susanne Venn
Consultant Urologist
St Richards Hospital
Chichester, UK

Eva H Wanderås
Senior Consultant
Department of Medical
Oncology and Radiotherapy
The Norwegian Radium Hospital
Oslo, Norway

Richard D Williams
Professor & Head
Department of Urology
University of Iowa
Iowa City, IA, USA

Christopher Woodhouse
Consultant Urologist
Royal Marsden Hospital
London, UK

Neville B Wright
Consultant Paediatric
Radiologist
Royal Liverpool Childrens
Hospital
Liverpool, UK

Preface

Any reader in search of 'novelties', whose scanning eyes notice the title of our book on a shelf will undoubtedly wonder why, yet again, there is another publication on urologic cancer. Indeed, bookshelves and medical libraries are inundated with oncologic textbooks, references and other literature by prestigious authors. Very few, however, give short concise information and practical updated, state-of-the-art advice on how to manage patients in day-to-day routine urologic practice, away from the highly specialized oncologic institutions. In recent years, as a result of the rapid expansion of knowledge in oncology, and growing controversies in the managment of certain malignancies, the production of a book which would appeal to a broad readership has become an increasingly difficult task, if not a real challenge. Such a work becomes either too detailed for busy clinicians, or too superficial for those who are closely concerned with the subject. In routine daily practice, the general urologist is frequently faced with patients suffering from a urologic malignancy and has to initiate appropriate investigations and treatment. Whilst in some countries, the office urologist will decide to refer the patient to an appropriate oncologic center for specialized treatment, many general urologists will prefer to manage the patient themselves.

This book is not intended to be a textbook, nor is it meant to be a reference for 'difficult cases'. It is dedicated to the 'urologist' across the world. Our ambition is to provide pragmatic, up-to-date information about the various common malignancies encountered in day to day practice in urology, and how the authors believe they should be optimally managed, with views from either side of the Atlantic.

To satisfy the different levels of interest and readership, a number of simple management algorithms are provided for individual conditions which are further expanded in the text, and a comprehensive list of references is included to enable the reader to continue in-depth study with the source literature, if they so wish. We would be pleased if this work achieves its goal to help as many readers as possible in making the best informed decisions when managing their cancer patients.

F C Hamdy
J W Basler
D E Neal
W J Catalona

February 2002

PART ONE
Bladder cancer

Chapter 1
Incidence, etiology, epidemiology and genetics

Chapter 2
Natural history

Chapter 3
Pathology

Chapter 4
Bladder carcinoma presentation, diagnosis and staging

Chapter 5
Treatment of superficial transitional cell carcinoma

5.1 Surgical treatment of superficial transitional cell carcinoma

5.2 Intravesical treatment of superficial transitional cell carcinoma

5.3 The follow up of superficial bladder cancer

Chapter 6
Treatment of carcinoma in situ

Chapter 7
Treatment of invasive transitional cell carcinoma

7.1 Surgical ablation of invasive transitional cell carcinoma of the bladder

7.2 Urinary diversion and bladder replacement

7.3 Bladder preserving treatment for muscle invasive bladder cancer

7.4 Systemic chemotherapy for transitional cell carcinoma of the urinary tract

7.5 Radiotherapy in the management of bladder cancer

Chapter 8
Adenocarcinoma of the bladder

Chapter 9
Squamous tumors of the urinary bladder

1 Incidence, etiology, epidemiology and genetics

M A Knowles

Incidence

In the United Kingdom, bladder cancer accounts for 12 700 new cancer cases per annum and 5300 deaths. This represents 4.2% of all new cancer cases registered and 3.3% of cancer deaths[1]. Similar statistics have been reported from the United States[2]. In men bladder cancer is now the fourth most common cancer, representing 6% of new cancers. In women, bladder cancer represents 2% of cancers diagnosed. Peak prevalence is in the sixth and seventh decades of life and both incidence and prevalence are rising[3,4]. In Northern Europe and North America, the majority (>90%) of bladder tumors are transitional cellcarcinomas (TCC) and the remainder are squamous cell carcinoma, adenocarcinoma and undifferentiated carcinoma[5].

In regions of endemic schistosomiasis (bilharzia), a very different situation exists. In Egypt for example, where schistosomiasis is hyperendemic, more than 20% of the population are infected[6,7] and bladder cancer is the most common cancer, representing 30% of all recorded cases[8]. Schistosomiasis-associated bladder cancer shows an earlierpeak incidence, in the fourth and fifth decades of life, and there is a preponderance of squamous cell carcinoma rather than TCC[9,10].

Etiology and epidemiology

Although there is evidence for a familial association in some cases[11,] the vast majority of patients with bladder cancer have no obvious family history. However, the contribution of environmental risk factors is clear cut. Bladder cancer is the best known example of a human cancer linked to occupational exposure to environmental carcinogens. Dyestuff production, rubber manufacturing, the textile and leather industries, printing, the metal industry and work involving exposure to petroleum products have all been clearly implicated[12,13]. Several chemicals associated with these occupations including 4-aminobiphenyl, 2-naphthylamine, benzidine, 4,4´-methylenebis(2-chloroaniline) and o-toluidine are considered to be human carcinogens[14]. Cigarette smoking is also a significant risk factor for TCC[15,16]. Schistosomiasis, smoking and recurrent urinary tract infections are implicated as risk factors for squamous cell carcinoma of the bladder[17,18]. The association with smoking is supported by the presence of aromatic amines in cigarette smoke[19,] the finding of high levels of mutagenic compounds in the urine of smokers[20] and the finding of higher levels of aromatic amine DNA adducts in smokers than in non-smokers[21]. Several other risk factors have been suggested, including use of dietarysweeteners, coffee drinking and excessive use of phenacetin-containing analgesics. Apart from use of phenacetin[22] the role of these factors remains controversial. The contribution of the various risk factors to the total number of new bladder cancer cases per annum is not entirely clear but it has been estimated that 50% of bladder tumors in men and 25% in women are smoking-attributable[16] and that 10–50% may be related to occupational exposure[23]. Thecarcinogenic activity of arylamines is generated followingN-hydroxylation to N-hydroxyarylamines and subsequent O-acetylation (for review see [24]). These compounds may also be N-acetylated which effectively competes with the N-oxidation pathway and provides a means of detoxification. In man, interindividual variability in the metabolism of arylamines has been

3

identified and attributed to genetic differences at one of the N-acetyltransferase loci (NAT2). A series of mutant alleles of NAT2 have been characterized which give rise to so-called 'slow' and 'fast' acetylator phenotypes. Several studies link the 'slow' acetylator phenotype which is present in 50% of individuals to a higher risk of bladder cancer[25,26]. It seems likely that other inherited variations in the ability to activate or detoxify other types of carcinogen may also have considerable impact.

In schistosomiasis-associated bladder cancer, whilst the link between infection and cancer development is clear, the mechanisms involved are not fully understood[27]. The infection induces chronic inflammation in the bladder due to the deposition of large numbers of eggs in the sub-epithelial tissues. This eventually leads to fibrosis, stenosis and urinary retention which is commonly associated with recurrent bacterial infections. The urine of infected individuals has been shown to contain higher levels of N-nitroso compounds than that from uninfected individuals[28,29]. These may be exogenous in origin (e.g. from diet) or may be produced endogenously through the action of bacteria or inflammatory cells.

Carcinogenesis is a multistep process involving the sequential acquisition of a series of genetic alterations. The role of mutagens in this process is clear. However, in addition to the effect of increasing the dose or the duration of exposure to mutagenic compounds, it can be envisaged that factors which increase cell turnover in the urothelium are likely to affect tumor development. Both urinary tract infection and schistosomiasis may have this effect, as may various other benign pathologies. For more detailed discussion on the epidemiology of bladder cancer, see [11,12,30,31].

Genetics

Many genetic changes have now been described in carcinoma of the bladder[32,33]. These include alterations to known proto-oncogenes and tumor suppressor genes and some non-random alterations (mostly deletions or amplifications of specific chromosomal regions) which are likely to identify the location of hitherto unknown tumor suppressor genes or proto-oncogenes (Tables 1.1 and 1.2). Since most studies have been carried out in Europe and the United States, the tumors examined are largely TCCs. Only a small amount of information is available concerning schistosomiasis-associated squamous cell carcinomas (see below).

There are also numerous reports of alterations in gene expression in bladder cancer which are beyond the scope of this discussion. These probably represent downstream consequences of primary genetic events, several of which may be very useful prognostic markers (e.g. expression of E-cadherin and EGFR[34,35]).

TCC: proto-oncogenes

Oncogenic activation of several genes has been described in TCC. Although the first identification of a mutated HRAS gene was in a bladder tumor cell line, the absolute frequency of RAS-gene mutation in bladder tumor tissues is not clear. Estimates range from 6–36%[36,37]. No association of RAS-gene mutation with specific tumor histopathology or clinical outcome has been demonstrated.

ERBB2 encodes a receptor-like protein with homology with the epidermal growth factor receptor (EGFR). This gene is amplified in approximately 14% of TCCs at presentation resulting in expression of high levels of the pro-

Table 1.1   Oncogenes genetically altered in TCC

Gene	Observation in tumors	Association with clinical parameters	References
HRAS	mutated in 6–44%	grade	36, 90, 91
ERBB2	amplified in 10–14%	grade/stage recurrence	38–40, 92, 93
CCND1	amplified in 10–20%	no association with grade and stage	41, 42, 94
(MYC) or another 8q gene	8q gain MYC overexpression	grade/stage	95, 96
1q22–24	amplification	grade/stage	45, 46
3p24	amplification	grade/stage	44, 45
6p22	amplification	grade/stage	43–45
8q21–22	amplification	grade/stage	43, 45
10p13–14	amplification	grade/stage	43–45
10q22–23	amplification	grade/stage	46
12q15	amplification	grade/stage	43–45
20q	amplification	grade/stage	43, 45, 46

Table 1.2   Tumor suppressor genes and predicted suppressor gene loci implicated in transitional cell carcinoma

Gene/cytogenetic location	Frequency of deletion/mutation	Association with clinical parameters	References
RB (13q14)	30%	high stage progression reduced survival	56–58
TP53 (17p13)	10–70%	grade and stage (≥T2 50–70%) progression reduced survival	50, 52, 97, 98
INK4A (p16) (9p21) p14/ARF (9p21) INK4B (p15) (9p21)	20–45%	? in vivo immortalization in vitro	72, 73
PTEN (10q23)	10–30%	high stage	84, 85
PTCH (9q22)	LOH in ~50% mutation identified in 2/54 tumors	none	76
TSC1 (9q34)	LOH in ~50% mutation identified in some cases	none	75
DBCCRI (9q32–33)	LOH in 50% no mutations identified DNA hypermethylation	none	74
18q (DCC/SMAD4)	no mutation analysis done to date	high stage	81
3p	48%	stage	78
4p	22%	none	99, 100
4q	24%	grade/stage	100
8p	23%	grade/stage	77, 101, 102
11p	40%	grade	80, 103, 104
11q	15%	?	80, 105
14q	10–40%	stage	79

tein product. The majority of tumors with amplification are of high grade and stage, suggesting that this may represent a useful prognostic indicator[38–40]. This has not yet been adequately assessed.

Approximately 20% of TCCs have amplification of a region of the long arm of chromosome 11 (11q13)[41]. Discontinuity in the amplified sequences indicates that more than one critical gene may be present. The majority of the amplicons focus on the cyclin D1 (*CCND1*) and *EMS1* genes and tumors with amplification over-express the protein products[42]. *CCND1* plays a critical role in regulating progression from G1 to S phase in the cell cycle and over-expression would be predicted to result in deregulation of the cell cycle.

It is difficult to carry out a comprehensive search for activated oncogenes, since activation may occur by diverse mechanisms (e.g. mutation, gene amplification or over-expression following genetic translocation). Other proto-oncogenes may therefore play a role. Recent results using comparative genomic hybridization (CGH), a technique in which the representation of all genomic sequences in tumor DNA is assessed, pinpoint several additional regions of DNA amplification in bladder tumors (Table 1)[43–46].

TCC: tumor suppressor genes

Most genetic alterations identified in TCC to date involve inactivation of known tumor suppressor genes or non-random deletions which are believed to identify the locations of as yet unknown tumor suppressor genes (Table 1.2). Several of these are reflected by cytogenetic findings[47]. Inactivation of the function of tumor suppressor genes including the retinoblastoma gene *RB*, commonly involves deletion or mutation of both alleles. In sporadic tumors such as TCC, this can be identified by loss of heterozygosity (LOH), i.e. deletion of one parental allele in particular regions of the genome. The characterization of thousands of common genetic polymorphisms in recent years has greatly facilitated the process of identifying and precisely mapping regions of LOH[48]. In the case of *RB* and *TP53*, a gross deletion of one allele (LOH) is generally associated with an inactivating mutation within the gene on the retained allele.

TP53 on chromosome 17p is the most frequently mutated gene in human cancers. Deletion of 17p and mutation of *TP53* have been frequently reported in TCC. The frequency of 17p LOH is significantly higher in tumors of high grade and/or stage and in muscle invasive TCC has been found in 50% to 70% of cases[49,50]. Single strand conformation polymorphism (SSCP) analysis and/or sequence analysis have been used to determine the frequency of *TP53* gene mutation. In general, mutations are found in tumors with 17p LOH. Particular attention has been paid to the mutational spectrum found, since this may reflect the nature of the inducing carcinogens[51]. Given the known association with cigarette smoking, it might be expected that specific mutations would be present in the tumors of smokers compared with non-smokers. Overall, the spectrum of point mutations found is intermediate between that for lung cancer and colorectal cancer[50,52]. This may reflect the known effect of smoking but also suggests that other mutagens or mechanisms of mutation are involved.

The association between *TP53* mutation and tumor grade and stage appears to be of potential prognostic significance. The ease with which mutant p53 with increased protein half-life can be detected by immunohistochemistry provides a simple means to detect mutations. Several studies have demonstrated a significant difference in the rate of progression of p53-positive and p53-negative staining cases[53–55].

Loss of function of *RB* has been demonstrated in TCC. LOH within the gene has been detected in 29% of tumors and is associated with high tumor grade and stage[56]. LOH correlates with loss of pRb protein expression and there is evidence that this may represent a useful prognostic indicator. Two studies have shown a poorer outcome in patients whose tumors lacked detectable pRb protein[57,58]. pRb negative regions in pRb positive tumors have been described[58]. indicating that this may be a late change during bladder tumor progression. Since pRb protein can be demonstrated with ease by immunocytochemistry, as for p53 this may be added to the routine histopathologic assessment of bladder tumors.

Recent elucidation of the control of cell cycle progression, particularly at the G1 checkpoint, has identified several molecules known to be involved in TCC which are implicated. These include p16, p14/ARF, pRB, p53 and cyclin D1, molecules involved in the so-called pRB and p53 pathways[59]. It is now known that p14/ARF and p53 provide a fail-safe mechanism for preventing progression from G1 to S phase in the presence of DNA damage or inappropriate expression of oncogenes and that this can operate even if the pRB pathway is damaged. Thus it can be predicted that inactivation of both p53 and pRB may have more serious consequences than inactivation of either gene alone. Several recent studies on TCC have now confirmed that tumors with inactivation of *TP53* and *RB* have a worse prognosis than tumors with alteration to either gene alone[60–62].

Several other common regions of LOH have been found. The most frequent are on chromosome 9[63]. LOH is commonly found at all chromosome 9 loci examined, indicating likely loss of an entire homologue. This is compatible with the finding of monosomy 9 by cytogenetic analysis[47]. The frequency of chromosome 9 deletion is high (~60%) and is similar in TCC of all grades and stages, indicating that this may represent an early genetic change in bladder cancer development. It is now thought that loss of the entire chromosome indicates the likely presence of tumor suppressor loci on both 9p and 9q[63–67] and the critical regions of deletion have been mapped. At least three regions exist on the long arm[68–70] and one on the short arm at 9p21[65,71]. Within this latter region, the genes *INK4A* (p16), *INK4B* (p15) and p14/*ARF* have been identified[72,73]. Unlike other tumor suppressor genes, inactivation of *INK4A* in virtually all bladder tumors involves deletion of both alleles (homozygous deletion) rather than deletion of one allele and localized mutation of the other allele. p15 and the unrelated cell cycle regulator p14/*ARF* have not been studied for mutation in TCC but, since both lie within the region of homozygous deletion in the majority of bladder tumors, it is possible that deletion of any or all of these genes may confer a growth advantage.

On 9q, candidate genes *DBCCR1* and *TSC1* have been identified at 9q32–33[69,74] and 9q34[75] respectively. In the most proximal region, the Gorlin syndrome gene *PTCH* represents a candidate and a small number of mutations have been identified within the gene[76]. Functional confirmation of the involvement of all these 9q genes is now awaited.

Other common regions of LOH include 3p, 4p, 4q, 8p, 10q 11p, 11q and 18q[77–83] (Table 1.2). The likely target of 10q deletion is the gene *PTEN*[84,85]. Possible targets of 18q deletion are *DCC* and *SMAD4*. Except in the case of chromosome 4, LOH of all these chromosome arms is significantly more common in tumors of high grade and stage. Muscle-invasive tumors often contain high numbersof inflammatory cells and dissection of tumor free of muscle is difficult so that DNA preparations commonly contain much more normal cell DNA than those from papillary tumors. Detection of LOH is more difficult in this material and the frequencies of involvement of genes on 3p, 8p, 11p and 18q are probably higher than our current estimates. Contamination of extracted papillary tumor DNA with normal DNA is less of a problem. It seems therefore that only chromosome 9 LOH is common in these, the majority of all bladder cancers. Undoubtedly, other genetic alterations exist in these tumors but their identification may require novel approaches.

Genetic alterations in schistosomiasis-associated bladder cancer

The molecular genetic events underlying tumor progression in schistosomiasis-associated bladder cancer are not well characterized. Four studies have examined *TP53* mutation in a total of 126 tumors and found an overall mutation frequency of 42%[50,86-88]. Three tumors in a series of 21 examined by Ramchuuren *et al.*[87] contained *HRAS* mutations, a frequency similar to that in TCC. We have recently examined a series of 80 bladder tumors from Egypt for LOH on chromosome arms commonly deleted in TCC[89]. This partial allelotype revealed similar frequencies of LOH on 3p, 4p, 4q, 8p, 11p, 13q, 17p and 18q to those found in muscle invasive TCC. However, LOH on 9p was more frequent than in TCC and that on 9q significantly less frequent.

Potential use of genetic markers in bladder cancer

Since the phenotype of a tumor is almost certainly dictated to a great extent by its genotype, specific genetic information should greatly improve our understanding of the diverse clinical phenotypes of human bladder cancers. Already it is clear that PCR-based analysis can identify small numbers of tumor cells in urine. Undoubtedly this will lead to improvements in diagnosis, screening of at-risk populations and predicting prognosis. It may also provide a useful non-invasive follow up screen in patients post-resection. Finally it can be envisaged that the identification of commonly altered genes, e.g. *CDKN2*, will provide the basis for development of novel therapeutic regimens.

References

1. HMSO. *Cancer registration statistics*. England and Wales. 1994.
2. Boring CC, Squires TS, Tong T. Cancer Statistics CA 1993; 43:7–26.
3. Feldman AR, Kessler L, Myers MH, Naughton MD. The prevalence of cancer: estimates based on the Connecticut Tumor Registry. *N Engl J Med* 1986;3115:1394–1397.
4. Davies JM. Occupational and environmental factors in bladder cancer. In: Chisholm G and Innes Williams D (eds) *Scientific foundations of urology*, 2nd edn. London: Heinemann, 1982, pp. 723–727.
5. Koss LG. *Tumors of the urinary bladder*. Atlas of Tumor Pathology, 2nd Series. Fascicle 11. Washington D.C.: Armed Forces Institute of Pathology, 1975.
6. World Health Organisation. Progress in assessment of morbidity due to *Schistosoma haematobium* infection. A review of recent literature. Geneva: WHO, 1987.
7. World Health Organisation. *The control of schistosomiasis*. Report of a WHO Expert Committee. Geneva: WHO, 1985.
8. Ibrahim S. Site distribution of cancer in Egypt: twelve years experience (1970–1981). In: Gjorgove A and Ismail A (eds) *Cancer prevention in developing countries*. Oxford: Pergamon Press, 1986. pp. 45–50.
9. El-Bolkainy MN, Mokhtar NM, Ghoneim MA, Hussein MH. The impact of schistosomiasis on the pathology of bladder carcinoma. *Cancer* 1981; 48:2643–2648.
10. IARC. *Schistosomes, liver flukes and* Helicobacter pylori. Lyon: International Agency for Research on Cancer, 1994.
11. Kantor AF, Hartge P, Hoover RN, Fraumeni JF, Jr. Familial and environmental interactions in bladder cancer risk. *Int J Cancer* 1985; 35:703–706.
12. BAUS Subcommittee on Industrial Bladder Cancer. Occupational bladder cancer: A guide for clinicians. *Br J Urology* 1988; 61:183–191.
13. Cole P, Hoover R, Friedell GH. Occupation and cancer of the lower urinary tract. *Cancer* 1972; 29:1250–1260.
14. Tomatis L, Agthe C, Bartsch H, Huff J, Montesano R, Saracci R et al. Evaluation of the carcinogenicity of chemicals: a review of the Monograph Program of the International Agency for Research on Cancer (1971 to 1977). *Cancer Res* 1978; 38:877–885.
15. Armstrong B, Doll R. Bladder cancer mortality in England and Wales in relation to cigarette smoking and saccharin consumption. *Br J Prev Soc Med* 1974; 28:233–240.
16. IARC. Mongraphs on the evaluation of carcinogenic risk of chemicals to humans: tobacco smoking. Geneva: World Health Organisation, 1986.
17. Kantor AF, Hartge P, Hoover RN, Narayana AS, Sullivan JW, Fraumeni Jr JF. Urinary tract infection and risk of bladder cancer. *Am J Epidemiol* 1984; 119:510–515.
18. Kantor AF, Hartge P, Hoover RN, Fraumeni Jr JF. Epidemiological characteristics of squamous cell carcinoma and adenocarcinoma of the bladder. *Cancer Res* 1988; 48:3853–3855.
19. Patrianakos C, Hoffmann D. Chemical studies of tobacco smoke. LXIV. On the analysis of aromatic amines in cigarette smoke. *J Anal Chem* 1979; 3:150–154.
20. Connor TH, Ramanujam VMS, Ward Jr JB, Legator MS. The identification and characterisation of a urinary mutagen resulting from cigarette smoke. *Mutat Res* 1983; 113:161–172.
21. Bryant M, Skipper PL, Tannenbaum SR, Maclure M. Hemoglobin adducts of 4-aminobiphenyl in smokers and non-smokers. *Cancer Res* 1987; 47:602–608.
22. McCredie M, Stewart JH, Ford JM, MacLennan RA. Phenacetin-containing analgesics and cancer of the bladder in women. *Br J Urology* 1983; 55:220–224.
23. Higginson J. Chronic toxicology – an epidemiologist's approach to the problem of carcinogenesis. *Essay Toxicol* 1976; 77:29–72.
24. Kadlubar FF, Butler MA, Kaderlik KR, Chou H-C, Lang NP. Polymorphisms for aromatic amine metabolism in humans: relevance for human carcinogenesis. *Env Health Persp* 1992; 98:69–74.
25. Cartwright RA, Glashan RW, Rogers HJ, Ahmod RA, Barham-Hall D, Higgins E, et al. The role of N-acetyltransferase in bladder carcinogenesis: a pharmacogentic epidemiological approach to bladder cancer. *Lancet* 1982; ii:842–846.
26. Risch A, Wallace DMA, Bathers S, Sim E. Slow N-acetylation genotype is a susceptibility factor in occupational and smoking related bladder cancer. *Hum Mol Genet* 1995; 4:231–236.
27. World Health Organisation. Possible basic mechanisms of carcinogenesis in schistosomiasis and other trematode infections. 1983. Technical Report Series WHO/83. 74. WHO, Geneva.
28. El-Merzabani MM, El-Aaser AA, Zakhary NI. A study on the aetiological factors of bilharzial bladder cancer in Egypt: 1. Nitrosamines and their precursors in urine. *Eur J Cancer* 1979; 15:287–291.
29. Tricker AR, Mostafa MH, Speiglhalder B, Preussmann R. Urinary excretion of nitrate, nitrite and N-nitroso compounds in schistosomiasis and bladder cancer patients. *Carcinogenesis* 1989; 10:547–552.
30. Wynder EL, Goldsmith R. The epidemiology of bladder cancer: a second look. *Cancer* 1977; 40:1246–1268.
31. Thompson IM, Fair WR. The epidemiology of bladder cancer. *AUA Update Ser* 1989; 8:210–215.
32. Knowles MA. Genetics of transitional cell carcinoma: progress and potential clinical application. *B. J. U. Int.* 1999; 84:412–427.
33. Knowles MA. Molecular genetics of bladder cancer: pathways of development and progression. In: Oliver RTD and Coptcoat MJ (eds) *Bladder cancer*. Cold Spring Harbor: Cold Spring Harbor Press, 1998.
34. Bringuier PP, Umbas R, Schaafsma E, Karthaus HFM, Debruyne FMJ, Schalken JA. Decreased E-cadherin immunoreactivity correlates with

poor survival in patients with bladder tumors. *Cancer Res* 1993; **53**:3241–3245.

35. Neal DE, Sharples L, Smith K, Fenelly J, Hall RR, Harris AL. The epidermal growth factor receptor and the prognosis of bladder cancer. *Cancer* 1990; **65**:1619–1625.

36. Knowles MA, Williamson M. Mutation of H-ras is infrequent in bladder cancer: confirmation by single-strand conformation polymorphism analysis, designed restriction fragment length polymorphisms, and direct sequencing. *Cancer Res* 1993; **53**(1):133–139.

37. Czerniak B, Deitch D, Simmons H, Etkind P, Herz F, Koss LG. Ha-*ras* gene codon 12 mutation and DNA ploidy in urinary bladder carcinoma. *Br J Cancer* 1990; **62**:762–763.

38. Sauter G, Moch H, Moore D, Carroll P, Kerchmann R, Chew K *et al.* Heterogeneity of *erb*B-2 gene amplification in bladder cancer. *Cancer Res* 1993; **53**:2199–2203.

39. Coombs LM, Pigott DA, Sweeney E, Proctor AJ, Eydmann ME, Parkinson C *et al.* Amplification and over-expression of c-erbB-2 in transitional cell carcinoma of the urinary bladder. *Br J Cancer* 1991; **63**(4):601–608.

40. Sato K, Moriyama M, Mori S, Saito M, Watanuki K, Terada E *et al.* An immunohistologic evaluation of c-erbB-2 gene product in patients with urinary bladder carcinoma. *Cancer* 1992; **70**:2493–2498.

41. Proctor AJ, Coombs LM, Cairns JP, Knowles MA. Amplification at chromosome 11q13 in transitional cell tumors of the bladder. *Oncogene* 1991; **6**:789–795.

42. Bringuier PP, Tamimi Y, Schuuring E, Schalken J. Expression of cyclin D1 and EMS1 in bladder tumors: relationship with chromosome 11q13 amplification. *Oncogene* 1996; **12**:1747–1753.

43. Kallioniemi A, Kallioniemi O-P, Citro G, Sauter G, DeVries S, Kerschmann R *et al.* Identification of gains and losses of DNA sequences in primary bladder cancer by comparative genomic hybridisation. *Genes, Chromosomes and Cancer* 1995; **12**:213–219.

44. Richter J, Jiang F, Gorog JP, Sartorius G, Egenter C, Gasser TC *et al.* Marked genetic differences between stage pTa and stage pT1 papillary bladder cancer detected by comparative genomic hybridization. *Cancer Res* 1997; **57**(14):2860–2864.

45. Richter J, Beffa L, Wagner U, Schraml P, Gasser TC, Moch H *et al.* Patterns of chromosomal imbalances in advanced urinary bladder cancer detected by comparative genomic hybridization. *Am J Pathol* 1998; **153**(5):1615–1621.

46. Hovey RM, Chu L, Balazs M, DeVries S, Moore D, Sauter G *et al.* Genetic alterations in primary bladder cancers and their metastases. *Cancer Res* 1998; **58**(16):3555–3560.

47. Sandberg AA, Berger CS. Review of chromosome studies in urological tumors. II. Cytogenetics and molecular genetics of bladder cancer. *J Urol* 1994; **151**:545–560.

48. Knowles MA. Localisation of tumor suppressor genes by loss of heterozygosity and homozygous deletion analysis. In: Adolph KW (Ed.) *Human molecular genetics.* New York: Academic Press, 1996, pp. 113–136.

49. Fujimoto K, Yamada Y, Okajima E, Kakizoe T, Sasaki H, Sugimura T *et al.* Frequent association of p53 gene mutation in invasive bladder cancer. *Cancer Res* 1992; **52**:1393–1398.

50. Habuchi T, Takahashi R, Yamada H, Ogawa O, Kakehi Y, Ogura K *et al.* Influence of cigarette smoking and schistosomiasis on p53 gene mutation in urothelial cancer. *Cancer Res* 1993; **53**:3795–3799.

51. Greenblatt MS, Bennett WP, Hollstein M, Harris CC. Mutations in the p53 tumor suppressor gene: clues to cancer etiology and molecular pathogenesis. *Cancer Res* 1994; **54**:4855–4878.

52. Spruck CH, III, Rideout WM, III, Olumi AF, Ohnesit, PF *et al.* Distinct pattern of p53 mutations in bladder cancer: relationship to tobacco usage. *Cancer Res* 1993; **53**:1162–1166.

53. Soini Y, Turpeenniemi-Hujanen T, Kamel D, Autio-Harmainen H, Risteli J, Risteli L *et al.* p53 immunohistochemistry in transitional cell carcinoma and dysplasia of the urinary bladder correlates with disease progression. *Br J Cancer* 1993; **68**:1029–1035.

54. Sarkis AS, Zhang Z-F, Cordon-Cardo C, Melamed J, Dalbagni G, Sheinfeld J *et al.* p53 nuclear overexpression and disease progression in Ta bladder carcinoma. *Intl J Oncology* 1993; **3**:355–360.

55. Esrig D, Elmajian D, Groshen S, Freeman JA, Stein JP, Chen S-C *et al.* Accumulation of nuclear p53 and tumor progression in bladder cancer. *N Engl J Med* 1994; **331**:1259–1264.

56. Cairns P, Proctor AJ, Knowles MA. Loss of heterozygosity at the *RB* locus is frequent and correlates with muscle invasion in bladder carcinoma. *Oncogene* 1991; **6**:2305–2309.

57. Cordon-Cardo C, Wartinger D, Petrylak D, Dalbagni G, Fair WR, Fuks Z *et al.* Altered expression of the retinoblastoma gene product: prognostic indicator in bladder cancer. *J Natl Cancer Inst* 1992; **84**:1251–1256.

58. Logothetis CJ, Xu H-J, Ro JY, Hu S-X, Sahin A, Ordonez N *et al.* Altered expression of retinoblastoma protein and known prognostic variables in locally advanced bladder cancer. *J Natl Cancer Inst* 1992; **84**:1256–1261.

59. Paulovich AG, Toczyski DP, Hartwell LH. When checkpoints fail. *Cell* 1997; **88**(3):315–321.

60. Grossman HB, Liebert M, Antelo M, Dinney CP, Hu SX, Palmer JL *et al.* p53 and RB expression predict progression in T1 bladder cancer. *Clin Cancer Res* 1998; **4**(4):829–834.

61. Cote RJ, Esrig D, Groshen S, Jones PA, Skinner DG. p53 and treatment of bladder cancer. *Nature* 1997; **385**:123–125.

62. Cordon-Cardo C, Zhang Z-F, Dalbagni G, Drobnjak M, Charytonowicz E, Hu S-X *et al.* Cooperative effects of p53 and pRB alterations in primary superficial bladder tumors. *Cancer Res* 1997; **57**:1217–1221.

63. Linnenbach AJ, Pressler LB, Seng BA, Simmel BS, Tomaszewski JE, Malkowicz SB. Characterization of chromosome 9 deletions in transitional cell carcinoma by microsatellite assay. *Human Mol Gen* 1993; **2**(9):1407–1411.

64. Keen AJ, Knowles MA. Definition of two regions of deletion on chromosome 9 in carcinoma of the bladder. *Oncogene* 1994; **9**(7):2083–2088.

65. Cairns P, Tokino K, Eby Y, Sidransky D. Homozygous deletions of 9p21 in primary human bladder tumors detected by comparative multiplex polymerase chain reaction. *Cancer Res* 1994; **54**:1422–1424.

66. Miyao N, Tsai YC, Lerner SP, Olumi AF, Spruck CH, III, *et al.* Role of chromosome 9 in human bladder cancer. *Cancer Res* 1993; **53**:4066–4070.

67. Ruppert JM, Tokino K, Sidransky D. Evidence for two bladder cancer suppressor loci on human chromosome 9. *Cancer Res* 1993; **53**:5093–5095.

68. Habuchi T, Devlin J, Elder PA, Knowles MA. Detailed deletion mapping of chromosome 9q in bladder cancer: evidence for two tumor suppressor loci. *Oncogene* 1995; **11**:1671–1674.

69. Habuchi T, Yoshida O, Knowles MA. A novel candidate tumor suppressor locus at 9q32-33 in bladder cancer: localisation of the candidate region within a single 840kb YAC. *Human Mol Gen* 1997; **6**:913–919.

70. Simoneau M, Aboulkassim TO, LaRue H, Rousseau F, Fradet Y. Four tumor suppressor loci on chromosome 9q in bladder cancer: evidence for two novel candidate regions at 9q22.3 and 9q31 [In Process Citation]. *Oncogene* 1999; **18**(1):157–163.

71. Devlin J, Keen AJ, Knowles MA. Homozygous deletion mapping at 9p21 in bladder carcinoma defines a critical region within 2cM of *IFNA*. *Oncogene* 1994; **9**:2757–2760.

72. Williamson MP, Elder PA, Shaw ME, Devlin J, Knowles MA. p16 (*CDKN2*) is a major deletion target at 9p21 in bladder cancer. *Human Mol Gen* 1995; **4**:1569–1577.

73. Orlow I, Lacombe L, Hannon GJ, Serrano M, Pellicer I, Dalbagni G *et al.* Deletion of the p16 and p15 genes in human bladder tumors. *J Natl Cancer Inst* 1995; **87**:1524–1529.

74. Habuchi T, Luscombe M, Elder PA, Knowles MA. Structure and methylation-based silencing of a gene (DBCCR1) within a candidate bladder cancer tumor suppressor region at 9q32-q33. *Genomics* 1998; **48**(3):277–288.

75. Hornigold N, Devlin J, Davies AM, Aveyard JS, Habuchi Y, Knowles MA. Mutation of the 9q34 gene *TSC1* in bladder cancer. *Oncogene* 1999; **18**:2657–2661.

76. McGarvey TW, Maruta Y, Tomaszewski JE, Linnenbach AJ, Malkowicz SB. PTCH gene mutations in invasive transitional cell carcinoma of the bladder. *Oncogene* 1998; **17**(9):1167–1172.

77. Knowles MA, Elder PA, Williamson M, Cairns JP, Shaw ME, Law MG. Allelotype of human bladder cancer. *Cancer Res* 1994; **54**(2):531–538.

78. Presti JC, Jr, Reuter VE, Galan T, Fair WR, Cordon-Cardo C. Molecular genetic alterations in superficial and locally advanced human bladder cancer. *Cancer Res* 1991; **51**(19):5405–5409.

79. Chang WY-H, Cairns P, Schoenberg MP, Polascik TJ, Sidransky D. Novel suppressor loci on chromosome 14q in primary bladder cancer. *Cancer Res* 1995; **55**:3246–3249.

80. Shaw ME, Knowles MA. Deletion mapping of chromosome 11 in carcinoma of the bladder. *Genes, Chromosomes and Cancer* 1995; **13**:1–8.

81. Brewster SF, Gingell JC, Browne S, Brown KW. Loss of heterozygosity on chromosome 18q is associated with muscle-invasive transitional cell carcinoma of the bladder. *Br J Cancer* 1994; **70**:697–700.

82. Kagan J, Liu J, Stein JD, Wagner SS, Babkowski R, Grossman BH *et al*. Cluster of allele losses within a 2.5 cM region of chromosome 10 in high-grade invasive bladder cancer. *Oncogene* 1998; **16**(7):909–913.

83. Cappellen D, Gil Diez de Medina S, Chopin D, Thiery JP, Radvanyi F. Frequent loss of heterozygosity on chromosome 10q in muscle-invasive. *Oncogene* 1997; **14**(25):3059–3066.

84. Aveyard JS, Skilleter A, Habuchi T, Knowles MA. Somatic mutation of *PTEN* in bladder carcinoma. *Br J Cancer* 1999; **80**:904–908

85. Cairns P, Evron E, Okami K, Halachmi N, Esteller M, Herman JG *et al*. Point mutation and homozygous deletion of PTEN/MMAC1 in primary bladder cancers. *Oncogene* 1998; **16**(24):3215–3218.

86. Warren W, Biggs PJ, El-Baz M, Ghoneim MA, Stratton MR, Venitt S. Mutations in the p53 gene in schistosomal bladder cancer: a study of 92 tumors from Egyptian patients and a comparison between spectra from schistosomal and non-schistosomal urothelial tumors. *Carcinogenesis* 1995; **16**:1181–1189.

87. Ramchuuren N, Cooper K, Summerhayes IC. Molecular events underlying schistosomiasis-related bladder cancer. *Int J Cancer* 1995; **62**:237–244.

88. Gonzalez-Zulueta M, Shibata A, Ohneseit PF, Spruck C H, III, Busch C *et al*. High frequency of chromosome 9p allelic loss and *CDKN2* tumor suppressor gene alterations in squamous cell carcinoma of the bladder. *J Natl Cancer Inst* 1995; **87**:1383–1393.

89. Shaw ME, Elder PA, Abbas A, Knowles MA. Partial allelotype of schistosomiasis-associated bladder cancer. *Int J Cancer* 1998;80:656–661

90. Malone PR, Visvinathan KV, Ponder BAJ, Shearer RJ, Summerhayes IC. Oncogenes and bladder cancer. *Br J Urol* 1985; **57**:664–667.

91. Levesque P, Ramchuuren N, Saini K, Joyce A, Libertino J, Summerhayes IC. Screening of human bladder tumors and urine sediments for the presence of H-*ras* mutations. *Int J Cancer* 1993; **55**:785–790.

92. Underwood M, Bartlett J, Reeves J, Gardiner S, Scott R, Cooke T. C-*erbB*-2 gene amplification: a molecular marker in recurrent bladder tumors? *Cancer Res* 1995; **55**:2422–2430.

93. Mellon JK, Lunec J, Wright C, Horne CH, Kelly P, Neal DE. C-erbB-2 in bladder cancer: molecular biology, correlation with epidermal growth factor receptors and prognostic value [see comments]. *J Urol* 1996; **155**(1):321–326.

94. Shin KY, Kong G, Kim WS, Lee TY, Woo YN, Lee JD. Overexpression of cyclin D1 correlates with early recurrence in superficial bladder cancers. *Br J Cancer* 1997; **75**(12):1788–1792.

95. Lipponen PK. Expression of c-myc protein is related to cell proliferation and expression of growth factor receptors in transitional cell bladder cancer. *J Pathol* 1995; **175**(2):203–210.

96. Sauter G, Carroll P, Moch H, Kallioniemi A, Kerschmann R, Narayan P *et al*. c-myc copy number gains in bladder cancer detected by fluorescence in situ hybridization. *Am J Pathol* 1995; **146**(5):1131–1139.

97. Sidransky D, von Eschenbach A, Tsai YC, Jones P, Summerhayes I, Marshall F *et al*. Identification of p53 gene mutations in bladder cancers and urine samples. *Science* 1991; **252**:706–709.

98. Williamson MP, Elder PA, Knowles MA. The spectrum of *TP53* mutations in bladder carcinoma. *Genes, Chromosomes and Cancer* 1994; **9**:108–118.

99. Elder PA, Bell SM, Knowles MA. Deletion of two regions on chromosome 4 in bladder carcinoma: definition of a critical 750kB region at 4p16.3. *Oncogene* 1994; **9**(12):3433–3436.

100. Polascik TJ, Cairns P, Chang WYH, Schoenberg MP, Sidransky D. Distinct regions of allelic loss on chromosome 4 in human primary bladder carcinoma. *Cancer Res* 1995; **55**:5396–5399.

101. Knowles MA, Shaw ME, Proctor AJ. Deletion mapping of chromosome 8 in cancers of the urinary bladder using restriction fragment length polymorphisms and microsatellite polymorphisms. *Oncogene* 1993; **8**:1357–1364.

102. Takle LA, Knowles MA. Deletion mapping implicates two tumor suppressor genes on chromosome 8p in the development of bladder cancer. *Oncogene* 1996; **12**(5):1083–1087.

103. Fearon ER, Feinberg AP, Hamilton SH, Vogelstein B. Loss of genes on .the short arm of chromosome 11 in bladder cancer. *Nature* 1985; **318**:377–380.

104. Tsai YC, Nichols PW, Hiti AL, Williams Z, Skinner DG, Jones PA. Allelic losses of chromosomes 9, 11, and 17 in human bladder cancer. *Cancer Res* 1990; **50**:44–47.

105. Rosin MP, Cairns P, Epstein JI, Schoenberg MP, Sidransky D. Partial allelotype of carcinoma in situ of the human bladder. *Cancer Res* 1995; **55**:5213–5216.

2 Natural history

D E Neal and T R L Griffiths

Introduction

The natural history of bladder cancer can be classified as follows:

- no further recurrence
- local recurrence – which can occur on a single occasion or on multiple occasions; it can involve single or multiple tumor recurrences, but recurrent tumors are usually of the same stage and grade as the primary tumor
- local progression – an increase in local stage with time
- the appearance of distant metastases (which usually presages death)

Whilst the prediction of these events currently depends strongly on the presenting stage and grade of the primary tumor, it is presently inaccurate in estimation of risk in individual patients (as opposed to populations). The addition of molecular markers may well improve prediction of tumor behavior in the future.

Tumor stage

The TNM staging system provides the basis for assessing the future behavior of a newly diagnosed tumor (Table 2.1)[1]. In superficial tumors (pTa and pT1), good data on the pT category should be obtained from histologic examination of resection biopsies, although if deep muscle is not included accurate staging will be impossible ~5% of cases). On examination under anesthesia (EUA), a soft palpable mass may be present before resection in T1 tumors.

On the basis of resection biopsies, the pathologist can only state that muscle invasion is present or absent. True tumor category in muscle invasive tumors depends on pathologic examination of a radical cystectomy specimen. However, a careful examination under anesthesia (EUA) can determine clinical stage and tumor size, but it will understage about 40% to 50% of T2 and T3a tumors. Some disagreement has been demonstrated among pathologists in the detection of lamina propria and even

Table 2.1 TNM staging system: bladder carcinoma

Tx		Primary tumor cannot be assessed
T0		No evidence of primary tumor
Ta		Non-invasive papillary carcinoma
Tis		Carcinoma in situ
T1		Tumor invades sub-epithelial connective tissue
	T1a	Basement membrane penetration
	T1b	Lamina propria invasion
T2		Tumor invades the detrusor muscle
	T2a	Superficial (inner half) muscle invasion
	T2b	Deep (outer half) muscle invasion
T3		Tumor invades the perivesical tissue
	T3a	Microscopic invasion
	T3b	Macroscopic invasion (extravesical mass)
T4		Tumor invades any of the following:
	T4a	Prostate*, uterus, vagina
	T4b	Pelvic wall, abdominal wall

(* Current evidence suggests that only invasion of prostatic stroma worsens clinical outcome.)

Nx	Regional nodes not assessed
N0	No regional lymph node metastases
N1	Single nodal metastases (<2 cm)
N2	Single or multiple nodal metastases (none >2–5 cm)
N3	Nodal metastases (>5 cm)
Mx	Distant metastases not assessed
M0	No distant metastases
M1	Distant metastases

of muscle invasion[2]. There is certainly considerable discrepancy between clinical and pathological stage (Table 2.2)[3]. In practice the presence of a palpable mass following endoscopic resection biopsy (clinical T3) indicates a much worse outcome than a muscle invasive tumor which is identified on histological examination but which is associated on EUA after resection with no mass (clinical T2).

Tumor grade

Considerable disagreement has been shown among pathologists in the interpretation of histological grade[4]

11

Table 2.2 Relationship between clinical stage estimated by EUA versus pathologic stage following cystectomy[3]

Clinical stage	Number	Understage (%)	Overstage (%)	Agreement (%)
T1 + Tis	74	26 (35%)	12 (16%)	36 (49%)
T2	87	48 (55%)	20 (23%)	19 (22%)
T3	81	6 (8%)	31 (38%)	44 (54%)
T4	19	none	2 (11%)	17 (89%)
Totals	261	80 (31%)	65 (25%)	116 (44%)

Table 2.4 Risk of recurrence based on tumor behaviour

Prognostic groups	Cystoscopic findings
Group 1	Solitary tumor at presentation; no tumor recurrence at 3 months (20% risk of recurrence at 1 year)
Group 2	Solitary tumor at presentation; tumor recurrence at 3 months Multiple tumors at presentation; no tumor recurrence at 3 months (40% risk of recurrence at 1 year)
Group 3	Multiple tumors at presentation; tumor recurrence at 3 months (90% risk of recurrence at 1 to 2 years)

Group 1: followed up by means of outpatient flexible cystoscopy at annual intervals.
Group 2: should be followed up 3 monthly by flexible cystoscopy for the first year.
Group 3: three monthly rigid cystoscopic assessment under general anesthesia.

both between pathologists at the same sitting and within the same pathologist on a later occasion. This variation may amount to 30% to 40% even in the definition of the important pT1 G3 tumor. There are several grading systems in use, but there is no evidence that any one system is better than another; it is more important that the pathologist is familiar with one system.

Tumor size

Tumors >5 cm in diameter are known to have a worse prognosis[5]. Most muscle invasive tumors are <5 cm in size, but the interpretation of size is somewhat subjective. Superficial tumors less than 2 cm in size have a significantly lower risk of recurrence (Table 2.3). Parmar and colleagues[6] and Hall and colleagues[7] have proposed stratifying risks of recurrence on the basis of size, multifocality and recurrence at 3 months (Table 2.4).

Table 2.3 Risk of recurrence in superficial tumors[38]

Tumor status	Number	Recurrence rate (+ ve cystoscopies per 100 patient months)
Primary	190	5.2
Recurrent	118	10.4
Number of prior recurrences per year		
Primary tumors (none)	190	5.2
1 or less	38	5.6
1 to 2	28	12.7
>2	42	12.8
Number of tumors		
1	161	4.8
2 to 3	71	7.8
>3	68	12.3
Diameter of largest (cm)		
<2	201	6.4
>3	95	7.9
Grade		
1	241	6.4
2 to 3	60	8.9

Abnormalities of urothelium distant from primary lesion

Urologists should be aware of the imprecision in interpreting biopsies from normal appearing bladder mucosa. In one study, consensus usually could be reached on severe dysplasia and carcinoma in situ (*cis*), but in milder forms of dysplasia pathologists only managed to reproduce their own assessment in 62% of cases[8]. Urine cytology may detect *cis* which has not been found by random mucosal biopsies because surface urothelial cells are not adherent in *cis*. In patients with marked irritative symptoms such as bladder pain, urethral irritation and dysuria, but no abnormal clinical findings, the cytological examination of several specimens of urine is recommended. The yield of cells is often higher in bladder washings than from urine cytology[9]. When ploidy is compared by multivariate analysis with other prognostic factors, it has no clinical advantage over conventional stage and grade[10].

Prognostic factors and natural history

Bladder cancer can be classified into superficial and muscle-invasive tumors, but most urologists now prefer to separate pT1 and pTa tumors. Of patients presenting with transitional cell carcinomas (TCC), 70% have superficial tumors (50% pTa and 20% pT1) not invading detrusor muscle and 25% have muscle-invasive tumors. The latter group account for the majority of deaths from bladder cancer and such patients have an overall survival of 50% at 5 years. Of newly diagnosed superficial bladder tumors, approximately 30% are multifocal at presentation[11], 60% to 70% will recur[12] and 10% to 20% will undergo stage progression to muscle-invasive or metastatic disease[11]. Of newly-diagnosed muscle-invasive tumors, 50% have occult metastases which manifest themselves within 12 months. Few patients with metastatic disease survive more than 2 years.

Superficial tumors

Ta disease

In 425 patients with Ta disease, Fitzpatrick *et al.*[13] found that after 5 to 10 years of follow up, 50% of patients had no recurrence. Twenty per cent had only one recurrence and 30% had more than one recurrence. Recurrence at 3 months follow up is highly predictive of further recurrence (90% continue to recur), whereas absence of recurrence at this time is predictive of a clear bladder (only 21% of such patients recur later). The longer the bladder is free from recurrent tumor, the smaller is the probability of future recurrence. Small papillary tumors have a significantly lower risk of recurrence (30%) compared with multifocal or large sessile tumors (80%; Table 2.3).

Among patients with Ta tumors who develop recurrence, about 15% progress, although these patients comprise only 7% of the total group with Ta disease[5,11,14–16]. In most instances Ta disease is a benign disease posing little threat to the patient. The survival of patients with Ta G1/G2 disease is similar to that of an age and sex matched control population[17].

T1 disease

About 20% of patients with T1 disease will die from bladder cancer within 5 years[5,11,14,15]. Many authors have reported that pTa and pT1 tumors have similar risks of recurrence. True recurrence is recurrence at the site of the original tumor and new occurrence is recurrence at sites distant from the original tumor. True recurrence may be due to tumor tissue not having been removed at the initial operation[18], unresected lymphatic vessel invasion[15] or *cis* adjacent to the tumor. The presence of *cis* near the site of the initial tumor is associated with a greater risk of tumor progression[19]. The survival of patients with early recurrence at the site of the initial T1 tumor is poor, being similar to patients with muscle invasive cancer which may indicate that some of these tumors are understaged.

Table 2.5   Risk of progression

Ta	10%
T1	24%
T1 (recurrent)	56%
Solitary versus multiple	
Ta single	5%
Ta multiple	20%
T1 single	33%
T1 multiple	46%
Grade	
pTa grade 1	none
pTa grade 2	6%
pTa grade 3	25%
pT1 grade 2	25%
pT1 grade 3	50%

Grade

Despite inaccuracies in grading, most authors report that tumor grade has a pronounced influence on progression (Table 2.5)[5] and in particular a number of authors[2,20–22] have stressed the very poor prognosis of T1 Grade 3 tumors (50% progression rate if accompanied by *cis*). These reports are consistent with that of Fitzpatrick *et al.*[13] who found that 70% of patients presenting with a superficial tumor of grade 3 progressed. Several authors have found that tumor grade is the second most important independent variable predicting outcome despite lacking reproducibility[16,23].

Grade 2 tumors are a heterogeneous group, including both non-invasive (Ta) and invasive (T1) disease. On standard histopathologic evaluation it is not possible to identify grade 2 tumors that are likely to progress and those that are not. Grade 3 tumors have a high risk of progression to muscle invasion (35% to 50%), particularly if accompanied by *cis*.

Others have proposed systems based on morphometry[4,10,24] which has been shown to have prognostic significance. These morphometric measurements correlate well with tumor grade[25]. Flow-cytometric DNA analysis correlates in general with grade, recurrence rate, risk of progression and survival[26–28] and represents an objective method which may be used to improve the reproducibility of tumor characterization. However, it is unclear whether such objective assessments improve prediction over conventional grading.

Carcinoma in situ (*cis*)

Carcinoma in situ is usually classified into primary and secondary *cis*. In primary *cis*, there is no history of previous or concurrent tumor. The term concomitant *cis* is used when a tumor is present at the same time.

Primary *cis*

Patients presenting with bladder pain and dysuria and positive cytology have primary *cis* which is a serious risk to life, around 50% of patients dying of metastatic bladder cancer within a year or two if aggressive treatment with intravesical therapy is not instituted.[29] Patients failing to respond to an initial course of bacille Calmette Guèrin (BCG) may respond to second courses, but an early decision to perform cystectomy is vital if death is to be averted. Some patients with *cis* have a more prolonged course[30].

Secondary *cis*

This can be demonstrated by carrying out random or pre-selected site biopsies in patients with bladder cancer. However most authors have found that random biopsies of apparently normal urothelium does not add prognostic information.

Concomitant *cis*

Concomitant *cis* can be demonstrated in around 40% of patients[31]. In a group of 209 patients, 87% of those with *cis* or dysplasia developed recurrence[32]. Its presence is highly predictive of recurrent disease[5,33]. Concomitant *cis* also predicts progression of superficial bladder cancer[19,34]. Fifty per cent of those with *cis* or severe dysplasia progress to muscle invasion[34]. There is a good case to be made for carrying out near and far biopsies of urothelium at initial tumor presentation to detect unsuspected *cis*.

Muscle invasive disease

Over 50% of patients with muscle invasive disease have occult systemic or nodal metastatic disease at presentation; its presence is strongly related to initial tumor stage being most frequent in T4 disease. A larger tumor (>5 cm) is associated with a poor outcome, stage for stage and grade for grade. Other non-specific features of poor prognostic import include systemic signs such as anemia, renal failure and performance status.

Squamous tumors generally are of a higher stage and have a worse outcome as do those transitional cell tumors containing squamous elements. The presence of upper tract dilatation in muscle invasive disease is associated with increased risks of lymph node metastases, systemic spread and a worse clinical outcome[35].

Tumor stage at presentation is the most useful prognostic indicator associated with outcome (Table 2.6). The presence of lymph node metastases is clearly related to tumor stage, a gradually increasing proportion of lymph node metastases being found with increasing stage (Table 2.7)[36]. In most series, few patients with even N1 disease

Table 2.6   Effect of pathologic stage on survival after cystectomy

T1	80%
T2	50%
T3a	35%
T3b	25%
T4a	15%
T4b	5%

Table 2.7   Association between pathologic stage and lymph node metastasis

cis	
PTa	<2%
PT1	5%
T2	25%
T3a	30%
T3b	50%
T4	60%

Data from Skinner *et al.*[36]

survive following radical cystectomy (~10%), although some have reported 20% survival rates following extensive pelvic lymphadenectomy.

The option of orthotopic reconstruction of the urinary bladder after cystectomy remains controversial mainly because of the risk of urethral recurrences. Many series of cystectomies have shown that the risk of urethral recurrence is about 5% to 10% at 5 years[37]. Various factors are associated with an increased risk of urethral recurrence, but the major factor is the presence of stromal invasion of the prostate or carcinoma in situ change in the urethra. This item is discussed further in the chapter on urinary diversion and bladder reconstruction (chapter 7.2).

References

1. Union Internationale Contre le Cancer. The TNM classification of tumors. 1992.
2. Abel PD, Henderson D, Bennett MK, Hall RR, Williams G. Differing interpretations by pathologists of the pT category and grade of transitional cell cancer of the bladder. *Br J Urol* 1988;**62**:339–342.
3. Pagano F, Bassi P, Galetti TP, Meneghini A, Milani C, Artibani W, Garbeglio A. Results of contemporary radical cystectomy for invasive bladder cancer: a clinicopathological study with an emphasis on the inadequacy of the tumor, nodes and metastases classification. *J Urol* 1991;**145**:45–50.
4. Ooms EC, Anderson WA, Alons CL, Boon ME, Veldhuizen RW. Analysis of the performance of pathologists in the grading of bladder tumors. *Human Path* 1983;**14**:140–143.
5. Heney NM, Ahmed S, Flanagan MJ, Frable W, Corder MP, Hafermann MD, Hawkins IR. Superficial bladder cancer: progression and recurrence. *J Urol* 1983;**130**:1083–1086.
6. Parmar MK, Freedman LS, Hargreave TB Tolley DA. Prognostic factors for recurrence and followup policies in the treatment of superficial bladder cancer: report from the British Medical Research Council Subgroup on Superficial Bladder Cancer (Urological Cancer Working Party). *J Urol* 1989;**142**:284–288.

7. Hall RR, Parmar MK, Richards AB, Smith PH. Proposal for changes in cystoscopic follow up of patients with bladder cancer and adjuvant intravesical chemotherapy [see comments]. *BMJ* 1994; **308**:257–260.

8. Richards B, Parmar MK, Anderson CK, Ansell ID, Grigor K, Hall RR, Morley AR et al. Interpretation of biopsies of 'normal' urothelium in patients with superficial bladder cancer. MRC Superficial Bladder Cancer Sub Group. *Br J Urol* 1991;**67**:369–375.

9. Mellon K, Shenton BK, Neal DE. Is voided urine suitable for flow cytometric DNA analysis? *Br J Urol* 1991;**67**:48–53.

10. Lipponen PK, Eskelinen MJ, Nordling S. Progression and survival in transitional cell bladder cancer: a comparison of established prognostic factors, S-phase fraction and DNA ploidy. *Eur J Cancer* 1990;**27**:877–881.

11. Lutzeyer W, Rubben H, Dahm H. Prognostic parameters in superficial bladder cancer: an analysis of 315 cases. *J Urol* 1982;**127**:250–252.

12. Greene LF, Hanash KA, Farrow GM. Benign papilloma or papillary carcinoma of the bladder? *J Urol*, 1973;**110**:205–207.

13. Fitzpatrick JM, West AB, Butler MR, Lane V, O'Flynn JD. Superficial bladder tumors (stage pTa, grades 1 and 2): The importance of recurrence pattern following initial resection. *J Urol* 1986;**135**:920–922.

14. Pryor JP. Factors influencing the survival of patients with transitional cell tumours of the urinary bladder. *Br J Urol* 1973;**45**:586–592.

15. Anderstrøm C, Johansson S, Nilsson S. The significance of lamina propria invasion on the prognosis of patients with bladder cancer. *J Urol* 1980;**124**:23–26.

16. Hendry WF, Rawson NBS, Turney L, Dunlop A, Whitfield HN. Computerisation of urothelial carcinoma records: 16 years experience with the TNM system. *Br J Urol* 1990;**65**:583–588.

17. Olsen PR, Wolf H, Schrøder T, Fischer A, Højgaard K. Urothelial atypia and survival rate of 500 unselected patients with primary transitional-cell tumor of the urinary bladder. *Scand J Urol Nephrol* 1988;**22**:257–263.

18. Klan R, Loy V, Huland H. Residual tumor discovered in routine second transurethral resection in patients with T1 transitional cell carcinoma of the bladder. *J Urol* 1991;**146**:316–318.

19. Flamm J, Havelec L. Factors affecting survival in primary superficial bladder cancer. *Eur Urol* 1990;**17**:113–115.

20. Jakse G, Loidl W, Sieber G, Hofstadter F. Stage T1 grade G3 transitional cell carcinoma of the bladder: an unfavourable tumor? *J Urol* 1987;**137**:39–43.

21. Jenkins BJ, Nauth-Misir RR, Martin JE, Fowler CG, Hope-Stone HF, Blandy JP. The fate of G3 pT1 bladder cancer. *Br J Urol* 1989;**64**:608–610.

22. Kaubisch S, Lum BL, Riese J, Freiha F, Torti FM. Stage T1 bladder cancer: Grade is the primary determinant for risk of muscle invasion. *J Urol* 1991;**146**:28–31.

23. Malmstrøm P-U, Norlen BJ, Andersson B, Busch C. Combination of blood group ABH antigen status and DNA ploidy as independent prognostic factors in transitional cell carcinoma of the bladder. *Br J Urol* 1989;**64**:49–55.

24. Desanctis PN, Concepcion NB, Tannenbaum M, Olsson C. Quantitative morphometry measurement of transitional cell bladder cancer nuclei as indicator of tumor aggression. *Urology* 1987;**24**:322–324.

25. Nielsen K, Colstrup H, Nilsson T, Gundersen H]G. Stereological estimate of nuclear volume correlated with histopatholocal grading and prognosis of bladder tumor. *Virchow Arch (Cell Pathol)* 1986;**52**:41–54.

26. Gustafson H, Tribukait B, Eposti PL. DNA pattern, histological grade and multiplicity related to recurrence rate in superficial bladder tumors. *Scand J Urol Nephrol* 1982;**16**:135–139.

27. Hofstadter F, Jakse G, Lederer B, Mikuz G, Delgado R. Biological behavior and DNA cytophotometry of urothelial bladder carcinomas. *Br J Urol* 1984;**56**:289–295.

28. Tribukait B. Flow cytometry in assessing clinical aggressiveness of genito-urinary neoplasms. *World J Urol* 1987;**5**:108–122.

29. Utz DC and Farrow GM. The management of carcinoma in situ of the urinary bladder: the case for surgical management. *Urol Clin N Am* 1981;**7**:160–164.

30. Riddle PR, Chisholm GD, Trott PA, Pugh RCB. Flat carcinoma in situ of the bladder. *Br J Urol* 1975;**47**:829–833.

31. Wolf H, Olsen PR, Fischer A, Højgaard K. Urothelial atypia concomitant with primary bladder tumor. Incidence in a consecutive series of 500 unselected patients. *Scand J Urol Nephrol* 1987;**21**:33–38.

32. Wolf H, Højgaard K. Urothelial dysplasia concomitant with bladder tumors as a determinant factor for future new occurrences. *Lancet* 1983;**ii**:134–136.

33. Smith G, Elton RA, Beynon LL et al. Prognostic significance of biopsy of normal-looking mucosa in cases of superficial bladder cancer. *Br J Urol* 1983;**55**:665–669.

34. Smith G, Elton RA, Chisholm GD, Newsan JE, Hargreave TB. Superficial bladder cancer: Intravesical chemotherapy and tumor progression to muscle invasion or metastases. *Br J Urol* 1986;**58**:659–663.

35. Greiner R, Skaleric C, Veraguth P. The prognostic significance of ureteral obstruction in carcinoma of the bladder. *Int J Rad Oncol Biol Phys* 1977;**2**:1095–1100.

36. Skinner DG, Tift JP and Kaufman JJ. High dose, short course pre-operative radiation therapy and immediate single stage radical cystectomy with pelvic nose dissection in the management of bladder cancer. *J Urol* 1982;**127**:671–674.

37. Stöckle M, Gökcebay E, Riedmiller H, Hohenfellner R. Urethral tumor recurrences after radical cystoprostatectomy: the case for primary cystoprostatourethrectomy. *J Urol* 1990;**143**:41–43.

38. Dalesio O, Schulman CC, Sylvester R, De Pauw M, Robinson M, Denis L, Smith P, Viggiano G. Prognostic factors in superficial bladder tumors. A study of the European Organization for Research on Treatment of Cancer: Genitourinary Tract Cancer Cooperative Group. *J Urol* 1983;**129**:730–733.

3 Pathology

M C Robinson

Microanatomy of the normal bladder

The urinary bladder is lined by a unique transitional epithelium or urothelium, which is five to seven cells in thickness in the contracted bladder, but only three to four cells in thickness when the bladder is distended[1] (Figure 3.1). The cells of the superficial layer of epithelium are large and dome-shaped with a scalloped surface and have been called 'umbrella' cells. They are sometimes binucleate and may contain small amounts of mucin. The underlying intermediate and basal cells are smaller and regular with glycogen rich cytoplasm[2]. They show ovoid nuclei, with the long axis oriented at right-angles to the surface and show fine nuclear chromatin and an inconspicuous nucleolus. A thin basal lamina separates the urothelium from the underlying connective tissue of the lamina propria, which contains vessels, lymphatics and nerve fibres. Small islands of urothelium (the nests of von Brunn), which are focally connected to the overlying epithelium, may be seen in the superficial part of the lamina propria[1]. There is often a definable, but usually discontinuous layer of thin smooth muscle bundles, forming a muscu-

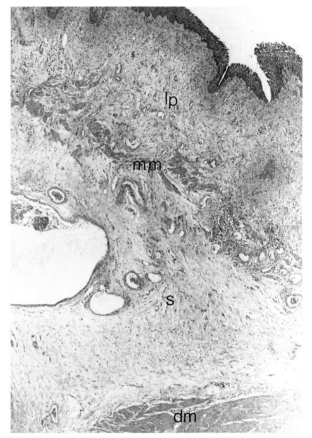

Fig. 3.2 Bladder wall demonstrating lamina propria (lp), muscularis mucosae (mm), submucosa (s) and detrusor muscle (dm).

laris mucosae in the sub-epithelial connective tissue[3] (Figure 3.2). The muscularis mucosae is associated with a layer of medium sized vessels and subdivides the sub-epithelial connective tissue into the lamina propria, between the epithelium and muscularis mucosae, and the

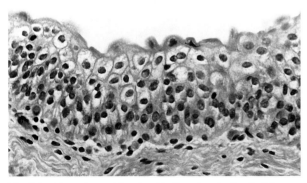

Fig. 3.1 Normal transitional epithelium (urothelium) of the urinary bladder.

submucosa, between the muscularis mucosae and the detrusor muscle[3–5]. The detrusor muscle consists of much larger interlacing bundles of smooth muscle, which are more densely packed and thicker at the bladder neck. Adipose tissue is sometimes present within detrusor muscle bundles, and its presence in a small biopsy does not necessarily indicate perivesical tissue[6].

Histological classification of urinary bladder tumors

Tumors of the bladder epithelium may be subdivided into transitional, squamous, glandular and undifferentiated subtypes[7]. Transitional cell papilloma and inverted transitional cell papilloma are rare and benign[7,8]. Transitional cell carcinoma (TCC), also known as urothelial carcinoma, is the most common bladder tumor, making up 92% of epithelial tumors[9].

The most common histological variants of transitional cell carcinoma (TCC) are those containing foci of squamous or glandular de-differentiation, or both[10]. Rarer variants include microcystic carcinoma[11], sarcomatoid carcinoma[12] and tumors with trophoblastic differentiation[10]. Squamous tumors include pure squamous carcinoma, which comprises no more than 5% of bladder cancer in the USA and Great Britain[10], but is more commonly seen in countries where schistosomiasis is endemic[13], and the rare verrucous variant of squamous carcinoma. Also uncommon are tumors of glandular morphology including villous adenoma and adenocarcinoma (0.5–2%)[10] and undifferentiated carcinomas including small cell carcinoma, (0.5–1%)[14].

Non-epithelial tumors of the bladder are rare and for detailed information the reader is directed to larger pathology texts[15]. Benign tumors include leiomyoma, hemangioma and neurofibroma. Malignant mesenchymal tumors include rhabdomyosarcoma, which is the most frequent tumor of the bladder in childhood, and leiomyosarcoma, the most common sarcoma of the bladder in adults. Malignant lymphoma in the bladder is usually secondary to systemic disease[15].

Transitional cell (urothelial) papilloma

There has been much controversy as to the existence of a benign transitional cell papilloma of the urinary tract. Many urologists have been reluctant to accept the entity of benign 'papilloma' at all, preferring to regard all well differentiated papillary transitional tumors as low-grade carcinomas, because of their unpredictable clinical course, with no means to determine which will recur or progress

to invasion[16]. The long history of the papilloma–papillary carcinoma debate has been comprehensively reviewed by Eble and Young[17].

In the World Health Organization classification of bladder tumors (1973)[7], transitional cell papilloma is strictly defined as 'a papillary tumour with a delicate branching fibrovascular stalk, covered by a regular transitional cell epithelium, indistinguishable from that of the normal bladder and not more than 6 cell layers in thickness. There is no cellular anaplasia. Nuclei are of uniform size and show normal chromatin distribution. Mitoses are rare or absent and the superficial "umbrella" cell layer is preserved'. The recent WHO and International Society of Urological Pathology (ISUP) Consensus Classification of urothelial neoplasms describes a urothelial papilloma as a rare benign condition, typically occurring as a small isolated growth, commonly, but not exclusively, in younger patients and has slightly modified the above definition to 'a discrete exophytic papillary growth with a central fibrovascular core lined by urothelium of normal thickness and cytology', without the need to specify the number of cell layers[18].

Inverted transitional cell papilloma

Inverted transitional cell papilloma[19, 20] is an uncommon tumor comprising less than 1% of transitional cell neoplasms[21]. It is most often situated at the trigone or bladder neck where it projects from the mucosal surface as a solitary polyp with a lobulated or smooth surface, usually measuring 3 cm or less, but occasionally as large as 8 cm[21] (Figure 3.3). It is covered by a normal or attenuated surface urothelium, from which anastomosing cords and islands of urothelial cells extend downwards to invaginate the lamina propria of the polyp[21]. The peripheral cells

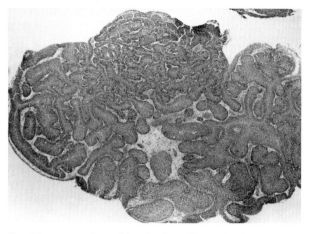

Fig. 3.3 Inverted transitional cell papilloma showing a smoothly lobulated polyp.

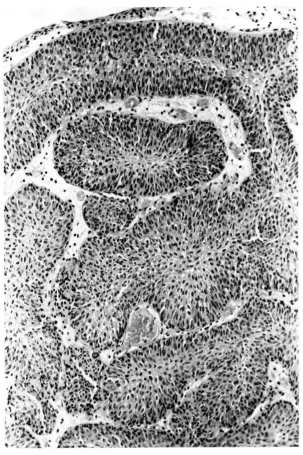

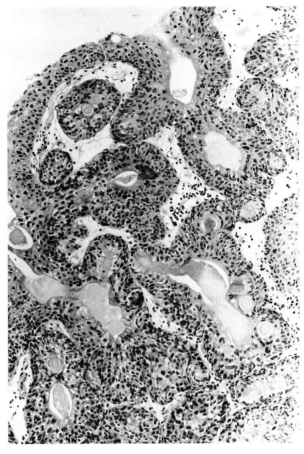

Fig. 3.4A Trabecular variant of inverted transitional papilloma.

Fig. 3.4B Glandular variant of inverted papilloma showing glandular differentiation within the cell nests.

of these islands lie perpendicular to the surrounding basement membrane, which is continuous with that of the surface epithelium; the more central cells lie in a horizontal position. There is no mitotic activity, but minor, focal degrees of cellular atypia are acceptable[22]. Kunze *et al.*[23] described trabecular and glandular variants of inverted papilloma, the former (Figure 3.4A) showing the typical appearances described above; the latter showing glandular differentiation within the cell nests (Figure 3.4B). Inverted papilloma is considered to have a low risk of recurrence when correctly diagnosed and completely excised. Rare cases of recurrence[24,25] and co-existence with TCC[25–28] have been reported, either at separate locations or growing together as a single lesion, but some of these cases may have represented TCC with an inverted growth pattern[17,22,29]. In TCC there are thicker, more variable cell columns, with transition to solid areas. The peripheral palisading and orderly maturation of an inverted papilloma are lacking in TCC, which shows cellular atypia, with nuclear pleomorphism and appreciable mitotic activity[22].

Transitional cell (urothelial) carcinoma

Pattern of tumor growth and macroscopic appearances

Transitional cell carcinoma may be described as papillary (non-invasive), invasive, both papillary and invasive, or as flat carcinoma in situ (non-papillary and non-invasive)[1]. Well and moderately differentiated urothelial carcinomas show an exophytic papillary pattern, which is seen macroscopically as fine pinkish grey villous fronds, projecting into the bladder lumen. Tumors may be single or multiple and may extend over large areas of the mucosal surface, showing a diffuse fronded velvety appearance. On cystoscopic examination, the differential diagnosis includes papillary cystitis, catheter cystitis, nephrogenic metaplasia and villous adenoma of the bladder. More poorly differentiated tumors appear less papillary and more nodular, with coarser, closely packed fronds, or may lack

19

a papillary component altogether and from inception show solid white invasive growth, often with surface necrosis and ulceration. Carcinoma in situ is often multifocal and the affected mucosa may appear normal or show a raised red velvety appearance, simulating inflammatory change.

Grading of transitional cell carcinoma

An ideal grading system is one in which the grades accurately reflect the biological behavior of the tumor and are independent indicators of prognosis. Several grading systems for transitional cell tumors based on cytological features have previously been proposed, the most well known of which are those of Bergvist[30], Koss[1], Mostofi[7] and Murphy[21].

The grading system proposed by Mostofi et al., and adopted by the World Health Organization[7], is widely used and incorporates three grades of transitional cell carcinoma which are defined as: Grade 1 – tumors with the least degree of anaplasia compatible with a diagnosis of malignancy, Grade 3 – tumors with the most severe degree of cellular anaplasia and Grade 2 – tumors that lie in between. The histologic criteria for each grade were not more exactly specified, although the cytologic features

were well illustrated in the accompanying atlas[7]. Alternative grading systems of Bergvist[30] and Murphy[21] are compared with the WHO classification in Table 3.1, but exact extrapolation between grading systems is difficult to achieve[21,31]. Ayala and Ro have summarized the histologic features of the individual WHO grades[9].

Grade I transitional cell carcinoma (Figure 3.5) is a papillary tumor with a branching fibrovascular stroma, covered by urothelium with an increased number of cell layers. The tumor cells show slight nuclear enlargement and pleomorphism and slightly abnormal nuclear polarization. Nuclei show evenly dispersed chromatin and small or absent nucleoli. Mitoses are rare and the cell cytoplasm shows reduced or absent glycogen content. Superficial umbrella cells are usually preserved.

Grade 1 tumors have been reported to be solitary in 68% of cases[32] and are usually non-invasive[33], although one study described lamina propria invasion in 6% of grade 1 tumors at first diagnosis[34]. Recurrences are common and there may be progression to a higher grade[32,34,35].

Grade 2 papillary TCC (Figure 3.6A and 3.6B) shows papillary stalks covered by urothelium of variable thickness, with a moderate increase in nuclear size, moderate

Table 3.1   A comparison of grading systems for urothelial tumors

	Bergvist* (1965)[30]	WHO** (1973)[9]	Murphy (1993)[21]
Urothelial tumor Grade 0* or **Papilloma	Urothelium of normal thickness. Cellular pattern identical with normal urothelium.	Regular epithelium, indistinguishable from normal. Not more than six cell layers.	Papilloma
Urothelial tumor Grade 1*	Urothelium slightly and irregularly thickened. No appreciable cellular deviations from normal.		
Carcinoma Grade 1**		Tumors with the least degree of anaplasia compatible with a diagnosis of malignancy	
			Low-grade urothelial carcinoma
Grade 2	Definite thickening of the epithelium. Moderate cellular deviations. Some variation in size of cells and nuclei. Tendency to loss of cellular polarity	Tumors with a degree of anaplasia that lies in between grades 1 and 3	
			High-grade urothelial carcinoma
Grade 3	Considerable cellular abnormality. Great variation in size and shape of cells and nuclei	Tumors with the most severe degree of anaplasia	
Grade 4	Severe cellular abnormalities (anaplasia) with complete loss of the urothelial pattern	Undifferentiated carcinoma	

Exact extrapolation between grading systems cannot be achieved. The category of 'low-grade' urothelial carcinoma in Murphy's classification includes some grade 1 and approximately 25% of grade 2 tumors in the WHO classification [117].
The category of 'high-grade' urothelial carcinoma in Murphy's classification includes WHO grade 3 tumors and approximately 75% of grade 2 tumors [117].

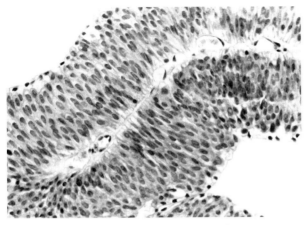

Fig 3.5   Grade 1 Papillary transitional cell carcinoma.

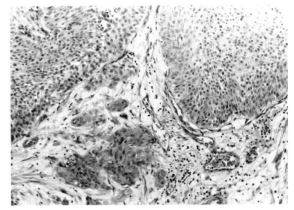

Fig. 3.6C   Grade 2 TCC showing disordered nuclear polarity and evidence of lamina propria invasion.

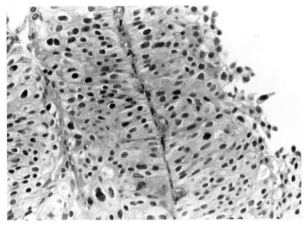

Fig. 3.6A   Grade 2 transitional cell carcinoma.

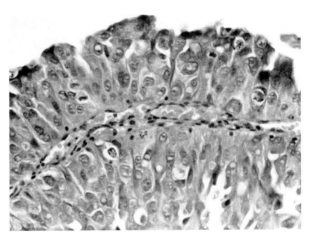

Fig. 3.7A   Grade 3 papillary TCC showing marked nuclear anaplasia.

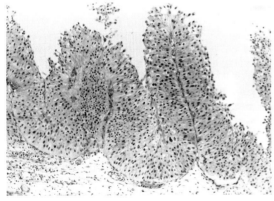

Fig. 3.6B   Grade 2 TCC with a low papillary pattern. The basement membrane is clearly intact and there is no evidence of invasion.

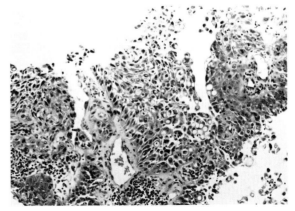

Fig. 3.7B   Grade 3 TCC showing poorly formed papillary structures and complete lack of nuclear polarization.

nuclear pleomorphism and hyperchromatism, more coarsely granular chromatin and disordered nuclear polarity. Mitoses may be identified and superficial umbrella cells are usually lost[9,36]. The tumor is predominantly papillary, but may invade lamina propria (Figure 3.6C) and detrusor muscle.

In Grade 3 TCC superficial umbrella cells are lost. The tumor cells show greatly increased nuclear size, marked nuclear pleomorphism and hyperchromatism, complete loss of nuclear polarity and prominent mitoses (Figure 3.7A). Increasing grade is associated with a diminution of papillary features (Figure 3.7B) and many grade 3 tumors are sessile, white nodular masses showing evidence of invasion at presentation[21,36]. While there may be remnants of papillary architecture at the surface, invasive tumor consists of nests, islands or solid sheets of pleomorphic cells with abundant cytoplasm and large pleomorphic nuclei with prominent nucleoli. Tumor necrosis is common and islands of tumor may be surrounded by a desmoplastic fibrous stromal reaction, with a variable inflammatory infiltrate.

Grade and prognosis

Tumor grade at presentation is an important biological predictor of disease behavior[34,37–39] and there is a general correlation of increasing histologic grade with increasing tumor stage[33,40,41]. Other factors associated with a poorer prognosis are high tumor stage[33,42,43], multiple tumors at presentation[32,34,38,44–46], size of the largest tumor[32,34,45,46], more than 10 g of tumor fragments[44], associated dysplasia or carcinoma in situ in the bladder epithelium[34,38,39], and the presence of tumor at 3 month follow up cystoscopy[44–46].

Reproducibility of grading

The differentiation of a tumor may vary within the tumor and some pathologists use intermediate grades to describe a tumor with a small component of a higher grade[47]. Other workers assign only the highest grade present[7,48]. It is recommended that tiny areas of a higher grade are ignored when assigning an overall grade[18]. There may be significant inter- and intra-observer variation in the grading of tumors[49–51]. Ooms et al.[50] found that in almost 50% of cases, tumors were graded differently on a subsequent occasion, by the same pathologist using the WHO classification, although another study using analysis by kappa statistics concluded that pathologists can determine grade with a 'fair to good' degree of reproducibility[52]. In a superficial bladder cancer trial, Witjes et al. reported that review pathology caused considerable changes in the pathology results in 40% of patients, but did not actually change the results of treatment and hardly altered the results of a prognostic factor analysis in a randomized study[53].

Alternative grading systems

An alternative grading system was proposed by Murphy in the Armed Forces Institute of Pathology fascicle 11, 1994[21], in which many of the transitional tumors with the cellular morphology of WHO grade 1 papillary carcinoma were designated transitional cell 'papilloma' and were considered to be benign, because almost 50% of patients had no tumor recurrence after primary resection and recurrences were usually low-grade non-invasive papillary lesions, similar to the primary tumor[54]. In a study by Jordan et al.[55], patients diagnosed with a grade 1 TCC showed 10 and 20 year survivals of 98% and 93% respectively. Nevertheless, 4.4% of these patients died of bladder cancer due to development of a grade 3 tumor and progression to grade 3 occurred in a further 3.3%. A further study of non-invasive grade 1 papillary TCC showed progression to a more advanced grade in 16% of patients and invasion developed in 4.5%[32].

At present we are unable to predict with certainty which of the patients with a well differentiated papillary urothelial tumor will *not* develop tumor recurrence or progression over a lifetime of follow up and many pathologists prefer to limit the term 'papilloma' to the very small number of tumors conforming to the strict definition of the original WHO classification (see above)[7], for which a more confident prognosis of benign behavior can be offered[1,9,15,47,56].

However, the Bladder Consensus Conference Committee of the WHO and ISUP has recently suggested that papillary urothelial lesions with an orderly arrangement of cells, showing minimal architectural abnormality, minimal nuclear atypia and infrequent mitoses, but differing from a papilloma by showing urothelial thickening and/or nuclear enlargement (i.e. many of the tumors which are classified as grade 1 TCC in the WHO classification), should be designated 'papillary urothelial neoplasms of low malignant potential' and not 'carcinoma'[18]. The committee recommends that pathologists include a statement in the biopsy report that 'patients with these tumors are at risk of developing new bladder tumors (recurrences), usually of a similar histology' and that 'occasionally these subsequent lesions manifest as urothelial carcinoma, such that follow-up of the patient is warranted'[18]. Perhaps an easier solution to avoid the label 'carcinoma' would be to use the term 'grade 1 papillary urothelial tumor'.

A further problem in the grading of urothelial tumors is that there is a tendency among pathologists to identify only the best differentiated lesions as low grade and the most anaplastic as high grade, therefore allocating most tumors to WHO grade 2, which is therefore a large and heterogeneous group, both in clinical and histologic terms[48]. Attempts have been made to split grade 2 tumors into more useful prognostic groups[48,57]. Pauwels et al.[57] subdivided pTa/pT1 WHO grade 2 tumors into: grade 2a – tumors with thickened epithelium showing slight variation in the size of cells and nuclei and normal cellular polarity; and grade 2b – tumors with thickened epithelium showing clear variation in nuclear and cellular size, evident hyperchromasia and a tendency to loss of normal cellular polarity. Tumor progression occurred in 4% of grade 2a and 33% of grade 2b tumors. Grade 2a and grade 1 tumors showed no significant difference in recurrence and progression and it was concluded that these could be grouped together as 'low' grade. Grade 2b carcinomas were classified as 'intermediate' grade, with grade 3 tumors unchanged as 'high' grade.

Carbin et al.[48] subdivided grade 2 into two groups, with regard to variation in nuclear size and number of mitoses: grade IIa – tumors showing slight to moderate variation in nuclear size, with less than a twofold variation in each diameter at the same axis among adjacent cells, smooth nuclear membrane, even fine chromatin pattern and few mitoses; and grade IIb – tumors showing moderate to strong variation in nuclear size, with at least a twofold variation in each diameter among adjacent cells, prominent nuclear membrane, fine hyperchromatic chromatin pattern, increased nucleo- cytoplasmic ratio and mitoses easily found. The 5 year survival was 92% for patients with grade IIa TCC compared with 43% for patients with grade IIb tumors[58].

The WHO/ISUP Consensus Committee has proposed a new classification of 'Low grade' and 'High grade' Papillary Urothelial Carcinoma, with distinction between these categories made on the basis of both architectural features (predominantly ordered organization of cells versus predominant or total disorder) and cytologic abnormalities (mild cytologic atypia versus moderate to marked pleomorphism)[18]. The new 'Low grade' category includes approximately 10% of tumors at the upper end of WHO grade 1 combined with the lower 40% of WHO grade 2 tumors. The 'High grade' category includes the remaining 50–60% of WHO grade 2 tumors and all grade 3 tumors[59]. Whether use of the new classification will improve observer variability or will be of proven benefit to urologists and pathologists in routine practice remains to be validated in clinical trials. The WHO classification has gained wide acceptance among urologists, oncologists and pathologists over the years and the potential introduction of a new grading system will require considerable retraining for all of them[56].

Additional prognostic factors

Additional factors which have been reported to be of prognostic value for prediction of disease behaviour in bladder cancer include DNA ploidy[60], morphometric analysis of nuclear features[61], assessment of cellular proliferation,[62,63] and expression of class I histocompatibility antigens[64]. Tumor markers with prognostic significance include decreased expression of the retinoblastoma gene product in high-grade and high-stage tumors[65] and p53 oncoprotein overexpression, which is associated with an increased risk of tumor progression[66–68].

Variants of transitional cell carcinoma

The most common variants of TCC are those showing squamous or glandular de-differentiation or both. These account for approximately 10% of bladder cancers and usually occur within moderately or poorly differentiated invasive tumors[10]. Squamous de-differentiation requires the presence of squamous cells showing intercellular bridges or keratinization[9]. The term glandular de-differentiation should be restricted to the formation of true glandular structures in an otherwise typical TCC and not used for an occasional mucin containing vacuole or pseudoglandular space, formed by individual cell necrosis[10] (Figure 3.8A and 3.8B). In the WHO classification, these tumors are grouped as variants of TCC with squamous and glandular metaplasia, respectively. It has been suggested that tumors exhibiting a truly mixed appearance, with more than one differentiation prominent, should be classified by their separate components in order to gain more meaningful information on their behavior[36]. Martin et al. reported that tumors with squamous de-differentiation are more resistant to radiotherapy than pure TCC[69], however another study did not find this to be of predictive value.[70] Logothetis et al. (71) reported that TCC with admixtures of other histologic types showed a poorer response to systemic chemotherapy, but found this to be attributable to the presence of glandular rather than squamous elements.

Small (oat) cell carcinoma is less commonly seen in association with TCC or with adenocarcinoma, but may be a further avenue of differentiation for urothelial carcinoma[10]. It is recommended that a small cell component in a TCC should be reported as a separate histologic type[10], but the prognostic implications are at present unclear, due to the small number of cases and limited clinical data available[72].

The sarcomatoid variant of urothelial carcinoma is a transitional cell carcinoma merging imperceptibly with a spindle cell carcinomatous component (Figure 3.9), which may resemble leiomyosarcoma, malignant fibrous histiocytoma or fibrosarcoma[12]. Sarcomatoid carcinoma may

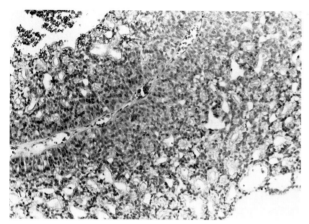

Fig. 3.8A Grade 2 papillary TCC showing glandular metaplasia.

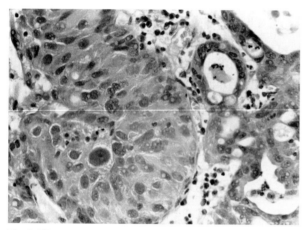

Fig. 3.8B Invasive grade 3 TCC showing glandular metaplasia.

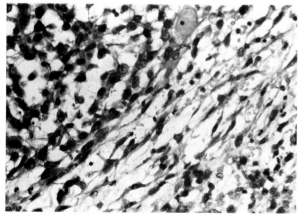

Fig. 3.9 Sarcomatoid variant of TCC. The spindle cell component merges imperceptibly with the epithelial component.

be distinguished from a true sarcoma by the presence of an accompanying epithelial component, either TCC or CIS, or by at least focal positivity with immunohistochemical markers for cytokeratin in the spindle cells[12]. The differential diagnosis is carcinosarcoma, in which there are discrete, but intimately admixed areas of malignant epithelial and mesenchymal tumor. The clinical usefulness of separately distinguishing sarcomatoid carcinoma and carcinosarcoma of the bladder is debatable[15,73], as both are highly aggressive malignancies with a similar outcome, regardless of histologic findings and treatment. Pathologic stage is reported to be the best predictor of survival[73].

A further rare variant is TCC with trophoblastic de-differentiation[10]. Poorly differentiated TCC may show isolated syncytiotrophoblastic giant cells, which contain beta hCG[74]. The cells of morphologically typical TCC may also contain beta hCG[10,75] and this feature may indicate tumor resistance to radiotherapy[75]. There are several reports of choriocarcinoma in association with poorly differentiated TCC in the bladder[76–78] and cases which were previously reported as pure choriocarcinoma of bladder[79,80] may actually have represented TCC with overgrowth of a de-differentiated trophoblastic component[10].

Pathologic staging of bladder tumors

The pathologic stage of the tumor is the degree of penetration into the bladder wall or beyond the confines of the bladder and is the primary basis upon which therapeutic decisions are made. The Tumour Nodes Metastasis (TNM) staging classification of the International Union against Cancer (UICC)[81], which is applicable to biopsies and cystectomy specimens, is commonly used[81] (Table 3.2). Approximately 80% of urothelial cancers are clinically 'superficial' tumors[82]. This confusing term includes non-invasive papillary tumor (pTa), flat in situ tumor (pTis) and invasive tumor infiltrating sub-epithelial connective tissue (pT1). Two-thirds of these tumors are at risk of local recurrence (actually new occurrence) but never become invasive, and the remaining third will progress to invasion[82]. The remaining 20% to 30% of transitional cell tumors are clinically referred to as 'invasive cancer'. This term is applied to tumor invading either the inner half of the detrusor muscle, also known as 'superficial' muscle (pT2a), or the outer half of the detrusor muscle, i.e. 'deep muscle' (pT2b), or extending into perivesical fat, either microscopically (pT3a) or macroscopically (pT3b) or involving contiguous organs (pT4). More than 80% of TCC that infiltrate detrusor muscle, do so at presentation, with no previous history of superficial disease[83].

Table 3.2   TNM staging of carcinoma of the urinary bladder (1997)

	T – Primary tumor
TX	Primary tumor cannot be assessed
T0	No evidence of primary tumor
Ta	Non-invasive papillary carcinoma
Tis	Carcinoma in situ: 'flat tumor'
T1	Tumor invades subepithelial connective tissue
T2	Tumor invades muscle
	T2a Tumor invades superficial muscle (inner half)
	T2b Tumor invades deep muscle (outer half)
T3	Tumor invades perivesical tissue
	T3a microscopically
	T3b macroscopically (extravesical mass)
T4	Tumor invades any of the following: prostate, uterus, vagina, pelvic wall, abdominal wall
	T4a Tumor invades prostate or uterus or vagina
	T4b Tumor invades pelvic wall or abdominal wall
	N – Regional lymph nodes
NX	Regional lymph nodes cannot be assessed
N0	No regional lymph node metastasis
N1	Metastasis in a single lymph node, 2 cm or less in greatest dimension
N2	Metastasis in a single lymph node, more than 2 cm but not more than 5 cm in greatest dimension; or multiple lymph nodes, none more than 5 cm in greatest dimension.
N3	Metastasis in a lymph node, more than 5 cm in greatest dimension.

Assessment of lamina propria invasion

Many workers have reported that lamina propria invasion indicates a worse prognosis[37,41,42,83]. Farrow and Utz noted that 'microinvasion' of 5 mm or less into the lamina propria was associated with a significantly increased risk of metastatic carcinoma[84]. A number of factors complicate the assessment of lamina propria invasion, leading to observer variation in interpretation[22,49]. Cross cutting of the base of tumor fronds may mimic invasion. Non-invasive papillary tumors may show complex papillary infoldings into the lamina propria, which may be difficult to distinguish from superficial invasion[9,47]. Amin et al. have described urothelial carcinomas with an endophytic growth pattern, showing broad front extension pushing into the lamina propria, but this does not constitute invasion as long as the basement membrane is intact around large rounded tumor nests and the surrounding stroma is normal[22]. True invasion is seen as small infiltrative tongues of tumor cells, sometimes of a higher grade than the overlying tumor, breaching the basement membrane (Figure 3.10), and sometimes surrounded by a fibroblastic stromal response[22,47]. Occasionally, invasive transitional cell carcinomas may be misdiagnosed as benign due to bland cytologic features and inconspicuous individual cell infiltration[85].

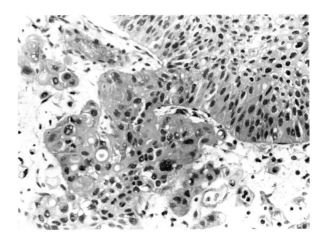

Fig. 3.10 Microinvasion of the lamina propria. There is penetration of the basement membrane by infiltrative tongues of tumor cells.

Level of the muscularis mucosae

Attempts have been made to subdivide the T1 category into prognostic groups using the level of the muscularis mucosae. Younes et al. reported that patients with tumors invading through the muscularis mucosae into submucosa, but not involving muscularis propria had a 5 year survival of 11%, which was comparable with that of patients with detrusor muscle invasion, whereas patients with tumors invading the lamina propria above, or reaching to the level of the muscularis mucosae, had a 75% 5 year survival[4]. Angulo et al. found it possible to distinguish tumor invasion confined to the lamina propria (pT1A) from tumor infiltrating the submucosa (pT1B) in 58% of transurethral resection biopsies[5]. Five year survival was reported to be 86% in pT1A tumors and 52% in group pT1B. The depth of sub-epithelial connective tissue invasion in pT1 grade 2 transitional cell carcinomas was an independent prognostic factor ($P < 0.05$) in a multivariate analysis[5]. Unfortunately, accurate distinction between lamina propria and submucosa is not always possible in a small, poorly oriented biopsy specimen and sub-staging of the T1 category is not routinely practiced.

Invasion of the wispy smooth muscle bundles of the muscularis mucosae should not be confused with invasion of the large thick rounded bundles of the detrusor muscle (Figure 3.11). Pathologists must not refer to strands of muscularis mucosae as superficial muscle in the biopsy report, as the term 'superficial muscle' is usually applied to the inner half of the detrusor muscle and a serious error of overstaging may ensue. In small biopsies, it is not always possible to distinguish with certainty between muscularis mucosae and detrusor muscle,

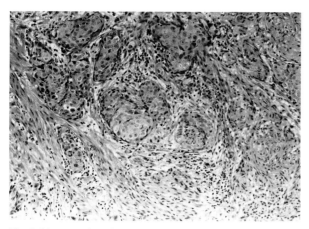

Fig. 3.11 Invasion of large muscle bundles of the detrusor muscle by poorly differentiated TCC.

particularly when there has been previous resection, or there is a desmoplastic stromal response around invasive tumor and this difficulty should be stated in the biopsy report[22].

Detrusor muscle invasion

Assessment of muscle invasion is crucial in determining therapy and prognosis and pathologists should routinely record the presence or absence of detrusor muscle in transurethral biopsy specimens and whether or not this is invaded by tumor. In practice, pathologists are not able to substage the depth of muscularis propria invasion in a small biopsy, although urologists may attempt to sample the deep muscle and send this separately, in order to obtain more accurate staging. It should be noted that invasion of adipose tissue in a small biopsy is not necessarily an indicator of perivesical extension of tumor, as adipose tissue may be present within detrusor muscle[6].

Prostatic involvement by transitional cell carcinoma

Secondary prostatic involvement by transitional cell carcinoma has been estimated to occur in approximately 30% of cystoprostatectomy specimens for TCC of bladder, whereas primary transitional cell carcinoma of the prostate is relatively rare[86,87]. TCC in the prostate may be considered in three loco-regional subgroups: 1) papillary tumor or CIS confined to the prostatic urothelium; 2) extension of papillary tumor or CIS into the prostate ducts and acini, but limited by the basement membrane; and 3) prostate stromal invasion[88]. To define separate prognostic categories, it is necessary to consider whether the prostate

tumor is a primary prostatic TCC or is secondary to bladder cancer and, in the latter case, to distinguish whether prostate stromal invasion has occurred from within the prostatic urethra or ducts, or by direct extension from the bladder, through the bladder wall, traversing the prostate capsule[87,89,90]. The 1997 revision of the TNM classification has introduced a separate staging for transitional cell carcinoma arising within the prostatic urethra[81] (Table 3.3).

In patients with bladder cancer, non-invasive TCC and CIS confined to the prostatic urethral mucosa and periurethral ducts are reported not to alter survival predicted by primary bladder stage alone[86,87]. Prostatic stromal invasion arising from TCC or CIS in the prostatic urethra or ducts has been reported significantly to decrease survival, when compared with tumors without stromal invasion, and significantly to decrease survival predicted by the primary bladder stage[87,91]. The extent of loco-regional spread has been reported to be the strongest predictor of patient survival outcome in patients with prostatic TCC in the absence of invasive bladder cancer[92]. In the study of Cheville et al. the 5 year disease specific survival rate for patients with CIS of the prostatic urethra or of the prostatic ducts and acini was 100%, in comparison with 45% for patients with urethral submucosal and prostatic stromal invasion by TCC[92]. In patients with extraprostatic extension and seminal vesicle involvement, the 5 year survival rate was 0%.

Papillary urothelial tumors and CIS in the prostatic urethra may be single or multifocal. Within the prostate ducts, papillary fronds of TCC tend to be compressed and stromal cores may be less easily distinguishable. CIS may be seen in the prostatic urethra and filling and expanding the prostate ducts, at first growing between intact prostatic luminal epithelial cells and the basal cell layer[93] (Figure 3.12A), and later filling the ducts and acini, which often show central comedonecrosis[94] (Figure 3.12B). The pathologist must clearly differentiate between prostate ductal involvement by CIS and prostate stromal invasion which carries a worse prognosis. CIS confined within the

Table 3.3 TNM staging of urethra

	Transitional cell carcinoma of prostate (prostatic urethra)
Tis pu	Carcinoma in situ, involvement of prostatic urethra
Tis pd	Carcinoma in situ, involvement of prostatic ducts
T1	Tumor invades subepithelial connective tissue
T2	Tumor invades any of the following: prostatic stroma, corpus spongiosum, periurethral muscle
T3	Tumor invades any of the following: corpus cavernosum, beyond prostatic capsule, bladder neck (extraprostatic extension)
T4	Tumor invades other adjacent organs (invasion of bladder)

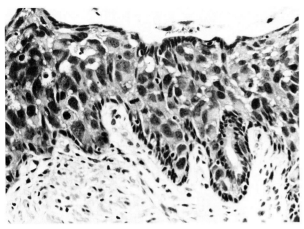

Fig. 3.12A Carcinoma in situ in the prostatic urethra. The dysplastic cells have grown between the intact prostate luminal epithelial cells and the basal layer.

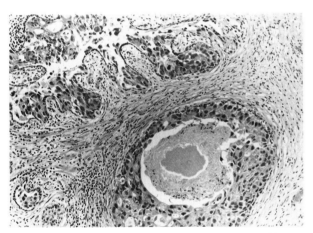

Fig. 3.12B Carcinoma in situ within prostate ducts with comedonecrosis. There is no penetration of the basement membrane of the involved ducts.

ducts and acini is seen as well circumscribed, smooth edged nests, with an intact basement membrane and no surrounding desmoplastic stromal response[94] (Figure 3.12B). Larger cell masses of invasive tumor breach the basement membrane of the ducts and show irregular borders, with a surrounding fibrous stromal reaction and often associated chronic inflammation.

The distinction between high-grade invasive TCC infiltrating the prostate and poorly differentiated prostatic adenocarcinoma is sometimes difficult. Immunohistochemical staining for prostate-specific antigen and prostatic acid phosphatase is usually helpful, but both markers are negative in approximately 1.6% of high-grade prostate cancers[95].

Vascular invasion

Angiolymphatic invasion has been shown to be important in the prediction of tumor progression in stage T1 bladder cancer[41,96], but the depths of vascular and/or lymphatic invasion (which may be greater than the depth of invasion of the tumor) are not taken in to account when determining tumor stage[7]. Lopez and Angulo reported that vascular invasion, verified by immunocytochemistry, was present in 10% of T1 tumors[96]. Five year survival was 81% for cases without vascular invasion, compared with 44% survival for those showing vascular invasion. In a multivariate analysis, vascular invasion was an independent prognostic factor. Another study reported reduced survival in patients with muscle invasive TCC, without nodal involvement when small vessel invasion was present[42]. Assessment of vascular invasion may be made difficult by retraction artefact around tumor islands, simulating invasion of vascular spaces. Endothelial markers have been reported to be of value to identify true vascular invasion[97,98].

Hyperplasia, reactive atypia, dysplasia and urothelial carcinoma in situ

In simple urothelial hyperplasia, which may be seen in association with local irritation and chronic inflammation, the urothelium is markedly thickened, superficial umbrella cells are preserved and there is no associated cytologic atypia[36]. Papillary urothelial hyperplasia is defined as an undulating urothelium arranged into thin non-branching mucosal folds of varying heights, lined by urothelium of variable thickness, lacking atypia[18,99]. It may be seen in the mucosa adjacent to papillary tumors and is considered to be a potential precursor lesion of low-grade papillary neoplasms[36,99]. Neovascularization in the connective tissue stalk of hyperplastic papillary fronds may represent the earliest evidence of papillary tumor formation[100]. Reactive urothelial atypia is associated with bladder inflammation or irritation and may follow intravesical chemotherapy. Urothelial nuclei are uniformly enlarged and vesicular with a central prominent nucleolus and mitotic figures may be frequent[18].

In urothelial dysplasia, the urothelium is flat and may be attenuated, of normal thickness or thicker than normal. Dysplasia is recognized at low magnification by decreased or absent cytoplasmic clearing of urothelial cells and nuclear clustering[21]. Nagy *et al.* described the cytologic changes in mild, moderate and severe dysplasia as corresponding to the epithelial changes seen in the fronds of transitional cell carcinoma, WHO grades 1, 2 and 3, as if the tumor fronds were to be flattened out[101]. Low-grade dysplasia may be difficult to distinguish from reactive

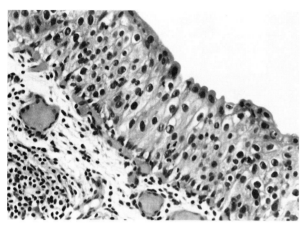

Fig. 3.13 Urothelial dysplasia. There is disordered nuclear polarity and variation in nuclear size. Some nuclei show enlarged nucleoli. Superficial cells are retained.

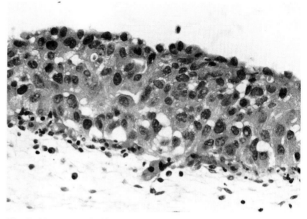

Fig. 3.14A Urothelial CIS. There are severe full thickness cellular abnormalities and loss of cell cohesion.

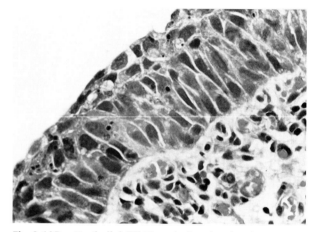

Fig. 3.14B Urothelial CIS. There is disordered nuclear polarity and marked nuclear pleomorphism and hyperchromatism.

atypia and several studies have reported a lack of reproducibility in the grading of urothelial dysplasia and CIS, when several diagnostic categories are used[52,101–103]. A reduction in the number of categories of dysplasia has been recommended in order to achieve interobserver reproducibility[18,52,102,104].

In mild/moderate dysplasia (Figure 3.13), the basal and intermediate cells of the urothelium are larger than those in adjacent normal areas[104]. Their nuclei are large and more spherical than ovoid, so that there appears to be some loss of cellular polarization. There is nuclear crowding and irregularity of nuclear borders. Nuclear chromatin is more granular and small nucleoli may be identified. Mitoses may be present, but are not a distinguishing feature of dysplasia. Superficial cells form a continuous layer over the surface.

Severe dysplasia shows more severe cytologic abnormalities, similar to those of CIS and grade 3 TCC. There is markedly altered nuclear polarity, marked nuclear enlargement, prominent nuclear irregularity, coarsely granular and irregularly distributed nuclear chromatin and large irregular nucleoli. In severe dysplasia, superficial umbrella cells are preserved and there is no loss of cell cohesion.

In carcinoma in situ (Figures 3.14A and 3.14B) the urothelium is replaced by crowded cells, similar to those seen in severe dysplasia. There is complete loss of nuclear polarity, mitoses are common and may be atypical. The full thickness of the urothelium may be involved with loss of the superficial umbrella cells, but it is the severe cytologic abnormalities that are important for the diagnosis of CIS and many authors now consider that full thickness mucosal involvement is unnecessary[15,105]. After reviewing existing reported information on dysplasia and CIS, a workshop of pathologists and clinicians agreed that marked dysplasia and CIS could be combined in one category for clinicopathological correlation[105]. The WHO/IUCC consensus classification recommends use of the terms 'high-grade intra-urothelial neoplasia' (CIS) for lesions previously designated as either severe dysplasia or CIS and 'low-grade intra-urothelial neoplasia' (dysplasia) for urothelium with appreciable cytologic and architectural changes, yet falling short of the diagnostic threshold for CIS[18].

In CIS, there is often loss of cell cohesion and dysplastic cells are shed from the surface, a process described as 'denuding cystitis'[106]. The underlying lamina propria shows capillary proliferation and congestion and an associated lymphocytic infiltrate. Direct microinvasion of single tumor cells into the lamina propria should be carefully sought and may be camouflaged by the inflammation.

Biopsies of 'red patches' may reveal only inflamed lamina propria, with a few residual atypical basal cells on the biopsy surface. In this situation, CIS may be detected in Von Brunn's nests, either as atypical cells infiltrating between normal urothelial cells or completely replacing the epithelium[82,107]. Urine cytology is useful to identify dysplastic epithelial cells shed into the urine from CIS and to monitor the response to therapy.

In the pagetoid variant of CIS, the dysplastic cells show abundant pale cytoplasm, large nuclei and prominent nucleoli and infiltrate singly and in clusters between normal urothelial cells[107], or undermine normal urothelium causing it to slough[82]. This variant does not occur without conventional CIS elsewhere in the urothelium. A small cell variant of CIS is also recognized[1].

Carcinoma in situ and dysplasia tend to be multifocal[108]. Ninety per cent of cases are found in association with urothelial cancer, usually of high grade[39,109], whereas primary CIS accounts for only 10% of cases. It is well established that patients with dysplasia or CIS accompanying their bladder cancer are more likely to suffer tumor recurrences and to progress to invasion, than those with normal mucosa[110–114], but there are conflicting opinions as to the biological significance of CIS and dysplasia. Many authors regard CIS as an aggressive cancer, that has the capacity to evolve into a solid muscle invasive tumor[110–112,115,116]. Others believe that CIS is an indolent lesion, that appears in situ because it lacks the capacity for invasion[117–119]. Primary and secondary CIS are histologically indistinguishable[117], but opinions are divided as to whether primary CIS[39,115,116], or secondary CIS[111] has a less favorable clinical course or whether there is no difference in prognosis[120]. Norming et al. reported progression in 59% of cases of primary CIS and found that the occurrence of multiple aneuploid cell populations was a sign of high aggressiveness[121]. On reviewing the literature, Hudson and Herr have suggested the possibility of predicting 'low' and 'high' risk forms of CIS, using factors such as multifocality, prostatic urethral involvement, DNA aneuploidy, p53 status and expression of various tumor associated or proliferative antigens[122].

Little is known about the natural history of dysplasia in the absence of urothelial carcinoma[123]. Zuk et al. described progression to CIS in 15% of 15 patients with primary urothelial dysplasia[124]. Cheng et al. followed 36 untreated patients with primary urothelial dysplasia (mean follow up 8.2 years) and found development of CIS and invasive urothelial cancer in 19%[123]. There is no doubt that patients with urothelial dysplasia require careful follow up, but it is not known whether a dysplastic focus can regress or progress, or remains the same. Murphy and Soloway have suggested that mild/moderate dysplasia is not in itself malignant, but represents a cellular response to various unknown events occurring in genetically susceptible individuals, which may mark patients with an increased risk of developing bladder cancer[104].

Squamous carcinoma

Squamous carcinoma is defined as a malignant epithelial tumor of one cell type with cells forming keratin or showing intercellular bridges[7]. Squamous carcinoma is variably reported as comprising 3–7% urothelial malignancies in the USA and in England[1,125,126], but is much more common in countries where schistosomiasis is endemic, comprising 75% of an Egyptian series of urothelial malignancies[13]. Patients may have a long history of irritation of the bladder mucosa due to chronic bacterial infection, lithiasis, calcified schistosoma ova, infected diverticula and indwelling catheters. There is often associated keratinizing squamous metaplasia of the urothelium (Figure 3.15), which appears macroscopically as white plaques and may show dysplastic maturation[127,128,129] (Figure 3.16). Benson and co-workers reported that 22% of patients with

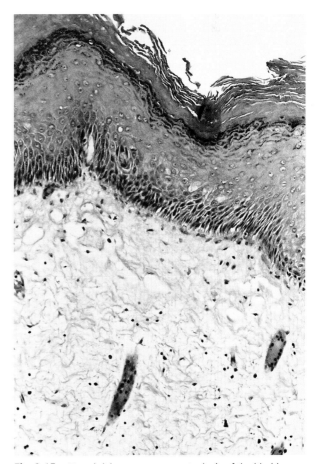

Fig. 3.15 Keratinizing squamous metaplasia of the bladder mucosa.

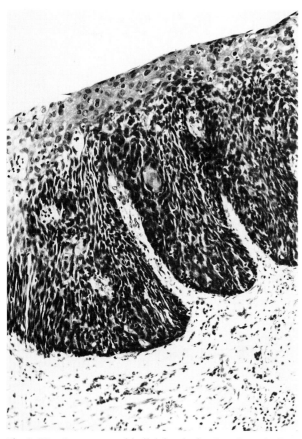

Fig. 3.16 Squamous epithelial dysplasia. There is marked crowding and hyperchromatism of cells in the lower two-thirds of the epithelium.

bladder leukoplakia (which they defined as squamous metaplasia with dysplastic maturation) had coexisting bladder cancer (either squamous carcinoma or TCC) and that 21% of patients with leukoplakia of the bladder suffered bladder carcinoma at a later date, after a mean interval of 11 years[128]. Conversely, another study reported that the majority of squamous tumors appear to develop from apparently normal urothelium[126]. Squamous carcinoma may also develop from extensive squamous de-differentiation in a pre-existing TCC[127].

It should be noted that keratinizing squamous metaplasia is distinct from the normal non-keratinizing vaginal type squamous epithelium present at the trigone in pre-menopausal women[127,128].

The macroscopic appearances of squamous carcinoma vary from a sessile, solitary ulcerative mass to a papillary, polypoid or nodular tumor, sometimes with a shaggy white necrotic surface and often deeply invasive at presentation[10]. Keratin flakes in the urine occasionally give a snowstorm appearance at cystoscopy. Squamous cell carcinoma is graded according to the amount of keratiniza-

tion and the degree of nuclear pleomorphism of tumor cells[1,21,36,126]. Well differentiated squamous cell carcinoma is composed of islands and sheets of polygonal cells, with well defined borders and intercellular bridges. At the periphery of the islands, there are fairly uniform basaloid cells which keratinize as they progress centrally or to the surface, with varying degrees of individual cell keratinization and keratin pearl formation. Nuclei are bland with only mild pleomorphism. Moderately differentiated tumors (Figure 3.17A and 3.17B) show greater nuclear pleomorphism, but still show well developed keratinization. Poorly differentiated squamous carcinoma shows pronounced nuclear pleomorphism and mitotic activity, with reduced keratinization. Non-keratinizing areas of a squamous tumor cannot be reliably distinguished from high-grade TCC.

The differential diagnosis of squamous carcinoma in the bladder includes TCC with squamous de-differentiation[69,127] and secondary extension of squamous carcinoma from the female genital tract.

Verrucous carcinoma is an extremely rare low-grade variant of squamous carcinoma, with only a few single cases, unassociated with schistosomiasis reported in the literature[130,131], but comprising 3% of a large Egyptian series of bladder cancer, almost all of which showed schistosome eggs in the surgical specimen[132]. Verrucous carcinoma is a large papillary exophytic tumor, with a white, warty surface, shedding friable keratinous debris. On microscopic examination there is marked hyperkeratosis, papillomatosis and acanthosis of squamous epithelial cells, which form bulbous, rounded, downgrowths with a 'pushing' margin and minimal cytologic atypia. Mitoses are limited to the basal layer. A superficial biopsy will include only bland squamous cells and may be erroneously interpreted as benign. Diagnostic biopsies require the full thickness of the tumor, including the growing edge[130]. Many otherwise typical squamous carcinomas show areas with a verrucous pattern and the diagnosis of verrucous carcinoma can only be made with certainty after examination of the whole tumor[10].

Glandular epithelial tumors

Villous adenoma of the bladder is a rare neoplasm showing a tubulovillous configuration similar to that of tumors in the large bowel[133,134,135]. Papillary fronds are covered by intestinal type columnar epithelium, which may show epithelial dysplasia. Caution is advised in the interpretation of a superficial biopsy of a tubulovillous neoplasm, particularly when there is a cribriform glandular pattern or high-grade nuclear atypia, as this may represent the surface of a papillary adenocarcinoma and the base of the tumor should be sampled to exclude invasion[10].

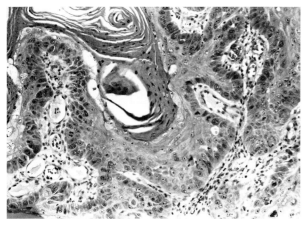

Fig. 3.17A Squamous carcinoma of the bladder. There is prominent surface keratinization.

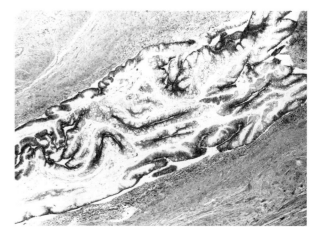

Fig. 3.18A Villous adenoma of the urachus.

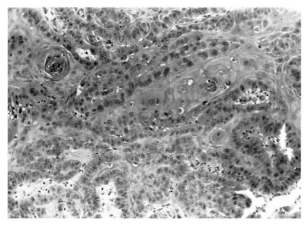

Fig. 3.17B Squamous carcinoma with keratin pearls and cytoplasmic keratinization at the center of cell islands.

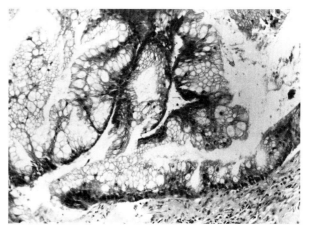

Fig. 3.18B Mucin secreting epithelium of villous adenoma showing mild dysplasia.

Villous adenoma also occurs in the urachus, where it forms a cystic mass at the bladder dome, with mucin-filled locules which may rupture[136]. The lining epithelium is of tall columnar mucus secreting goblet cells which may simply line the locules or may cover villous fronds[136] (Figures 3.18A and 3.18B). The presence of infiltrative growth through the cyst wall is indicative of malignancy.

Primary adenocarcinoma of the bladder

Primary bladder adenocarcinoma is an uncommon tumor, comprising 0.5–2% of primary urothelial tumors[137]. Approximately two-thirds of adenocarcinomas arise from the bladder mucosa[138] and these include a small number of cases associated with exstrophy[139], schistosomiasis[140] and endometriosis[141]. The remain-

ing third of adenocarcinomas arise from the urachus and make up 90% of urachal carcinomas[136]. Pathologic criteria for the diagnosis of an urachal origin are: 1) location in the bladder dome, 2) absence of cystitis glandularis and cystitis cystica in the bladder mucosa, 3) predominant invasion of the muscularis or deeper tissues, with a sharp demarcation between the tumor and normal surface epithelium, 4) presence of a urachal remnant in association with the neoplasm and 5) upward extension to the space of Retzius, anterior abdominal wall or umbilicus[142]. The most critical features are considered to be location in the bladder wall of the dome or anteriorly, a sharp demarcation between the tumor and surface epithelium and exclusion of a primary adenocarcinoma elsewhere[143]. Secondary adenocarcinoma in the bladder usually represents direct extension from adjacent structures by tumor of colonic, prostatic or ovarian origin[137].

31

Adenocarcinomas are usually solitary tumors and are often advanced at diagnosis. There may be obvious mucin production, leading to mucusuria, but the macroscopic appearances are otherwise seldom diagnostic. In the signet ring form of adenocarcinoma there may be diffuse thickening of the bladder wall with a linitis plastica-like appearance[144]. Signet ring cell adenocarcinoma has been reported to behave very aggressively[145], but a recent study of primary vesical adenocarcinoma found tumor stage, grade and lymph node involvement to be the only significant prognostic factors[146].

Five histologic subtypes of adenocarcinoma are described[10,138] and tumors may show one or more patterns.

1. Enteric, with architectural and cytologic features resembling typical colonic adenocarcinoma (Figure 3.19);
2. Mucinous (colloid), with single cells or nests of cells, floating in lakes of extracellular mucin;
3. Signet ring, composed of single tumor cells, distended with mucin and a diffusely infiltrating growth pattern (Figure 3.20);
4. Clear cell, varying from cells with abundant, clear glycogen rich cytoplasm to flattened and hobnail cells, arranged in tubulocystic, papillary and diffuse growth patterns;
5. Adenocarcinoma, not otherwise specified, when the pattern does not fit any of these categories.

All of these histologic types may occur in primary vesical and urachal adenocarcinomas, with the exception that clear cell adenocarcinoma has not been reported arising in the urachus or in the exstrophic bladder[10]. It may be difficult to distinguish between primary vesical

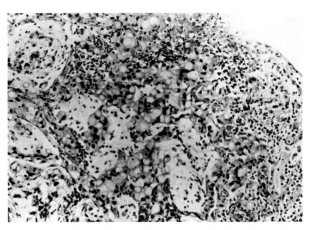

Fig. 3.20 Primary adenocarcinoma of the bladder: signet ring cell type.

adenocarcinoma and urachal cancer, as 15% of non-urachal adenocarcinomas are located at the dome and diagnosis requires correlation of clinical and pathologic findings.

The high frequency of adenocarcinoma in exstrophy appears to be related to the presence of metaplastic glandular epithelium in the exstrophic bladder and it has been suggested that extensive areas of colonic type mucosa in the urinary bladder (Figure 3.21) are a significant risk factor for subsequent carcinoma[147]. However, in a recent study of 53 cases of intestinal metaplasia of the bladder followed for 10 years, none of the patients developed bladder adenocarcinoma[148].

Undifferentiated carcinoma

Small cell carcinoma

Small cell carcinoma comprises 0.5–1% of bladder neoplasms[14,21,149] and shows an aggressive course similar to that of small cell undifferentiated carcinoma of lung, to which it is histologically and ultrastructurally similar[149,150]. Blomjous et al. reported that 78% of patients died of their tumor after a mean follow up period of 9.4 months[14]. Combination chemotherapy[14], surgical resection with adjuvant systemic multidrug chemotherapy[72], or chemotherapy and adjuvant radiotherapy[151] have been advocated for treatment, but there are insufficient cases to determine the best therapeutic strategy[72]. Paraneoplastic syndromes are uncommon, but hypercalcemia, hypophosphatemia and ectopic adrenocorticotrophic hormone production have been reported[152–154]. Tumors are broad-based solid, nodular and ulcerated masses with deep invasion into the muscular wall or beyond at presentation[14].

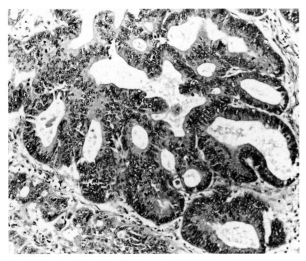

Fig. 3.19 Primary adenocarcinoma of the bladder: intestinal type.

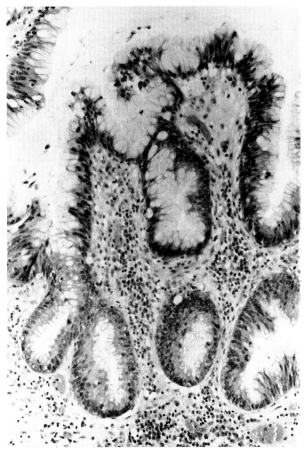

Fig. 3.21 Colonic type metaplasia with dysplasia in the bladder.

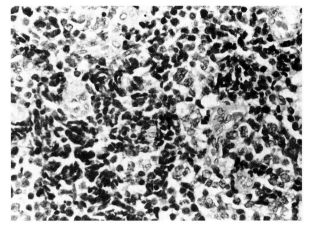

Fig. 3.22 Small cell undifferentiated (oat cell) carcinoma of the bladder.

with variable reports of chromogranin[72] and synaptophysin positivity[14]. Electron microscopic analysis shows dense core neurosecretory granules, but these may be sparse and difficult to find[14,152,153].

Small cell carcinoma of the bladder must be differentiated from malignant lymphoma and metastatic small cell carcinoma or from direct extension by small cell carcinoma of prostate[72].

The histogenesis of small cell carcinoma of the bladder is unknown[10]. The tumor may arise from multipotential stem cells that represent the common precursors of various types of bladder cancer[150], or may arise from malignant transformation of neuroendocrine cells which occur sporadically in the bladder mucosa[14].

Light microscopy shows sheets of closely packed small tumor cells, which are separated by fibrovascular stroma with a sparse lymphocytic infiltrate. Necrosis is common and there may be much crush artefact. Tumor cells show small hyperchromatic, round to oval nuclei, with dispersed chromatin, inconspicuous nucleoli and scanty cytoplasm (Figure 3.22). There is nuclear moulding and DNA encrustation of vessels[72]. Mitotic figures are common. Tumors may be divided into three groups as defined by the WHO: 1) oat cell carcinoma type, 2) intermediate cell type, and 3) combined carcinoma type, in which the tumor combination may include TCC, squamous carcinoma, adenocarcinoma or urothelial carcinoma in situ with small cell carcinoma[155]. There is no recorded difference in survival between these histologic subtypes[72].

The diagnosis may be confirmed by demonstration of neuroendocrine features by immunohistochemistry or by electron microscopy. Blomjous *et al.* found neuroendocrine features in 78% of cases[14]. The most sensitive neuroendocrine marker is neuron-specific enolase[14,72,149,150],

References

1. Koss LG. *Tumors of the urinary bladder, Atlas of tumor pathology* (2nd series Fascicle 11), Armed Forces Institute of Pathology, Washington 1975.
2. Kissane JM. Development and structure of the urogenital system. In: Murphy WM (Ed.) *Urological pathology*. WB Saunders, Philadelphia, 1989, pp. 1–33.
3. Ro JY, Ayala AG, El-Naggar A. Muscularis mucosae of the urinary bladder, importance for staging and treatment. *Am J Surg Pathol* 1987;**11**:668–673.
4. Younes M, Sussman J, True LD. The usefulness of the level of the muscularis mucosae in the staging of invasive transitional cell carcinoma of the urinary bladder. *Cancer* 1990;**66**:543–548.
5. Angulo JC, Lopez JI, Grignon DJ, Sanchez-Chapado, M. Muscularis mucosa differentiates two populations with different prognosis in stage T1 bladder cancer. *Urology* 1995;**45**:47–53.
6. Murphy WM. ASCP survey on anatomic pathology examination of the urinary bladder. *Am J Clin Pathol* 1994;**102**:715–723.
7. Mostofi FK, Sobin HL, Torloni H. *Histological typing of urinary bladder tumors* (International Histological Classification of Bladder Tumors, No. 10). World Health Organization, Geneva, Switzerland, 1973.
8. Miller A, Mitchell JB, Brown NJ. The Bristol bladder tumour registry. *Br J Urol* 1969;**41**(Suppl):1–64.

9. Ayala AG and Ro JY. Pre-malignant tumours of the urothelium and transitional cell tumours. In Young RH (Ed.) *Pathology of the urinary bladder*. Churchill Livingstone, New York, 1989; pp. 65–101.

10. Young RH, Eble JN. Unusual forms of carcinoma of the urinary bladder. *Hum Pathol* 1991;**22**:948–965.

11. Young RH, Zukerberg LR. Microcystic transitional cell carcinoma of the urinary bladder: a report of four cases. *Am J Clin Pathol* 1991;**96**:635–639.

12. Young RH, Wick MR, Mills SE. Sarcomatoid carcinoma of the urinary bladder, a clinicopathologic analysis of 12 cases and review of the literature. *Am J Clin Pathol* 1988;**90**:653–661.

13. el-Bolkainy MN, Mokhtar NM, Ghoneim MA, Hussein MH. The impact of schistosomiasis on the pathology of bladder carcinoma. *Cancer* 1981;**48**:2643–2648.

14. Blomjous EM, Vos W, De Voogt J, Van der Valk P, Meijer CJLM. Small cell carcinoma of the urinary bladder. *Cancer* 1989;**64**:1347–1357.

15. Grignon DJ. Neoplasms of the urinary bladder. In Bostwick DG and Eble JE (eds) *Urologic surgical pathology*. Mosby, St Louis, 1997; pp. 214–305.

16. Ash JE. Epithelial tumours of the bladder. *J Urol* 1940;**44**:135.

17. Eble JN, Young RH. Benign and low-grade papillary lesions of the urinary bladder: a review of the papilloma-papillary carcinoma controversy and a report of five typical papillomas. *Sem Diagn Pathol* 1989;**6**:351–371.

18. Epstein JI, Amin MB, Reuter VR, Mostofi KM and the Bladder Consensus Conference Committee. The World Health Organization/International Society of Urological Pathology Consensus Classification of Urothelial (Transitional Cell) Neoplasms of the Urinary Bladder. *Am J Surg Path* 1998;**22**:1435–1448.

19. Paschkis R: Über adenome der Harnblase. *J Urol Chir* 1927;**21**:315–325.

20. Potts AF, Hirst E. Inverted papilloma of the bladder. *J Urol* 1963;**90**:175–179.

21. Murphy WM, Beckwith JB, Farrow GM. *Tumours of the kidney, bladder and related urinary structures, Atlas of tumour pathology* (3rd series Fascicle 11), Armed Forces Institute of Pathology, Washington, 1994.

22. Amin MB, Gómez JA, Young RH. Urothelial transitional cell carcinoma with endophytic growth patterns. *Am J Surg Pathol* 1997;**21**:1057–1068.

23. Kunze E, Schauer A, Schmitt M. Histology and histogenesis of two different types of inverted urothelial papillomas. *Cancer* 1983;**51**:348–358.

24. De Meester LJ, Farrow GM, Utz DC. Inverted papillomas of the urinary bladder. *Cancer* 1975;**36**:505–513.

25. Renfer LG, Kelley J, Belville WD. Inverted papilloma of the urinary tract: histogenesis, recurrence and associated malignancy. *J Urol* 1988;**140**:832–834.

26. Stein BS, Rosen S, Kendall R. The association of inverted papilloma and transitional cell carcinoma of the urothelium. *J Urol* 1984;**131**:751–752.

27. Whitesel JA. Inverted papilloma of the urinary tract: malignant potential. *J Urol* 1982;**127**:539–540.

28. Lazarevic B, Garret R. Inverted papilloma and papillary transitional cell carcinoma of the urinary bladder. *Cancer* 1978;**42**:1904–1911.

29. Witjes JA, van Balken MR, van der Kaa CA. The prognostic value of a primary inverted papilloma of the urinary tract. *J Urol* 1997;**158**:1500–1505.

30. Bergvist A, Ljuungqvist A, Moberger G. Classification of bladder tumours based on the cellular pattern. *Acta Chir Scand* 1965;**130**:371–378.

31. Olsen S. Urothelium and urothelial neoplasia. In: *Tumors of the kidney and urinary tract*. Munksgaard, Copenhagen, 1984, p. 125–135.

32. Prout GR, Barton BA, Griffin PP and Friedell GH for the National Bladder Cancer Group. Treated history of non-invasive grade 1 transitional cell carcinoma. *J Urol* 1992;**148**:1413–1419.

33. Kern WH. The grade and pathological stage of bladder cancer. *Cancer* 1984;**53**:1185–1189.

34. Heney NM, Ahmed H, Flanagan MJ, Frable W, Corder MP, Hafermann MD and Hawkins IR for National Bladder Cancer Collaborative Group A. Superficial bladder cancer: progression and recurrence. *J Urol* 1983;**130**:1083–1086.

35. Gilbert HA, Logan JL, Kagan AR *et al*. The natural history of papillary transitional cell carcinoma of the bladder and its treatment in an unselected population on the basis of histologic grading. *J Urol* 1978;**119**:488–492.

36. Eagan JW, Jr. Urothelial neoplasms: Pathologic anatomy. In: Hill GS (Ed.) *Uropathology*, vol. 2. Churchill Livingstone, New York, 1989, pp. 719–782.

37. Kaubisch S, Lum BL, Reese J, Freiha F, Torti FM. Stage T1 bladder cancer: grade is the primary determinant for risk of muscle invasion. *J Urol* 1991;**146**:28–31.

38. Kiemeney LA, Witjes JA, Heijbroek RP, Verbeek AL, Debruyne FM. Predictability of recurrent and progressive disease in individual patients with primary superficial bladder cancer. *J Urol* 1993;**150**:60–64.

39. Birch BRP, Harland SJ. The pT1 G3 bladder tumour. *Br J Urol* 1989;**64**:109–116.

40. Jewett HJ, King LR and Shelley WJ. A study of 365 cases of infiltrating bladder cancer: relation of certain pathological characteristics to prognosis after extirpation. *J Urol* 1964;**92**:668–678.

41. Anderstrom C, Johansson S and Nilsson S. The significance of lamina propria invasion on the prognosis of patients with bladder tumours. *J Urol* 1980;**124**:23–26.

42. Heney NM, Proppe K, Prout GR, Griffin PP, Shipley WU. Invasive bladder cancer: tumor configuration, lymphatic invasion and survival. *J Urol* 1983;**130**:895–897.

43. Jewett HJ, Strong GH. Infiltrating carcinoma of the bladder: relation of depth of penetration of the bladder wall to incidence of local extension and metastases. *J Urol* 1946;**55**:366–372.

44. Fitzpatrick JM, West AB, Butler MR, Lane V, O'Flynn JD. Superficial bladder tumours (stage pTa, grades 1 and 2). The importance of recurrence pattern following initial resection. *J Urol* 1986;**135**:920–922.

45. Dalesio O, Schulman CC, Sylvester R, and Members of the EORTC, Genitourinary Tract Cancer Cooperative Group. Prognostic factors in superficial bladder tumors. A study of the European Organization for Research on Treatment of Cancer. *J Urol* 1983;**129**:730–733.

46. Parmar MKB, Freedman LS, Hargreave TB, Tolley DA. Prognostic factors for recurrence and followup policies in the treatment of superficial bladder cancer: Report from the British Medical Research Council Subgroup on superficial bladder cancer (Urological Cancer Working Party). *J Urol* 1989;**142**:284–288.

47. Brodsky GL. Pathology of bladder carcinoma. *Hematol Onco Clin North Am* 1992;**6**(1):59–80.

48. Carbin BE, Ekman P, Gustafson H, Christiensen NJ, Sandstedt B, Silfversward C. Grading of human urothelial carcinoma based on nuclear atypia and mitotic frequency. I. Histological description. *J Urol* 1991;**145**:968–971.

49. Abel P. Differing interpretations by pathologists of pT category and grade. *Br J Urol* 1988;**62**:339–342.

50. Ooms ECM, Blok APR, Veldhuizen RW. The reproducibility of a quantitative grading system of bladder tumours. *Histopathology* 1985;**9**:501–509.

51. Sorensen F, Sasaki M. Fukuzawa, Yamabe H, Olsen S, Yoshida O. Qualitative and quantitative histopathology in transitional cell carcinomas of the urinary bladder. An international investigation of intra- and interobserver reproducibility. *Lab Invest* 1994;**70**:242–254.

52. Robertson AJ, Swanson Beck J, Burnett RA *et al*. Observer variability in histopathological reporting of transitional cell carcinoma and epithelial dysplasia in bladders. *J Clin Pathol* 1990;**43**:17–21.

53. Witjes JA, Kiemeney LALM, Schaafsma HE, Debruyne FMJ, and the members of the Dutch South East Cooperative Urological Group. The influence of review pathology on study outcome of a randomized multicentre superficial bladder cancer trial. *Br J Urol* 1994;**73**:172–176.

54. Murphy WM. Diseases of the urinary bladder, urethra, ureters and renal pelvis. In: Murphy WM (Ed.) *Urological pathology*. Philadelphia: WB Saunders, 1989, pp. 34–146.

55. Jordan AM, Weingarten J, Murphy WM. Transitional cell neoplasms of the urinary bladder. Can biologic potential be predicted from histological grading? *Cancer* 1987;**60**:2766–2744.

56. Amin MB, Young RH. Intraepithelial lesions of the urinary bladder with a discussion of the histogenesis of urothelial neoplasia. *Sem Diagn Pathol* 1997;**14**:84–97.

57. Pauwels RPE, Schapers RFM. Smeets AWGB, Detomynetis J, Geraedts JPM. Grading in superficial bladder cancer. (1) Morphological criteria. *Br J Urol* 1988;**61**:129–134.

58. Carbin BE, Ekman P, Gustafson H, Christiensen NJ, Silfversward C. and Sandstedt B. Grading of human urothelial carcinoma based on nuclear atypia and mitotic frequency. II. Prognostic importance. *J Urol* 1991;**14**:972–997.

59. Lapham RL, Grignon D, Ro JY. Pathologic prognostic parameters in bladder urothelial biopsy, transurethral resection and cystectomy specimens. *Sem Diagn Pathol* 1997;**14**:109–122.

60. Wheeless LL, Badalement RA, de Vere White RW, Fradet Y, Tribukait B. Consensus review of the clinical utility of DNA cytometry in bladder cancer. *Cytometry* 1993;**14**:478–481.

61. Lipponen PK, Eskelinen MJ, Kivranta J *et al.* Prognosis of transitional cell bladder cancer. A multivariate prognostic score for improved prediction. *J Urol* 1991;**146**:1535–1540.

62. Lipponen PK, Eskelinen MJ, Jauhiainen K, Terho R, Nordling S. Proliferation indices as independent factors in papillary Ta-T1 transitional cell bladder tumours. *Br J Urol* 1993;**72**:451–457.

63. Cohen MB, Waldman FM, Carroll PR *et al.* Comparison of five histopathological methods to assess cellular proliferation in transitional cell carcinoma of the urinary bladder. *Hum Pathol* 1993; **24**:772–778.

64. Levin I, Klein T, Goldstein J *et al.* Expression of class I histocompatibility antigens in transitional cell carcinoma of the urinary bladder in relation to survival. *Cancer* 1991;**68**:2591–2594.

65. Cordon-Cardo C, Wartinger D, Petrylak D *et al.* Altered expression of the retinoblastoma gene product, prognostic indicator in bladder cancer. *J Natl Cancer Inst* 1988;**88**:1251–1256.

66. Esrig D, Elmajian D, Groshen S *et al.* Accumulation of nuclear p53 and tumor progression in bladder cancer. *N Engl J Med* 1994;**331**:1259–1264.

67. Sarkis AS, Dalbagni G, Cordon-Cardo C *et al.* Nuclear overexpression of p53 protein in transitional cell bladder carcinoma: a marker for disease progression. *J Natl Cancer Inst* 1993;**85**:53–59.

68. Kuczyk MA, Bokemeyer C, Serth J *et al.* P53 overexpression as a prognostic factor for advanced stage bladder cancer. *Eur J Cancer* 1995;**31A**:2243–2247.

69. Martin JE, Jenkins BJ, Zuk RJ, Blandy JP, Baithun SI. Clinical importance of squamous metaplasia in invasive transitional cell carcinoma of the bladder. *J Clin Path* 1989;**42**:250–253.

70. Vale JA, A'Hern RP, Liu K *et al.* Predicting the outcome of radical radiotherapy for invasive bladder cancer. *Eur Urol* 1993;**24**:48–51.

71. Logothetis CJ, Dexeus FH, Chong C *et al.* Cisplatin, cyclophosphamide and doxorubicin chemotherapy for unresectable urothelial tumors: the M.D. Anderson experience. *J Urol* 1989;**141**:33–37.

72. Grignon DJ, Ro JY, Ayala AG *et al.* Small cell carcinoma of the urinary bladder. *Cancer* 1992;**69**:527–537.

73. Lopez-Beltran A, Pacelli A, Rothenberg HJ *et al.* Carcinosarcoma and sarcomatoid carcinoma of the bladder: clinicopathological study of 41 cases. *J Urol* 1998;**159**:1497–1503.

74. Grammatico D, Grignon DJ, Eberwein P *et al.* Transitional cell carcinoma of the renal pelvis with choriocarcinomatous differentiation: Immunohistochemical and immunoelectron microscopic assessment of human chorionic gonadotrophin production by transitional cell carcinoma of the urinary bladder. *Cancer* 1993;**71**:1835–1841.

75. Jenkins BJ, Martin JE, Baithun SI, Zuk RJ, Oliver RTD, Blandy JP. Prediction of response to radiotherapy in invasive bladder cancer. *Br J Urol* 1990;**65**:345–348.

76. Norton KD, Burnett RA. Choriocarcinoma arising in transitional cell carcinoma of the bladder: a case report. *Histopathology* 1988; **12**:325–328.

77. Gallagher L, Lind R, Oyasu R. Primary choriocarcinoma of the bladder in association with undifferentiated carcinoma. *Hum Pathol* 1984; **15**:793–795.

78. Tinkler SD, Roberts JT, Robinson MC, Ramsden PD. Primary choriocarcinoma of the urinary bladder: a case report. *Clin Oncol* 1996;**8**:59–61.

79. Ainsworth RW, Cresham GA. Primary choriocarcinoma of the urinary bladder in a male. *J Pathol Bacteriol* 1960;**79**:185–192.

80. Weinberg T. Primary chorionepithelioma of the urinary bladder in a male patient: a report of a case. *Am J Pathol* 1939;**15**:783–795.

81. International Union against Cancer, *TNM Atlas* (4th edn 1997). Illustrated guide to the TNM/pTNM Classification of Malignant Tumours. Springer-Verlag.

82. Ro JY, Staerkel GA, Ayala AG. Cytologic and histologic features of superficial bladder cancer. *Urol Clin North Amer* 1992;**3**:435–453.

83. Abel PD Prognostic indices in transitional cell carcinoma of the bladder. *Br J Urol* 1988;**62**:103–109.

84. Farrow GM, Utz DC. Observations on microinvasive transitional cell carcinoma of the urinary bladder. *Clin Oncol* 1982;**1**:609–614.

85. Young RH, Oliva E. Transitional cell carcinomas of the urinary bladder that may be underdiagnosed. *Am J Surg Pathol* 1996;**20**:1448–1454.

86. Matzkin H, Soloway MS, Hardeman S. Transitional cell carcinoma of the prostate. *J Urol* 1991;**146**:1207–1212.

87. Esrig D, Freeman JA, Elmajian DA *et al.* Transitional cell carcinoma involving the prostate with a proposed staging classification for stromal invasion. *J Urol* 1996;**156**:1071–1076.

88. Hardeman SW, Perry A, Soloway MS. Transitional cell carcinoma of the prostate following intravesical therapy for transitional cell carcinoma of the bladder. *J Urol* 1988;**140**:289–292.

89. Hudson MA. Editorial: A new staging system for transitional cell carcinoma involvement of the prostate and reconfirmation studies of intravesical therapy for superficial bladder cancer. *J Urol* 1996;**156**:972–974.

90. Pagano F, Bassi P, Ferrante GL, Piazza N, Abatangelo G, Pappagallo GL, Garbeglio A. Is stage pT4a (D1) reliable in assessing transitional cell carcinoma involvement of the prostate in patients with a concurrent bladder cancer? A necessary distinction for contiguous or noncontiguous involvement. *J Urol* 1996;**155**:244–247.

91. Solsona E, Iborra I, Ricos JV, Monrós JL, Casanova JL, Almenar S. The prostate involvement as prognostic factor in patients with superficial bladder tumors. *J Urol* 1995;**154**:1710–1713.

92. Cheville JC, Dundore PA, Bostwick DG *et al.* Transitional cell carcinoma of the prostate. *Cancer* 1998;**82**:703–707.

93. Mahadevia PS, Koss LG, Tar IJ. Prostatic involvement in bladder cancer. *Cancer* 1986;**58**:2096–2102.

94. Epstein JI. Transitional cell carcinoma. In: *Prostatic biopsy interpretation* (2nd edn). Lipincott-Raven, Philadelphia 1995, pp. 211–234.

95. Bostwick DG. Neoplasms of the prostate. In: Bostwick DG, Eble JN (eds) *Urologic surgical pathology.* Mosby, St Louis, 1997, pp. 342–421.

96. Lopez JI, Angulo JC. The prognostic significance of vascular invasion in stage T1 bladder cancer. *Histopathology* 1995;**27**:27–33.

97. Ramani P, Birch BRP, Harland SJ, Parkinson MC. Evaluation of endothelial markers in detecting blood and lymphatic channel invasion in pT1 transitional cell carcinoma of the bladder. *Histopathology* 1991;**19**:551–554.

98. Larsen NP, Steinberg GD, Brendler CB *et al.* Use of the *Ulex europaeus* agglutinin 1 (UEA1) to distinguish vascular and pseudovascular invasion in transitional cell carcinoma of bladder with lamina propria invasion. *Mod Pathol* 1990;**3**:83–88.

99. Taylor DC, Bhagavan BS, Larsen MP, Cox JA, Epstein JI. Papillary urothelial hyperplasia: a precursor to papillary neoplasms. *Am J Surg Pathol* 1986;**20**:1481–1488.

100. Sarma KP. Genesis of papillary tumours: histological and microangiographic study. *Br J Urol* 1981;**53**:228–236.

101. Nagy GK, Frable WJ, Murphy WM. Classification of premalignant urothelial abnormalities. A Delphi study of the National Bladder Cancer Collaborative Group A. *Path Ann* 1982;**17**:219–233.

102. Richards B, Parmar MKB, Anderson CK *et al.* and the MRC Superficial Bladder Cancer Sub Group. Interpretation of biopsies of 'normal' urothelium in patients with superficial bladder cancer. *Br J Urol* 1991;**67**:369–375.

103. Sharkey FE, Sarosdy MF. The significance of central pathology review in clinical studies of transitional cell carcinoma in situ. *J Urol* 1997;**157**:68–71.

104. Murphy WM, Soloway MS. Urothelial dysplasia. *J Urol* 1982;**127**:849–854.

105. Friedell GH, Soloway MS, Hilgar AG, Farrow GM. Summary of workshop of carcinoma in situ of the bladder. *J Urol* 1986;**136**:1047–1048.

106. Elliott GB, Moloney PJ, Anderson GH. 'Denuding cystitis' and in situ urothelial carcinoma. *Arch Pathol* 1973;**96**:91–94.

107. Orozco RE, Vander Zwaag R, Murphy WM. The pagetoid variant of urothelial carcinoma in situ. *Hum Pathol* 1993;**24**:1199–1202.

108. Melicow MM Histological study of vesical urothelium intervening between gross neoplasms in total cystectomy. *J Urol* 1952;**68**:261–278.

109. Kakizoe T, Matumoto K, Nishio Y, Ohtani M, Kishi K. Significance of carcinoma in situ and dysplasia in association with bladder cancer. *J Urol* 1985;**133**:395–398.

110. Wolf H, Højgaard K. Urothelial dysplasia concomitant with bladder tumours as a determinant factor for future new occurrences. *Lancet* 1983;**ii**:134–136.

111. Vicente J, Laguna MP, Duarte D, Algaba F, Chéchile G. Carcinoma in situ as a prognostic factor for G3pT1 bladder tumours. *Br J Urol* 1991; **68**:380–382.

112. Althausen AF, Prout GR, Daly JJ. Non-invasive papillary carcinoma in situ. *J Urol* 1976;**166**:575–560.

113. Smith G, Elton RA, Beynon LL, Newsam JE, Chisolm GD, Hargreave TB. Prognostic significance of biopsy results of normal-looking mucosa in cases of superficial bladder cancer. *Br J Urol* 1983;**55**:665–669.

114. Mufti GR, Singh M. Value of random mucosal biopsies in the management of superficial bladder cancer. *Eur Urol* 1992;**22**:288–293.

115. Prout GR, Jr, Griffin PP, Daly JJ, Heney NM. Carcinoma in situ of the urinary bladder with and without associated vesical neoplasms. *Cancer* 1983;**52**:524–532.

116. Fukui I, Yokokawa M, Sekine H *et al.* Carcinoma in situ of the urinary bladder. *Cancer* 1987;**59**:164–173.

117. Orozco RE, Martin AA, Murphy WM. Carcinoma in situ of the urinary bladder. *Cancer* 1994;**74**:115–122.

118. Solsona E, Iborra I, Ricós JV, Monrós JL, Dumont R, Casanova J *et al.* Carcinoma in situ associated with superficial bladder tumor. *Eur Urol* 1991;**19**:93–96.

119. Farrow GM, Utz DC, Rife CC, Greene LF. Clinical observations on sixty-nine cases of in situ carcinoma of the urinary bladder. *Cancer Res* 1977;**37**:2794–2798.

120. van Gils-Gielen RJM, Debruyne FMJ, Witjes WPM *et al.* Risk factors in carcinoma in situ of the urinary bladder. *Urology* 1995;**45**:581–586.

121. Norming U, Tribukait B, Gustafson H *et al.* Deoxyribonucleic acid profile and tumor progression in primary carcinoma in situ of the bladder: a study of 63 patients with grade 3 lesions. *J Urol* 1992;**147**:11–15.

122. Hudson MA, Herr HW. Carcinoma in situ of the bladder. *J Urol* 1995;**153**:564–572.

123. Cheng L, Cheville JC, Neumann RM, Bostwick DG. Natural history of urothelial dysplasia of the bladder. *Am J Surg Pathol* 1999;**23**:443–447.

124. Zuk RJ, Rogers HS, Martin JE, Baithun SI. Clinicopathological importance of primary dysplasia of bladder. *J Clin Pathol* 1988;**41**:1277–1280.

125. Petersen RO. Urinary bladder. In: Petersen RO (Ed.) *Urologic Pathology*. JB Lippincott, Philadelphia 1986, pp. 279–416.

126. Rundle JSH, Hart AJL, McGeorge A, Smith JS, Malcolm AJ, Smith PM. Squamous cell carcinoma of the bladder. A review of 114 patients. *Br J Urol* 1982;**54**:522–526.

127. Sakamoto N, Tsuneyoshi M, Enjoji M. Urinary bladder carcinoma with a neoplastic squamous component: a mapping study of 31 cases. *Histopathology* 1992;**21**:135–141.

128. Benson RC, Swanson SK, Farrow GM. Relationship of leukoplakia to urothelial malignancy. *J Urol* 1984;**131**:507–511.

129. Morgan RJ, Cameron KM. Vesical leukoplakia. *Br J Urol* 1980;**52**:96–100.

130. Horner SS, Fisher HAG, Barada JH *et al.* Verrucous carcinoma of the bladder. *J Urol* 1991;**145**:1261–1263.

131. Walther M, O'Brien D, III, Birch HW. Condylomata acuminata and verrucous carcinoma of the bladder. *J Urol* 1986;**135**:362–365.

132. el-Sebai I, Sherif M, el-Bolkainy MN, Mansour MA, Ghoneim MA. Verrucose squamous carcinoma of the bladder. *Urology* 1974;**4**:407–410.

133. Assor D. A villous tumour of the bladder. *J Urol* 1978;**119**:287–288.

134. Channer JL, Williams JL, Henry L. Villous adenoma of the bladder. *J Clin Pathol* 1993;**46**:450–452.

135. Miller DC, Gang DL, Gavris V, Alroy J, Ucci AA, Parkhurst EC. Villous adenoma of the urinary bladder: a morphologic or biologic entity? *Am J Clin Pathol* 1983;**79**:728–731.

136. Eble JN. Abnormalities of the urachus. In: Young RH (Ed.) *Pathology of the urinary bladder*. Churchill Livingstone, New York, 1989, pp. 213–243.

137. Thomas DG, Ward AM, Williams JL. A study of 52 cases of adenocarcinoma of the bladder. *Br J Urol* 1971;**43**:4–15.

138. Grignon DJ, Ro JY, Ayala AG, Johnson DE, Ordóñez NG. Primary adenocarcinoma of the urinary bladder. *Cancer* 1991;**67**:2165–2172.

139. Abeshouse BS. Exstrophy of the bladder, complicated by adenocarcinoma of the bladder and renal calculi. *J Urol* 1943;**49**:254–289.

140. Makar N. Some observation on pseudoglandular proliferation in the bilharzial bladder. *Acta Unio Internationalis contra cancrum* 1962;**18**:599–607.

141. Al Izzi MS, Horton LWL, Kelleher J *et al.* Malignant transformation in endometriosis of the urinary bladder. *Histopathology* 1989;**14**:191–198.

142. Sheldon CA, Clayman RV, Gonzalez R, Williams RD, Fraley EE. Malignant urachal lesions. *J Urol* 1984;**131**:1–8.

143. Johnson DE, Hogan JM, Ayala AG. Primary adenocarcinoma of the urinary bladder. *South Med J* 1972;**65**:527–530.

144. Kamat MR, Kulkarni JN, Tongaonkar HB. Adenocarcinoma of the bladder: study of 14 cases and review of the literature. *Br J Urol* 1991;**68**:254–257.

145. Grignon DJ, Ro JY, Johnson DE. Primary signet-ring carcinoma of the urinary bladder. (Review) *Am J Clin Path* 1991;**95**:13–20.

146. el-Mekresh MM, el-Baz MA, Abol-Enein H, Ghoneim MAC Primary adenocarcinoma of the urinary bladder: a report of 185 cases. *Br J Urol* 1998;**82**:206–212.

147. Bullock PS, Thoni DE, Murphy WM. The significance of colonic mucosa (intestinal metaplasia) involving the urinary tract. *Cancer* 1987;**57**:2086–2090.

148. Corica FA, Husmann DA, Churchill BM *et al.* Intestinal metaplasia is not a strong risk factor for bladder cancer: study of 53 cases with long-term follow-up. *Urology* 1997;**50**:427–431.

149. Lopez JI, Angulo JC, Flores N, Toledo JD. Small cell carcinoma of the urinary bladder. A clinicopathological study of six cases. *Br J Urol* 1994;**73**:43–49.

150. Podesta A, True L. Small cell carcinoma of the bladder. *Cancer* 1989;**64**:710–714.

151. Bastus R, Caballero JM, Gonzalez G *et al.* Small cell carcinoma of the urinary bladder treated with chemotherapy and radiotherapy: Results in five cases. *Eur Urol* 1999;**35**:323–326.

152. Reyes CV, Soneru I. Small cell carcinoma of the urinary bladder with hypercalcemia. *Cancer* 1985;**56**:2530–2533.

153. Cramer SF, Aikawa M, Cebelin M. Neurosecretory granules in small cell invasive carcinoma of the bladder. *Cancer* 1981;**47**:724–730.

154. Partanen S, Asikainen U. Oat cell carcinoma of the urinary bladder with ectopic adrenocorticotrophic hormone production. *Hum Pathol* 1985;**16**:313–315.

155. World Health Organisation. The World Health Organisation histological typing of lung tumors. *Am J Clin Pathol* 1982;**77**:123–136.

4 Bladder carcinoma presentation, diagnosis and staging

J W Basler and C Magee

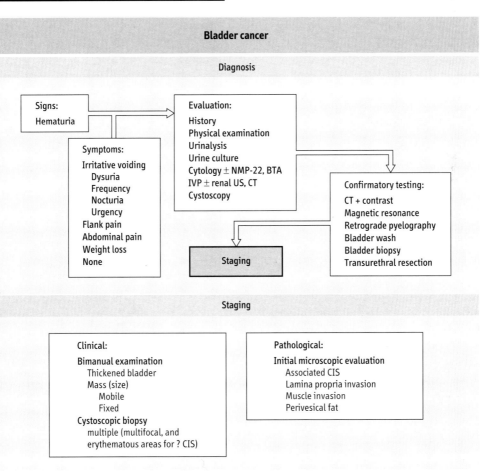

Presentation

Most bladder tumors are discovered during a routine evaluation for haematuria or irritative voiding symptoms (frequency, urgency, nocturia, dysuria) although many remain asymptomatic for months prior to discovery. Eighty per cent of patients with bladder cancer have painless, intermittent hematuria as the primary symptom[1]. Often the initial episodes of intermittent gross hematuria were either not evaluated or were treated as presumed urinary tract infections or 'passed' stones. Unfortunately, in some cases urinary tract infections or stone disease may co-exist and confuse or delay the diagnosis. The amount of hematuria varies from microscopic to frank blood but is not reliably related to amount of tumour, therefore, all hematuria warrants thorough investigation (see Hematuria algorithm). Irritative voiding symptoms such as dysuria, urgency or frequency may be associated with CIS or invasive cancer. For tumors overlying the ureteral orifice the presenting symptom may be flank pain or pyelonephritis from obstruction. These findings are also suggestive of invasive cancer. Symptoms of advanced disease such as pain, abdominal mass or weight loss may be present as well. The differential diagnosis includes urinary calculi, urinary tract infections (including tuberculosis), benign prostatic hypertrophy, prostate cancer, trauma and renal tumors.

Diagnosis

The standard evaluation for hematuria and irritative voiding includes urine culture, cytology, intravenous urography (IVU) and cystoscopy. In some patients with renal insufficiency, significant proteinuria or contrast allergy, a renal ultrasound and cystoscopy with retrograde pyelography is indicated. Recent studies of immediate 'day-case' outpatient screening of patients with hematuria have demonstrated that renal ultrasound and cystoscopy alone may be adequate evaluation leaving IVU and other imaging modalities in a confirmatory role [2]. While spiral CT and MRI imaging may be helpful for finding gross lesions or differentiating soft tissue masses from stones, their role in the initial management should be limited due to their insensitivity to subtle urothelial lesions. A new technique utilizing MR (MR urogram) may eventually be useful for evaluating urothelium, especially in dilated ureters and full bladders.

Interpreting the test results

While usually negative, a positive urine culture should not necessarily preclude further evaluation with upper tract imaging and cystoscopy after the urine has been sterilized with antibiotic therapy. Cytologic evaluation can be helpful and guide further work if positive but may fail to predict the presence of well to moderately differentiated tumors. False positive cytology occurs occasionally especially if obtained after contrast agents have been instilled into the urinary tract. Other urine-based tests (Table 4.1) are not indicated for initial evaluation but may be helpful in follow up of patients treated for transitional cell carcinoma of the bladder.

Filling defects on IVU not corresponding to calcifications on plane films (Figure 4.1) are differentiated into: bladder tumor, clot, fungal ball, lucent stones (urate), etc. A filling defect over a ureteral orifice with obstruction of the ureter suggests muscle invasive disease around the trigone and possibly ureteral tumors[3].

Table 4.1   Partial list of some currently available tests for detection of bladder cancer

Test	Measures	Indication
Cytology	Nuclear morphology	Diagnosis, Follow up
BTA	Bladder tumor associated analyte	Follow up
BTAstat	Compliment factor H-related protein	Follow up
BTA trak	Bladder tumor antigen	Follow up
NMP-22	Nuclear matrix protein	Follow up

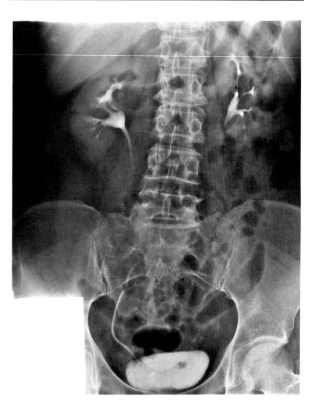

Fig. 4.1   IVU demonstrating filling defect in the bladder that was later found on cystoscopy to be a small pedunculated bladder tumor. Tumors in the bladder are best detected on drainage films and often appear as dark defects with a rim of contrast surrounding them.

In general, ultrasonography is insensitive to all but the most prominent bladder tumors, but recent advances in technology may cause this to change. A finding of hydronephrosis should be further evaluated with IVU and/or retrograde pyelography.

Cystoscopic evaluation is usually carried out in the office setting unless there is evidence on IVU that biopsy or transurethral resection of bladder tumor may be needed. Cystoscopy using a rigid 17Fr cystoscope or a flexible cystoscope with 2% lidocaine jelly as a local anesthetic should be performed on all patients with hematuria. The flexible cystoscope is more comfortable for the patient and allows for better inspection of the dome and bladder neck; however, visibility is poor when there is gross hematuria. In these cases the rigid cystoscope using 30° and 70° lenses and sterile water irrigant provides better visualization of the bladder mucosa. It is important to inspect the mucosa in a systematic fashion so that small papillary tumors or areas of potential CIS are not overlooked. Patients with other identified causes of hematuria (stones, UTI, etc.) should still undergo cystoscopy to look for concominant disease. Patients found to have tumors should then be scheduled for resection. If no cause for the hematuria can be identified, urinalysis is performed at 3–6 months and complete evaluation repeated if hematuria persists.

Cystoscopy may reveal the classic flat velvety lesion of carcinoma in situ (CIS) (Figure 4.2a) or easily distinguished frondular transitional cell carcinoma (Figure 4.2b). Often, CIS and papillary lesions coexist (Figure 4.2c). Invasive carcinomas will often have a sessile appearance with infiltration into the surrounding bladder wall (Figure 4.3). Diagnosis is made by cold-cup biopsy or transurethral resection of the lesion(s). Additionally, biopsies of other suspicious bladder lesions as well as the prostatic fossa (male) should be made. The utility of 'random' or site-directed biopsies of normal appearing areas of mucosa is not well supported but is advocated by some. Some other benign lesions such as squamous metaplasia, cystitis cystica, cystitis glandularis and unusual tumors such as nephrogenic adenoma and inflammatory pseudotumor are sometimes confused with carcinoma. Adenocarcinoma, carcinosarcoma and other unusual bladder malignancies are usually discrete sessile lesions. Prostatic carcinoma may be visualized as a diffuse infiltrative lesion originating at the bladder base often with a nodular, friable surface causing anatomical distortion and may invade the trigone and obstruct the ureter as it invades along the ureteral sheath.

Staging

There is not a uniformly accepted staging regimen for all types of bladder tumors. Superficial tumors and CIS

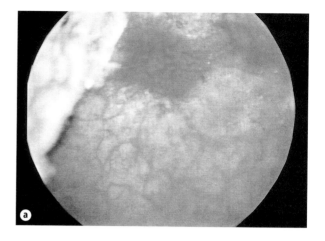

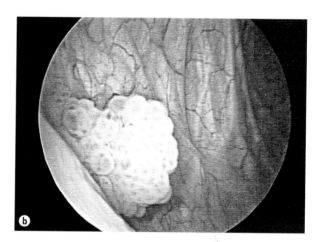

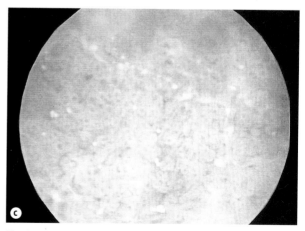

Fig. 4.2 a. Velvety patch of carcinoma in situ. b. Multiple frondular tumor excrescences along the bladder base. c. Frondular transitional cell carcinoma with a few satellite lesions.

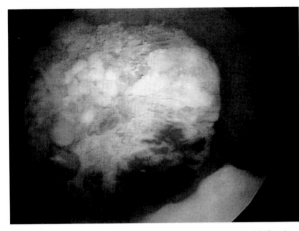

Fig. 4.3   A large sessile transitional cell carcinoma with fresh and old superficial areas of hemorrhage.

Table 4.2   TNM classification system[4]

TIS		Carcinoma in situ
Ta		Papillary tumor not invading lamina propria
T1	T1a	Papillary tumor invading basement membrane
	T1b	Papillary tumor invading true lamina propria
T2	T2a	Tumor invading superficial (inner half) detrusor
	T2b	Tumor invading deep (outer half) detrusor
T3	T3a	Tumor invading perivesical fat microscopically
	T3b	Tumor invading perivesical fat macroscopically
T4	T4a	Tumor invading prostate stroma, vagina, uterus
	T4b	Tumor invading pelvic or abdominal sidewall
Nx		Not assessed
N0		No nodal metastases
N1		Single nodal metastasis (<2 cm)
N2		Multiple nodal metastases (<5 cm)
N3		Multiple nodal metastases (>5 cm)
Mx		Presence of distant metastases not assessed
M0		No distant metastases
M1		Distant metastases

System used for all histologic types of bladder cancer (transitional cell, squamous cell, adenocarcinoma, other carcinoma) but not tumors that invade or metastasize to the bladder secondarily (prostate, lymphoma, etc.) Primary vesical melanoma or pheochromocytoma without other extravesicle lesions are rare exceptions.

generally require only the findings at cystoscopy, the results of upper tract imaging and the pathologic evaluation of the specimen. However, general guidelines for evaluation of invasive tumors would include the findings at cystoscopy, pathologic findings, examination under anesthesia, upper tract imaging and, depending on the depth of penetration of the tumor, CT scan of the chest, abdomen and pelvis. Bone scan may be helpful in situations where metastases are suspected due to an elevated serum alkaline phosphatase (an unproven but widely used indicator of bone activity) or bony pain. MRI may be helpful for determining the depth of penetration of the tumor and to assess the regional lymph nodes but usually offers little advantage over CT scan. If invasive tumor is suspected, CT or MRI imaging may be more useful for staging purposes prior to resection to eliminate the post-resection inflammatory artefact that may produce bladder wall thickening and perivesical inflammation. The TNM classification system for bladder carcinoma is presented in Table 4.2.

References

1. Cummings KB, Barone JG, Ward WS. Diagnosis and staging of bladder cancer. *Urologic Clinics of N Am* 1992; **3**: 455–465.
2. Yip S, Peh W, Tam P, Li J, Lam H. Day case hematuria diagnostic service: use of ultrasonography and flexible cystoscopy. *Urology* 1998; **52** (5):762–766.
3. Haleblian G, Skinner E, Dickinson M, Lieskovsky G, Boyd S, Skinner D. Hydronephrosis as prognostic indicator in bladder cancer patients. *J Urol* 1998;**160**(6 part 1):2011–2014.
4. Fleming ID *et al*: AJCC Cancer Staging Manual / American Joint Committee on Cancer, 5th edn. Philadelphia: Lippincott-Raven, 1997.

5 Treatment of superficial transitional cell carcinoma

Algorithm

Superficial papillary transitional cell carcinoma

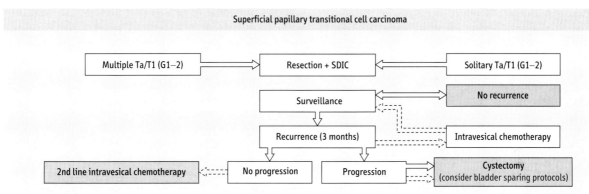

(SDIC) single dose intravesical chemotherapy = mitomycin-C/epirubicin/thiotepa
Surveillance: cystoscopy (with optional cytology, BTA, NMP, Flow cytometry) every 3 months x 24 months, then every 6 months x 24 months, then annually. or: follow Parmar's Prognostic criteria after first check at 3 months.

5.1 Surgical treatment of superficial transitional cell carcinoma

J Carbone, C Magee and J W Basler

There are many options available for the surgical treatment of superficial bladder cancer. Transurethral resection, electrosurgical and laser fulguration, partial cystectomy and total cystectomy have all been used successfully. The type of treatment used should be individualized for each patient. The indications for each method and potential complications are discussed below.

Transurethral resection

Transurethral resection (TUR) plays a unique role in the treatment of superficial transitional cell cancer (TCC) of the bladder. In addition to being the therapeutic intervention of choice for removal of superficial tumors (Ta/T1), it serves as the primary means of diagnosing and staging bladder cancers[1]. Cystoscopic evaluation may suggest the differential diagnosis of carcinoma in situ (CIS) *vs.* superficial bladder cancer *vs.* invasive bladder cancer, but only pathologic examination of specimens obtained by cold-cup biopsy or TUR of the lesion confirms the diagnosis. Superficial bladder tumors will present as a solitary lesion 70% of the time while multiple tumors will be present in 30%. Of these superficial tumors, 70% will be confined to the mucosa (Ta) while the remaining 30% will invade the lamina propria (T1). Superficial tumors have approximately a 50% lifetime risk of recurrence; however, this risk increases to nearly 75% when there are multiple previous recurrences. Patients with superficial TCC can be counseled to expect a 75–90% 5 year overall survival rate when treated by TUR alone with only 10–15% ultimately requiring more aggressive therapy[2]. Several prognostic factors are currently being investigated which may provide insight into which subset of patients are more likely to experience disease progression[3].

Carcinoma in situ, when present, significantly alters the clinical course and risk of progression of bladder cancer. It appears cystoscopically as focal or diffuse areas of velvety erythema or occasionally as a thickened whitish lesion similar to squamous metaplasia. A majority of the cases of CIS (90%) are associated with other papillary tumors, but it may appear *de novo* (10%)[4]. When found in conjunction with papillary tumors, the risk of muscle invasion is greatly increased (50–70%) and more aggressive treatment is usually recommended.

Resection, fulguration and cold-cup biopsy are all painful procedures with potential complications and are best performed under general or regional anesthesia. Patients with recurrent low-grade tumors undergoing laser fulguration may do well with only local intravesical anes-

thesia (liquid lidocaine, dyclonine, etc.) or conscious sedation. These methods, however, carry the risk of bladder perforation and extravesical spillage of tumor cells if the patient makes any sudden movements due to pain from inadequate anesthesia or obturator nerve stimulation during resection of lateral wall tumors. Local obturator nerve block or general anesthesia with paralysis will help prevent this from occurring[5]. Patients with spinal cord lesions at T6 level and above with sensory neurogenic bladders are at risk for autonomic dysreflexia and should have regional or general anesthesia with careful intraoperative monitoring to prevent this potentially dangerous complication. The type of anesthesia used ultimately depends on the patient's overall state of health and concominant medical problems.

Before starting a TUR, endoscopic evaluation using 30° and 70° lenses through a rigid cystoscope should be performed. Thorough inspection of the mucosa is necessary to identify any lesions which may have been overlooked during initial cystoscopy. Areas of erythema or lesions suspicious for CIS can be biopsied with cold-cup forceps prior to resection of larger papillary or sessile tumors. The surgical objectives when performing TUR of bladder tumors are to obtain tissue for pathologic diagnosis and staging as well as complete excision of all lesions without perforating the bladder wall. TUR is performed with the patient in lithotomy positioning under appropriate anesthesia as previously described. A blended cutting-coagulating current is typically used unless resecting near or over the ureteral orifices where pure cutting current is appropriate to prevent coagulation injury to the ureter. The irrigating fluid must be sterile, non-toxic and have a low coefficient of electrical conductivity. Sterile water is the preferred irrigation fluid for two reasons: 1) hypotonic water will lyse red blood cells and provide better visualization should bleeding be encountered; 2) it may also lyse or significantly injure tumor cells and could decrease the chance of tumor implantation elsewhere in the bladder or extravesically in the case of bladder perforation. During resection, the bladder should be sufficiently distended to prevent the bladder wall from folding back on itself. However, overdistension may stretch and thin the bladder wall increasing the risk of perforation. Using a continuous flow resectoscope will provide improved vision when bleeding is encountered and help keep the bladder from becoming overdistended.

When the bladder tumor is small, simple removal of the tumor via cold-cup biopsy may suffice. For larger exophytic tumors, the resection should proceed in an organized fashion beginning usually on the superior or lateral aspect of the tumor field. Resection progresses in a superior to inferior and lateral to medial direction with care being taken to control bleeding as it occurs. When a large stalk is encountered, removal of the more superficial tumor initially may be wise in order to prevent hemorrhage from the larger vessels in the pedicle and to avoid the difficulty of having to remove large tumor fragments that may lodge in the resectoscope. Once the exophytic portion has been removed, resection/biopsy of the deep tissue is performed. This specimen should include part of the detrusor muscle to allow for accurate surgical staging After the base of the tumor has been resected along with the muscular biopsy, the bed of the resected area should be fulgurated along with a 1 cm rim of normal mucosa surrounding the tumor bed. The superficial and deep specimens should be sent separately for pathologic examination. When multiple tumors are to be addressed, complete hemostasis by fulguration of the initial tumor site is recommended before proceeding to the next tumor.

Special situations

There are a few situations encountered when performing TUR of bladder tumors which warrant special mentioning:

1. When there are recurrent low grade tumors which have been pathologically diagnosed and staged during previous resections, they may be treated with laser fulguration without obtaining additional specimens for pathologic examination. Laser fulguration is frequently less painful and provides better hemostasis than electrocautery resection. The risk of complications, specifically bladder perforation, is still present if inadequate anesthesia is provided.
2. If the patient has a history of CIS on prior resections then random biopsies and biopsies of any suspicious lesions should be obtained. Biopsies should be performed prior to resection of larger papillary tumors with hemostasis obtained prior to starting the resection.
3. Tumors overlying or entering a ureteral orifice may be resected completely using pure cutting current without regard for the orifice. Once resected, fulguration of the bed of the tumor should not be done since this may lead to scarring and stricturing of the ureteral orifice. A ureteral stent may be placed prior to resection but this may interfere with resection of all the tumor. Postoperative edema around the ureteral orifice may lead to obstruction requiring drainage of the kidney via placement of a percutaneous nephrostomy. Alternatively, a ureteral stent may be placed after the tumor has been completely resected. There is a risk of developing vesicoureteral reflux, however resection is still warranted.
4. When a tumor is located within a diverticulum, the preferred treatment is an open partial or total cystectomy due to high incidence of perforation with TUR.
5. When the pathologist is unable to accurately determine the presence or depth of tumor invasion due to inadequate sampling or lack of muscle in the tumor specimen then a repeat resection under anesthesia should be performed.

Concurrent urologic problems

Occasionally the patient will have concurrent urologic problems which need to be addressed either prior to, during, or after a TUR.

Stricture disease
If the patient suffers from urethral strictures, a meatotomy and/or visual internal urethrotomy (VIU) may be carried out to allow passage of the resectoscope into the bladder. Alternatively, in cases of severe obstruction or malformation, a perineal urethrostomy or percutaneous transvesicle approach is warranted. The latter approaches should be 'last resort' efforts since the chances of seeding the tracts may be significant.

Stone disease
Renal and ureteral stones should be managed when the risk of tumor implantation can be minimized. When there is an associated urinary obstruction, percutaneous nephrostomy may be used to temporize until the bladder is cleared of multiple or higher grade tumors. However, a solitary, low-grade superficial (e.g. Ta) lesion may not be an absolute contraindication if it can be resected and cleared from the system prior to ureteral manipulation. If the stone is non-obstructing, it is best to perform the TUR first then address the stone at a subsequent setting. Bladder stones often require destruction (e.g. holmium laser, lithoclast, etc.) and removal at time of TUR. It is important to minimize mucosal trauma from bouncing stone fragments if this is performed concurrent with TUR.

Retrograde pyelography
An atraumatic retrograde study performed with an occlusive catheter (e.g. Rutner catheter) can usually be carried out without the risk of upper tract seeding as long as tumors are not in the immediate vicinity of the ureteral orifice. However, catheterization with guidewires and/or open-ended catheters may lead to tumor implants in the ureter and should probably be delayed until the bladder is cleared of viable TCC.

BPH
When obstructive uropathy due to benign prostatic hypertrophy is encountered and a TURP is required, it can be safely performed after clearing the bladder of low-grade superficial (e.g. Ta) TCC. Concurrent limited TUR biopsy of the prostatic fossa is a usual procedure during resection of larger TCC but extensive resection is probably unwise.

There is a significant risk of opening sinuses and allowing intravascular dissemination of TCC during a formal TURP.

Complications

There are many documented complications resulting from transurethral resection of bladder tumors. The most common are infection (24%), hemorrhage requiring transfusion (13%) and bladder perforation (5%)[6]. The risk of perioperative mortality is less than 1%.

Infection following resection is usually attributed to untreated urinary tract infection at time of resection. When present, the infection may progress to pyelonephritis and be a significant cause of morbidity and possible mortality. Infection may be prevented by obtaining preoperative urine culture and sensitivity to document infection and guide preoperative antibiotics for sterilization of urine at time of resection. Post-operative free urinary drainage via catheter will also help prevent infection.

Hemorrhage is nearly impossible to prevent during a TUR. The patient should be screened for coagulopathies prior to surgery and these corrected when found. Careful resection with attention to detail is the other key to limiting operative bleeding. Resection of superficial portions of the tumor first with control of bleeding maintained after each individual resection will help minimize the amount of bleeding encountered.

Bladder perforations are the most feared complication and may be extraperitoneal or intraperitoneal. These are more likely to occur when the tumors are located on the lateral walls or the dome respectively. They are also more likely to occur when the bladder becomes overdistended with thinning of the bladder wall. Perforation may allow spillage of tumor cells into the perivesical tissue with subsequent development of metastatic disease. It also increases the risk of postoperative infection and associated morbidity. When bladder perforation is suspected, any remaining tumor fragments within the bladder should be immediately removed, followed by control of any associated bleeding. Many perforations are easily recognized by identification of perivesical fat. If there are any doubts about perforation, a cystogram may be performed by instilling 300–400 cc of dilute contrast under gravity and obtaining flat and oblique plain films followed by a drainage film. When no perforation is identified, cautious resection of the tumor may resume. When an extraperitoneal perforation is identified, any remaining tumor should be fulgurated and the patient treated with continuous catheter drainage for 5–7 days or until follow-up cystogram shows resolution of extravasation. The role of external beam radiation therapy in this situation to decrease the chance of extravesical tumor development has been debated, however its use may complicate any future treatment of the bladder cancer. When an intraperitoneal perforation is identified, immediate exploration via laparotomy should be performed.

TUR syndrome of hyponatremia due to extravasation of hypotonic irrigating solution is rare but has been reported following tumor resections[7]. Its treatment is identical to that encountered during TUR of the prostate for benign prostatic hypertrophy, namely, correction of electrolytes and supportive care of associated symptoms.

Laser fulguration

Laser fulguration of bladder tumors has its advantages and drawbacks. It may be performed using a flexible cystoscope using only local intravesical anesthesia which is beneficial when the patient has other medical conditions which would make them a poor candidate for general or regional anesthesia. As previously mentioned, it is useful for the patient who has had multiple papillary low-grade recurrences[1]. Laser fulguration in these cases provides adequate tumor vaporization with little bleeding due to its coagulative properties. The problem with using lasers for the treatment of bladder tumors is that little if any tissue is obtained for histologic evaluation. Therefore transurethral resection and not laser fulguration should be used for first time tumors which have not been properly staged. A possible complication of using lasers is small bowel injury without any apparent bladder mucosal injury. Limiting the power output to 35 W for 3 s has been shown to keep the temperature of the outer bladder wall below 60 °C thereby reducing the risk of thermal damage to adjacent structures[8]. Treatment of any bowel injury should consist of exploratory laparotomy with resection of the injured segment of bowel.

Partial cystectomy

The main indication for performing a partial cystectomy would be for a tumor located within a bladder diverticulum where the bladder wall is very thin and risk of perforation is greatly increased for transurethral resection. Other indications are superficial tumors which are inaccessible to TUR or high-grade solitary lesions which do not respond to intravesical chemotherapy[9]. Selective mucosal biopsies should show no evidence of CIS or atypical cells. Perioperative intravesical chemotherapy with thiotepa or mitomycin-C is recommended in these cases to decrease the risk of tumor cell spillage into the perivesical tissues. Debulking of the tumor by transurethral resection may help prevent tumor cell spillage at the time of partial cystectomy. The incision in the bladder should be located several centimeters away from the tumor and a 2 cm margin of normal urothelium removed with the tumor. Suprapubic drainage should be avoided. Please refer to Chapter 7.3 on management of invasive bladder cancer for more details on partial cystectomy.

Total cystectomy

Total cystectomy with urinary diversion is indicated for the treatment of superficial bladder cancer in the following instances: extensive bladder involvement not accessible to transurethral resection and fulguration; rapidly recurring tumors which show increase in grade, especially T1G3 tumors; diffuse CIS unresponsive to intravesical chemotherapy; invasion of prostatic urethra; and presence of squamous cell carcinoma or adenocarcinoma[9]. Please refer to the treatment of invasive bladder cancer for more details on total cystectomy.

References

1. Smith JA. Surgical management of superficial bladder cancer (Stages Ta/T1/CIS). *Semin Surg Oncol* 1997;**13**:328–334.
2. Messing EM, Catalona W. Urothelial tumors of the urinary tract. In: Walsh PC, Retik AB, Vaughan ED Jr, Wein AJ (eds) *Campbell's Urology*, 7th edn. W.B Saunders Company, Philadelphia, 1998, pp. 2327–2410.
3. deVere White RW, Stapp E. Predicting prognosis in patients with superficial bladder cancer. *Oncology* 1998;**12**:1717–1723.
4. Hudson MA, Herr HW. Carcinoma in situ of the bladder. *J Urol* 1995;**153**:564–572.
5. Deliveliotis C, Alexopoulou K, Picramenos D, Econornacos G, Goulandris N, Kostakopoulos A. The contribution of the obturator nerve block in the transurethral resection of bladder tumors. *Acta Urologica Belgica* 1995;**63**:51–54.
6. Dick A, Barnes R, Hadley H, Bergman RT, Ninan CA. Complications of transurethral resection of bladder tumors: prevention, recognition and treatment. *J Urol* 1980;**124**:810–811.
7. Hahn RG. Transurethral resection syndrome after transurethral resection of bladder tumors. *Can J Anaesthesia* 1995;**42**:69–72.
8. Hofstetter A, Frank F, Keiditsch E, Bowering B. Endoscopic neodymium:YAG laser application for destroying bladder tumors. *Eur Urol* 1981;**7**:278–282.
9. Soloway MS. The management of superficial bladder cancer. *Cancer* 1980;**45**:Suppl, 1856–1865.

M F Sarosdy

Bladder cancer is the fourth most common cancer in American males, with more than 50 000 new cases of bladder cancer diagnosed annually in the USA[1]. The majority are superficial, and will never result in serious morbidity or mortality. However, many patients will have recurrences and some will progress to higher stage, with risk of eventual cystectomy. Thus, adjuvant therapy to prevent recurrences in patients at risk after surgical resection is very reasonable.

Early attempts to reduce recurrences used intravesical chemotherapy, and a host of literature supports its bene-fit[2–11]. Immunotherapy with bacillus Calmette-Guérin (BCG) has become the primary treatment for Tis, and also has been shown to prevent superficial tumor recurrence[12–16]. Due to the efficacy of BCG, one author has suggested that intravesical chemotherapy is now contraindicated[17]. However, some patients are unable to tolerate BCG and other patients fail to respond to it. Intravesical chemotherapy still has a role in the treatment of superficial bladder cancer, and a rational interpretation of the literature may allow an individualized and optimal treatment plan for each patient, using either chemotherapy or immunotherapy.

Measures of efficacy of chemotherapy and BCG

Chemotherapy

The commonly used chemotherapeutic agents – Thiotepa, doxorubicin, mitomycin-C and, in Europe, Epirubicin, have all been shown to have efficacy against existing, residual disease, which is a relatively straightforward endpoint to measure. Responding percentages of patients who had marker tumors or in which residual disease regress completely with treatment are shown in Table 5.2.1. While there may be considerable variation in the percentage responding between individual studies for each drug, the range of responses for each of the drugs is surprisingly similar at roughly 40% to 60%. The wide ranges of percentages responding for each drug individually are explained by the variability of tumor grade and stage between studies, as well as differing schedules and doses of drugs used. Clearly, however, these drugs do have anti-cancer activity against existing disease when used in that fashion.

A scientifically valid measure of efficacy in the use of chemotherapy to prevent recurrence after resection of papillary tumors is difficult to arrive at, and most clinical trials have not used adequate endpoints[20]. The use of *time to first recurrence* as an endpoint leaves out much relevant information, such as progression rates and additional

Table 5.2.1   Response in patients with residual disease

Drug	Authors	Efficacy (%)
Thiotepa	Koontz *et al.*[3]	47
	Veenoma *et al.*[5]	37
	Nocks *et al.*[6]	55
	Heney *et al.*[18]	47
Doxorubicin	Boffioux *et al.*[19]	38
Mitomycin	Heney *et al.*[18]	63
	Bouffioux *et al.*[19]	43
Epodyl	Bouffioux *et al.*[19]	42
Epirubicin	Bouffioux *et al.*[19]	56

recurrences. Use of the *percent with tumor recurrence* is heavily dependent upon the time chosen, and valid comparison between studies is not possible due to the use of differing time-points in different studies. Even if *percent with tumor recurrence at a particular time* is chosen, the problem of censoring and variable lengths of time on study for all patients makes comparisons difficult. For these reasons, the *recurrence rate* is thought to represent the most accurate measure of efficacy, defined as the number of tumor recurrences divided by the total duration of follow up for all patients in a treatment group. Unfortunately, many otherwise knowledgeable investigators incorrectly use the term recurrence rate when actually referring to percentage of patients with recurrence, the most commonly used endpoint, even for large, recent multicenter studies, including most of the Southwest Oncology Group studies. A final factor that makes comparison of the results of different trials invalid is the differing distribution of risk factors among populations in different studies, often not even specified, including stage, grade, prior therapies, and prior numbers and frequencies of recurrences[21].

However, with those caveats in mind, most studies of the prevention of tumor recurrence by intravesical chemotherapy demonstrate positive results which overall are also strikingly close for different drugs. In large series compiled from reviews or major trials (Table 5.2.2), prevention of recurrences were seen in 36–70% of Thiotepa-treated patients, 55–68% of doxorubicin-treated patients and in 49–74% of mitomycin-C-treated patients. Control or untreated patients were free of recurrences in those series listed in 21–40% of the Thiotepa studies, 29–38% of the doxorubicin studies, and 35–50% of the mitomycin-C studies. Thus, there does appear to be a benefit in terms of time to first recurrence in all of these studies using percentage with recurrence as a measure, and the effect appears to be roughly equivalent for all of the drugs used. Therefore, it should not be surprising that the limited number of comparative studies evaluating two or three different drugs for prophylaxis or treatment of residual disease have failed to show that one agent is superior to any other, particularly since most such studies are statistically underpowered to do so[8,9,18,31,33,34].

Single dose chemotherapy immediately after tumor resection

A use for which intravesical chemotherapy has distinct and proven potential while BCG does not is the single, immediate, instillation of an agent following resection of a tumor. The postulated mode of action is prevention of implantation of viable cancer cells into raw, denuded mucosa. Burnand *et al.* reported recurrences in 58% of non-randomized patients treated with a single dose of Thiotepa compared with 98% in non-treated patients[35]. However, this percentage of recurrences is higher than one would normally expect in untreated patients after TUR alone. A randomized, blinded study also reported recurrences in 30% of doxorubicin-treated patients compared with 71% of observed patients[11]. In a large, prospective, contemporary trial involving 431 patients, the EORTC tested the prophylactic value of a single dose of the doxorubicin analogue epirubicin immediately after resection of a single Ta or T1 tumor[32]. The recurrence rate was decreased in all patients by almost 50%, and in those with a primary, first occurrence tumor by exactly 50%. This trend was seen in all subgroups by grade and stage. Based upon all these data, the use of a single dose of chemotherapy immediately after resection should be more accepted and widespread than currently is practised in the USA.

Doses and regimen

The mechanism of action of intravesical chemotherapy is not completely understood, nor is the optimal dose and schedule known, for any of the chemotherapeutic agents used. From the National Bladder Cancer Cooperative Group studies of the 1970s and early 1980s, it is clear that the efficacy of chemotherapy, at least Thiotepa, may be limited to low- and intermediate grade tumors[7]. The long-term use of chemotherapy in a 'maintenance' fashion has not been evaluated, with most studies stopping therapy empirically after one year in treated patients in comparative trials. That any beneficial effect of chemotherapy might disappear after stopping the drug is not surprising and, in fact, it appears that the same may be true in BCG-treated patients, even those treated with one commonly used maintenance regimen.

Commonly used chemotherapy regimen supported by clinical trial data are shown in Table 5.2.3.

Table 5.2.2   prophylaxis of recurrent tumors

Drug	Authors	Free of recurrence (%)
Thiotepa	Prout *et al.*[7]	36
	Zincke *et al.*[8]	70
	Byar *et al.*[22]	53
	Nocks *et al.*[6]	50
	Asahi *et al.*[23]	60
	Schulman *et al.*[24]	41
Doxorubicin	Zinke *et al.*[8]	68
	Niijima *et al.*[25]	55
	Martinez-Pineiro *et al.*[26]	57
Mitomycin-C	Witjes *et al.*[27]	74
	Huland *et al.*[28]	57
	Niijima *et al.*[25]	49
	Tolley *et al.*[29]	
Epodyl	Kurth *et al.*[30]	72
Epirubicin	DaSilva *et al.*[31]	
	Oesterlink *et al.*[32]	71

Table 5.2.3   Commonly used regimen

Drug	Dose	Schedule
Thiotepa	30 mg in 30 ml NS	weekly x 6–8, then monthly
Mitomycin-C	40 mg in 40 ml NS	weekly x 6, then monthly
Doxorubicin	50 mg in 50 ml NS	weekly x 6, then monthly
Epodyl	1.13 g in 100 ml sterile water	weekly x 4, then monthly

Bacillus Calmette-Guérin

While chemotherapeutic agents do have activity against superficial tumors, the benefit of BCG is superior. BCG also is effective in the treatment of residual, unresected papillary tumor; eradication of residual papillary disease can be expected in one- to two-thirds of such patients (Table 5.2.4). It is also of value against papillary tumor recurrence. Such tumor prophylaxis is the major use of BCG in superficial bladder cancer, with recent approval by the US Food and Drug Administration for that purpose. BCG also decreases progression in stage of tumors that do recur, from 30% to around 6% to 7%[14,46]. These figures represent the risk of stage progression seen in patients with T1 tumors with or without CIS who were treated with aggressive amounts of BCG, usually two or more 6-week courses.

Trials of BCG versus intravesical chemotherapy

In all but two clinical trials comparing BCG with chemotherapy, BCG has been found to be superior, and therapeutic equivalence was shown in those two remaining studies. BCG was superior to intravesical Thiotepa in two studies[47,48], and superior to doxorubicin in the SWOG

Table 5.2.4   BCG efficacy: per cent free of papillary recurrence or with resolution of residual tumors

Residual disease	Responding (%)
Morales et al.[45]	67
Lamm et al.[46]	61
Brosman[47]	60
deKernion et al.[48]	36
Schellhammer et al.[49]	55
Kavoussi et al.[50]	41
Papillary disease	**Free of recurrence (%)**
Martinez-Pinero et al.[26]	87
Lamm et al.[51]	80
Herr et al.[52]	58
Cookson and Sarosdy[14]	91
Haaf et al.[53]	90
Kelley et al.[54]	94

trial comparing BCG with doxorubicin[12]. In the latter trial, 127 patients with rapidly recurrent papillary tumors were treated for prophylaxis after resection of all visible tumor. Papillary tumors recurred in 53 (79%) of 67 doxorubicin-treated patients but in only 34 (57%) of 60 BCG-treated patients ($P = 0.005$). In the SWOG trial of BCG versus mitomycin-C, patients with rapidly recurring superficial tumors without CIS were treated with either 50 mg Tice BCG or mitomycin-C 20 mg in 20 ml normal saline weekly for 6 weeks, then monthly to complete 1 year. Recurrent papillary tumors were seen in 37 (19.4%) of 190 treated with BCG compared with 61 (32.6%) of 187 treated with mitomycin-C ($P = 0.00052$)[42].

Two Dutch reports found equivalence between BCG and mitomycin-C, but both used a higher (30 mg) dose of mitomycin-C and less intense BCG consisting of a single 6 week course[27,49]. In one of the studies, with an average follow up of only 12 months, 30% of BCG-treated patients experienced tumor recurrence compared with 25% of mitomycin-C-treated patients[41].

The optimal course of BCG – that which provides the most benefit with least morbidity – likewise has not been determined. A single 6 week course may be effective in preventing tumor recurrences in many patients, but it is clear that many patients require and will respond to additional courses of BCG (Table 5.2.5). One reasonable option is to give an initial 6 week course, and after a 6 week period of rest followed by the surveillance cystoscopy, repeat a second 6 week course, especially if tumor recurred and resection was repeated. This may be the most agreed upon clinical principle in recent years[50]. Twelve consecutive weekly treatments is also possible, but the toxicity is not warranted by the response[51].

Despite the very large Southwest Oncology Group trial investigating the role of maintenance BCG, the issue of maintenance remains largely unresolved from a scientific standpoint[52]. This is because the non-maintenance patients in that trial received only a single 6 week course, while the maintenance group received substantial additional therapy, consisting of seven 3 week courses over the remaining 2.75 years (six versus 27 treatments). A significant delay in recurrence was seen with maintenance, but

Table 5.2.5   Six weeks of BCG is less than optimal

Authors	Use	Success and No. of 6 week courses		
		1	2	3
Kelley et al.[45]	BT	11/17 (65%)	16/17 (94%)	
Haaf et al.[44]	BT	20/29 (69%)	26/29 (90%)	
Haaf et al.[44]	CIS	8/19 (42%)	13/19 (68%)	
Sarosdy and Lamm[13]	BT/CIS	64/82 (78%)	70/82 (85%)	73/82 (89%)

BT = prophylaxis for papillary tumor, CIS = carcinoma in situ.

the toxicity was much more frequent and intense when it did occur. Grade 3 toxicity (that which requires stopping or withholding therapy, dose reduction, or INH therapy) occurred in 9% during induction, but in 26% of those on maintenance[53]. Furthermore, more than 10% failed to complete maintenance therapy because of toxicity[53].

Choice of agent and course of therapy

With all of this knowledge in mind, it would seem reasonable to base the choice of agent, and whether or not to use any adjuvant therapy, on the disease characteristics of the initial tumor for those with primary tumors, and upon those characteristics and frequency of recurrences in patients with recurrent tumors. Table 5.2.6 shows a simplified grouping of favorable and unfavorable characteristics of primary tumors. It also defines descriptors for recurrent tumors based upon tumor characteristics and recurrence frequency, ranging from nuisance, to troublesome, to dangerous. Nuisance tumors would include those with favorable characteristics but single occurrence or infrequent recurrences. Troublesome tumors have similar characteristics, but require more frequent endoscopic resection or fulguration. Dangerous tumors are those which have unfavorable characteristics, even at the first occurrence. A clear example of the latter is a grade III, T1 tumor with random distant biopsies showing CIS.

Since 40% to 50% of initial tumors with favorable characteristics will not recur after resection, it is reasonable to give no adjuvant therapy at all, or at most, to provide a single, immediate postoperative dose only. Patients with such favorable first tumors which do eventually recur, whether early or late, may reasonably be treated with a course of intravesical chemotherapy. Since no agent is superior to any other, choice should be based upon cost, familiarity with the drug, and ability to watch for and treat side effects (see below).

Table 5.2.6   Practical classification of superficial bladder cancers

A. By initial superficial tumor characteristics:

Favorable	Unfavorable
Single tumor	Multiple tumors
Stage Ta	Stage T1
Low grade	High grade
No field changes	Atypia or dysplasia
Diploid	Aneuploid
Negative cytology	Positive cytology

B. By characteristics and recurrence history:

Nuisance:	Favorable characteristics, single occurrence or infrequent recurrences
Troublesome:	Favorable characteristics but frequent recurrences
Dangerous:	Unfavorable characteristics, any occurrence, or recurrences

Some patients' initial tumors have favorable histologic characteristics, but with multiple tumors, placing them at low risk for progression but high risk of recurrence. In such patients, it is reasonable to employ adjuvant intravesical chemotherapy at the outset, particularly with multiple or large volume of tumor(s). Regardless of the regimen or drug chosen, it also would be prudent to give the first dose immediately postoperatively, if possible.

Patients with unfavorable characteristics such as T1 grade 2 or 3 with or without associated Tis have a high risk of progression to invasive disease. The treatment of choice is BCG. Immunocompromised patients or those who do not tolerate BCG should be given a trial of mitomycin-C. While it is statistically inferior to BCG, mitomycin-C has the most activity against Tis of the intravesical chemotherapeutic agents, particularly with 30 mg weekly for 4 weeks and then monthly for 5 months[19].

With BCG, it also seems reasonable to tailor the regimen to the individual patient according to the disease characteristics and tolerance of side effects[54]. For many with recurrent nuisance tumors who have failed chemotherapy, a single 6 week course of BCG followed by observation may be adequate. On the other hand, for a patient with a dangerous process consisting of grade 2 or 3 T1 tumors with or without CIS, aggressive BCG should be used, consisting of two 6 week courses followed by maintenance therapy if the toxicity experienced is acceptable. Recurrences that are of lower grade and lower stage may be controlled with resection, but some sort of additional adjuvant therapy might be considered. For a dangerous disease process with no disease present after two 6 week courses, the benefits and risks of maintenance BCG should be discussed with the patient. If severe side effects have not been seen, it may be reasonable to employ maintenance therapy. However, some prefer not to receive additional BCG without additional indications such as recurrent disease or positive cytology.

Definitions of failure of intravesical therapy

Patients who have a papillary recurrence immediately after weekly chemotherapy should be switched different chemotherapy drug or to BCG. Patients who have a recurrent tumor or persistent CIS after only a single 6 week course of BCG have a 65% probability of responding to a second course, and should not be considered BCG failures after that one course[13,44,45]. Likewise, patients who remain disease-free during a year of chemotherapy or BCG, but later relapse during year 2 or 3, particularly if not on maintenance, should not necessarily be considered a failure to the previous therapy. If the recurrence is no worse than previous disease, a repeat induction course may result in disease-free status, and may be entirely reasonable. However, patients with persistent CIS or continued recurrences of dangerous T1 tumors immediately after two courses of BCG or while receiving maintenance therapy (3 weekly treatments every 6 months) should be considered for investigational therapy or cystectomy[55].

Potential chemotherapeutic toxicity: prevention and recognition

Thiotepa

Thiotepa has a low molecular weight (189 daltons), and therefore is readily absorbed across the urothelium. Myelosuppression is the most common toxicity of Thiotepa, and this is highly dependent on dosage[56]. It occurs with an incidence of up to 12% at doses of 60 mg weekly, but less than 5% if the dosage is limited to 30 mg weekly[7]. White blood cell counts should be checked prior to each treatment during weekly therapy, although this is not necessary for patients who are on a monthly schedule. The second common toxicity of Thiotepa is chemical cystitis, but this is very rare at a dosage of 30 mg. A very rare, but fatal, delayed complication of intravesical Thiotepa is acute non-lymphocytic leukemia–myelodysplastic syndrome[56]. Six cases have been reported. The average cumulative dose for those six patients was 1366 mg, likely playing some role in the etiology of this complication.

Doxorubicin

With a high molecular weight of 580 daltons, there is essentially no absorption of doxorubicin, and therefore, no systemic toxicity. Its major toxicity is chemical cystitis, seen in approximately 28% of patients[56]. This cystitis may be quite severe, but is self-limited and resolves when the drug is voided from the bladder. Despite this, doxorubicin was found to have less toxicity than BCG in the randomized SWOG study comparing it with intravesical BCG[12].

Mitomycin-C

The molecular weight of mitomycin-C is intermediate (329 daltons), so it is slightly absorbed. A death from myelosuppression was reported in a patient who received 80 mg of mitomycin-C immediately after resection of a tumor, but in a review of 11 series with 613 patients, leukopenia and thrombocytopenia occurred in only four patients[56]. The major toxicity of mitomycin-C is chemical cystitis, ranging in frequency from 6% to 41%. Drug-like skin reactions are common, and generally may involve the palms but may also involve the feet and genitalia. These may be so severe as to cause vesicular eruptions, seen in up to

10%. A contact dermatitis may also occur, so it is important to prevent spillage onto the skin of the genitalia. Both systemic drug reactions and contact reactions are self-limited, with prompt resolution. Two prospective trials comparing mitomycin-C with BCG found the incidence of side effects with mitomycin-C to be significantly less than with BCG[58].

Epirubicin

This anthracycline drug was synthesized with the intent of improved antitumor activity and decreased toxicity compared with doxorubicin. In a trial in which 205 patients received epirubicin 50 mg in 50 ml sterile water for one dose only immediately after resection, cystitis was seen in only 24 (11.7%) and a skin reaction in only two (1%)[32]. Cystitis was seen in 14% of 911 patients receiving eight weekly treatments of 50 mg in 50 ml. All reactions were self-limited.

Potential BCG toxicity

Despite the overall superior efficacy of BCG compared with chemotherapeutic agents, toxicity and side effects are common and generally play a role in the decision whether or not to employ BCG, and if so, whether or not to employ maintenance in patients who appear to benefit. Mild to moderate toxicity occurs in up to 90%, and severe or life-threatening toxicity is seen in less than 5%[56,58,59]. Most patients have mild side effects, but these mild, frequent symptoms often increase in intensity and incidence with repeated courses. Making the distinction between intense, harmless symptoms and severe, life-threatening symptoms is important.

Cystitis and dysuria occur in up to 90% of patients, usually after the third or fourth treatment, and both may intensify substantially with further therapy[56,58]. Both can be expected to resolve spontaneously within 24 hours in most cases. Hematuria may occur in 20% to 35%[56]. BCG administration should be withheld in patients having gross hematuria, as absorption may lead to systemic complications. It is not necessary to withhold BCG for microscopic hematuria.

Mild, constitutional symptoms such as malaise, fatigue, and lethargy occur in approximately 20% of patients[56]. Low-grade fever (<101°F) may occur in 10–15%, and usually resolves spontaneously in <24 h.

The sudden onset of severe fever >103 °F shortly after treatment heralds such systemic infection, which has been reported in 3% of patients[56]. This extreme temperature distinguishes this life-threatening complication, from the mild or moderate symptoms which most patients experience. Early, appropriate intervention results in prompt defervescence and overall improvement[60,61].

49

Failure to recognize this or a delay in initiation of effective antituberculous therapy can result in progressive sepsis, including vascular collapse and multiple organ failure. Several deaths from BCG sepsis have been reported[61].

Treatment and prevention of BCG toxicity

Patients having mild symptoms require no support or, at most, acetaminophen, pyridium or anticholinergic therapy[62]. Local or mild symptoms which do not resolve spontaneously in 12 to 24 h or more intense, local symptoms may be controlled with Isoniazid (INH) administered around the time of BCG treatment only[62]. Most commonly used is INH 300 mg daily for three consecutive days, starting 1 day prior to subsequent treatment, thereby avoiding prolonged daily administration.

Patients with temperature >103 °F should be admitted and aggressive systemic therapy started[60–63]. Routine bacteriologic cultures including urine and blood should be obtained immediately. Cultures for Acid Fast Bacillus and urinary AFB stains are not required. In addition to antibacterial antibiotics, cycloserine 250–500 mg p.o. twice daily should be administered starting immediately. Less ill patients may respond to INH 300 mg and rifampicin 600 mg daily, but these two drugs require 1 week to produce an antibacillus effect.

Patients with high fever should not be given additional BCG until the fever has resolved. Immunotherapy with BCG then may be restarted at one-half strength with 3 day INH coverage initiated 1 day prior to therapy. For patients with life-threatening sepsis, the current recommendation is that they should not receive additional BCG.

New agents

Some patients will not appear to respond to either chemotherapy or BCG, and some patients who do respond may not have a durable benefit, even with maintenance BCG treatments. For those with infrequent nuisance tumors, continued surgical ablation remains a reasonable option. However, some patients will have frequent recurrences of nuisance tumors, and others may harbor frankly dangerous disease processes for which cystectomy may be warranted. Fortunately, clinical investigations of new agents continue to expand the number of options for adjuvant therapy.

Interferon

Interferons (IFNs) are naturally occurring glycoproteins with antiviral and antiproliferative properties. The IFN which is most active is interferon alpha (IFNα[64]). A multicenter Phase III trial comparing 10 to 100 mU weekly confirmed activity in CIS, including some patients who had failed prior BCG therapy[65]. The efficacy of IFNα against existing tumors or for prophylaxis has not been studied sufficiently, although one prospective trial in prophylaxis is underway. In interim reports, Calais daSilva et al. have reported what appears to be similar efficacy of 60 and 100 mU dose schedules in preventing superficial tumor recurrence, although no placebo or control arm is included in the trial design[66]. Continued investigation, though, appears warranted.

Bropirimine

Bropirimine is an immunostimulatory agent originally designed and synthesized to function as an inducer of endogenous IFN. In addition to that trait, it also stimulates a wide range of both cellular and humoral components of the immune system. It has been found to be active against CIS of the bladder in both newly diagnosed and BCG-failed patients[67,68]. It has not been evaluated adequately as an adjuvant therapy against superficial tumor recurrence, but bropirimine does have activity in patients with secondary bladder CIS, including those with associated papillary disease.

Keyhole limpet hemocyanin

Keyhole limpet hemocyanin (KLH) is a pigment protein of *Megathura crenulata*, a mollusk, and is highly immunogenic. Olsson et al. first reported a reduction of papillary bladder tumor recurrences in patients who were immunized subcutaneously with KLH as a test of their immunologic status[69]. Subsequently, a small prospective study confirmed this effect, and no toxicity was noted[70]. Jurincic et al. reported a small comparative study in which superficial tumor recurrences were seen in three (14%) of 21 patients receiving KLH (1 mg intradermally followed by 10 mg intravesically) compared with nine (39%) of 23 patients receiving intravesical mitomycin-C[71]. Further investigation into the adjunctive value of KLH is needed.

Other investigational drugs

Additional new agents are undergoing clinical trials at a number of centers, and many have potential as successful adjuvant agents. Included are novel compounds such as the immunotoxin conjugate TP-40 and the anthracycline AD-32[72,73]. Patients with nuisance tumors that appear to be refractory to the standard agents should be considered for potential inclusion in such trials that might be available to them and their physician.

References

1. Parker SL, Wingo PA, Tong T, Bolden S. Cancer statistics. *Am Cancer J Clin* 1996;**46**:5–27.

2. Jones HC, Swinney J. Thiotepa in the treatment of tumours of the bladder. *Lancet* 1961;**2**:615–618.

3. Koontz WW Jr, Prout GR Jr, Smith W, Frable WJ, Minnis JE. The use of intravesical Thio-tepa in the management of non-invasive carcinoma of the bladder. *J Urol* 1981;**125**:307–312.

4. Abassian A, Wallace DM. Intracavity chemotherapy of diffuse non-infiltrating papillary carcinoma of the bladder. *J Urol* 1966;**96**:461–465.

5. Veenema RJ, Dean AL Jr, Uson AC *et al.* Thiotepa bladder instillations therapy and prophylaxis for superficial bladder tumors. *J Urol* 1969;**101**:711–715.

6. Nocks BN, Nieh PT, Prout GR Jr. A longitudinal study of patients with superficial bladder carcinoma successfully treated with weekly intravesical thio-tepa. *J Urol* 1979;**122**:27–29.

7. Prout GR Jr, Koontz WW Jr, Coombs LJ, Hawkins IR, Friedell GH. Long-term fate of 90 patients with superficial bladder cancer randomly assigned to receive or not to receive thiotepa. *J Urol* 1983;**130**:677–680.

8. Zincke H, Utz DC, Taylor WF, Myers RP, Leary FJ. Influence of Thiotepa and Doxorubien instillation at the time of transurethral surgical treatment of bladder cancer on tumor recurrence: a prospective, randomized double-blind, controlled trial. *J Urol* 1983;**129**:505–509.

9. Zincke H, Benson RC Jr, Hilton JF, Taylor WF. Intravesical Thiotepa and mitomycin-C treatment immediately after transurethral resection and later for superficial (stages ta and tis) bladder cancer; a prospective, randomized, stratified study with crossover design. *J Urol* 1985;**134**:1110–1114.

10. Akaza H, Isaka S, Koiso K *et al.* Comparative analysis of short-term and long-term prophylactic intravesical chemotherapy of superficial bladder cancer. *Cancer Chemother Pharmacol* 1987;**20**:91–96.

11. Flamm J. Long-term versus short-term doxorubicin hydrochloride instillation after transurethral resection of superficial bladder cancer. *Eur Urol* 1990;**17**:119–124.

12. Lamm DL, Blumenstein BA, Crawford ED *et al.* A randomized trial of intravesical doxorubicin and immunotherapy with bacillus Calmette-Guérin for transitional cell carcinoma of the bladder. *N Engl J Med* 1991;**325**:1205–1209.

13. Sarosdy MF, Lamm DL. Long-term results of intravesical Bacillus Calmette-Guérin therapy for superficial bladder carcinoma. *J Urol* 1989;**142**:719–722.

14. Cookson MS, Sarosdy MF. Management of stage T1 superficial bladder cancer with intravesical BCG therapy. *J Urol* 1992;**148**:797–801.

15. Morales A, Nickel JC, Wilson JWL. Dose-response of bacillus Calmette-Guérin in the treatment of superficial bladder cancer. *J Urol* 1992;**147**:1256–1258.

16. Nadler RB, Catalona WJ, Hudson MA, Ratliff TL. Durability of the tumor-free response for intravesical bacillus Calmette-Guérin therapy. *J Urol* 1994;**152**:367–373.

17. Lamm DL, Riggs DR, Traynelis CL, Nseyo UO. Apparent failure of current intravesical chemotherapy prophylaxis to influence the long-term course of superficial transitional cell carcinoma of the bladder. *J Urol* 1995;**153**:1444–1450.

18. Heney NM, Koontz WW, Barton B *et al.* Intravesical Thiotepa versus Mitomycin-C in patients with Ta, T1 and Tis transitional cell carcinoma of the bladder: a phase iii prospective randomized study. *J Urol* 1988;**140**:1390–1393.

19. Bouffioux C, Meijden A vd, Kurth KH *et al.* Objective response of superficial bladder tumors to intravesical treatment (including review of response of marker lesions). *Prog Clin Biol Res* 1992;**378**:29–42.

20. Kaihara S, Dalesio O, Freedman L *et al.* Statistical analysis/sample size determination for clinical trials of treatments of bladder cancer. In: Niijima T, Aso Y, Koontz W, Prout G, Denis L (eds). *Consensus development in clinical bladder cancer research.* SCI, Paris, 1993, pp. 5–8.

21. Sylvester R, Barton B, Hisazumi H *et al.* Prognostic factors for randomization, stratification, and endpoints for the evaluation of bladder trials. In: Niijima T, Aso Y, Koontz W, Prout G, Denis L (eds). *Consensus development in clinical bladder cancer research.* SCI, Paris, 1993, pp. 17–26.

22. Byar D, Blackard D. Comparisons of placebo, pyridoxine, and topical thiotepa in preventing recurrence of stage I bladder cancer. *Urology* 1977;**10**:556–561.

23. Asahi T, Matsumura Y, Tanahashi T *et al.* The effects of intravesical instillation of thiotepa on the recurrence rate of bladder tumors. *Acta Med Okayama* 1980;**34**:43–49.

24. Schulman CC, Robinson M, Denis L *et al.* for EORTC. Prophylactic chemotherapy of superficial transitional cell bladder carcinoma: an EORTC randomized trial comparing thiotepa, VM-26 and TUR alone. *Eur Urol* 1982;**8**:207–212.

25. Niijima T, Akaza H, Koisok K, and the Japanese Urologic Cancer Research Group for Adriamycin. Randomized clinical trial on chemoprophylaxis of recurrence in cases of superficial bladder cancer. *Cancer Chemother and Pharm* 1983;**11**(Suppl.):79–82.

26. Martinez-Pineiro JA, Leon JJ, Martinez-Pineiro L Jr, *et al.* Bacillus Calmette-Guérin versus Doxorubicin versus Thiotepa; a randomized prospective study in 202 patients with superficial bladder cancer. *J Urol* 1990;**143**:502–506.

27. Witjes JA, Meijden APM vd, Witjes WPJ. A randomised prospective study comparing intravesical instillations of mitomycin-C, BCG-Tice, and BCG-RIVM in pTa-pT1 tumours and primary carcinoma in situ of the urinary bladder. *Eur J Cancer* 1993;**29A**(12):1672–1676.

28. Huland H, Otto U. Mitomycin-C instillation to prevent recurrence of superficial bladder carcinoma. *Eur Urol* 1983;**9**:84–86.

29. Tolley DA, Hargreave TB, Smith PH *et al.* Effect of intravesical mitomycin-C on recurrence of newly diagnosed superficial bladder cancer: an interim report from the Medical Research Council Subgroup on Superficial Bladder Cancer. *Br Med J* 1988;**296**:1759–1761.

30. Kurth KH, Debruyne FJM, Senge T *et al.* Adjuvant chemotherapy of superficial transitional cell carcinoma: an EORTC randomized trochloride, ethoglucide, and TUR alone. In: Debruyne FMJ, Denis L, Meijden ADPM van der (eds) *Superficial bladder cancer.* New York, Alan R Liss, 1989; pp. 145.

31. DaSilva FC, Ferrito F, Brandao T, Santos A. 4-Epidoxorubicin versus Mitomycin-C intravesical chemoprophylaxis of superficial bladder cancer. *Eur Urol* 1992;**21**:42–44.

32. Oosterlinck W, Kurth KH, Schroder F, Buttinck J, Hammond B, Sylvester R. A prospective European Organization for Research and Treatment of Cancer Genitourinary Group randomized trial comparing transurethral resection followed by a single intravesical instillation of epirubicin or water in single stage Ta, T1 papillary carcinoma of the bladder. *J Urol* 1993;**149**:749–752.

33. Kurth KH, Schroeder FH, Tunn U *et al.* Adjuvant chemotherapy of superficial transitional cell bladder carcinoma: preliminary results of a European Organization for Research on Treatment of Cancer randomized trial comparing doxorubicin hydrochloride, ethoglucid and transurethral resection alone. *J Urol* 1984;**132**:258–262.

34. Flanigan RC, Ellison MF, Butler KM *et al.* A trial of prophylactic thiotepa or mitomycin-C intravesical therapy in patients with recurrent or multiple superficial bladder cancers. *J Urol* 1986;**136**:35–37.

35. Burnand KG, Boyd PJR, Mayo ME, Shuttleworth KED, Lloyd-Davies RW. Single dose intravesical Thiotepa as an adjuvant to cystodiathermy in the treatment of transitional cell bladder carcinoma. *Br J Urol* 1976;**48**:55–59.

36. Morales A, Eidinger D, Bruce AW. Intracavity bacillus Calmette-Guérin in the treatment of superficial bladder tumors. *J Urol* 1976;**116**:180–183.

37. Lamm DL, Thor DE, Stogdill VD, Radwin HM. Bladder cancer immunotherapy. *J Urol* 1982;**128**:931–935.

38. Brosman SA. Experience with bacillus Calmette-Guérin in patients with superficial bladder cancer. *J Urol* 1982;**128**:27–30.

39. DeKernion JB, Huang M-Y, Lindner A, Smith RB, Kaufman JJ. The management of superficial bladder tumors and carcinoma in situ with intravesical bacillus Calmette-Guérin. *J Urol* 1985;**133**:598–601.

40. Schellhammer PF, Ladaga LE, Fillion MB. Bacillus Calmette-Guérin for superficial transitional cell carcinoma of the bladder. *J Urol* 1986;**135**:261–264.

41. Kavoussi LR, Torrence RJ, Gillen DP *et al.* Results of 6 weekly intravesical Bacillus Calmette-Guérin instillations on the treatment of superficial bladder cancer. *J Urol* 1988;**139**:935–940.

42. Lamm DL, Blumenstein BA, Crawford ED *et al.* Randomized intergroup comparison of Bacillus Calmette-Guérin immunotherapy and mitomycin-C chemotherapy prophylaxis in superficial transitional cell carcinoma of the bladder. *Urol Onc* 1995;**1**:119.

43. Herr HW, Landone VP, Badalament RA *et al.* Experience with intravesical BCG therapy of superficial bladder tumors. *Urology* 1985;**25**:119.

44. Haaf EO, Dresner SM, Ratliff TL *et al.* Two courses of intravesical Bacillus Calmette-Guérin for transitional cell carcinoma of the bladder. *J Urol* 1986;**136**:820–824.

45. Kelley DR, Ratliff TL, Catalona WJ *et al.* Intravesical Bacillus Calmette-Guérin therapy for superficial bladder cancer: effect of Bacillus Calmette-Guérin viability on treatment results. *J Urol* 1985;**134**:48–53.

46. Eure GR, Ladaga LE, Schellhammer PF. BCG therapy for stage T1 superficial bladder cancer. *J Urol* 1990;**143**:341A.

47. Brosman SA. Experience with Bacillus Calmette-Guérin in patients with superficial bladder cancer. *J Urol* 1982;**128**:27–30.

48. Netto NR Jr, Lemos GCA. A comparison of treatment methods for prophylaxis of recurrent superficial bladder tumors. *J Urol* 1983;**129**:33–34.

49. Debruyne FMJ, Van der Meijden APM. BCG (RIVM) versus mitomycin-C intravesical therapy in superficial bladder cancer. First results of randomized prospective trial. *Urol* 1988;**31**:20–25.

50. Morales A, Nickel JC, Wilson JWL. Dose-response of bacillus Calmette-Guérin in the treatment of superficial bladder cancer. *J Urol* 1992;**147**:1256–1258.

51. Brosman SA. The use of Bacillus Calmette-Guérin in the therapy of bladder carcinoma in situ. *J Urol* 1985;**134**:36–39.

52. Lamm DL, Blumenstein BA, Crissman JD et al. Maintenance BCG immunotherapy in recurrent TA, T1, and carcinoma in-situ transitional cell carcinoma: a randomized Southwest Oncology Group Study. *J Urol* 2000; **163**:1124–1129.

53. Blumenstein BA. Personal communication, 1996.

54. Sarosdy MF. Principles of intravesical chemotherapy and immunotherapy. *Urol Clin North Am* 1992;**19**(3):509–519.

55. Catalona WJ, Hudson Ma, Gillen DP, Andriole GL, Ratliff TL. Risks and benefits of repeated course of intravesical bacillus Calmette-Guérin therapy for superficial bladder cancer. *J Urol* 1987;**137**:220–224.

56. Thrasher JB, Crawford ED. Complications of intravesical chemotherapy. *Urol Clin North Am* 1992;**19**:529–539.

57. Lamm DL, Stogdill VD, Stogdill BJ *et al.* Complications of Bacillus Calmette-Guérin immunotherapy in 1,278 patients with bladder cancer. *J Urol* 1985;**135**:272–274.

58. Doesburg W, Schaafsma HE, Debruyne FMJ. A randomized prospective study comparing intravesical instillations of Mitomycin-C, BCG-Tice, and BCG-RIVM in pTa-pT1 tumors and primary carcinoma in situ of the urinary bladder. Intravesical instillations in superficial bladder cancer. *Eur J Cancer* 1993;**29A**:1672–1676.

59. Lamm DL, Steg A, Boccon-Gibod L *et al.* Complications of bacillus Calmette-Guérin immunotherapy: review of 2,602 patients with comparison of chemotherapy complications. *Prog Clin Biol Res* 1989;**310**:335–355.

60. DeHaven JL, Traynellis C, Riggs DR, Ting E, Lamm DL. Antibiotic and steroid therapy of massive systemic Bacillus Calmette-Guérin toxicity. *J Urol* 1992;**147**:738–742.

61. Rawls WH, Lamm DL, Lowe BA *et al.* Fatal sepsis following intravesical BCG administration for bladder cancer: a Southwest Oncology Group Study. *J Urol* 1990;**144**:1328–1330.

62. Lamm DL, Meijden APM van der, Morales A. Incidence and treatment of complications of bacillus Calmette-Guérin intravesical therapy in superficial bladder cancer. *J Urol* 1992;**147**:596–600.

63. Lamm DL. Complications of Bacillus Calmette-Guérin immunotherapy. In: Lamm DL (Ed.) *Urologic clinics of North America.* Philadelphia, PA, WB Saunders, 1992;**19**(3):565–572.

64. Christophersen IS, Jordal R, Osther K, Lindenberg J, Pedersen PH, Berg K. Interferon therapy in neoplastic disease. *Act Med Scan* 1978;**204**:471–476.

65. Glashan R. A randomized controlled study of intravesical α-2b-interferon in carcinoma in situ of the bladder. *J Urol* 1990;**144**:658–661.

66. Da Silva FC. Interferon Alpha 2b 60 millions vs 100 million in intravesical prophylaxis of superficial bladder cancer. *J Urol* 1993;**149**:282A.

67. Sarosdy MF, Lowe BA, Schellhammer PF *et al.* Bropirimine immunotherapy of bladder CIS: Positive phase II results of an oral interferon inducer. *J Urol* 1994;**13**:304A.

68. Sarosdy MF, Lowe BA, Schellhammer PF *et al.* Oral bropirimine immunotherapy of carcinoma in situ of the bladder: results of a phase II trial. *Urology* 1996;**48**:21–27.

69. Olsson CA, Rao C, Menzoian J *et al.* Immunologic unreactivity in bladder cancer patients. *J Urol* 1972;**107**:607–609.

70. Olsson CA, Chute R, Rao C. Immunologic reduction of bladder cancer recurrence rate. *J Urol* 1974;**111**:173–176.

71. Jurincic CD, Engelman V, Gasch J, Klippel KF. Immunotherapy in bladder cancer with Keyhole-Limpet Hemocyanin: a randomized study. *J Urol* 1988;**139**:723–726.

72. Goldberg MR, Heimbrook DC, Russo P *et al.* Phase I cal study of the recombinant Oncotoxin TP40 in superficial bladder cancer. *Clin Cancer Res* 1995;**1**:57–61.

73. Greenberg R, O'Dwyer P, Patterson L *et al.* Intravesical AD 32 (N-Trifluoroacetyladriamycin-14-Valerate) in the treatment of patients with refractory bladder carcinoma – clinical efficacy, pharmacology, and safety. *J Urol* 1995;**153**:233A.

5.3   The follow up of superficial bladder cancer

R R Hall

Introduction

Patients with superficial bladder cancer undergo regular cystoscopic follow up in the belief that this reduces the risk of dying from the disease. As an American urologist reportedly once observed, his secretary's typewriter was an essential instrument for the management of bladder cancer. Although never tested by randomized trial, common sense dictates that long-term regular follow up cystoscopies must be beneficial. On one hand, the majority of tumors found at routine follow up are small and asymptomatic; on the other, many bladder cancers cause no symptoms until they are large or invasive. Thus, by routine follow up cancers are prevented from becoming invasive. Furthermore, although recurrent tumors need to be removed, the resection is more likely to be completed as a simple day case procedure and the need for hospital admission over a number of years will be diminished.

Frequency of cystoscopic follow up

In the past most urologists have treated all Ta/T1 bladder tumors similarly, according to a common follow up schedule; 3 monthly cystoscopies for 1, 2 or even 3 years, then 6 monthly and finally annually, but returning to 3 monthly examinations if tumor recurs. Others have adjusted the frequency of cystoscopy according to their assessment of the individual patient's risk based on known prognostic factors such as the number, size and grade of tumor and the frequency of previous recurrences. However, in general all patients have undergone three or four cystoscopies during the first year and between two and four during the second year irrespective of their tumor type.

The case for a single cystoscopy about 3 months after the treatment TUR is self-evident. The need for frequent cystoscopies thereafter, especially for good risk patients, is less convincing. Residual Ta/T1 tumors 'missed' by the previous TUR will be found at the first follow up examination and can be dealt with. Similarly, local 'relapse' at the site of the previous TUR, due to previous incomplete resection, understaging or a genuinely aggressive cancer will be recognized and the treatment plan modified accordingly. Genuinely new occurrences of tumor at a new site in the bladder will also be seen and the need for adjuvant intravesical treatment may be considered. All of these will be assessed and can be dealt with at the first 3 month cystoscopy. Some colleagues recognize that the first two of these features happen more commonly than we may wish to think and perform a 'second look' cystoscopy and repeat TUR as routine practice. This is usually done after 2 or 3 weeks rather than 3 months and is really an extension of the initial therapeutic TUR rather than for follow up in the usual sense. It is certainly advisable for T1 G3 cancers[1] and for patients with many tumors, where lesions on the anterior bladder wall or just inside the bladder neck may be overlooked.

In addition to its therapeutic role we now know that a first follow up cystoscopy at 3 months has very useful prognostic value. Parmar et al.[2] demonstrated that the presence of Ta or T1 tumor at the 3 month cystoscopy was an independent prognostic factor for future superficial recurrence. Furthermore, if this factor was combined with the number of tumors seen at diagnosis, patients could be separated into three prognostic groups for whom subsequent cystoscopic follow up could be different. The best risk (Group 1) patients had solitary tumors at diagnosis and no relapse at 3 months. Medium risk (Group 2) patients had multiple tumors at diagnosis and no relapse at 3 months or solitary tumors at diagnosis, but recurrence at 3 months. Poor risk patients (Group 3) had both multiple tumors at diagnosis and recurrence at 3 months. Most importantly, 60% of all new Ta, T1 transitional cell carcinomas were found to be solitary at diagnosis and tumor free at 3 months and thus were considered to be good risk and were predicted to be suitable for annual cystoscopic follow up only. If this latter suggestion could be confirmed, many patients would avoid between four and six cystoscopies over 2 years (depending on their urologist's usual practice) which would amount to a considerable saving for providers of health care and a welcome reduction in discomfort, inconvenience, anxiety and cost for many patients. Reading et al.[3] confirmed the feasibility of Parmar's prognostic grouping but, being a retrospective

survey, were unable to test the safety of a schedule of fewer cystoscopies. For medium and poor risk patients less frequent cystoscopic follow up cannot be recommended. Patients with frequently recurring multiple tumors are at greatest risk of muscle invasion as well as superficial recurrence and frequent cystoscopic follow up is essential to determine the choice and assess the efficacy of bladder preserving therapy. Prospective audit of reduced frequency follow up for good risk patients with superficial bladder cancer will be necessary to demonstrate its safety but, if confirmed, the quality of life of many bladder cancer patients will be improved. It is important to note that this management policy for good risk superficial bladder tumors will be enhanced by the instillation of a single dose of intravesical chemotherapy (Mitomycin-C or Epirubicin) within a few hours of transurethral resection. The rationale for this has been discussed elsewhere[4,5].

Flexible or rigid cystoscopy?

Flexible cystoscopy[6] is not entirely free of discomfort but is preferred to rigid cystoscopy[7] by most if not all patients who have experienced both procedures. For the purposes of follow up both are equally effective. The endoscopic view is, if anything, better with the flexible instrument. Cold-cup biopsies may be taken with both instruments and small tumors (up to about 5 mm) can be destroyed using diathermy without anesthesia in all but the most apprehensive of patients. Vigorous bladder barbotage for bladder washing cytology is not feasible with the flexible instrument, but is not likely to be welcomed by any unsedated patient. For the routine cystoscopic follow up of bladder tumors, the flexible cystoscope is the ideal instrument. However, it is not suitable for patients with pT1 G3 or muscle invasive cancers, nor for the early follow up of carcinoma in situ (CIS), for all of whom careful bimanual palpation, TUR biopsies, multiple mucosal biopsies and/or bladder washings may be necessary.

Random mucosal biopsies

With the exception of patients with CIS the taking of random biopsies from endoscopically normal looking bladder mucosa is not necessary during follow up[8–10]. Even for patients with known CIS it is of doubtful value if the urothelium looks normal. Quite often, intravesical BCG or chemotherapy cause inflammatory changes that are difficult to distinguish from persistent or recurrent CIS. In this situation biopsies are essential, but it should be remembered that the abnormal cells of CIS tend to fall off the urothelium and if a biopsy is deemed necessary, it should always be accompanied by the cytologic examination of bladder washings or voided urine.

Imaging

Ultrasound, CT and MR scanning of the bladder add nothing to the follow up of superficial bladder cancer that cannot be detected by cystoscopy with cytology, bimanual palpation and TUR biopsies as necessary. In individual hands the combination of ultrasound and cytology may offer a very reliable method for follow up, but in the large majority of institutions the sensitivity of both examinations is poor and inferior to cystoscopy. The routine imaging of the ureters and kidneys by intravenous urography (IVU) or ultrasound is another issue. Some urologists suggest that IVU is not necessary in the follow up of superficial bladder cancer because the overall incidence of upper tract tumors is so low. Others argue the reverse on the basis of a small but nonetheless important detection rate for tumors of the upper tract. Patients with CIS are particularly at risk[11]. Ultrasound is preferred to IVU by some colleagues for the diagnostic work up of patients with hematuria[12] but the needs of follow up are different. The purpose is to detect unsuspected tumors of the ureter or renal pelvis and for this purpose IVU is usually superior. At the present time a definitive statement applying to all patients with superficial bladder carcinoma is inappropriate and clinical discretion is advised. For patients with a history of CIS an IVU every year is a wise precaution for the first few years. Any patient with tumor adjacent to a ureteric orifice or any patient with malignant urine cytology but normal cystoscopy should have an IVU. For all other patients, an IVU every 2 to 3 years will rarely cause harm and may detect unsuspected upper tract pathology. Furthermore, patients who have had tumors resected or fulgurized very close to a ureteric orifice may develop fibrotic ureteric obstruction. For both reasons IVU as part of their routine follow up is a wise precaution.

Urine cytology

Although voided urine cytology is used by many urologists in the follow up of patients with superficial bladder cancer, its sensitivity is generally very poor. Recent studies have reported the sensitivity of voided urine cytology for Ta/T1 transitional cell carcinoma to vary between 25 and 47%[10]. On this basis it is difficult to justify the use of urine cytology in addition to cystoscopy, except for patients with previous CIS, abnormal areas of mucosa yielding denuded urothelium on biopsy, or those with an IVU showing possible upper tract tumor. The specificity of urine cytology is very high but despite this, its low sensitivity precludes this examination as a substitute for cystoscopy, especially since the advent of the flexible cystoscope.

Barbotage of the bladder may provide a more cellular specimen[13,14] for cytology and is preferable to a voided urine sample, if the patient has to undergo rigid cyst-oscopy. However, the sensitivity of bladder wash cytology will inevitably fall far short of 100% because the surface cells of well differentiated transitional cell carcinoma, and some moderately differentiated tumors also, appear normal on light microscopy when examined in isolation. As barbotage requires catheterization (or rigid cystoscopy) there is no advantage over flexible cystoscopy.

Alternative diagnostic tests

Flow cytometry for the measurement of the DNA content of exfoliated cell nuclei[15,16], using quantitative fluorescent image analysis[17] or fluorescence in situ hybridization (FISH)[18], or to measure cytokeratin[19] or blood group antigens[20] have all been shown to be more sensitive than voided urine cytology. However, all these tests have a significant proportion of false negative results which has limited their practical usefulness.

The *NMP 22 urinary immunoassay* is a quantitative test that measures a nuclear matrix protein from urothelial cells[21,22]. Its sensitivity has been reported to be 61% compared with 33% for voided urine cytology[23]. Despite this low sensitivity (and a high false-positive rate of up to 36%)[22] the test has been proposed as a predictor of the likelihood of tumour recurrence; Soloway *et al.*[24] proposed that raised levels of urinary NMP 22 following TUR of superficial bladder cancer could 'prompt more aggressive management'. Long-term evidence to support this notion is awaited.

Telomerase is a ribonucleoprotein enzyme present in most cancer cells but not in benign tissue. It can be measured in the urine[25,26] and pilot studies have reported a 90% association with bladder cancer, including well differentiated tumors. The latter would be of particular interest if confirmed.

The urinary *BTA dipstick test* (Bladder Tumour-associated Analyte test)[27] has been evaluated in much larger numbers of patients. It has revealed poor sensitivity for Ta or G1 (well differentiated) tumors, but more than 80% sensitivity for muscle invasive or poorly differentiated cancers[28,29]. Although initially encouraging the BTA test has been superseded by the BTA STAT measurement of complement factor H-related protein[30] in urine, and the BTA TRAK quantitative urine assay for urinary bladder tumor antigen[29]. The sensitivity of these latter two tests has been reported to be higher than for the BTA dipstick test[28,29,31] and all three are superior to urine cytology.

Those clinicians who have used cytology as part of their routine investigation or follow up of transitional cell carcinoma would be advised to consider using one of the foregoing tests instead of cytology, on the basis of the published comparisons. However, those who seek to avoid unnecessary investigations (and expense) would question the role of any of these tests in routine practice, including cytology, given their inability to replace flexible cystoscopy as the most reliable means of diagnosing recurrent bladder cancer.

Conclusions

The cystoscopic follow up of patients with superficial bladder cancer is an essential part of their long-term management. By using two simple prognostic criteria (the number of tumors at diagnosis and the findings of the first follow up cystoscopy) it may be possible to rationalize and reduce the frequency of cystoscopy for many patients. Voided urine cytology and recently developed alternative urine diagnostic tests are not as reliable as flexible cystoscopy for the diagnosis of tumor recurrence. With the exception of patients with carcinoma in situ or pT1 G3 tumors none of these tests, nor routine mucosal biopsies, CT or MR imaging are necessary for the regular follow up of superficial bladder tumors. Infrequent but regular intravenous urography is advisable as it will detect upper tract tumors or ureteric obstruction in occasional patients.

The inconvenience, discomfort, cost and anxiety caused by follow up cystoscopy should not be underestimated. The necessity for follow up cystoscopy may be turned to extra advantage by using the opportunity provided to talk with patients about the nature of their disease and respond to unanswered questions or fears about its long-term prognosis[32].

References

1. Hall RR. Transurethral resection and staging of bladder cancer. In: Hall RR (Ed.) *Clinical Management of Bladder cancer.* London: Arnold; 1998.
2. Parmar KB, Friedman LS, Hargreave *et al.* Prognostic factors for recurrence and follow up policies in the treatment of superficial bladder cancer: report from the British Medical Research council Subgroup on superficial bladder cancer (Urological Cancer Working Party). *J Urol* 1989;**142**:284–288.
3. Reading J, Hall RR, Parmar MKB. The application of a prognostic factor analysis for Ta.T1 bladder cancer in routine urological practice. *Br J Urol* 1995;**75**:604–607.
4. Hall RR, Parmar MKB, Smith PH. Proposals for change in cystoscopic follow-up of patients with bladder cancer and adjuvant intravesical chemotherapy. *Br Med J* 1994;**308**:257–260.
5. Smith PH, Hall RR. Prognostic factors, treatment options and follow up of Ta and T1 bladder tumours. In: Hall RR (Ed.) *Clinical Management of Bladder cancer.* London: Arnold; 1998.
6. Powell PH, Manohar V, Ramsden PD *et al.* A flexible cystoscope. *Br J Urol* 1994;**56**:622–624.
7. Flannagan GM, Gelister JSK, Noble JG *et al.* Rigid versus flexible cystoscopy. A controlled trial of patient tolerance. *Br J Urol* 1988;**62**:537–540.
8. Witjes JA, Kiemeney LALM, Verbeek *et al.* Random biopsies and the risk of recurrent superficial bladder cancer: a prospective study in 1026 patients. *World J Urol* 1992;**10**:231–234.

9. Richards B, Parmar MKB, Anderson CK *et al.* Interpretation of biopsies of 'normal' urothelium in patients with superficial bladder cancer. *Br J Urol* 1991;**67**:369–375.
10. Hall RR. The diagnosis of bladder cancer. In: Hall RR (Ed.) *Clinical Management of Bladder cancer.* London: Arnold; 1998.
11. Jakse G. Carcinoma in situ of the bladder. In: Hall RR (Ed.) *Clinical Management of Bladder cancer.* London: Arnold; 1998.
12. Starling JF, Camerer A, Tiwari A *et al.* Ultrasonography vs intravenous pyelography in the initial evaluation of patients with haematuria. *J Urol* 1997;**157**:124#485.
13. Trott PA, Edwards L. Comparison of bladder washings and urine cytology in the diagnosis of bladder cancer. *J Urol* 1973;**110**:664
14. Kurth KH. Diagnosis and treatment of superficial transitional cell carcinoma of the bladder: facts and perspectives. *Eur Urol* 1997; (suppl 1): 10–19.
15. De Vere White RW, Baker WC. Use of flow cytometric analysis of urine in the diagnosis of bladder cancer. *J Urol* 1987;**137**:216A #451.
16. Badalament RA, Hermansen DK, Kimmel M *et al.* The sensitivity of bladder wash flow cytometry, bladder cytology and voided cytology in the detection of bladder carcinoma. *J Urol* 1987;**137**:215A #447.
17. Carter HB, Amberson JB, Bander MH *et al.* Newer diagnostic techniques for bladder cancer. *Urol Clin N Am* 1987;**14**:763
18. Shankey V, Stankiewicz, Waters B *et al.* Fluorescence in-situ hybridisation analysis of bladder washings as a means to detect genetic changes in the urothelium in transitional cell bladder cancers. *J Urol* 1997;**339**:#1325.
19. Klein A, Zemer R, Buchumensky V *et al.* Detection of bladder carcinoma: a urine test, based on cytokeratin expression. *J Urol* 1997;**157**:339#1326.
20. Fradet Y, Tardif M, Bourget L *et al.* Clinical cancer progression in urinary bladder tumours evaluated by multiparameter flow cytometry with monoclonal antibodies. *Cancer Res* 1990;**30**:432
21. Carpinito GA, Stadler WM, Briggman JV *et al.* Urinary nuclear matrix protein as a marker for transitional cell carcinoma of the urinary tract. *J Urol* 1996;**156**:1280–1285.
22. Miyanage N, Akaza H, Ishikawa S *et al.* Clinical evaluation of nuclear matrix protein 22 (NMP 22) in urine as a novel marker for urothelial cancer. *Eur Urol* 1997;**31**:163–168.
23. Akaza H, Miyanga N, Tsukamoto T *et al.* Evaluation of matrix protein 22 (NMP 22) as a diagnostic marker for bladder cancer: a multicentre trial in Japan. *J Urol* 1997;**157**:337#1315.
24. Soloway MS, Briggman JV, Carpinito GA *et al.* Use of new tumour marker, urinary NMP 22, in the detection of occult or rapidly recurring transitional cell carcinoma of the urinary tract following surgical treatment. *J Urol* 1996;**156**:363–367.
25. Kavaler E, Schu WP, Chang Y *et al.* Detection of human bladder cancer cells in voided urine samples by assaying the presence of telomerase activity. *J Urol* 1997; 157:**338**#1321.
26. Lance RS, Aldous WK, Blaser J *et al.* Telomerase activity in solid transitional cell carcinoma (TCC) and bladder washings. *J Urol* 1997;**338**:#1320.
27. Sarosdy MF, de Vere White RW, Soloway MS *et al.* Results of a multicentre trial using the BTA test to monitor for and diagnose recurrent bladder cancer. *J Urol* 1995;**154**:379–383.
28. Leyh H, Hall RR, Mazeman E *et al.* Comparison of the BARD BTA test with voided urine and bladder wash cytology in the diagnosis and management of cancer of the bladder. *Urology* 1997;**50**:49–53.
29. Ishak LM, Enfield DL, Sarosdy MF *et al.* Detection of recurrent bladder cancer using a new quantitative assay for bladder tumor antigen. *J Urol* 1997;**158**:337 #1317.
30. Kinders RJ, Root R, Jones T *et al.* Complement factor H-related proteins are expressed in bladder cancers. *Proc Am Ass Can Res* 1997;**38**:29 #189.
31. Sarosdy MF, Hudson MA, Ellis WJ *et al.* Detection of recurrent bladder cancer using a new one-step for bladder tumor antigen. *J Urol* 1997;**157**:337#1318.
32. Hall RR, Charlton M and Ongena P. Talking with patients about bladder cancer. In: Hall RR (Ed.) *Clinical Management of Bladder cancer.* London: Arnold; 1998.

6 Treatment of carcinoma in situ

K H Kurth

Algorithm

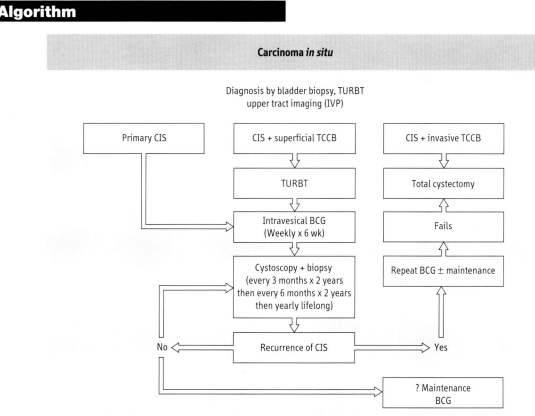

Carcinoma *in situ*

Diagnosis by bladder biopsy, TURBT
upper tract imaging (IVP)

Primary CIS

CIS + superficial TCCB

CIS + invasive TCCB

TURBT

Total cystectomy

Intravesical BCG
(Weekly x 6 wk)

Fails

Cystoscopy + biopsy
(every 3 months x 2 years
then every 6 months x 2 years
then yearly lifelong)

Repeat BCG ± maintenance

No ⟵ Recurrence of CIS ⟶ Yes

? Maintenance
BCG

[TURBT, transurethral resection of bladder tumor]

Introduction

Carcinoma *in situ* (CIS) of the bladder, first described by Melicow in 1952, is the precursor of invasive cancer and may coexist with non-invasive papillary cancer[1]. The term transitional CIS is limited to flat lesions with enough cellular anaplasia to be recognized as carcinomas[2]. Such lesions should be graded as Grade 2 or Grade 3. The majority will be classified as Grade 3.

The classic endoscopic appearance of flat CIS, which may be focal or diffuse, is usually a patchy, serpiginous or granular, slightly raised, velvety lesion with poorly defined margins[3]. The critical diagnostic features involve the recognition of cytologic anaplastic abnormalities in individual cells and alteration in the normal cell relationships within the bladder epithelium. The anaplasia of the epithelium is not part of a papillary structure and there is no infiltration of the underlying connective tissue. The term dysplasia is used to cover changes in the epithelium which fall short of the diagnostic threshold for CIS[4].

Diagnostic assessment

Most patients with either primary (no other bladder neoplasm) or secondary CIS (concurrent with – or subsequent other bladder neoplasm) present with symptoms such as urgency, dysuria, frequency and hematuria. The irritative symptoms may be misinterpreted as being caused by cystitis or prostatic disease in elderly men leading to a protracted time-lapse from the onset of symptoms to diagnosis of CIS. In a report from Farrow *et al.*[5] the mean duration of symptoms in men was 19 months with a range of 0–99 months. Asymptomatic patients may be diagnosed by urine cytology during follow up cystoscopy after previous papillary Ta/T1 bladder carcinoma. Patients with irritative symptoms of the lower urinary tract and a negative urine culture should have cystoscopy and cytologic examination from barbotage specimen[6].

Selected site biopsies

When increased vascularity of the bladder mucosa and erythematous zones without clearly defined margins are seen, or when exfoliative epithelium from a barbotage specimen contains cancer cells, cold-cup biopsies of suspicious areas and from preselected sites are indicated. The commonly affected sites are the trigone or floor of the bladder, the periureteral areas and the bladder neck. The posterior and lateral walls and the bladder dome are also frequently involved. In situ carcinoma is seldom found on the anterior wall[5]. If mucosal biopsies from areas other than the obvious neoplasm contain severe dysplasia or CIS, there is as much greater likelihood of subsequent tumor development[7]. Biopsy from the prostatic urethra is best done with a cutting loop of a resectoscope at the five and seven o'clock position and must be deep enough to include the mucosa of the prostatic urethra, together with underlying ducts, glands and stroma[8]. In the pathology report, in situ involvement of the prostatic ducts by transitional cell carcinoma (TCC) must be differentiated from prostatic stromal invasion because the prognosis is different[9]. CIS involving the prostate is notoriously silent. The incidence of prostatic involvement in association with bladder CIS in two consecutive series from the Mayo Clinic was 26% and 62% respectively[10]. The incidence of primary TCC of the prostate varies between 1% and 4%[10]. Thus, routine biopsy of the prostate in patients with CIS of the bladder is mandatory. The main site for involvement is the verumontanum area, as most prostatic ducts open into this region[11]. CIS can also involve the urethra and peri-urethral glands[12,13].

Non-urothelial mucosa in the urinary tract can be involved by Tis. Sites involved are the seminal vesicles, ejaculatory epithelium, urethral meatus and the collecting ducts of the kidney[13,14]. Guidelines as to the indications for mucosal biopsies are given in Table 6.1.1. All visible changes of the bladder mucosa are recorded on a diagram.

Although there is significant discrepancy between pathologists in the classification of papillary tumors Ta/T1 and grading[15], pathologists were in excellent agreement on the classification of CIS. Richards *et al.*[16] reported that consensus was reached on all biopsies which showed either severe dysplasia or CIS by a group of six pathologists having a special interest in urological pathology

Cytology

Cytology is most effective in the identification of high grade tumors. Urine specimens should be immediately fixed for later processing. A sample of 50 ml of urine is regarded as sufficient; the patient can be best provided with a container already filled with 50 ml of the fixative

Table 6.1.1   Indications for mucosal biopsies

- Abnormal looking areas of urothelium seen in association with exophytic tumor or at cystoscopic follow up
- Urine cytology showing malignant cells in the absence of an exophytic tumor in the urinary tract
- Presence of high-grade papillary tumor to detect or to exclude concurrent CIS
- Symptoms from the lower urinary tract not explained by urinary infection or obstruction.

(50% ethanol). The presence of cancer cells should be reported as 'positive for malignant cells'. Abnormal cells should be reported as 'suspicious for malignant tumor'. Atypical cells, thought to represent non-neoplastic epithelium, should be reported as 'atypical cells present'. The cytologists should report 'negative for malignant cells' when a specimen does not contain malignant or atypical cells.

A specimen is reported unsatisfactory if the quality of the preservation is poor. All cytologic diagnosis of bladder cancer must be confirmed by biopsy prior to therapy in patients seen for the first time. In patients with a known history of CIS positive cytology heralds the appearance of CIS inside or outside the bladder. The accuracy of urinary cytology in detecting CIS of the bladder exceeds 80% for all lesions, and identifies more than 90% of multifocal diffuse lesions in symptomatic patients[17].

Bladder washing

The superiority of bladder washing over voided urine cytology has recently been confirmed and has been recommended[18]. Iso-osmotic fluid preserving cellular integrity is mandatory for bladder irrigation. Bladder washing will yield abundant, well preserved cellular material. Information submitted together with the specimens for cytologic examination are given in Table 6.1.2.

Imaging studies

Intravenous pyelogram should be carried out on a routine basis to exclude upper urinary tract tumor and should be repeated annually for 10 years in patients with CIS of the bladder. In selected cases retrograde pyelograms and ureteroscopy may be necessary.

Staging carcinoma in situ

Completed diagnostic assessment should allow proper identification of CIS. It requires close cooperation of the urologists, pathologists and cytologists. The pathologists should note the presence and characteristics of flat epithelial lesions and classify the tumor as shown in Table 6.1.3.

Table 6.1.2   Information for the cytopathologist

- Patient identification and demographic data
- Clinical history including exposure to carcinogens
- Known or suspected urinary tract calculi
- Alteration and other inflammatory processes in the urinary tract
- Type of specimen (voided, catheterized, catheterized after cystoscopy, bladder irrigation via catheter or cystoscope, ureteral urine or irrigation)
- Type of treatment (immunotherapy or chemotherapy)

Treatment of carcinoma in situ of the bladder

Transurethral resection

Biopsy and fulguration alone would not be regarded as appropriate treatment for CIS. Most patients treated by resection alone are at risk of developing invasive disease[19,20].

Intravesical chemotherapy and immunotherapy

Cytostatics applied intravesically, immunotherapy with bacillus Calmette-Guérin (BCG), the cytokines Interferon[21] and Interleukin-2[22] and the BRM KLH (Keyhole-Limpet Hemocyanin)[23] were also used for the treatment of CIS. The Interferon-inducer Bropirimine given orally has activity against both bladder and upper tract CIS[24]. Experience is limited.

Local intravesical treatment, whether with chemotherapeutic or immunotherapeutic agents, is evaluated by the rate of complete remission. In addition the duration of complete remission, the prevention of local progression to muscle invasive disease or metastasis and the success in delaying or avoiding cystectomy are important measures of successful treatment.

Immunotherapy with bacillus Calmette-Guérin (BCG)

The precise mechanisms of action by which BCG inhibits tumor growth are at present unknown, but evidence suggests an immunologically mediated effect[25]. A requirement for BCG effect is direct contact with the urothelium. Areas of urothelium remote from BCG contact, i.e. upper tracts, will not respond to treatment with intravesical BCG.

BCG instillation generates a chronic, granulomatous inflammation within the bladder[26,27]. Patients become immunized to BCG antigen as demonstrated by the development of a cutaneous delayed type hypersensitivity response to PPD. BCG generates a local immunological

Table 6.1.3   Tis tumor classification

Tis*	location
b	bladder
u	ureter (one or both)
pu	prostatic urethra
pd	prostatic ducts (prostatic acini)
	(ps – prostatic stroma = T4 not Tis)
fu	female urethra

* The suffix 'm' should be added to indicate multiple lesions and the suffix 'is' can be added to any T category to indicate concurrent CIS (e.g. T2G2 + Tis).

reaction as demonstrated by the identification of cytokines in the urine[27,28]. The mycobacteria induce a strong T-lymphocyte dependent immune response[29], but which components of this response are essential for the induction of antibladder tumor activity is unclear[25]. BCG immunotherapy has been confirmed by investigators all over the world to be effective in the treatment of CIS. The average complete response rate is about 70% (Table 6.1.4).

A number of schedules have produced a complete response. Herr and associates[20] reported resolution of the CIS in 68% of the patients with a mean follow up of 3 years after a 6 week intravesical therapy program. Several authors treated patients not achieving complete remission after one 6 week course with a second 6 week course[30,31]. Lamm presented the interim results of a randomized prospective South-West Oncology Group study investigating maintenance BCG immunotherapy of superficial bladder cancer[32]. Patients received 6 weekly intravesical instillations of 120 ml Connaught BCG. Those who attained a complete response were randomized to observation or 3 weekly BCG instillations at 3 months and 6 months and every 6 months to 3 years. In the CIS subgroup of 121 patients the advantage of maintenance BCG was significant at $P = 0.04$.

Although the aforementioned study has clearly shown the superiority of maintenance over a 6 week course only, the optimal schedule has not been determined. The viability of BCG may have an impact on therapeutic efficacy as reported by Kelley and associates[33]. Patients who failed initial therapy with a low viability lot of BCG responded favorably to retreatment with a higher viability lot. The BCG strain used may not be important for the final outcome[34].

Several authors have been unable to demonstrate more favorable results when intravesical BCG therapy was combined with percutaneous BCG injections[20,35,36]. Patients with CIS of the bladder should have control cystoscopy, selected site biopsy and bladder barbotage 8–10 weeks after initiation of the induction course. Patients who still have positive cytology after the induction treatment of 6 weekly instillation are at high risk for either overlooked concurrent or recently developed invasive disease. Merz et al.[37] observed that among patients with primary CIS not responding to a 6 week BCG-Pasteur 3/25 had either CIS of both ureters, CIS of the prostatic urethra or invasive bladder tumor (pT3). Among patients with secondary CIS early failure was observed in 20/90 patients. Four had invasive bladder tumor (>pT2), three upper urinary tract CIS and four involvement of the prostatic urethra. Orsola et al.[38] reported complete remission (CR) in 81% (21/26 patients) after weekly intravesical BCG for 6 weeks and progression to ≥T2 in three out of five no responding patients in a period of 6 months. Thus both the development of invasive disease or CIS of the upper urinary tract should be excluded in patients with early failure.

None of the large studies investigating BCG in carcinoma in situ of the bladder is mature enough to be analyzed for a possible decrease in disease progression and an increase in survival duration. In the SWOG studies, reported by Lamm et al. differences in survival were not significant in patients treated by either Mitomycin-C, doxorubicin or BCG[39,40]. Similar observations were reported by other authors[41,42,43]. However significant improvement in survival from 68% to 86% has been reported in a randomized prospective comparison of

Table 6.1.4   BCG responses in Cis*

Author	No. of patients	CR (%)	Relapse following CR on BCG				FU for CR patients
			Tis	Ta/T1	≥T2	N+M+	
Harland[30]	53	28 (53)	9	no	3	no	32 months (median)
Kavoussi[31]	32	25 (78)	3	no	no	1	21.4 months (mean)
Merz[37]	115	92 (80)	8	14	no	no	40 months (median)
Lamm[39]	64	45 (70)	19/45*	(42%)* na	stage relapse	na	65 months (median)
Lamm[40]	31	17 (55)					30 months (median)
Herr[†]	180	105 (58)	11*		7	1	≥5 years
van Gils-Gielen[‡]	37	25 (66)	2	6	4	2	45 months (mean)
Brosman[§]	48	34 (71)	stage relapse	na		9	35 months (mean)
Takashi[**]	30	25 (83)	3	no	3	no	56 (median)
Jakse[63]	103	77 (75)	7*		7	16	7.6 years (median)
Lamm[32]	116 no maintenance vs. 117 maintenance	97 (84)	not separately reported for Tis Points				91.4 months (median)

*Different treatment schedules and BCG strains were used; * these numbers were shared between the Tis and Ta/T1 categories; CR=complete response; na=not available; †1993, personal communication; ‡*Urology* 1995; **45**: 581–586; § *Prog Clin Biol Res* 1989; **310**:193–205; ** *Int Urol Nephrol* 1997;**29**:557–563.

transurethral resection alone with surgery plus BCG in 86 patients[44].

Treatment of carcinoma in situ involving the prostatic urethra

Stromal invasion of the prostate (T4) contraindicates treatment with BCG. Whether ductal involvement should preclude intravesical therapy requires further study. Instillations begin as soon after transurethral resection as irritative symptoms permit, the treatment schedule and follow up are identical to that for carcinoma *in situ* of the bladder.

Schellhammer[45] treated 17 patients with a positive pretreatment prostatic urethral biopsy for CIS. In none of the 17 patients was acinar or stromal tumor invasion identified. Eleven patients had a concurrent bladder CIS. 12/17 (70%) of patients had no evidence of tumor in the prostatic urethra after treatment with BCG.

Bretton *et al.*[46] reported 23 patients presenting with multifocal superficial bladder cancer and concurrent *in situ* transitional cell carcinoma of the prostatic urethra (mucosal in 19, ductal in four). Of the 23 patients 13 (56%) had a complete response with a median follow up of 43.7 months without recurrence. In seven patients cystectomy was performed for progression or residual disease in the bladder; in all patients the prostatic urethra was negative for transitional cell carcinoma.

Such favorable results have not been achieved with intravesical chemotherapy[47]. The contact time of an intravesical chemotherapeutic agent may be insufficient to allow absorption within the cell to produce a lethal event. Generally, the situation differs from intravesical BCG because of the documented BCG attachment to urothelium[25].

Hardeman and Soloway[48] defined the risk of subsequent urethral occurrence based on initial prostatic urethral biopsy. In patients with stromal invasion the risk of recurrence was 64%. If ductal involvement was present, the risk was 25%. The risk was less than 5% if the prostatic urethra was negative or only mucosal involvement present.

Interferon for the treatment of CIS

Using alpha 2b interferon intravesical instillations Torti *et al.* reported a 32% complete response rate among 19 patients with CIS[49]. A dose–response relationship for interferon was studied in a prospective randomized trial comparing the effect of low dose (10×10^6 units) of alpha 2b interferon with high dose (100×10^6 units) as primary therapy for CIS in 87 patients[21]. Patients were treated weekly $\times$ 12 then monthly for up to 1 year. A 43% com-

plete response rate was obtained using the high dose vs. a 5% complete response rate using the low dose ($P \leq 0.0001$). In the same study the high dose of interferon was used as a rescue therapy for nine patients who had relapsed after BCG therapy. Two of nine patients had a complete response. Side effects from interferon instillation were minimal and consisted of mild to moderate flu-like symptoms.

Oral bropirimine immunotherapy in CIS

CR of CIS was seen in 21 of 65 patients, including 14 (30%, confidence interval (CI) 17% to 43%) of BCG-resistant, and seven (39%, CI 16% to 61%) of 18 BCG-intolerant patients. Most BCG-resistant patients were failures to BCG without relapse, and had received 12 to 36 (median 12) BCG treatments. Response duration ranged from 65 to 810 days, with median not yet reached (but greater than 12 months). Progression to invasive or metastatic disease either during or immediately after therapy was documented in four patients (6%), all non-responders. Overall, by intent-to-treat analysis CR was seen in 21 (24%) of 86 subjects. Thirteen (15%) of 86 stopped Bropirimine due to toxicity (similar to that seen with administration of exogenous interferon)[50]. In a report of Bropirimine treatment for upper tract CIS 10/21 (48%) had their positive cytology converted to negative[51].

Chemotherapy in CIS

Several groups showed that organ conservation is possible by means of different intravesically instilled chemotherapeutic drugs (Table 6.1.5). In the only large-scale randomized trial comparing chemotherapy with immunotherapy (BCG) it became evident that doxorubicin in the schedule used was inferior to BCG[39]. The complete remission rate was 34% vs. 70%. However, the doxorubicin was only used in a schedule recommended for adjuvant treatment[55].

Table 6.1.5 Complete remission of *in situ* cancer after intravesical chemotherapy

	CR	%	Recur	CR-dur (months)	DOD	Follow up (months)
DOX[52]	34/56	75	17/35	28	4	54
DOX[39]	23/67	34	11/23	10	na	65
EPI[53]	16/22	73	8/16	24	0	35
MMC[54]	15/19	79	6/15	na	0	49

CR = complete remission; recur = recurrence; CR-dur=duration of complete remission; DOD = dead of disease; na = not available.

Treatment of CIS of the bladder by cystectomy

The management of CIS has changed considerably with time. In patients with symptomatic CIS not associated with prior or concurrent bladder tumors[17], early radical cystectomy deserves consideration[6]. This is justified by the association of microinvasive carcinoma in as many as 34% of these patients and the occurrence of metastatic disease despite early cystectomy in 6% or more of the patients[1]. Intravesical bacillus Calmette-Guérin therapy has clearly revolutionized the treatment of CIS. It has not been demonstrated that an initial trial of BCG immunotherapy compromises overall survival compared with immediate cystectomy[39].

Cystectomy is indicated for the treatment of patients with CIS who have not responded to intravesical therapy within a 6 month period, because the development of invasive carcinoma or lymph node metastases has been seen in approximately 50% of patients with CIS followed for longer intervals[56]. Patients with stromal invasion of the prostate or extensive intraductal involvement are best managed by cystoprostatectomy initially.

Five year overall survival rates without and with stromal invasion in men treated by radical cystoprostatectomy were 71% and 36% respectively[57].

Photodynamic therapy for CIS

The experimental treatment modality, known as photodynamic therapy (PDT), uses an interaction between absorbed light and a photosensitizer in the presence of oxygen to destroy tissue. Hematoporphyrin derivative (HPD) was the initial photosensitizer used but over the past decade most clinical treatments have used a purified combination of ethers and esters known as Photofrin II[R]. A new, experimentally used potent photosensitizer is aminolevulinic acid (ALA)[58].

Transitional cell carcinoma of the bladder is responsive to PDT with better responses generally seen in treatment of CIS.

D'Hallewin et al.[59] reported on the preliminary results of 12 patients with multifocal CIS of the bladder treated with whole bladder wall photodynamic therapy. CR was achieved in 9/12 patients (average follow up 11.5 months).

Jocham et al.[60] evaluated 28 patients with CIS 12–60 months after whole bladder PDT in which nine sustained complete responses were noted.

Manyak et al.[61] have evaluated the use of a soybean emulsion solution to scatter light equally throughout the bladder in patients with CIS resistant to intravesical treatment with chemotherapy and bacille Calmette-Guérin. Out of 17 patients a complete response was observed in six (35%). At present PDT remains experimental.

Conclusions

CIS of the bladder is a high-grade lesion recognized as a morphologic entity. Bladder irritability is the leading symptom in patients with primary CIS. Exfoliative urinary cytology is the most important diagnostic tool. Biopsies have to be taken from suspicious areas, preselected sites in the bladder and from the prostatic urethra. While cystectomy was the initial treatment of choice, the high response rate to intravesical BCG justifies a more conservative approach to management. The complete response rate with BCG immunotherapy is ≥70%. Patients not responding to BCG immunotherapy without evidence of progression may be treated with alternative immunotherapies such as alpha-2b interferon, keyhole limpet hemocyanin (KLH) or bropirimine, with intravesical chemotherapy or photodynamic therapy. If treatment is ineffective, cystectomy should not be delayed for more than 6 months. Further studies with long-term observation will be warranted to elucidate the natural history and to identify prognostic factors of CIS of the bladder. Because of the lifelong risk for either recurrence of Tis, Ta/T1 or invasive bladder tumor patients with preserved bladder must be followed and controlled lifelong[62,63].

References

1. Utz DC, Farrow GM. Carcinoma in situ in the urinary tract. *Urol Clin N Am* 1984;**11**:735–749.
2. Friedell G, Kotake T, Barlebo H, Jakse G, Fukushima S, Melamed M, Cohen S et al. Transitional cell carcinoma in situ. In: Niijima T, Aso Y, Koontz W, Prout G, Denis L (eds) *Consensus development in clinical bladder cancer research.* Proceedings of the second and third international consensus development symposia. Ivry/France: Digital Print, 1993: pp. 55–64.
3. Utz DC, Farrow GM. Management of the carcinoma in situ of the bladder: a case for the surgical management. *Urol Clin North Am* 1980;**7**:533–541.
4. Murphy WM, Soloway MS. Urothelial dysplasia. *J Urol* 1982;**127**:849–854.
5. Farrow GM, Utz DC, Rife CC, Greene LF. Clinical observations on 69 cases of in situ carcinoma of the urinary bladder. *Cancer Res* 1977;**37**:2794–2798.
6. Lamm DL. Carcinoma in situ. *Urol Clin North Am* 1992;**19**:499–508.
7. Wolf H, Hojgaard K. Urothelial dysplasia concomittant with bladder tumors as a determinant factor for future new occurrences. *Lancet* 1983;**16**:134–136.
8. Wood DP Jr, Montie JE, Pontes JE, Vanderbrug Medendorp S, Levin HS. Transitional cell carcinoma of the prostate in cystoprostatectomy specimens removed for bladder cancer. *J Urol* 1989;**141**:346–349.
9. Schellhammer PF, Bean MA, Whitmore WF Jr. Prostatic involvement by transitional cell carcinoma: pathogenesis, patterns and prognosis. *J Urol* 1977;**118**:399–403.
10. Zincke H, Utz DCH, Farrow GM. Review of Mayo Clinic experience with carcinoma in situ. *Urology* 1985;**26** (suppl):39–46.
11. Ro JY, Staerkel GA, Ayala AG. Cytologic and histologic features of superficial bladder cancer. *Urol Clin North Am* 1992;**19**:435–453.
12. Schellhammer PF, Whitmore WF Jr. Transitional cell carcinoma of the urethra in men having cystectomy for bladder cancer. *J Urol* 1976;**115**:56–60.
13. Tomaszewski JE, Korat OC, LiVolsi VA, Connor AM, Wein A. Paget's disease of the urethral meatus following transitional cell carcinoma of the bladder. *J Urol* 1986;**135**:368–370.

14. Ro JY, Ayala AG, El-Naggar A, Wishnow I. Seminal vesicle involvement by in situ and invasive transitional cell carcinoma of the bladder. *Am J Surg Pathol* 1987;**11**:951–958.

15. Kurth KH, Denis L, Bouffioux Ch, Sylvester R, Debruyne FMJ, Pavone-Macaluso M, Oosterlinck W. Factors affecting recurrence and progression in superficial bladder tumours. *Eur J Cancer* 1995;**31A**(11):1840–1846.

16. Richards B, Parmar MKB, Anderson CK, Ansell ID, Grigor K, Hall RR, Morley AR et al. and the MRC Superficial Bladder Cancer Sub Group. Interpretation of biopsies of 'normal' urothelium in patients with superficial cancer. *Br J Urol* 1991;**67**:369–375.

17. Herr HW. Carcinoma in situ of the bladder. *Sem Urol* 1983;**1**:15–22.

18. Matzkin H, Moinuddin SM, Soloway MS. Value of urine cytology versus bladder washing in bladder cancer. *Urology* 1992;**39**:201–203.

19. Prout GR Jr, Griffin PP, Daly JJ. The outcome of conservative treatment of carcinoma in situ of the bladder. *J Urol* 1987;**138**:766–770.

20. Herr HW, Pinsky CM, Whitmore WF Jr, Sogani PC, Oettgen HF, Melamed MR. Long-term effect of intravesical bacillus Calmette-Guérin on flat carcinoma in situ of the bladder. *J Urol* 1986;**135**:265–267.

21. Glashan RW. A randomized controlled study of intravesical α-2b-interferon in carcinoma in situ of the bladder. *J Urol* 1990;**144**:658–661.

22. Cockett ATK, Davis RS, Cos LR, Wheeless LL Jr. Bacillus Calmette-Guérin and Interleukin-2 for treatment of superficial bladder cancer. *J Urol* 1991;**146**:766–770.

23. Jurincic-Winkler C, Metz KA, Beuth J, Sippel J, Klippel KF. Effect of Keyhole Limpet Hemocyanin (KLH) and bacillus Calmette-Guérin (BCG) instillation on carcinoma in situ of the urinary bladder. *Anticancer Res* 1995;**15**(6B):2771–2776.

24. Sarosdy MF. A review of clinical studies of Bropirimine immunotherapy of carcinoma in situ of the bladder and upper urinary tract. *Eur Urol* 1997;**31**:20–26.

25. Ratliff TL. Mechanisms of action of BCG in superficial bladder cancer. In: *EORTC Genitourinary Group Monograph 11: Recent progress in bladder and kidney cancer*. Wiley-Liss, New York. *Progr Clin Biol Res*, 1992;**378**:103–109.

26. Torrence RJ, Kavoussi LR, Catalona WJ, Ratliff TL. Prognostic factors in patients treated with intravesical bacillus Calmette-Guérin for superficial bladder cancer. *J Urol* 1988;**139**:941–944.

27. Schamhart DHJ, Kurth KH, De Reijke ThM, Vleeming R. BCG treatment and the importance of an inflammatory response. *Urol Res* 1992;**20**:199–203.

28. Böhle A, Nowc CH, Ulmer AJ, Musehold J, Gerdes J, Hofstetter AG. Elevations of cytokines interleukin-1, interleukin-2, and tumor necrosis factor in the urine of patients after intravesical bacillus Calmette-Guérin immunotherapy. *J Urol* 1990;**144**:59–64.

29. De Boer EC, De Jong WH, Van der Meijden APM, Steerenberg PA, Witjes JA, Vegt PDJ et al. Presence of activated lymphocytes in the urine of patients with superficial bladder cancer after intravesical immunotherapy with bacillus Calmette-Guérin. *Cancer Immunol Immunother* 1991;**33**:411–416.

30. Harland SJ, Charig CR, Highman W, Parkinson MC, Riddle PR. Outcome in carcinoma in situ of bladder treated with intravesical bacille Calmette-Guérin. *Br J Urol* 1992;**70**:271–275.

31. Kavoussi LR, Torrence RJ, Gillen DP, Hudson MA, Haaff EO, Dresner SM, Ratliff TL, Catalona WJ. Results of 6 weekly intravesical bacillus Calmette-Guérin instillations on the treatment of superficial bladder tumors. *J Urol* 1988;**139**:935–939.

32. Lamm DL, Blumenstein BA, Crissman JD, Montie JE, Gottesman JE, Lowe BA, Sarosdy MF, Bohl RD, Grossman HB, Beck TM, Leimert JT, Crawford ED. Maintenance bacillus Calmette-Guerin immunotherapy for recurrent TA, T1 and carcinoma in situ transitional cell carcinoma of the bladder: a randomised Southwest Oncology Group Study. *J Urol* 2000;**163**(4):1124–9.

33. Kelley DR, Ratliff TL, Catalona WJ, Shapiro A, Lage JM, Bauer WC, Haaff EO et al. Intravesical bacillus Calmette-Guérin therapy for superficial bladder cancer: effect of bacillus Calmette-Guérin viability on treatment results. *J Urol* 1985;**134**:48–53.

34. Mukherjee A, Persad R, Smith JB. Intravesical BCG treatment for superficial bladder cancer: long-term results using two different strains of BCG. *Br J Urol* 1992;**69**:147–150.

35. Lamm DL, DeHaven JI, Shriver J, Sarosdy MF. Prospective randomized comparison of intravesical with percutaneous bacillus Calmette-Guérin versus intravesical bacillus Calmette-Guérin in superficial bladder cancer. *J Urol* 1991;**145**:738–740.

36. Witjes JA, v d Meijden AP, Sylvester LC, Debruyne FM, van Aubel A, Witjes WP. Long-term follow-up of an EORTC randomized prospective trial comparing intravesical bacille Calmette-Guerin-RIVM and mitomycin C in superficial bladder cancer. EORTC GU Group and the Dutch South East Cooperative Urological Group. European Organisation for Research and Treatment of Cancer Genito-Urinary Tract Cancer Collaborative Group. *Urology*. 1998;**52**(3):403–10.

37. Merz VW, Marth D, Kraft R, Ackermann DK, Zingg EJ, Studer UE. Analysis of early failures after intravesical instillation therapy with bacille Calmette-Guérin for carcinoma in situ of the bladder. *Br J Urol* 1995;**75**:180–184.

38. Orsola A, Palou J, Xavier B, Algaba F, Salvador J, Vicente J. Primary bladder carcinoma in situ: Assessment of early BCG response as a prognostic factor. *Eur Urol* 1998;**33**:457–463.

39. Lamm DL, Blumenstein BA, Crawford ED, Montie JE, Scardino P, Grossmann H B, Stanisic TH et al. A randomized trial of intravesical Doxorubicin and immunotherapy with bacillus Calmette-Guérin for transitional cell carcinoma of the bladder. *New Eng J Med*, 1991;**325**:1205–1209.

40. Lamm DL, Blumenstein BA, Crawford ED, Crissman JD, Lowe BA, Smith JA Jr, Sarosdy MF et al. Randomized intergroup comparison of bacillus Calmette-Guérin immunotherapy and mitomycin-C chemotherapy prophylaxis in superficial transitional cell carcinoma of the bladder. *Urol Oncol* 1995;**1**:119–126.

41. Krege S, Giani G, Meyer R, Otto T, Rübben H and participating clinics. A randomized multicenter trial of adjuvant therapy in superficial bladder cancer: transurethral resection only versus transurethral resection plus Mitomycin-C versus transurethral resection plus bacillus Calmette-Guérin. *J Urol* 1996;**156**:962–966.

42. Lundholm C, Norlen BJ, Ekman P, Jahnson S, Lagerkvist M, Lindeborg T, Olsson JO et al. A randomized prospective study comparing long-term intravesical instillations of Mitomycin-C and Bacillus Calmette-Guérin in patients with superficial bladder carcinoma. *J Urol* 1996;**156**:372–376.

43. Vegt PDJ, Witjes JA, Witjes WPJ, Doesburg WH, Debruyne FMJ, Van der Meijden APM. A randomized study of intravesical Mitomycin-C, Bacillus Calmette-Guérin Tice and Bacillus Calmette-Guérin RIVM treatment in pTa-pT1 papillary carcinoma and carcinoma in situ of the bladder. *J Urol* 1995;**153**:929–933.

44. Herr HW, Laudone VP, Badalament RA, Oettgen HF, Sogani PC, Freedman BD, Melamed MR, Whitmore WF Jr. Bacillus Calmette-Guérin therapy alters the progression of superficial bladder cancer. *J Clin Oncol* 1988;**6**:1450–1455.

45. Schellhammer PF, Ladaga LE, Moriarty RP. Intravesical bacillus Calmette-Guérin for the treatment of superficial transitional cell carcinoma of the prostatic urethra in association with carcinoma in situ. *J Urol* 1995;**153**:53–56.

46. Bretton PR, Herr HW, Whitmore WF Jr, Badalament RA, Kimmel M, Provet J, Oettgen HF et al. Intravesical bacillus Calmette-Guérin therapy for in situ transitional cell carcinoma involving the prostatic urethra. *J Urol* 1989;**141**:853–856.

47. Lockhart JL, Chaikin L, Bondhus MJ, Politano VA. Prostatic recurrences in the management of superficial bladder tumors. *J Urol* 1983;**130**:256–257.

48. Hardeman SW, Soloway MS. Urethral recurrence following radical cystectomy. *J Urol* 1990;**144**:666–669.

49. Torti FM, Shortliffe LD, Williams RD, Pitts WC, Kempson RL, Ross IC, Palmer J et al. Alpha-interferon in superficial bladder cancer: a Northern California Oncology Group study. *J Clin Oncol* 1988;**6**:476–483.

50. Sarosdy MF, Manyak MJ, Sagalowsky AI, Belldegrun A, Benson MC, Bihrle W, Carroll PR et al. Oral Bropirimine immunotherapy of bladder carcinoma in situ after prior intravesical Bacille Calmette-Guérin. *Urology* 1998;**51**:226–231.

51. Sarosdy MF, Pisters LL, Carroll PR, Benson MC, Moon TD, Lamm DL, Hudson MA et al. Bropirimine immunotherapy of upper urinary tract carcinoma in situ. *Urology* 1996;**48**:28–32.

52. Jakse G, Hofstädter F, Marberger H. Topical doxorubicin hydrochloride therapy for carcinoma in situ of the bladder: a followup. *J Urol* 1984;**131**:41–42.

53. Kurth KH, Vd Vijgh WJF, Ten Kate FWJ, Bogdanowicz JF, Carpentier PJ, Van Reyswoud I. Phase 1/2 study of intravesical epirubicin in patients with carcinoma in situ of the bladder. *J Urol* 1991;**146**:1508–1513.

54. Stricker PD, Grant ABF, Hosken BM, Taylor JS. Topical Mitomycin-C therapy for carcinoma in situ of the bladder: a follow-up. *J Urol* 1990;**143**:34–35.

55. Kurth KH, Tunn U, Ay R, Schröder FH, Pavone-Macaluso M, Debruyne F, ten Kate F, De Pauw M, Sylvester R and members of the European Organization for Research and Treatment of Cancer. Genitourinary. Adjuvant chemotherapy of superficial transitional cell bladder carcinoma: long-term results of a European Organization for Research and Treatment of Cancer randomized trial comparing Doxorubicin, Ethoglucid and transurethral resection alone. *J Urol* 1997;**158**:378–384.

56. Whitmore WF Jr. Management of bladder cancer. *Curr Prob Cancer* 1979;**4**:1–48.

57. Esrig D, Freeman JA, Elmajian DA, Stein JP, Chen SC, Groshen S, Simoneau A *et al.* Transitional cell carcinoma involving the prostate with a proposed staging classification for stromal invasion. *J Urol* 1996;**156**:1071–1076.

58. Stenzl A, Eder I, Kostron H, Klocker H, Bartsch G. Electromotive diffusion (EMD) and photodynamic therapy with delta-aminolevulinic acid (delta-ALA) for superficial bladder cancer. *J Photochem Photobiol B – Biology* 1996;**36**(2):233–236.

59. D'Hallewin MA, Baert L, Marijnissen JPA, Star WM. Whole bladder wall photodynamic therapy with in situ light dosimetry for carcinoma in situ of the bladder. *J Urol* 1992;**148**:1152–1155.

60. Jocham D, Baumgartner R, Stepp H, Unsöld E. Clinical experience with the integral photodynamic therapy of bladder carcinoma. *J Photochem Photobiol*, 1990;**6**:183–187.

61. Manyak MJ. Photodynamic therapy: principles and urological applications. *Sem Urol* 1991;**9**:192–202.

62. Jakse G, Hall R, Bono A, Holtl W, Carpentier P, Spaander JP, van Der Meijden AP, Sylvester R. Intravesical BCG in Patients with Carcinoma in situ of the Urinary Bladder: Long-Term Results of EORTC GU Group Phase II Protocol 30861. *Eur Urol* 2001;**40(2)**:144–50.

63. Herr HW, Sogani PC. Does early cystectomy improve the survival of patients with high risk superficial bladder tumors? *J Urol* 2001;**166(4)**:1296–9.

7 Treatment of invasive transitional cell carcinoma

Bladder cancer

Invasive transitional cell carcinoma (T2)

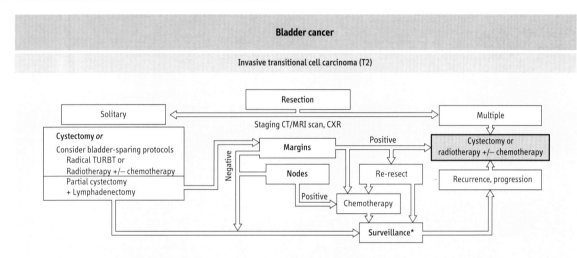

*Surveillance: every 3 months 3 x 24 months, then every 6 months 3 x 24 months, then anually: cystoscopy + examination under anesthesia

Invasive transitional cell carcinoma (T3)

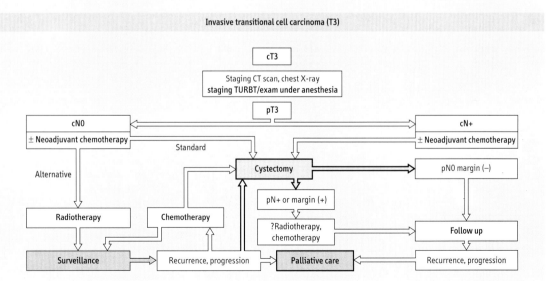

65

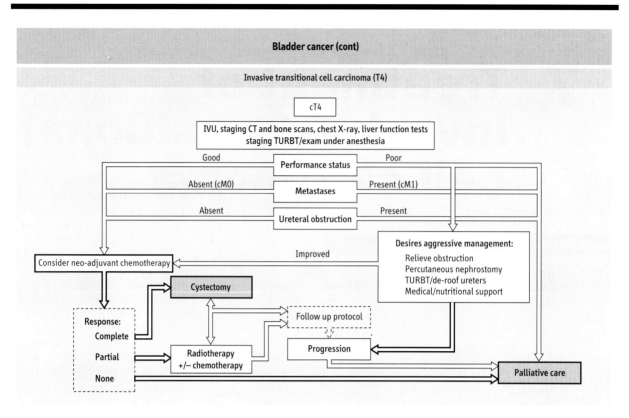

Bladder cancer (cont)

Invasive transitional cell carcinoma (T4)

cT4

IVU, staging CT and bone scans, chest X-ray, liver function tests
staging TURBT/exam under anesthesia

Good   Performance status   Poor

Absent (cM0)   Metastases   Present (cM1)

Absent   Ureteral obstruction   Present

Desires aggressive management:
Relieve obstruction
Percutaneous nephrostomy
TURBT/de-roof ureters
Medical/nutritional support

Improved

Consider neo-adjuvant chemotherapy

Cystectomy

Response:
Complete

Partial

None

Radiotherapy
+/– chemotherapy

Follow up protocol

Progression

Palliative care

7.1 Surgical ablation of invasive transitional cell carcinoma of the bladder

J P Stein and D G Skinner

Introduction

Transitional cell carcinoma of the bladder is the second most common malignancy of the genitourinary tract, and the second most common cause of death of all genitourinary tumors. In 1998, it is estimated that 54 400 new cases of the disease will be diagnosed, with 12 500 of these patients projected to die from the disease[1]. Approximately 75% to 85% of patients with primary transitional cell carcinoma of the bladder present with low-grade tumors confined to the superficial mucosa. The risk of superficial recurrence in patients with bladder tumors confined to the mucosa is 75%, with the majority of these cancers amenable to initial transurethral resection and selected administration of intravesical immuno- or chemotherapy[2–4]. However, 20% to 40% of all patients with transitional cell carcinoma of the bladder will either initially present with, or develop an invasive carcinoma of the bladder. Furthermore, nearly 50% of these patients treated locally for invasive bladder tumors die of metastatic disease within 2 years of therapy[3]. This clearly underscores a malignant subset of invasive bladder tumors which may be most effectively treated by early aggressive radical therapy.

Invasive bladder cancer includes a spectrum of tumors ranging from infiltration of the superficial lamina propria, to extension into and through the muscularis propria. Traditionally, tumor invasion of the bladder muscularis has been the indication for aggressive radical therapy. In addition, there is sufficient evidence to suggest that high-grade tumors that invade the lamina propria (T1) are at high risk for muscularis propria invasion, and tumor progression[4–11], which may also warrant an early aggressive management scheme. Furthermore, superficial bladder tumors with lymphovascular invasion[7,12], those with prostatic urethral involvement[13], or those which are associated with carcinoma in situ[14,15], in conjunction with a poor response to repeated transurethral resection and intravesical therapy[11], may also adversely affect the natural history of a superficial bladder tumor, and require similar aggressive therapy.

Currently, radical cystectomy provides the optimal result with regard to accurate pathologic staging, prevention of local recurrence and overall survival. In addition, radical cystectomy may influence the decision for adjuvant chemotherapy based upon pathologic criteria. In contemporary series, the best long-term survival rates for invasive bladder cancer have been achieved with radical cystectomy[4,16–18]. This may be a result of the natural history of high-grade invasive bladder tumors. Invasive bladder tumors tend progressively to invade from their superficial origin in the mucosa, to the lamina propria, and sequentially into the muscularis propria, perivesical fat and contiguous pelvic organs, with an increasing incidence of lymph node involvement at each site[18–20]. Furthermore, despite recent advances in radiographic imaging techniques, error in clinical staging of the primary bladder tumor is very common[21,22]. Radical cystectomy, however, provides accurate pathologic staging of the primary bladder tumor and regional lymph nodes, which may serve to influence the decision of adjuvant treatment strategies.

With improvements over the past several decades in medical, surgical and anesthetic techniques, the morbidity and mortality associated with radical cystectomy has dramatically decreased. Prior to 1970, the perioperative complication rate of radical cystectomy was reportedly close to 35%, with a mortality rate of nearly 20%. This has dramatically diminished to a less than 10% complication rate and 2% mortality rate reported in contemporary series[3]. In addition, radical cystectomy with en bloc pelvic lymphadenectomy provides optimal local control of the tumor. Pelvic recurrence rates in patients undergoing radical cystectomy are less than 10% for patients with node-negative bladder tumors, and 10–20% for patients with resected pelvic nodal metastases[17,20,23–25]. Furthermore, transitional cell carcinoma is generally resistant to radiation therapy even at high doses, and chemotherapy alone or as adjuvant therapy, coupled with bladder sparing surgery, has yet to demonstrate equivalent recurrence and long-term survival rates compared with radical cystectomy alone[26].

With a better understanding of the anatomic innervation to the corpora cavernosa, coupled with the evolution of orthotopic lower urinary tract reconstruction, the social, sexual and psychological implications following radical cystectomy have improved. In 1982, Walsh and Donker demonstrated that impotence following radical prostatectomy involved injury to the nerve supply to the corpora cavernosa[27]. This important anatomical discovery has subsequently been applied to the technique of cystoprostatectomy in order to improve potency results following surgery[28]. In addition, improvements in urinary diversion now provide most men and women the opportunity safely to undergo orthotopic lower urinary tract reconstruction following cystectomy[29–32]. This form of urinary diversion most closely resembles the original bladder in both location and function, provides a continent means to store urine, and allows volitional voiding per urethra. A dedicated effort has been made to improve the technique of radical cystectomy, and provide an acceptable form of urinary diversion without compromise of a sound cancer operation, in a hope that patients may undergo earlier aggressive therapy when the potential for cure is highest.

Definition

Radical cystectomy implies the en bloc removal of the pelvic organs anterior to the rectum: the bladder, urachus, prostate, seminal vesicles, and visceral peritoneum in men; the bladder, urachus ovaries, Fallopian tubes, uterus, cervix, vaginal cuff and the anterior pelvic peritoneum in women. The perivesical fat, pelvic and iliac lymph nodes are also removed en bloc with the specimen. Certain technical issues regarding the surgical technique of a radical cystectomy are critical in order to minimize local recurrence and positive surgical margins, and maximize cancer-specific survival. In addition, attention to surgical detail is important to the success of orthotopic diversion in order to maintain the rhabdosphincter mechanism and optimize urinary continence in these patients.

Pre-operative evaluation

The majority of patients with bladder cancer present with hematuria or irritative voiding symptoms. After excluding a urinary tract infection, an excretory urogram (IVP) is usually performed to evaluate the upper urinary tract. Cystoscopy and urine cytology are then performed. Any filling defect identified on the IVP can be further assessed at the time of cystoscopy with a retrograde ureteropyelogram. When a bladder wall filling defect is seen on IVP, associated with ipsilateral hydronephrosis it is highly suggestive of an invasive lesion and can be further evaluated with computerized tomography (CT) prior to transurethral resection.

When a bladder tumor is identified cystoscopically, or abnormal cells reported on urine cytology, a careful bimanual examination and transurethral resection (or deep biopsy of the tumor) is performed under general anesthsia to establish a pathologic diagnosis with determination of depth of tumor invasion. This should include directed bladder biopsies of adjacent and normal appearing bladder mucosa remote from the primary tumor. Complete resection of an obvious invasive bladder tumor, particulaly when radical cystectomy is anticipated, should be avoided. In men, transurethral biopsy of the prostatic urethra and stroma should be performed for complete staging purposes. In women, particular attention should be directed toward the anterior vaginal wall on bimanual pelvic examination. If the primary bladder tumor is a deeply invasive posterior lesion with involvement of the anterior vaginal wall, the bladder should be removed en bloc with the anterior vaginal wall. This may require vaginal reconstruction if sexual function is desired post-

operatively. In addition, women with anterior vaginal wall involvement with tumor are at increased risk of urethral tumor involvement which may preclude orthotopic urinary diversion[33]. Furthermore, all women should undergo cystoscopic evaluation of the bladder neck (vesico-urethral junction) to evaluate for bladder neck tumor involvement which may preclude orthotopic reconstruction in a female patient[33,34].

Complete clinical staging for bladder cancer should evaluate the most common metastatic sites including the lungs, liver and bone. A chest X-ray, liver function tests and serum alkaline phosphatase should be obtained routinely. Patients with an elevated serum alkaline phosphatase or with complaints of bone pain should undergo a bone scan. A CT scan of the chest is obtained when pulmonary metastases are suspected by history, or because of an abnormal chest X-ray. A CT scan of the abdomen/pelvis is not routinely performed as it is neither sensitive nor specific enough to evaluate the degree of bladder wall tumor invasion, or accurately determine pelvic lymph node involvement with tumor[21,35]. However, a CT scan of the abdomen/pelvis may be performed in patients with suspected metastases, elevated liver functions tests, a bladder tumor associated with ipsilateral hydronephrosis, or in patients with a T4 primary bladder tumor, the results of which may impact upon the decision for neoadjuvant therapy.

Pre-operative radiation therapy

The rationale for pre-operative radiation therapy for invasive bladder cancer has been based upon three assumptions: 1) pre-operative radiation may reduce the primary tumor burden, impacting systemic metastases, and improving survival rates; 2) pre-operative radiation may improve local control by decreasing microscopic or macroscopic tumor extension and the positive surgical margin rate; and 3) pre-operative radiation may make radical cystectomy technically easier by reducing the overall primary tumor burden. However, these presumptions are not supported by data from contemporary series. Pre-operative radiation is not an effective adjuvant therapy to cystectomy with regard to survival, compared with surgery alone for the treatment of invasive bladder cancer[16,36–38]. In addition, per-operative radiation therapy has not been found to improve local recurrence rates compared with cystectomy alone[16,36]. Furthermore, although pre-operative radiation of less than 5000 rads has little significant impact on the operation in terms of complications, or the ability to performa successful procedure, this dose is generally ineffective against bladder cancer. However, radiation doses in excess of 6000 rads is associated with increased surgical morbidity and mortality[39]. Currently, the only sound indication for pre-operative radiation therapy in the management of invasive bladder cancer is in the event of an inadvertent tumor spill. Wound implantation with tumor may occur in 10–20% of these patients[40], and can be prevented by a high-dose, short course of pre-operative radiation[41].

En bloc radical cystectomy and pelvic-iliac lymphadenectomy: surgical technique in the male and female patient

Pre-operative preparation

Pre-operative evaluation and counseling by the enterostomal therapy nurse is a critical component to the successful care of all patients undergoing cystectomy and urinary diversion. Currently, approximately 90% of male and 80% of female patients requiring cystectomy for bladder cancer undergo orthotopic diversion at our institution[30,31]. Patients determined to be appropriate candidates for orthotopic reconstruction are instructed how to catheterize per urethra should it be necessary post-operatively. Furthermore, all patients are site marked for a cutaneous stoma, instructed in the care of a cutaneous diversion (continent or incontinent form), and instructed in proper catheterization techniques should medical or technical factors preclude orthotopic reconstruction.

Patient positioning

The patient is placed in the hyperextended supine position with the iliac crest located just below the fulcrum of the operating table. The legs are abducted so that the heels are positioned near the corners of the foot of the table. In the female patient considering orthotopic diversion, the modified frogleg position is employed allowing access to the vagina. Care should be taken to ensure that all pressure points are well padded. Reverse Trendelenberg position levels the abdomen parallel with the floor. A nasogastric tube is placed, and the patient is prepped from nipples to mid-thigh. In the female patient the vagina is fully prepped. After the patient is draped, a 20 F Foley catheter is placed in the bladder, and left open to gravity. A right-handed surgeon stands on the patient's left-hand side of the operating table.

Incision

A vertical midline incision is made extending from the pubic symphysis to the cephalad aspect of the epigastrium. The incision should be made lateral to the umbilicus on the contralateral side of the marked cutaneous stoma site. The anterior rectus fascia is incised, the rectus muscles retracted laterally, and the posterior rectus sheath and

peritoneum entered in the superior aspect of the incision. As the peritoneum and posterior fascia are incised inferiorly to the level of the umbilicus, the urachal remnant (median umbilical ligament) is identified, circumscribed, and removed en bloc with the cystectomy specimen. This maneuver prevents early entry into a high-riding bladder, and ensures complete removal of all bladder remnant tissue. Care is taken to remain medial and avoid injury to the inferior epigastric vessels (lateral umbilical ligaments) which course posterior to the rectus muscles. If the patient has had a previous cystotomy or segmental cystectomy, the cystotomy tract and cutaneous incision should be circumscribed full-thickness and excised en bloc with the bladder specimen. The medial insertion of the rectus muscles attached to the pubic symphysis are then incised, maximizing pelvic exposure throughout the operation.

Abdominal exploration

A careful systematic intra-abdominal exploration is performed to determine the extent of disease, and to evaluate for any hepatic metastases, or gross retroperitoneal adenopathy.

Bowel mobilization

The bowel is mobilized starting with the right colon. A large right-angle Richardson retractor elevates the right abdominal wall. The cecum and ascending colon are then reflected medially to allow incision of the lateral peritoneal reflection along the avascular/white line of Toldt. The mesentery to the small bowel is then mobilized off its retroperitoneal attachments cephalad (toward the ligament of Treitz) until the retroperitoneal portion of the duodenum is exposed. Combined sharp and blunt dissection facilitates mobilization of this mesentery along a characteristic avascular fibroareolar plane.

The left colon and sigmoid mesentery are then mobilized to the region of the lower pole of the left kidney by incising the peritoneum lateral to the colon along the avascular/white line of Toldt. The sigmoid mesentery is then elevated off the sacrum, iliac vessels and distal aorta up to the origin of the inferior mesenteric artery. This maneuver provides a mesenteric window through which the left ureter may pass (without angulation or tension) for the ureteroenteric anastomosis to the urinary reservoir, and also facilitates retraction of the sigmoid mesentery while performing the lymph node dissection. Care should be taken to dissect along the base of the mesentery which prevents injury to the mesenteric blood supply to the colon.

Following mobilization of the bowel, a self-retaining retractor is placed. The right colon and small intestine are carefully packed into the epigastrium with three moist lap pads, followed by a moistened towel rolled to the width of the abdomen. The descending and sigmoid colon are not packed, and left as free as possible, providing the necessary mobility required for the ureteral and pelvic lymph node dissection. Successful packing of the intestinal contents is an art and prevents their spillage into the operative field. Packing begins by sweeping the right colon and small bowel under the surgeon's left hand along the right sidewall gutter. A moist open lap pad is then swept with the right hand along the palm of the left hand, under the viscera along the retroperitoneum and sidewall gutter. In similar fashion, the left sidewall gutter is packed ensuring not to incorporate the descending or sigmoid colon. The central portion of the small bowel is packed with a third lap pad. A moist rolled towel is then positioned horizontally below the lap pads, but cephalad to the bifurcation of the aorta.

Ureteral dissection

The ureters are most easily identified in the retroperitoneum just cephalad to the common iliac vessels. They are dissected into the deep pelvis several centimeters beyond the iliac vessels and divided between two large hemoclips. The ureter is then mobilized cephalad and tucked under the rolled towel to prevent inadvertent injury. Frequently, an arterial branch from the common iliac artery or the aorta needs to be divided to provide adequate ureteral mobilization. In addition, the rich vascular supply emanating from the gonadal vessels should remain intact and undisturbed. Leaving the proximal hemoclip on the divided ureter during the exenteration allows for hydrostatic ureteral dilation, and facilitates the ureteroenteric anastomosis.

Pelvic lymphadenectomy

A meticulous pelvic lymph node dissection is routinely performed en bloc with radical cystectomy. When performing a salvage procedure following definitive radiation treatment (greater then 5000 rads) a pelvic lymphadenectomy is usually not performed because of the significant risk of iliac vessel and obturator nerve injury[39].

All fibroareolar and lymphatic tissue is dissected caudally off the aorta, vena cava, and common iliac vessels over the sacral promontory into the deep pelvis.

Ligation of the lateral vascular pedicle to the bladder

Following dissection of the obturator fossa and dividing the obturator vessels, the lateral vascular pedicle to the bladder is isolated and divided. Developing this plane isolates the lateral vascular pedicle to the bladder which is a critical maneuver in performing a safe cystectomy with proper vascular control. The inferior vesicle vein serves as an excellent landmark as the endopelvic fascia is just distal to this structure. The endopelvic fascia just lateral

to the prostate may then be incised which helps identify the distal limit of the lateral pedicle.

Ligation of the posterior pedicle to the bladder

Following division of the lateral pedicles, the bladder specimen is retracted anteriorly exposing the cul-de-sac (pouch of Douglas). The surgeon elevates the bladder with a small gauze sponge under the left hand, while the assistant retracts on the peritoneum of the rectosigmoid colon in a cephalad direction. This provides excellent exposure to the recess of the cul-de-sac, and places the peritoneal reflection on traction which facilitates proper division. The peritoneum lateral to the rectum is incised, and extended anteriorly across the cul-de-sac to join the incision on the contralateral side. It must be emphasized that the anterior and posterior peritoneal reflections converge in the cul-de-sac to form Denonvilliers' fascia, which extends caudally to the urogenital diaphragm. This is an important anatomic boundary in the male, separating the prostate and seminal vesicles anterior to the rectum posterior. The plane between the prostate and seminal vesicles, and the anterior sheath of Denonvilliers' will not develop easily. However, the plane between the rectum and the posterior sheath of Denon villiers' (Denonvilliers' space) should develop easily with blunt dissection. Therefore, the peritoneal incision in the cul-de-sac must be made on the rectal side rather than the bladder side. This allows proper and safe development of Denonvilliers' space between the anterior rectal wall and the posterior sheath of Denonvilliers' fascia. Employing a posterior sweeping motion of the fingers, the rectum can be swept off the seminal vesicles, prostate and bladder in men, and off the posterior vaginal wall in women. This motion helps to thin and develop the posterior pedicle which appears like a collar emanating from the lateral aspect of the rectum. Care should be taken as this posterior plane is developed more caudally as the anterior rectal fibers often are adherent to the specimen, and can be difficult to dissect bluntly. In the region just proximal to the urogenital diaphragm, sharp dissection may be required to dissect off the anterior rectal fibers in order to prevent rectal injury.

Particular mention should be made concerning several situations which may impede the proper development of this posterior plane. Most commonly, when the incision in the cul-de-sac is made too far anteriorly, it prevents proper entry into Denonvilliers' space. Improper entry can occur in between the two layers of Denonvilliers' fascia, or even anterior to this, making the posterior dissection difficult, increasing the risk of rectal injury. Furthermore, posterior tumor infiltration, or previous high-dose pelvic irradiation can obliterate this plane making the posterior dissection difficult. To prevent injury to the rectum in these situations, dissection of this plane can be facilitated by combining an initial perineal approach (see salvage cystectomy) from below with sharp dissection from above. If a rectotomy occurs, a two or three layer closure is recommended. A diverting proximal colostomy is not routinely required unless gross contamination occurs, or if the patient has received previous pelvic radiation therapy. If orthotopic diversion or vaginal reconstruction is planned, an omental interposition is recommended to prevent fistulization between suture lines.

Once the posterior pedicles have been defined, they are clipped and divided to the endopelvic fascia in the male patient. The endopelvic fascia is then incised (if not done previously) to facilitate the apical dissection. In the female patient, the posterior pedicles including the cardinal ligaments are divided 4 to 5 cm beyond the cervix. With cephalad pressure on a previously placed vaginal sponge stick, the apex of the vagina can be identified, and opened posteriorly just distal to the cervix. The vagina is then circumscribed anteriorly with the cervix attached to the cystectomy specimen. If there is concern about an adequate surgical margin at the posterior or base of the bladder, then the anterior vaginal wall should be removed en bloc with the bladder specimen, subsequently requiring vaginal reconstruction post-operatively if sexual function is desired. We prefer to spare the anterior vaginal wall if orthotopic diversion is planned. This eliminates the need for vaginal reconstruction, and helps maintain the complex musculofascial support system to the proximal urethra which may be an important component to the continence mechanism in these women. The anterior vaginal wall is then sharply dissected off the posterior bladder down to the region of the bladder neck (vesicourethral junction) which is identified by palpating the Foley catheter balloon. At this point, the specimen is attached only at the apex in men and vesicourethral junction in women.

Anterior apical dissection in the male patient

Attention is now directed anteriorly. All fibroareolar connections between the anterior bladder wall, prostate and undersurface of the pubic symphysis are divided. The superficial dorsal vein is identified, ligated and divided. With tension placed posteriorly on the prostate, the puboprostatic ligaments are identified, and divided just beneath the pubis, and lateral to the dorsal venous complex which courses in between these ligaments. Following transection of the puboprostatic ligaments the levator muscle fibers are mobilized laterally off the prostate. The apex of the prostate and membranous urethra now becomes palpable. In the past, under direct vision, we

passed an angled clamp beneath the dorsal vein complex, anterior to the urethra. The venous complex was then ligated with a 2-0 absorbable suture, and divided close to the apex of the prostate. The urethra was then incised just beyond the apex of the prostate and a series of 2-0 polyglycolic acid sutures placed in the urethra circumferentially, carefully incorporating the edge of the rhabdosphincter and levator muscle laterally and recto-urethralis muscle posteriorly or the caudal extent of Denonvilliers' fascia. The Foley catheter is then clamped with a curved Kocher clamp and transected distal to the specimen removed.

We have recently modified this technique of apical dissection in men undergoing orthotopic diversion based on the excellent functional results observed in female patients undergoing the same form of diversion. These women retain their continence mechanism almost immediately following removal of the urethral catheter which we attributed to the limited dissection performed anterior to the urethra along the pelvic floor. We believe the continence mechanism in men may also be maximized if dissection in the region of the anterior urethra is minimized. This has led to a slight modification in the technique of the apical dissection in the male patient undergoing orthotopic reconstruction.

Currently, the dorsal venous complex is sharply transected without dividing the puboprostatic ligaments or without securing vascular control. Cephalad traction on the prostate elongates the proximal and membranous urethra, and allows the urethra to be skeletonized laterally by dividing the so-called 'lateral pillars' which are extensions of the rhabdosphincter. The anterior two-thirds of the urethra is divided, exposing the urethral catheter. The urethral sutures are then placed under direct vision. Six 2-0 polyglycolic acid sutures are placed equally spaced into the urethral mucosa and lumen anteriorly. The rhabdosphincter, the edge of which acts as a hood overlying the dorsal vein complex, is included in these sutures if the venous complex was sharply incised. This maneuver serves to enhance urinary continence, and compresses the dorsal vein complex against the urethra for hemostatic purposes. The urethral catheter is then drawn through the urethrotomy, clamped on the bladder side and divided. Cephalad traction on the bladder side with the clamped catheter occludes the bladder neck, prevents tumor spill from the bladder, and provides exposure to the posterior urethra. Two additional sutures are placed in the posterior urethra incorporating the recto-urethralis muscle or distal Denonvilliers' fascia. The posterior urethra is then divided and the specimen removed. The urethral sutures are appropriately tagged to identify their location and placed under a towel until the urethroenteric anastomosis is performed. Bleeding from the dorsal vein is usually

71

minimal at this point. If additional hemostasis is required, one or two anterior urethral sutures can be tied to stop the bleeding. Frozen section analysis of the distal urethral margin of the cystectomy specimen is then performed to exclude tumor involvement.

Anterior dissection in the female

When considering orthotopic diversion in female patients undergoing cystectomy, several technical issues are critical to the procedure in order to maintain the continence mechanism in these women.

When developing the posterior pedicles in women, the posterior vagina is incised at the apex just distal to the cervix. This incision is carried anteriorly along the lateral and anterior vaginal wall forming a circumferential incision. The anterior lateral vaginal wall is then grasped with a curved Kocher clamp. This provides counter traction, and facilitates dissection between the anterior vaginal wall and the bladder specimen. Development of this posterior plane and vascular pedicle is best performed sharply with the use of hemoclips, and carried just distal to the vesicourethral junction. Palpation of the Foley catheter balloon assists in identifying this region. This dissection effectively maintains a functional vagina. Furthermore, an intact anterior vaginal wall helps support the proximal urethra through a complex musculofascial support system that extends from the anterior vagina. The vagina is then closed at the apex and suspended to Cooper's ligament to prevent vaginal prolapse or the development of an enterocele post-operatively.

Alternatively, in the case of a deeply invasive posterior bladder tumor with concern of an adequate surgical margin, the anterior vaginal wall should be removed en bloc with the cystectomy specimen. After dividing the posterior vaginal apex, the lateral vaginal wall subsequently serves as the posterior pedicle and is divided distally. This leaves the anterior vaginal wall attached to the posterior bladder specimen. Again, the Foley catheter balloon facilitates identification of the vesicourethral junction. The surgical plane between the vesicourethral junction and the anterior vaginal wall is then developed distally at this location. A 1 cm length of proximal urethra is mobilized while the remaining distal urethra is left intact with the anterior vaginal wall. Vaginal reconstruction by a clam shell (horizontal) or side-to-side (vertical) technique is required. Other means of vaginal reconstruction may include: a rectus myocutaneous flap, detubularized cylinder of ileum, a peritoneal flap, or an omental flap. Regardless, a well vascularized omental pedicle graft is placed between the reconstructed vagina and neobladder, and secured to the levator ani muscles to separate the suture lines and prevent fistulization.

It is important that no dissection be performed anterior to the urethra along the pelvic floor in women considering orthotopic diversion. This prevents injury to the rhabdosphincter region and corresponding innervation which is critical in maintaining the continence mechanism.

When the posterior dissection is completed (ensuring to dissect just distal to the vesicourethral junction), a Statinski vascular clamp is placed across the bladder neck. With gentle traction the proximal urethra is divided anteriorly, distal to the bladder neck and clamp. The anterior urethral sutures are placed as described in the male patient. The distal portion of the catheter is then drawn into the wound through the urethrotomy and divided. The Statinski vascular clamp placed across the catheter at the bladder neck prevents any tumor spill from the bladder. Gentle cephalad traction on the clamped catheter allows placement of the posterior urethral sutures. The posterior urethra is then transected and the specimen is removed. Frozen section analysis is performed on the distal urethral margin of the cystectomy specimen to exclude tumor.

Following removal of the cystectomy specimen, the pelvis is irrigated with warm sterile water. The presacral nodal tissue previously swept off the common iliac vessels and sacral promontory into the deep pelvis is collected, and sent separately for pathologic evaluation. All nodal tissue in the presciatic notch anterior to the sciatic nerve is also sent for histologic analysis. Hemostasis is obtained and the pelvis is packed with a lap pad while attention is directed to the urinary diversion. The pelvis is drained by a 1-inch Penrose drain for 3 weeks, and a large suction hemovac drain for 24 hours. A gastrostomy tube 18 French Foley catheter is routinely placed utilizing the Stamm technique. This provides a simple means to drain the stomach, and prevents the need for an uncomfortable nasogastric tube while the post-operative ileus resolves.

Management of the urethra in patients with bladder cancer

Indications for urethrectomy in the female patient

In the past, urethrectomy was routinely performed in all women undergoing cystectomy. However, with a better understanding of the continence mechanism in women[45], coupled with sound pathologic criteria in which safely to select appropriate female candidates for orthotopic diversion[33], urethrectomy is currently performed in those female patients who are not suitable candidates for an orthotopic reservoir, or who would prefer an alternative form of diversion. Currently, over 80% of women undergoing cystectomy at our institution undergo orthotopic diversion[31,32]. The clinical and functional results in these women undergoing orthotopic urinary diversion has been excellent.

Urethrectomy is performed at the time of cystectomy in women with a high risk for urethral tumor involvement, with known urethral tumor involvement, or in patients who prefer a cutaneous form of diversion. From an extensive analysis of female cystectomy specimens removed for transitional cell carcinoma of the bladder, we have demonstrated that tumor involving the bladder neck is an important risk factor for urethral tumor involvement[23]. All cystectomy specimens with carcinoma involving the urethra had concomitant tumor involvement at the bladder neck. However, not all specimens with tumor involving the bladder neck demonstrated urethral tumor involvement. This is an important issue because, although bladder neck involvement with tumor is a risk factor for urethral tumor involvement, approximately 50% of patients with tumor at the bladder neck will have a urethra free of tumor. In this situation, the female patient may be considered an appropriate candidate for orthotopic diversion.

We have recently found intraoperative pathologic evaluation of the proximal urethra to be the most critical determinant for orthotopic diversion in women[32]. We demonstrated that intraoperative frozen section analysis of the distal cystectomy margin (proximal urethra) to be an accurate and reliable method prospectively to evaluate the proximal urethra for tumor involvement. Furthermore, because of the potential risk of injuring the continence mechanism with a pre-operative biopsy of the bladder neck and urethra in women, coupled with a reliable method to evaluate the proximal urethra intraoperatively; we now rely primarily upon intraoperative frozen section analysis of the proximal urethra for proper patient selection in women considering orthotopic lower urinary tract reconstruction.

Indications for urethrectomy in the male patient

With the increasing familiarity and application of orthotopic diversion, the management of the urethra in the male patient undergoing cystectomy for bladder cancer is of particular importance[30]. Urethral recurrences develop in approximately 10% of male patients following cystectomy for bladder cancer[47]. The greatest risk factor for urethral recurrence is tumor involvement of the prostate in the radical cystectomy specimen, with prostatic stromal invasion more ominous then either ductal or mucosal involvement. Patients considering orthotopic diversion have traditionally undergone pre-cystectomy screening of the prostate by means of a deep transurethral biopsy at the 5 and 7 o'clock position adjacent to the verumontanum, which has been suggested to be the most common site of involvement of the prostatic urethra, ducts and stroma with transitional cell carcinoma[48,49].

Recently, we have evaluated the incidence of urethral recurrence in male patients undergoing a cutaneous form of diversion, and compared it with the urethral recurrence rate in men undergoing an orthotopic diversion[50]. Interestingly, the estimated probability of a urethral recurrence at 5 years following cystectomy was significantly increased in male patients with a cutaneous diversion, compared with those undergoing an orthotopic diversion (10% compared with 4% respectively, $P=0.015$). Even those patients with high-risk pathology (prostate involvement), diverted by means of an orthotopic diversion, had a lower probability of urethral recurrence compared with patients with similar pathology undergoing a non-orthotopic form of diversion. The 5 year risk of recurrence in those patients with prostate involvement was 5% in the orthotopic group compared with 24% for the non-orthotopic group ($P=0.05$). Although the exact etiology is unknown, it has been suggested that the orthotopic form of diversion may provide some protective effect, perhaps by the mucus or some other secretory product of the intestine, that prevents the development of cancer in the retained urethra[51].

We believe that the current indication for urethrectomy (contraindication to orthotopic diversion) in male patients include those demonstrating carcinoma in situ or overt carcinoma of the urethral margin detected on intraoperative frozen section analysis. En bloc urethrectomy is performed at the time of cystectomy in those male patients with known tumor involving the urethra. A delayed urethrectomy is performed in patients with prostatic stromal tumor involvement demonstrated on final pathologic examination of the cystectomy specimen who have undergone a cutaneous form of urinary diversion. Those patients with prostatic stromal involvement of tumor demonstrated in the cystectomy specimen, who underwent an orthotopic diversion are closely monitored postoperatively with urethral wash cytology for recurrence purposes.

Salvage cystectomy

Salvage cystectomy by definition is an anterior exenteration (radical cystectomy) following definitive radiation therapy for a pelvic malignancy, or those with crippling irritative bladder symptoms following radiation therapy. Patients undergoing this procedure require a meticulous metastatic evaluation prior to surgery.

To minimize the morbidity associated with a salvage cystectomy specific mention should be made concerning several technical issues of the operative procedure. Some patients develop an intense desmoplastic fibrotic reaction to high-dose radiation therapy. In these patients, an initial perineal approach facilitates dissection of the prostate off the anterior rectal wall under direct vision rather than performing this part of the dissection deep in the pelvis through the abdominal incision. If a rectotomy occurs at any time during the salvage cystectomy it should be closed in multiple layers with silk suture, and protected with a diverting proximal colostomy.

The classic radical cystectomy is generally not feasible in patients receiving greater than 5000 rads pre-operatively because of the fibrotic reaction produced by these higher doses of radiation[39]. Skeletonization of the vessels and removal of the lymph nodes is generally not possible, and may result in a higher incidence of vascular injury as a result of the severe desmoplastic reaction.

Post-operative care

A meticulous, team-oriented approach to the care of these generally elderly patients undergoing radical cystectomy helps reduce perioperative morbidity and mortality. All patients are monitored in a surgical intensive care unit for at least 24 hours or until stable. Third space fluid loss in these patients can be tremendous and very deceiving. A combination of crystalloid and colloid fluid replacement is given on the night of surgery, and converted to crystalloid on post-operative day 1. Prophylaxis against stress ulcer is initiated with an H_2 blocker. Intravenous broad spectrum antibiotics are continued, and converted to orals as the diet progresses. Pulmonary toilet is encouraged with incentive spirometry, deep breathing and coughing.

Prophylaxis against deep vein thrombosis is important in these patients undergoing extensive pelvic operations for malignancies. Anticoagulation is initiated in the recovery room with 10 mg of sodium warfarin via the nasogastric or gastrostomy tube. The daily dose is adjusted to maintain a prothrombin time in the range of 18 to 22 s. If the prothrombin time exceeds 22 s, 2.5 mg of vitamin K is administered intramuscularly to prevent bleeding. Pain control is maintained with either an epidural catheter, or a patient-controlled analgesic system, or a combination of the two. Patient comfort enhances deep breathing, and early ambulation. If digoxin was given pre-operatively, it is continued until discharge. The gastrostomy tube is removed on post-operative day 7, or later if bowel function is delayed. The catheter and drain management is specific to the form of urinary diversion.

Complications specific to radical cystectomy

Advances in medical, surgical and anesthetic techniques have reduced the morbidity and mortality associated with radical cystectomy. Early complications attributed solely to the radical cystectomy are difficult, if not impossible to separate from the complications related to the urinary diversion. A recently reported series of 295 consecutive male patients undergoing radical cystectomy and orthotopic diversion attempted to distinguish these early complications[30]. Early complications in this series were categorized to those related to the radical cystectomy (pouch unrelated) and those related to the urinary diversion (pouch related). A total of 52 early complications occurred in 46 patients (15.7%); 21 pouch unrelated and 31 pouch related. The most common early complications associated with the radical cystectomy in this series included: a prolonged ileus in seven patients (2.4%), deep venous thrombosis in four patients (1.4%), upper gastrointestinal bleeding in three patients (1.0%), and intraabdominal bleeding in three patients (1.0%). Late complications reported in this study were primarily related to the urinary diversion. The most common late complication associated with the cystectomy was an incisional hernia in three patients (1.0%). In addition, we have found that age alone does not independently increase the risk of morbidity or mortality from radical cystectomy, and should not be a contraindication for definitive surgical therapy for invasive bladder carcinoma[54,55].

Conclusions

The technique of en bloc radical cystectomy with bilateral pelvic lymphadenectomy has provided superior survival rates with lower pelvic recurrence rates compared with other forms of therapy for invasive bladder cancer[23]. Survival following radical cystectomy is dependent on the pathologic stage of the primary bladder tumor, and the status of the pelvic lymph nodes[20,24]. Survival at 5 years for stages P0, Pis, P1, P2, P3 and P4 node negative bladder cancers is approximately 95%, 85%, 80%, 76%, 44% and 35% respectively[12,16]. Survival of patients with node-positive disease is dependent on the stage of the primary tumor and the extent of nodal involvement[56]. Survival in node-positive patients is 50% at 5 years if the primary bladder tumor is confined to the bladder (<P3b), compared with an 18% 5 year survival if the tumor demonstrates extravesical extension (≥P3b) The 5 year survival in node positive patients with less than six nodes involved is 35% compared with a 17% 5 year survival if greater than six nodes are involved with tumor. These data suggest that en bloc radical cystectomy, along with a meticulous node dissection, can provide accurate staging information with good survival even in a select group of patients with metastatic disease to the pelvic nodes.

Since radical cystectomy has become the primary form of therapy for invasive bladder cancer, emphasis has been directed to the quality of life issues, and reconstruction of the genitourinary tract following the ablative surgery. Potency preserving radical cystectomy has been advocated by some for selected patients[52, 57] but the efficacy appears to be significantly less than that reported for nerve-sparing radical prostatectomy. In addition, it remains to be determined what the pelvic recurrence rates will be following nerve-sparing surgery for high-stage bladder tumors. Since pre-operative staging correlates poorly with the final pathologic extent of disease, one should be cautious about the broad application of this technique. Furthermore, with the established options of vacuum erection devices, improved penile prostheses, along with use of intracorporal pharmacotherapy, and with oral medications on the horizon for the treatment of impotence, we currently feel that the nerve-sparing radical cystectomy should be reserved for very highly selected patients and not considered an option for those men with high-grade muscle invasive transitional cell carcinoma.

Advances in lower urinary tract reconstruction have increased both patient and physician acceptance of radical cystectomy. One recent report indicated that the option for orthotopic diversion led to an earlier acceptance of cystectomy compared with those offered a cutaneous form of diversion, and that cystectomy improved survival[58]. Modern urologic reconstructive techniques now allow for creation of a urinary reservoir (orthotopic neobladder) with similar characteristics of the native bladder – large capacity, low pressure, non-refluxing, continent reservoir – that allows volitional voiding per urethram[59]. This eliminates the need for a cutaneous stoma, and the need for catheterization, relying on the striated external sphincter for continence. We believe these advances which allow patients to return to a near normal lifestyle, with a positive self-image, will encourage earlier treatment for invasive bladder tumors when the potential for cure is highest.

References

1. Lanois SH, Murray T, Bolden S et al. Cancer statistics, 1998. Cancer J Clin 1988;48:6–29.

2. Crawford ED, Davis MA. Nontransitional cell carcinomas of the bladder. In: Genitourinary cancer management. de Kernian JB, Paulson DF (eds), Lea & Febiger, Philadelphia, chap. 4, 1987, pp. 95–105.

3. Skinner DG, Lieskovsky G. Management of invasive and high-grade bladder cancer. In: Skinner DG and Lieskovsky G (eds) Diagnosis and management of genitorurinary cancer. W. B. Saunders Co. Philadelphia, vol. 1, chap. 16, 1988. pp. 295–312.

4. Droller MJ. Individualizing the approach to invasive bladder cancer. Contemp Urol 1990; July/August: 54–61.

5. Trasher JB, Crawford ED. Minimally invasive transitional cell carcinoma (T1 and T2). In: Resnick MI and Kursh E (eds) Current therapy in genitourinary surgery (2nd edn). BC, Decker St Louis 1992, pp. 74–78.

6. Freeman JA, Esrig D, Stein JP, Simoneau AR, Skinner EC, Chen, S-C, Groshen S et al. Radical cystectomy for high risk patients with superficial bladder cancer in the era of orthotopic urinary reconstruction. Cancer 1995;76:833–839.

7. Anderstrom C, Johansson S, Nilsson S. The significance of lamina propria invasion on the prognosis of patients with bladder tumors. J Urol 1980;124:23–26.

8. Heney NM, Ahmed S, Flanagan MJ, Frable W, Corder MP, Hafermann MD, Hawkins IR. Superficial bladder cancer: progression and recurrence. J Urol 1983;130:1083–1086.

9. Dalesio O, Schulman CC, Sylvester R, DePauw M, Robinson M, Denis L, Smith P, Viggiano G. Prognostic factors in superficial bladder tumors. A study of the European Organization for Research on Treatment of Cancer: Genitourinary Tract Cancer Cooperative Group. J Urol 1983;129:730–733.

10. Herr HW, Jakse G, Sheinfeld J. The T1 bladder tumor. Sem Urol 1990;8:254–261.

11. Fitzpatrick JM. The natural history of superficial bladder cancer. Sem Urol 1993;11:127–136.

12. Malkowicz SB, Nichols P, Lieskovsky G, Boyd SD, Huffman J, Skinner DG. The role of radical cystectomy in the management of high grade superficial bladder cancer (PA, P1, PIS and P2). J Urol 1990;144:641–645.

13. Schellhammer PF, Bean MA, Whitmore WF, Jr. Prostatic involvement by transitional cell carcinoma: pathogenesis, patterns, and prognosis. J Urol 1977;118:399–403.

14. Prout GR, Jr, Griffin PP, Daly JJ, Henery NM. Carcinoma in situ of the urinary bladder with and without associated vesical neoplasms. Cancer 1983;52:524–532.

15. Utz DC, Farrow DM. Management of carcinoma in situ of the bladder: a case for surgical management. Urol Clin N Am 1980;7:533–540.

16. Skinner DG, Lieskovsky G. Contemporary cystectomy with pelvic node dissection compared to preoperative radiation therapy plus cystectomy in management of invasive bladder cancer. J Urol 1984;131:1069–1072.

17. Montie JE, Strafton RA, Stewart BH. Radical cystectomy without radiation therapy for carcinoma of the bladder. J Urol 1984;131:477–482.

18. Frazier HA, Robertson JE, Dodge RK, Paulson DF. The value of pathologic factors in predicting cancer-specific survival among patients treated with radical cystectomy for transitional cell carcinoma of the bladder and prostate. Cancer 1993;71:3993–4001.

19. Skinner DG, Tift JP, Kaufman JJ. High dose, short course preoperative radiation therapy and immediate single stage radical cystectomy with pelvic node dissection in the management of bladder cancer. J Urol 1982;127:671–674.

20. Lerner SP, Skinner DG, Lieskovsky G, Boyd SD, Groshen SL, Ziogas A, Skinner EC et al. The rationale for en bloc pelvic lymph node dissection for bladder cancer patients with nodal metastases: long-term results. J Urol 1993;149:758–765.

21. Soloway MS, Lopez AE, Patel J, Lu Y. Result of radical cystectomy for transitional cell carcinoma of the bladder and the effect of chemotherapy. Cancer 1994;73:1926–1931.

22. Voges GE, Tauschke E, Stockle M, Alken P, Hohenfellner R. Computerized tomography: an unreliable method for accurate staging of bladder tumors in patients who are candidates for radical cystectomy. J Urol 1989;142:972–974.

23. Wishnow KI, Dmochowski R. Pelvic recurrence after radical cystectomy without preoperative radiation. J Urol 1988;140:42–43.

24. Roehrborn CG, Sagalowsky AI, Peters PC. Long-term patient survival after cystectomy for regional metastatic transitional cell carcinoma of the bladder. J Urol 1991;146:36–39.

25. Mathur VK, Krahn HP, Ramsey EW. Total cystectomy for bladder cancinoma. J Urol 1981;125:784–786.

26. Thrasher JB, Crawford ED. Current management of invasive and metastatic transitional cell carcinoma of the bladder. J Urol 1993;149:957–972.

27. Walsh PC, Donker PJ. Impotence following radical prostatectomy: insight into etiology and prevention. J Urol 1982;128:492–497.

28. Schlegel PN, Walsh PC. Neuroanatomical approach to radical cystoprostatectomy with preservation of sexual function. J Urol 1987;138:1402–1406.

29. Elmajian DA, Stein JP, Skinner DG. Orthotopic urinary diversion: the Kock ileal neobladder. World J Urol 1996;14:40–46.

30. Elmajian DA, Stein JP, Esrig D, Freeman JA, Skinner EC, Boyd SD, Lieskovsky G, Skinner DG. The Kock ileal neobladder: update experience in 295 male patients. J Urol ;156(3):920–5.

31. Stein JP, Stenzl A, Esrig D, Freeman JA, Boyd SD, Lieskovsky G, Cote RJ et al. Lower urinary tract reconstruction following cystectomy in women using the

Kock ileal reservoir with bilateral ureteroileal urethrostomy: initial clinical experience. *J Urol* 1994;**152**:1404–1408.

32. Stein JP, Grossfeld G, Freeman JA, Esrig D, Elmajian DA, Boyd SD, Lieskovsky G, Skinner DG. Orthotopic lower urinary tract reconstruction in women using the Kock ileal neobladder: updated experience in 27 patients. *J Urol* 1996;**155**(2):399A (abstract 353).

33. Stein JP, Cote RJ, Freeman JA, Esrig D, Elmajian DA, Groshen S, Skinner EC *et al*. Indications for lower urinary tract reconstruction in women after cystectomy for bladder cancer: a pathological review of female cystectomy specimens. *J Urol* 1995;**154**:1329–1333.

34. Stenzl A, Draxl H, Posch B, Colleselli K, Falk M, Bartsch G. The risk of urethral tumors in female bladder cancer: can the urethra be used for orthotopic reconstruction of the lower urinary tract? *J Urol* 1995;**153**:950–955.

35. Pagano F, Bassi P, Galetti TP, Meneghini A, Milani C, Artibani W, Garbeglio A. Results of contemporary radical cystectomy for invasive bladder cancer: a clinicopathological study with an emphasis on the inadequacy of the tumor, nodes and metastases classification. *J Urol* 1991;**145**:45–50.

36. Crawford ED, Das S, Smith JA, Jr. Preoperative radiation therapy in the treatment of bladder cancer. *Urol Clin N Am* 1987;**14**:781–787.

37. Anderstrom C, Johansson S, Nilsson S, Unsgaard B, Wahlqvist LA. A prospective randomized study of preoperative irradiation with cystectomy or cystectomy alone for invasive bladder carcinoma. *Eur Urol* 1983;**9**:142–147.

38. Smith JA Jr, Crawford ED, Blumenstein BL, Paradelo J, Herschman BR. Pre-operative irradiation plus radical cystectomy versus surgery alone for invasive bladder cancer: final results of a randomized prospective Southwest Oncology Group study. *J Urol* 1993;**149**(2): 316A (abstract 415).

39. Crawford ED, Skinner DG. Salvage cystectomy after radiation failure. *J Urol* 1980;**123**:32–34.

40. Magri J. Partial cystectomy: review of 104 cases. *Br J Urol* 1962;**34**:74–87.

41. van der Werf-Messing B. Carcinoma of the bladder treated by suprapubic radium implants: the value of additional external irradiation. *Eur J Urol* 1969;**5**:277–281.

42. Nichols RL, Broido P, Condon RE, Gorbach SL, Nyhus LM. Effect of preoperative neomycin-erythromycin intestinal preparation on the incidence of infectious complications following colon surgery. *Ann Surg* 1973;**178**:453–462.

43. Pinaud MLJ, Blanloeil YAG, Souron RJ. Preoperative prophylactic digitalization of patients with coronary artery disease – a randomized echocardiographic and hemodynamic study. *Anesth Analg* 1983;**62**:685–689.

44. Burman SO. The prophylactic use of digitalis before thoracotomy. *Ann Thorac Surg* 1972;**14**:359–368.

45. Colleselli K, Strasser H, Moriggl B, Stenzl A, Poisel S, Bartsch G. Hemi-Kock to the female urethra: anatomical approach to the continence mechanism of the female urethra. *J Urol* 1994;**151**(2):500A, (abstract 1089).

46. Grossfeld GD, Stein JP, Bennett CJ, Ginsberg DA, Boyd SD, Lieskovsky G, Skinner DG. Lower urinary tract reconstruction in the female using the Kock ileal reservoir with bilateral ureteroileal urethrostomy: update of continence results and flurourodynamic findings. *Urology* [In Press].

47. Freeman JA, Esrig D, Stein JP, Skinner DG. Management of the patient with bladder cancer. Urethral recurrence. *Urol Clin N Am* 1994;**21**(4):645–651.

48. Sakamoto N, Tsuneyoshi M, Naito S, Kumazawa J. An adequate sampling of the prostate to identify prostatic involvement by urothelial carcinoma in bladder cancer patients. *J Urol* 1993;**149**:318–321.

49. Wood DP, Jr, Montie JE, Pontes JE, Levin HS. Identification of transitional cell carcinoma of the prostate in bladder cancer patients: a prospective study. *J Urol* 1989;**142**:83–85.

50. Freeman JA, Tarter TA, Esrig D, Stein JP, Elmajian DA, Chen S-C, Groshen S *et al*. Urethral recurrence in patients with orthotopic ileal neobladders. *J Urol* 1996;**156**:1615–9.

51. Crocitto LE, Simpson J, Wilson TG. Bladder augmentation in the prevention of cyclophosphamide induced hemorrhagic cystitis in the rat model. *J Urol* 1994;**151**(2):379A (abstract 608).

52. Brendler CB, Schlegel PN, Walsh PC. Urethrectomy with preservation of potency. *J Urol* 1990;**144**:270–273.

53. Van-Poppel H, Strobbe E, Baert L. Prepubic urethrectomy. *J Urol* 1989;**142**:1536–1537.

54. Skinner EC, Lieskovsky G, Skinner DG. Radical cystectomy in the elderly patient. *J Urol* 1984;**131**:1065–1068.

55. Leibovitch I, Avigad I, Ben-Chaim J, Nativ O, Goldwasser B. Is it justified to avoid radical cystoprostatectomy in elderly patients with invasive transitional cell carcinoma of the bladder? *Cancer* 1993;**71**:3098–3101.

56. Lerner SP, Skinner E, Skinner DG. Radical cystectomy in regionally advanced bladder cancer. *Urol Clin N Am* 1992;**19**(4):713–723.

57. Brendler DC, Steinberg GD, Marshall FF, Mostwin JL, Walsh PC. Local recurrence and survival following nerve-sparing radical cystoprostatectomy. *J Urol* 1990;**144**:1137–1141.

58. Hautmann RE, Paiss T. Does the option of the ileal neobladder stimulate patient and physician decision towards earlier cystectomy? *J Urol* 1996;**155**(2):437A (abstract 508).

59. Hautmann RE, Paiss T, Petriconi R. The ileal neobladder in women: 9 years of experience with 18 patients. *J Urol* 1996;**155**:76–81.

7.2   Urinary diversion and bladder replacement

D E Neal

Introduction and historical development

For over a century, urologic surgeons have grappled with the problem of how to replace the function of the lower urinary tract when it has to be removed or when it has been rendered useless or dangerous by disease. The solutions have ranged from simple anastomosis of the ureters to the rectosigmoid, the creation of various intestinal conduits to the skin and, more recently, to the reconstruction of the bladder with various intestinal segments or the formation of continent diversions.

Uretero-intestinal anastomosis

Critical to the success of any urinary diversion is the creation of a safe uretero-intestinal anastomosis that is prone neither to leakage nor stricture. Early experimental studies demonstrated that creation of a freely refluxing anastomosis could lead to dilatation in the presence of phasic intestinal contractions – a conclusion supported by more recent physiological studies[1]. Coffey[2,3] developed an antireflux technique, but it was soon realized that stricture formation could complicate this type of anastomosis and Nesbitt[4] suggested the use of interrupted sutures to reduce ischemia if non-refluxing anastomoses were being performed. The use of a direct mucosa to mucosa technique was popularized by Leadbetter[5], the antireflux procedure being performed externally by laying the ureter into an incision of the colonic taeniae or internally by opening the lumen of the bowel and the creation of a sub-mucosal tunnel[6].

The submucosal tunnel technique is not possible in the small intestine since the mucosal layer is too thin. Kock and colleagues[7] described the formation of an afferent intussuscepted small bowel nipple valve to prevent reflux. This procedure proved to be highly effective in an extensive series reported by Skinner and colleagues[8,9], but most surgeons find the technique complicated and an additional 10 cm length of ileum is required. An easier approach was described[10] in which the ileal mucosa is incised for 3 cm. At one end of this incision the ureter is brought into the lumen and placed into the sulcus between the mucosal edges where it is fixed by interrupted absorbable sutures. This technique was also used in a series of 100 consecutive patients undergoing bladder replacement[11]; the reflux rate was less than 5% whilst obstruction was reported in 8%. It has been reported[12] that the deleterious effect of reflux can be eliminated by implantation of the ureters into an afferent, tubular, isoperistaltic 20 cm length of ileum.

The rate of stricture formation following these techniques is clearly dependent on surgical skill and the use of well vascularized ureter. In most series with long-term follow up, the stricture rate is in the region of 5% to 10% even in straightforward ileal conduit diversion[13,14]. If an antireflux procedure is performed, then reflux will be prevented in about 85% of patients.

Pre-operative assessment and counselling

Quite apart from counselling patients about cystectomy with its associated risks and benefits compared with other treatments, patients require accurate information about the options that are available for urinary diversion. Currently, this requires surgeons performing radical cystectomy to be conversant with the various types of urinary diversion including orthotopic bladder replacement, continent diversion and conduit diversion. It is unacceptable for patients simply to be offered conduit diversion. Booklets, videos and the involvement of a committed stoma therapist play important roles in enabling patients to make an informed choice. Patients also need to be told about the long-term implications of urinary diversion.

Careful pre-operative staging of the tumor is vital. This should include biopsies of the bladder, the bladder neck and prostatic urethra. The reason is to classify the risk of long-term urethral recurrence into high, medium and low (see below): patients in the first group should undergo urethrectomy and an alternative form of urinary diversion. Patients should also be advised that on occasion it still may be necessary to form an ileal diversion on the basis of per-operative findings. The pros and cons of each method should be discussed. A stoma therapist should counsel the patient regarding the management of an ileal conduit, even if a continent technique is planned. The patient may wish to meet others who have had similar procedures carried out. The age, motivation and the potential compliance of the patient with intermittent catheterization must be taken into consideration for selection of the most appropriate technique.

Understandably, many patients prefer the construction of a orthotopic neo-bladder allowing natural micturition. However, the chance of cancer cure should not be compromised. The option of orthotopic reconstruction after cystectomy is now well accepted, though one concern is the risk of late urethral recurrences. Many series of cystectomies have shown that the risk of urethral recurrence increases with length of follow up, but is about 5% to 10% at 5 years[15]. Various factors are associated with an increased risk of urethral recurrence. In situ change in the urethra was found in 19% of men with multifocal papillary disease who died of bladder cancer[16]; being found only rarely in patients with solid solitary tumors. It might seem that multifocal tumors and carcinoma in situ of the bladder (cis) would represent a significant risk, but one recent study showed that prostatic stromal involvement poses the major risk of subsequent urethral recurrence[17]. However, in this paper, most men with a previous history of cis or multifocal disease underwent a prophylactic urethrectomy. In another series of men who had rather heavily been pre-treated with intravesical chemotherapy[18], urethral recurrence was also associated with prostatic tumor; 11 of 30 such men (37%) developed a urethral recurrence and 20 of these 30 men also had multifocal disease or cis. Only one of 29 patients (3%) with tumor at the bladder neck or with multifocal tumor or cis, but without prostatic involvement developed a urethral recurrence and only one of 27 patients with a solitary tumor away from the bladder neck developed a urethral tumor. This is helpful information in deciding whether to preserve the urethra or to carry out a urethrectomy. It is of interest that Skinner considers that the only contra-indication to bladder reconstruction after cystectomy is the presence of urethral tumor, or tumor or carcinoma in situ involving the prostate; carcinoma in situ of the bladder apparently not being regarded as a contra-indication[9]. Reddy et al.[19] excluded patients with a history of significant cis, multifocal tumor growth or involvement of the prostatic urethra from bladder replacement. The greatest risk of urethral recurrence is encountered in cases of prostatic stromal or ductal involvement and such patients should undergo simultaneous urethrectomy.

Gastrointestinal diseases may determine the choice of intestinal segment. Use of the ileocecal segment or ileum is not recommended in those with malabsorption or diarrhea. In patients who have undergone pre-operative high-dose irradiation of the pelvis, transverse colon may be suitable for bladder replacement or continent diversion.

Metabolic and electrolyte disturbance after diversion

Electrolyte disturbances

Hyperchloremic acidosis

The incidence of electrolyte and acid–base problems is greater in patients with impaired renal function before operation (GFR < 30 ml/min; creatinine > 150μ mol/L). The use of ureterosigmoidostomy was historically associated with a high occurrence of clinically apparent electrolyte and acid–base problems, although the precise prevalence of more subtle abnormalities depends on how carefully they are searched for. Some impairment of ability to rid the body of hydrogen ions can usually be identified if an acid load is given and blood gas measurement is carried out. For instance, using these techniques most patients with ileal conduits, continent diversions and bladder reconstruction have been found to have a mild compensated acidosis[20–22], often with decreased bicarbonate and increased chloride levels. This magnitude of the metabolic acidosis is a consequence of the absorptive function of the bowel, the segment used, its surface area and the duration of contact between urine and the mucosa.

On the cell membrane of luminal gastrointestinal cells is a sodium/hydrogen pump and a bicarbonate/chloride exchanger. Often the transfer of electrolytes is linked by the need to maintain electrochemical equilibrium, but movements of electrolytes and water are also dependent on osmotic gradients. In the normal intact gut, one hydrogen ion is secreted into the lumen for the absorption of one sodium ion and one bicarbonate ion secreted into the lumen in exchange for the absorption of one chloride ion. In the presence of urine in the lumen of gut (with high levels of ammonium ions), certain of these processes are reversed resulting in loss of sodium and effectual absorption of hydrogen ions (due to the metabolism of ammonium) along with absorption of chloride and loss of bicarbonate: these processes are the explanation for the metabolic acidosis found in ileal conduits and ureterosigmoidostomies. Key to an understanding of the etiology of hyperchloremic acidosis has been the finding that transfer of ammonium ions is the basis for the acidosis (ammonium after combination with carbon dioxide to form urea is metabolized by the liver via the ornithine cycle leaving a residual acid load). Ammonia, but not the ammonium ion, can be absorbed through epithelium by passive diffusion, although active transport of ammonium ions can occur. Urinary ammonium ions in the gut compete with sodium for the sodium/hydrogen pump which allows the inward transfer of ammonium ions, leaving sodium in the lumen. Chloride ions are absorbed along with the ammonium ion leading in effect to the absorption of an ammonium chloride load into the blood.[23] Severe fluid depletion is also found in patients with an uncompensated hyperchloremic acidosis.

Potassium depletion also occurs in some such patients in part because of sub-clinical renal tubular damage leading to impairment of potassium conservation and in part because of its loss into the intestinal segment. Potassium depletion may be so severe as to cause a flaccid paralysis, particularly if an acidosis is corrected suddenly by bicarbonate infusion. Hyperchloremic acidosis is the feature of colonic and ileal interpositions.

The mainstay of treatment of hyperchloremic acidosis is repletion of fluid and electrolytes (0.9% NaCl with potassium supplements), oral bicarbonate can be given when the nausea resolves. Only rarely is correction of acidosis required and this should be done slowly. The precipitating factor often is urinary infection and this will require appropriate antibiotic treatment.

Jejunal conduits

Jejunal conduits are associated with different metabolic problems characterized by marked losses of sodium and water. Very rapid movements of water and electrolytes occur across the jejunal conduits because of the osmotic gradient found between urine and blood and the facility with which water and sodium can cross the jejunal mucosa. This can lead to increased urine outputs from the conduits, even if ureteric urine outputs are normal. The jejunal mucosa also actively secretes sodium in exchange for hydrogen and potassium ions, chloride moves with the sodium and the patient becomes dehydrated and hyperkalemic. Hypovolemia can occur which results in increased serum renin which in turn stimulates aldosterone secretion. The aldosterone conserves urinary sodium at the expense of potassium. High levels of potassium impair the ability of the distal tubule to secrete hydrogen ions which worsens the acidosis. The low levels of sodium in the urine in the conduit further stimulate loss of sodium across the jejunal osmotic gradient in exchange for hydrogen, worsening the acidosis and loss of water and sodium. The patient presents with nausea, vomiting, hypovolemia and eventual prostration[24].

Gastric reservoirs

The use of gastric segments may be associated with aciduria and a metabolic alkalosis due to losses of acid in the urine. Severe dysuria and urethral or peri-stomal erosion can occur because of the high acid content[25,26].

Magnesium and calcium

Rarely, severe losses of magnesium and calcium occur as the result of leaching from bone. These cations are released when the systemic acid load is buffered by carbonate, a large amount of which is found in bone. Renal losses of calcium are increased because the acidosis inhibits renal reabsorption and because sulfate which is absorbed from the intestinal segment also inhibits renal tubule absorption of calcium.

Hyperammonemia

The ammonium load found in patients with urinary diversions is cleared by hepatic metabolism through the hepatic ornithine cycle so that no change in serum ammonia is found. Patients with pre-existing hepatic disease can develop hyperammonemia and as a consequence develop encephalopathy[27].

Metabolic and bowel problems

Gastrointestinal function and nutritional status may be severely affected after urinary diversion, depending on the bowel segment used. Bile salts as well as vitamin B_{12} are absorbed in the ileum. The critical length for the development of B_{12} deficiency in the short term seems to be around 50 cm[28], but longer-term studies have shown that even taking a short segment of ileum out of gastrointestinal continuity can result in impaired B_{12} absorption[29]. Removal of the ileal segment from intestinal continuity may also lead to the onward passage of unabsorbed bile salts into the colon resulting in diarrhea because they are irritant to the colonic mucosa. On removal of more than 100 cm of ileum, the loss of bile salts may exceed the capacity of the liver for re-synthesis, resulting in fat malabsorption, steatorrhea, hypovitaminosis A and D and increased colonic re-absorption of oxalate which eventually results in urolithiasis. Gallstones can also occur because of altered bile composition. Normally, the function of the ileo-cecal valve is integrated with that of the terminal ileum to form an ileal 'brake' mechanism which controls the transit of distal small bowel content. Ileal resection, particularly if accompanied by loss of the ileocecal valve, can result in uncontrolled flow pof bowel content including irritative bile acids into the colon, resulting in diarrhea[30]. Reflux of colonic content may also cause bacterial colonization of the small bowel after resection of the ileo-cecal valve with resultant malabsorption. Severe diarrhea is more common in neuropathic patients with pre-existing bowel dysfunction and in patients with idiopathic detrusor instability, many of whom have pre-existing disturbances in colonic motility[31]. Severe diarrhea is found in 10% and moderate diarrhea is found in 27% of patients following urinary diversion, being most severe in the neuropathic patients or those with detrusor instability, in those who have lost the ileo-cecal valve and in those who have had more than 40 cm of bowel taken out of continuity[32].

Bone is an organic vascularized complex of mineralized collagen in which a variety of cells are embedded.

Even in patients with normal renal function, the constant mild compensated acidosis following urinary diversion can result in impaired bone growth, decreased height and rickets in children and osteomalacia in adults[21,33,34]. Bone contains 99% of the body's calcium, 85% of its phosphorus, 80% of its carbon dioxide in the form of bicarbonate and carbonate and no less than 50% of its sodium and magnesium. A proportion of bone mineral is easily accessible for hydrogen ion exchange and buffering. As a result bone becomes de-mineralized, but because bone mineral is constantly turning over, impairment of active mineralization is equally important. Normally, conversion of calcium phosphate to hydroxyapatite $(Ca_{10}(PO)_4(OH)_2)$ occurs at the mineralization front in bone and acidosis appears to inhibit this process. As a consequence, some patients with urinary diversions in the long term show decreased bone mass, decreased apposition of cortical bone and an increased proportion of trabecular bone. The role of vitamin D and its metabolites is unclear, but acidosis impairs the production of 1,25-dihydroxy-cholecalciferol. It should be pointed out that other studies have been unable to demonstrate any major abnormalities of bone metabolism in adults undergoing ileal conduit diversion or Kock continent diversion[35].

There is an increased production of upper tract stone in patients with urinary diversion and in the formation of stones in the reservoir, but this is mainly a consequence of stasis and infection with urease forming organisms.

Risk of tumor formation

The danger of tumor formation after uretero-sigmoidostomy has been realized for over 50 years, adenocarcinomas being found in around 10% to 15%[36] in the long term which is a 500-fold increased risk compared with controls. Most tumors are adenocarcinomas situated at the site of ureteric entry. Recent surveillance programs have demonstrated that the incidence of adenomas – which are likely to predate malignant transformation – is around 30% in the long term[37]. Tumors occurring in ileal conduits are excessively rare; four cases having been reported, only two of which were malignant. Similarly only three malignant tumors have been found in patients with colonic conduits. We do not yet know the true incidence of tumors in bladder reconstructions or continent diversions, but so far 14 have been reported which is a concern. These tumors were mainly found in patients who had poor bladder emptying and a long history of chronic infection. However, it may well be that patients undergoing enterocystoplasty occupy an intermediate position of risk between uretero-sigmoidostomy and ileal conduit diversion and it would seem wise to counsel younger patients that there may be some increased risk of tumor formation in the longer term.

Conclusions

Despite this formidable array of potential metabolic problems, most older adults undergoing cystectomy for cancer with satisfactory pre-operative renal function develop few problems other than mild compensated hyperchloremic acidosis. However, a vigilant watch should be kept in the long term. How serious these complications will be in practice is as yet unclear. A greater concern is whether these complications will be a major problem in younger adults and children undergoing these procedures for neuropathic and congenital disorder in whom there is greater time for the development of these complications. It may be that children should receive prophylactic bicarbonate treatment, although we do not know whether this will prevent later osteomalacia.

Conduit diversion

Despite the increasing use of orthotopic urinary diversion and continent diversion after cystectomy, there are patients in whom a straightforward ileal or colonic conduit diversion is preferable (Table 7.2.1).

The ileal conduit was developed by Eugene Bricker in 1950[38] and has been little altered since then. The technique is well described in standard texts. Careful positioning of the intended site of the stoma is important. The terminal ileum is the usual segment chosen; some surgeons avoid the terminal 60 cm of ileum in order to minimize post-operative bile acid malabsorption, but whether this prevents the problem is unclear. If pre-operative radiotherapy has affected the ileum it is probably better to use transverse colon rather than very proximal small bowel because of the electrolyte problems that may be encountered if jejunum is utilized[39].

Care taken with the formation of the stoma is vital to minimize later problems. Preservation of good vascularity will ensure that early ischemia and venous congestion are avoided. The long-term problems of external urinary diversion include (Table 7.2.2[13,40]):

Table 7.2.1   Considerations weighing in favor of a conduit diversion

- unwillingness to consider intermittent self-catheterization and patient choice
- poor renal function (GFR < 30 ml/min)
- obesity, age and co-morbidity
- patients who have received high-dose pelvic radiotherapy
- extensive gastrointestinal disease
- intra-operative problems including untoward intra-operative events (severe bleeding and cardiovascular problems) or those in whom it is not possible for an intestinal reservoir to reach the urethra (uncommon)
- patient requiring urethrectomy who do not want to incur the increased risk of further surgery for post-operative complications associated with a continent reservoir.

Table 7.2.2   Long-term complications following ileal conduit diversion

- stomal stenosis (30% in children; 5–10% in adults)
- stomal retraction (5%)
- prolapse (2%)
- leakage around the appliance (usually related to stomal retraction or poor siting of the stoma) leading to excoriation
- narrowing and fibrosis of the aperture in the abdominal wall (10%)
- peri-stomal herniation (15% – higher in obese patients)
- long term changes in the conduit including severe fibrosis and the formation of mucosal webs (1%)
- recurrent infection (20%)
- upper tract dilatation caused by stenosis or reflux in the presence of distal conduit obstruction (20%)
- upper tract stone formation (10%)
- deterioration in renal function (20%)
- metabolic problems related to malabsorption of B_{12} and bile acids
- electrolyte disturbance including hyperchloremic acidosis

Current evidence suggests that the use of colonic conduits is not associated with a lower risk of long-term complications[41].

Follow up of patients with diversions

Regular follow up is mandatory to check stomal function, electrolyte function, serum B12 levels and upper tract status. Increasing upper tract dilatation suggests uretero-ileal stenosis, distal conduit obstruction or radiolucent stone formation. These can usually be distinguished by careful examination, IVU and loopogram. Sometimes pressure studies of the conduit can be helpful[1,42] in demonstrating functional obstruction at the level of the abdominal wall when the static loopogram has failed to demonstrate any abnormality.

Continent diversion and bladder reconstruction

Features of the reservoir

Almost every part of the gut from stomach[43] to rectum has been used for urinary reservoir formation. Geometric considerations suggest that configuration of a given length of bowel to a spherical pouch produces the highest volume per unit length[44,45]. Because of the Laplace relationship, mural tension at constant pressure increases with the radius; pouches with a larger radius will be subjected to greater wall tension than tubular reservoirs with a smaller diameter but since the bowel wall is visco-elastic, they will accommodate a greater volume. De-tubularization of intestinal segments does not prevent peristaltic contraction, but when the de tubularized bowel is folded in a complex manner the contractile activity becomes discontinuous and disorganized. This prevents increases in intratubular pressure resulting from synchronized circular contraction. Indeed several investigators have pointed out that even short segments of tubularized bowel segments proximal to the urethral sphincter may cause incontinence in patients with a neobladder anastomosed to the urethra[8,46]. Regardless of the bowel segment used for reservoir formation, results are satisfactory as long as the bowel is de-tubularized and a spherical-shaped reservoir created. Most surgeons have abandoned techniques using non de-tubularized bowel for construction of urinary reservoirs.

The continence mechanism in bladder replacement

Obviously in orthotopic reconstruction reliance is placed on the distal sphincter mechanism. In the male careful dissection of the apex of the prostate is essential and experience of radical prostatectomy proves useful. Eversion of the intestinal mucosa at the site of the urethral anastomosis will diminish the risk of stenosis. In women, the urethra should be transected no further than just beyond the bladder neck if continence is to be preserved. Recent experience of orthotopic replacement has rather surprisingly shown that women are more likely to develop impaired bladder emptying than men, particularly if colposuspension is performed.

The continence mechanism in continent diversion

A non-refluxing continence mechanism through which the pouch can be catheterized is required. The commonest techniques include:

- an invaginated nipple valve (the Kock technique[47]),
- the Mitrofanoff principle using the appendix or a 'neo-appendix' made from tubularized ileum or colon which is then implanted in a submucosal tunnel[48–51],
- imbricated ileum[52].

Nipple valve

Intussusception of the bowel to create a continent nipple valve was described by Kock[47] for the formation of a continent ileostomy. Later, other surgeons successfully employed this technique for a continent urinary diversion. Initially, complications such as nipple necrosis, incontinence or nipple sliding were common and the rate of re-operation for nipple revision was over 30%. The technique has been modified and the revision rate has declined to about 10% in some hands[53]. The final length of the intussuscepted segment should be at least 3 cm long, stripping of the mesentery at the site where the bowel is intussuscepted is important and fixation of the valve with three rows of staples and polyglycolic acid mesh to the base of the nipple prevents sliding of the nipple valve. Late complications were reported in only 3% of patients in a recent

series.[9] However, the nipple technique is still a time-consuming and technically demanding operation which most surgeons find so difficult and unsatisfactory that they have eagerly taken up other methods.

Tapered efferent loop

Plication of the ileum to form the efferent loop in techniques utilizing the ileocecal region as a reservoir has been described by several investigators as a reliable and safe continence mechanism[52,54–56]. The advantage is that it is easier to construct than the invaginated nipple valve. Short-term follow up reveals similar urinary continence results, but long-term results are not yet available and difficulties with catheterization have been reported.

The Mitrofanoff principle

Mitrofanoff[49] originally used the isolated appendix to create a continent vesicostomy in patients with neurogenic bladder dysfunction or those with a severely damaged urethra. The basic objective is the use of a narrow, catheterizable outlet which is implanted into the reservoir by means of an antireflux technique. This principle was successfully utilized for construction of an effective continence mechanism for continent diversion. Barker[57] used the detubularized ileocecal segment for construction of the reservoir. The appendix was divided, mobilized at the mesentery and the tip re-implanted into the cecum so that a portion of 3 cm was in a mucosal gutter and the base of the appendix was brought to the skin. Continence rates have been most satisfactory, but catheterization difficulties are a problem. A different procedure using the appendix was described by Riedmiller and colleagues[50]. In a modification of the Mainz pouch, the appendix was not divided but submucosally embedded into a 3 to 4 cm longitudinal incision of the cecal tenia. The tip of the appendix was placed to the lower right abdominal wall or alternatively an umbilical stoma was fashioned. Continence was reported in 100% of patients, although one of 13 patients required re-operation for stomal stenosis. Higher re-operation rates than these have been reported by most surgeons in the longer term[48,51]. A potential hazard of all techniques of continent diversion is urinary leakage when the pouch is full; however, sustained high pressures can lead to perforation. Patients must be encouraged to empty the reservoir at intervals not exceeding 6 hours. In most surgeons' hands, the re-operation rate in continent diversion is high, being in the order of 25% to 30%. The reasons include stenosis and failure of the continence mechanism. If the appendix is missing, short segments of ileum or colon can be used to fashion a 'neo-appendix' by excision of the antimesenteric section of the gut over a 14 FG catheter.

Emptying of the reservoir and reconstructed bladder

The proportion of patients needing to perform intermittent self-catheterization following orthotopic reconstruction varies in different series from 20% to 70%; the remaining patients learn to recognize when the neo-bladder is full and strain to void. The technique of ISC is well tolerated[57-59]. It may be that patients with orthotopic reconstruction using non de-tubularized segments of right colon are less likely to require ISC following operation compared with de-tubularized ileal and ileocecal pouches. Nevertheless it is good practice to ensure that patients before operation understand that ISC may be needed afterwards. All patients with continent diversion will need to practice ISC.

Kock pouch

The technical details have been well described by Skinner et al.[53] Briefly, an 80 cm segment of ileum is isolated on its mesentery. The 44 cm middle portion is folded to a U-shape and de-tubularized for construction of the reservoir. The intact proximal and distal ends are then intussuscepted into the reservoir for creation of nipple valves: the afferent valve prevents ileo-ureteral reflux and the efferent ensures stomal continence. However, nipple construction is technically demanding and complications include necrosis, leakage, nipple sliding or malfunction as well as stone formation. Re-operation is still necessary in 10% to 15% of patients, even in the best hands[53]. Since 1986, Skinner et al.[9] have performed bladder replacement using a modified Kock reservoir. The pouch was constructed without an efferent nipple and directly anastomosed to the urethral stump. Day and night continence was achieved in 94% and 85% respectively.

Ulm bladder

A different technique of lower urinary tract reconstruction using an ileal reservoir was described by Hautmann et al.[60] A 70 cm ileal segment is mobilized 15 cm proximal to the ileo-cecal valve and completely de-tubularized. The ileal plate is W- or M-shaped and a spherical reservoir is formed. The ureters are implanted by a non-refluxing technique as described by Le-Duc and Camey (1979)[10] and the reservoir anastomosed to the urethra by means of a buttonhole in the bowel. A review of the first 100 cases showed no peri-operative mortality, re-operation was necessary in 13 patients and day- and night-time continence was achieved in 82%[11]. However, continence was strongly dependent on patient age – 50% of patients over the age of 70 were incontinent at night.

Ileo-cecal Pouches

Various methods have been described using the ileo-cecal segment for construction of a continent urinary reservoir. The basic idea was to use the cecum as a reservoir and the terminal ileum as an efferent outlet. The continence mechanism was provided by the natural ileo-cecal valve. This technique did not become common practice because continence rates were poor. When de-tubularization was defined as an important principle in bladder replacement it became possible to achieve continence by various techniques; utilization of the ileo-cecal segment then regained interest.

Current techniques vary with respect to the extent of colonic or ileal segment to be utilized. Thüroff et al.[46] described a surgical procedure for construction of a urinary reservoir using 15 cm of de-tubularized cecum and ascending colon together with two, longitudinally split ileal loops of the same length. The pouch is fashioned by arranging the de-tubularized bowel in the shape of an N; a bowel plate is created by ceco-ileal and ileo-ileal side-to-side anastomosis. The ileo-cecal valve is spared if a continent stoma is to be achieved. The efferent valve utilizes an additional 15 cm segment of intact ileum which is left attached to create an intussuscepted nipple valve. For further stabilization, the nipple is pulled through the ileocecal valve and stabilized by two rows of staples. A uretero-cecal anastomosis is accomplished by a submucosal tunnel technique, the reservoir is closed and an umbilical stoma than fashioned. For bladder re-construction, no efferent nipple is created, instead, a buttonhole incision is made into the cecal pole of the reservoir which is anastomosed to the membranous urethra. This procedure provides a low-pressure reservoir with a mean capacity of more than 600 ml and incontinence rates are 4% to 7%[46]. Alternatively, the appendix or a tube of bowel may be utilized according to the Mitrofanoff principle and anastomosed to the umbilicus[50]. The use of a tapered ileal valve has been discussed above.

A de-tubularized ileo-ceçal reservoir is very versatile, being able to be used as a continent diversion using the appendix or as a reservoir in orthotopic reconstruction. Fifteen cm of cecum and a single limb of 15 cm of ileum give a de-tubularized reservoir with sufficient capacity for orthotopic reconstruction. However, the pressure characteristics of the sigmoid are less favorable than ileum showing low compliance and increased phasic activity.

Sigmoid neo-bladder

The sigmoid colon has some advantages over small bowel or ileo-cecal segments. It is located in the pelvis so correct positioning of the reservoir is easily accomplished. The ileo-cecal valve and the terminal ileum are not excluded from the gut and non-refluxing ureteral anastomoses are easily achieved.

In the usual technique, a 35 cm sigmoid segment is isolated on its mesenteric pedicle. The segment is folded to a U-shape and the ureters are anastomosed into the lateral tenia. De-tubularization is accomplished along the medial tenia and a spherical reservoir is fashioned. A small incision is made at the lowest point of the reservoir which is anastomosed to the urethral stump. The average capacity is 600 ml and 67% of patients were continent day and night.[19]

Uretero-sigmoidostomy

Somewhat surprisingly uretero-sigmoidostomy, despite its historically high rate of late post-operative complications such as metabolic acidosis and recurrent pyelonephritis, is regaining some popularity in patients who require a urethrectomy. One reason is the high re-operation rate in patients with continent diversion and the need in some countries to avoid appliances and external stomas.

Hohenfellner and colleagues have described a variation of the classical Goodwin uretero-sigmoidostomy which is based on modern concepts of de-tubularization[62]. Essentially a standard uretero-sigmoidostomy is performed, but this is followed by a side-to-side sigmoid entero-enterostomy which results in a low pressure region in the recto-sigmoid. This reduces the incidence of high pressure reflux which causes recurrent pyelonephritis and of fecal frequency and incontinence. In most series of uretero-sigmoidostomy the rate of nocturnal frequency (>3) is more than 70% and a third suffer from bouts of incontinence[63]. The Mainz II pouch is associated with better results. Incontinence was found in 2% with minor degrees of stress leakage in 6%. The frequency of daytime voiding was 5 (range 2 to 8) and nocturnal voiding was 1 (range 0 to 4).

Functional results and urinary continence

In general, continence after continent urinary diversion and bladder replacement is satisfactory. Most series show an incontinence rate of less than 10%. The voiding interval averages 5 hours.

The definition of continence after bladder replacement or reconstruction diverges greatly in the literature. The length of time between emptying of the reservoir to ensure dryness when the bladder is full is one criterion. Camey[64] defined continence as an interval of more than 2 hours. A more stringent definition was given by Reddy et al.[19], who defined enuresis if patients needed to empty the reservoir more than twice per night to ensure dryness. Continence

in some men may only be achieved by two to three voids per night. An adequate reservoir capacity is a prerequisite for continence, this will usually be around 500 ml (range 300 to 700 ml). Wenderoth et al.[11] reported a 50% rate of incontinence in men aged over 70 compared with 11% in younger patients. As a normal sensation of bladder filling is not experienced after bladder replacement with intestinal segments, patients may suffer from overflow incontinence at night. However, two other mechanisms have been proposed. Jakobsen and colleagues[61] indicated that the tone of the external sphincter decreases during sleep and secondly contractions of the neo-bladder are not accompanied by reflex contraction of the distal sphincter mechanism. Finally the high osmotic gradient generated by the concentrated urine leads to a fluid shift into the reservoir with subsequent increases in urine volumes[21].

Patients with incontinence can be treated with oral or topical anticholinergics to inhibit extensive bowel contractions. However, a controlled study evaluating the effect of these drugs is not yet available.

Another criteria is patient satisfaction. This value is subjective and chiefly depends on the attitude taken by each individual, making comparison between series rather difficult, although there is evidence that continent techniques achieve better results than conduits[66]. Good quality of life data are still needed in patients who have undergone bladder reconstruction and continent diversion.

References

1. Neal DE. Urodynamic investigation of the ileal conduit: upper tract dilatation and the effects of revision of the conduit. *J Urol* 1989;**142**:97–100.
2. Coffey RC. Physiologic implantation of the severed ureter or common bile-duct into the intestine. JAMA 1911;**56**:397–403.
3. Coffey RC. Transplantation of the ureters into large intestine in the absence of a functioning bladder. *Surg Gynecol Obstet* 1921;**32**:382–391.
4. Nesbit RM. Uretero-sigmoid anastomosis by direct eliptical anastomosis. *J Urol* 1949;**61**:628.
5. Leadbetter WF. Consideration of problems incident to performance of uretero-sigmoidostomy: report of a technique. *J Urol* 1950;**65**:818–830.
6. Goodwin WE, Harris AP, Kaufman JJ, Beal JM. Open transcolonic ureterointestinal anastomosis: a new approach. *Surg Gynecol Obstet* 1953;**97**:295–300.
7. Kock NG, Norlén LJ, Philipson BM, Åkerlund S. The continent ileal reservoir (Kock pouch) for urinary diversion. *World J Urol* 1985;**3**:146–151.
8. Skinner DG, Lieskovsky G, Boyd S. Continent urinary diversion. *J Urol* 1989;**141**:1323–1327.
9. Skinner DG, Boyd SD, Lieskovsky G, Bennett C, Hopwood B. Lower urinary tract reconstruction following cystectomy: experience and results in 126 patients using the Kock ileal reservoir with bilateral ureteroileal urethrostomy. *J Urol* 1991;**146**:756–760.
10. Le Duc A, Camey M. Un procédé d'implantation urétéroiléale antireflux dans l'entéro-cystoplastie. *J Urol Néphrol* 1979;**85**:449–454.
11. Wenderoth UK, Bachor R, Egghart G, Frohneberg D, Miller K, Hautmann RE. The ileal neobladder: experience and results of more than 100 consecutive cases. *J Urol* 1990;**143**:492–496: discussion 49.
12. Studer UE, Spiegel T, Casanova GA, Springer J, Gerber E, Ackermann DK, Gurtner F, Zingg EI. Ileal bladder substitute: antireflux nipple or afferent tubular segment? *Eur Urol* 1991;**20**:315–326.

13. Neal DE. Complications of ileal conduit urinary diversion in adults with cancer followed up for at least 5 years. *Br Med J* 1985;**290**:1695–1697.

14. Sullivan JN, Grabstaldt H, Whitmore WF. Complications of of ureteroileal conduit with radical cystectomy. *J Urol* 1980;**124**:797–801.

15. Stöckle M, Gökcebay E, Riedmiller H, Hohenfellner R. Urethral tumor recurrences after radical cystoprostatectomy: the case for primary cystoprostatourethrectomy. *J Urol* 1990;**143**:41–43.

16. Hendry WF, Gowing NFC, Wallace DM. Surgical treatment of urethral tumors associated with advanced bladder cancer. *Proc Roy Soc Med* 1974;**67**:304–307.

17. Levinson AK, Johnson DE, Wishnow KI. Indications for urethrectomy in an era of continent urinary diversion. *J Urol* 1990;**144**:73–75.

18. Hardeman SW, Soloway MS. Urethral recurrence following radical cystectomy. *J Urol* 1990;**144**:666–669.

19. Reddy PK, Lange PH, Fraley EE. Total bladder replacement using detubularized sigmoid colon: technique and results. *J Urol* 1991;**145**:51–55.

20. Hall MC, Koch MO, McDougal WS. Metabolic consequences of urinary diversion through intestinal segments. *Urol Clin North Am* 1991;**18**:725–735.

21. Koch MO, McDougal WS. Reddy PK, Lange PH. Metabolic alterations following continent urinary diversion through colonic segments. *J Urol* 1991;**145**:270–273.

22. Nurse DE, Mundy AR. Metabolic complications of cystoplasty. *Br J Urol* **63**:165.

23. Koch MO, Gurevitch E, Hill DW, McDougal WS. Urinary solute transport by intestinal segment. A comparative study of ileum and colon in rats. *J Urol* 1990;**143**:1275.

24. Golimbu M, Morales P. Jejunal conduits: techniques and complications. *J Urol* 1975;**113**:787.

25. Nguyen DH, Ganesan GS, Mitchell. Lower urinary tract reconstruction using stomach tissue in children and young adults. *World J Urol* 1992;**10**:76–79.

26. Nguyen DH, Bain MA, Samuelson KL *et al.* The syndrome of dysuria and hematuria in pediatric urinary reconstruction with stomach. *J Urol* 1993;**150**:707–709.

27. Silbermanm R. Ammonia intoxication following ureterosigmoidostomy in a patient with liver disease. *Lancet* 1958;**ii**:937

28. Pannek J, Haupt G, Schulze H, Senge T. Influence of continent ileal urinary diversion on vitamin B12 absorption. *J Urol* 1996;**155**:1206–1208.

29. Kinn A, Lantz B. Vitamin B12 deficiency after irradiation for bladder carcinoma. *J Urol* 1984;**131**:888.

30. Barrington JW, Fern-Davies H, Adams RJ, Evans WD, Woodcock JP, Stephenson TP. Bile acid dysfunction after clam cystoplasty. *Br J Urol* 1995;**76**:169–171.

31. Thorpe AC, Roberts JP, Williams NS, Blandy JP, Badenoch DF. Pelvic floor physiology in women with fecal incontinence and urinary symptoms. *Br J Surg* 1995;**82**:173–176.

32. Mark SD, Webster GD. Bowel dysfunction following entero-cystoplasty. In Webster GD and Goldwasser B (eds) *Urinary diversion: scientific foundations and clinical practice*, ch 11. Isis Medical Media, Oxford, 1995, pp 121–124.

33. Graversen PH, Gasser TC, Friedman AL, Bruskewitz RC. Surveillance of long term metabolic changes after urinary diversion. *J Urol* 1988;**140**:818.

34. Wagstaff KE, Woodhouse CRJ, Rose GA, Duffy PG, Ransley PGL. Blood and urine analysis in patients with intestinal bladders. *Br J Urol* 1991;**68**:311.

35. Campanello M, Herlitz H, Lindstedt G, Mellström D, Wilske J, Åkerlund S, Jonsson O. Bone mineral and related biochemical variables in patients with kock ileal reservoir or Bricker conduit for urinary diversion. *J Urol* 1996;**155**:1209–1213.

36. Silverman SH, Woodhouse CR, Strachen JR, Cumming J, Keighley MRB. Long-term management of patients who have had urinary diversion into urine. *Br J Urol* 1986;**58**:634–639.

37. Stewart M, McCrae FA, Williams CB. Neoplasia and ureterosigmoidostomy: a colonoscopic survey. *Br J Surg* 1982;**69**:414–416.

38. Bricker EM. Bladder substitution after pelvic evisceration. *Surg Clin N Am* 1950;**30**:1511–1521.

39. Kosko JW, Kursh ED, Resnick MI. Metabolic complications of urologic intestinal substitutes. *Urol Clin N Amer* 1986;**13**:193.

40. Pitts WR Jr, Muecke EC. A 20 year experience of ileal conduits: the fate of the kidneys. *J Urol* 1979;**122**:154–157.

41. Elder DD, Moisey CV, Rees RWM. A long term followup of the colonic conduit operation in children. *Br J Urol* 1979;**51**:462.

42. Neal DE, Hawkins T, Gallaugher AS, Essenhigh DM, Hall RR. Pressure and flow in ileal conduits: a comparison of patients with normal and dilated upper tracts. *Br J Urol* 1985;**57**:520–524.

43. Leong CH. Use of the stomach for bladder replacement and urinary diversion. *Ann R Coll Surg Engl* 1978;**60**:283–289.

44. Hinman-F Jr. Selection of intestinal segments for bladder substitution: physical and physiological characteristics. *J Urol* 1988;**139**:519–523.

45. Colding-Jorgensen M, Poulsen AL, Steven K. Mechanical characteristics of tubular and detubularized bowel for bladder substitution: theory, urodynamics and clinical results. *Br J Urol* 1993;**72**:586–593.

46. Thüroff JW, Alken P, Riedmiller H, Jacobi GH, Hohenfellner R. 100 cases of Mainz pouch:continuing experience and evolution. *J Urol* 1988;**140(2)**:283–288.

47. Kock NG. Intra abdominal 'reservoir' in patients with permanent ileostomy. Preliminary observations on a procedure resulting in fecal 'continence' in five ileostomy patients. *Arch Surg* 1969;**99**:223–231.

48. Hasan ST, Marshall C, Neal DE. Continent urinary diversion using the Mitrofanoff principle. *Br J Urol* 1994;**74**:454–459.

49. Mitrofanoff P. Cystostomie continente trans-appendiculaire dans le traitement des vessies neurologiques. *Chir Pediatr* 1980;**21**:297–305.

50. Riedmiller H, Burger R, Muller S, Thüroff J, Hohenfellner R. Continent appendix stoma: a modification of the MAINZ pouch technique. *J Urol* 1990;**143**:1115–1117.

51. Woodhouse CR, Malone PR, Cumming J, Reilly TM. The Mitrofanoff principle for continent diversion. *Br J Urol* 1989;**63**:53.

52. Rowland RG, Mitchell ME, Bihrle R, Kahnoski RJ, Piser JE. Indiana continent urinary reservoir. *J Urol* 1987;**137**:1136–1139.

53. Skinner DG, Boyd SD, Lieskovsky G. An update on the Kock pouch for continent urinary diversion. *Urol Clin North Am* 1987;**14(4)**:789–795.

54. Lockhart JL. Remodeled right colon: an alternative urinary reservoir. *J Urol* 1987;**138**:730–734.

55. Lockhart JL, Pow Sang JM, Persky L, Kahn P, Helal M, Sanford E. A continent colonic urinary reservoir: the Florida pouch. *J Urol* 1990;**144**:864–867.

56. Bejany DE, Politano VA. Stapled and nonstapled tapered distal ileum for construction of a continent colonic urinary reservoir. *J Urol* 1988;**140**:491–494.

57. Barker SB. Continent diversion with an appendix conduit and an ileocecal bladder. *J Urol* 1991;**146**:754–755.

58. Lapides J, Diokno AC, Silber SJ, Lowe BS. Clean intermittent self catheterization in the treatment of urinary tract disease. *J Urol* 1972;**107**:458–461.

59. Webb RL, Lawson AL, Neal DE. Clean intermittent self-catheterisation in adults. *Br J Urol* 1990;**65**:20–23.

60. Hautmann RE, Egghart G, Froheberg G, Miller K. The ileal neobladder. *J Urol* 1988;**139**:39–42.

61. Jakobsen H, Steven K, Stigsby B, Klarskov P, Hald T. Pathogenesis of nocturnal urinary incontinence after ileocaecal bladder replacement. Continuous measurement of urethral closure pressure during sleep. *Br J Urol* 1987;**59**:148–152.

62. Fisch M, Wammack R, Müller SC, Hohenfellner R. The Mainz pouch II (sigma rectum pouch). *J Urol* 1993;**149**:258–263.

63. McConnel JB, Stewart WK. The long-term management and social consequences of ureterosigmoid anastomosis. *Br J Urol* 1975;**47**:607–612.

64. Camey M. Bladder replacement by ileocystoplasty following radical cystectomy. *World J Urol* 1985;**3**:161–166.

65. Mansson A, Johnson G, Mansson W. Quality of life after cystectomy. Comparison between patients with conduit and those with continent caecal reservoir urinary diversion. *Br J Urol* 1988;**62**:240–245.

66. Svare J, Walter S, Kristensen JK, Lund F. Ileal conduit urinary diversion – early and late complications. *Eur Urol*, 1985; **11**: 83–86.

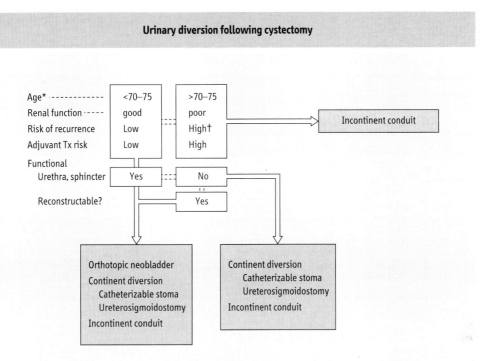

Urinary diversion following cystectomy

*Able to self catheterize if necessary; † Multifocal CIS, prostatic urethral involvement.

7.3 Bladder preserving treatment for muscle invasive bladder cancer

R R Hall

Introduction

The curative principles of radical surgery for cancer were enunciated by William Halsted in 1894[1]. It has taken most of the intervening 104 years for surgeons to heed the views of women and the results of clinical trials that radical mastectomy should and could be avoided for many women with breast cancer; organ preserving treatment is now accepted as optimal therapy for the majority[2]. For carcinoma of the larynx and osteosarcomas, organ and limb preserving treatments are receiving increasingly serious consideration. For rectal cancer, national guidance has been issued that seeks to maximize the preservation of normal bowel function on the grounds that this can be achieved without compromising survival[3]. At the same time, the importance of meticulous radical dissection has been re-emphasized by a

number of studies demonstrating superior survival following mesorectal excision and histologically confirmed negative surgical margins[3].

In the case of bladder cancer the results of meticulous radical pelvic lymphadenectomy combined with cystectomy exemplify the crucial role truly radical surgery can play[4]. The cost to the patient is the loss of a critical organ which, although acceptable, can be justified only so long as the survival advantages are demonstrable, significant and maintained. The problem concerns mainly patients with T2, T3 and T4a bladder cancer[5]. The alternatives to cystectomy are external beam radiotherapy, interstitial irradiation (brachytherapy), partial cystectomy, transurethral resection and systemic chemotherapy. In most institutions world-wide, cystectomy is regarded as the preferred treatment option and the extent to which the alternatives are even considered is very variable. Over the past decade cystectomy has received great attention as a consequence of the improvements in continent urinary diversion and bladder substitution. The perceived 'near normal' quality of life after cystectomy has enhanced a general view of cystectomy as the effective panacea for all invasive bladder cancer. This, however, is not the case. For urologists treating invasive bladder cancer, the question that has yet to be resolved is which patients may and which should not be advised to retain their bladders.

In the first place, cystectomy is not an option for many patients because of old age or co-morbidity. Reports of successful cystectomy in octogenarians not withstanding[6], the very few population based studies[7,8] reveal that two-thirds of patients presenting with muscle invasive bladder cancer are not candidates for cystectomy. In the international trial of neo-adjuvant CMV for invasive bladder cancer[9], patients who chose or were selected for cystectomy were of considerably better performance status than those treated by radiotherapy. The regular cystectomist almost inevitably develops a selected and limited view of the relevance of radical surgery. Secondly, despite the undoubted ability of cystectomy to cure some invasive bladder cancers, the impact of cystectomy on the overall survival of patients with muscle invasive tumors is small. In the study of Holmang[8] the overall 5 year survival for T2 to T4 cancers was 13% despite the use of radical surgery whenever possible: 'a sobering reminder of the lethal nature of muscle invasive bladder cancer as it presents in the population'[10]. Thirdly, the cure rates achieved by cystectomy are not as impressive as many published reports would suggest. Patient selection inflates survival rates[11]. Reviews of cystectomy based on less selective referral patterns have revealed that current best surgery fails in more than half of our patients[8,9,12].

Considering the numerous publications on innovative forms of bladder substitution and the success of nerve sparing cystectomy, readers may be forgiven for concluding that 'cystectomy is the cornerstone of treatment' for muscle invasive bladder cancer[13]. In reality it is of limited application and successful in only a fortunate few. The need for alternative more effective treatments than cystectomy has not diminished since Whitmore observed 'the limitations of radical cystectomy justify, indeed demand, considering exploration of other hopeful methods either alone or in combination with surgery'[14], a need that has been largely ignored by urology over the past three decades. From the patient's point of view the fact that alternative treatments preserve normal bladder function is an important, additional advantage provided, of course, that their use does not jeopardize the chance of cure for the few that would benefit from cystectomy, and cystectomy alone.

Radiotherapy

External beam radiotherapy and brachytherapy are both very effective bladder conserving treatments for appropriately selected patients. Both have been reviewed recently elsewhere[15,16].

Transurethral resection and partial cystectomy

TUR and partial cystectomy are complementary forms of surgery that aim to cure without sacrificing bladder function. They complement each other in that TUR is most suitable for tumours invading on the base, lateral and lower posterior bladder walls, and partial cystectomy is accomplished most easily for tumours of the dome, anterior and upper posterior walls where TUR is not indicated. The selection criteria for both are similar: solitary, freely mobile, T2[5] cancers up to 5 cm in diameter without concomitant carcinoma in situ[17,18]. Few such tumors occur at the bladder dome and consequently partial cystectomy is not frequently indicated.

In the past the inappropriate use of partial cystectomy has been associated with a high local relapse rate[18] and iatrogenic metastasis in the lower abdominal wall, both of which can be avoided by very careful patient selection and surgical technique. For partial cystectomy to be successful it is essential that a wide margin of normal bladder is removed with the tumor, a minimum of 3 cm of the undistended bladder. To prevent tumor implantation, the incision margins should be covered throughout the operation, tumor spillage avoided and the wound and pelvis washed thoroughly with sterile water before closure. Up to 30% of T2 tumors may be associated with microscopic pelvic lymph node metastases. As has been shown by several authors, pelvic lymphadenectomy can be curative in this situation[4,19] and there is a strong case to combine bilateral pelvic lymphadenectomy with partial cystectomy if the latter is the treatment of choice.

Transurethral resection (TUR) alone is not generally accepted to be adequate definitive treatment for muscle invasive bladder cancer although the reasons for this are not clear. Reviews have repeatedly drawn attention to the good survival rates following TUR alone in selected patients[18,20]. The most recent report of Solsona et al.[17] demonstrated 80.5% 5 year and 74.5% 10 year disease specific survival for 133 patients with T2 transitional cell carcinoma treated by TUR alone. All tumors were confined to the bladder wall (T2) and TUR was shown to be complete by confirming negative biopsies from the floor and margins of the resection. Fifty-three per cent were poorly differentiated tumors; 26% had associated carcinoma in situ. Intravesical BCG was used subsequently if CIS became apparent clinically. The completeness of the TUR was undoubtedly crucial. Such resections require endoscopic skill and a determination to explore with the patient the feasibility of bladder preserving surgery, two factors that are decreasingly evident in many urology departments.

Systemic chemotherapy

Bladder cancer is widely considered to be a chemosensitive tumor. Compared with most other solid cancers response rates of 70% for phase II studies of metastatic bladder cancer and pathologically confirmed complete responses in more than 20% of primary invasive cancers are very high. Cisplatin containing chemotherapy, with no other treatment, achieved durable complete remission in 18% of T2 and T3 bladder cancers at 3 years[22]. While this finding is of great interest it is of no direct clinical value; chemotherapy is less than half as effective as radiotherapy against primary invasive cancers, and as monotherapy has no therapeutic role in this situation. However, chemotherapy activity has generated a wide expectation of benefit if used as adjuvant treatment. In terms of contributing to local tumor control, a short-term 20% pathologic complete response rate and long-term 18% clinical complete response rate would never make a great impact, but if combined with TUR or partial cystectomy could extend the curative role of these conservative procedures to include more extensive, more invasive or more aggressive cancers. To this effect chemotherapy may be given first and partial or complete responses consolidated by TUR or partial cystectomy. Alternatively these operations may be performed first and the presumed residual microscopic disease treated with chemotherapy. Which would be the more appropriate approach is debatable, but the principle is to achieve long-term, local tumor control by combining 'lumpectomy' with chemotherapy, irrespective of any systemic effect that chemotherapy may have on distant metastases. The published experience to date has been reviewed in detail by Roberts[23] and others[18,25]. In summary, 10 different studies involving more than 338 patients with T2, T3 or T4a bladder cancer have demonstrated 3 year disease-specific survival up to 56–70%.

In view of the results that can be achieved by TUR alone, the value of adding chemotherapy may be questioned, particularly when the complete response rate of current combination chemotherapy is only modest. The answer lies in the patient selection of the studies discussed above. Those using TUR alone were successful in patients with smaller cancers that could be confirmed to have been resected completely, and with no extravesical invasion. Those studies that used TUR or partial cystectomy with chemotherapy included many patients with larger tumors, a larger proportion of G3 cancers, and included some with extravesical or prostatic invasion. For the latter group of patients TUR alone is not recommended and the fact that significant long-term tumor control can be achieved certainly suggests that the addition of chemotherapy is beneficial.

Follow up and risk of recurrence

One main advantage of cystectomy is that recurrence of invasive cancer within the bladder wall or the development of new bladder tumors is impossible. The likelihood of these occurring and the need for lifelong cystoscopic follow up are important considerations when discussing bladder preserving treatments with the patient. Following TUR alone for T2 cancers[17] or following TUR plus systemic chemotherapy[23,26] approximately one-quarter of patients develop new Ta/T1 bladder tumors during follow up, and another 25% develop recurrent muscle invasive cancer or extension into the prostate. A few of the subsequent invasive cancers develop at new sites within the bladder[26]. Any patient who undergoes TUR, partial cystectomy, radiotherapy, chemotherapy or any combination of these as initial treatment of muscle invasive bladder cancer must be followed assiduously with cystoscopies at 3 monthly intervals for the first 2 years and 6 monthly for the next 2 or 3 years. If their bladder remains free of invasive cancer at 5 years annual cystoscopy is almost certainly appropriate thereafter. If at any stage Ta or T1 tumors, or carcinoma in situ should develop, these may be treated by endoscopic resection with or without intravesical chemotherapy or BCG. The development of such superficial recurrence is not necessarily an indication for cystectomy.

Conclusions

Given the uncertainties of patient selection inherent in all non-randomized studies, and the absence of any randomized comparison of these bladder preserving treatments with cystectomy, no definite conclusions can be reached. The foregoing brief review indicates, nonetheless, that a significant proportion of patients with muscle invasive bladder cancer can be cured by bladder preserving surgery either by itself or in combination with chemotherapy. Neither alone or in combination can these treatments be considered optimal, but nor can radical cystectomy. Everybody recognizes that a new form of systemic therapy for bladder cancer is required[27]. When this has been identified, it is reasonable to expect that it will be equally efficacious against small amounts of residual microscopic cancer remaining after 'debulking' surgery as against microscopic disseminated disease. Thus the principle of 'lumpectomy plus systemic therapy' will displace radical surgery and organ preserving treatment will become the norm. Until then, randomized trials and prospective studies of subsets of patients with invasive bladder cancer are required to determine which patients require cystectomy and which may be served equally well by bladder preserving alternatives.

'While addressing these clinical endpoints represents a significant challenge, our own behavioural patterns and clinical dogma may pose even greater obstacles. Despite objections, some of which are valid, there are no insurmountable obstacles to evaluating and perhaps achieving the goal of bladder preservation.'[13]

References

1. Halsted WM. Results of operations for the care of carcinoma of the mamma. *Hopkins Hospital Review* 1964;**4**:297–350.
2. NHS Executive Cancer Guidance Subgroup of the Clinical Outcomes Group 1996. Improving outcomes in breast cancer – the manual. UK Department of Health, 96CC00 21.
3. NHS Executive Cancer Guidance Subgroup of the Clinical Outcomes Group 1997. Improving outcomes in colorectal cancer – the research evidence. UK Department of Health 97CC01200.
4. Lerner SP, Skinner DG. Radical cystectomy for bladder cancer. In: NJ Vogelsang, PT Scardino, WU Shipley, DS Coffey (eds) *Comprehensive textbook of genitourinary oncology*. Williams and Wilkins, Baltimore, 1996, pp. 442–463.
5. Sobin LH, Wittekind C. UICC TNM classification of malignant tumours. Wiley-Liss, New York, 1997, pp 187–190.
6. Stroumbakis N, Herr HW, Cookson MS, Fair WR. Radical cystectomy in the octogenarian. *J Urol* 1997;**158**:2113–2117.
7. Waehre H, Ous S, Klevmark B *et al.* A bladder cancer multi-institutional experience with total cystectomy for muscle-invasive bladder cancer. *Cancer* 1993;**72**:3044–3051.
8. Holmang N, Hedelin H, Anderstrom C, Johansson SL. Long term follow up of all patients with muscle invasive (stages T2, T3 and T4) bladder carcinoma in a geographical region. *J Urol* 1997;**158**:389–392.
9. International collaboration of trialists. Neoadjuvant CMV chemotherapy for muscle invasive bladder cancer: result of the international trial BA06 (MRC) 30894 (EORTC). 1998.
10. Schellhammer PF. Editorial: a world-wide view of bladder cancer. *J Urol* 1997;**158**:406–407.
11. Studer UE, Bacchi M, Biedermann C *et al.* Adjuvant cisplatin chemotherapy following cystectomy for bladder cancer: results of a prospective randomized trial. *J Urol* 1994;**152**:81–84.
12. Pagano F, Bassi P, Galetti TP *et al.* Results of contemporary radical cystectomy for invasive bladder cancer: a clinicopathological study with an emphasis of the tumor common nodes and metastases classification. *J Urol* 1991;**145**:45–50.
13. See WA. Editorial: radical cystectomy – cornerstone or millstone? *J Urol* 1996;**155**:504–505.
14. Whitmore WF, Marshall VF. Radical total cystectomy for cancer of the bladder: 230 consecutive cases five years later. *J Urol* 1962;**87**:853–868.
15. Gospodarowicz MK, Warde P, Bristow R. Radiotherapy for bladder cancer. In: Hall R R (Ed.) *Clinical Management of Bladder Cancer*. London: Arnold; 1998
16. Moonen LMF. Radiotherapy for bladder cancer: brachytherapy. In: RR Hall (Ed.) *The clinical management of bladder cancer*. Chapman & Hall, 1998.
17. Solsona E, Iborra I, Ricos JV *et al.* Feasibility of transurethral resection for muscle infiltrating carcinoma of the bladder: long term follow up of a prospective study. *J Urol* 1998;**159**:95–99.
18. Sternberg CN, Pansadoro V. Bladder preserving treatments: chemotherapy and conservative surgery. In: MJ Vogelsang, PT Scardino, WU Shipley, DS Coffey (eds). Comprehensive Textbook of Genitourinary Oncology. Williams and Wilkins, Baltimore, 1996, pp 522–533.
19. Ghoneim MA, El-Mekresh MM, El-Baz MA *et al.* Primary radical cystectomy for carcinoma of the bladder: critical evaluation of the results of 1026 cases. *J Urol* 1997;**158**:393–399.
20. Herr HW. Conservative management of muscle infiltrating bladder cancer: prospective experience. *J Urol* 1987;**138**:1162–1163.
21. Raghavan D. Systemic chemotherapy for metastatic cancer of the uroepithelial tract. In: Hall R R (Ed.) *Clinical Management of Bladder Cancer*. London: Arnold; 1998.
22. Hall RR, Roberts JT. Neoadjuvant chemotherapy, a method to conserve the bladder? *Eur J Can* 1991;**27** (suppl. 2): S29, #144.
23. Roberts JT. Bladder preservation in muscle invasive bladder cancer. In: Hall R R (Ed.) *Clinical Management of Bladder Cancer*. London: Arnold; 1998.
24. Hall RR. The role of transurethral surgery alone and with combined modality therapy. In: NJ Vogelsang, PT Scardino, WU Shipley, DS Coffey (eds) *The comprehensive textbook of genitourinary oncology*. Williams and Wilkins, Baltimore, 1996, pp. 509–513.
25. Angulo JC, Sanchez-Chapado M, Lopez JI, Flores N. Primary cisplatin methotrexate and vinblastine aiming at bladder preservation in invasive bladder cancer: multivariate analysis on prognostic factors. *J Urol* 1996;**155**:1897–1902.
26. Thomas DJ, Roberts JT, Hall RR, Reading J. Radical TUR and chemotherapy in the treatment of muscle invasive bladder cancer: long term follow up. In press
27. Roth BJ, Bajorin DF. Advanced bladder cancer: the need to identify new agents in the post-MVAC (methotrexate, vinblastine, doxorubicin and cisplatin) world. *J Urol* 1995;**153**:894–900.

7.4 Systemic chemotherapy for transitional cell carcinoma of the urinary tract

J T Roberts

Introduction

Before the middle of the 1980s transitional cell carcinoma (TCC) of the bladder was regarded as a chemoresistant entity. There had been a reluctance to combine the renally excreted and potentially nephrotoxic drugs cisplatin and methotrexate, particularly in this elderly population in whom cancer is often accompanied by other pathologies, of which renal impairment is only one. The results of phase II studies of combinations of the two drugs, as a doublet or combined with vinblastine (CMV) or vinblastine and adriamycin (M-VAC), were exciting. High response rates with substantial proportions of complete responses encouraged the belief that TCC might become a reliably chemocurable malignancy or, at the very least, that the addition of chemotherapy combinations to routine radical treatments might result in worthwhile improvements in survival. The reality is somewhat more disappointing. The translation of combinations from the single institution to the multicenter setting has been accompanied by the inevitable fall in response rate that has been observed in the context of other cancers. Palliative responses are commonly seen and individual palliative benefit is often worthwhile. However, survival benefit is often modest and long-term survivors with metastatic disease are extremely uncommon. No chemotherapy regimen has, so far, emerged as superior to M-VAC or CMV. No neoadjuvant or adjuvant study involving the use of combination chemotherapy before or after conventional definitive treatment has convincingly shown a survival benefit. However, there is evidence that the addition of concomitant cisplatin to radiotherapy significantly improves local control. While attempts to improve on the chemotherapy regimens of the past decade have proved frustrating, new agents are emerging as candidates for inclusion in chemotherapy regimens that may allow improvements in response and, it is to be hoped, in survival. They at least offer the prospect of similar response rates with reduced toxicity and, because of their lack of nephrotoxicity, the possibility of treating more patients with renal impairment.

Metastatic disease

In phase II studies single agent cisplatin produces a response rate of approximately 35% overall with a range of 26 to 65%. Complete responses are unusual[1–10]. In phase III trials the results of single agent cisplatinum are less good[11–15] and in only one such did the overall response rate exceed 10%[14]. Doses of cisplatin varied in these studies but there is no evidence of a dose–response curve for cisplatin over the dose range 50–120 mg/m^2.

Its lack of nephrotoxicity makes carboplatin an attractive potential alternative to cisplatin in this group of patients, in whom renal function is frequently compromised. However, overall and complete response rates are lower than with cisplatin[16] and its greater myelotoxicity decreases its usefulness as a component of drug combinations.

Methotrexate has a single agent response rate of approximately 30% but with responses of short duration and only anecdotal reports of complete responses[17–21].

Adriamycin (doxorubicin) produces an overall response rate of approximately 17% with short responses[22–26] and, in one study, a suggestion of a fairly steep dose–response curve[23]. Although vinblastine is frequently-incorporated into drug regimens used in the treatment of transitional cell carcinoma there are very few data on its single agent use. In one phase II study the overall response rate was 18% (22% in non-pre-treated patients) and response duration was short[27]. Cisplatin and methotrexate have been combined in a variety of schedules designed to reduce the nephrotoxicity of the combination. In phase II studies, these combinations have produced response rates between 45% and 68% overall, with CR rates between 9% and 21%[28–31]. However response duration was generally short; in one case only 21 weeks[30]

The Northern California Oncology Group reported a three drug combination of cisplatin, methotrexate and vinblastine (CMV)[32] which produced an overall response rate of 56%, with 28% CR. The median survival for treated patients was only 8 months but, at the time of the report, 14 of the CR patients remained disease-free at intervals of 6+ to 35+ months, suggesting the possibility of long-term survival benefit for some patients.

The initial report of the combination of methotrexate, vinblastine, adriamycin and cisplatin (M-VAC) appeared in the same year[33]. A response rate of 71% with a CR rate of 50% was observed. Remarkably, the median duration of response exceeded 9.5 months and encouraged the enthusiasm that transitional cell carcinoma might emerge as a reliably chemocurable malignancy[34]. However, in subsequent reports from the same center, while the overall response rate was maintained at 72% the CR rate with chemotherapy alone was only 18%, 68% of clinical CRs relapsed and only 20% of the CRs remained disease free long term[35,36]. In other phase II and phase III studies response rates and complete response rates have generally been less than those obtained in the original study group[11,37–40]). The median survival obtained in these different studies is remarkably similar (10–13.4 months) despite wide differences in overall and complete survival rates.

M-VAC has been shown to be superior to single agent cisplatin[11] and to CisCA (cisplatin, cyclophosphamide and adriamycin)[40]; no randomized comparison of M-VAC with CMV has ever been conducted.

The inclusion of cisplatin in chemotherapy combinations adds considerably to toxicity and necessitates inpatient treatment. Attempts to substitute carboplatin in combinations have produced results generally inferior to those obtained with cisplatin-based regimens[41–44]. Similarly the substitution of a less-toxic anthracycline or anthracenedione for adriamycin has generally resulted in poorer response and survival figures[42,43,45,46].

The use of recombinant hematopoetic growth factors to increase doses of individual drugs in the M-VAC combination or to shorten the cycle length and hence to escalate dose intensity has not resulted in any improvement in efficacy[47–50].

Rescheduling and dose intensification of the drug combinations that have now been standard for more than a decade has failed to produce improvements in either response rates or survival and any advances in the treatment of transitional cell carcinoma must therefore await the identification of new active agents.

The role of chemotherapy in locally advanced bladder cancer

Adjuvant and neoadjuvant chemotherapy

The use of adjuvant chemotherapy in other, more common, cancers such as breast and bowel has become routine in groups of patients at high risk of metastatic relapse. Chemotherapy regimens which, in the setting of palliation of metastatic disease, produce response rates lower than those seen in metastatic TCC, when given after conventional radical treatment add modest but statistically significant and clinically worthwhile survival benefit. The high rate of metastatic relapse after local therapy for muscle-invasive bladder cancer prompted the exploration of the effect of adding systemic chemotherapy to conventional, radical therapies. The high response rates and particularly the high rate of complete response observed in phase II studies of cisplatin-based regimens in metastatic disease encouraged the belief that the addition of systemic chemotherapy to cystectomy or radiotherapy would result in a clinically worthwhile improvement in survival.

Randomized trials of non-cisplatin-containing chemotherapy regimens given in addition to conventional radical treatment have failed to demonstrate a survival advantage[51,52]. Similarly, single agent cisplatin, given prior to radiotherapy, produced no improvement in the actuarial survival at 3 years when two similarly designed trials were analysed together[53]. The dramatic results of phase II studies of combination chemotherapy in metastatic disease produced preconceptions about the likely benefits of such combinations in the adjuvant setting that were cited as among the reasons for early closure. Other randomized comparisons of radical surgery alone, or followed by three cycles of single agent cisplatin have closed early with numbers too small reliable to detect even quite large survival differences[54,55].

Since the superiority of combination chemotherapy over single agent cisplatin in the context of metastatic disease has been established[11] the hope remains that combination chemotherapy may confer worthwhile benefit when given in an adjuvant or neoadjuvant setting.

Non-randomized comparisons with historical control series have been made in patients at high risk of relapse[56,57] and suggest benefit for the addition of chemotherapy. However, the conclusions need to be interpreted in the knowledge of the potential biases associated with non-randomized comparisons. Several randomized trials in which platinum-based combinations have been given as adjuvant therapy (after conventional definitive treatment) suggest, but fail to prove, a survival benefit (Table 7.4.1). These studies have been criticized, for example for containing only small patient numbers and for major flaws in trial design and execution which call to question the validity of their conclusions[62–65]. Cisplatin-based combination chemotherapy given before definitive treatment is generally well tolerated, relieves symptoms due to cancer in the majority of patients[66–68] and has significant activity against the primary tumor, with objective tumor response in the majority of patients and significant

downstaging, as evinced by the significant increase over the expected T_0 rate in cystectomy specimens after chemotherapy over that expected. In cystectomy series the percentage of patients with muscle-invasive cancer free of tumor in the cystectomy specimen after initial staging TUR is approximately 10%, whereas the figure after initial platinum based chemotherapy is typically 20–40%[69,70]. It is therefore disappointing that the largest randomized trial ever conducted in locally advanced muscle-invasive bladder cancer[70], which included more than 900 patients randomized to conventional radical treatment (cystectomy, with or without radiotherapy, or definitive radiotherapy) alone, or preceded by four cycles of chemotherapy with CMV, failed to demonstrate a clinically worthwhile improvement in survival with the addition of chemotherapy. A Nordic study of neoadjuvant chemotherapy prior to cystectomy has been interpreted as showing a survival benefit for the use of initial chemotherapy in patients with T3b disease[71]. However, this interpretation depends on the analysis of a subgroup, with retrospective, rather than prospective stratification, and the study overall showed no benefit for neoadjuvant chemotherapy. The successor study, 'Nordic2' has now been reported, at least in abstract form. This study was confined to the subgroup of patients who apparently derived benefit from neoadjuvant chemotherapy in the original study, omitted preoperative radiotherapy and substituted methotrexate for adriamycin. Despite a substantial downstaging effect no survival benefit was evident. With a median follow up of 3.4 years the crude 5 year survivals were 50% in each arm[71a].

In a recently reported randomized study, conducted in Egypt, 196 patients were randomized to radical cystectomy alone, or preceded by two cycles of chemotherapy with a combination of carboplatin, methotrexate and vinblastine. With a median follow up of only 32 months the estimated 5 year survival for the chemotherapy group was 59.1% compared with 41.6% in the cystectomy only group[72]. This was however a small study with short follow up and the results must be interpreted with appropriate caution. The North American Intergroup are examining the impact of three cycles of M-VAC, prior to cystectomy, in a prospective randomized trial. Recruitment has been extremely slow and, while the results are eagerly awaited, it is difficult to conceive that with less than 300 patients randomized it will possess the statistical power to enable robust conclusions to be drawn.

Chemotherapy as a component of a bladder conserving strategy

The significant response rate of primary bladder tumors to cisplatin-containing chemotherapy combinations has encouraged investigators to examine the effectiveness of chemotherapy as the sole treatment of muscle invasive bladder cancer.

Several series have been reported in which patients with muscle invasive disease have been treated with M-VAC for three or four cycles and then assessed, either with TURB or open biopsy of the bladder, with or without lymph node dissection. Definitive treatment (surgery or radiotherapy) has not then been given. Of patients who were rendered apparently tumor free in the bladder, 43–77% are reported to remain disease free, albeit with relatively short follow up. The relatively small proportion of patients rendered durably disease free in the bladder is less than one would expect with radical radiotherapy alone. Nevertheless, there is no other adult cancer where chemotherapy 'cures' are observed in such a substantial minority of patients. While this makes the all the more surprising failure of chemotherapy given in addition to conventional radical treatments to make any major impact on outcome it has encouraged the use of chemotherapy as a component of various bladder conserving strategies. Based on an initial observation that the combination of high-dose methotrexate and partial cystectomy produced excellent results in a series of patients with bladder cancer[73], others have explored the use of systemic chemotherapy and either thorough TUR[74–77] or partial cystectomy[78,79]. Survival and disease free survival in these (selected) series compare favorably with conventionally treated series.

While chemotherapy given before or after radical radiotherapy confers no advantage, a number of phase II series have suggested that the use of concurrent chemoradiotherapy is safe and that local control rates and survival are superior to historical radiotherapy only series[80–82]. Only one randomized controlled trial has compared radiotherapy alone with combined chemoradiotherapy[83]. In this multicenter Canadian study patients received definitive or pre-operative radiotherapy with, or without, concurrent cisplatin. No survival benefit was apparent but the numbers in the study were small and it lacked the power reliably to detect a true survival benefit of 10–15%. The pelvic recurrence rate was, however, reduced by some 25%.

Future developments

The current 'Gold Standard' chemotherapy regimens, M-VAC and CMV, are toxic, poorly tolerated by many and simply not applicable to a large number of patients. The average age of presentation with bladder cancer in the UK is 67 and, at this age, renal impairment, which precludes the use of cisplatin, is common. Many patients have other concurrent disease processes which themselves prevent the safe administration of aggressive chemotherapy combinations. The palliative benefits of chemotherapy in metastatic disease are short-lived and survival benefit usually modest. Furthermore, robust evidence for the benefit of adding chemotherapy to standard treatments for localized disease is lacking. There is therefore a need to develop chemotherapy combinations that are more widely applicable, that are better tolerated and more active than those currently used. Such regimens will need to be compared with M-VAC in fitter patients with metastatic disease and with combinations such as M-V in the less fit. The taxanes paclitaxel and docetaxel have both demonstrated activity in phase II studies, as has gemcitabine[84]. Paclitaxel has been successfully combined with gemcitabine and cisplatin in an escalating dose phase I–II study (J Baselga personal communication) and a similar combination but with docetaxel rather than paclitaxel is being piloted in the UK. Paclitaxel has also been combined with ifosfamide[85] and with ifosfamide and cisplatin[86]. Phase II results of the doublet combination of gemcitabine and cisplatin have been presented[87,88]. A large multinational, multicenter randomized phase III study is currently recruiting, comparing a combination of gemcitabine and cisplatin with classic M-VAC.

If new combinations prove superior to M-VAC, either because of increased activity or better tolerability this will improve the lot of patients with metastatic disease and provide the impetus to conduct further studies of adjunctive therapy. Even if no regimen emerges as a candidate to replace M-VAC there is a need to conduct a randomized trial of sufficient size to establish the role of adjuvant chemotherapy in bladder cancer or to allow us to omit 4 months of toxic and dangerous treatment from the routine management of patients with poor risk localized disease.

Conclusions

For patients with metastatic transitional cell carcinoma, combination chemotherapy offers a significant chance of response and palliation of symptoms to those fit enough to tolerate M-VAC. The survival benefit afforded such patients who do respond is generally modest, being measured in months rather than years. Long-term survivors with metastatic disease are those with nodal, rather than visceral, disease.

Many patients are unfit for M-VAC or similar regimens. While combinations such as MV may offer palliation to some, response rates are lower, as is response duration. Although M-VAC remains the standard against which newer regimens must be tested, patients with metastatic disease should, in general, be offered the opportunity to participate in clinical trials. Patients and clinicians may be assured that the benefits of conventional chemotherapy are not such that patients will be significantly disadvantaged by such participation. There is the real possibility that less toxic and perhaps more active regimens will soon emerge as a result of such studies.

There is insufficient evidence of benefit to recommend the routine use of adjuvant chemotherapy in patients with bladder cancer. A large, convincing study is required to allow such practice to become standard or routine. If newer agents allow the creation of chemotherapy combinations which are either more active or less toxic or both, then these new regimens will be the natural candidates for such studies. If not, it is imperative that one or more studies, which will avoid the shortcomings of those studies published or about to be published, are carried out.

References

1. Yagoda A. Phase II trials in patients with urothelial tumors: Memorial Sloan-Kettering Cancer Centre. *Cancer Chemother Pharmacol* 1983;**11**(Suppl):9–12.
2. Herr HW. *Cis*-Diamminedichloride platinum II in the treatment of advanced bladder cancer. *J Urol* 1980;**123**:853–857.
3. Peters PC, O'Neill MR. *Cis*-Diamminedichloroplatinum as a therapeutic agent in metastatic transitional cell carcinoma. *J Urol* 1980;**123**:375–377.
4. Merrin C. Treatment of advanced bladder cancer with *cis*-Diamminedichloroplatinum II: a pilot study. *J Urol* 1978;**119**:493–495.
5. Soloway MS, Ikard M, Ford K. *Cis*-Diamminedichloroplatinum (II) in locally advanced and metastatic urothelial cancer. *Cancer* 1981;**47**:476–480.
6. DeLena M, Lorusso V, Iacobellis U, Marzullo F, Maiello E, Crammarossa A. *Cis*-Diamminedichloroplatinum activity in bidimensionally measurable metastatic lesions of bladder carcinoma. *Tumori* 1984;**70**:85–88.
7. Oliver RTD, Newlands ES, Wiltshaw E, Malpas JS. A Phase II study of *cis*-platinum in patients with recurrent bladder carcinoma. *Br J Urol* 1981;**53**:444–447.
8. Rossof AM, Talley RW, Stephens RL *et al.* Phase II evaluation of *cis*-dichlorodiammineplatinum (II) in advanced malignancies of the genitourinary and gynaecological organs: a Southwest Oncology Group study. *Cancer Treat Rep* 1979;**63**:1557–1564.
9. Fagg SL, Dawson-Edwards P, Hughes MA, Latief TN, Rolfe EB, Fielding JWL. *Cis*-Diamminedichloroplatinum (DDP) as initial treatment of invasive bladder cancer. *Br J Urol* 1984;**56**:296–300.
10. Raghavan D, Pearson B, Duval P *et al.* Initial intravenous *cis*-platinum therapy: improved management for invasive high-risk bladder cancer. *J Urol* 1985;**133**:399–402.
11. Loehrer PJ, Einhorn LH, Elson PJ *et al.* A randomised comparison of cisplatin alone or in combination with methotrexate, vinblastine and doxorubicin in patients with metastatic urothelial carcinoma: a co-operative group study. *J Clin Oncol* 1992;**10**:1066–1073.
12. Khandekar JD, Elson PJ, DeWys WD, Slayton RE, Harris DT. Comparative activity and toxicity of *cis*-diamminedichloroplatinum (DDP) and a combination of doxorubicin, cyclophosphamide and DDP in disseminated transitional cell carcinoma of the urinary tract. *J Clin Oncol* 1985;**3**:539–545.
13. Soloway MS, Einstein A, Corder MP, Bonney W, Prout GR, Coombes J. A comparison of cisplatin and the combination of cisplatin and cyclophosphamide in advanced urothelial cancer. *Cancer* 1983;**52**:767–772.
14. Hillcoat BL, Raghavan D, Matthews J *et al.* A randomised trial of cisplatin versus cisplatin plus methotrexate in advanced cancer of the urothelial tract. *J Clin Oncol* 1989;**7**:706–709.
15. Troner M, Birch R, Omura GA, Williams S. Phase III comparison of cisplatin alone versus cisplatin, doxorubicin and cyclophosphamide in the treatment of bladder (urothelial) cancer: a Southeastern Cancer Study Group Trial. *J Urol* 1987;**137**:660–662.
16. Mottet-Auselo KC, Bons-Rosset, Costa P, Louis JF, Navrati H. Carboplatin and urothelial tumors. *Oncology* 1993;**50**:28–36.
17. Turner AG, Hendry WF, Williams GB, Bloom HJG. The treatment of advanced bladder cancer with methotrexate. *Br J Urol* 1977;**49**:673–678.
18. Hall RR, Bloom HJG, Freeman JR, Nawrocki A, Wallace DM. Methotrexate treatment for advanced bladder cancer. *Br J Cancer* 1977;**35**:40–51.
19. Gad-el-Mawla NH, Hamsa R, Cairns J, Anderson T, Ziegler JL. Phase II analysis of methotrexate in carcinoma of the bilharzial bladder. *Cancer Treat Rep* 1978;**62**:1075–1076.
20. Natale RB, Yagoda A, Watson RC, Whitmore WF, Blumenrich M, Braun DW. Methotrexate: an active drug in bladder cancer. *Cancer* 1981;**47**:1246–1250.
21. Turner AG. Methotrexate for advanced bladder cancer. *Cancer Treat Rep* 1981;**62**:183–186.
22. Pavone-Macaluso M. EORTC Genitourinary Cooperative Group A. Single drug chemotherapy of bladder cancer with Adriamycin, VM-26, or bleomycin. *Eur Urol* 1976;**2**:138–141.
23. O'Bryan RM, Baker LH, Gottlieb JE *et al.* Dose-response evaluation of Adriamycin in human neoplasm. *Cancer* 1977;**39**:1940–1948.
24. Yagoda A, Watson RC, Whitmore WF, Grabstalt H, Middleman MF, Krakoff HI. Adriamycin in advanced urinary tract cancer: experience in 42 patients and review of the literature. *Cancer* 1977;**39**:279–285.
25. Knight EW, Pagand EM, Hahn RG, Horton J. Comparison of 5-FU and doxorubicin in the treatment of carcinoma of the bladder. *Cancer Treat Rep* 191983;**67**:514–515.
26. Gagliano R, Levin H, El-Bolkainy MN *et al.* Adriamycin versus Adriamycin plus *cis*-dichlorodiammineplatinum (II) in advanced transitional cell bladder carcinoma: a Southwest Oncology Group study. *Am J Clin Oncol* 1983;**6**:215–218.
27. Blumenreich MS, Yagoda A, Natale RB, Watson RC. Phase II trial of vinblastine sulfate for metastatic urothelial tract tumours. *Cancer* 1982;**50**:435–438.
28. Stoter G, Splinter TAW, Child JA *et al.* Combination chemotherapy with cisplatin and methotrexate in advanced transitional cell cancer of the bladder. *J Urol* 1987;**137**:663–667.
29. Oliver RTD. Chemotherapy of invasive carcinoma of the bladder. *Aust NZ J Surg* 1985;**55**:249–252.
30. Oliver RTD, Kwok HK, Highman WJ, Waxman J. Methotrexate, cisplatin and carboplatin as single agents and in combination for metastatic bladder cancer. *Br J Urol* 1986;**58**:31–35.
31. Carmichael J, Cornbleet MA, MacDougall FH *et al.* Cis-platin and methotrexate in the treatment of transitional cell carcinoma of the urinary tract. *Br J Urol* 1985;**57**:299–302.
32. Harker WG, Meyers FJ, Freiha FS *et al.* Cisplatin, methotrexate and vinblastine (CMV): an effective treatment for for metastatic transitional cell carcinoma of the urinary tract: a Northern California Oncology Group study. *J Clin Oncol* 1985;**3**:1463–1470.
33. Sternberg CN, Yagoda A, Scher HI *et al.* Preliminary results of M-VAC (methotrexate, vinblastine, doxorubicin and cisplatin) for transitional cell carcinoma of the urothelium. *J Urol* 1985;**133**:461–469.
34. Waxman J. Chemotherapy for bladder cancer. Is there new hope? *Br J Urol* 1990;**65**:1–6.
35. Sternberg CN, Yagoda A, Herr HW *et al.* M-VAC (methotrexate, vinblastine, doxorubicin and cisplatin) for advanced carcinoma of the urothelium. *J Urol* 1988;**139**:461–469.
36. Sternberg CN, Yagoda A, Scher HI *et al.* Methotrexate, vinblastine, doxorubicin and cisplatin for advanced transitional cell carcinoma of the urothelium: efficacy and patterns of response and relapse. *Cancer* 1989; **64**:2448–58.
37. Tannock I, Gospodarawicz M, Connolly J, Jewett M. M-VAC (methotrexate, vinblastine, doxorubicin and cisplatin) chemotherapy for transitional cell carcinoma: the Princess Margaret Hospital experience. *J Urol* 1989;**142**:289–292.
38. Igawa M, Ohkuchi T, Ueki T, Ueda M, Okada K, Usui T. Usefulness and limitations of methotrexate, vinblastine, doxorubicin and cisplatin for the treatment of advanced urothelial cancer. *J Urol* 1990;**144**:662–665.

39. Boutan-Laroze A, Mahjoubi M, Droz JP et al. M-VAC (methotrexate, vinblastine, doxorubicin and cisplatin) for advanced carcinoma of the bladder. Eur J Cancer 1991;27:1690–1694.

40. Logothetis CJ, Dexeus FH, Finn L, Sella A, Amato RJ, Ayala AG, Kilbourn RG. A prospective randomised trial comparing MVAC and CISCA chemotherapy for patients with metastatic urothelial tumours. J Clin Oncol 1990;8:1050–1055.

41. Klocker J, Pont J, Schumer J, Prüger J, Kienzer H. Carboplatin, methotrexate and vinblastine (Carbo-MV) for advanced urothelial cancer: a phase II trial. Am J Clin Oncol 1991;14:328–330.

42. Bellmunt J, Albanell J, Vicente P, Gallego OS, Carulla J, Sole Calvo LA. A prospective randomised trial comparing MVAC with MCAVI (methotrexate, carboplatin, doxorubicin and vinblastine) in patients with bladder cancer. Proc Am Soc Clin Oncol 1993;12:237.

42. Waxman J, Abel P, Farah JN et al. New combination chemotherapy programme for bladder cancer. Br J Urol 1989;19:21–25.

43. Waxman J, Barton C. Carboplatin-based chemotherapy for bladder cancer. Cancer Treat Rev 1993;19:21–25.

44. Lorusso V, Berardi F, Catino A, De Lena M. Methotrexate, vinblastine, epidoxorubicin and carboplatin (M-VECA) in the treatment of advanced bladder cancer. Proc Am Soc Clin Oncol 1992;11:212.

45. Goldfarb A, Negro A, Coimbra F et al. Methotrexate, vinblastine, epidoxorubicin and cisplatin (M-VEC) for stage II-IV bladder cancer final results. Proc Am Soc Clin Oncol 1992;11:210.

46. Passalcqua R, Cocconi G, Macaluso G et al. M-VAC versus the same combination using epirubicin at double dose in locally invasive bladder cancer: a prospective study. Proc Am Soc Clin Oncol 1992;11:210.

47. Sternberg CN, de Mulder PHM, van Oosterom AT, Fossà SD, Giannarelli D, Soederman JR. Escalated M-VAC chemotherapy and recombinant human granulocyte-macrophage colony-stimulating factor (rhGM-CSF) in patients with advanced urothelial tract tumours. Ann Oncol 1993;4:403–407.

48. Logothetis C, Finn LD. Escalated MVAC with or without recombinant human granulocyte-macrophage colony-stimulating factor for the initial treatment of advanced malignant urothelial tumours: results of a randomised trial. J Clin Oncol 1995;13:2272–7.

49. Moor MJ, Iscoe N, Tannock IF. A phase II study of methotrexate, vinblastine, doxorubicin and cisplatin plus recombinant human granulocyte-macrophage stimulating factors in patients with advanced transitional cell carcinoma. J Urol 1993;150:1131–1134.

50. Loehrer PJ, Elson P, Dreicer R, Hahn R, Nichols CR, Williams R, Einhorn LH. Escalated doses of methotrexate, vinblastine, doxorubicin and cisplatin plus recombinant human granulocyte colony stimulating factor in advanced urothelial cancer: an Eastern Co-operative Oncology Group trial. J Clin Oncol 1994;12:483–488.

51. Richards B, Bastable JRG, Freedman L et al. Adjuvant chemotherapy with doxorubicin (adriamycin) and 5-fluorouracil in T3, Nx, M0 bladder cancer treated with radiotherapy. Br Urol 1983;55:386–391.

52. Shearer RJ, Chilvers CED, Bloom HJG et al. Adjuvant chemotherapy in carcinoma of the bladder. A prospective trial preliminary report. Br J Urol 1988;62:558–564.

53. Wallace DMA, Raghavan D, Kelly KA et al. Neo-adjuvant (pre-emptive) cisplatin therapy in invasive transitional cell carcinoma of the bladder. Br J Urol 1991;67:608–615.

54. Martinez-Pineiro JA, Martin MG, Arocena F et al. Neoadjuvant cisplatin therapy before radical cystectomy in invasive transitional cell carcinoma of the bladder: CUETO study 84005. In: Villavicenio H, Fair WR (eds) Societé International d'Urologie Reports: Evaluation of chemotherapy in bladder cancer. Churchill Livingstone, Edinburgh, 1992; pp. 103–108.

55. Studer VE, Hering F, Jaeger P et al. Adjuvant cisplatin chemotherapy following cystectomy for bladder cancer (SAKK 09/84). J Urol 1991;145:335A (abstract).

56. Logothetis CJ, Johnson DE, Chong C et al. Adjuvant cyclophosphamide, doxorubicin and cisplatin chemotherapy for bladder cancer: an update. J Clin Oncol 1988;6:1590–6.

57. Fradet Y, Chin JL, Carrier S et al. Adjuvant MVAC after radical cystectomy for invasive bladder cancer. J Urol 1992;147:446A (abstract).

58. Skinner DG, Daniels JR, Russell CA et al. The role of adjuvant chemotherapy following cystectomy for invasive bladder cancer: a prospective trial. J Urol 1991;145:459–467.

59. Stockle M, Meyenburg W, Wellek S et al. Advanced bladder cancer (stages pT3b, pT4a,pN1 and pN2): improved survival after radical cystectomy and three adjuvant cycles of chemotherapy. Results of a controlled prospective study. J Urol 1992;148:302–307.

60. Freiha FS, Reese J, Torti F. A randomised trial of radical cystectomy versus radical cystectomy plus cisplatin, vinblastine, and methotrexate chemotherapy for muscle invasive bladder cancer. J Urol 1996;155:495–500.

61. Studer UE, Bacchi M, Biedermann C et al. Adjuvant cisplatin chemotherapy following cystectomy for bladder cancer: results of a prospective randomised trial. J Urol 1994;152:81–84.

62. Droller MJ. Adjuvant chemotherapy following cystectomy for invasive bladder cancer. J Urol 1991;145:465 (Editorial).

63. Raghavan D. Adjuvant chemotherapy following cystectomy for invasive bladder cancer. J Urol 1991;145:465 (Editorial).

64. Raghavan D, Shipley WU, Hall RR and Ritchie JP. Biology and management of invasive badder cancer. In: Raghavan D, Scher HI, Leibel SA and Lange P (eds) Principles and practice of genitourinary oncology. Phildelphia: Lippincott- Raven, 1996.

65. Roberts JT, Hall RR. The role of chemotherapy in the treatment of bladder cancer. In: Neal DE (Ed.) Tumours in urology. London. Springer-Verlag, 1994, pp. 80–90.

66. Howard GCW, Cornbleet MA, Whillis D et al. Neoadjuvant chemotherapy with methotrexate and cisplatin prior to radiotherapy for invasive transitional carcinoma of the bladder. Assessment of feasibility and toxicity. Br J Urol 1991;68:490–494.

67. Fossà SD, Harland SJ, Kaye SB et al. Initial combination chemotherapy with cisplatin, methotrexate and vinblastine in locally advanced transitional cell carcinoma of the bladder – response rate and pitfalls. Br J Urol 1992;70:161–168.

68. Roberts JT, Fossà SD, Richards B et al. Results of a medical research council phase II study of low dose cisplatin and methotrexate in the primary treatment of locally advanced (T3 and T4) transitional cell carcinoma of the bladder Br J Urol 68:162–168.

69. Seidman AD, Scher HI. The evolving role of chemotherapy for muscle-infiltrating bladder cancer. Sem Oncol 1991;18:585–595.

70. Hall RR for MRC advanced bladder cancer working party et al. Neo-adjuvant CMV chemotherapy plus cystectomy and or radiotherapy in muscle-invasive bladder cancer: first analysis of an MRC/EORTC intercontinental collaborative trial. Proc Asco 1996;15:244. Abstr 612.

71. Malmström P-U, Rintala E, Wahlqvist R et al. Five year follow-up of a prospective trial of radical cystectomy and neoadjuvant chemotherapy: Nordic cystectomy trial I. J Urol 1996;155:1903–1906.

71a. Malmström P-U, Rintala E, Wahlqvist R et al. Neoadjuvant cisplatin-methotrexate chemotherapy of invasive bladder cancer. Nordic Cystectomy Trial 2. Eur Urol 1999;35(Suppl 2):60 (Abstr 238).

72. Abol-Enoin H, E1-Mekresh M, E1-Bar M, Ghonheim MA. Neo adjuvant chemotherapy in treatment of invasive transitional bladder cancer: a controlled prospective randomised study. Br J Urol 1997;80(Suppl 2):49, 191 (Abstract).

73. Soquet Y. Combined surgery and adjuvant chemotherapy with high-dose methotrexate and folinic acid rescue (HDMTX-CF) for infiltrating tumours of the bladder. Br J Urol 1981;53:439–443.

74. Hall RR, Newling DW, Ramsden PD, Richards B, Robinson MR, Smith PH. Treatment of invasive bladder cancer by local resection and high dose methotrexate. Br J Urol 1984;56:668–672.

75. Martinez-Pineiro JA, Jiminez L, Martinez-Pineiro L Jr. Aggressive TURB combined with systemic chemotherapy for locally invasive TCC of the urinary bladder. Eur J Cancer 1991;27(Suppl 2): 5104 (Abstract 605).

76. Nogueira March JL (1991) Radical TUR and M-VAC in the treatment of infiltrating bladder tumours. Proceedings of the 22nd Congress, Societé Internationale d'Urologié, Seville, Spain. (Abstract 215).

77. Amiel J, Quintens H, Thyss, Caldani, C, Schneider M, Toubol J. Combination transurethral resection and systematic chemotherapy as primary treatment

of infiltrating bladder tumour (pT2-pT4 Nx,M0). [Fre. Eng Abs] *J Urol* (Paris) 1985;**94**:333–336.

78. Hatcher PA, Hahn RG, Richardson RL, Zincke H. Neoadjuvant chemotherapy for invasive bladder carcinoma: disease outcome and bladder preservation and relationship to local tumour response. *Eur Urol* 1994;**25**:209–215.

79. Herr HW, Scher HJ. Neoadjuvant chemotherapy and partial cystectomy for invasive bladder cancer. *Cancer Treat Res* 1992;**59**:99–103.

80. Housset M, Maulard C, Chretien Y *et al.* Combined radiation and chemotherapy for invasive transitional cell carcinoma of the bladder; a prospective study. *J Clin Oncol* 1993;**11**:2150–2157.

81. Kaufman DS, Shipley WU, Griffin PP, Heney NM, Althausen AF, Efird JT. Selective bladder preservation by combination treatment of invasive bladder cancer. *N Eng J Med* 1993;**329**:1377–1382.

82. Tester W, Porter A, Absell S, Coughlin C, Heaney J, Krall J *et al.* Combined modality programme with possible organ preservation for invasive bladder carcinoma: results of RTOG protocol 85–12. *Int J Radiat Oncol Biol Phys* 1993;**25**:783–790.

83. Coppin C, Gospodarowicz MK, Keith J *et al.* Improved local control of invasive bladder cancer by concurrent cisplatin and preoperative or definitive radiation. *J Clin Oncol* 1996;**14**:2901–2907.

84. Stadler W, Kuzel T, Roth B, Raghavan D, Dorr A. Phase II study of single-agent gemcitabine in previously untreated patients with metastatic urothelial cancer. *J Clin Oncol* 1997;**15**:3394–3398.

85. McCaffrey JA, Hilton S, Mazumdar M *et al.* A phase II trial of ifosfamide, paclitaxel and cisplatin (ITP) in patients with transitional cell carcinoma. *Proc ASCO* 1997;**16**:324a (Abstract 1154).

86. Roth BJ, Finch DE, Birhle R *et al.* A phase II trial of ifosfamide + paclitaxel in advanced transitional cell carcinoma of the urothelium. *Proc ASCO* 1997;**16**:324a (Abstract 1156).

87. Stadler W, Murphy B, Kaufman D, Raghavan D, Voi M. Phase II trial of gemcitabine plus cisplatin in metastatic uroyhelial cancer. *Proc ASCO* 1997;**16**:323a (Abstract 1152).

88. von der Maase H, Anderson L, Crino L, Weissbach L, Dogliotti L. A phase II study of gemcitabine and cisplatin in patients with metastatic transitional cell carcinoma of the urothelium. *Proc ASCO* 1997;**16**:324a (Abstract 1155).

7.5 Radiotherapy in the management of bladder cancer

J T Roberts

Radiotherapy is an established technique for the radical treatment of muscle invasive bladder cancer. It offers a viable organ-conserving alternative to radical cystectomy. There are no adequate, modern, randomized comparisons of radiotherapy and surgery. However, when allowance is made for selection bias in single center studies, radiotherapy produces comparable survival figures to cystectomy. Selection bias for radiotherapy, as opposed to cystectomy, was apparent in the recently published report of a large, multi-national, randomized investigation of the role of neoadjuvant chemotherapy in muscle-invasive bladder cancer. Patients receiving radiotherapy generally were of poorer performance status than those undergoing a cystectomy[1].

Modern techniques involve the use of CT planned radiotherapy. Treatment is given over a four to seven week period using three or more fields to deliver a high dose to the bladder and a 1.5 to 2 cm safety margin. There is a clear dose-response relationship[2,3] The majority of patients will experience mild to moderate short-term urinary and bowel symptoms. With modern radiotherapy only a small minority of patients will experience significant long term toxicity. The prejudice that the use of radical radiotherapy is associated with long term distressing bowel symptoms appears not to be founded[4,5]. It would appear that even the irradiated urinary bladder functions better than a surgically constructed neo-bladder. Following radical radiotherapy 50–70% of patients obtain a complete response. A number of these will subsequently relapse, either with a recurrence of the original tumor or with development of a second transitional cell carcinoma within the intact bladder. Any patient not cured by radiotherapy will require a salvage cystectomy. The morbidity of salvage cystectomy after radical radiotherapy is somewhat greater than in the unirradiated patient. There is controversy over the possibility of bladder reconstructive surgery following radical radiotherapy. However, reports of successful bladder reconstruction following radical pelvic radiotherapy exist.

Patient selection for radiotherapy will have an effect upon outcome. There are contra-indications to radiotherapy, such as inflammatory bowel disease, extensive prior pelvic surgery, previous radiotherapy or severe irritative bladder symptoms. There are other relative contraindications to radiotherapy such as the presence of concomitant carcinoma in situ, a large primary tumor[6,7,8] or ureteric obstruction[9,10]. The ability to achieve a full transurethral resection has also been associated a favourable outcome after radiotherapy[11,12].

The acute and long term morbidity of pelvic radiotherapy is decreased by the use of modern, computer-based, treatment planning and delivery. It has been demonstrated that 3D conformal radiotherapy results in a reduced incidence of acute and of long term side effects[13].

A number of approaches have been used in an attempt to improve the results of radiotherapy. These have included alteration of traditional radiotherapy fractionation, attempts to overcome hypoxia and, recently, investigation of chemo-radiotherapy.

Following observations that breaks in treatment are associated with impaired outcome and that bladder cancers may have a short potential doubling time accelerated fractionation has been explored with a suggestion of improved local control in a pilot Phase II study. Despite this promising data, a recently completed randomized trial comparing 60.8 Gy in 32 fractions, treating twice daily with standard treatment of 64 Gy in 34 daily fractions failed to show any improvement in local control while at the same time showing an enhancement of acute toxicity.

Transitional cell carcinoma of the bladder is a tumor in which hypoxia has been shown to be clinically important. Twelve trials, including more than 700 patients, have studied the effects of modifying hypoxia, either with hyperbaric oxygen or hypoxic cell sensitizers. These trials show an overall trend for an improvement associated with modification of hypoxia, despite a low efficacy of sensitization. After head and neck cancer bladder cancer seems to be the second most promising site for hypoxic modification. A recently published Phase II study of Carbogen (95% O2, 5% CO2), delivered during radiotherapy showed a significant improvement in local control, disease free survival and overall survival for patients treated with radiotherapy and Carbogen when compared with a historical control group. This regimen (ARCON) is now being tested in a multi-center Phase III study in the UK and Europe.

The acute toxicity of radiotherapy for bladder cancer is dominated by urinary dysfunction. Retrospective studies have shown that the side effects of radical bladder radiotherapy are directly related to the volume irradiated. Interstitial radiotherapy, using radioactive implants inserted into the bladder at the time of surgery has produced good local control rates with a favourable toxicity profile. A small pilot study at the Royal Marsden Hospital has demonstrated that reducing the high dose volume in selected patients may reduce bladder toxicity. This approach is to be tested in a Phase III study (Huddart R personal communication). If it can be demonstrated that toxicity is reduced by a reduction of the high dose volume the next step would be, as with prostate cancer, to escalate the dose to the reduced volume in the hope of improving local control.

Attempts to improve outcomes for muscle invasive bladder cancer by the addition of neoadjuvant or adjuvant chemotherapy to standard, radical, local treatment have proved disappointing. A number of phase II studies have examined the effect of concomitant chemotherapy on response rate and local control. The majority of those in which a platinum compound, either alone or in combination, was given concomitantly with radiotherapy show an increased local control rate, compared with historical controls. These results need to be treated with caution since at least one Canadian single center study appears to demonstrate that patient selection can have an equally strong effect on this measure of treatment outcome[14]. There is one randomized controlled study, comparing radiotherapy (+/− cystectomy) alone with radiotherapy with concomitant Cisplatin. This Canadian study demonstrated an improvement in response rate and local control for the chemo-radiotherapy group. No survival benefit was demonstrated. However, the study was small and was not powered reliably to detect even a 15% improvement in survival[15].

A number of clinical parameters can be used to select patients more likely to benefit from radical radiotherapy. These include performance status, haemoglobin concen-

tration, size of tumor, presence or absence of squamous differentiation, ureteric obstruction, presence of concomitant CIS and the ability, or otherwise, of the urologist to perform a complete transurethral resection of the tumor. Molecular techniques may allow the selection of those tumors which will best respond to radiotherapy and, hence, patients who should be directed towards this organ conserving technique. An alternative approach is to use the early response to chemotherapy and/or radiotherapy to select patients for organ conservation. Patients responding poorly are selected for early surgical salvage.

In summary, radiotherapy remains an important modality in the management of patients with muscle invasive bladder cancer. A number of alternative avenues are being evaluated which may improve further the therapeutic ratio for such patients. Selection, physical modification (3D CRT), altered fractionation, sensitization of hypoxic cells and chemo-radiotherapy are among these.

References

1. Neoadjuvant cisplatin, methotrexate, and vinblastine chemotherapy for muscle-invasive bladder cancer: a randomised controlled trial. International collaboration of trialists. *Lancet* 1999; **354**: 150–6.
2. Morrison R. The results of treatment of the bladder: a clinical contribution of radiobiology. *Clin Radiol* 1975; **76**: 67–78.
3. Parsons JT, Thar TL, Bova FJ, Million RR. An evaluation of split-course radiation for pelvic malignancies. *Int J Radiat Oncol Biol Phys* 1980; **6**: 175–81.
4. Lynch WJ, Jenkins BJ, Fowler CG, Hope-Stone HF, Blandy JP. The quality of life after radical radiothgerapy for bladder cancer. *Br J Urol* 1992; **70**: 519–521.
5. Mommsen S, Jakobsen A, Sell A. Quality of life in patients with advanced bladder cancer. A randomized study comparing cystectomy and irradiation–the Danish Bladder Cancer Study Group (DAVECA protocol 8201). *Scand J Urol Nephrol Suppl* 1989; **125**: 115–20.
6. Goffinet DR et al. Bladder cancer: results of radiation therapy in 384 patients. *Radiology* 1975; **117**: 149–53.
7. Van der Werf-Messing. Carcinoma of the urinary bladder category T3 Nx M0 treated by the combination of radium implant and external irradiation. *Int J Radiat Oncol Biol Phys* 1983; **9**: 177–80.
8. Yu WS, Sagerman RH, Chung CT, Dalad PS, King GA. Bladder cancer: experience with radical and pre-operative radiotherapy in 421 patients. *Cancer* 1985; **56**: 1293–9.
9. Greiner R, Skaleric C, Veraguth P. The prognostic significance of ureteral obstruction in carcinoma of the bladder. *Int J Radiat Oncol Biol Phys* 1977; **2**: 1095–100.
10. Pre-operative irradiation followed by cystectomy to treat carcinoma of the urinary bladder category T3NxM0. *Int J Radiat Oncol Biol Phys* 1983; **5**: 394–401.
11. Shipley WU, Rose MA, Perrone TL, Mannix CM, Heney NM, Prout GR Jr. Full-dose irradiation for patients with invasive bladder carcinoma: clinical and histological factors prognostic of improved survival. *J Urol* 1985; **134**(4): 679–83.
12. Megavoltage radiation for bladder carcinoma: alone, postoperative, or preoperative. 1973, Proceedings of the 7th national Cancer Conference. pp. 771–82. Lippincott, Philadelphia, PA.
13. Nutting C, Dearnaley DP, Webb S. Intensity modulated radiotherapy: a clinical review. *Br J Radiol* 2000; **73**: 459–469.
14. Gospodarowicz MK, Rider WD, Keen CW, Connolly JG, Jewett MA, Cummings BJ, Duncan W, Warde P, Chua T. Bladder-cancer long-term follow-up results of patients treated with radical radiation. *Clin Oncol (R Coll Radiol)* 1991; **3**(3): 155–61.

15.   Coppin CM, Gospodarawicz MK, Tannock IF, Zee B, Carson J, Pater J,
      Sullivan LD. Improved Local Control of invasive bladder cancer by
      concurrent cisplatin and preoperative or definitive radiation. The National
      Cancer Institute of Canada Clinical Trials Group. *J Clin Oncol*, 1996; **11**:
      2901–7.

Ad nocarcinoma of the bladder

J Catto & F C Hamdy

Adenocarcinoma of the bladder is a rare tumor with a poor prognosis. It is best divided into three types: primary tumors arising in the urachal remnant, primary non-urachal tumors and secondary tumors metastasizing from other viscera[1]. Whilst urachal and non-urachal tumors are both primary adenocarcinomas, they may have different etiologies, behaviors and modes of treatment, and so have historically been considered separately. Adenomatous regions can be found in transitional cell carcinomas, but these behave as transitional cell tumors[2] and are best treated as such.

Incidence

In 1992 there were 12 012 new bladder cancers registered in England and Wales[3]. The incidence of primary non-urachal adenocarcinoma comprises 0.5–2.0% of all bladder cancers[4–6]. The incidence increases in regions with endemic bilharzia, with 10% of bladder cancers in Egypt being adenocarcinomas[7–9]. Non-urachal adenocarcinoma is the commonest primary bladder tumor in exstrophic bladders[10]. Urachal adenocarcinomas are rarer, with an estimated annual incidence in the general population of one in 5 million[11] or 0.01% of all adult cancers[12]. They have been found to comprise either 1/1400[13], 0.17%[11] or 0.34%[14] of all bladder cancers. Secondary metastatic adenocarcinomas are much more common, comprising 50–88% of bladder adenocarcinomas[2,15,16].

Age and sex distribution

Most series have found differences in the populations affected by each tumor. Urachal tumors tend to affect younger patients (mean age 49 years)[8,10,15,17–19], with an equal sex distribution[8,19–21]. Non-urachal tumors affect older patients (mean age 61 years)[2,15,19,22,23], with a male preponderance (2–3:1 ratio)[15,17,19–23]. Metastatic tumors also affect the older patients (mean of 65 years[15]), with a male preponderance reflecting the importance of prostatic and colonic cancer.

Etiology and pathogenesis

Urachal adenocarcinomas are thought to arise by one of two methods[17,20]. Either previously arrested sequestrated primitive cloacal cells undergo neoplastic degeneration, or urothelial cells, which have kept the totipotential ability of primitive cloacal cells, undergo adenomatous metaplasia with malignant transformation. The former, while less accepted, would explain the younger patient age and the initial subepithelial growth that is typical of these tumors. The latter is more widely accepted and is similar to the theory proposed for non-urachal adenocarcinomas. Cases of urachal carcinoma in situ have been described[19,24], indicating a pre-invasive state exists.

It is believed that non-urachal adenocarcinomas are produced when unstable transitional cell epithelium undergoes metaplasia[25–29]. This occurs in response to chronic infection, irritation and obstruction[1,5,25,26,30,31]. This explains the association with exstrophic bladders[10,32], chronic urinary tract infections and bilharzia. Exstrophic bladders are known to have normal urothelium at birth, which is gradually replaced by glandular epithelium as a result of chronic inflammation[33]. Anderstrom et al.[34] found 10% of their cases had chronic UTIs prior to the development of adenocarcinoma. Mostofi[28] hypothesized two distinct methods of this transformation. Either hyperplastic epithelium invaginates into nests (von Brunn's), thus forming cystitis cystica with regions of the pre-malignant cystitis glandularis[26,30], or the metaplasia occurs in flat sheets along the bladder mucosa, without invagination of the cells.

Primary adenocarcinomas have been described in several augmented bladders[35]. These tumors usually occur either on the enterovesical anastomotic line or on the enteric mucosa. There is debate as to the actual significance of these cases. While it is accepted that urine mixed with stool, in the case of ureterosigmoidostomy, is carcinogenic[35], there is less evidence to show urine alone exerts a carcinogenic effect on bowel mucosa, and in 20 excised ileal conduits no dysplasia or pre-malignant features were found[36].

Metastatic adenocarcinoma usually occur by direct invasion of adjacent tumors. The commonest primary sites are colonic (53%), prostatic (39%) and from the female genital tract (8%)[16,22]. Hematogenous spread is much less common, although there are case reports of breast, stomach and pancreatic adenocarcinomas spreading to the bladder[37]. Klinger[38] found only 0.26% of metastatic cancers had secondary deposits only in the bladder. Renal adenocarcinomas have been described as metastasizing to the bladder via the urine[37].

Pathology

Primary adenocarcinomas are usually solitary tumors at presentation[27]. They are less inclined to multifocality and bladder mucosal recurrence than transitional cell tumors[34]. They are often poorly differentiated tumors[18,19,34]. Urachal and non-urachal adenocarcinomas can not be distinguished by histology alone, therefore criteria have been produced to classify them separately.

Non-urachal adenocarcinomas usually occur on the base (25–40%) or lateral walls (75%) of the bladder[15,17,22]. Macroscopically they are more often ulcerative and infiltrative (75–90%) than papillary (8–25%)[15–22]. They are mostly mucus secreting[20]. Microscopically Anderstrom[34] classified these tumors into five varieties: 1) glandular, not otherwise specified, 2) colloidal carcinoma, 3) papillary adenocarcinoma, 4) signet cell carcinoma and 5) clear cell carcinoma, with 1) and 3) being commonest and 4) and 5) rarest. However, there is little evidence that prognosis varies amongst these groups. The simplest and most useful classification is to divide them into those of signet ring cells (worse prognosis, which deposit their mucus intracellularly, hence they resemble a signet ring) and those secreting mucus (thought to have a slightly better prognosis)[2,16,18,19,34]. Usually the adjacent epithelium contains areas of glandular metaplasia[2,16] and a transition zone from normal urothelium to tumor is present[23].

Mostofi et al.[27] defined a urachal adenocarcinoma as one arising from the bladder dome (or rarely the anterior bladder wall) with no other primary bladder tumor present. There is an abrupt change in epithelium between the tumor and the adjacent urothelium, which should not contain glandular metaplasia. They arise intramurally and have deep ramifications into the bladder wall. They grow by invading deep into the bladder wall, into the perivesical fat in the retropubic space of Retzius, up to the umbilicus and even onto the anterior abdominal wall. At surgery 7% of tumors involve the umbilicus[20]. These tumors are always solid, not papillary, arising intramurally with the overlying epithelium initially appearing normal (hence the risk of a false negative cystoscopy) although ulceration does occur later.

Following the initial localized growth phase, there is intra-abdominal spread with peritoneal, mesenteric and small bowel metastases[18,21]. Recurrence post-surgery is most likely to be locally (51%) with 30% involving the regional nodes. Later, distant metastases spread to the lungs (23–40%), liver (14–37%) and skeleton (13–37%)[21,34].

Presentation and investigation

Usually adenocarcinoma of the bladder presents at an advanced stage with macroscopic hematuria (0–71%)[2,15,19,20,23,34]. Irritative bladder symptoms (i.e. urgency, frequency and dysuria) are also common. These symptoms are non-specific and may also occur in benign diseases, thus hindering diagnosis.

Metastatic and primary non-urachal adenocarcinomas often have irritative symptoms[19,23], lying on the bladder trigone, than urachal lesions. Urachal tumors, subepithelial and situated at the dome, are often silent until local invasion causes symptoms, therefore a suprapubic mass may be present at presentation[20]. Adenocarcinomas are usually mucus secreting and while mucousuria is a rare symptom, it suggests glandular epithelium, and always requires full investigation. Mucousuria often precedes hematuria while the tumor is still subepithelial. Rarely urachal carcinomas can present with a mucous or bloody discharge from the umbilicus. Metastatic tumors presented to the urologist do so with urinary symptoms. Hematuria and irritative symptoms are the commonest presenting complaints, but obstruction can occur with adenocarcinoma of the prostate[16].

Urine cytology may show abnormal cells in up to 50% of cases[15]. These abnormal cells may be diagnostic of primary or metastatic adenocarcinoma in 39%[37].

Urachal tumors are initially subepithelial. Therefore, both cystoscopy and contrast radiology (IVU) may give false negative results. Several authors have found 67–75% of IVUs performed at presentation may be normal[6,15,21]. Non-urachal adenocarcinomas more commonly grow as exophytic lesions, thus IVU and cystoscopy are more sensitive (100% abnormal IVU[6,15]). Whilst there are few specific diagnostic features of adenocarcinoma seen cystoscopically, up to 88% of examinations are abnormal[20]. Endoscopically these usually appear as infiltrative masses, possibly with a bloody discharge from a sinus; less commonly they are papillary exophytic lesions[18,20]. The diagnosis is usually confirmed when a transurethral biopsy shows adenocarcinoma. CT or MRI can then be used to help in staging. An examination under anesthetic is important to assess resectability. Most tumors have a residual mass after transurethral resection, hence stage T2 or T3.

It is important to distinguish primary from secondary adenocarcinomas. A full clinical evaluation should be made of all other possible primary sites. This should include the breasts, gastrointestinal and genital tracts. It can be difficult to differentiate a primary bladder tumor growing into the prostate and a primary prostate tumor growing into the bladder. Whilst a serum PSA, histology or imprint immunohistochemistry with antisera to PSA on the specimen can be diagnostic, 10–15% of poorly differentiated prostatic tumors will be negative for PSA[39]. Pantuck et al.[40] found the antibody 7E12H12 to differentiate the primary tumor with 100% specificity. Torenbeek et al.[41] found a panel of CEA, PSA, OC15 and vimentin antibodies applied to the specimen correctly diagnosed the source of the primary tumor in 70–91% of cases.

Grading and staging

The grading and staging classifications are similar for all bladder cancers. The previously accepted Jewett–Strong staging classification (A to D) has been replaced by the TNM classification devised by the International Union Against Cancer (UICC)[42]. The tumor stage varies between Ta and T4 depending upon invasion. Unlike transitional cell carcinomas most adenocarcinomas are at an advanced stage at the time of diagnosis. Most are muscle invasive (T2 or T3a) or have invaded the perivesical fat (T3b). Nodal and metastatic scores are calculated from the degree of spread.

Mostofi et al.[43] produced the most accepted tumor grading classification in 1973. A grade between I (well differentiated) and III (poorly differentiated) is assigned by the degree of anaplasia. A strong correlation exists between the tumor grade and stage at diagnosis. Most adenocarcinomas are moderately (II) or poorly (III) differentiated tumors.

Treatment

The rarity of these tumors has made it difficult to develop optimum treatment guidelines. There are no centers with sufficient incidence prospectively to randomize matched patients. Most published series have been collected over decades with different surgeons, pathologists, variable clinical records and historical controls. Several authors have reviewed the literature to assess treatment trends[2,8,15,18–21,34]. Surgery has remained the main stay of treatment in the majority of series. Mostly authors have separated urachal and non-urachal primary adenocarcinoma in the belief their treatment may be different.

Surgery for non-urachal primary adenocarcinoma

Radical cystectomy

Most authors are agreed that radical cystectomy should be performed for this disease, where possible. The tumors are usually located around the bladder base and therefore not accessible to segmental bladder resections. The largest single series by El-Mekresh et al.[8] has 185 primary adenocarcinomas, collected over 25 years, for which radical cystectomy and urinary diversion was performed. Most of their tumors were stage 3a (55%) and well differentiated (52%). They routinely perform a radical pelvic lymphadenectomy[44]. Their 5 year disease-free survival was 55% and is better than other published series, 19–30%/ 5 year[2,16,22,45]. It should be noted that they had a surprisingly high rate (52%) of well differentiated tumors; perhaps the endemic bilharzia changes the tumor profile. Whilst other series have shown less impressive cure rates, they have detailed a prolongation in survival time of several months[6,15,22]. This probably represents survival with recurrence by the removal of the possibility of death from bilateral ureteric obstruction.

Transurethral resection (TUR)

Usually this is the method of diagnosis. Several authors have shown that it is unsatisfactory as the main treatment modality, even with radiotherapy. Unless it is an early superficial tumor, there is little chance of successful clearance, hence the high recurrence and low survival rates[5,22,46]. TUR does have a role in palliation of symptoms in unresectable tumors.

Surgery for urachal primary adenocarcinoma

There is debate about which is the most appropriate surgical procedure for urachal adenocarcinomas. With respect to the umbilicus, most authors agree that en bloc excision of the urachal tract and umbilicus is necessary, although some advocate a margin of rectus sheath, peritoneum and anterior abdominal wall (20). With respect to the bladder there are two views, either partial bladder resection or radical cystectomy and urinary diversion.

Partial cystectomy

Whilst several series have shown improved survival with partial versus radical cystectomy[15,18,34,45] and Kakizoe's[21] review of 154 urachal tumors concluded that the best remission rates were produced by extended partial cystectomy, most authors advocate radical cystectomy. The poor survival rates for radical cystectomy in these series indicate a selected population with advanced disease at the time of surgery. Partial cystectomy can be recommended in an early well differentiated tumor. If a partial cystectomy is undertaken, due to the infiltrative nature of urachal adenocarcinomas, it is vital to perform adequate clearance. Abenoza and Gill[2,15] have advocated intra-operative frozen section histology of the margins to ensure complete removal. Others[6,20] have performed a salvage cystectomy in cases of positive tumor margins after partial cystectomy, with good results. Burnett and Sheldon[16,20] recommended partial cystectomy should not be used in cases of the aggressive signet ring and all poorly differentiated adenocarcinomas.

Radical cystectomy

Urachal adenocarcinomas are submucosal, intramurally infiltrative and invade locally into the perivesical tissues. After partial cystectomy 50% of recurrences occur locally, 18% in the bladder and 37% in the pelvic lymph nodes. These features make radical cystectomy seem a more logical cancer operation. Whilst Wilson[6] found radical cystectomy leads to improved cure rates, few other published series have done so. Most authors believe that the better results of partial cystectomy in most series reflects patient selection, and results could be improved further with radical surgery to this population[19]. Mostofi et al.[19] found urachal carcinoma had a worse prognosis than non-urachal carcinoma, perhaps reflecting the widespread practice of radical surgery in the latter group. The authors of the two largest reviews[20,21] both advocate radical cystectomy in their conclusions.

Radiotherapy

Radiotherapy has been used extensively in the literature. Whilst some authors have used it on advanced inoperable tumors, with little effect[5,15,20,22,23], others have used it as an adjunct to surgery[5,22]. Most authors have found no improvement in survival and conclude that bladder adenocarcinomatous cells are not radiosensitive and therefore there is little use for radiotherapy[5,15,22]. Signet cell tumors are known to be particularly radioresistant[16,20]. However, there are a few case reports of good results with radiotherapy[47], which justify further investigation of this modality. In Kakizoe's[21] review adjuvant radiotherapy was associated with shorter survival than no radiotherapy, perhaps reflecting patient selection.

Chemotherapy

As with radiotherapy there have been no randomized trials with chemotherapy and bladder adenocarcinoma. Logothetis[48] looked at eight cases of advanced metastatic disease. Little response was found to cisplatin-based chemotherapy, however five of eight responded to doxorubicin, mitomycin-C and 5-fluorouracil (5-FU), with one in complete remission at 9 months. Nevin[49], in 1974, commented that three-quarters of adenocarcinomas have some response to 5-FU. Hatch[50] reported a case of metastatic colon adenocarcinoma successfully treated by 5-FU. However, most authors have not found a reproducible significant benefit from adjuvant chemotherapy.

Metastatic secondary adenocarcinomas

Most metastatic tumors are often beyond curative treatment at diagnosis. Locally invasive tumors may be suitable to en bloc excision and pelvic exenteration, in the hope of cure. The aim of treatment in most cases will be palliative. Limited TUR resection or diathermy may be used to limit hemorrhage. Fistulas can be controlled with catheterization. Rarely, cystectomy can be used to palliate severe irritative symptoms in the younger patient. However, it must be remembered that the patient's best interests may be to do the minimum needed to return some quality of life.

Colon

Gill[15] treated four of 12 patients with colonic resection and total cystectomy to good effect (all alive at 3 years), while those treated by partial cystectomy faired less well, with only three of 12 patients alive at 18 months. Burnett[16] had similar results with colonic resection and either total and partial cystectomy, all with radiotherapy.

Prostate

The disease at presentation is metastatic and therefore not suitable to radical surgery. Most groups have tried either hormonal manipulation or radiotherapy to control the disease[15,16] with little success, only one in 14 of the described patients alive at 2 years. The only 5 year survivor had a radical cystoprostatectomy, despite having a Gleason sum 9 tumor.

Female genital tract

Several ovarian tumors have been described as invading the bladder[15,16]. Both radiotherapy and surgery have been used as treatment. In the surgical case a partial cystectomy was combined with a bilateral salpingo-oophorectomy, however the patient was lost from follow up. Most cervical and uterine tumors described have been treated with hysterectomy and local bladder resection, with poor results.

Prognosis

The combination of a poorly differentiated tumor and a late presentation lead to a poor prognosis. The best results have been achieved with radical surgery in well differentiated tumors, 55% 5 year survival[8]. Mostofi[28] suggested that the prognosis was worse than a stage and grade matched transitional cell carcinoma, Wilson et al.[6] confirmed this when they compared the 3 year survival rates (TCC 62% versus adeno. 48%). Most series have found 5 year survival rates between 0% and 61%[2,8,17,19,22,23,34], actual disease free rates are thought to be lower. Prognosis does not seem to vary consistently between matched urachal and non-urachal primary adenocarcinomas, although urachal tumors often present later. Several large series have shown stage and grade of the tumor to be the most accurate predictors of prognosis[2,8,17,19,22,23,34]. Kramer et al.[22] found those with Stage A disease to have a 67% 5 year survival, compared with 8–20% 5 year survival for stage D. El-Mekresh et al.[8] found lymph node status to be an independent prognostic indicator, 60% versus 12% 5 year survival. Signet cell tumors have been found universally to have a poorer prognosis.

Conclusions

Bladder adenocarcinoma has a poor prognosis. It presents non-specifically and the diagnosis may be missed until too late. Primary and secondary tumors must be correctly distinguished as their treatments differ widely. Radical surgery appears to offer the best hope of cure, although in a well differentiated, localized urachal tumor a partial cystectomy may be adequate. Future trials should be organized to assess the best treatment of urachal tumors and the role of adjuvant therapy.

References

1. Wheeler JD, Hill WT. Adenocarcinoma involving the urinary bladder. *Cancer* 1954;**7**:468–476.
2. Abenoza P, Manivel C, Fraley EE. Primary adenocarcinoma of urinary bladder. *Urology* 1987;**39**:9–14.
3. Cancer statistics registration. Office of National Statistics. Series MB1; No. 25: 1998.
4. Thomas DG, Ward AM, Williams JL. A study of 32 cases of adenocarcinoma of the bladder. *Br J Urol* 1972;**42**:4–15.
5. Malek R, Rosen J, O'Dea M. Adenocarcinoma of the bladder. *Urology* 1983;**21**:357–359.
6. Wilson TG, Rand Pritchett T, Lieskovsky G et al. Primary adenocarcinoma of the bladder. *Urology* 1991;**38(3)**:223–226.
7. Ghoneim MA, El-Mekresh MM, El-Baz MA et al. Radical cystectomy for carcinoma of the bladder: critical evaluation of the results in 1,026 cases. *J Urol* 1997;**158(2)**:393–399.
8. El-Mekresh MM, El-Baz MA, Abol-Enein H et al. Primary adenocarcinoma of the urinary bladder: a report of 185 cases. *Br J Urol* 1998;**82**:206–212.
9. El-Bolkainy MN, Ghoneim MA, Mansour MA et al. Carcinoma of the bilharzial bladder in Egypt: clinical and pathological features. *Br J Urol* 1972;**44**:561–570.
10. Culp DA. The histology of the extrophied bladder. *J Urol* 1964;**91**:538–548.
11. Ohman U, von Garrelts B, Moberg A. Carcinoma of the urachus. Review of the literature and report of two cases. *Scand J Urol Nephrol* 1971;**5**:91.
12. Cornil C, Reynolds CT, Kickham CJE. Carcinoma of the urachus. *J Urol* 1967;**98**:93.
13. Beck AD, Gaudin HJ, Bonham DG. Carcinoma of the urachus. *Br J Urol* 1970;**42**:555.
14. Yu HHY, Leong LH. Carcinoma of the urachus: report of one case and a review of the literature. *Surgery* 1974;**77**:726.
15. Gill HS, Dhillon HK, Woodhouse CRJ. Adenocarcinoma of the urinary bladder. *Br J Urol* 1989;**64**:138–142.
16. Burnett AL, Epstein JI, Marshall FF. Adenocarcinoma of urinary bladder: classification and management. *Urology* 1991;**37**:315–321.
17. Bennett JK, Wheatley JK, Walton KN. 10-year experience with adenocarcinoma of the bladder. *J Urol* 1984;**131**:262–263.
18. Kamat MR, Kulkarni JN, Tongaonkar HB. Adenocarcinoma of the bladder: study of 14 cases and review of the literature. *Br J Urol* 1991;**68**:254–257.
19. Grignon DJ, Ro JY, Ayala A et al. Primary adenocarcinoma of the urinary bladder. A clinicopathologic analysis of 72 cases. *Cancer* 1990;**67**:2165–2172.
20. Sheldon CA, Clayman RV, Gonzalez R et al. Malignant urachal lesions. *J Urol* 1984;**131**:1–8.
21. Kakizoe T, Matsumoto K, Andoh M et al. Adenocarcinoma of the urachus. *Urology* 1983;**21**:360–366.
22. Kramer SA, Bredael J, Crocker BP et al. Primary non-urachal adenocarcinoma of the bladder. *J Urol* 1979;**121**:278–281.
23. Jones WA, Gibbons RP, Correa RJ et al. Primary adenocarcinoma of bladder. *Urology* 1980;**15**:119–122.
24. Paul AB, Hunt CR, Harney JM et al. Stage 0 mucinous adenocarcinoma in situ of the urachus. *J Clin Pathol* 1998;**51(6)**:483–484.
25. Allen TD, Henderson BW. Adenocarcinoma of the bladder. *J Urol* 1965;**93**:50–56.
26. Shaw JL, Gislason GJ, Imbriglia JE. Transition of cystitis glandularis to primary adenocarcinoma of the bladder. *J Urol* 1958;**79**:815.
27. Mostofi FK, Thompson RV, Dean AL. Mucous adenocarcinoma of the urinary bladder. *Cancer* 1955;**8**:741–758.
28. Mostofi FK. Potentialities of bladder epithelium. *J Urol* 1954;**71**:705–714.
29. Patch FS, Rhea LJ. The genesis and development of Brunn's nests and their relation to cystitis, cystitis glandularis and primary adenocarcinoma of the bladder. *Canad Med Ass J* 1935;**33**:597.
30. Kittredge WE, Henthorne JC, Whitehead M. Glandular metaplastic malignancy in the urinary tract: report of four cases. *J Urol* 1947;**58**:282.
31. Darcia PJ, MacKenzie F, Reed RJ et al. Primary adenovillous carcinoma of the bladder. *J Urol* 1976;**115**:41.
32. O'Kane HOJ, Megaw JMcI. Carcinoma in the exstrophied bladder. *Br J Surg* 1968;**55**:631.
33. Formiggini B. Contributo allo studio istologico della mucosa vesicale extrofica. *La Riforma Medica* 1920;**36**:252–254.
34. Anderstrom C, Johansson SL, von Schultz L. Primary adenocarcinoma of the urinary bladder. A clinicopathologic and prognostic study. *Cancer* 1983;**52**:1273–1280.
35. Filmer RB, Spencer JR. Malignancies in bladder augmentations and intestinal conduits. *J Urol* 1990;**143**:671–676.
36. Deane AM, Woodhouse CRJ, Parkinson MC. Histological changes in ileal conduits. *J Urol* 1984;**132**:1108.
37. Bardales RH, Pitman MB, Stanley et al. Urine cytology of primary and secondary urinary bladder adenocarcinoma. *Cancer* 1998;**84(6)**:335–343.
38. Klinger ME. Secondary tumours in the genito-urinary tract. *J Urol* 1951;**42**:555.
39. Gallee MPW, Visser-de-Jong E, van der Korput JAGM et al. Variation of prostate specific antigen expression in different tumour growth patterns in prostatectomy specimens. *Urol Res* 1990;**18**:181–187.

40. Pantuck AJ, Murphy DP, Amenta PS *et al.* The monoclonal antibody 7E12H12 can differentiate primary adenocarcinoma of the bladder and prostate. *Br J Urol* 1998;**82(3)**:426–430.
41. Torenbeek R, Lagendijk JH, Van Diest PJ *et al.* Value of a panel of antibodies to identify the primary origin of adenocarcinomas presenting as bladder carcinoma. *Histopathology* 1998;**32**:20–27.
42. Harmer MH. *Classification of malignant tumours* (3rd edn). International Union Against Cancers (UICC), Geneva, 1978:**113**.
43. Mostofi FK, Sobin LH, Torloni H. *Histological typing of urinary bladder tumours.* International Histological Classification of Tumours, no. 10. World Health Organisation, Geneva.
44. Ghoneim MA, El-Hammady SM, El-Bolkainy MN *et al.* Radical cystectomy for carcinoma of bilharzial bladder. Technique and results. *Urology* 1976;**8**:547–552.
45. Dandekar NP, Dalal AV, Tongaonkar HB *et al.* Adenocarcinoma of bladder. *Eur J Surg Oncol* 1997;**23(2)**:157–160.
46. Loening SA, Jacobo E, Hawtrey CE *et al.* Adenocarcinoma of the urachus. *J Urol* 1978;**119(1)**:68–71.
47. Jakse G, Schneider HM, Jacob GH. Urachal signet ring cell carcinoma, a rare variant of vesical adenocarcinoma: incidence and pathological criteria. *J Urol* 1978;**120**:764.
48. Logothetis CJ, Samuels ML, Ogden S. Chemotherapy for adenocarcinomas of bladder and urachal origin: 5-Fluorouracil, doxorubicin and mitomycin-C. *Urology* 1985;**26**:252–255.
49. Nevin JE *et al.* Advanced carcinoma of the bladder: treatment using hypogastric arterial infusion with 5-Fluorouracil, either as a single agent or in combination with bleomycin or adriamycin and supervoltage radiation. *J Urol* 1974;**112**:752.
50. Hatch TR, Fuchs EF. Intra-arterial infusion of 5-Fluorouracil for recurrent adenocarcinoma of bladder. *Urology* 1989;**33**:311–312.

9 Squamous tumors of the urinary bladder

M A Ghoneim

Squamous cell tumors can develop either in non-bilharzial or bilharzial bladders. The incidence, epidemiology and possibly the natural history of these two subpopulations are different; therefore, it is scientifically safer to discuss them independently.

Squamous cell carcinoma in the non-bilharzial bladder

Primary squamous cell carcinoma in non-bilharzial bladders is uncommon. Out of 1500 cases collected in the Bristol Bladder Tumour Registry, 24 were documented as squamous tumors (1.6%)[1]. Johnson and associates reviewed the records of 2010 patients with bladder tumors and found squamous tumors in 90 (4.5%)[2]. In Glasgow, 119 out of 3889 patients with bladder tumors were reported to have squamous cell carcinoma, an incidence of (3%)[3].

The disease presents relatively more often in female patients than transitional cell carcinoma. The reported male/female ratio varies from 1.25:1 to 1.8:1[1–3]. Because urinary tract infection is more common in women, a relation between squamous metaplasia, leukoplakia and the development of squamous cell carcinoma was proposed by Connery[4] and Holly and Mellinger[5]. In a series of 20 patients with long-standing leukoplakia, O'Flynn and Mullaney observed the development of five cases of squamous carcinoma[6]. Although these observations suggest an association between squamous metaplasia and squamous carcinoma, other studies indicate that the tumor arises more frequently from normal transitional epithelium[2,3,7].

Clinically, these tumors are usually solitary and are invariably invasive at the time of diagnosis. A correlation of the clinical and the pathologic stage of the disease usually reveals a tendency for understaging of the pathologic extent of the disease[7].

Miller and colleagues described the tumor as a viciously malignant one showing little response to treatment[1]. The reported results after treatment by definitive external irradiation are uniformly poor[3,8]. Surgical treatment appears to provide a better therapeutic yield. Richie and associates reported 5 year survival in 12 out of 33 patients treated by radical cystectomy[7]. Partial cystectomy also produced relatively good results. Sarma reported a 5 year survival of (50%) in eight patients[9]. Utz and colleagues reported a 5 year survival of 25% in 20 patients[10]. These results, however should be interpreted with extreme caution because they represent a highly selected category of cases.

Johnson and co-workers employed integrated pre-operative radiation therapy followed by cystectomy and reported a 5 year survival of 34%[2]. Swanson and colleagues reported their results using the same approach[11]. The actuarial overall survival rate was 50% at 5 years. Survival correlated to the stage of the disease and was highest among patients with a T_2 disease. Furthermore, survival was better for patients whose tumors were down staged by pre-operative radiation than for those who showed no downstaging.

Although it appears that integrated pre-operative radiation therapy followed by cystectomy offers the best chances of cure for such cases, because the tumor is rare, only a few cases are available for study. It would be extremely difficult to conduct well controlled prospective studies to achieve objective conclusions.

Squamous cell carcinoma in the bilharzial bladder

Carcinoma of the urinary bladder contributed to 27.6% of all cancer cases treated at the Cancer Institute of Cairo University[12]. It is the most common solid tumor occurring in men in Egypt. A causal relation between urinary bilharziasis and cancer of the bladder was first reported by Fergusson[13], and has since been supported by studies from Egypt[14], Zimbabwe[15] and Iraq[16,17].

There is good evidence from animal models that the biogenesis of bladder cancer is a multistage phenomenon that involves initiation by a carcinogen followed by promotion and propagation of tumor growth by other factors, which need not be carcinogenic[18]. Bilharzial bladder cancer may be initiated by exposure to an environmentally or locally produced chemical carcinogen that excreted in urine reacts with the mucosal surface of the bladder to produce an irreversible and potentially carcinogenic change in the DNA of some urothelial cells. Chronic bacterial infection, commonly complicating urinary bilharziasis, has been implicated in the production of nitrosamines, well known and potent carcinogens, from their precursors in urine[19,20]. Mechanical irritation of the urothelium by the erupting bilharzial eggs then encourages tumor growth into clinically detectable masses.

Clinicopathological features

The association of bladder cancer with urinary bilharziasis determines a distinct clinico-pathological behavior. The peak age incidence is between the third and fifth decades[13,21]. The male/female ratio is 4:1, the average age of incidence is 46.7 years in men and 46.3 years in women[21].

Presentation is frequently with symptoms of cystitis, painful micturition, frequency and hematuria. Urography usually reveals an extensive irregular filling defect in its cystographic phase. The diagnosis depends upon cystoscopy, biopsy and careful bimanual examination under anesthesia.

The disease usually presents when in an advanced stage, and 25% of cases when first seen may be considered inoperable[21]. It is probable that late presentation is due to the overlapping of symptoms of simple bilharzial cystitis with early malignant cystitis. In a study by Ghoneim and colleagues, the results of clinical staging were compared with the pathologic findings in 135 cases[22]. The clinical error in this study was 37.2% with a tendency for underestimation of the extent of the disease. Various factors may contribute to this clinical understaging: 1) certain sites were

difficult to palpate, such as tumors of the vault or anterior wall; 2) endoscopic biopsy was performed to establish the diagnosis but not to evaluate the depth of muscle infiltration; and 3) the regional lymph nodes were inaccessible for clinical assessment. In this series, most tumors were in an advanced stage, with infiltration of deeper muscles in 56.3% of cases, and extravesical spread in 12.8%.

Grossly, the tumors are generally of the nodular fungating type and occupy the vault, posterior or lateral walls of the bladder. Histologically, two-thirds of cases show evidence of squamous cell carcinoma, most of low-grade malignancy. Careful examination of cystectomy specimens revealed the presence of multicentric lesions in 22% of cases, and associated squamous metaplasia in 65%[23].

The frequency of lymph node involvement and distant metastasis is relatively low. In cases treated by radical cystectomy, the incidence of lymph node metastases varied from 15% to 17%[22,24].

In an autopsy series distant metastasis were encountered in only 3%[25]. Similar low figures were reported after radical cystectomy by El-Sebai[13] and Ghoneim and colleagues[26].

This tendency to slow and late dissemination may be due to the extensive mural fibrosis in addition to the low-grade malignancy of carcinoma in the bilharzial bladder. Other factors, undefined, related to tumor behavior or host response, may also play a role.

Treatment
Conservative resection
Endoscopic resection In view of the bulk and advanced stage of these tumors, transurethral resection is inappropriate for definitive treatment, and there are no reports on results with the procedure in bilharzial bladder malignancy. Endoscopic resection is limited to obtaining biopsy material for histopathological diagnosis and evaluation.

Segmental resection The physiological and social inconvenience of urinary diversion, the inevitable loss of sexual potency, and the relatively high mortality of radical cystectomy, render segmental resection an attractive alternative. Local resection is only feasible in certain conditions: 1) if the tumor is solitary, does not involve the trigone, and its size allows excision with an adequate safety margin, and 2) if the rest of the bladder is free of any associated pre-cancerous lesion. Few patients with carcinoma of the bilharzial bladder satisfy these conditions. Of 190 patients with clinically resectable bladder cancer, only 19 (10%) were judged suitable for segmental resection in a series reported by El-Hammady and colleagues[27]. Augmentation cystoplasty was required to supplement residual bladder capacity in five of these patients. The post-operative mortality was 5% and the 5 year survival was 26.5%. Patients with low-grade tumors on histology had roughly double the survival rate of those with high-grade tumors. On the other hand, less favorable results were reported by Omar in a series of 22 cases[28]. Follow up data were only available in 14 cases and all but one patient developed recurrence within 2 years. The discrepancy in these reported results probably reflects a wide variability in selection criteria.

Radical cystectomy

In view of the pathology and natural history of the disease, radical cystectomy and some form of urinary diversion provides the logical surgical approach to most cases with resectable tumors[24,26]. The extent of operation in these studies was to remove the bladder, perivesical fat, peritoneal covering, the prostate, seminal vesicles and distal common iliac, internal iliac and external iliac lymph nodes. In the women, the bladder, urethra, uterus and upper two-thirds of the vagina with the pelvic cellular tissue and the aforementioned lymph nodes are removed.

In a series of 138 cases, Ghoneim and associates reported a post-operative mortality of 13.7%[26]. The main causes of fatality in the post-operative period were peritonitis and adhesive intestinal obstruction. Cardiovascular and pulmonary complications were uncommon among this relatively young group of patients. The 5 year direct survival was 32.6%. An analysis of survival data relative to the tumor stage and grade showed a 5 year survival of 43% in patients with superficial tumor (P_1 and P_2) and of 30% in patients with deeply infiltrating tumors (P_3, P_4). Similarly, low-grade tumors showed better survival (46%) than high-grade ones (21%). Involvement of the regional lymph nodes reduced the probability of 5 year survival to 20%. It was also observed that most treatment failures were due to local recurrences in the pelvis which developed within 24 months after cystectomy.

Based on these data, Ghoneim and associates concluded that an operation alone, despite being radical, was inadequate to deal with the extent of the pathology[29]. Accordingly, they suggested that adjuvant treatment directed to the pelvis might improve survival and proposed pre-operative radiation therapy as a logical approach.

Radiation Therapy

The growth characteristics of carcinoma of the bilharzial bladder have been studied to evaluate its potential radio-responsiveness[30]. Two growth features were disclosed: 1) a relatively high cell mitotic rate corresponding to a potential doubling time of 6 days and 2) an extensive cell loss factor. Tumors with such growth character-

istics are expected to exihibit a prompt radiation response[31].

Nevertheless, early experiences with external beam therapy for definitive control of these tumors were disappointing[32]. Two sets of factors interfered with the efficiency of radiation treatment in these cases: 1) coexisting bilharzial urologic lesions interfere with the local tissue tolerance, and 2) the probability of local tumor control is reduced as a result of their considerable bulk. Furthermore, the presence of a substantial population of radio-resistant hypoxic tumor cells is suspected in view of the capillary vascular pattern of this cancer[33].

Adjuvant pre-operative radiation

Problems related to large tumor volumes do not pertain to pre-operative radiation. In this setting the aim of radiation treatment is to sterilize smaller cell burdens in the deep infiltrating parts of the tumor as well as microextensions into the perivesical tissues and lymphatics. Such foci are expected to have a better radiation response because they are more highly oxygenated and are composed of a relatively small number of cells with a high mitotic index.

Motivated by these biologic factors and by the fact that most of the treatment failures after radical cystectomy were due to local recurrences, trials using pre-operative radiation therapy have been implemented in a number of Egyptian centers. Awaad and associates compared the results of cystectomy after pre-operative administration of 4000 cGy of irradiation with a control group treated by cystectomy only[34]. The reported 2 year survival rates demonstrated significant improvement in the irradiated group. In another randomized trial, Ghoneim and colleagues compared the results of cystectomy after pre-operative irradiation using 2000 cGy rad with those of cystectomy only[35] (Table 9.1). The post-operative mortality and morbidity were similar in both groups. Patients were followed up for 60 months. Although patients who received pre-operative radiations had better survival rates, this improvement did not approach statistical significance. Survival data were further correlated to some pathological features of the tumor (Table 9.2). With low-stage tumors and irrespective of grade, survival appeared to be uninfluenced by pre-operative irradiation. On the other hand, patients with high-stage tumors in whom pre-operative radiation was used, improved survival was noted in each grade category.

This concentrated regimen of pre-operative irradiation has the potential advantage of being applicable on a large scale because the required logistics are fairly simple. Nevertheless, the expected therapeutic value with such a concentrated regimen may be compromised by the presence of a large proportion of hypoxic cells. This could, in

Table 9.1   Five year survivals

	Cystectomy	2000 Rad and cystectomy
Total number	49	43
Died post-operatively	5	4
Died from disease	17	14
Died cause unknown	3	4
Living with disease	7	4
Unfollowed	1	0
Free of disease $\geq$ 5 year	16	17
% Survival	32	39

Table 9.2   Five year survival relative to the pathologic stage and grade

	Cystectomy	2000 rad and cystectomy
Superficial disease (P1 + P2):		
Low grade	9/13	5/10
High grade	1/02	2/03
Infiltrating disease (P3 + P4):		
Low grade	6/21	7/13
High grade	0/10	2/08
Metastatic disease		
Low grade	0.01	0.03
High grade	0/02	1/06

Table 9.3   Comparison of five year survival

	Cystectomy	2000 rad and cystectomy	Misonidazole cystectomy 2000
Total number	35	34	28
Died post-operatively	–	–	–
Died from disease	1	2	0
Died cause unknown	11	4	7
Living with disease	9	8	4
Unfollowed	–	–	–
Free of disease $\geq$ 5 years	14	20	17
% Survival	40	58	60

Chemotherapy

Several chemotherapeutic agents have been evaluated in bladder cancer patients at the Cancer Institute of Cairo University. All these were phase II trials using a single agent. The most promising results were obtained with epirubicin[37]. Clinical trials with this agent as a neoadjuvant chemotherapy was started in patients with T_3 lesions. Evaluation of these trials is not completed at this date.

Conclusions

Radical cystectomy with some form of urinary diversion still remain the cornerstone in the treatment of squamous cell carcinoma of the bladder. Pre-operative irradiation offers some advantages to a certain subpopulation of patients. Adjuvant chemotherapy is still under investigation. Efforts must be directed toward early detection of this tumor to improve the therapeutic yield of the available treatment modalities. Urine cytology shows promising results in the screening of rural populations at high risk in endemic bilharzial areas. In a screening campaign involving three villages around Mansoura, 3366 people were examined with urine cytology, carcinoma was detected in seven, all of whom were farmers 20 years of age or older (a yield value of two per 1000 population). Of these, four tumors were at an early stage of development (PIS and PI). Recently cytokeratin shedding in urine was used as a possible biological marker for early detection of squamous tumors[38]. Cytokeratins in urine were measured using an enzyme-linked immunosorbent assay with promising results. Early detection of patients with bladder cancer may improve the results of existing methods of treatment or allow the adoption of fewer radical surgical procedures with their attending social stigma and functional handicap.

part, explain the modest improvements after this regimen. In an attempt to enhance the therapeutic value of this short-course high-dose radiation treatment, misonidazole, a hypoxic cell sensitizer, was given before the delivery of the radiation regimen. Patients eligible for cystectomy were randomized into three treatment groups: 1) cystectomy only, 2) 2000 cGy of pre-operative radiation followed by cystectomy, or 3) 2000 cGy of pre-operative radiation and misonidazole followed by radical cystectomy. Misonidazole was given orally in a dose of 2 g/m^2 3 hours before radiation treatment. According to Denekamp and colleagues, an enhancement ratio of 1.7 is expected after this regimen[36].

The 5 year survival of this trial is outlined in Table 9.3. The addition of misonidazole did not provide any additional benefit to patients receiving pre-operative irradiation. There was no difference of statistical significance among the three treatment groups although the survival figures of patients receiving pre-operative radiation with or without misonidazole were better than those treated by cystectomy only. Improvements in survival figures over the previous trial were largely due to elimination of post-operative fatalities.

References

1. Miller A, Mitchell JP, Brown NN. The Bristol Bladder Tumour Registry. *Br J Urol* 1969;**52**:511.
2. Johnson DE, Schoenwald MB, Ayala AG, Miller LS. Squamous cell carcinoma of the bladder. *J Urol* 1976;**115**:542.
3. Rundle JSH, Hart AJL, McGeorge A, Smith JS, Malcolm AJ, Smith PM. Squamous cell carcinoma of bladder. A review of 114 patients. *Br J Urol* 1982;**54**:522.
4. Connery DB, Leukoplakia in the urinary bladder and its association with carcinoma. *J Urol* 1953;**69**:121.
5. Holly PS, Mellinger GT. Leukoplakia of the bladder and carcinoma. *J Urol* 1961;**86**:235.
6. O'Flynn JD, Mullaney J. Vesical leukoplakia progressing to carcinoma. *Br J Urol* 1974;**46**:31.
7. Richie JP, Waisman J, Skinner DG, Dretler SP. Squamous carcinoma of the bladder: treatment by radical cystectomy. *J Urol* 1976;**115**:670.
8. Bessette PL, Abell MR, Herwig KR. A clinicopathologic study of squamous cell carcinoma of the bladder. *J Urol* 1974;**112**:66.
9. Sarma KP. Squamous cell carcinoma of the bladder. *Internat Surg* 1970;**53**:313.
10. Utz DC, Schmitz, SE, Fugelso PD, Farrow GM. A clinico-pathological evaluation of partial cystectomy for carcinoma of the urinary bladder. *Cancer* 1973;**11**:1075.
11. Swanson DA, Liles A, Zagars GK. Pre-operative irradiation and radical cystectomy for stages T_2 and T_3 squamous cell carcinoma of the bladder. *J Urol* 1990;**143**:37.
12. El-Sebai I, El-Bolkainy MN, Hussein MH. Cancer Institute Registry. *Med Cairo Univ* 1973;**41**:175.
13. Fergusson AR. Associated bilharziasis and primary malignant diseases of the urinary bladder with observations on a series of 40 cases. *J Pathol Bacteriol* 1991;**16**:76.
14. El-Sebai I. Cancer of the bladder in Egypt. Kasr-El-Aini. *J Surg.* 1961;**2**:180.
15. Gelfand M, Weinberg RW, Castle WM. Relation between carcinoma of the bladder infestation with *Schistosoma haematobium*. *Lancet* 1967;**i**:1249.
16. Shamma AH. Schistosomiasis and cancer in Iraq. *Am J Clin Pathol* 1955;**52**:1283.
17. Halawani A, Al-Waidh M, Said SM. Serology in the study of relationship between *Schistosoma haematobium* and cancer of the urinary bladder. *Br J Urol* 1970;**42**:580.
18. Hicks RM. Multistage carcinogenesis in the urinary bladder *Br Med Bull* 1980;**36**:39.
19. Hicks RM, Walters CL, El-Sebai I, El-Aaser AA, El-Merzabni MM, Gough TA. Demonstration of nitrosamines in human urine: Preliminary observations on a possible aetiology for bladder cancer in association with chronic urinary tract infections. *Proc Roy Soc Med* 1977;**70**:413.
20. El-Merzabani MM, El-Aaser AA, Zakhary NT. A study on the etiological factors of bilharzial bladder cancer in Egypt. Nitrosamines and their precursors in urine. *Eur J Cancer* 1979;**15**:287.
21. El-Bolkainy MN, Ghoneim MA, Mansoura MA. Carcinoma of the bilharzial bladder in Egypt. Clinical and pathological features. *Br J Urol* 1972;**44**:561.
22. Ghoneim MA, Mansour MA, El-Bolkainy MN. Staging of carcinoma of the bilharzial bladder. *Urology* 1974;**3**:40.
23. Khafagy MM, El-Bolkainy MN, Mansour MA. Carcinoma of the bilharzial urinary bladder. A study of the associated lesions in 86 cases. *Cancer* 1972;**30**:150.
24. Ghoneim MA, Awaad HK. Results of treatment in carcinoma of the bilharzial bladder. *J Urol* 1980;**123**:850.
25. Mohamed AS. Association of bilharziasis and malignant disease in urinary bladder, pathogenesis of bilharzial cancer in the urinary bladder. *J Egypt Med Assn* 1954;**37**:1066.
26. Ghoneim MA, Ashamallah AG, Hammady S, Gaballah MA, Soliman HS. Cystectomy for carcinoma of the bilharzial bladder: 138 cases 5 years later. *Br J Urol* 1979;**51**:541.
27. El-Hammady SM, Ghoneim MA, Hussein ES, Ashamallah AG, El-Bolkainy MN. Segmental resection for carcinoma of the bladder. *Mansoura Med Bull* 1975;**3**:191.
28. Omar SM. Segmental resection for carcinoma of the bladder. *Egypt Med Assn* 1969;**52**:975.
29. Ghoneim MA, El-Bolkainy MN, Mansour MA, El-Hammady SM, Ashamallah AG. Radical cystectomy for carcinoma of the bilharzial bladder: Technique and results. *Urology* 1977;**51**:541.
30. Awad HK, Hegazy M, Ezzat S, El-Bolkainy MN, Burgers MV. Cell proliferation of carcinoma in bilharzial bladder: an autoradiology study. *Cell Tissue Kinetics* 1979;**12**:513.
31. Denekamp J. The relationship between the cell loss factor and the immediate response to radiation in animal tumours. *Eur J Cancer* 1972;**8**:118.
32. Awaad HK. Radiation therapy in bladder cancer. *Alex Med J Cancer* 1958;**4**:118.
33. Omar AH, Shalaby MA, Ibrahim AH. On the capillary vascular bed in carcinoma of the urinary bladder. *East Afr Med J* 1975;**51**:34.
34. Awaad HK, Abdel Baki H, El-Bolkainy N, Burgers MV, El-Badawi S, Mansour M. Pre-operative irradiation of t3-carcinoma in bilharzial bladder. *Int J Radiation, Oncol, Biol Phys* 1979;**5**:787.
35. Ghoneim MA, Ashamallah AK, Awaad HK, Whitmore WF. Randomized trial of cystectomy with or without pre-operative radiotherapy for carcinoma of the bilharzial bladder. *J Urol* 1985;**134**:266.
36. Denekamp J, McNally NJ, Fowler JF, Joiner MC. Misonidazole in fractionated radiotherapy. Are many small fractions best? *Br J Radiol* 1980;**53**:981.
37. Gad El-Mawla N, Hamza MR, Zikri Z Kh, El-Serafi M, El-Khodary A, Khaled H, Abdel-Wareth A. Chemotherapy in invasive carcinoma of the bladder. A review of phase II trials in Egypt. *Acta Oncologica* 1989;**28**:73.
38. Basta MT, Attallah AM, Seddek MN, El-Mohamady H, Al-Hilaly ES, Atwaan N, Ghoneim MA. Cystokeratin shedding in urine: a biological marker for bladder cancer. *Br J Urol* 1988;**61**:116.

PART TWO
Prostate cancer

Chapter 10
Epidemiology and etiology

Chapter 11
The natural history

Chapter 12
Pathology

Chapter 13
Presentation and diagnosis

Chapter 14
Staging

Chapter 15
Treatment of early organ-confined disease

15.1 Issues and options: patient and tumor factors

15.2 Watchful-waiting

15.3 Prostate cancer treatment: radical prostatectomy for early organ-confined disease

15.4 Radiotherapy for organ-confined prostate cancer

Chapter 16
Treatment of locally advanced disease

16.1 Hormonal downstaging: myth or reality?

16.2 Surgery: Is there a rationale?

16.3 Radiation Therapy

16.4 Locally advanced prostate cancer - hormonal treatment

Chapter 17
Treatment of metastatic prostate cancer

17.1 Endocrine therapy

17.2 Immediate versus deferred treatment

17.3 Radiation therapy

17.4 Strontium[89] in metastatic disease

17.5 The use of bisphosphonates in prostate carcinoma metastatic to the skeleton

17.6 The role of monoclonal antibody imaging in the management of prostate cancer

17.7 Chemotherapy in patients with androgen independent prostate cancer

Chapter 18
Management of sequelae, voiding dysfunction and renal failure

10 Epidemiology and etiology

D W Keetch

Incidence

Adenocarcinoma of the prostate is the most common non-cutaneous malignancy in American men. Over the past several years, the incidence of prostate cancer has increased dramatically. In the United States, an estimated 198 100 men will be diagnosed with prostate cancer in 1998 and it will account for 31 500 deaths[1]. Combining the projected incidence rates with the aging population of the United States, Carter and Coffey[2] have estimated a 90% increase in the total number of prostate cancers diagnosed between the early 1980s and the year 2000. The lifetime risk that a man will develop clinical prostate cancer has been estimated to be between 9.5% and 12.5%[3]. Across the world, the incidence of clinical prostate cancer varies widely from country to country. It is relatively high in North American and Northern European countries, intermediate in Southern European, Central and Southern American countries and low in Asian countries[5].

The rising estimates of prostate cancer incidence in the United States (number of new cases diagnosed) must be viewed with caution. New evidence suggests that the incidence of prostate cancer may have peaked and is beginning to decline. Stephenson *et al.*[4] reported that the Utah Tumor Registry (one of nine participating Surveillance, Epidemiology and End Results [SEER] Program registries) had recorded a rise in age-adjusted prostate cancer incidence from 116.9 per 100 000 in 1985 to 235.5 per 100 000 in 1992. However, the age-adjusted prostate cancer incidence in 1993 had fallen significantly to 180.3 per 100 000. Stanford and associates[6] analysed the trends in prostate cancer incidence in the Seattle-Puget Sound region (also a SEER participant). They found that the age-adjusted incidence of prostate cancer increased an average of 3.4% per year between 1974 and 1984. After 1984, the incidence began to rise dramatically and peaked in 1991 with an overall age-adjusted rate of 459 per 100 000 men. Following this peak in 1991, the rate began to decline and, by 1993, the rate was 34% lower than that observed in 1991.

This rise and subsequent fall in prostate cancer incidence may be due to several factors but the most important one is the increased prostate cancer detection secondary to the use of serum PSA testing. The widespread use of serum PSA testing initially resulted in more cases of prostate cancer. However, as men with prostate cancer were identified and culled from the population, the pool of remaining individuals with detectable prostate cancer became smaller, resulting in fewer cases and a lower prostate cancer incidence. This phenomenon has been observed in screening studies at Washington University where during the third and fourth years of repetitive PSA evaluation, cancer detection rates are similar to those observed for age-matched men in the pre-PSA era. Moreover, when using a currently accepted definition of a histologically significant cancer (i.e. one that is larger than 0.5 cc and Gleason sum 5 or greater) the large majority of cancers detected during the second, third and fourth years of screening are significant tumors. Based on these considerations, the widespread use of PSA based screening does not appear to have 'manufactured' a prostate cancer epidemic.

Prevalence

The exact prevalence of prostate cancer remains difficult to quantify. Numerous autopsy studies have demonstrated a high prevalence of prostate cancer in men who die from other causes. The presence of microscopic prostate cancer is age dependent. In a review of eight autopsy studies, Coley and colleagues[7] found the overall prevalence of prostate cancer to increase with decade of life. Fifteen per cent of men aged 50 to 59 years, 22% of men 60 to 69 years, 39% of men 70 to 79 years and 43% of men older than 80 years demonstrate foci of prostate cancer. Overall, it is estimated that 30% of men older than 50 years with no clinical evidence of prostate cancer will harbor microscopic foci of disease[8]. Although the clinical incidence of cancer of the prostate varies from country to country, the frequency of microscopic cancer of the prostate at autopsy is remarkably similar. By age 80, approximately 60% to 70% of men have evidence of histologic prostate cancer[9–14]. Even though difficult to quantity, the overall higher incidence of prostate cancer (compared with other cancers) combined with the prevalence of sub-clinical disease occurring at autopsy allows one to implicate prostate cancer as the most prevalent non-cutaneous malignancy in men.

Mortality

As the incidence of prostate cancer has increased so has the mortality rate, albeit at a slower rate. Prostate cancer is currently the second leading cause of cancer death among American men and has risen from 32 378 prostate cancer deaths in 1990 to an estimated 39 200 in 1998[1]. The lifetime probability that a man will die as a result of prostate cancer is estimated to be 3% to 4.5%[3]. Carter and Coffee have estimated a 37% increase in prostate cancer related deaths among American men between the early 1980s and the year 2000[2]. The average lifeyears lost due to premature death from prostate cancer is an estimated 9 years[15,16]. The prostate cancer death rate is higher among African-American men compared with Caucasian men[1]. The likelihood of a white American man dying of prostate

cancer was 2% in 1975, 2.3% in 1980 and 2.6% in 1985 compared with 2.6%, 3.4% and 4.3%, respectively, for African-American men[3]. In addition, the death rates from clinical prostate cancer vary dramatically from country to country (Figure 10.1). Asian countries have the lowest death rates while the Scandinavian countries have the highest.

Risk factors

Race and nationality

Racial differences in the incidence and mortality rates of prostate cancer have been well described. The highest incidence rates in the world occur among African-American men while the lowest rates occur among mainland Chinese[1,17]. African-American men are more likely to develop prostate cancer, more often present with advanced disease and more often die as a result of the prostate cancer when compared with white American men[18]. Data from the SEER programme reveals that African-American men living in the United States have a higher incidence rate of clinical prostate cancer than do white men of similar socioeconomic and educational status[19]. There is a relatively low incidence of prostate cancer among Hispanic groups[20] and Orientals[21] while the incidence is relatively high among Scandinavian men. It is unclear if the differences in the incidence and mortality rates for prostate cancer from country to country are due to racial or environmental factors or a combination of both. However, migration studies have shown that men tend to take on the incidence of their host country[22,23]. This fact, combined with the similar histologic prevalence of prostate cancer among different nationalities suggests that environmental factors play a significant role in the transition of occult to clinical prostate cancer.

Dietary fat

The amount of dietary fat consumed appears to be a significant risk factor for the development of clinical prostate cancer. The diet of Japanese men has a much lower fat content than that of men in the United States correlating with the lower incidence of clinical prostate cancer in Japanese men compared with American men. Rose and associates[24] found that prostate cancer death rates from different countries were significantly related to total dietary fat intake and that the association was limited to animal fat and not vegetable fat intake. Giovannucci et al.[25] reported that the increased risk for prostate cancer was primarily due to animal fat and the strongest association was with red meat intake. The relative risk for developing prostate cancer in men with high dietary fat intake has been reported to be 1.6 to 1.9[26,27].

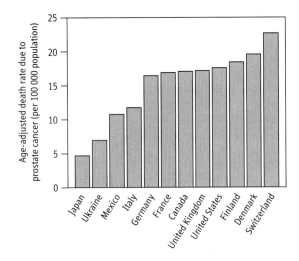

Fig. 10.1 Age-adjusted death rates due to prostate cancer. (From Greenlee and associates[1])

Vitamins

The results of studies relating vitamin deficiency or excess with prostate cancer have been mixed. Vitamin A excess has been implicated in increasing the risk for prostate cancer[28,29]. These studies must be interpreted with caution, however, as vitamin A from plant sources may decrease the risk while vitamin A from animal sources may increase the risk[30]. Whether the increased risk is actually due to excess vitamin A or due to higher levels of animal fat intake remains to be determined.

Lower levels of vitamin D, which has potent antitumor properties, may increase the risk for prostate cancer. Hanchette and Schwartz[31] reported that geographic areas with the highest sunlight exposure have the lowest frequency of prostate cancer. They suggest that this may be due to the effect of vitamin D on human prostate cancer cells. They also suggest that a lower rate of vitamin D synthesis in the skin of African-American men may be linked to the higher rates of prostate cancer in this population.

Hormone status

Several factors point to a role for testosterone in the development of prostate cancer. Testosterone and its main metabolite, dihydrotestosterone, are the principal hormones regulating the normal growth and function of the prostate[32,33]. Prostate cancer rarely develops in castrated men and prolonged administration of high levels of testosterone has induced prostate cancer in rats[34]. Some human studies have documented elevated serum testosterone levels in prostate cancer patients compared with normal controls[35-37]. Other studies, however, have found no difference in circulating testosterone levels in men with prostate cancer compared with controls[38,39]. Ross and associates[40] found that African-American men had serum testosterone levels that were 15% higher than that of white counterparts and have suggested that this difference is sufficient to explain the increased risk for prostate cancer in African-American men.

Vasectomy

It has been suggested that vasectomy may increase the risk for prostate cancer. Sidney[41] followed 5332 vasectomized men, each matched with three non-vasectomized controls, and found no increased risk for prostate cancer in men who had undergone vasectomy. Other studies have also shown no association between vasectomy and prostate cancer[42-44]. However, in men having undergone vasectomy, Mettlin and associates[45] reported a relative risk of 1.7 for developing prostate cancer. Giovannucci et al. have also reported a positive association between vasectomy and prostate cancer. In a prospective study, 10 055 vasectomized men showed a relative risk of 1.85 over 37 800 non-vasectomized men for developing prostate cancer[46]. In a retrospective analysis[47,] a relative risk of 1.56 was associated with vasectomy.

Currently, the available data are insufficient to determine if vasectomy causes an increased risk for prostate cancer. In addition, no plausible mechanism has been established. Because of this, current recommendations advocate no change in the use of vasectomy for sterilization[48].

Occupation

No strong associations exist between environmental factors and prostate cancer although several have been implicated. Cadmium is a trace mineral found in cigarette smoke and alkaline batteries and may be antagonistic to zinc in the prostate gland[49]. Most data suggest that cadmium exposure may increase the risk for prostate cancer[50].

In a review of the literature, Blair and Zahm[51] reported a positive association between farming and prostate cancer. The proposed mechanism is the exposure to pesticides and herbicides.

Prospective studies have demonstrated a positive association between smoking and prostate cancer with relative risks ranging from 1.5 to 2[52,53]. Most studies, however, show no such association[50,54].

Benign prostatic hyperplasia

The association between benign prostatic hyperplasia (BPH) and prostate cancer remains unclear. Studies by Armenian et al.[55] and Mishina and colleagues[56] have found that men with a diagnosis of BPH have an increased relative risk for developing prostate cancer. However, Greenwald et al.[57] found no association between BPH and prostate cancer. It has been, and will most likely remain, difficult to determine whether BPH is a risk factor for prostate cancer because both are such common entities in elderly men.

Sexual activity and marital status

Several studies have investigated the relationship between sexual practices and prostate cancer. Early age at onset of sexual activity, increased number of sexual partners, frequency of sexual activity, and extramarital sexual relations have all shown a possible association with prostate cancer[58-60]. Studies have shown mixed results with regard to marital status and the risk for prostate cancer.[61,62] Overall, it remains unclear if sexual activity has any relationship to prostate cancer risk.

Viral factors

The association between infectious agents and prostate cancer remains unclear. One study showed that men with prostate cancer had higher titers of herpes virus and cytomegalovirus[63]. Other studies have shown no association between sexually transmitted diseases and prostate cancer[64,65]. None of the studies to date have used current viral technology and as such, this issue should be revisited.

Family history

Several studies have demonstrated a clustering of prostate cancer cases in certain families[60,66–71]. Between 13 and 26% of prostate cancer probands have at least one other affected male relative[67,68,70]. Familial prostate cancer is the simple clustering of disease within families. Hereditary prostate cancer is believed to be a subtype of familial prostate cancer, and is characterized by either three successive generations being affected with the disease, a clustering of three or more men with prostate cancer in a nuclear family, or two men with early age at onset of disease (younger than 55 years) in the same family. The hereditary form of prostate cancer has been reported to comprise only 5% to 6% of all prostate cancer cases[67,70]. It usually occurs 10 years earlier than sporadic prostate cancer, and is believed to be transmitted in a Mendelian pattern of inheritance by a highly penetrant, autosomal dominant gene[72]. It is also believed to account for 43% of all early onset prostate cancers[71,72].

Clinical and pathologic analysis has revealed few differences between cases of hereditary prostate cancer and sporadic prostate cancer in men undergoing radical prostatectomy[73,74]. However, these pathologic changes occur at earlier ages in men with hereditary prostate cancer. Germline DNA alterations in genes involved in cellular growth and differentiation that control the promotion and/or inhibition of aberrant cellular growth are most likely the basis for this early expression of disease in these select cases. Carter and associates[75] examined allelic loss in prostate cancer specimens and found that 54% of clinically localized cancers and 100% of metastatic tumors showed loss of heterozygosity on at least one chromosome, with chromosomes 10q and 16q demonstrating the highest frequency of mutation. Environmental factors may or may not influence these apparent genetic abnormalities. Further studies characterizing possible genetic aberrations are needed.

Conclusions

Prostate cancer has become and will most likely remain the most common non-cutaneous malignancy among men. The mortality rate from prostate cancer has also demonstrated a steady rise, albeit at a slower pace compared with incidence. Given the similar prevalence rates of prostate cancer at autopsy, environmental factors most likely play a significant role in the development of many cases of prostate cancer, although a straightforward explanation of the etiology of prostate cancer does not exist. Further epidemiologic research is needed for a better understanding of the role of environmental factors in the development of prostate cancer with the hope of providing prevention strategies. Cases of hereditary prostate cancer may be due to a specific genetic abnormality, the delineation of which may provide further insight into the cause of sporadic prostate cancer in general.

References

1. Geenlee RT, Hill-Harmon MB, Murray T, Thur M. Cancer Statistics, 2001. CA 2001; **51**:15.
2. Carter HB, Coffey DS. The prostate: An increasing medical problem. *Prostate* 1990;**16**:39.
3. Seidman H, Mushinski MH, Gelb SK et al. Probabilities of eventually developing or dying of cancer: United States. *Cancer* 1985;**35**:36.
4. Stephenson RA, Smart CR, Mineau GP, James BC, Janerich DT, Dibble RL. The fall in incidence of prostate carcinoma. On the down side of a prostate specific antigen induced peak in incidence – Data from the Utah Cancer Registry. *Cancer* 1996;**77**:1342.
5. Catalona WJ. Prostate cancer. *Curr Prob Surg* 1990;**27**:389.
6. Stanford JL, Wicklund KG, Blumenstein BA, Brawer MK. The changing epidemiology of prostate cancer in the Seattle-Puget Sound region, 1974–1993. *J Urol* 1995;**153**:504A.
7. Coley CM, Barry MJ, Fleming C, Wasson JH, Fahs MC, Oesterling JE. Should Medicare provide reimbursement for prostate-specific antigen testing for early detection of prostate cancer? Part II: Early detection strategies. *Urol* 1995;**46**:125.
8. Scardino PT, Weaver R, Hudson MA. Early detection of prostate cancer. *Hum Pathol* 1992;**23**:211.
9. Andrews GS. Latent carcinoma of the prostate. *J Clin Pathol* 1954;**2**:197.
10. Lundberg S, Berge T. Prostate carcinoma: an autopsy study. *Scand J Urol Nephrol* 1970;**4**:93.
11. Holund B. Latent prostatic cancer in a consecutive autopsy series. *Scan J Urol Nephrol* 1980;**14**:29.
12. Oota K. Latent carcinoma of the prostate among the Japanese. *Acta Un Int Cancer* 1961;**17**:952.
13. Halpert B, Sheehan E, Schmalhorst W, Scott R. Carcinoma of the prostate: A survey of 5000 autopsies. *Cancer* 1963;**16**:737.
14. Yamabe H, ten Kate FJ, Gallce MP, Schroeder FH, Oisha K, Okada K et al. Stage A prostatic cancer: a comparative study in Japan and the Netherlands. *World J Urol* 1986;**4**:136.
15. Kramer BS, Brown ML, Prorok PC, Potosky AL, Gohagan JK. Prostate cancer screening: what we know and what we need to know. *Ann Intern Med* 1993;**119**:914.
16. Horm JW, Sondik EJ. Person-years of life lost due to cancer in the United States, 1970 and 1984. *Am J Public Health* 1989;**79**:1490.
17. Waterhouse J, Muir C, Shaumugaratnam K. Cancer incidence in five continents. In: *Cancer incidence*. Lyon, France: International Agency for Research in Cancer 1982; publication 42, Vol. 6.
18. Morton RA. Racial differences in adenocarcinoma of the prostate in North American men. *Urology* 1994;**44**:637.
19. Bauet CR, Horm JW, Gibbs T, Greenwald P. Socioeconomic factors and cancer incidence among Blacks and whites. *J Natl Cancer Inst* 1991;**83**:551.
20. Menck HR, Henderson BE, Pike MC et al. Cancer incidence in the Mexican-American. *J Natl Cancer Inst* 1975;**55**:531.
21. Fraumeni JR Jr, Mason TJ. Cancer mortality among Chinese-Americans, 1950–1969. *J Natl Cancer Inst* 1974;**52**:659.

22. Meikle AW, Smith JA. Epidemiology of prostate cancer. *Urol Clin North Am* 1990;**17**:709.

23. Haenszel W, Kuriboro M. Studies of Japanese migrants. *J Natl Cancer Inst* 1968;**40**:43.

24. Rose DP, Boyar AP, Wynder EL. International comparisons of mortality rates for cancer of the breast, ovary, prostate and colon, and per capita food consumption. *Cancer* 1986;**58**:2363.

25. Giovannucci E, Rimm EB, Colditz GA, Stampfer MJ, Ascherio A, Chute CC, Willett WC. A prospective study of dietary fat and risk of prostate cancer. *J Natl Cancer Inst* 1993;**85**:1571.

26. Graham S, Haughey B, Marshall J, Priore R, Byers T, Rzepka T *et al.* Diet in the epidemiology of carcinoma of the prostate gland. *J Natl Cancer Inst* 1983;**70**:687.

27. West DW, Slattery JL, Robison LM, French TK, Mahoney AW. Adult dietary intake and prostate cancer risk in Utah: a case-control study with special emphasis on aggressive tumors. *Cancer Causes Control* 1991;**2**:84.

28. Kolonel LN, Yoshizawa CN, Hankin JH. Diet and prostate cancer: a case-control study in Hawaii. *Am J Epidemiol* 1988;**127**:999.

29. Heshmat MY, Kaul L, Kovi J, Jackson MA, Jackson AG, Jones GW *et al.* Nutrition and prostate cancer: a case-control study. *Prostate* 1985;**6**:7.

30. Mettlin C, Selenskas S, Natarajan N, Huben R. Beta-carotene and animal fats and their relationship to prostate cancer risk. A case-control study. *Cancer* 1989;**64**:605.

31. Hanchette CL, Schwartz GG. Benign and malignant neoplasms of the prostate. Geographic patterns of prostate cancer mortality: Evidence for a protective effect of ultraviolet radiation. *JAMA* 1993;**269**:1328.

32. O'Malley BW. Mechanism of action of steroid hormones. *N Engl J Med* 1971;**284**:370.

33. Wilson JD. Recent studies on the mechanism of action of testosterone. *N Engl J Med* 1972;**287**:1284.

34. Noble RL. The development of prostatic adenocarcinoma in NB rats following prolonged sex hormone administration. *Cancer Res* 1977;**37**:1929.

35. Hovenian MS, Deming CL. The heterologous growth of cancer of the human prostate. *Surg Gynecol Obstet* 1948;**86**:29.

36. Ghanadian R, Puah CM, O'Donoghue EPN. Serum testosterone and dihydrotestosterone in carcinoma of the prostate. *Br J Cancer* 1979;**39**:696.

37. Drafta D, Proca E, Zamfir V, Schindler AE, Neacsu E, Stroe E. Plasma steroids in benign prostatic hypertrophy and carcinoma of the prostate. *J Steroid Biochem* 1982;**17**:689.

38. Wright F, Poizat R, Bongini M, Bozzolan F, Doukani A, Mauvais-Jarvis P. Decreased urinary 95 α-androstane-3α, 17β-diol flucuronide excretion in patients with benign prostatic hyperplasia. *J Clin Endocrinol Metab* 1985;**60**:294.

39. Hammond GL, Kontturi M, Vihko R. Serum steroids in normal males and patients with prostatic diseases. *Clin Endocrinol* 1978;**9**:113.

40. Ross RK, Bernstein L, Judd H, Hanisch R, Pike M, Henderson B. Serum testosterone levels in healthy young black and white men. *JNCI* 1986;**76**:45.

41. Sidney S. Vasectomy and the risk of prostatic cancer and benign prostatic hypertrophy. *J Urol* 1987;**138**:795.

42. Nienhuis H, Goldacre M, Seagroatt V, Leicester G, Vessey M. Incidence of disease after vasectomy: a record linkage retrospective cohort study. 1992;**304**:743.

43. John EM, Whittemore AS, Wu AH *et al.* Vasectomy and prostate cancer: results from a multiethnic case-control study. *J Natl Cancer Inst* 1995;**87**:662.

44. Niehuis H, Goldacre M, Seagroatt V *et al.* Incidence of disease after vasectomy: a record linkage retrospective cohort study. *Br Med J* 1992;**304**:743.

45. Mettlin C, Natarajan N, Huben R. Vasectomy and prostate cancer risk. *Am J Epidemiol* 1990;**132**:1056.

46. Giovannucci E, Ascherio A, Rimm EB, Colditz GA, Stampfer MJ, Willett WC. Prospective cohort study of vasectomy and prostate cancer in US men. *JAMA* 1993;**269**:873.

47. Giovannucci E, Tosteson TD, Speizer FE, Ascherio A, Vessey MP, Colditz G. A retrospective cohort study of vasectomy and prostate cancer in US men. *JAMA* 1993;**269**:878.

48. Howards SS, Peterson HB. Vasectomy and prostate cancer, chance, bias, or a causal relationship? *JAMA* 1993;**269**:913.

49. Feuatel A, Wenrich R, Steiniger D *et al.* Zinc and cadmium concentration in prostatic carcinoma of different histological grading in comparison to normal tissue and adenofibromyomatosis (BPH). *Urol Res* 1982;**10**:301.

50. Pienta KJ, Esper PS. Risk factors for prostate cancer. *Ann Intern Med* 1993;**118**:793.

51. Blair A, Zahm SH. Cancer among farmers. *Occup Med* 1991;**6**:335.

52. Hsing AW, McLaughlin JK, Hrubec Z *et al.* Tobacco use and prostate cancer: 26-year follow-up of US veterans. *Am J Epidemiol* 1991;**133**:437.

53. Hsing AW, McLaughlin JK, Schuman LM *et al.* Diet, tobacco use, and fatal prostate cancer: results from the Lutheran Brotherhood Cohort Study. *Cancer Res* 1990;**50**:6836.

54. Nomura AM, Kolonel LN. Prostate cancer: a current perspective. *Epidemiol Rev* 1991;**13**:200.

55. Armennian NK, Lilienfeld AM, Diamond EL, Bross IDJ. Relation between benign prostatic hyperplasia and cancer of the prostate: a prospective retrospective study. *Lancet* 1974;**ii**:115.

56. Mishina T, Watanabe H, Araki H, Nakao M. Epidemiological study of prostatic cancer by matched-pair analysis. *Prostate* 1985;**6**:423.

57. Greenwald P, Kirmss V, Polan AK, Dick VS. Cancer of the prostate among men with benign prostatic hyperplasia. *JNCI* 1974b;**53**:335.

58. Schuman LM, Mandel J, Blackard C, Bauer H, Scarlett J, McHugh R. Epidemiologic study of prostatic cancer: preliminary report. *Cancer Treat Rep* 1977;**61**:181.

59. Steele R, Lees REM, Kraus AJ, Rao C. Sexual factor in the epidemiology of cancer of the prostate. *J Chronic Dis* 1971;**24**:29.

60. Cannon L, Bishop DT, Skolnick M, Hunt S, Lyon JL, Smart CR. Genetic epidemiology of prostate cancer in the Utah Mormon genealogy. *Cancer Surveys* 1983;**1**:47.

61. Wynder EL, Mabuchi K, Whitmore WF Jr. Epidemiology of cancer of the prostate. *Cancer* 1971;**28**:344.

62. Schuman LM, Mandel J, Blackard C, Bauer H, Scarlett J, McHugh R. Epidemiologic study of prostatic cancer: preliminary report. *Cancer Treat Rep* 1977;**61**:181.

63. Schuman LM, Mandel JS, Radke A *et al.* Some selected features of the epidemiology of prostate cancer. Minneapolis-St Paul, Minnesota case-control study, 1976–1979. In: Magnus K (Ed.) *Trends in cancer incidence: Causes and practical implications.* Washington, D.C., Hemisphere Publishing Corp, 1982, pp. 345.

64. Armstrong B, Doll R. Environmental factors and cancer incidence and mortality in different countries, with special reference to dietary practices. *Int J Cancer* 1975;**15**:617.

65. Winkelstein W Jr, Ernster VL. Epidemiology and etiology. In Murphy GP (Ed.) *Prostatic cancer.* Littleton, MA: PSG Publishing Company, 1979.

66. Woolf CM. An investigation of the familial aspects of carcinoma of the prostate. *Cancer* 1960;**13**:739.

67. Steinberg GS, Carer BS, Beaty TH, Childs B, Walsh PC. Family history and the risk of prostate cancer. *Prostate* 1990;**17**:337.

68. Spitz MR, Currier RD, Fueger JJ, Babaian RJ, Newell GR. Familial patterns of prostate cancer: a case-control analysis. *J Urol* 1991;**146**:1305.

69. Aprikian AG, Bazinet M, Plante M, Meshref A, Trudel C, Aronson S, Nachabe M *et al.* Family history and the risk of prostatic carcinoma in a high risk group of urological patients. *J Urol* 1995;**154**:404.

70. Keetch DW, Rice JP, Suarez BK, Catalona WJ. Familial aspects of prostate cancer: a case control study. *J Urol* 1995;**154**:2100.

71. Carter BS, Bova GS, Beaty TH, Steinberg GD, Childs B, Isaacs WB, Walsh PC. Hereditary prostate cancer: epidemiological and clinical features. *J Urol* 1993;**150**:797.

72. Carter BS, Beaty TH, Steinberg GD, Childs B, Walsh PC. Mendelian inheritance of familial prostate cancer. *Proc Natl Acad Sci* 1992;**89**:3367.

73.   Keetch DW, Humphrey PA, Smith DS, Stahl D, Catalona WJ. Clinical and pathological features of hereditary prostate cancer. *J Urol* 1996;**155**:1841.

74.   Bastacky SI, Wojno KJ, Walsh PC, Carmichael MJ, Epstein JI. Pathological features of hereditary prostate cancer. *J Urol* (part 2) 1995;**153**:987.

75.   Carter BS, Ewing CM, Ward WS, Trieger FB, Aalders TW, Schalken JA, Epstein JI, Isaacs WB. Allelic loss of chromosomes 16q and 10q in human prostate cancer. *Proc Natl Acad Sci USA* 1990;**87**:8751f.

11 Natural history

P Stattin and J Damber

Introduction

No sufficiently large randomized study has compared curative procedures with conservative therapy. Consequently, while awaiting the results of such studies[5,6], the natural history of prostate cancer continues to be a baseline with which the outcome of active therapy is compared. However, comparisons between new treatment modalities and historical controls yield significantly more positive results than studies with randomized controls[7].

Natural history

Definition

The natural history of prostate cancer may be defined as the evolving clinical manifestations of the disease in the untreated host [8]. However, since the introduction of androgen deprivation for prostate cancer, virtually all patients with progressive disease have sooner or later during the course of disease been treated with androgen depletion.

Early versus late therapy

In Scandinavia, an interesting comparison can be made between, on the one hand, Sweden, where the incidence is high, and, on the other hand, Denmark where the incidence is low due to little effort used to detect asymptomatic disease. During the time period 1983–87, the age-adjusted incidence rate (patients diagnosed/100 000 men) was 50 in Sweden and 30 in Denmark[9], i.e. differing by 60%. In contrast, the age-adjusted mortality rate (deaths due to prostate cancer/100 000 men) is remarkably similar, 18 in Sweden and 17 in Denmark[10]. Accordingly, no obvious survival benefit could be observed for early compared with late androgen deprivation in the VACURG studies[11]. Conversely, a recent study showed an advantage for early

endocrine treatment[12]. However, it appears that the difference between early and late endocrine deprivation is relatively small, and it still seems justified to use studies on deferred endocrine treatment in an attempt to describe the natural history of prostate cancer.

Observational studies of deferred treatment in clinically detected prostate cancer in the pre-PSA era

Requirements for informative studies

To obtain optimal information on the natural history from observational studies, data on cancer grade, stage, patient age, co-morbidity, as well as the selection criteria for inclusion of patients has to be provided. Cancer stage and grade are very strong prognostic factors in determining outcome[13,14], and host factors such as age and co-morbidity are also important[15]. Patient age significantly affects cause-specific mortality since patients younger than 60 years at diagnosis had an 80% risk of dying of prostate cancer, compared with 49% for the patients older than 80 years[16]. On the other hand, the relative survival was almost equal in all ages, indicating that the biological aggressiveness of the tumour is independent of age[16], and that age-related co-morbidity is an important determinant for cause-specific survival. Furthermore, co-morbidity was shown to be an important prognostic factor for survival in another recent study[15]. Finally, follow up has to be long due to the slow progression rate for many tumors. Ten year progression-free survival has been proposed as an end-point. However, it is difficult to evaluate progression correctly and, as the time from symptomatic metastasis to death is usually 2–3 years, 15 year cause-specific survival seems to be a more useful end-point[17]. Only a few studies meet these criteria. Moreover, most patients in this overview probably had a more advanced disease at the time of diagnosis than men currently diagnosed by PSA testing. Thus, a lead time bias is introduced, so these studies are probably not comparable with series recruited today.

Single institution series

In a widely cited population-based series collected by Johansson and co-workers, patients with prostate cancer were prospectively recruited from March 1977 to February 1984[18–20]. At the time of diagnosis, all patients underwent bone scan, but neither lymph node staging nor PSA testing was performed. At the end of the observation period 541 (84%) of the patients had died, prostate cancer accounted for 37% of all deaths, including 159 patients with metastatic disease at diagnosis (Figure 11.1).

Localized disease

Patients with localized disease were included in a surveillance protocol if the following criteria were fulfilled. During the first 2 years of the study, only patients with well differentiated tumors (grade 1)[14] were allocated to the protocol. After February 1979, patients with a localized tumor were given deferred treatment if they were older than 75 years, or had a grade 1 tumor. The patients were randomized to either radiotherapy or surveillance if they had an intermediate (grade 2), or a poorly differentiated (grade 3) tumor. Thus, 223 patients with a localized tumor were put on a surveillance protocol. There were 66% grade 1, 30% grade 2, and only 4% grade 3 tumors in this group. Tumour stage was T0 localized in 32%, T0 diffuse in 15%, T1 in 6% and T2 in 47%[21]. The majority

of these patients with palpable tumors were asymptomatic, as only 13% of them required a TUR during subsequent follow up. After a mean follow up of 14 years, 25% of these patients were alive. The disease had become generalized in 13% of these patients, and 11% of the deaths in this group were due to prostate cancer. Six per cent of the patients with well differentiated tumors, 17% of those with intermediately differentiated tumors, and 56% of those with poorly differentiated tumors succumbed to prostate cancer. Other studies, similar in character, have essentially confirmed these results[22–30].

Overview analysis of deferred treatment

In an overview analysis of six studies[19,22,28–31], Chodak *et al.* reanalyzed primary data on 828 patients[31]. In this study, 10 year survival was 87% both for the patients with grade 1 (n = 492) and grade 2 (n = 265) tumors. The corresponding figure was only 34% for patients with grade 3 tumours (n = 62) (Table 11.1). Ten years after diagnosis, metastasis had occurred in 19%, 42% and 74% of the men with grade 1, grade 2 and grade 3 cancer, respectively.

The main objection to a generalization of the results from these studies is that there was a high ratio of well differentiated tumors and few poorly differentiated tumors in these series, due to various selection criteria applied. In most registry-based studies, the number of well differentiated tumors has been considerably lower (18–30%), and the number of poorly differentiated tumors has been considerably higher (17–18%)[1,32,37]. Furthermore, the

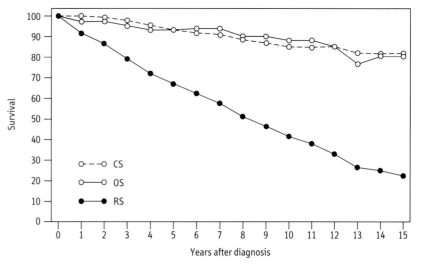

Fig. 11.1 Cause-specific survival among patients with localized disease with (n = 77) and without (n = 223) initial treatment, and those with locally advanced (n = 183) and metastatic disease (n = 159). (From Johansson J-E, Holmberg L, Johansson S, Bergström R, Adami H-O. Fifteen-year survival in prostate cancer, a prospective, population-based study in Sweden. *JAMA* 1997;277:467–471. © 1997, by the American Medical Association)[20].

Table 11.1 Studies on deferred endocrine treatment of prostate cancer

Author	Type of study	Follow up (years)	No. of patients	Cause specific survival (%) 10-years	15-years
Localized					
Johansson *et al.*[24–26]	population-based, prospective	12.5	223	all grades: 85 G1: 91[a] G2: 85 G3[b]	all grades 81
Chodak *et al.*[37]	overview	10	828	G1: 87 G2: 87 G3: 84	
Albertsen *et al.*[21]	registry, retrospective	15.5	451	G1[c]: 2–4 91 Gl: 5–7 76 G1: 8–10 54	G1 2–4 91 G1 5–7 72 G1 8–10 49
Lu-Yao *et al.*[3]	registry, retrospective	10	59 876	G1: 93 G2: 77 G3: 45	
All stages					
Helgesen *et al.*[47]	registry, retrospective	10 years	80 901	all grades: 45[d]	29 at 20 years[d]
Johansson *et al.*[26]	prospective	15 years	642	all grades: 60	all grades: 54
Stattin *et al.*[45]	retrospective[e]	10 years	186	all grades: 45 G1: 84 G2: 41 G3: 18	

[a] Grade 1 highly differentiated, grade 2 intermediately differentiated, grade 3 poorly differentiated
[b] Data not available because of small sample size
[c] Gleason score
[d] Relative survival
[e] Locally symptomatic requiring transurethral resection

mean age of the patients was higher than in many early detection programs[34–36].

Registry-based studies

In a population-based retrospective cohort study from Connecticut, USA, 451 patients with localized prostate cancer were identified[15]. Ten per cent of the tumors were Gleason score 2–4, 35% were Gleason 5–7, 29% were Gleason 8–10, and for 26% of the tumors no Gleason score was reported. After a mean follow up of 15.5 years, 9% of the patients were alive, 34% had died of prostate cancer, 41% had died of other causes, and in 8% the cause of death was unknown. Tumor grade and co-morbidity were both powerful predictors for outcome. The 15 year cause-specific survival was 91% for patients with Gleason score 2–4 tumors; 72% for Gleason score 5–7, and 49% for patients with Gleason score 8–10 (Figure 11.2 and Table 11.1). In a registry-based study in Northern

Sweden, mortality in 6514 patients diagnosed with prostate cancer in all stages during 1971–87 was investigated[37]. The cause-specific mortality was 55%. Local tumor stage and presence of metastasis were unknown. Once again, grade was a significant predictor of outcome. The 15 year cause-specific mortality was 40%, 54% and 72% for grade 1, 2 and 3 tumors respectively. Patients younger than 60 years at the time of diagnosis had an 80% cause-specific mortality which was significantly higher than for older patients.

Data on 59 876 men was compiled from the Surveillance, Epidemiology and End Results (SEER) program in a recent study[38]. Patients treated with prostatectomy, radiotherapy and conservative therapy were included according to the intention to treat. For grade 1 tumors, 10 year cancer-specific survival was 94% for prostatectomy, 90% for radiotherapy, and 93% for conservative therapy. The corresponding figures for grade 2 tumors were 87%,

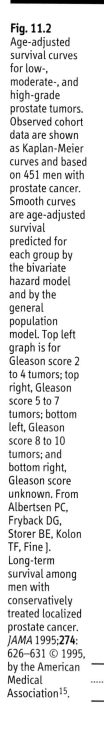

Fig. 11.2
Age-adjusted survival curves for low-, moderate-, and high-grade prostate tumors. Observed cohort data are shown as Kaplan-Meier curves and based on 451 men with prostate cancer. Smooth curves are age-adjusted survival predicted for each group by the bivariate hazard model and by the general population model. Top left graph is for Gleason score 2 to 4 tumors; top right, Gleason score 5 to 7 tumors; bottom left, Gleason score 8 to 10 tumors; and bottom right, Gleason score unknown. From Albertsen PC, Fryback DG, Storer BE, Kolon TF, Fine J. Long-term survival among men with conservatively treated localized prostate cancer. *JAMA* 1995;**274**: 626–631 © 1995, by the American Medical Association[15].

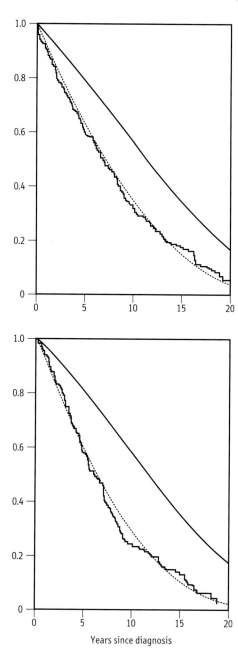

76% and 77%, and for grade 3 tumors 67%, 53% and 45%. The risk of dying of grade 3 prostate cancer was 10 times higher that of dying of grade 1 disease after 10 years irrespective of treatment. Interestingly, the patients with grade 3 tumors seemed to have the largest benefit of surgery in this study.

Locally symptomatic cancer

In a series of 186 consecutive prostate tumors, diagnosis was made in tissue obtained from transurethral resection (TUR) of the prostate[39]. The patients were previously untreated, and TUR was performed because of voiding symptoms. The examination of the resected tissue either revealed a cancer in patients with a non-palpable tumor, or confirmed a clinically suspected tumor in patients with a palpable nodule. Histological evaluation showed 47 grade 1, 87 grade 2, and 52 grade 3 tumors. Bone scan performed at the time of diagnosis was negative in 94 patients, showed metastatic disease in 23 patients, and in 69 patients no bone scan was done. The patients were put on surveillance after surgery, and after 13–21 years of follow up 43% of the patients had died of prostate cancer. Stage, grade and presence of metastasis were all independent predictors of outcome (Figure 11.3). In this series, 97 patients had clinically localized disease. Comparing these 97 patients with voiding symptoms with the series of Johansson et al.[19], and stratifying for tumor stage, 42% of the patients with T1–T2 and voiding symptoms died of prostate cancer as compared with 7% of the patients with the same clinical stage without symptoms. When stratified for grade, prostate cancer was the cause of death in 28% of the patients with a grade 2 tumor and voiding symptoms, compared with 11% of the asymptomatic patients with grade 2 tumors. This difference suggests that patients presenting with voiding symptoms have a worse prognosis than asymptomatic patients of the same stage and grade. This study confirms the adverse influence of obstructive symptoms on prognosis observed in an earlier study that compared the risk of distant metastasis after TUR versus needle biopsy[40]. However, this difference is not accounted for by present staging systems.

Results beyond 15 years of observation

Survival beyond 15 years of follow up has recently been described in several papers. In a nation-wide population-based study of 80 901 men diagnosed with prostate cancer during the period 1960 to 1988 in Sweden, Helgesen and co-workers found that the relative survival rate leveled off after about 18 years after diagnosis[41]. Furthermore, it was found that the loss of life expectancy had decreased by more than 50% in all age groups from 1960–64 to 1985–88. In another Scandinavian study of 1896 patients with prostate cancer surviving more than 10 years after diagnosis, Adolfsson et al. also found that the excess mortality leveled off at 18 years[42]. Conversely, Aus and co-workers, in a study criticized for its methodological flaws, reported that the death rate from prostate cancer increased after 10 years[43].

High mortality

The mortality for clinically detected prostate cancer is high, approximately 50% in many series[1,7,8,15–17,37,39], and is actually higher than for breast cancer, although the incidence is about the same[2]. Once a prostate tumor has become locally advanced, metastatic or de-differentiated, the outcome is very poor.

Early diagnosis and prognostic markers

PSA detection of early cancer

Screening with PSA and digital rectal examination has been shown to detect tumors in approximately 2–4% of a screened population[34–36]. A large proportion of the prostate cancers detected by screening is over 0.5 cc in volume, a limit that has been judged to be a threshold for clinical significance[44–46]. Studies of archived serum for PSA values from men in whom prostate cancer was subsequently diagnosed has provided valuable information regarding PSA in the early development of prostate cancer. In a longitudinal study, Carter and co-workers showed that PSA was significantly elevated 15 years before the diagnosis of metastatic disease[47] (Figure 11.4). In a nested case-control study of 22 071 male physicians, serum PSA values in 366 men later diagnosed with prostate cancer were compared with matched controls[48]. The sensitivity for detection of all prostate cancer cases was 73% during a 10 year follow up, and the specificity was 91%. In addition, men with a PSA level above 3 ng/ml had a five-fold increased relative risk to be diagnosed with prostate cancer compared with men with PSA below 1.0. Thus, it appears that in most cases PSA detected prostate cancer is clinically relevant, and not merely cases of latent cancer known to exist in a high frequency[49–52]. Unfortunately, even in a highly medicalized cohort[48] half of the tumors were locally advanced or of poor differentiation at the time of diagnosis. However, it remains to be shown that an earlier time of diagnosis will decrease cancer mortality. Interestingly, the incidence of prostate cancer in the

Fig. 11.3 Kaplan-Meier analysis of cancer specific survival for 186 patients with prostate cancer treated with TUR and surveillance. Stratification according to tumor stage, grade and metastasis[39].

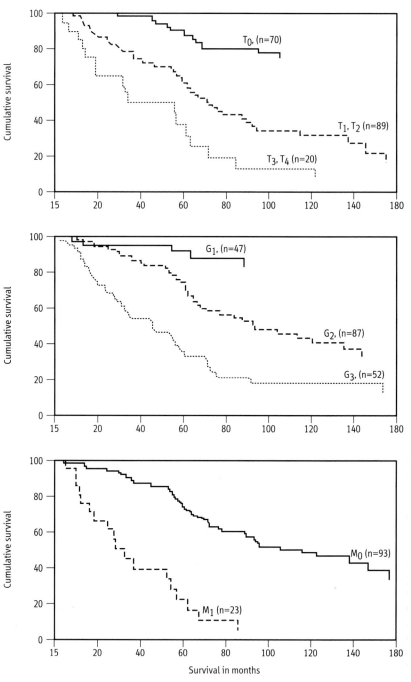

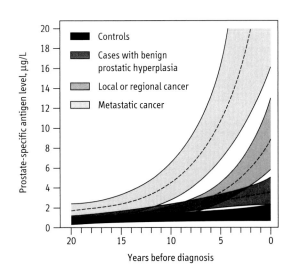

Fig. 11.4 Longitudinal evaluation of prostate specific antigen (PSA) levels in men with prostate disease in controls. Average curves (±95% confidence intervals) of PSA levels as a function of years before diagnosis for three diagnostic groups estimated from a mixed-effects model assuming an age of diagnosis of 75 years. (From Carter HB, Pearson JD, Metter EJ *et al.* Longitudinal evaluation of prostate-specific antigen levels in men with and without prostate disease. *JAMA* 1992;**267**:2215–2220. © 1992, by the American Medical Association)[47].

USA is now decreasing, as is the number of metastatic patients[53–55].

Putative prognostic markers

Much effort has been invested in the search for markers that could predict the natural history of prostate cancer. In a recent inventory on putative prognostic markers, DNA ploidy and histopathologic markers for proliferation, apoptosis, microvessel density, cellular adhesion, neuroendocrine differentiation and nuclear morphometry were considered to be of interest for future studies[56]. It is encouraging that these rather crude methods based on immunohistochemistry and morphometry appear to add information on prognosis. Hopefully more sophisticated methods will add further information about the progression pattern of an individual tumor. Molecular investigation techniques such as RT-PCR for PSA in peripheral blood may become useful prognostic markers[57]. Unfortunately, prognostic information on the natural history of the disease does not necessarily entail predictive information (i.e. information about whether a given therapy will be effective[58]).

Conclusion and discussion

Highly variable outcome

In conclusion, investigations of deferred treatment, recruited before early case-finding and screening became widespread, show that the natural history of prostate cancer entails a high mortality. The natural history is highly dependent on tumor grade, stage, co-morbidity and patient age. A dramatic increase in the detection rate of early prostate cancer and frequency of curatively intended procedures has been seen in the last decade. However, because of the lead and length time bias introduced, the prostate cancer patients detected by screening cannot yet be compared with older studies of deferred treatment.

Future studies

No randomized study to date provides valid information on the difference in outcome of curative procedures and conservative therapy. Consequently, this critical issue needs to be considered in randomized studies in order to provide the next generation of urologists and their patients with well-founded scientific evidence, on which to base rational treatment decisions in prostate cancer[59]. The Scandinavian Prostate Cancer Group (SPCG) study IV which compares radical prostatectomy with surveillance[5], has recruited more than 600 patients. The Prostate Intervention Versus Observation Treatment (PIVOT) study, similar in design, is at present ongoing in the USA[6]. Hopefully these and other studies will provide some scientific facts so eagerly sought for.

Conclusions

The clinical outcome of deferred endocrine treatment of prostate cancer has been used to elucidate the natural history of the disease. The natural history is highly dependent on stage, grade, co-morbidity and age of the patient. The cancer mortality in clinically detected prostate cancer is high, approximately 50%. PSA screening appears to detect clinically relevant prostate cancer in an early stage. However, the natural history of these early detected cancers is at present unknown, and it remains to be shown that mortality is reduced by early detection and therapy. These issues are currently being addressed by a number of important and ongoing studies, including the European Randomised Study of Screening in Prostate Cancer (ERSPC), the North American Prostate, Lung, Colon and Ovary (PLCO) screening study in the US, the Scandinavian randomised trial of treatment, the PIVOT (Prostate cancer intervention versus observation trial) in the United States, and the ProtecT (Prostate testing for cancer and Treatment) study in the United Kingdom. Results of these studies will start to emerge by the year

2008, and are awaited eagerly by patients and clinicians alike[1–3].

References

1. Wilt TJ, Brawer MK. The prostate cancer intervention versus observation trial: a randomised trial comparing radical prostatectomy versus expectant management for the treatment of clinically localised prostate cancer. *J Urol* 1994;**152**:1910–14.

2. de Koning HJ, Auvinen A, Berenguer Sanchez A, Calais Da Silva F, Ciatto S, Denis L, Gohagan JK, Hakama M, Hugosson J, Kranse R, Nelen V, Prorok PC, Schroder FH. Large-scale randomized prostate cancer screening trials: Program performances in the European randomized screening for prostate cancer trial and the prostate, lung, colorectal and ovary cancer trial. *Int J Cancer* 2002;**97**:237–244.

3. Donovan JL, Frankel SJ, Neal DE, Hamdy FC. Screening for prostate cancer in the UK. Seems to be creeping in by the back door. *BMJ* 2001;**323**:763–4.

5. Norlén BJ. Swedish randomized trial of radical prostatectomy versus watchful waiting. *Can J Oncol* 1994;**4**(suppl 1):38–42.

6. Wilt TJ, Brawer MK. The Prostate Intervention Versus Observation Trial: a randomized trial comparing radical prostatectomy versus expectant management for the treatment of clinically localized prostate cancer. *J Urol* 1994;**152**:1910–1914.

7. Sacks H, Chalmers TC, Smith H Jr. Randomized versus historical controls for clinical trials. *Am J Med* 1982;**72**:233–240.

8. Whitmore WF Jr. The natural history of prostatic cancer. *Cancer* 1973;**32**:1104–1112.

9. Engeland A, Haldorsen T, Tretli S *et al*. Prediction of cancer incidence in the Nordic countries up to the years 2000 and 2010. *APMIS* 1993;**101**(suppl 38):1–124.

10. Engeland A, Haldorsen T, Tretli S *et al*. Prediction of cancer mortality in the Nordic countries up to the years 2000 and 2010. *APMIS* 1995;**103**(suppl 49):1–163.

11. Byar DP. The Veterans Administration Cooperative Research Group's studies of cancer of the prostate. *Cancer* 1973;**32**:1126–1130.

12. The Medical Research Council Prostate Cancer Working Party Investigator Group. Immediate versus deferred treatment for advanced prostatic cancer: initial results of the Medical Research Council trial. *Br J Urol* 1997;**79**:235–246.

13. Gleason DF, Mellinger GT. The Veterans Administration Cooperative Urological Research Group. Prediction of prognosis for prostatic adenocarcinoma by combined histological staging and clinical staging. *J Urol* 1974;**111**:58–63.

14. Mostofi FK, Sesterhenn I, Sobin LH. *International histological classification of tumours of the prostate*. World Health Organization, 1981.

15. Albertsen PC, Fryback DG, Storer BE, Kolon TF. Fine J. Long-term survival among men with conservatively treated localized prostate cancer. *JAMA* 1995;**274**:626–631.

16. Grönberg H, Damber J-E, Jonsson H, Lenner P. Patient age as a prognostic factor in prostate cancer. *J Urol* 1994;**152**:892–895.

17. Aus G, Hugosson J, Norlén L. Long-term survival and mortality in prostate cancer treated with noncurative intent. *J Urol* 1995;**154**:460–465.

18. Johansson J-E, Adami H-O, Andersson S-O, Bergström R, Krusemo UB, Kraaz W. Natural history of localised prostatic cancer. A population-based study in 223 untreated patients. *Lancet* 1989;**i**:799–803.

19. Johansson J-E, Adami H-O, Andersson S-O, Bergström R, Holmberg L, Krusemo UB. High 10-year survival rate in patients with early, untreated prostatic cancer. *JAMA* 1992;**267**:2191–2196.

20. Johansson J-E, Holmberg L, Johansson S, Bergström R, Adami, H-O. Fifteen-year survival in prostate cancer, a prospective, population-based study in Sweden. *JAMA* 1997;**277**:467–471.

21. Union International Contre le Cancer. *TNM classification of malignant tumors* (3rd edn). Geneva: UICC, 1978.

22. Adolfsson J, Carstensen J, Lowhagen T. Deferred treatment in clinically localized prostatic carcinoma. *Br J Urol* 1992;**69**:183–187.

23. Rana A, Chisholm GD, Christodoulou S, McIntyre MA, Elton RA. Audit and its impact in the management of early prostatic cancer. *Br J Urol* 1993;**71**:721–727.

24. George NJR. Natural history of localised prostatic cancer managed by conservative therapy alone. *Lancet* 1988;**i**:494–497.

25. Stenzl A, Studer UR. Outcome of patients with untreated cancer of the prostate. *Eur Urol* 1993;**24**:1–6.

26. Handley R, Carr TW, Travis D, Powell PH, Hall RR. Deferred treatment for prostate cancer. *Br J Urol* 1988;**62**:249–253.

27. Moskovitz B, Nitecki A, Richter Levin D. Cancer of the prostate: is there a need for aggressive treatment? *Urol Int* 1987;**42**:49–52.

28. Goodman CM, Busuttil A, Chisholm GD. Age, and size and grade of tumour predict prognosis in incidentally diagnosed carcinoma of the prostate. *Br J Urol* 1988;**62**:576–580.

29. Jones GW. Prospective conservative management of localized prostate cancer. *Cancer* 1992;**70**(suppl):307–310.

30. Whitmore WF Jr, Warner JA, Thompson IM Jr. Expectant management of localized prostatic cancer. *Cancer* 1991;**67**:1091–1096.

31. Chodak GW, Thisted RA, Gerber GS *et al*. Results of conservative management of clinically localized prostate cancer. *N Engl J Med* 1994;**330**:242–248.

32. Lu-Yao GL, Potosky AL, Albertsen PC, Wasson JH, Barry MJ, Wennberg JE. Follow-up prostate cancer treatments after radical prostatectomy: a population-based study. *J Natl Cancer Inst* 1996;**88**:166–173.

33. Lu-Yao GL, Yao S-L. Population-based study of long-term survival in patients with clinically localised prostate cancer. *Lancet* 1997;**349**: 906–910.

34. Richie JP, Ratliff TL, Catalona WJ *et al*. Effect of patient age on early detection of prostate cancer with serum prostate-specific antigen and digital rectal examination. *Urology* 1993;**42**:365–374.

35. Catalona WJ, Smith DS, Ratliff TL *et al*. Measurement of prostate-specific antigen in serum as a screening test for prostate cancer. *N Engl J Med* 1991;**324**:1156–1161.

36. Gustafsson O, Norming U, Almgàrd L-E *et al*. Diagnostic methods in the detection of prostate cancer: a study of a randomly selected population of 2,400 men. *J Urol* 1992;**148**:1827–1831.

37. Grönberg H, Damber L, Jonsson H, Damber J-E. Prostate cancer mortality in northern Sweden, with special reference to tumor grade and patient age. *Urology* 1997;**49**:374–378.

38. Lu-Yao GL, Yao S-L. Population-based study of long-term survival in patients with clinically prostate cancer. *Lancet* 1997;**349**:906–910.

39. Stattin P, Bergh A, Karlberg L, Tavelin B, Damber J-E. Long-term outcome of conservative therapy in men presenting with voiding symptoms and prostate cancer. *Eur Urol* 1997;**32**:404–409.

40. Meacham RB, Scardino PT, Hoffman GS, Easley JD, Wilbanks JH, Carlton CE Jr. The risk of distant metastasis after transurethral resection of the prostate versus needle biopsy in patients with localized prostate cancer. *J Urol* 1989;**142**:320–325.

41. Helgesen F, Holmberg L, Johansson, J-E, Bergström R, Adami H-O. Trends in prostate cancer survival in Sweden, 1960 through 1988: Evidence of increasing non-lethal tumors. *J Natl Cancer Inst* 1996;**88**:1216–1221.

42. Adolfsson J, Rutqvist LE, Steineck G. Prostate carcinoma and long-term survival. *Cancer* 1997;**80**:748–752.

43. Aus G, Hugosson J, Norlen L. Long term survival and mortality in prostate cancer treated with non-curative intent. *J Urol* 1995;**154**:4605.

44. Stamey TA, Freiha FS, McNeal JE, Redwine EA, Whittemore AS, Schmid H-P. Localized prostate cancer: relationship of tumor volume to clinical significance for treatment of prostate cancer. *Cancer* 1993;**71**:933–938.

45. Villers A, McNeal JE, Freiha FS, Stamey TA. Multiple cancers in the prostate: morphologic features of clinically recognized versus incidental tumors. *Cancer* 1992;**70**:2313–2318.

46. Brendler CB. Characteristics of prostate cancer found with early detection regimens. *Urology* 1995;**46**(suppl 3A):71–76.

47. Carter HB, Pearson JD, Metter EJ *et al.* Longitudinal evaluation of prostate-specific antigen levels in men with and without prostate disease. *JAMA* 1992;**267**:2215–2220.

48. Gann PH, Hennekens CH, Stampfer MJ. A prospective evaluation of plasma prostate-specific antigen for detection of prostatic cancer. *JAMA* 1995;**273**:289–294.

49. Breslow N, Chan CW, Dhom G *et al.* Latent carcinoma of prostate at autopsy in seven areas. *Int J Cancer* 1977;**20**:680–688.

50. Guileyardo JM, Johnson WD, Welsh RA, Akazaki K, Correa P. Prevalence of latent prostate carcinoma in two U.S. populations. *J Natl Cancer Inst* 1980;**65**:311–316.

51. Hølund B. Latent prostatic cancer in a consecutive autopsy series. *Scand J Urol Nephrol* 1980;**14**:29–35.

52. Lundberg S, Berge T. Prostatic carcinoma. An autopsy study. *Scand J Urol Nephrol* 1970;**4**:93–97.

53. Schwartz KL, Severson RK, Gurney JG, Montie JE. Trends in the stage specific incidence of prostate carcinoma in the Detroit metropolitan area. *Cancer* 1996;**78**:1260–1266.

54. Mettlin CJ, Murphy GP, Hor: Menck H. R, The national cancer data base report on longitudinal observations on prostate cancer. *Cancer* 1996;**77**:2162–2166.

55. Stephenson RA, Smart CR, Mineau GP, James BC, Janerich DT, Dibble RL. The fall in incidence of prostate carcinoma. On the down side of a prostate specific antigen induced peak in incidence – Data from the Utah Cancer Registry. *Cancer* 1995;**77**:342–348.

56. Eschenbach von AC, Brawer MK, di Sant'Agnese PA, Humphrey PA, Mahran H, Murphy GP, Sebo TJ, Veltri R. Exploration of new pathologic factors in terms of potential for prognostic significance and future applications. *Cancer* 1996;**78**:372–381.

57. Katz AE, de Vries GM, Begg MD *et al.* Enhanced reverse transcriptase-polymerase chain reaction for prostate specific antigen as an indicator of true pathologic stage in patients with prostate cancer. *Cancer* 1995; **75**:1642–1648.

58. Steineck G, Adolfsson J, Scher HI, Whitmore WF Jr. Distinguishing prognostic and treatment-predictive information for localized prostate cancer. *Urology* 1995;**45**:610–615.

59. Horton R. Surgical research or comic opera: questions, but few answers. *Lancet* 1996;**347**:984–985.

12 Pathology

D G Bostwick

Introduction

Although most prostatic cancers are relatively slow growing and will not become manifest during a man's lifetime, the clinical course is often unpredictable in its speed of progression, perhaps due to the marked heterogeneity and other factors which influence tumor growth.

Prostate cancer is rare before 40 years of age, but the incidence rises quickly thereafter. Autopsy studies of thoroughly evaluated prostates from men without clinical evidence of cancer have shown an extraordinarily high level of clinically-undetected cancer, increasing from about 10% at 50 years of age to as high as 80% by the age of 80 (Figure 12.1)[1]. Interestingly, the prevalence of latent histologic cancer is similar in different geographic groups despite wide variation in clinical incidence.

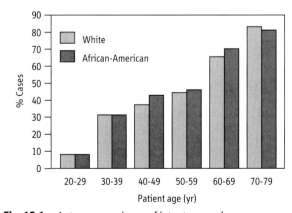

Fig. 12.1 Autopsy prevalence of latent cancer in totally-embedded prostates from the Detroit Medical Examiners Office. Data from Sakr W *et al. Eur Urol* 1996;**30**:138.

Examination of biopsies

The introduction of the automated spring-loaded 18-gauge core-biopsy gun in the last decade began a new era in the sampling of the prostate for histologic diagnosis. The main disadvantage of the 18-gauge biopsy is that it provides about 36% of the amount of tissue per needle core of the traditional biopsy. When compared with matched prostatectomy specimens, needle core biopsy underestimates tumor grade in 33–45% of cases and overestimates grade in 4–32%[2]. Grading errors are greatest in biopsies with small amounts of tumor and low-grade tumors, and are probably due to tissue sampling error, tumor heterogeneity and undergrading of needle biopsies. There is no correlation of biopsy grading error and clinical staging error. Gleason score should be reported in all needle biopsies, even in those with small amounts of tumor.

Needle biopsy usually samples tissue from the peripheral zone of the prostate, unlike TURP specimens, which sample tissue from the transition zone, urethra, periurethral area, bladder neck and anterior fibromuscular stroma. Studies of radical prostatectomies performed after TURP reveal that the resection does not usually include tissue from the central or peripheral zones, and not all of the transition zone is removed.

Well-differentiated cancer found incidentally in TURP chips usually represents cancer that has arisen in the transition zone. These tumors are frequently small and may be completely resected by TURP. Conversely, poorly differentiated cancer in TURP chips usually represents part of a larger tumor that has invaded the transition zone after arising in the peripheral zone. The optimal number of chips to submit for histologic evaluation from a TURP specimen remains controversial, with some advocating complete submission even with large specimens that require many tissue cassettes.[2] The College of American Pathologists recommends a minimum of six cassettes for

127

the first 30 g of tissue and 1 cassette for every 10 g thereafter[3].

Prostatic intraepithelial neoplasia

Prostatic intraepithelial neoplasia (PIN) represents the putative pre-cancerous end of the morphologic continuum of cellular proliferations with prostatic ducts, ductules and acini[4]. Two grades of PIN are identified (low-grade and high-grade), and high-grade PIN is considered the pre-invasive stage of invasive carcinoma (Figure 12.2). The continuum which culminates in high-grade PIN and early invasive cancer is characterized by basal cell layer disruption, progressive loss of markers of secretory differentiation, increasing nuclear and nucleolar abnormalities, increasing proliferative potential and increasing variation in DNA content (aneuploidy). PIN predates carcinoma by 10 years or more, with low-grade PIN first emerging in men in the third decade of life[5]. PIN is often found in the vicinity of carcinoma, and its identification in biopsy specimens of the prostate warrants further search for concurrent invasive carcinoma.

The term PIN replaces other synonymous terms used in the literature, including intraductal dysplasia, large acinar atypical hyperplasia, atypical primary hyperplasia, hyperplasia with malignant change, marked atypia, and duct-acinar dysplasia. PIN is divided into two grades (low-grade and high-grade) to replace the previous three grade system (PIN 1 is considered low grade, and PIN 2 and 3 are considered high grade). A recent consensus conference sponsored by the World Health Organization declared PIN the most likely precursor of prostate cancer[6].

In low-grade PIN (formerly PIN 1), the cells within ducts and acini are heaped up, crowded, and irregularly spaced with marked variation in nuclear size (anisonucleosis). Elongate hyperchromatic nuclei and small nucleoli are also observed, but these are not usually prominent features. The diagnosis of PIN requires a combination of both cytologic and architectural abnormalities, and lesions displaying some but not all of these changes are considered atypical but not dysplastic. High-grade PIN (formerly PIN 2 and 3) exhibits features similar to low-grade PIN, although cell crowding and stratification are usually more pronounced, with less variability in nuclear size because the majority of nuclei are enlarged; the presence of prominent nucleoli, often multiple, is of greatest diagnostic value.

There are four architectural patterns of high-grade PIN: tufting, micropapillary, cribriform and flat. The patterns often merge with each other, although fields with only a single pattern may be present, and familiarity with these patterns aids in recognition of PIN and avoids potential diagnostic pitfalls.

The peripheral zone of the prostate, the area in which the majority of prostatic carcinomas occur (70%), is also the most common location for PIN[7]. Cancer and PIN are usually multifocal in the peripheral zone, indicating a 'field' effect similar to the multifocality of transitional cell carcinoma of the bladder. The transition zone and periurethral area, the anatomic areas in which nodular hyperplasia occurs, account for about 20–25% of prostate cancers, and harbor foci of PIN in only 8% of cases.

Increasing grades of PIN are associated with progressive disruption of the basal cell layer. Antibodies directed against high molecular weight keratins (e.g. clone 34 β-E12) selectively label the prostatic basal cell layer[8]. Tumor cells consistently fail to react with this antibody, whereas normal prostatic epithelium is invariably stained, with a continuous intact circumferential basal cell layer observed in most instances. Basal cell layer disruption is present in 56% of cases of high-grade PIN, more commonly in glands adjacent to invasive carcinoma than in distant glands. Also, the amount of disruption increases with increasing grades of PIN, with loss of more than one-third of the basal cell layer in 52% of foci of high-grade PIN. Early invasive carcinoma occurs at sites of glandular out-pouching and basal cell disruption (Figure 12.3).

The frequency of PIN in prostates with cancer is significantly increased when compared with prostates without cancer. PIN was present in 82% of step-sectioned prostates with cancer, but in only 43% of benign prostates

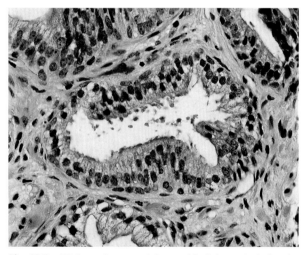

Fig. 12.2 High-grade prostatic intraepithelial neoplasia (PIN) involving a single acinus. The epithelial cells show moderate nuclear and nucleolar enlargement.

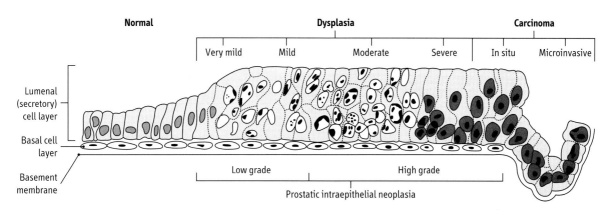

Normal | Dysplasia | Carcinoma

| Very mild | Mild | Moderate | Severe | In situ | Microinvasive |

Lumenal (secretory) cell layer

Basal cell layer

Basement membrane

Low grade | High grade

Prostatic intraepithelial neoplasia

Fig. 12.3 Morphologic continuum from normal prostatic epithelium through increasing grades of PIN to early invasive carcinoma, according to the disease-continuum concept. Low-grade PIN (grade 1) corresponds to very mild to mild dysplasia. High-grade PIN (grades 2 and 3) correspond to moderate to severe dysplasia and carcinoma in situ. The precursor state ends when malignant cells invade the stroma; this invasion occurs where the basal cell layer is disrupted. The dysplastic changes occur in the superficial (luminal) secretory cell layer, perhaps in response to lumenal carcinogens. Disruption of the basal cell layer accompanies the architectural and cytologic features of high-grade PIN, and appears to be a necessary prerequisite for stromal invasion. The basement membrane is retained with high-grade PIN and early invasive carcinoma. (Modified with permission from Bostwick DG, Brawer MK. Prostatic intraepithelial neoplasia and early invasion in prostate cancer. *Cancer* 1987;**59**:788–794.)

from patients of similar age. PIN was more extensive in amount in lower stage tumors, presumably due to 'overgrowth' or obliteration of PIN by larger high-stage tumors. The severity of PIN in prostates with cancer was significantly increased when compared with prostates without cancer.

The prevalence of PIN in prostates with cancer increases with age. Sakr *et al.* studied young men and found PIN in 8% and 23% of men in their twenties and thirties, respectively; most foci of PIN in young males were low-grade, with increasing frequency of high-grade PIN with advancing age[5]. The prevalence of PIN was similar in blacks and whites. Lee *et al.* studied 256 ultrasound-guided biopsies of hypoechoic lesions of the prostate, and identified 103 cancers and 27 cases of PIN; the mean age of those with PIN (65 years) was significantly lower than those with cancer (70 years)[9].

Virtually all measures of phenotype and nuclear abnormality by computer-based image analysis reveal that PIN and cancer are similar, in contrast with normal and hyperplastic epithelium[4,10]. Nuclear changes include area, DNA content, chromatin content and distribution, perimeter, diameter and roundness. Also, most measures of nucleolar abnormality show the similarity of PIN and cancer, in contrast with normal epithelium. These cumulative data indicate that the continuum from PIN to cancer is characterized by progressive nuclear and nucleolar changes. These morphologic changes are accompanied by progressive changes in DNA ploidy.

Biopsy remains the definitive method for detecting PIN and early invasive cancer. A retrospective case-control study of high-grade PIN without carcinoma in needle biopsy specimens revealed cancer in 36% of study cases on subsequent biopsy, compared with 15% in the control cases (Figure 12.4)[11]. There was a greater likelihood of finding cancer in patients with PIN undergoing more than one follow up biopsy (44%) than in those with only one biopsy (36%). These results indicate that the identification of PIN on needle biopsy is strongly predictive of

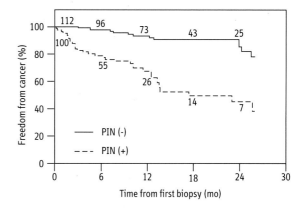

Fig. 12.4 Freedom from cancer from time of first biopsy according to the presence or absence of high grade PIN. (With permission from Davidson D *et al. J Urol* 1995;**154**:1295–1299.)

adenocarcinoma in a significant number of cases, and that PIN is a significant histologic risk factor for cancer.

If all procedures fail to identify coexistent carcinoma, close surveillance and follow up appear to be indicated. Follow up is suggested at 6 monthly intervals for 2 years, and thereafter yearly for life. The identification of pre-malignant lesions in the prostate should not influence or dictate therapeutic decisions. PIN also offers promise as an intermediate end-point in studies of chemoprevention of prostatic carcinoma.

Pathologic diagnosis of adenocarcinoma

Gross identification of prostate cancer may be difficult or impossible, and definitive diagnosis requires microscopic examination. In TURP specimens, cancer is rarely identified grossly unless it is abundant due to the confounding macro-scopic features of BPH. In prostatectomies, cancer tends to be multifocal, with a predilection for the peripheral zone. Grossly apparent tumor foci are at least 5 mm, and appear yellow-white with a stony-hard consistency due to stromal desmoplasia. Some tumors appear as yellow granular mass-es which contrast sharply with the normal spongy prostatic parenchyma. These could resemble lesions caused by tuber-culosis, granulomatous prostatitis, and extensive acute and chronic inflammation.

Microscopically, prostatic adenocarcinoma usually con-sists of a proliferation of small acini with multiple patterns (Figure 12.5). Evaluation of small acinar proliferations of

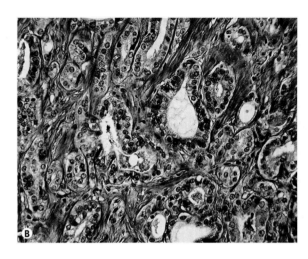

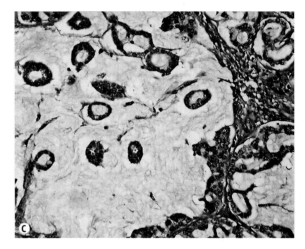

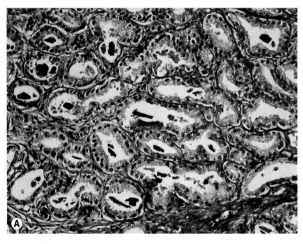

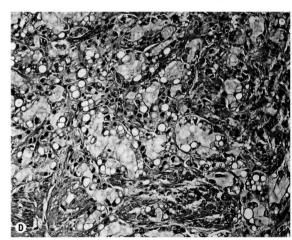

Fig. 12.5   Prostatic adenocarcinoma. A: Gleason grade 1. Note the uniform size and spacing of the acini, as well as the presence of intraluminal crystalloids; B; Gleason grade 3 adenocarcinoma, showing variation in acinar size, shape, and spacing; C: Gleason grade 4 adenocarcinoma with prominent mucin production; the malignant acini are swimming in mucin pools; D: Gleason grade 5 adenocarcinoma with prominent signet-ring cell pattern.

the prostate can be a diagnostic challenge, particularly when the specimen or suspicious focus is small[12]. Diagnosis relies on a combination of architectural and cytologic findings, and may be aided by ancillary studies such as immunohistochemistry. Architectural features are assessed at low to medium power magnification, and include irregular glandular contours which deviate from the smoothly sculpted rounded contours of normal prostatic glands. The arrangement of the glands is useful; malignant glands often exhibit an irregular haphazard arrangement, sometimes with splitting or distortion of muscle fibers in the stroma. Variation in gland size can also be of value, particularly when there are small irregular abortive glands with primitive lumens, usually at the periphery. Comparison with the adjacent uninvolved prostatic glands is always of value.

Cytologic features of cancer such as nuclear and nucleolar enlargement are also important for the diagnosis of malignancy. Enlargement is seen in the majority of the suspicious cells. It is important to remember that every cell has a nucleolus, so one searches for 'prominent' nucleoli, which are at least 1.50 microns in diameter or larger. The identification of more than one nucleolus is virtually diagnostic of malignancy, according to Helpap; also, the nucleoli of cancer cells are frequently eccentrically located in the nucleus, although this is often a difficult feature to evaluate objectively[13].

The basal cell layer is critical in the diagnosis of adenocarcinoma. Compressed stromal fibroblasts can mimic basal cells, but are usually only seen focally at the periphery of the glands; an intact basal cell layer is present at the periphery of benign glands, whereas carcinoma lacks a basal cell layer entirely[14]. Sometimes, small foci of adenocarcinoma cluster around larger glands which have an intact basal cell layer, compounding the difficulty. In problematic cases, it may be useful to employ monoclonal antibodies directed against high molecular weight keratin (e.g. 34β-E12) to evaluate the basal cell layer.

Other ancillary histologic features may aid in the diagnosis of adenocarcinoma. Perineural invasion is common in cancer, and represents strong presumptive evidence of malignancy, but is not pathognomonic because it has been rarely reported with benign glands. However, circumferential impingement on nerves or intraneural invasion is only seen with malignancy. Perineural invasion often indicates tumor spread along planes of least resistance which accompany intraprostatic nerves, but does not represent lymphatic invasion as originally suggested; further, it is not an important predictor of extraprostatic spread[15]. Acidic sulfated and non-sulfated mucin is produced in the majority of cancers, appearing as wispy faintly basophilic luminal material on hematoxylin and eosin-stained sec-

tions. This mucin stains with alcian blue, pH 2.5, whereas the normal prostatic epithelium contains periodic acid Schiff-reactive neutral mucin. Acidic mucin is not specific for carcinoma, and has been identified in PIN, atypical adenomatous hyperplasia, sclerosing adenosis, and rarely in benign prostatic hyperplasia. Crystalloids are needle-like brightly eosinophilic sharp-edged structures which are often present in the lumens of well differentiated and moderately differentiated carcinoma. Ultrastructurally they are composed of electron-dense material that lacks the periodicity of crystals; thus, the term crystalloids rather than crystals is appropriate. X-ray microanalysis has demonstrated uniform high sulfur peaks with small sodium peaks. Their pathogenesis is uncertain, but is probably related to abnormal protein and mineral handling by malignant glands. Crystalloids are not specific for carcinoma, and have been found in PIN, atypical adenomatous hyperplasia, benign prostatic hyperplasia and normal prostatic epithelium. Collagenous micronodules are an incidental finding in mucin-producing prostatic adenocarcinoma, consisting of microscopic nodular masses of paucicellular eosinophilic fibrillar stroma which impinge on gland lumens; they probably result from extravasation of acidic mucin into the stroma. Despite being present in less than 13% of cancers, collagenous micronodules are found exclusively in association with cancer, and are not present in benign epithelium, hyperplasia or PIN. Microvascular invasion is a strong indicator of malignancy and its presence has been directly correlated with histologic grade, although it is sometimes difficult to distinguish from fixation-associated retraction artifact of glands.

Tumor within adipose tissue is indicative of extraprostatic extension, although this is an unusual finding in biopsy specimens. Inflammation is important to note when evaluating small glandular proliferations, particularly when the architectural features are equivocal and one is relying on the cytologic findings of nucleomegaly and nucleolomegaly for the diagnosis of carcinoma. Reactive atypia within glands may result from inflammation, radiation, infarction and other insults to the prostate. Also, granulomatous prostatitis is a vexing problem, and caution is warranted in the interpretation of biopsies with such a finding.

Grading

The histologic pattern of prostate cancer correlates significantly with biological malignancy, a finding exploited by more than 30 grading systems proposed in this century. All systems successfully identify well differentiated cancer which progresses slowly and poorly differentiated cancer which progresses rapidly; however, they are less successful in subdividing the great majority of moderately differentiated cancers which have an intermediate clinical and biologic potential. The Gleason grading system, based on the Veterans Administration Cooperative Urological Research Group (VACURG) study of more than 4000 patients between 1960 and 1975, is the de facto grading standard in the United States and other parts of the world.

The Gleason grading system is based on the degree of glandular differentiation, reflecting tumor heterogeneity by assigning a primary pattern for the dominant grade and a secondary pattern for the non-dominant grade; the histologic score is derived by adding these two patterns together. The success of the Gleason system is due to four factors: 1) histologic patterns are identified by their degree of glandular differentiation without relying on morphogenetic or histogenetic models; 2) a simplified and standardized drawing was created by Gleason (Figure 12.6); 3) the Veterans Administration Cooperative Urologic Research Group study provided invaluable prospective information that allowed objective development of this self-defining grading system; and 4) unlike any other grading system in the body, the Gleason system provides for tumor heterogeneity by identifying primary and secondary patterns.

Gleason noted that greater than 50% of cancers contained two or more patterns. Similarly, Aihara *et al.* recently found an average of 2.7 different Gleason grades (range 1–5) in a series of 101 totally embedded prostatectomies, and more than 50% of cancer contained at least three different grades; also, the number of grades increased with greater cancer volume, and the most common finding was high-grade cancer within the core of a larger well or moderately differentiated cancer (53% of cases)[16].

Interobserver and intraobserver variability have been reported with the Gleason grading system and other grading systems[17,18]. The subjective nature of grading precludes absolute precision, no matter how carefully the system is defined, yet the significant correlation of prostate cancer grade with virtually every outcome measure attests

Fig. 12.6   Gleason grading system.

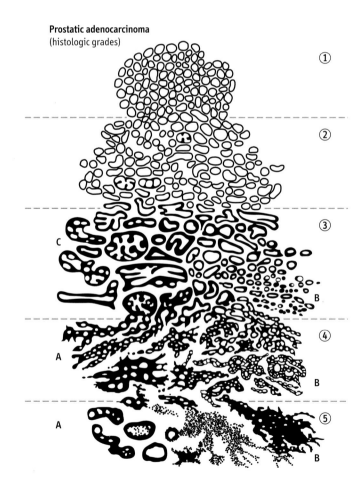

Prostatic adenocarcinoma
(histologic grades)

to the predictive strength and utility of grading in the hands of most investigators. Gleason himself noted exact reproducibility of score in 50% of needle biopsies and +1 score in 85%, similar to the findings of others.

Grade is one of the strongest predictors of biologic behavior in prostate cancer, including invasiveness and metastatic potential, but is not sufficiently reliable when used alone in predicting pathologic stage or patient outcome for individual patients. Grade is included among other prognostic factors in therapeutic decision making, including patient age and health, clinical stage and serum PSA level. Virtually every measure of recurrence and survival is strongly correlated with cancer grade, including crude survival, tumor-free survival following treatment or watchful waiting, metastasis-free survival, cause-specific survival, and time of recurrence after radical prostatectomy. Changes in grade after therapy are discussed later in this chapter.

Histological variants of prostate cancer

Many interesting and unusual morphologic variants of prostatic carcinoma have been identified, but account for less than 10% of cases (Table 12.1; Figure 12.5). It is important to recognize and diagnose accurately special variants, and understand the criteria that distinguish these from benign mimics. Unusual tumors arising in the prostate raise questions of tumor origin, particularly whether the tumor represents metastasis from another site. Also, the clinical behavior of morphologic variants may differ from usual prostatic adenocarcinoma, carrying a better or worse prognosis, but data are limited. These tumors are usually associated with typical acinar adenocarcinoma, rarely occurring in pure form.

Table 12.1   Variants of prostatic carcinoma

Adenocarcinoma and associated tumors	Gleason primary pattern
Ductal carcinoma (endometrioid carcinoma)	3 (no necrosis); 5 (necrosis)
Mucinous carcinoma	4
Signet ring cell carcinoma	5
Sarcomatoid carcinoma	5
Adenocarcinoma with neuroendocrine cells	Variable
Neuroendocrine carcinoma	5 (small cell carcinoma)
Squamous and adenosquamous carcinoma	Variable; usually high-grade
Adenocarcinoma with oncocytic features	Variable
Lymphoepithelioma-like carcinoma	5
Adenoid cystic carcinoma/basal cell carcinoma	Variable; usually high-grade

(With permission from Bostwick DG, Dundore PA. *Biopsy pathology of the prostate* Chapman and Hall Medical, London, 1997.)

Prostatectomy

The completeness of pathological sectioning of prostatectomies can affect the determination of pathologic stage. One study compared the results of limited sectioning (sections of palpable tumor and two random sections of apex and base) with complete sectioning (whole organ step sectioning procedure) and found a significant increase in positive surgical margins (12% vs. 59%, respectively) and pathologic stage with the complete approach. Also, the presence and extent of extraprostatic extension in clinical stage T2 cancer (and hence clinical staging error) is related to the number of prostate slices submitted.

Careful submission of tissue for histologic evaluation allows the following: 1) unequivocal orientation of specimen and tumor (left, right; transition zone, peripheral zone; anterior, mid, posterior; apex, base, etc.); 2) thorough evaluation of the extent and location of positive surgical margins; 3) thorough assessment and quantitation of the extent and location of capsular perforation and seminal vesicle invasion; 4) quality control data for the surgeon, particularly in regard to surgical margins in nerve-sparing prostatectomy; 5) post-operative measurement of tumor volume for correlation with imaging studies, etc.; 6) complete evaluation of tumor for grading (% poorly differentiated cancer, etc.); 7) Fulfilment of all recommendations by the College of American Pathologists; and 8) comparison of results with published prostatectomy studies[5].

Definition of extraprostatic extension (EPE)

Extension of cancer beyond the edge or capsule of the prostate is diagnostic of EPE. There are three criteria for EPE depending on the site and composition of the extraprostatic tissue: 1) cancer in adipose tissue (Figure 12.7); 2) cancer in perineural spaces of the neurovascular bundles; and 3) cancer in anterior muscle.

Cancer in adipose tissue

EPE is easily diagnosed when malignant acini are in contact with adipose tissue. There is no adipose tissue within the prostate, so this constitutes unequivocal EPE; it is useful in biopsy specimens and in poorly oriented sections from a prostatectomy. Adipose tissue is usually present adjacent to the lateral, posterolateral and posterior surfaces of the prostate.

Difficulty is occasionally encountered when cancer has provoked a dense desmoplastic response in the extraprostatic tissue, particularly in cases treated by androgen deprivation therapy. We resolve this uncommon problem by

133

Fig. 12.7 Extraprostatic extension of prostate cancer. Note the malignant acinus (centrally) surrounded by adipose tissue.

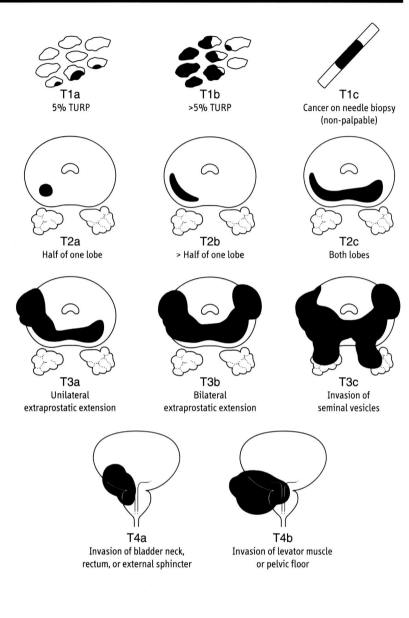

T1a
5% TURP

T1b
>5% TURP

T1c
Cancer on needle biopsy
(non-palpable)

T2a
Half of one lobe

T2b
> Half of one lobe

T2c
Both lobes

T3a
Unilateral
extraprostatic extension

T3b
Bilateral
extraprostatic extension

T3c
Invasion of
seminal vesicles

T4a
Invasion of bladder neck,
rectum, or external sphincter

T4b
Invasion of levator muscle
or pelvic floor

scanning the smooth rounded external contour of the prostate to determine if the focus of concern has breached this contour and is enmeshed within an extraprostatic nodule of fibrous tissue.

Cancer in perineural spaces of the neurovascular bundles

The neurovascular bundles are a path of least resistance for cancer to escape from the prostate. These bundles are clustered in the posterolateral corners of the prostate (at about 5 o'clock and 7 o'clock in transverse sections), and are best appreciated at scanning magnification in whole mount sections of non-nerve sparing radical prostatectomies. Although cancer may not be in contact with adipose tissue, involvement of perineural spaces of the neurovascular bundles represents EPE.

Perineural invasion alone does not constitute EPE, and there are often large nerve twigs within the prostate which may be mistaken for neurovascular bundles. Accordingly, it is best to diagnose cancer within the neurovascular bundles (and thus EPE) only when the malignant acini are present beyond the reasonable contour (edge) of the prostate.

Cancer in anterior muscle

This is a very uncommon site of EPE, and is only observed with large bulky cancers within the transition zone. The anterior fibromuscular stroma of the prostate interdigitates with external smooth muscle and skeletal muscle adjacent to the pubic bone, and there is usually insufficient adipose tissue in this area to define the extraprostatic tissue; consequently, it may be difficult to identify EPE. We diagnose EPE at this site only when there is unequivocal evidence of cancer extending beyond the reasonable confines of the prostatic edge into skeletal muscle and beyond the rounded interface between the fibromuscular stroma and skeletal muscle.

Biopsy findings after therapy

Biopsy after radiation therapy

For about 12 months after external beam irradiation, needle biopsy is of limited value due to the delayed and continuing tumor cell death[19]. After this period, however, biopsy is the best method for assessing local tumor control with a low level of sampling error which is minimized by obtaining multiple specimens[19–24]. Histopathologic changes of radiation injury in the prostate include acinar atrophy, shrinkage and distortion, marked cytologic abnormalities of the epithelium, basal cell hyperplasia, stromal fibrosis and decreased ratio of acini to stroma. Vascular sclerosis is also prominent, and may involve small and large vessels. Recent results with interstitial brachytherapy reveal negative biopsies in 80%, indeterminate in 17%, and positive in 3%; as follow up time increased, many of the indeterminate cases converted to negative on repeat biopsy[25].

No definitive method exists for assessment of tumor viability after irradiation. PSA and PAP expression persist, suggesting that tumor cells capable of protein production probably retain the potential for cell division and consequent metastatic spread[26]. Keratin 34βE12 expression also persists after radiation therapy, and is often of value in separating treated adenocarcinoma and some of its mimics. If prostatic carcinoma is not histologically ablated by external beam radiotherapy after 12 months, it is probably biologically active. Pre-treatment PSA serum concentration and post-treatment PSA nadir are the most important predictors of outcome[27].

Cancer grading after radiation therapy has yielded conflicting results, with some observers[19] noting no difference from pre-therapy grade, and others[23,24] finding an increase in grade. There may also be a shift towards aneuploid DNA content in up to 31% of pre-treatment diploid tumors, indicating increasing histologic and biologic tumor aggressiveness[23]. Consensus opinion is that grading should not be relied upon after radiation therapy[28].

Biopsy after androgen deprivation therapy

Androgen deprivation is used for pre-operative tumor shrinkage and treatment of prostatic hyperplasia, and may be effective for cancer prophylaxis, although this remains speculative. Androgen deprivation of normal, hyperplastic and dysplastic epithelial cells causes acceleration of programmed cell death of single cells (apoptosis), with fragmentation of tumor DNA, emergence of apoptotic bodies, and inhibition of cell growth.

Characteristic involutional changes occur in the prostate after androgen deprivation therapy. Benign acini show marked lobular and acinar atrophy, epithelial vacuolation, basal cell hyperplasia, squamous metaplasia, transitional metaplasia and acinar rupture with extravasation of secretions[29]. Androgen deprivation therapy also causes a marked reduction in the presence and extent of high-grade prostatic intra-epithelial neoplasia[30,31]. Cancer shows an increase in Gleason grade and a substantial reduction in nuclear and nucleolar size, accompanied by prominent cytoplasmic clearing[29–38]. These changes are rarely seen in benign acini and untreated carcinoma, and the combination of features following therapy is sufficiently distinctive to allow recognition of this morphologic change.

Androgen deprivation therapy causes an apparent increase in the Gleason grade of the tumor which is accompanied by nuclear size reduction, loss of recognizable nucleoli, chromatin condensation, nuclear pyknosis and cytoplasmic vacuolation ('nucleolus-poor clear cell adenocarcinoma')[38]. This uncoupling of the architectural and cytologic pattern is vexing due to the presence of small shrunken nuclei within malignant acini, particularly in lymph nodes submitted for frozen section evaluation. Grading after therapy is potentially misleading and is not recommended[28,34].

Immunohistochemical studies for PSA, PAP, and basal cell-specific keratin 34βE12 are useful in identifying carcinoma following therapy. PSA and PAP are retained in tumor cells after therapy, and keratin 34βE12 remains negative, indicating an absent basal cell layer. No differences are found in expression of neuroendocrine differentiation markers such as chromogranin, neuron-specific enolase, B-HCG, and serotonin. Proliferative activity according to proliferating cell nuclear antigen (PCNA) immunoreactivity falls after androgen deprivation therapy[34].

135

Biopsy after cryosurgery

Following cryosurgery, the prostate shows areas of complete tissue ablation as well as other areas with typical features of tissue repair, including marked stromal fibrosis and hyalinization, basal cell hyperplasia with epithelial regeneration, squamous metaplasia, and stromal hemorrhage and hemosiderin deposition[39–42]. Coagulative necrosis is present between 6 and 30 weeks of therapy, but patchy chronic inflammation is more common. Focal granulomatous inflammation is associated with epithelial disruption due to corpora amylacea. Dystrophic calcification is infrequent, and usually appears in areas with the greatest reparative response. Atypia and PIN are not seen in areas that otherwise show changes of post-cryoablation therapy.

Diagnostic and prognostic markers in prostate cancer

PSA is the most important, accurate and clinically useful biochemical marker in the prostate because it is, for all practical purposes, produced by and specific for prostatic tissue. Immunohistochemical expression of PSA is diagnostically helpful for the pathologist in distinguishing high-grade prostate cancer from transitional cell carcinoma, colonic carcinoma, granulomatous prostatitis, lymphoma and other histologic mimics. It also allows identification of site of tumor origin in metastatic adenocarcinoma. PSA expression is generally greater in low grade tumors than in high-grade tumors, but there is significant heterogeneity from cell to cell. Up to 1.6% of poorly differentiated cancers do not express PSA or prostatic acid phosphatase. At present, serum PAP has little or no clinical utility, but this marker is valuable for staining when used in combination with stains for PSA.

Androgen receptors are present within androgen-responsive and androgen-unresponsive cells in prostate cancer. These receptors are widely distributed in the normal prostate and in BPH, and can be identified in localized and metastatic prostatic carcinoma. The percentage of cancer cells with androgen receptors was not able to predict the time to progression after androgen-deprivation therapy; however, greater heterogeneity of androgen receptor immunoreactivity was seen in cancers which responded poorly to therapy.

Neuroendocrine cells may be present in large numbers in cancer. The presence of these cells may indicate a poor prognosis, perhaps due to insensitivity to hormonal growth regulation, but this has been refuted. The progressive loss of markers of neuroendocrine differentiation with increasing grades of PIN and cancer indicates that there is progressive impairment of cell differentiation and regulatory control with advancing stages of prostatic carcinogenesis. Aprikian and associates found neuroendocrine cells in 77% of untreated prostate cancers, 60% of hormone-refractory cancers, and 52% of metastases, with a small number of dispersed positive cells in each of these cases[43]. Berner et al. found no difference in neuron specific enolase expression in pre- and post-treatment specimens from 47 cases of hormone-resistant prostate cancer[44]. Neuroendocrine differentiation is down-regulated in prostatic carcinogenesis, with intermediate levels of expression in PIN compared with normal cells and carcinoma. Further studies are needed to evaluate the function and prognostic utility of neuroendocrine cells in the normal and neoplastic prostate.

Peptide growth factors appear to control development of normal and neoplastic prostatic epithelium by acting as paracrine mediators of epithelial-stromal interaction and growth[13]. The epidermal growth factor (EGF) family of peptides includes EGF, TGF-alpha (transforming growth factor alpha), and other factors which act through the same transmembrane glycoprotein receptor and tyrosine kinase. Prostate cancer cells induce synthesis of TGF-alpha, and this stimulates epithelial and fibroblastic proliferation. The transforming growth factor beta (TGF-beta) family of peptides, including TGF-beta 1 and TGF-beta2, appear to be regulators of cell differentiation and proliferation. Expression of the TGF-beta receptor appears to be under negative androgenic regulation, suggesting that TGF-beta plays a role in cell death following androgen deprivation. The TGF-beta binding protein is produced in benign and hyperplastic tissue but not in malignant tissue.

There are numerous other investigational tumor markers in prostate cancer. The antigen recognized by monoclonal antibody 7E11-C5 (PSM or PSMA) is a mixture of unique glycoproteins expressed on normal and neoplastic prostatic tissues, with greatest intensity in carcinoma and metastases[45]. This antigen is not affected by androgen deprivation therapy; currently, clinical trials are evaluating the utility of this marker for radioimmunodetection and radioimmunotherapy of prostate cancer. hK2 is a protein with 80% homology with PSA which may also be clinically useful[46].

Molecular biology of PIN and prostate cancer

DNA content analysis of prostate cancer by flow cytometry and static image analysis may provide independent prognostic information which supplements histopathologic examination. Patients with diploid tumors have a more favorable outcome than those with aneuploid tumors; for example, among patients with lymph node metastases treated with radical prostatectomy and androgen deprivation therapy, those with diploid tumors may survive 20 years or more, whereas those with aneuploid tumors die within 5 years. However, the ploidy pattern of prostate cancer is often heterogeneous, creating potential problems with sampling error. An international DNA Cytometry Consensus Conference reviewed the literature and concluded that the clinical significance and biologic basis of DNA ploidy needs further investigation[47].

Allelic loss is a common finding in prostatic adenocarcinoma, present in more than 50% of cases on chromosomes 8p, 10q, and 16q (Figure 12.8).[10] One or more tumor suppresser genes appear to be present on 8p which may be involved in carcinogenesis. Allelic loss appears to be more common in high-grade tumors. Fluorescent in situ hybridization (FISH) studies with centromere-specific probes for chromosomes 7, 8, 11, and 12 have shown that gains of chromosomes 7 and 8 are consistent numerical alterations and may be markers of tumor aggressiveness and prognosis.

Inactivation of p53, a tumor suppressor gene on chromosome 17p, is present in up to 25% of advanced prostate cancers, but is rare in early cancers, suggesting that it may play a role in late progression[48]. Another tumor suppressor gene, DCC, shows allelic deletion and loss of expression in 45% of cases, indicating that it is a frequent feature of prostate cancer. Loss of expression of the retinoblastoma gene on chromosome 13q is seen in a minority of prostate cancers, usually in advanced stages. Activated oncogenes such as ras and c-erbB-2 (HER-2/neu) appear to be infrequent in early prostate cancer.

Oncogenesis probably occurs through the selection of several genetic changes, each modifying the expression or function of genes controlling cell growth or differentiation. Genetic alterations in colon cancer have been extensively studied and a model has been proposed in which the activation of oncogenes and loss of function of tumor suppressor genes is correlated with progressive clinical and histopathologic changes observed during carcinogenesis. Although little is currently known about the molecular basis of prostatic carcinoma, a similar process of progressive genetic changes is thought to occur[49].

References

1. Bostwick DG, Cooner WH, Denis L, Jones GW, Scardino PT, Murphy GP. The association of benign prostatic hyperplasia and cancer of the prostate. *Cancer* 1992;**70**:291–301.

2. Bostwick DG, Myers RP, Oesterling JE. Staging of prostate cancer. *Sem Surg Oncol* 1994;**10**:60–73.

3. Henson DE, Hutter RVP, Farrow GM. Practice protocol for the examination of specimens removed from patients with carcinoma of the prostate gland. A publication of the Cancer Committee, College of American Pathologists. *Arch Pathol Lab Med* 1994;**118**:779–783.

4. Bostwick DG. Prospective origins of prostate carcinoma. Prostatic intraepithelial neoplasia and atypical adenomatous hyperplasia. *Cancer* 1996;**78**:330–336.

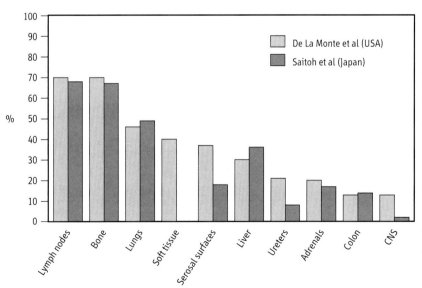

Fig. 12.8 Genetic changes and other changes associated with progression of prostate cancer. Some biomarkers show upregulation or gain (indicated by + sign), whereas others are downregulated or lost (− sign). There is a prominent clustering of changes in expression for many biomarkers between benign epithelium and high grade PIN, indicating that this is an important threshold for carcinogenesis in the prostate. A small number of other changes are introduced in the progression from high-grade PIN to localized cancer, metastatic cancer and hormone-refractory cancer. The model indicates the initial change in expression of a biomarker; most of these changes become magnified in subsequent steps. This model is based chiefly on studies of human prostatic tissue, and excludes many biomarkers that have not been evaluated in PIN or different stages of cancer (With permission from Bostwick DG, Pacelli A, Lopez-Beltran A. Molecular biology of prostatic intraepithelial neoplasia. *Prostate* 1996;**29**:117–134.)

5. Sakr WA, Grignon DJ, Haas GP, Heilbrun LK, Pontes JE, Crissman JD. Age and racial distribution of prostatic intraepithelial neoplasia. *Eur Urol* 1996;**30**:138–144.

6. Montironit R Bostwick DG, Bonkhoff H *et al.* Origins of prostate cancer. *Cancer* 1996;**78**:362–365.

7. Qian J, Wollan P, Bostwick DG. The extent and multicentricity of high grade prostatic intraepithelial neoplasia in clinically localized prostatic adenocarcinoma. *Hum Pathol* 1997; **28**: 143–8

8. Brawer MK, Peehl DM, Stamey TA, Bostwick DG. Keratin immunoreactivity in benign and neoplastic human prostate. *Cancer Res* 1985;**45**:3665–3669.

9. Lee F, Torp-Pedersen ST, Carroll JT, Siders DB, Christensen-Day C, Mitchell AE. Use of transrectal ultrasound and prostate-specific antigen in diagnosis of prostatic intraepithelial neoplasia. *Urology* (suppl) 1989;**24**:4–8.

10. Bostwick DG, Pacelli A, Lopez-Beltran A. Molecular biology of prostatic intraepithelial neoplasia. *Prostate* 1996;**29**:117–134.

11. Davidson D, Bostwick DG, Qian J *et al.* Prostatic intraepithelial neoplasia is a risk factor for adenocarcinoma: Predictive accuracy in needle biopsies. *J Urol* 1995;**154**:1295–1299.

12. Bostwick DG, Dundore PA. *Biopsy interpretation of the prostate.* Chapman & Hall, 1997.

13. Helpap B. Observations on the number, size, and localization of nucleoli in hyperplastic and neoplastic prostatic disease. *Histopathol* 1988; **13**:203–211.

14. Bonkhoff H. Role of the basal cells in premalignant changes of the human prostate: A stem cell concept for the development of prostate cancer. *Eur Urol* 1996;**30**:201–205.

15. Egan AJM, Bostwick DG. Prediction of extraprostatic extension of prostate cancer based on needle biopsy findings: Perineural invasion lacks significance on multivariate analysis. *Am. J Surg Pathol* 1997; **21**: 1496–500.

16. Aihara M, Wheeler TM, Ohori M, Scardino PT. Heterogeneity of prostate cancer in radical prostatectomy specimens. *Urology* 1994;**43**:60–66.

17. Cintra ML, Billis A. Histologic grading of prostatic adenocarcinoma: Intraobserver reproducibility of the Mostofi, Gleason and Bocking grading systems. *Int Urol Nephrol* 1991;**23**:449–454.

18. di Loreto C, Fitzpatrick B, Underhill S, Kim DH, Dytch HE, Galera-Davidson H, Bibbo M. Correlation between visual clues, objective architectural features and interobserver agreement in prostate cancer. *Am J Clin Pathol* 1991;**96**:70–75.

19. Bostwick DG, Egbert BM, Fajardo LF. Radiation injury of the normal and neoplastic prostate. *Am J Surg Pathol* 1982;**6**:541–548.

20. Dugan TC, Shipley WU, Young RH *et al.* Biopsy after external beam radiation therapy for adenocarcinoma of the prostate: correlation with original histological grade and current prostate specific antigens levels. *J Urol* 1991;**146**:1313–1316.

21. Helpap B, Koch V. Histological and immunohistochemical findings of prostatic carcinoma after external or interstitial radiotherapy. *J Cancer Res Clin Oncol* 1991;**117**:608–614.

22. Kabalin JN. Biopsy after external beam radiation therapy for adenocarcinoma of the prostate: correlation with original histological grade and current prostate specific antigen levels. *J Urol* 1992;**148**:1565–1566.

23. Siders DB, Lee F. Histologic changes of irradiated prostatic carcinoma diagnosed by transrectal ultrasound. *Hum Pathol* 1992;**23**:344–351.

24. Wheeler JA, Zagars GK, Ayala AG. Dedifferentiation of locally recurrent prostate cancer after radiation therapy. *Cancer* 1993;**71**:3783–3787.

25. Prestidge BR, Hoak DC, Grimm PD *et al.* Posttreatment biopsy results following interstitial brachytherapy in early-stage prostate cancer. *Int J Rad Oncol Biol Physics* 1997;**37**:31–39.

26. Crook JM, Bahadur YA, Robertson SJ *et al.* Evaluation of radiation effect, tumor differentiation, and prostate specific antigen staining in sequential prostate biopsies after external beam radiotherapy for patients with prostate carcinoma. *Cancer* 1997;**79**:81–89.

27. Crook JM, Bahadur YA, Bociek RG *et al.* Radiotherapy for localized prostate carcinoma. The correlation of pretreatment prostate specific antigen and nadir prostate specific antigen with outcome as assessed by systematic biopsy and serum prostate specific antigen. *Cancer* 1997;**79**:328–336.

28. Algaba F, Epstein JI, Aldape HC *et al.* Workgroup 5. Assessment of prostate carcinoma in core needle biopsy – definition of minimal criteria for the diagnosis of cancer in biopsy material. *Cancer* 1996;**78**:376–381.

29. Tetu B, Srigley JR, Boivin J, Dupont A, Monfette G, Pinault S, Labrie F. Effect of combination endocrine therapy (LHRH agonist and flutamide) on normal prostate and prostatic adenocarcinoma. *Am J Surg Pathol* 1991;**15**:111–120.

30. Ferguson J, Zincke H, Ellison E *et al.* Decrease of prostatic intraepithelial neoplasia (PIN) following androgen deprivation therapy in patients with stage T3 carcinoma treated by radical prostatectomy. *Urology* 1994;**44**:91–95.

31. Vaillancourt L, Tetu B, Fradet Y, Dupont A, Gomez J, Cusan L, Suburu ER *et al.* Effect of neoadjuvant endocrine therapy (combined androgen blockade) on normal prostate and prostate carcinoma. A randomized study. *Am J Surg Pathol* 1996;**20**:86–93.

32. Murphy WM, Soloway MS, Barrows GH. Pathologic changes associated with androgen deprivation therapy for prostate cancer. *Cancer* 1991;**68**:821–828.

33. Hellström M, Häggman M, Brändstedt S *et al.* Histopathological changes in androgen-deprived localized prostatic cancer. A study in total prostatectomy specimens. *Eur Urol* 1993;**24**:461–465.

34. Armas OA, Aprikian AG, Melamed J *et al.* Clinical and pathobiological effects of neoadjuvant total androgen ablation therapy on clinically localized prostatic adenocarcinoma. *Am J Surg Pathol* 1994;**18**:979–991.

35. Montironi R, Magi Galluzzi C, Muzzonigro G *et al.* Effects of combination endocrine treatment on normal prostate, prostatic intraepithelial neoplasia, and prostatic adenocarcinoma. *J Clin Pathol* 1994;**47**:906–913.

36. Smith DM, Murphy WM. Histologic changes in prostate carcinomas treated with Leuprolide (Luteinizing Hormone-Releasing Hormone effect). Distinction from poor tumor differentiation. *Cancer* 1994;**73**:1472–1479.

37. Civantos F, Marcial MA, Banks ER *et al.* Pathology of androgen deprivation therapy in prostatic carcinoma. A comparative study of 173 patients. *Cancer* 1995;**75**:1634–1641.

38. Ellison E, Chuang SS, Zincke H *et al.* Prostate adenocarcinoma after androgen deprivation therapy: a comparative study of morphology, morphometry, immunohistochemistry, and DNA ploidy. *Pathol Case Reviews* 1996;**1**:37–47.

39. Shabaik A, Wilson S, Bidair M, Masson D, Schmidt J. Pathologic changes in prostate biopsies following cryoablation therapy of prostate carcinoma. *J Urol Pathol* 1995;**3**:183–194.

40. Borkowski P, Robinson MJ, Poppiti RJ Jr, Nash SC. Histologic findings in postcryosurgical prostatic biopsies. *Mod Pathol* 1996;**9**:807–811.

41. Falconieri G, Lugnani F, Zanconati F *et al.* Histopathology of the frozen prostate. The microscopic bases of prostatic carcinoma cryoablation. *Path Res Pract* 1996;**192**:579–587.

42. Shuman BA, Cohen JK, Miller RJ Jr *et al.* Histological presence of viable prostatic glands on routine biopsy following cryosurgical ablation of the prostate. *J Urol* 1997;**157**:552–555.

43. Aprikian AG, Cordon-Cardo C, Fair WR, Reuter VE. Characterization of neuroendocrine differentiation in human benign prostate and prostatic adenocarcinoma. *Cancer* 1993;**71**:3952–3965.

44. Berner A, Nesland JM, Waehre H, Silde J, Fossa SD. Hormone resistant prostatic adenocarcinoma. An evaluation of prognostic factors in pre- and post-treatment specimens. *Br J Cancer* 1993;**68**:380–384.

45. Bostwick DG, Pacelli A, Blute M *et al.* Prostate specific membrane antigen expression in prostatic intraepithelial neoplasia and adenocarcinoma: study of 184 cases. *Cancer* 1998; **82**: 2256–61.

46. Darson MF, Pacelli A, Roche P *et al.* Human glandular kallikrein 2 (hK2) expression in prostatic intraepithelial neoplasia and adenocarcinoma: a novel prostate cancer marker. *Urology* 1997;**49**:857–862.

47. Shankey TV, Jin JK, Dougherty S *et al.* DNA ploidy and proliferation heterogeneity in human prostate cancers. *Cytometry* 1995;**21**:30–39.

48. Salem CE, Tomasic NA, Elmajian DA *et al.* p53 protein and gene alterations in pathological stage C prostate carcinoma. *J Urol* 1997;**158**:510–514.

49. Cheng L, Song S, Pretlow TG *et al.* Independent origin of multiple tumors from prostate cancer patients. *Cancer Res* 1998; **90**: 233–7.

13 Presentation and diagnosis

M M Ahmed and J E Oesterling

Algorithm

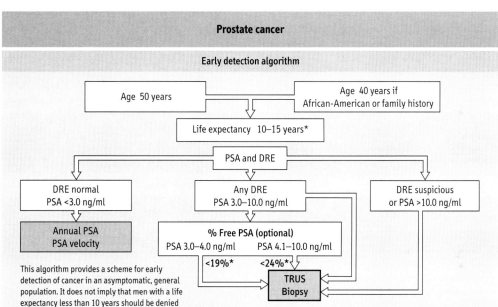

Prostate cancer

Early detection algorithm

Age 50 years

Age 40 years if African-American or family history

Life expectancy 10–15 years*

PSA and DRE

DRE normal
PSA <3.0 ng/ml

Any DRE
PSA 3.0–10.0 ng/ml

DRE suspicious
or PSA >10.0 ng/ml

Annual PSA
PSA velocity

% Free PSA (optional)
PSA 3.0–4.0 ng/ml   PSA 4.1–10.0 ng/ml

<19%*   <24%*

TRUS
Biopsy

This algorithm provides a scheme for early detection of cancer in an asymptomatic, general population. It does not imply that men with a life expectancy less than 10 years should be denied detection and treatment of prostate cancer. *These figures are based on published literature using specific assays and clinicians must validate their own assays prior to clinical decision. TRUS, transrectal ultrasound.

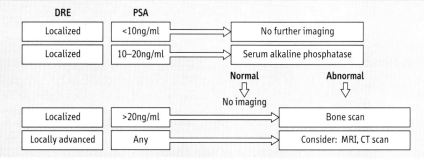

Clinical staging algorithm

DRE	PSA		
Localized	<10ng/ml	No further imaging	
Localized	10–20ng/ml	Serum alkaline phosphatase	

Normal   Abnormal

No imaging

| Localized | >20ng/ml | Bone scan |
| Locally advanced | Any | Consider: MRI, CT scan |

Prostate adenocarcinoma is a leading cause of death in men. In 2001, 31 500 men are expected to die of prostate cancer, and more than 198 000 men will be diagnosed with this condition in the United States[1]. Paradoxically, it is also the leading neoplasm noted incidentally at autopsy, seen in 50% of men aged 80 or older. The challenge of prostate cancer is to identify those in whom the neoplasm will be clinically significant. This chapter will review the tools at a urologist's disposal for the diagnosis of prostate cancer, evaluate screening strategies for prostate cancer, and discuss an algorithm for the diagnosis of early, curable prostate cancer.

Patient history

A good patient history is the first step in any evaluation for prostate cancer. In the history, risk factors for prostate cancer should be identified. Patient age, race and a family history (both maternal and paternal) significant for prostate cancer are the three generally accepted risk factors. An age above 50 years in individuals with no family history of prostate cancer or 40 years in Blacks and individuals with a family history of prostate cancer increases the risk of developing prostate cancer. Although the incidence of prostate cancer found at autopsy is approximately the same in men world-wide, clinically relevant prostate cancer appears to be more prevalent amongst Blacks and least prevalent among Asians[2,3]. These risk factors are discussed in the previous chapter.

There are no clear clinical signs that seem to correlate well with the presence of early, organ-confined prostate cancer. Complaints of prostatism can occur in over 50% of men above the age of 50 years[4]. Pain complexes, such as orchalgias and prostatdynia, have also been noted, although these symptoms are quite non-specific. The high incidence and non-specific symptoms illustrate the difficulty in detecting early stage prostate cancer based on history alone.

Advanced prostate cancer presents more frequently with symptoms, usually genitourinary obstruction, gross haematuria or bone pain. The presentation of advanced stage prostate cancer is declining in the United States, but this does not appear to be a world-wide phenomenon[5]. Of men with advanced stage disease, 20–40% are symptomatic as compared with 0% of the men who have only localized disease. Patient history is neither sensitive nor specific enough to be relied upon for detecting the vast majority of prostate cancer at an early organ-confined, curable stage.

Digital rectal examination

The digital rectal examination (DRE) plays an important role in the diagnosis of prostate adenocarcinoma. It has been recommended as early as 1940 to detect prostate cancer[6]. The position of the patient in which the examination is performed, the experience of the examiner, the sensitivity of the examining finger can all vary, making the DRE a decidedly subjective test.

In large screening studies, palpable abnormalities on DRE can be as high as 33%[7]. A number of series have estimated that the sensitivity of the DRE for PCa ranges from 69–89% and the specificity from 84–98%[8]. False-positives on DRE can be attributed to benign prostatic hyperplasia (BPH), granulomas, calcifications and cysts. False-negatives on DRE can also be attributed to several factors: tumor location, prostate gland volume and tumor density[9]. The overall detection rate for prostate cancer appears to range from 0.8–1.7% when the DRE alone is used in a screening setting[10].

The DRE has failed consistently to identify organ-confined, curable prostate cancer. Catalona and co-workers demonstrated 57% of patients diagnosed with prostate cancer following an abnormal DRE had advanced disease, and over 25% of patients diagnosed with a prostatic malignancy by DRE alone are understaged[11,12]. Although the DRE plays an important role in the evaluation of the urologic patient, it should be used in conjunction with other studies when evaluating the prostate for the presence of early, curable prostate cancer.

Imaging studies

Imaging of the prostate has improved significantly over the past decades. The most commonly utilized imaging modality is the transrectal ultrasound (TRUS). However, other technologies also can provide detailed images of the prostate. These will be briefly discussed.

MRI and CT scan

Magnetic resonance imaging (MRI) is now widely available and has been used to evaluate the prostate (Figure 13.1). With T-2 weighted images, the zones of the prostate can be visualized: the central and transition zones of the prostate are low signal and the peripheral zone has a higher signal. Prostate cancer is seen as a distinctly low signal area. However, in comparison with transrectal ultrasound, there does not appear to be a significant advantage to using the more expensive MRI[13]. The MRI scanner has also been adapted with a balloon mounted endorectal coil. While this may have some potential use in the future, further studies are needed.

CT scanners have also not attained the level of detail needed to identify prostate cancer (Figure 13.2)[14]. Both CT and MRI may play a role in the staging of select prostate cancers, but both modalities are too inefficient to be used for purposes of detecting early, curable prostate cancer.

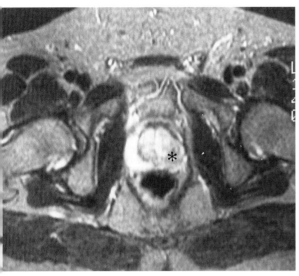

Fig. 13.1 MR of prostate cancer. A transverse T2 weighted image of the prostate demonstrates a large area of low signal intensity (asterisk) representing the neoplasm which is seen against the bright signal of the normal prostate (Courtesy of Robert L. Bree, M.D., University of Michigan Medical School.)

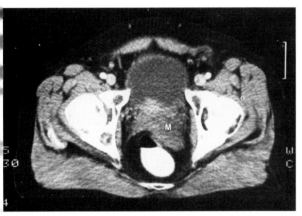

Fig. 13.2 CT of prostate cancer. CT image through the prostate demonstrates a mass (M) emanating from the left side of the gland appearing to extend into the periprostatic soft tissues. (Courtesy of Robert L. Bree, M.D., University of Michigan Medical School.)

TRUS

TRUS has been in vogue since the early 1980s. Initial studies were enthusiastic about its ability to evaluate prostatic anatomy and identify prostate cancer. Currently, TRUS probes use high frequency 7.0 to 7.5 MHz scanners. With these transducers, normal prostatic stroma appears isoechoic, with the peripheral zone, central zone and the seminal vesicles usually well visualized.[15] A fairly accurate

assessment of prostatic volume also can be obtained. Prostate cancer, when identifiable, appears as a hypoechoic area in over 50% of histologically examined specimens (Figure 13.3); higher-grade tumors or those outside of the peripheral zone can have more variability[16,17]. Color doppler ultrasonography can also image prostate cancer; focal peripheral zone hypervascularity is highly associated with malignancy[80].

Extensive experience with TRUS has revealed certain limitations. The sensitivity of TRUS alone has been reported to range from 48–100% and the specificity from 36–94%[10]. The more optimistic figures were reported earlier on in the TRUS experience and have not been duplicated. Most cancers missed by TRUS appear to be in the anterior and central regions of the prostate[18]. Since approximately 25% of the tumors occur in the heterogeneous transition zone, a substantial number of tumors can be missed. Studies which compare TRUS findings with the pathologic specimen in detail usually find a more modest sensitivity and specificity of 52% and 68%, respectively[19].

The assessment of tumor volume also can vary, since tumor diameter on TRUS appears to underestimate pathological tumor diameter by as much as 4.8 mm[20]. Determination of total prostatic volume is more consistent: a variability of 5.5 cc overall has been reported, with greatest variations occurring in glands over 50 cc[21].

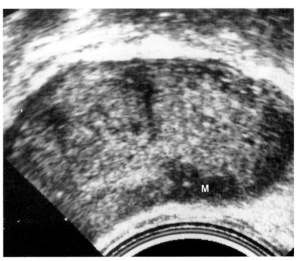

Fig. 13.3 Ultrasound of prostate cancer. Transrectal scan in the transverse plane of the prostate demonstrates a large hypoechoic mass (M) involving a large area of the peripheral zone. Biopsy revealed prostate cancer. (Courtesy of Robert L. Bree, M.D., University of Michigan Medical School.)

TRUS-guided sextant biopsy

The TRUS has significantly improved a urologist's ability to sample the prostate. Accurately guided biopsies from the peripheral and transition zones of the prostate can be taken when utilizing the TRUS (Figure 13.4). This has improved the yield of prostate biopsies. Systematic sampling of the prostate with 1.5 cm cores from the apex, midportion and base of the prostate bilaterally was able to detect prostate cancer in 53% of patients who previously underwent digitally guided biopsies with negative results. The theoretical probability of sampling a tumor 2.0 cc in size in a 40 g prostate with sextant biopsies is approximately 25%[22]. Patients who underwent systematic sextant sampling rather than directed biopsies only through hypoechoic regions had higher rates of prostate cancer detection[23]. Obtaining an additional sample from any suspicious regions (including extracapsular) has been shown significantly to improve the ability of the modified sextant biopsy to predict final pathological diagnosis[24]. There is now mounting evidence that sextant biopsies do not represent the optimal method of detecting early prostate, and that this should be increased to 10 or 12 cores routinely [81].

Performing a transrectal biopsy with an 18-gauge needle using a rapid-fire system carries a low morbidity rate. Infection can be seen in up to 6.2%, and less than 2% have significant bleeding, urinary retention or rectal injury[25]. A TRUS-guided sextant biopsy with additional sampling of suspicious areas has become the standard procedure for a definitive diagnosis of prostate cancer.

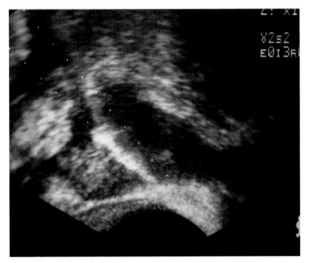

Fig. 13.4 Prostate biopsy. Sagittal image obtained during the performance of a transrectal ultrasound guided prostate biopsy. The needle is seen as a bright echo entering the prostate from the rectum. (Courtesy of Robert L. Bree, M.D., University of Michigan Medical School.)

Laboratory studies

The most significant advance in prostate cancer detection has been the discovery of the prostate-specific antigen (PSA). PSA has emerged to become the most useful tumor marker available for prostate cancer. Other laboratory markers, such as prostatic acid phosphatase (PAP), do not have the sensitivity or specificity needed to become viable tumor markers[26]. While PAP once played a role in evaluating metastatic prostate cancer, the superiority of the PSA has made the PAP essentially obsolete in 1996. Several additional prostate cancer markers are currently being investigated for correlation with prostate cancer, including TURP-27, PD41, 7E11-C5 and PR92. Nevertheless, their clinical utility still needs to be ascertained[27].

Prostate-specific antigen

Prostate-specific antigen was identified in the early 1970s, and recognized as a potential marker for prostate cancer by Wang and co-workers in 1979[28,29]. PSA that is measured in the serum is produced largely by the columnar epithelial cells in the prostate gland. Its primary biological role is to cleave certain seminal fluid proteins, which improves sperm motility and liquefaction of the seminal coagulum[30]. Although its production is decreased in high-grade malignancies, the overall increased prostate and tumor volume causes higher serum levels of PSA. Other causes of PSA elevation include BPH, transurethral procedures, prostatitis[31], infarction[32], ejaculation[33] and prostatic massage[34].

PSA exists in several molecular forms (see Table 13.1). Standard serum assays for PSA measure the total PSA (t-PSA) in the serum, which is a combination of all the molecular forms of PSA. The predominant forms of PSA in the serum, however, are f-PSA (free and unbound PSA comprising 5–30%), PSA-ACT (PSA complexed to alpha-1-antichymotrypsin comprising 60–95%) and PSA-MG (PSA complexed to alpha-2-macroglobulin). Currently available immunoasays are unable to detect PSA-MG. Thus, the total PSA will reflect the amount of free-PSA and PSA-ACT.

Total PSA has been extensively studied and characterized. High PSA values are strongly associated with prostate cancer. For a PSA of >10 ng/ml, 50–88% of men will have prostate cancer, and for those between 4–10 ng/ml, 20% will have PCa[35]. In a mass screening program involving over 5000 men, almost 10% had PSA values between 4 ng/ml and 10 ng/dl[36]. Since the PSA values which fall between 4.0–10 ng/ml are not as well correlated with the presence of prostate cancer, investigators have attempted to characterize PSA in a variety of different ways to optimize its sensitivity and specificity, for purposes of

Table 13.1   Molecular forms of PSA

PSA form	Description
Total PSA	All immunologic detectable forms of PSA, primarily consists of f-PSA and PSA-ACT
Free PSA	Unbound PSA, inactive in serum
PSA-ACT	PSA bound to alpha-1-antichymotrypsin, or 'complexed PSA'
PSA-MG	PSA bound to alpha-2-macroglobulin, not immunodetectable
PSA-PCI	PSA bound to protein-C inhibitor, not found in serum
PSA-AT	PSA bound to alpha-1-antitrypsin, trace amounts found in serum
PSA-ITI	PSA bound inter-alpha-trypsin inhibitor, trace amounts found in serum

(Table modified from McCormack RT *et al. Urology* 1995;**45**:729–744.)

distinguishing the men with early, curable cancer from the men with BPH only. These characterizations of PSA include age-specific reference ranges for PSA, PSA density (PSAD) and PSA velocity (PSAV).

Age-specific reference ranges for PSA

Utilizing a PSA value of 4.0 ng/ml or greater in screening for prostate cancer, large studies have found a cancer detection rate of 2.2–2.6%[37,38]. The sensitivity and specificity of a PSA value of 4.0 ng/dl alone in detecting prostate cancer range from 50–80% and 60–70%, respectively. For a PSA value between 4.0–10.0 ng/ml, the performance of PSA as a tumor marker falls considerably. Furthermore, up to 9–27% of prostate cancers occur in men with a PSA below 4.0[39,40].

Age-specific PSA limits were created in hopes of making the PSA a better predictor of cancer with the mildly elevated PSA levels (4.0–10.0 ng/ml). Several age-specific reference ranges have been proposed; the initial ranges by Oesterling *et al.* correlate fairly closely with others[41]. Oesterling and co-workers stratified the PSA results of 471 prospectively chosen men who were determined to be prostate cancer-free by DRE, TRUS and prostate biopsy (Figure 13.5). Subsequent studies of PSA values amongst men of varying races indicates that these reference ranges need to be made race-specific also (Table 13.2)[42,43].

Several investigators found age-specific ranges improve prostate cancer detection in younger men and reduce biopsy rates in older men. Reissigl *et al.* found that age-specific reference ranges detected 16 prostate cancers in men aged 40–49 with a PSA ranging from 2.5–4.0 ng/ml, all of which were organ confined by pathological staging, comprising 16% of all organ detected prostate cancer found in this prospective screening study of 21 078 Austrian men. These organ confined malignancies would have been missed by using the standard PSA cut-off of 4.0 ng/ml.[44] Other studies confirm this finding[45,46]. However, the lower sensitivity for prostate cancer amongst older men may be a concern. Age-specific reference ranges and DRE would have missed 16 cancers (8% of total detected) in men with a mean age of 73.5 years in the Reissigl study. Catalona *et al.* similarly reports 8% of otherwise detectable prostate cancer cases would be missed, and Bangma *et al.* reports a 12% loss in detection of clinically localized prostate cancer[47,48]. The long-term effect on morbidity and mortality when using this or other measures is not yet available.

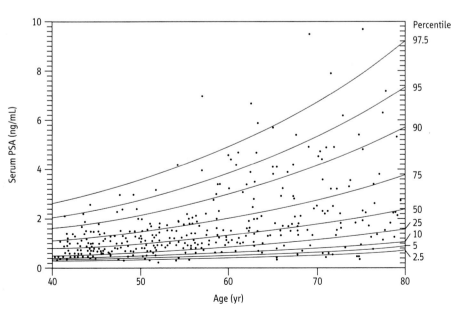

Fig. 13.5 Scattergram demonstrating the relationship between serum PSA and patient age among 471 men without prostate cancer. The curves identify the cutpoints for each serum PSA percentile. (Taken from JE Oesterling *et al.*, *JAMA* 1993;**270**:860–864. Copyright 1993, American Medical Association.)

Table 13.2 Age-specific ranges for PSA based on race

Age range	PSA references ranges		
	White	Black	Japanese
40–49	0.0–2.5	0.0–2.0	0.0–2.0
50–59	0.0–3.5	0.0–4.0	0.0–3.0
60–69	0.0–4.5	0.0–4.5	0.0–4.0
70–79	0.0–6.0	0.0–5.5	0.0–5.0

Table 13.3 Comparison of men with elevated and normal PSAD and age-specific PSA

Serum PSA	PSA density*		Total (%)
	Normal (%)	Elevated (%)	
Normal	441 (94)	7 (1)	448 (95)
Elevated	11 (2)	13 (3)	23 (5)
Total	425 (96)	19 (4)	471 (100)

* Defined by 95th percentile for both PSA and PSAD.
(Table modified from JE Oesterling *et al. Urol Clin North Am.* 1993;**20**: 671–680.)

The rise in PSA with age can be explained to some extent by prostate size. Prostate gland volume appears to correlate strongly to PSA (r = 0.55), and can be expected to rise approximately 1–2% a year. With each millilitre increase in prostate size, the PSA can be expected to rise 4%[49,50]. The relationship between PSA and volume can be further clarified with the concept of PSAD.

PSA density

The PSAD is defined as the ratio of PSA to the prostatic volume as assessed by TRUS. Benson *et al.* reported initially that this should be greater than 0.15 ng/ml/cc, and that this can be used in men with a PSA between 4.0–10.0 ng/ml for better detection of cancer[21,51]. Large series have used PSAD with some success: Seaman and co-workers reported on 3140 men, 426 of whom underwent a biopsy because the PSA was between 4.0 and 10.0 ng/ml[52]. While the mean PSA between the positive and negative biopsy group was not statistically different, the mean PSAD between these two groups (0.285 ± 0.147 and 0.199 ± 0.108, respectively) was significant (*P* < 0.00001). Figure 13.5 depicts the relationship between PSAD and probability of prostate cancer based on these data.

Not all investigators have found PSAD to be useful. Catalona's large prostate cancer screening study found that using PSAD in men with a PSA between 4–10 ng/ml missed almost half of identified prostate cancers[53]. Further refinements of the PSAD have been proposed, specifically, using the transition zone volume to calculate PSAD instead of total gland volume or measuring changes in PSAD over time; none of these, however, appear to add significant clinical information[21,54]. Investigators have been able to demonstrate that the clinical information derived from PSAD is minimal when age-specific reference ranges are used. In a group of 471 prospectively selected men, only seven (1%) had an elevated PSAD (95th percentile) with a normal age-specific PSA (Table 13.3)[55]. There is currently no compelling reason to continue widespread use of PSAD in place of other markers.

PSA velocity

PSA velocity (change in PSA over time) also has been shown significantly to improve the specificity of PSA.

Initial reports were based on a review of 57 men followed for seven to 25 years[56]. Here, it was found that men who were eventually diagnosed with cancer had a higher rate of PSA increase compared with men with BPH, which in turn was greater than men without any detectable prostatic disease (Figure 13.6). A PSA increase of more than 0.75 ng/ml per year had a 90% specificity for prostate cancer over BPH. A larger series involving 701 patients with a repeat PSA 1 year later found 260 (37%) with a 20% rise in PSA, of which 82 (31%) elected to undergo a biopsy[57]. Amongst these 82 men, 14 cancers were found (17% detection). Most of these cancers were in men below the age of 70 (64%), and in men with a PSA of less than 4.0 ng/ml (92%). An additional study of 951 screened patients with at least two serial PSA reports found a PSA increase of 0.6 ng/ml/yr is better than a PSA increase of 20%/yr (*P* < 0.05), and has a specificity of approximately 90% for cancer.[21]

The PSAV has several drawbacks. First, its sensitivity for prostate cancer ranges from 60–80%. The variability of PSA is also problematic. The probability that the PSA might rise 0.8 ng/ml in men with BPH ranged from 6–23% when one consecutive PSA measurement was made. However, this probability decreased to 1–4% with two consecutive PSA measurements[58]. Therefore, PSAV may be more useful when it is used in conjunction with other tests, and when at least three PSA assessments are made at least 12 to 18 months apart.

Trials comparing the ability of the various PSA characterizations to detect prostate cancer have not found an overall consistent advantage of any one modality than another[40]. These studies each have their own drawbacks, including selection biases and different screening strategies, as will be discussed shortly. Finally, there is no completed study at this time which makes any correlation between the various PSA characterizations and long-term cancer-specific patient survival.

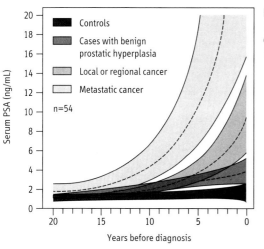

Fig. 13.6 Graph demonstrating the exponential rise of PSA in men with prostate cancer compared with men with BPH and the control group prior to diagnosis of each diagnostic group. (Taken from Carter *et al. JAMA* 1992;**267**:2215–2220. Copyright 1992, American Medical Association.)

Molecular PSA

The advent of molecular PSA has given the clinician more accuracy in diagnosing prostate cancer in those men with normal or mildly elevated PSA levels. PSA-ACT levels are significantly increased in men with prostate cancer compared with men with BPH, and the free-PSA/total-PSA (or per cent free-PSA) is lower[59,60]. The assays used to quantitate PSA-ACT have high variability, making its clinical utility difficult at this time. As a result, the per cent free-PSA appears to have the best clinical utility.

From a group of 422 randomly chosen men determined not to have prostate cancer, per cent free-PSA was determined to be age-independent[61]. Investigators have tried to determine the optimal per cent free-PSA cut-off point to distinguish malignant from benign disease. Luderer *et al.* found that for men with a PSA between 4.0–10.0 ng/ml (n = 57), per cent free-PSA of <0.25 had 31% specificity in detecting prostate cancer, compared with 0% specificity using a total PSA of > 4.0 ng/ml alone[62]. Outside of the PSA range of 4.0–10.0 ng/ml, the per cent free-PSA was not clinically useful. Similarly, Catalona *et al.* determined a 23% free-PSA cut-off will achieve a specificity of 38.1% in men with a PSA from 4.0–10.0 ng/ml[63].

More recently, Vashi *et al.* evaluated 413 men with total PSA ranging from 2.0–20.0 ng/ml (225 men had BPH and 188 men had PCa)[64]. Per cent free-PSA was found to be most useful when the total PSA ranged from 3.0–10.0 ng/ml – the 'reflex range'. This study suggested a per cent free-PSA cut-off point of 0.19 (values greater than 0.19 are normal) for PSAs ranging from 3.0–4.0 ng/ml would increase sensitivity (90%) to malignancy, whereas a per cent free-PSA cut-off point of 0.24 (values greater than 0.24 are normal) for PSAs ranging from 4.1–10.0 ng/ml would increase specificity (13%). This would allow greater detection of cancers amongst men likely to have organ-confined disease (3.0–4.0 ng/ml range), and decrease the number of negative biopsies amongst men with PSA ranging from 4.1–10.0 ng/ml.

All of the studies for per cent free-PSA have a relatively small number of patients and the evaluated population is not always consistent. While it is clear that the per cent free-PSA has clinical utility for a selected total PSA range, this range may vary with age, and the appropriate cut-off point for per cent free-PSA may vary according to age and/or prostate size.

Screening

Early detection of prostate cancer can be done amongst a variety of populations. When performed amongst men who present to a urologist's office, such early detection efforts have a much higher yield of prostate cancer than early detection efforts amongst a random selection of men in the community. Early detection of prostate cancer amongst non-selected men in the community, or screening, requires institutional coordination. It carries different implications of cost and efficacy than does early detection by urologists in their individual offices. This section will discuss the optimal combination of diagnostic tools used for the early detection of prostate cancer and review the controversies surrounding generalized screening of men.

Optimal use of diagnostic tools

A number of centers have performed large-scale screening studies of the general population. These are summarized in Table 13.4. These studies demonstrate a cancer detection rate ranging from 1.1–5.2%, using a various combination of screening tools to determine need for

Table 13.4   Detection rates for prostate cancer using screening tests by various authors

Author (Ref. No.)	No. men screened	Initial screening criteria for biopsy†	No. biopsies*	No. cancers	Detection rate in %
Bangma (67)	1726	PSA >4 or + DRE	308	67	3.9
Brawer (38)	1249	PSA >4	107	32	2.6
Catalona (35)	6630	PSA >4 or + DRE	1167	264	4.0
Catalona (11)	9629	PSA >4 and then if +DRE or +TRUS	860	296	3.1
Gustafsson (79)	1782	PSA >10, +DRE or +TRUS	371	65	3.6
Labrie (65)	8029	PSA >3 and then if +DRE or +TRUS‡	906	322	4.0
Mettlin (66)	2999	+DRE or +TRUS	–	156	5.2
Reissgl (39)	21 078	Age-specific PSA	778	197	3.7
Tsukamoto (68)	1639	PSA >3.6 or +DRE	83	18	1.1

* Includes only those consenting to a biopsy after recommendation was made.
† Lists the initial criteria sued to determine the need for biopsy.
‡ Biopsy also performed if PSA is 10% greater than predicted.

biopsy. Using primarily DRE and TRUS, Labrie noted a detection rate of 4.0% amongst a randomly chosen screening population[65]. An analysis of this population's PSA revealed that a PSA of > 3.0 ng/ml and a suspicious DRE would have detected most of the prostate cancers found with TRUS and DRE alone. The American Cancer Society's National Prostate Cancer Detection Project used serial screening with TRUS and DRE for a detection rate of 5.2%[66]. However, their detection rate with one-time initial screening was 3.7%.

Using PSA as an initial screening test, then performing a TRUS and DRE to determine the need for biopsy on those with a PSA above 4.0 ng/ml was a strategy used by Catalona and co-workers in several early studies[11,37]. The detection rate for such strategies ranged from 2.2–3.1%. When PSA was used as the sole criterion for biopsy, the detection rate for a PSA of greater than 4.0 ng/ml was only 2.6%[38]. Age-specific PSA cut-offs were used for initial screening in a large Austrian study[39]. Men with an elevated age-specific PSA underwent systematic sextant biopsies after a DRE and TRUS had been performed. The detection rate was 3.7%.

Combining PSA and DRE as the initial screening tool, and performing a biopsy on all those with abnormalities was a strategy employed in 6630 men to detect 4.0% prostate cancer in the population[35]. This well designed study minimized use of the time consuming and relatively expensive TRUS, limiting its role to that of an adjunctive test used primarily to perform sextant biopsies. A similar strategy employed in Europe had a detection

rate of 3.9%[67]. Here, the use of TRUS did not appear to improve the ability of the PSA and DRE in detecting prostate cancer. A Japanese study using these modalities demonstrated a detection rate of only 1.1%. This may be explained by demographic differences in prostate cancer incidence in Japan and study design, as its authors discuss[68]. These data show that PSA and DRE are effective enough to serve as primary screening modalities.

The cost of screening programs has been an important issue in determining their application on a large scale. While this discussion is beyond the scope of this chapter, some important points need to be noted. The cost of both a DRE and PSA is considerably lower than a TRUS. Minimizing the use of TRUS, yet maintaining the same level of prostate cancer detection will lower the overall costs. Moreover, the PSA is an objective and easily reproducible parameter, unlike the DRE and TRUS. Amongst the handful of studies evaluating cost-effectiveness, Gustafsson and co-workers determined the most cost-effective strategy in detecting prostate cancer involved initially obtaining a PSA and performing a DRE, followed by selective TRUS[25].

The various PSA modifications may optimize specificity for prostate cancer further. PSA density cannot be obtained without TRUS, and it has had mixed results as previously discussed. More study will be needed before it can be given a primary role in screening. The PSA velocity appears to be clinically useful when serial PSAs are obtained over the course of at least 2 years. For initial screening, however, PSA velocity can play no role.

The per cent free-PSA appears to provide independent information regarding the presence of neoplasm. To date optimal cutpoints have been proposed for per cent free PSA after evaluation of referral populations. These cut-off points still need to be validated in a prospective manner amongst a screening population.

Is mass screening effective?

Perhaps the most important measure of success of any screening program is its effect on mortality and morbidity from prostate cancer. Long-term studies currently underway to determine the effect of screening and intervention will take many years to complete[69]. In the interim, only inferences can be made from the available data.

The natural history of prostate cancer and its clinical course varies. It is currently difficult to predict with preoperative data which cancer will remain indolent and which will become clinically significant in an individual's lifetime[70]. Ideally, a screening program should identify only aggressive prostate cancer at a stage when it is curable, i.e. organ confined.

In order to evaluate the efficacy of screening tests in detecting organ-confined prostate cancer (Stage T2c or less), investigators have reviewed the pathologic specimens of patients who underwent RRP following a diagnosis of prostate cancer as part of a screening study. The results are summarized on Table 13.5; with PSA based screening, 57–71% of patients who were treated with RRP had organ-confined prostate cancer. This incidence of organ-confined disease is an improvement over non-screened populations who have organ-confined disease in only 43% of men undergoing RRP[11]. With the use of per cent free-PSA and similar modalities, it is hoped that the per cent of organ-confined disease found on detection can be further improved. By clinical staging, similar disproportions can be noted between PSA-tested populations and non-PSA tested populations. One such population in Minnesota saw the presentation of clinically advanced prostate cancer decline from 31% in 1986 to 17% in 1992 with widespread PSA use[71]. Prostate cancer detected during serial visits, following initial screening, are almost always organ-confined[21,65].

Screening tests have been criticized for overdiagnosing prostate cancer and finding prostate cancer that would not ordinarily be clinically manifest[72]. Such insignificant tumors can have negative effects upon patients, particularly if they are treated. These tumors can also falsely improve outcome data of prostate cancer screening and intervention trials. It is well established that such clinically insignificant tumors are low grade (Gleason 2–4) and low volume (less than 0.5 cc)[73]. These tumors incur no additional loss of life expectancy at 10 to 15 years follow up[74,75]. Use of life expectancy tables and estimated cancer doubling times has further enhanced the definition of 'clinically insignificant' tumor[70]. If these are the cancers detected by screening programs, no long-term benefits should be expected from their identification.

On the contrary, investigators are finding that prostate cancers detected by screening programs are typically larger than 0.5 cc and/or have Gleason scores above 4. Pathologic staging of 100 consecutive radical retropubic prostatectomy patients identified from a screening study found only 6% with a total Gleason score of 4 or less[76,77]. Similar results have been obtained after evaluation of men with stage T1c tumors[78]. Clearly, clinically significant, organ-confined tumors are being identified with PSA-based detection. Whether intervention for these tumors will actually translate into improved cancer-specific survival, as expected, remains to be definitively demonstrated.

Conclusions

Based on the preceding discussion, a flexible algorithm can be proposed for early detection of prostate cancer which incorporates our increasing knowledge about the utility of molecular PSA. Men with a family history of prostate cancer and those who are Black should begin assessment at age 40. All others should begin after the age of 50, providing they have a life expectancy of 10–15 years.

The initial assessment can be done by urologists or other clinicians: a DRE and a serum PSA. If the DRE is suspicious or the PSA is > 10.0 ng/ml, then one proceeds directly to a TRUS-guided biopsy. For those with a normal DRE and a PSA < 3.0 ng/ml, repeat annual screening is performed with calculation of PSA velocity.

Men with a PSA between 3.0–10.0 ng/ml fall within the 'reflex' range, where the serum is further analysed automatically in the laboratory to determine per cent free-PSA. For those men with a PSA between 3.0–4.0 ng/ml, TRUS and biopsy are recommended if the per cent free-PSA is less than 0.19. For those with a PSA between 4.1–10.0 ng/ml, TRUS and biopsy are recommended if the per cent free-PSA is less than 0.24.

This algorithm attempts to increase detection of organ-confined prostate cancer and decrease the number of negative prostate biopsies. Use of TRUS as an independent detection tool is minimized. This algorithm is most appropriate for early detection amongst a referral population to a urologist's office; it remains to be proven that this algorithm will be equally effective amongst a screening population.

Certainly, prostate cancer detection has undergone significant progress over the past decade. The various diagnostic modalities and their combinations continue to be evaluated in order to find an optimal prostate cancer detection strategy. Only through long-term investigation will efforts to affect morbidity and mortality from prostate cancer be realized. Results from large studies of screening such as the European Randomised Study of Screening in Prostate Cancer (ERSPC), due by 2008, are awaited eagerly.

Table 13.5 Number of organ-confined prostate cancers diagnosed through screening tests based on pathologic specimens

Author (Ref. No.)	No. cancers	No. undergoing RRP	No. (%) confined	No. (%) non-confined
Brawer (72)	32	16	9 (57)	7 (43)
Catalona (36)	264	160	114 (71)	46 (29)
Catalona (38)	296	244	153 (63)	91 (37)
Mettlin (66)	156	100	64 (64)	36 (36)
Reissgl (73)	197	135	95 (70)	40 (30)

References

1. Greenlee RT, Hill-Harmon MB, Murray T, Thun M. *Cancer statistics, 2001*. CA Cancer J Clin. 2001;**51(1)**:15–36.

2. Carter HB, Piantadosi S, Isaacs JT. Clinical evidence for and implications of the multistep development of prostate cancer. *J Urol* 1990;**143**:742.

3. Tsukamoto T, Kumamoto Y, Masumori N. Mass screening for prostate carcinoma: a study in Hokkaido, Japan. *Eur Urol* 1995;**27**:177–181.

4. Napalkov P, Boyle P, Maisoneuve P. Worldwide patterns of prevalence and mortality from BPH. *Urology* 1995;**46**(3A): 41.

5. Jacobsen SJ, Katusic SK, Bergsralh EJ, Oesterling JE et al. Incidence of prostate cancer diagnosis in the eras before and after serum PSA testing. *JAMA* 1995;**274**:1445–1449.

6. Young HH. *A surgeon's autobiography*. New York, Harcourt Brace 1940, p. 131.

7. Richie JP, Kavoussi LR, Ho GT et al. Prostate cancer screening: role of digital rectal examination and prostate specific antigen. *Ann Surg Onc* 1994; **1**:117–120.

8. Cupp MR, Oesterling JE. Prostate-specific antigen, digital rectal examination and transrectal ultrasonography: their roles in diagnosing early prostate cancer. *Mayo Clin Proc* 1993;**68**:297–306.

9. Brendler CB. Characteristics of prostate cancer found with early detection regimens. *Urology* 1995;**46**(3A):71–76.

10. Optenberg SA, Thompson IM. Economics for screening for carcinoma of the prostate. *Uro Clin N Am* 1990;**17**(4):719.

11. Catalona WJ, Smith DS, Ratliff TL, Basler JW. Detection of organ-confined prostate cancer is increased through PSA based screening. *JAMA* 1993;**270**:948–954.

12. Palken M, Cobb OE, Warren BH, Hoak DC. Prostate cancer: correlation of DRE, TRUS and PSA levels with tumor volumes in radical retropubic prostatectomy specimens. *J Urol* 1990;**143**:1155–1162.

13. Rifkin MD, Zerhouni EA, Gatsonis CA et al. Comparison of MRI and ultrasonography in staging early prostate cancer. *N Engl J Med* 1990;**323**:621–626.

14. Salo J, Kivsaari L, Ramilo S. Computerized tomagraphy and transrectal ultrasound in the assessment of local extension of prostatic cancer before radical retropubic prostatectomy. *J Urol* 1987;**137**:435–438.

15. Villerss A, Terris MK, McNeal JE, Stamey TA. Ultrasound anatomy of the prostate: the normal gland and anatomical variations. *J Urol* 1990;**142**:732–738.

16. Hernandez AD, Smith JA. Transrectal ultrasonagraphy for the early detection and staging of prostate cancer. *Urol Clin N Am* 1990;**17**(4):745–757.

17. Cooner WH, Mosley BR, Rutherford CL, Beard JH, Pond HS, Bass RB Jr, Terry WJ. Clinical application of transrectal ultrasound and PSA in the search for prostate cancer. *J Urol* 1988;**139**:758.

18. Stilmant MM, Kuligowska E. Transrectal ultrasonagraphic screening for prostate cancer with histopathologic correlations: factors affecting specificity. *Cancer* 1993;**71**(6):2041–2047.

19. Carter HB, Hamper UM, Sheth S, Sanders RC, Epstein JI, Walsh PC. Evaluation of transrectal ultrasound in the early detection of prostate cancer. *J Urol* 1989;**142**:1008–1010.

20. Cooner WH, Mosley BR, Rutherford CL et al. Prostate cancer detection in a clinical urologic practice by ultrasonography, digital rectal examination and PSA. *J Urol* 1990;**143**:1146–1154.

21. Littrup PJ, Kane RA, Mettlin CJ et al. Cost effective prostate cancer detection: reduction of low yield biopsies. *Cancer* 1994;**74**:3146–3158.

22. Stricker HJ, Ruddock LJ, Wan J, Belville WD. Detection of non-palpable prostate cancer: a mathematical and laboratory model. *Br J Urol* 1993;**71**:43–46.

23. Hodge KK, McNeal JE, Terris MK, Stamey TA. Random systematic versus directed ultrasound guided transrectal core biopsies of the prostate. *J Urol* 1989;**142**:71.

24. Narayan P, Gajendran V, Taylor SP et al. The role of transrectal ultrasound-guided biopsy based staging: Preoperative serum PSA, and biopsy gleason score in prediction of final pathologic diagnosis in prostate cancer. *urology* 1995;**46**:205–212.

25. Gustafsson O, Carlsson P, Norming U, Nyman CR, Svenson H. Cost effectiveness analysis in early detection of prostate cancer: an evaluation of six screening strategies in a randomly selected population of 2400 men. *Prostate* 1995;**26**:299–309.

26. Watson RA, Tang DB. The predictive value of prostatic acid phosphatase as a screening test for prostate cancer. *New Engl J Med* 1980;**303**:497.

27. Lee CT, Oesterling JE. Diagnostic markers of prostate cancer: Utility of PSA in diagnosis and staging. *Sem Surg Onc* 199511:23–35.

28. Wang MC, Valenzuela LA, Murphy GP et al. Purification of human prostate specific antigen. *Invest Urol* 1979; **17**:159–163.

29. Wang MC, Papsidero LD, Kuriyama M et al. Prostate antigen: a new potential marker for prostate cancer. *Prostate* 1981;**2**:89–96.

30. Lilja H, Oldbring J, Rannevik G et al. Seminal vesicle-secreted proteins and their reactions during gelation and liquifaction of human semen. *J Clin Invest* 1993;**80**:281–285.

31. Robles JM, Morell AR, Redorta JP et al. Clinical behavior of PSA and prostatic acid phosphatase: a comparative study. *Eur Urol* 1988;**14**:360–366.

32. Glenski WK, Malek RS, Myrtle JF, Oesterling JE. Sustained, substantially increased concentration of PSA in the absence of prostatic malignant disease: an unusual clinical scenario. *Mayo Clin Proc* 1992;**67**:249–252.

33. Tchetgen MB, Song JT, Strawderman M, Jacobsen SJ, Oesterling JE. Ejaculation increases the serum PSA concentration. *Urology* 1996;**47**:511–516.

34. Yuan JJJ, Coplen DE, Petros JA et al. Effects of rectal examination, prostatic massage, ultrasonagraphy and needle biopsy on serum PSA levels. *J Urol* 1992;**147**:810–814.

35. Catalona WJ, Richie JP, Ahmann FR et al. Comparison of DRE and serum PSA in the early detection of prostate cancer: Results of a multicenter clinical trial of 6,630 men. *J Urol* 1994;**151**:1283–1290.

36. Schwartz KL, Kau TY, Severson RK, Demers RY. PSA in a community screening program. *J Fam Pract* 1995;**41**(2):163.

37. Catalona WJ, Smith DS, Ratliff et al. Measurement of PSA in serum as a screening test for prostate cancer. *N Engl J Med* 1991;**324**:1156–1161.

38. Brawer MK, Chetner MP, Beatie J, Buchner DM, Vessella RL, Lange PH. Screening for prostatic carcinoma with PSA. *J Urol* 1992;**147**:841–845.

39. Reissigl A, Pointner J, Horninger W et al. Comparison of different PSA cutpoints for early detection of prostate cancer: results of a large screening study. *Urology* 1995;**46**:662.

40. Mettlin C, Littrup PJ, Kane RA et al. Relative sensitivity and specificity of serum PSA level compared with age-referenced PSA, PSA density, and PSA change. *Cancer* 1994;**74**(5):1615.

41. Oesterling JE, Jacobsen SJ, Chute CG et al. Serum PSA in a community-based population: Establishment of age-specific reference ranges. *JAMA* 1993;**270**:860–864.

42. Morgan TO, Jacobsen SJ, McCarthy WF, Jacobson DJ, McLeod DG, Moul JW. Age-specific reference ranges for PSA in African-American men. *N Engl J Med* 1996;**335**:345–6.

43. Oesterling JE, Kumamoto Y, Tsukamoto T et al. Serum PSA in a community based population of healthy Japanese men: lower values than for similarly aged white men. *Br J Urol* 1995;**75**:347–353.

44. Reissigl A et al. Comparison of different prostate-specific antigen cutpoints for early detection of prostate cancer: results of a large screening study. *Urology* 1995;**46**:662–665.

45. Oesterling JE, Jacobsen SJ, Cooner WH. The use of age specific reference ranges for serum PSA in men 60 years old or older. *J Urol* 1995;**153**:1160–1163.

46. El-Galley RES, Petros JA, Sanders WH et al. Normal range PSA versus age specific PSA in screening prostate adenocarcinoma. *Urology* 1995;**46**:200.

47. Catalona WJ, Hudson MA, Scardino PT, Richie JP, Ahmann FR, Flanigan FC, deKernion JB, Ratliff TL, Kavoussi LR, Dalkin BL et al. Selection of optimal prostate specific antigen cutoffs for early detection of prostate cancer: Receiver operated characteristic curves. *J Urol* 1994;**152**:2037–2042.

48. Bangma CH, Kranse R, Blijenberg BG, Schroder FH. The value of screening tests in the detection of prostate cancer. Part II: Retrospective analysis of free/total PSA ratio, age-specific reference ranges, and PSA density. *Urology* 1995;**46**:779–784.

49. Oesterling JE, Jacobsen SJ, Chute CG et al. Serum PSA in a community-based population: Establishment of age-specific reference ranges. JAMA 1993;**270**:860–864.

50. Collins GN, Lee RJ, McKelvie GB et al. Relationship between PSA, prostate volume and age in the benign prostate. Br J Urol 1993;**71**:445.

51. Benson MC, Whang IS, Olsson CA, McMahon DJ, Cooner WH. The use of PSA density to enhance the predictive value of intermediate levels of serum PSA. J Urol 1992;**147**:817–821.

52. Seaman E, Whang M, Olsson C et al. PSA density: Role in patient evaluation and management. Urol Clin N Am 1993;**20**:653–663.

53. Catalona WJ, Richie JP, DeKernion JB et al. Comparison of PSA concentration versus PSA density in the early detection of prostate cancer: Receiver operating characteristic curves. J Urol 1994;**152**:2031–2036.

54. Kalish J, Cooner WH, Graham SD Jr. PSA adjusted for volume of transitional zone is more accurate than PSA adjusted for total gland volume in detecting adenocarcinoma of the prostate. Urology 1994;**43**:601.

55. Oesterling JE, Cooner WH, Jacobsen SJ. Influence of patient age on the serum PSA concentration: an important clinical correlation. Urol Clin North Am 1993;**20**(4):671.

56. Carter HB, Pearson JD, Metter J et al. Longitudinal evaluation of PSA levels in men with and without prostate disease. JAMA 1992;**267**:2215–2220.

57. Brawer MK, Beatie J, Wener MH, Vessella RL, Preston SD, Lange PH. Screening for prostate carcinoma with prostate specific antigen: results of the second year. J Urol 1993;**150**:106–109.

58. Carter HB, Pearson JD, Wacliwew X, Metter EJ, Guess HA, Walsh PC. PSA variablity in men with BPH. (Abstract). J Urol 1994;**151**:312A.

59. Stenman UH, Leinonen J, Alfthan H et al. A complex between PSA and ACT-PSA is the major form of PSA in serum of patients with prostate cancer: assay of the complex improves clinical sensitivity for the cancer. Cancer Res 1991;**51**:222.

60. Christensson A, Bjork T, Nilsson O et al. Serum PSA complexed to ACT as an indicator of prostate cancer. J Urol 1993;**150**:100.

61. Oesterling JE, Jacobsen SJ, Klee GG et al. Free, complexed and total PSA: The establishment of appropriate reference ranges for their concentrations and ratios. J Urol 1995;**154**:1090.

62. Luderer AA, Thiel R, Carlson G, Cuny C, Soriano TF. Using proportions of free to total PSA to predict the possibility of prostate cancer. Urology 1996;**47**:518.

63. Catalona WJ, Smith DS, Wolfert RL et al. Evaluation of percentage free PSA to improve specificity of prostate cancer screening. JAMA 1995;**274**:1214–1220.

64. Vashi AR, Wojno KJ, Henricks WJ et al. Determination of the reflex range and appropriate age cutpoints for percent free PSA in 413 men referred for prostatic evaluation using the AxSYM system. Urology 1997; **49**:19–27.

65. Labrie F, Candas B, Cusan L et al. Diagnosis of advanced or noncurable prostate cancer can be practically eliminated by PSA. Urology 1996;**47**:212–217.

66. Mettlin C, Murphy GP, Lee F et al. Characteristics of prostate cancers detected in a multimodality early detection program. Cancer 1993;**72**:1701–1708.

67. Bangma CH, Kranse R, Blijenberg BG, Schroder FH. The value of screening tests in the detection of prostate cancer. Part I: Results of a retrospective evaluation of 1726 men. Urology 1995;**46**:773–778.

68. Tsukamoto T, Kumamoto Y, Masumori N. Mass screening for prostate carcinoma: a study in Hokkaido, Japan. Eur Urol 1995;**27**:177–181.

69. Rosen MA. Impact of PSA screening on the natural history of prostate cancer. Urology 1995;**46**:757–768.

70. Dugan JA, Bostwick DG, Myers RP, Qian J, Bergstralh EJ, Oesterling JE. The definition and preoperative prediction of clinically insignificant prostate cancer. JAMA 1996;**275**:288–294.

71. Jacobsen SJ, Katusic SK, Bergsralh EJ, Oesterling JE et al. Incidence of prostate cancer diagnosis in the eras before and after serum PSA testing. JAMA 1995;**274**:1445–1449.

72. Kramer BS, Brown ML, Prorok PC, Potosky AL, Gohagan JK. Prostate cancer screening: what we know and what we need to know. Ann Intern Med 1993;**119**:914–923.

73. Stamey TA, Freiha FS, McNeal JE, Redwine EA, Whittemore AS. Localized prostate cancer: Relationship of tumor volume to clinical significance for treatment of prostate cancer. Cancer 1993;**71**:933–938.

74. Albertsen PC, Fryback DG, Storer BE, Kolon TK, Fine J. Long-term survival among men with conservatively treated localized prostate cancer. JAMA 1995;**274**:626–631.

75. Chodak GW, Thisted RA, Gerber GS et al. Results of conservative management of clinically localized prostate cancer. NEJM 1994; **330**:242–248.

76. Humphrey PA, Keetch DW, Smith DS, Shepherd DL, Catalona WJ. Prospective characterization of pathological features of prostatic carcinomas detected via serum PSA based screening. J Urol 1996;**155**:816–820.

77. Stormont TJ, Farrow GM, Myers RP, Blute ML, Zincke H, Wilson TM, Oesterling JE. Clinical stage B0 or T1c prostate cancer: nonpalpable disease identified by elevated serum PSA concentration. Urology 1993;**41**:3.

78. Lerner SE, Seay TM, Blute ML, Bergstralh EJ, Barrett D, Zincke H. PSA detected prostate cancer (clinical stage T1c). An interim anaysis. J Urol 1996;**155**:821–826.

79. Gustafsson O, Norming U, Almgard LE et al. Diagnostic methods in the detection of prostate cancer: A study of a randomly selected population of 2,400 men. J Urol 1992;**148**:1827–1831.

80. Newman JS, Bree RL, Rubin JM. Prostate cancer: diagnosis with color doppler sonography with histologic correlation of each biopsy site. Radiology 1995;**195**:86–90.

81. Ismail M, Gomella LG. Ultrasound for prostate imaging and biopsy. Curr Opin Urol. 2001;**11**(5):471–7.

14 Staging

S D Graham Jr and W H Sanders

Clinical staging system (TNM 1997)			
Stage group	**Stage**		**Grade (Gleason score)**
	Tx	not assessed	–
	T0	no evidence of tumor	–
	Tis	PIN (not recognized as cancer)	–
	T1	clinically inapparent tumor	–
I	T1a	<5% resected tissue	1 (<5)
II			2–4 (5–10)
	T1b	>5% resected tissue	Any (any)
	T1c	detected by PSA	
	T2	palpable tumor	
	T2a	one lobe	
	T2b	both lobes	
III	T3	palpable extension	
	T3a	extracapsular	
	T3b	seminal vesicle invasion	
IV	T4	bladder neck, pelvis, rectum	

Nx not assessed
N0 no nodal metastases
N1 regional nodal metastases

Mx not assessed
M0 no distant metastases
M1a distant nodes
M1b bone
M1c other

Introduction

Adenocarcinoma of the prostate is the most common cancer among men in the United States. The America Cancer Society reduced their original estimate of 340 000 new cases in 1988 to 184 500 cases[1]. In assessing the potential therapeutic modalities available to the patient, the clinical stage of the cancer is among the most important of all factors since it helps to classify tumors according to the possible effectiveness of each therapy as well as providing some estimate of the prognosis. Organ confined cancers are generally amenable to a wide variety of definitive therapeutic interventions, such as radical prostatectomy or radiation therapy, whereas advanced disease is generally limited to palliative or hormonal therapy. The disease-specific survival of patients with organ confined prostate cancer approaches 90% at 10 years, while the disease-specific survival of patients with nodal metastases is poor.

Descriptive systems of staging

Whitmore/Jewett (USA)

The first systematic staging system for prostate cancer was proposed by Jewett and later modified by Whitmore and bases the classification upon physical examination and radiographic findings. Stage A is defined as a non-palpable lesion that is organ confined. This stage was subdivided into Stage A1 (minimal volume) and A2 (larger volume). Stage A1 tumors are defined as those which are low grade and comprise less than 5% of the tissue removed at TURP or open prostatectomy for benign disease. A stage designation of A1 is therefore dependent upon the amount of tissue resected, the degree of involvement of the transition zone, and the skill and diligence of the pathologist. Stage B is defined as an organ confined, palpable lesion. This stage is broken down into two or three substages dependent upon the size of the nodule and the laterality (unilateral vs. bilateral). The ability to assess a stage B tumor is dependent upon the experience of the examiner performing the digital rectal examination, the position and firmness of the nodule and the size of the prostate. Typically, the digital rectal examination underestimates the size of the cancer by 40% and the extent of the cancer (local vs. regional) by 50%. Stage C is defined as disease beyond the capsule, involving the seminal vesicles, or invading the bladder neck, rectum, or pelvic sidewall. Stage D disease implies distant disease, either confined to lymph nodes (D1) or involving other structures such as the skeleton (D2). The main problem with this staging schema is that it does not allow the clinician to describe both the local and distant involvement of the cancer. For example, involvement of the periprostatic tissue (Stage C) is associated with a 66% incidence of positive nodes.

UICC/AJCC (TNM)

The TNM system allows a description of the local (T) extent, the nodal involvement (N), and the distant (M) disease. Non-palpable disease is T1, with the same subclasses of T1a and T1b based upon the volume of the cancer vs. the volume of benign tissue resected (usually above or below 5%). Additionally, T1c is defined as a non-palpable tumor that is detected by PSA. T2 tumors are palpable and subclassified by the extent of the disease. T2a is less than half of 1 lobe, the T2b is unilateral, more than a half of a lobe, and T2c involves both sides. This assessment of local disease suffers from the same potential sources of error as the Jewett-Marshall system. Locally advanced disease is T3, involving the lateral sulci (T3a unilateral, T3b bilateral) or the seminal vesicle (T3c). Extension into the bladder neck (T4a) or pelvic sidewall (T4b) are the most advanced local stages. Nodal involvement is substaged into three categories: 1) N1 represents one local lymph node ≤ 2 cm; 2) N2 represents one local lymph node ≥ 2 cm but ≤ 5 cm, or more than one lymph node; 3) N3 represents a local lymph node > 5 cm. Distant metastases are designated as M1. Stage M1a tumors involve lymph nodes outside the pelvis. Stage M1b tumors involve the skeleton, and stage M1c tumors involve other soft tissue. A general comparison of the two staging systems is presented in Table 14.1.

Evaluation of local mass

The possible means of determining the clinical stage are assessments of both the local and distant extent of the cancer and employ many methods including

Table 14.1   Staging system comparisons. TNM vs. Whitmore/Jewett

Description	TNM (AJCC)	Whitmore/Jewett	Comment
Non-palpable, organ-confined tumors	T1*	A	Usually discovered on TURP, PSA test
Low volume (<5% of tissue)	Ta1*	A1	*=no pT1 stages in 1997 AJCC
Higher volume (>5% of tissue	T1b*	A2	
PSA/imaging detected tumor	T1c*		Not volume or PSA level dependent
Palpable, organ-confined tumors	T2	B	Heavily dependent on DRE, subjective
Discrete nodule, <half lobe	T2a	B1	
Discrete nodule, >half lobe	T2b	B2	
Discrete nodule, bilateral	T2c	B3	Palpability outweighs PSA in staging
Palpable, locally-extensive tumors	T3	C	Heavily dependent on DRE, subjective
Unilateral sulcus involvement	T3a		1997 AJCC T3a = uni- or bilateral ext.
Bilateral sulci involvement	T3b		1997 AJCC T3b = seminal vesicle ext.
Seminal vesicle	T3c		1997 AJCC does not utilize T3c
Bladder neck extension	T4a		1997 AJCC does not subdivide T4a/T4b
Pelvic sidewall or rectal extension	T4b		
Nodal involvement	Nx		Unable to assess nodes
No nodal disease	N0		Usually assessed by CT but unreliably
Local node (<1 cm)	N1	D1	Value of N subdivision debatable
Local node (>1 cm, <5 cm)	N2	D1	
Local node >5 cm	N3	D1	
Distant metastases	Mx, M0	D0	Assessment by PSA, acid phosphatase,
Extrapelvic nodal disease	M1a	D2	bone scan, CT, monoclonal antibody
Skeletal disease	M1b	D2	imaging. D0 is T1 or T2 with PSA>50
Soft-tissue/non-nodal metastases	M1c	D2	and/or elevated acid phosphatase.
Progression after hormone ablation		D3	

physical examination, biochemical determinations, imaging studies and pathologic features. The goal of clinical staging is to assign a relative biologic risk for the tumor, and there is no single parameter that is as predictive as a combination of multiple parameters. Thus all information should be collated and a clinical stage assigned based upon a complete evaluation.

Grade

The most important pathologic predictor of the clinical behavior of the tumor is the histologic grade. Though many systems for grading tumors have been described, based upon nuclear and cytoskeletal abnormalities as well as growth patterns, the most commonly utilized system is the Gleason sum which describes patterns of growth. Since its inception, the Gleason sum has been shown to predict the incidence of positive lymph nodes with a reliability that exceeds many imaging modalities. Initial reports of the correlation of grade with stage of disease showed that with increasing grade, the incidence of capsular involvement and positive nodes increased. Smith showed that the incidence of positive nodes in well differentiated carcinomas was 10%, while poorly differentiated carcinomas was 54% and later reports showed that the incidence of positive nodes was directly correlated with the Gleason sum[2].

Since 1980, the Gleason sum has become the relative standard for reporting histologic grade and has served in many studies to predict final pathologic stage. While there is general agreement that lower Gleason sums (1–6) indicate that the primary tumor is confined to the prostate and that the higher range (8–10) correlates with a higher incidence of advanced disease, the Gleason sum of 7 is controversial as a cut-off point for discriminating local from advanced disease. While some investigators have shown to have a rough correlation between the Gleason sum on the biopsy specimen and the final Gleason sum[3,4], others have shown significant discordance[5]. Poor correlation of biopsy Gleason score to final Gleason score is usually due to underestimation of Gleason score in the biopsy, secondary to a sampling effect.[6] Well-differentiated tumors are modestly predictive of organ confined disease, yet poorly-differentiated tumors are highly predictive of locally extensive disease.[7] Some patients with undifferentiated tumors do well with aggressive local therapy. The likelihood of an undetectable PSA at 5 years after radical prostatectomy in a patient with a Gleason score 8–10 and negative lymph nodes is 43–55%[8,9].

Digital rectal examination

The digital rectal examination is still useful in determining the local stage of disease. A non-palpable tumor is more likely to be organ confined than a palpable tumor[10]. As a single staging tool, it is neither a sensitive nor a specific predictor of extension beyond the capsule. Studies of patients with clinical stage T3 tumors could confirm extracapsular extension on pathologic evaluation of the specimen after radical prostatectomy in half the patients[11,12]. The digital rectal examination yields a poor estimate of tumor size and location.

Prostate-specific antigen

Prostate-specific antigen (PSA) has been useful in predicting pathologic stage. Increasing PSA correlates to some degree with increasing clinical stage. It has proved extremely useful in identifying patients who are unlikely to have metastases to the lymph nodes or to the skeleton. Patients with an initial diagnosis of prostate cancer, whose PSA levels are below 10 ng/ml, have a very small chance of a positive radionuclide bone scan. For this reason bone scans can be deferred in this group of patients[13]. PSA has been used in combination with Gleason score and with clinical stage to identify a group of patients with a very low likelihood of lymph node metastases[14,15]. Pelvic lymph node dissection is unnecessary prior to definitive local therapy in these patients. This work has been especially useful for patients undergoing perineal prostatectomy or radiation therapy. There is a poor correlation between serum PSA and tumor volume, and when used alone, PSA is only moderately predictive of organ confined disease[16]. Cancers which are confined to the transition zone of the prostate may be associated with very high levels of PSA without extending beyond the capsule[17].

PSA, the digital rectal examination, and Gleason score become more powerful predictors when used in combination. Several multivariate systems have been developed which allow urologists to predict the final pathologic stage. Partin has developed tables (Tables 14.2 and 14.3) in which the likelihood of organ-confined disease, established capsular penetration, seminal vesicle involvement and lymph node metastasis can be determined[11]. Similar algorithms have been derived to predict freedom from PSA recurrence after external beam radiation therapy[18]. These multivariate systems allow for a precise discussion of outcomes and success rates with a patient and his family prior to definitive local treatment of his prostate cancer.

Transrectal ultrasound

Transrectal ultrasound (TRUS) is similar to digital rectal examination in its ability to predict capsular penetration and seminal vesicle involvement[19]. While superior to CT or MRI, its sensitivity is inadequate to be useful in clinical decision making. It is unlikely that any imaging modality of gross architectural changes will detect

Table 14.2   Probability of organ-confined disease, based on PSA, clinical stage and Gleason score. Data adapted from Partin.

Gleason sum	PSA 0–4.0 ng/ml				PSA 4.1–10.0 ng/ml				PSA 10.1–20.0 ng/ml				PSA > 20.0 ng/ml			
	T1c	T2a	T2b	T3a	T1c	T2a	T2b	T3a	T1c	T2a	T2b	T3a	T1c	T2a	T2b	T3a
2–4	89	81	72	–	83	71	61	43	75	60	48	–	58	41	29	–
5	81	68	57	40	71	55	43	27	60	43	32	18	40	26	17	8
6	78	64	52	35	67	51	38	23	55	38	26	14	35	22	13	6
7	63	47	34	19	49	33	22	11	35	22	13	6	18	10	5	2
8–10	52	36	24	–	37	23	14	6	23	14	7	3	10	5	3	1

Table 14.3   Probability of lymph node involvement, based on PSA, clinical stage and Gleason score. Data adapted from Partin.[11]

Gleason Sum	PSA 0–4.0 ng/ml				PSA 4.1–10.0 ng/ml				PSA 10.1–20.0 ng/ml P				PSA 20.0 ng/ml			
	T1c	T2a	T2b	T3a	T1c	T2a	T2b	T3a	T1c	T2a	T2b	T3a	1c	T2a	T2b	T3a
2–4	0	0	0	–	0	0	1	1	0	1	1	-	1	1	3	-
5	0	0	1	2	0	1	2	3	1	2	4	7	3	3	7	11
6	0	1	2	5	1	2	4	9	3	4	10	18	7	8	16	26
7	1	2	5	9	3	4	9	15	8	9	17	26	14	14	25	32
8–10	4	5	10	–	8	9	16	24	16	17	29	37	24	24	36	42

the microscopic capsular penetration characteristic of prostate cancer. Tumors visible on TRUS are more likely to have capsular penetration than those tumors which are invisible[9]. Characteristics of sextant biopsy specimens obtained under ultrasound guidance have been used to predict tumor stage and behavior. The number of positive cores, the length of tumor in the biopsy cores, and the percentage of cancer in the biopsy specimens have been used to predict capsular penetration and seminal vesicle involvement[20–22]. These are continuous rather than dichotomous variables, so there is no strict upper limit, above which capsular penetration and seminal vesicle involvement are certain. Ultrasound-guided biopsy of the seminal vesicles is not routine, but may be useful if the physical examination suggests seminal vesicle extension or if the PSA is very high[23,24].

Magnetic resonance imaging

Magnetic resonance imaging (MRI), especially with the endorectal coil, produces images of the prostate with excellent tissue detail[25]. The ability of MRI to differentiate benign from malignant tissue within the prostate and to detect capsular penetration has been disappointing. Although some centres still find MRI provides superior detection of capsular penetration and seminal vesicle involvement compared with transrectal ultrasound, most have found that MRI lacks sufficient accuracy to use its a reason to defer radical prostatectomy in patients with apparently localized tumours[26, 27].

Volume

Tumor volume has been proposed as an important prognostic feature of prostate cancer. The larger the tumor, the more likely it has spread beyond the capsule and will recur after definitive local therapy. Tumors less than 0.5 cc in volume appear to be clinically insignificant. Urologists have spent a lot of energy demonstrating that most T1C prostate cancers are greater than 0.5 cc in volume and therefore clinically significant. The difficulty has been determining the volume of tumors prior to radical prostatectomy and step sectioning by pathology. Several strategies have been proposed. A microscopic focus of cancer on a single biopsy may signify a tumor less than 0.5 cc in volume. However, many clinically significant tumors are discovered as a microscopic focus of tumor in a single biopsy. Epstein has shown that a combination of a microscopic focus, a low PSA density and low-grade tumor represents a cancer less than 0.5 cc about 70% of the time[28].

The prostate cancer volume can be approximated using a formula to determine cancer-specific PSA, and dividing by the amount of PSA leak into the serum per cm^3 of prostate cancer[29]. The amount of PSA leak into the serum is a function of the Gleason grade. Gleason grades 1, 2, 3, 4, and 5 correspond to leakage of 20, 10, 4, 2, and 1 $ng/ml/cm^3$, respectively. The cancer-specific PSA is determined by subtracting the amount of PSA made by benign epithelial tissue from the total serum PSA. The PSA made by benign epithelial tissue is calculated by multiplying the epithelial fraction

(0.2) by the PSA leak per cm³ of epithelial tissue (0.33) by the volume of the entire prostate measured with transrectal ultrasound. The system is unwieldy, yet differentiates patients at high risk for recurrence from those with low risk much more precisely that the TNM system[30].

RTP-CR

Reverse transcription of prostate cell mRNA with amplification by the polymerase chain reaction has been used to detect small amounts of prostate cells in the circulation. Because RNA is degraded immediately after leaking from a cell by ubiquitous RNAses, any prostate-specific RNA detected means that prostate cells are present in the tissue. The presence of prostate-specific antigen RNA in the serum means that some prostate cells are leaving the prostate and circulating. This finding suggests that prostate cancer is no longer confined to the prostate. Investigators at Columbia have successfully used RTPCR to predict prior to radical prostatectomy which patients are likely to have extra-capsular extension[31]. They have found the predictive power of PCR to be greater than other clinical parameters. It has been difficult, however, to standardize the procedure for RTPCR. Investigators at other institutions have found poor sensitivity and specificity of the test[32,33]. While there is a correlation between a positive RTPCR and local extension, the test has no advantage over other indicators of extension[34].

Work on RTPCR has yielded important insights into the tumor biology of prostate cancer. A large proportion of patients undergoing radical prostatectomy have prostate cells in the lymph nodes that can be detected by RTPCR[35,36]. The vast majority of these patients had no pathologic evidence of cancer in the nodes. Transurethral resection of prostate and transrectal ultrasound can cause shedding of prostate cells into the circulation. RTPCR is more likely to be positive after those procedures[37]. These studies suggest that spread of prostate cancer cells into the blood and lymphatics occurs relatively early in the course of prostate cancer.

Evaluation of distant spread

Bone scan

The bone scan is the most sensitive test for detecting metastases to the skeleton. It is very useful in confirming metastatic disease in a patient with a very high PSA. Most investigators agree that patients with newly diagnosed prostate cancer who have a PSA < 10 ng/ml do not need a bone scan[13,38]. The consensus is not universal, however, as a report from Great Britain in 1992 found that 14.7% of patients with bone metastases had a PSA < 20 ng/ml[39].

Prostascint scan

Radionuclide scanning with Prostascint, an Indium labeled monoclonal antibody to prostate-specific membrane antigen (PSMA) has been used to detect soft tissue metastases[40]. It has also been used to differentiate local from distant recurrence when the PSA rises after radical prostatectomy[41]. Positive scans of primary tumors and local recurrence have been confirmed with ultrasound-guided biopsy. Positive scans outside the prostatic fossa have been difficult to confirm, because the Prostascint scan is a poor guide for needle biopsy. Nevertheless, this technology has potential, especially in the evaluation of PSA recurrence after radical prostatectomy[42].

Pelvic lymph node dissection

Pelvic lymph node dissection has been standard procedure immediately prior to radical prostatectomy[43]. The pelvic lymph nodes are set for frozen section evaluation, and the prostatectomy is performed only if there is no cancer in the lymph nodes. Several algorithms have been developed to determine which patients have such a low risk of lymph node involvement that it is reasonable to defer lymph node dissection[14,15,44]. Rees has suggested that pelvic lymph node dissection does not need to be performed in patients with: 1) PSA ≤ 5 ng/ml, or 2) Gleason score ≤ 5, or 3) a combination of a PSA ≤ 25 ng/ml, a Gleason score ≤ 7, and a negative digital rectal examination. Most urologists performing any kind of definitive local therapy for prostate cancer that does not involve a retropubic approach use this system, or a similar one to identify which patients do not require a lymph node dissection. Rogers et al.[45] reported that while PSA and biopsy Gleason sum were the most significant predictors of lymph node metastasis, they were not sufficiently sensitive to allow accurate prediction of lymph node metastasis in an individual patient.[45] He therefore recommends pelvic lymph node dissection in every patient undergoing radical prostatectomy. In patients with palpable tumours, the ipsilateral nodes should be sampled first, since they are the most likely to contain metastases[46].

Pelvic lymphadenectomy can be performed as a part of retropubic prostatectomy or as separate procedure. Laparoscopic lymph nodes dissection as popularized by Schuessler has lower morbidity than a standard open lymphadenectomy[47]. The operating time for the laparoscopic approach, however, is much greater. Recently, the technique of minilaparotomy for lymph node dissection has been developed[48]. A 6 cm midline incision, beginning 2 cm superior to the pubic arch, is made through the skin and the fascia. The lymph node dissection is completed through this small incision in the standard fashion. No pelvic drains are required. It is as efficacious as open and laparoscopic lymphadenectomy, has lower morbidity than open lymphadenectomy and requires less operative time[49,50].

References

1. Landis S, Murray T, Bolden S, Wingo P. Cancer statistics 1998. CA 1998;**48**(1):6–29.
2. Smith JA, Seaman JP, Gleidman JB, Middleton RG. Pelvic lymph node metastasis from prostatic cancer: influence of tumor grade and stage in 452 consecutive patients. J Urol 1983;**130**(2):290.
3. Catalona WJ, Stein AJ, Fair WR. Grading errors in prostatic needle biopsies: relation to the accuracy of tumor grade in predicting pelvic lymph node metastases. J Urol 1982;**127**(5):919.
4. Cookson MS, Fleshner NE, Soloway SM, Fair WR. Correlation between Gleason score of needle biopsy and radical prostatectomy specimen: accuracy and clinical implications. J Urol 1997;**157**(2):559.
5. Danziger M, Shevchuk M, Antonescu C, Matthews GJ, Fracchia JA. Predictive accuracy of transrectal ultrasound-guided prostate biopsy: correlations to matched prostatectomy specimens. Urology 1997;**49**:863.
6. Steinberg DM, Sauvageot J, Piantadosi S, Epstein JI. Correlation of prostate needle biopsy and radical prostatectomy Gleason grade in academic and community settings. Am J Surg Path 1997;**21**:566.
7. Fernandes ET, Sundaram CP, Long R, Soltani M, Ercole CJ. Biopsy Gleason score: how does it correlate with the final pathological diagnosis in prostate cancer? Br J Urol 1997;**79**(4):615.
8. Quinlan DM, Partin AW, Walsh PC. Can aggressive prostatic carcinomas be identified and can their natural history be altered by treatment? Urology 1995;**46**(3 suppl A):77.
9. Ohori M, Goad JR, Wheeler TM, Eastham JA, Thompson TC, Scardino PT. Can radical prostatectomy alter the progression of poorly differentiated prostate cancer? J Urol 1994;**152**(5 Pt 2):1843.
10. Ohori M, Wheeler TM, Scardino PT. The New American Joint Committee on Cancer and International Union Against Cancer TNM classification of prostate cancer. Clinicopathologic correlations. Cancer 1994;**74**(1):104.
11. Partin AW, Kattan M, Subong EN, Walsh PC, Wojno KJ, Oesterling JE, Scardino PT, Pearson JD. Combination of prostate-specific antigen, clinical stage, and Gleason score to predict pathological stage of localized prostate cancer. A multi-institutional update. JAMA 1997;**277**(18):1445.
12. Byar DP, Mostofi FK. Veterans Administration Cooperative Urological Research Group. Carcinoma of the prostate: prognostic evaluation of certain pathological features in 208 radical prostatectomies examined by the step-section technique. Cancer 1972;**30**:5.
13. Oesterling JE, Martin SK, Bergstralh EJ, Lowe FC. The use of prostate-specific antigen in staging patients with newly diagnosed prostate cancer. JAMA 1993;**269**(1):57.
14. Bluestein DL, Bostwick DG, Bergstralh EJ, Oesterling JE. Eliminating the need for bilateral pelvic lymphadenectomy in select patients with prostate cancer. J Urol 1994;**151**(5):1315.
15. Rees MA, Resnick MI, Oesterling JE. Use of prostate-specific antigen, Gleason score, and digital rectal examination in staging patients with newly diagnosed prostate cancer. Urol Clin North Am 1997;**24**(2):379.
16. Noldus J, Stamey TA. Limitations of serum prostate specific antigen in predicting peripheral and transition zone cancer volumes as measured by correlation coefficients. J Urol 1996;**155**(1):232.
17. Stamey TA, Dietrick DD, Issa MM. Large, organ confined, impalpable transition zone prostate cancer: association with metastatic levels of prostate specific antigen. J Urol 1993;**149**(3):510.
18. Pisansky TM, Kahn MJ, Bostwick DG. An enhanced prognostic system for clinically localized carcinoma of the prostate. Cancer 1997;**79**(11):2154.
19. Smith JA, Scardino PT, Resnick MI, Hernandez AD, Rose SC, Egger MJ. Transrectal ultrasound versus digital rectal examination for the staging of

20. carcinoma of the prostate: results of a prospective, multi-institutional trial. J Urol 1997;**157**(3):902.
20. Peller PA, Young DC, Marmaduke DP, Marsh WL, Badalament RA. Sextant prostate biopsies. A histopathologic correlation with radical prostatectomy specimens. Cancer 1995;**75**(2):530.
21. Bostwick DG, Qian J, Bergstralh E, Dundore P, Dugan J, Myers RP, Oesterling JE. Prediction of capsular perforation and seminal vesical invasion in prostate cancer. J Urol 1996;**155**(4):1361.
22. Dietrick DD, McNeal JE, Stamey TA. Core cancer length in ultrasound-guided systematic sextant biopsies: a preoperative evaluation of prostate cancer. Urology 1995;**45**(6):987.
23. Stone NN, Stock RG, Unger P. Indications for seminal vesicle biopsy and laparoscopic pelvic lymph node dissection in men with localized carcinoma of the prostate. J Urol 1995;**154**(4):1392.
24. Vallancien G, Bochereau G, Wetzel O, Bretheau D, Prapotnich D, Bougaran J. Influence of preoperative positive seminal vesicle biopsy on the staging of prostate cancer. J Urol 1994;**152**(4):1152.
25. Chelsky MJ, Schnall MD, Seidmon EJ, Pollack HM. Use of endorectal surface coil magnetic resonance imaging for local staging of prostate cancer. J Urol 1993;**150**(2 Pt 1):391.
26. Bates TS, Gillatt PM, Cavanagh PM, Speakman M. A comparison of endorectal magnetic resonance imaging and transrectal ultrasonography in the local staging of prostate cancer with histopathological correlation. Br J Urol 1997;**79**(6):927.
27. Perrotti M, Kaufman RP Jr, Jennings TA, Thaler HT, Soloway SM, Rifkin MD, Fisher HA. Endo-rectal coil magnetic resonance imaging in clinically localized prostate cancer: is it accurate? J Urol 1996;**156**(1):106.
28. Epstein JI, Walsh PC, Carmichael M, Brendler CB. Pathologic and clinical findings to predict tumor extent of nonpalpable (stage T1c) prostate cancer. JAMA 1994;**271**(5):368.
29. D'Amico AV, Chang H, Holupka E, Renshaw A, Desjarden A, Chen M, Loughlin KR, Richie JP. Calculated prostate cancer volume: the optimal predictor of actual cancer volume and pathologic stage. Urology 1997;**49**(3):385.
30. D'Amico AV, Whittington R, Schultz D, Malkowicz SB, Tomaszewski JE, Wein A. Outcome based staging for clinically localized adenocarcinoma of the prostate. J Urol 1997;**158**:1422.
31. Katz AE, Olsson CA, Raffo AJ, Cama C, Perlman H, Seaman E, O'Toole KM, McMahon D, Benson MC, Buttyan R. Molecular staging of prostate cancer with the use of an enhanced reverse transcriptase-PCR assay. Urology 1994;**43**(6):765.
32. de Cremoux P, Ravery V, Podgorniak MP, Chevillard S, Toublanc M, Thiounn N, Tatoud R, Delmas V, Calvo T, Boccon-Gibod L. Value of the preoperative detection of prostate-specific-antigen-positive circulating cells by nested RT-PCR in patients submitted to radical prostatectomy. Eur Urology 1997;**32**(1):69.
33. Goldman HB, Israeli RS, Lu Y, Lerner JL, Hollabaugh RS, Steiner MS. Can prostate-specific antigen reverse transcriptase-polymerase chain reaction be used as a prospective test to diagnose prostate cancer? World J Urol 1997;**15**(4):257.
34. Ignatoff JM, Oefelein MG, Watkin W, Chmiel JS, Kaul KL. Prostate specific antigen reverse transcriptase-polymerase chain reaction assay in preoperative staging of prostate cancer. J Urol 1997;**158**(5):1870.
35. Edelstein RA, Zietman AL, de las Morenas A, Krane RJ, Babayan RK, Dallow KC, Traish A, Moreland RB. Implications of prostate micrometastases in pelvic lymph nodes: an archival tissue study. Urology 1996;**47**(3):370.
36. Ferrari AC, Stone NN, Eyler JN, Gao M, Mandeli J, Unger P, Gallagher RE, Stock R. Prospective analysis of prostate-specific markers in pelvic lymph nodes of patients with high-risk prostate cancer. J Natl Cancer Inst 1997;**89**(20):1498.
37. Moreno JG, O'Hara SM, Long JP, Veltri RW, Ning X, Alexander AA, Gomella LG. Transrectal ultrasound-guided biopsy causes hematogenous dissemination of prostate cells as determined by RT-PCR. Urology 1997;**49**(4):515.
38. Wolff JM, Bares R, Jung PK, Buell U, Jakse G. Prostate-specific antigen as a marker of bone metastasis in patients with prostate cancer. Urol Int 1996;**56**(3):169.

39. Miller PD, Eardley I, Kirby RS. Prostate specific antigen and bone scan correlation in the staging and monitoring of patients with prostatic cancer. *Br J Urol* 1992;**70**(3):295.

40. Babaian RJ, Sayer J, Podoloff DA *et al*. Radioimmunoscintigraphy of pelvic lymph nodes with indium-labeled monoclonal antibody CYT-356. *J Urol* 1994;**152**:1952.

41. Sodee DB, Conant R, Chalfant M, Miron S, Klein E, Bahnson R, Spirnak JP, Carlin B, Bellon EM, Rogers B. Preliminary imaging results using In-111 labeled CYT-356 (Prostascint) in the detection of recurrence prostate cancer. *Clini Nuclear Med* 1996;**21**(10):759–767.

42. Kahn D, Haseman M, Libertino J, Manyak M, Maguire R and Williams R. Indium-111 capromab pendetide (ProstaScint) imaging of patients with rising PSA post-prostatectomy. Presented at the annual meeting of the American Urological Association in New Orleans, LA, April, 1997.

43. Olsson CA. Staging lymphadenectomy should be an antecedent to treatment in localized prostatic carcinoma. *Urology* 1985;**25**(2 suppl):4.

44. Campbell SC, Klein EA, Levin HS, Piedmonte MR. Open pelvic lymph node dissection for prostate cancer: a reassessment. *Urology* 1995;**46**(3):352.

45. Rogers E, Gurpinar T, Dillioglugil O, Kattan MW, Goad JR, Scardino PT, Griffith DP. The role of digital rectal examination, biopsy Gleason sum and prostate-specific antigen in selecting patients who require pelvic lymph node dissections for prostate cancer. *Br J Urol* 1996;**78**(3):419.

46. Harrison SH, Seale-Hawkins C, Schum CW, Dunn JK, Scardino PT. Correlation between side of palpable tumor and side of pelvic lymph node metastasis in clinically localized prostate cancer. *Cancer* 1992;**69**(3):750.

47. Schuessler WW, Vancaillie TG, Reich H, Griffith DP. Transperitoneal endosurgical lymphatonectomy in patients with localized prostate cancer. *J Urol* 1991;**145**(5):988.

48. Steiner MS, Marshall FF. Mini-laparotomy staging pelvic lymphadenectomy (Minilap). *Urology* 1993;**41**:201.

49. Herrell SD, Trachtenberg J, Theodorescu D. Staging pelvic lymphadenectomy for localized carcinoma of the prostate: a comparison of 3 surgical techniques. *J Urol* 1997;**157**(4):1337.

50. Lezin MS, Cherrie R, Cattolica EV. Comparison of laparoscopic and minilaparotomy pelvic lymphadenectomy for prostate cancer staging in a community practice. *Urology* 1997;**49**(1):60.

15 Treatment of early organ–confined disease

Algorithm

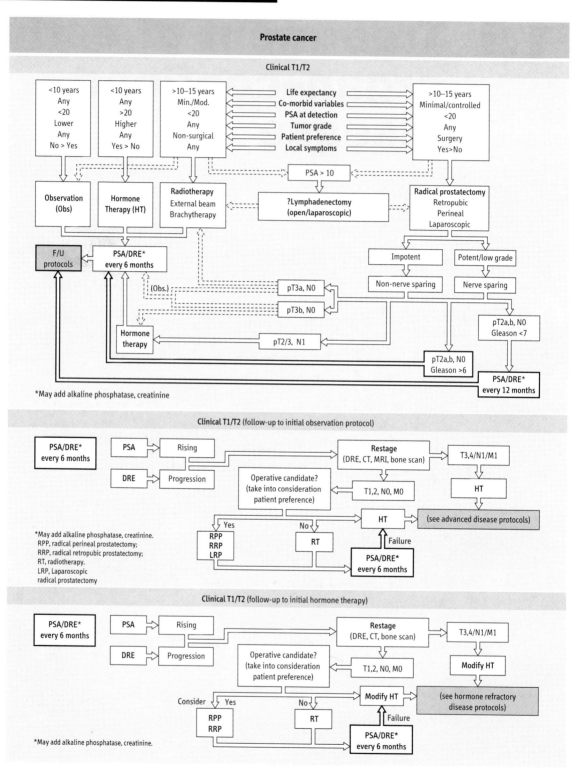

*May add alkaline phosphatase, creatinine

*May add alkaline phosphatase, creatinine.
RPP, radical perineal prostatectomy;
RRP, radical retropubic prostatectomy;
RT, radiotherapy.
LRP, Laparoscopic
radical prostatectomy

*May add alkaline phosphatase, creatinine.

Prostate cancer (cont)

Clinical T1/T2 (Follow up to initial radiotherapy)

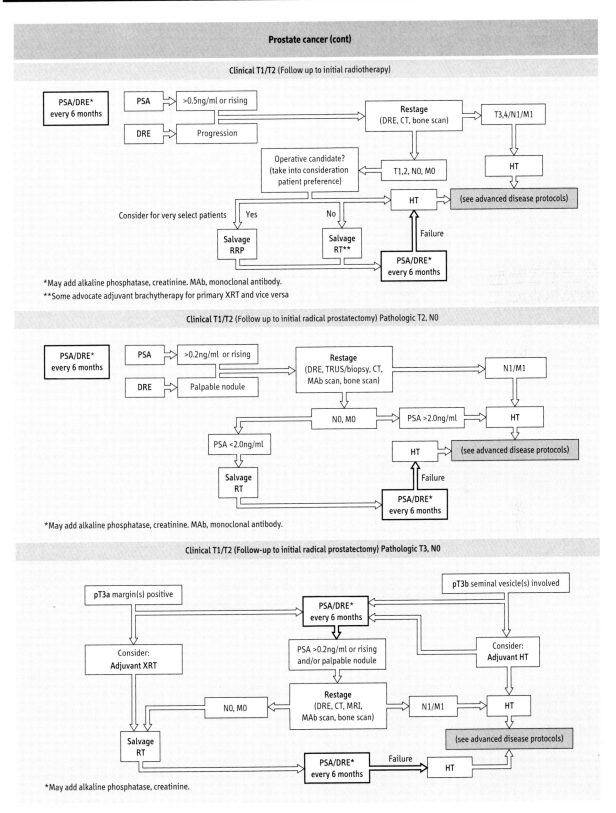

*May add alkaline phosphatase, creatinine. MAb, monoclonal antibody.
**Some advocate adjuvant brachytherapy for primary XRT and vice versa

Clinical T1/T2 (Follow up to initial radical prostatectomy) Pathologic T2, N0

*May add alkaline phosphatase, creatinine. MAb, monoclonal antibody.

Clinical T1/T2 (Follow-up to initial radical prostatectomy) Pathologic T3, N0

*May add alkaline phosphatase, creatinine.

161

15.1 Issues and options: patient and tumor factors

J W Basler

Tumor factors

The urologic literature is replete with reports of measurable elements, which can be associated with or predict more aggressive tumors. However, for the practising urologist, there are only a few readily available parameters that can give a reasonably accurate picture of the aggressiveness of an individual's prostate cancer. The tests, which are commonly available, are the clinical stage (including the results of the digital rectal examination (DRE) and bone scan), histology, Gleason score, ploidy analysis, prostatic acid phosphatase (PAP) and PSA. Graham and Sanders, Ahmed and Oesterling, and Bostwick present specific details of the value of these tests and pathologic staging in the previous chapters. A brief summary of important considerations that will help in discussing treatment options with patients is presented below.

The DRE is generally considered to be poorly reliable for detecting occult cancer but is still relied upon for crucial staging information. Findings of lateral induration, sidewall fixation or seminal vesicle induration and enlargement raise the suspicion that the cancer has invaded beyond the confines of the prostate. The incidence of nodal metastases in this situation can be as high as 50%. Histology of >90% of prostate cancers is adenocarcinoma but a smaller number of aggressive tumors turn out to be transitional cell carcinoma or small cell, neuroendocrine cancers that demand different treatment regimens. Gleason's scoring system relies upon patterns of glandular growth and thus provides quantitation to the appearance of the tumor. Low-grade (1) tumors are seen as small crowded glands that change to more bizarre patterns of branching and ingrowth (2, 3) ultimately to lose identity as gland tissue forming sheets of cells that send projections in and around the stromal components (4, 5). Tumors that demonstrate pattern 4 (having sums of 7 or greater) have apparently developed the 'invasive' phenotype and are thus associated with a higher likelihood of locally extensive disease or metastases. Ploidy analysis is becoming available in many areas as a routine analysis performed on pathologic specimens. While there remain some concerns about its ultimate clinical utility, several studies have suggested a correlation between aggressive behaviour and aneuploidy. In the pre-PSA era, PAP (enzymatic assay) was used extensively as a staging marker based on the findings that pre-operative elevations of PAP predicted treatment failure in over 80%[1]. This led to the concept of stage D0 cancer – any apparently localized tumor having an elevated PAP. When studied with respect to local tumor stage, elevations of PAP become apparent with stage C (T3) disease making it a helpful marker for clinical decision making[2]. This marker is still available today but has been largely supplanted by PSA, which is linearly related to tumor volume[2]. Nodal and bony metastases are rare in patients with PSA <10.0 ng/ml but become more prevalent with higher PSAs. Above a PSA of 50.0 ng/ml, metastases are common enough that this level redefines the D0 threshold. Pre-biopsy free/total PSA may also be an important predictor of cancer aggressiveness[3].

In summary, patients with smaller overall tumor burden, lower Gleason score adenocarcinoma and diploid DNA content will apparently do better with any management scheme on a stage-for-stage basis than those with poorer prognostic variables. The latter group may be best managed aggressively as early in the course of the disease as possible.

Patient factors

While age at diagnosis remains an important consideration in determining treatment options, a more important concept is that of life expectancy. Most patients will be able to understand the concept of 'average survival' and will likely be asking for these figures to help make treatment decisions. The accompanying chart of average life expectancy vs. age for American men based on recent census data[4] provides an important starting point for prostate cancer treatment discussions. (Fig. 15.1) A 73-year-old white male in the USA has an average of 10 years of life remaining. Relating this to survival with untreated cancer is somewhat difficult since data for untreated prostate cancer is sketchy and often limited by therapeutic interventions as the disease progresses. Additional confusion is generated by reporting methods for survival (median survival, mean survival, progression free survival, overall survival, etc.) which do not allow easy comparisons or conceptualization for the statistically naive lay person. However, the available data suggest that a man with localized prostate cancer and a reasonable 10-year life expectancy (e.g. 73-year-old) may benefit from aggressive local treatment. Unfortunately, the untreated patient with Stage C prostate cancer has about the same life expectancy as an 82-year-old (~5–6 yr) and untreated men with stage D disease can expect to survive less time than an 85–90 year old (median survival ~2.5–3 yr). (Fig. 15.2)[5,6] This underscores the need to identify cancers at a curable stage and develop new modalities for treatment of advanced tumors.

Physiologic age is also important in discussing treatment options. Consideration of co-morbid variables such as coronary disease, COPD, diabetes, hypertension, stroke and others must be an integral part of the

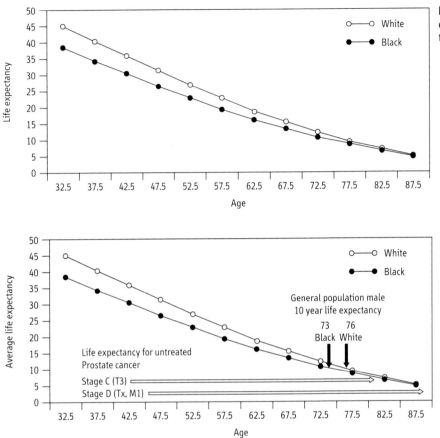

Fig. 15.1 Age vs. average life expectancy for blacks and whites in the US[4].

Fig.15.2 Average life expectancy for untreated prostate cancer plotted in the age vs. life expectancy plot for US blacks and whites[4, 5, 6].

pre-treatment evaluation of the prostate cancer patient. Some diseases have less of an impact on survival than the cancer (e.g. dementia, Parkinson's disease, paraplegia, psychosis, etc.) and may not be appropriate exclusionary criteria for aggressive local therapy in an otherwise healthy man.

Racial considerations may also be factored into the discussion of treatment options since black men in the United States tend to be diagnosed at more advanced stage and suffer a higher mortality rate than those of other ethnic groups[7]. Smith *et al.*[8] demonstrated that in comparing the pathologic features of prostatectomy specimens from two groups (10 black, 60 white) with similar pre-surgical PSAs (3.3 ng/ml vs. 3.1 ng/ml, $P = 0.03$), the black men were more likely to have pathologic stage T3 (40% vs. 18%, $P = 0.2$) and Gleason score 7 or greater (30% vs. 10%, $P = 0.1$). However, since both trends fall short of rigorous statistical significance, it may be premature to recommend more aggressive therapy for apparent localized disease based on race.

When considering aggressive treatment of advanced disease with hormonal, surgical or XRT one must keep in mind the risk vs. benefit analysis and incorporate this in discussions with the patient and his family. While most men are eager to proceed with any reasonable management protocol, some place a higher premium on further years of sexual activity and loathe the potential consequences of surgery (e.g. incontinence) or XRT (e.g. bowel, bladder dysfunction). To others, the stress caused by the knowledge of the cancer is enough to require psychiatric counseling. The latter group of men often request therapies that fly in the face of good judgement. Keeping an open mind to patient desires and expectations and an open line of communication will often alleviate this stress.

References

1. Whitesel JA, Donohue RE, Mani JH, Mohr S, Scanavino DJ, Augspurger RR, Biber RJ, *et al.* Acid phosphatase: its influence on the management of carcinoma of the prostate. *J Urol* 1984;**131**(1):70–72.
2. Stamey TA, Kabalin JN. Prostate specific antigen in the diagnosis and treatment of adenocarcinoma of the prostate. 1. Untreated patients. *J Urol* 1989;**141**(5):1070–1075.
3. Arcangeli CG, Humphrey PA, Smith DS, Harmon TJ, Shepherd DL, Keetch DW, Catalona WJ. Percentage of free serum prostate-specific antigen as a predictor

of pathologic features of prostate cancer in a screening population. *Urology* 1998;**51**(4):558–564.

4. Anderson RN. United States Abridged Life Tables, 1996, National Vital Statistics Reports, vol 47 (13) Dec. 1998.

5. Chodak GW, Thisted RA, Gerber GS, Johansson JE, Adolfsson J, Jones GW, Chisholm GD, *et al.* Results of conservative management of clinically localized prostate cancer. *N Engl J Med* 1994;**330**(4):242–248.

6. Blackard CE, Byar DP, Jordan WP Jr. Orchiectomy for advanced prostatic carcinoma. A re-evaluation. *Urology* 1973;**1**(6):553–560.

7. Parker SL, Davis KJ, Wingo PA, Ries LA, Heath CW Jr. Cancer statistics by race and ethnicity. *CA Cancer J Clin* 1998;**48**(1):31–48.

8. Smith DS, Carvalhal GF, Mager DE, Bullock AD, Catalona WJ. Use of lower prostate specific antigen cutoffs for prostate cancer screening in black and white men. *J Urol* 1998;**160**(5):1734–1738.

15.2   Watchful-waiting

J S Palmer and G W Chodak

Introduction

More than 90 years after Hugh Young performed the first radical prostatectomy[1], the management of localized prostate cancer continues to be controversial, partly due to a lack of randomized controlled trials. This is reflected by the wide fluctuation in rates of radical prostatectomy across the United States[2]. Contributing to this confusion is the wide disparity between the prevalence and mortality of this disease; only a small percentage of men actually die from prostate cancer[3] although the disease is present histologically in approximately 30% of 50-year-old men and over 50% of 80-year-old men. In addition, although modern diagnostic tests have led to earlier discovery, nearly 50% of cases are detected in men over age 70 where competing causes of death are increasingly common. Thus, the value of screening and treatment most likely diminishes with age. Factors which make management decisions problematic are the different rates of local and distant progression, the interval between diagnosis and death from cancer, and the inability to define accurately an individual's remaining life expectancy. Although prospective studies designed to evaluate the issue of early detection and treatment are currently being conducted, these controversies are unlikely to be settled soon. Therefore, physicians must present their patients with the outcomes from each management option based on current available data.

This growing controversy on therapeutic options for early organ-confined disease has also led to a changing role for the urologist. Whereas the traditional physician–patient relationship usually involved a recommendation for treatment followed by an agreement to proceed, increasingly the physician's role now is to present the relative risks and benefits of all options which is followed by a patient's informed choice of therapy. In order for a patient to make a truly informed choice, he needs detailed information about the probability of each favorable and unfavorable outcome that might result from each therapy rather than simply a list of the therapeutic options. This information is crucial to enable each patient to assess the relative value of each option in relation to his personal goals and fears and the risks he is willing to take.

Because many prostate cancers progress slowly, watchful waiting, also called expectant therapy, has received increased attention as an option for patients with early stage disease. Clearly, watchful waiting is not a curative therapy. However, it is an option for all men, especially if they expect that they are more likely to die of some other cause than prostate cancer. For some patients, the potential for and amount of improvement in survival that may result from local therapy may be more than offset by the adverse impact on one's quality of life. Patients who chose watchful waiting are more likely to value the quality rather than quantity of their life, because complications usually occur immediately after treatment and may be endured for the remainder of a patient's life. The benefits of treatment may not be realized until many years in the future. The focus of this chapter will be on the outcomes associated with this therapeutic option and how this information can be presented to patients with newly diagnosed prostate cancer so they may actively participate in the choice of therapy.

Management by watchful waiting

By definition, watchful waiting means not administering local therapy (radiation or surgery). Patients are treated expectantly which means they are treated if and when they develop clinical symptoms or signs of progression. Before the development of PSA, patients managed by watchful waiting would undergo some combination of a digital rectal examination, bone scan or bone X-rays and serum acid phosphatase at varying intervals. Local therapy such as a TURP was provided for symptoms such as urinary retention or voiding dysfunction and hormone therapy was used for ureteral obstruction or symptomatic metastatic disease. With the development of PSA, however, watchful waiting is now more likely to involve performing only a digital examination and PSA at regular intervals until high PSA levels occur. Some patients who initially choose watchful waiting may do so until the PSA reaches a 'critical' value, at which time local therapy may then be desired. Since there is no evidence for the benefit of delayed local therapy or for a particular critical PSA level at which local therapy is both necessary and beneficial, patients choosing watchful waiting need to understand that this option most likely means neither radiation therapy nor radical prostatectomy may ever be given. Although the natural history of this disease is quite variable, patients still should be told that prostate cancer will invariably grow and the PSA will rise at a variable rate. Since considerable patient and physician anxiety is likely to coincide with the rise in PSA, perhaps the best solution for now in the patients choosing watchful waiting may be to perform this test less often.

Benefits and risks of watchful waiting

In presenting patients with information about watchful waiting, the first question is what are the potential benefits. These may include maintaining one's immediate quality of life, which is usually quite good since most men are asymptomatic at diagnosis, and avoiding the potential complications that can occur following radiation or surgery. Another benefit of watchful waiting is that some men may avoid therapy entirely depending on the progression rate of their tumor and their remaining life expectancy. In addition, since no randomized clinical trial has yet demonstrated that surgery or radiation significantly reduces the morbidity and mortality of the disease, purists could argue that patients benefit by not undergoing a treatment of unproven value.

The risks of watchful waiting are quite obvious. First, patients may miss a chance to be cured of their disease. The cancer may then progress, eventually metastasize causing considerable pain and suffering, and ultimately cause death resulting in a loss of normal life expectancy. Although hormone therapy most often produces a clinical remission once metastases develop, men need to understand that most patients who develop metastases will ultimately die of their disease with at least the last 6 to 12 months almost invariably associated with a poor quality of life.

In addition to a potential reduction in life expectancy, another disadvantage of watchful waiting is progression of the cancer eventually resulting in the need for therapy. This may take the form of urinary obstruction requiring transurethral resection, ureteral obstruction causing renal impairment and requiring percutaneous nephrostomy, or bone metastases requiring hormone therapy, focal radiation therapy and/or narcotics for analgesia. The likelihood of receiving additional therapy in the pre-PSA era is approximately 25–30% for men managed by watchful waiting[4]. In contrast for men undergoing radical prostatectomy, the frequency of receiving additional cancer therapy ranged from 16% for well differentiated cancer to 41% for poorly differentiated disease[5]. Once again, the longer a patient survives, the greater the likelihood of requiring therapy for symptomatic progression.

Outcomes following watchful waiting

To date, only one randomized study comparing watchful waiting with local therapy has ever been performed[6], and the results are unreliable due to many methodological flaws. Therefore, the relative outcomes from this therapy compared with other treatments must be defined from uncontrolled studies. Over the past 10 years, several reports have appeared[4,7–11], however, three fundamental problems are associated with these reports which include patient selection bias, a larger proportion of men with low-grade disease than seen in men undergoing radical prostatectomy and an older age at diagnosis. Rather than focusing on any single paper with its inherent biases, the treatment guidelines panel of the American Urological Association attempted to compare treatments by performing a meta-analysis of the published literature[13]. This analysis revealed that the 95% confidence intervals for the 10 year cancer-specific survival rate could not be distinguished from the rates for radical prostatectomy or radiation therapy. These results led the panel to conclude that watchful waiting needed to be included in the presentation of choices when counseling patients with localized disease. Unfortunately, this meta-analysis did not stratify the outcomes of each treatment according to significant prognostic factors such as tumor grade because such a task was not really possible based on the data included in each report.

In an attempt to address some of the potential problems inherent in single institution reports, another attempt was made to compile the data from different watchful waiting studies into a 'pooled analysis' using original case data rather than published results[14]. A comparison of the results from a conventional meta-analysis and a pooled analysis has demonstrated that more reliable outcomes are obtained with a pooled analysis[15]. One major advantage of the pooled analysis is that it permits an assessment of the outcomes stratified for significant risk factors and the impact of specific biases on the outcomes.

The pooled analysis study included six non-randomized watchful waiting studies from four countries, published between 1985 and 1991[4,7–12,16]. Only patients with localized disease were included. Metastasis-free and cancer-specific survival were determined based on 828 patients followed for a median of 78 months. By 10 years after diagnosis, the disease-specific survival was 87%, 87% and 34%, and the metastasis-free survival was 81%, 58% and 26% for men with grade 1 (Gleason 2–4), grade 2 (Gleason 5–7), or grade 3 (Gleason 8–10) tumors, respectively. Importantly, when the data were analysed using current statistical methods, neither age, the use of delayed local therapy nor the inclusion of men with low-risk cancers had a significant impact on the above results.

Since this study was not based on randomized data, the findings must be interpreted cautiously. Perhaps the most significant deficiency in this study was the absence of a centralized review of the pathology. To compensate for this, a Cox regression analysis was performed to compare the outcomes from the six different centers to each other before combining the data together in order to minimize the possibility that the results would be unduly influenced by differences in pathology. Importantly, the results from only one of the reports differed from the other five and the overall results with and without these men did not differ significantly. These results not only provide support for the findings from each of the individual reports, but also clearly demonstrate that: 1) patients with grade 1 or 2 prostate cancer treated by watchful waiting have a relatively low risk while those with grade 3 disease have a very high risk of dying from prostate disease by 10 years after diagnosis; 2) metastatic rates are strongly correlated with tumor grade; and, 3) prostate cancer is a progressive disease when managed conservatively. Until a randomized study has been completed, these data can be useful for counseling patients with this disease.

These findings were partially substantiated by a subsequent report by Albertson[17] in which he reviewed the results for men aged 65–75 at diagnosis who were treated by watchful waiting in the state of Connecticut and followed long term. In this study, all specimens were re-reviewed by a single pathologist. The authors found that at 10 years, the cancer-specific survival was 91%, 76% and 52% for men with well, moderately and poorly differentiated cancers, respectively. An important feature of this study is that it provided the first reliable data on watchful waiting at 15 years after diagnosis. Cancer-specific survival was unchanged for men with well differentiated cancer, while it was 72% for patients with moderately differentiated cancers and 48% for those with poorly differentiated cancer. This analysis also permitted an estimate of the impact on life expectancy resulting from conservatively treated prostate cancer. The average number of years lost because of this management strategy was 0, 4–5 and 6–8, respectively, for the three tumor grades. There are two important points to recognize about these latter findings. First, this average means that some men are losing many more years of life while others are losing little or none. And second, these numbers represent the maximum potential gains from treatment; however, there is no evidence that all of these lost years can or will be regained by treatment.

One also must keep in mind that this patient population only included men between 65 and 75 at

diagnosis. Thus, for younger men who usually have a longer average life expectancy, the average number of years that might be lost following watchful waiting is almost certainly higher. Also, neither the pooled analysis nor the Connecticut study included men with stage T1C cancer who were diagnosed by PSA. Because of lead time bias, all of the above survival rates for men with either tumor grade are likely to be higher in patients with these cancers, regardless of treatment.

Having defined the best estimates of the outcomes from watchful waiting, the question is how these results compare with radical prostatectomy or radiation therapy? The criticisms suggested for the individual watchful waiting studies apply equally to the studies involving surgery or radiation. Until one of the ongoing randomized trials has been completed, the only valid method for comparing therapies is to perform a similar pooled analysis of the other treatments. A preliminary report of this methodology for radical prostatectomy was reported at the American Urological Association in 1995[18] and further analysis is now underway to make a comparison of similar groups of patients. One preliminary finding is that the non-cancer survival of the men treated by surgery (and radiation) is higher than that for men treated by watchful waiting. A second finding is that surgery appears to offer a survival advantage within 5 years of diagnosis for men with poorly differentiated cancers, an observation not previously substantiated in the literature.

Conclusions

Based on currently available information, how can physicians help patients come to a decision about whether to select watchful waiting or local therapy. First, patients need to be made aware of the relative risk of the cancer which primarily depends on tumor grade and life expectancy. For those with a life expectancy of 10 years or less, few men are likely to live longer as a result of local treatment unless they have a poorly differentiated cancer. Therefore, these men are clearly the best candidates for watchful waiting. For those diagnosed by PSA alone or those with a well or moderately differentiated cancer, a life expectancy of 13–15 years may be needed to derive a survival benefit from treatment because of the lead time of diagnosis. However, by 10 years, patients should recognize that watchful waiting may result in a greater chance of having metastatic disease.

The real dilemma about managing localized prostate cancer is the inability to identify which patients truly need local therapy and will also benefit from it. Consequently, for men hoping to maximize their survival and minimize their risks from prostate cancer, they must receive local therapy even though this will invariably result in treating some men unnecessarily. On the other hand, watchful waiting is best for men who are more concerned about their immediate quality of life, with the recognition that they might be deprived of several years of life expectancy and a poorer quality of life at the end of the life span. Since the quality of most men's lives is worse near the end of their life span than at the time of diagnosis of prostate cancer, many men may feel that the potential gain in survival is not worth the risks, and therefore watchful waiting should be selected. In the final analysis, this decision will be affected by the fears and goals of each patient and their family members, by cultural factors specific for each country and by the biases of counseling physicians. Hopefully, the ongoing clinical trials will provide even better information about the relative risks and benefits of surgery compared with watchful waiting.

References

1. Young HH. The early diagnosis and radical cure of carcinoma of the prostate. *Johns Hopkins Hosp Bull* 1904;**16**:315–320.
2. Lu-Yao GL, McLerran D, Wasson J, Wennberg JE and the Patient Outcomes Research Team. An assessment of radical prostatectomy – time trends, geographic variation, and outcomes. *JAMA* 1993;**269**:2633–2636.
3. Franks LM. Etiology, epidemiology and pathology of prostatic cancer. *Cancer* 1973;**32** (suppl): 1092–5.
4. Johansson JE, Adami HO, Andersson SO, Bergstrom R, Holmberg L, Krusemo UB. High 10-year survival rate in patients with early, untreated prostatic cancer. *JAMA* 1992;**267**:2191–2196.
5. Lu-Yao GL, Potosky AL and Albertsen PC. Secondary cancer treatments after radical prostatectomy among patients with prostate cancer. *J Urol* 1995;**153**:253A.
6. Madsen PO, Graversen PH, Gasser TC, Corle DK. Treatment of localized prostatic cancer: radical prostatectomy versus placebo: a 15 year follow-up. *Scan J Urol Nephrol* 1988;**110**(suppl):93–100.
7. Adolfsson J, Carstensen J, Lowhagen T. Deferred treatment in clinically localised prostatic carcinoma. *Br J Urol* 1992;**69**:183–187.
8. Jones GW. Prospective, conservative management of localized prostate cancer. *Cancer* 1992;**70** (suppl): 307–310.
9. Whitmore WF Jr, Warner JA, Thompson IM Jr. Expectant management of localized prostatic cancer. *Cancer* 1991;**67**:1091–1096.
10. George NJ. Natural history of localised prostatic cancer managed by conservative therapy alone. *Lancet* 1988;**i**:494–496.
11. Moskovitz B, Nitecki S, Levin DR. Cancer of the prostate: is there a need for aggressive treatment? *Urol Int* 1987;**42**:49–52.
12. Johansson JE, Adami HO, Andersson SO, Bergstrom R, Krusemok UB, Kraaz W. Natural history of localized prostatic cancer: a population-based study in 223 untreated patients. *Lancet* 1989;**i**:799–803.
13. Middleton RG, Thompson IM, Austerfeld MS et al. Prostate cancer clinical guidelines panel summary report – the management of clinically localized prostate cancer. *J Urol* 1995;**154**:2144–2148.
14. Chodak GW, Thisted RA, Gerber GS et al. Results of conservative management of clinically localized prostate cancer. *N Engl J Med* 1994;**330**:242–248.
15. Stewart LA, Parmar MKB. Meta-analysis of the literature or of individual patient data: is there a difference? *Lancet* 1993;**341**:418–422.
16. Goodman CM, Busuttil A, Chisholm GD. Age and size and grade of tumour predict prognosis in incidentally diagnosed carcinoma of the prostate. *Br J Urol* 1988;**62**:576–580.
17. Albertsen PC, Fryback DG, Stomer BG, Kolon TF, Fine J. Long-term survival among men with conservatively treated localized prostate cancer. *JAMA* 1995;**274**:626–631.
18. Gerber GS, Thisted RA, Chodak GW et al. Results of radical prostatectomy in men with clinically localized prostate cancer: multi-institutional analysis. *J Urol* 1995;**153**:252A.

15.3 Prostate cancer treatment: radical prostatectomy for early organ-confined disease

C E Bermejo Jr, D Shepherd and J W Basler

Introduction

At presentation, 56–60% of patients with prostate cancer will have clinically localized disease[1,2]. This percentage rises to 95–98% when populations are 'screened' with PSA and digital rectal examination[3]. Surgical extirpation, endeavouring completely to remove the prostate with its cancer would intuitively seem to be the best management for localized disease for several reasons: first, complete excision would leave no cancer cells in the body to spread later; secondly, unlike therapies that leave the treated prostate in place, removal prevents the later development of metachronous tumors in remnant benign tissues. These could theoretically be responsible for some of the 'late' local failures seen with radiotherapy. Third, local symptoms of bladder outlet obstruction related to tumor or BPH are readily controlled. Recent advances in laparoscopic surgery have led to the development of a laparoscopic radical prostatectomy technique that is gaining popularity as well[62–69].

Radical prostatectomy entails the total removal of the prostate, seminal vesicles, distal vasa and ejaculatory ducts as well as the prostatic urethra. Variations of the operation include: sparing the cavernosal nerves, proximal urethra, bladder neck, pubo-prostatic (vesical) ligament and apical urethra. The operation can be performed from the retropubic or perineal approaches and there are strong opinions about the relative efficacy and relative morbidity of each. The choice of approach generally is made based on surgeon preference. Suffice it to say that the two are nearly equal in their ability to render the patient free of prostate tissue and can be considered the 'Gold Standard' for treatment of localized disease. Evidence in favor of this statement comes through series from several institutions suggesting a long-term cure rate of up to 95% for low to intermediate grade disease that is confined to the surgical capsule[4–11].

Candidates for radical prostatectomy

The ideal candidate for radical prostatectomy would be a patient with organ confined disease, a life expectancy longer than the stage adjusted natural history of untreated prostate cancer and without risk factors that would jeopardize the patient during or after surgery. Some have argued that there may be no need for early definitive treatment, since conservative management of patients with clinically localized prostate cancer have a low risk of death from cancer within 10 to 15 years[12]. However, disease progression to incurability and significant morbidity may occur much earlier and after 10 years or longer, patients treated expectantly may have a significant excess mortality[13]. Since the mean survival of a 75-year-old American man is about 10 years and that for an 80 year old is about 7 years, patients who would likely benefit the most from a radical prostatectomy would be under 75 years of age and in good health[14]. However, conservative management (i.e. observation protocols) in patients with a small, organ confined, well differentiated cancer and life expectancy less than 10 years would not be unreasonable[15,16]. This does not mean that we should ignore the older patient since knowledge of the disease may allow prevention of the morbid sequellae even if curative therapy is not planned or possible.

Partin *et al.* have established that PSA and Gleason score from prostate biopsy samples, correlate directly with the likelihood of capsular penetration, seminal vesicle involvement and lymph node involvement in the radical prostatectomy specimen[17]. The probability, in this study, that a tumor detected with a PSA 0.0–4.0 ng/ml and Gleason score of 2–6 would be pathologically localized ranged from 50% to 90%. In this, as well as higher PSA ranges, lower Gleason scores were associated with a greater likelihood of organ confined disease. Table 15.3.1 summarizes some pertinent probabilities of organ confined disease for patients likely to be seen in clinical practice.

Pre-operative preparation

Younger patients without medical illnesses may proceed to surgery with only a minimal pre-operative evaluation (e.g. chest X-ray, ECG, serum chemistry, coagulation studies and CBC). However, given the potential for significant blood loss, those with a history of coronary artery disease, obstructive pulmonary disease, diabetes, hypertension, peripheral vascular disease, renal insufficiency, smoking, alcohol abuse or other potentially complicating diseases should undergo a pre-operative evaluation and 'tune-up' prior to anaesthetic. This will sometimes

Table 15.3.1   Prediction of organ confined disease[17]

PSA	Gleason score	Per cent correlation of clinical to pathological stage		
		cT1c	cT2a	cT2b
0–4.0 ng/ml	2–6	78–89	64–81	52–72
	7	63	47	34
	8–10	52	36	24
4.1–10 ng/ml	2–6	67–83	51–71	43–66
	7	49	33	22
	8–10	37	23	14
10.1–20 ng/ml	2–6	55–75	38–60	26–48
	7	35	22	13
	8–10	23	14	7
>20 ng/ml	2–6	35–58	22–41	13–29
	7	18	10	5
	8–10	10	5	3

Representative correlations between clinical (cTx) and ultimate pathologic stages based upon radical prostatectomy specimens. As an example, a clinical stage T1c tumor with a PSA of 12 and Gleason score of 7 has a 35% chance of being pathologic stage T1c. The full table has been published by Partin *et al.*[17]

uncover significant factors that could adversely affect the outcome of surgery and lead to another choice of therapy.

Patients may be admitted the morning of surgery unless there is a medical reason requiring inpatient monitoring. A full mechanical and antibiotic bowel cleansing, when judged necessary, is usually performed the day prior to surgery. Typically, however, a fleets enema the night prior to surgery is adequate. A broad spectrum antibiotic such as a fluoroquinolone is administered orally on the morning of surgery or intravenously 60 minutes pre-operatively. Oral cephalosporins are commonly started on post-operative day 1 and continued until pelvic drains are removed.

Since transfusion requirements vary by the approach used and experience of the surgeon, the decision to set up autologous or non-autologous blood pre-operatively should be made based on local needs. Maneuvers such as autologous hemodilution or the use of blood substitutes are intriguing new developments that may obviate the need for transfusion.

Anti-embolic pneumatic compression devices, low-dose heparin or warfarin have all been used in an attempt to prevent deep venous thrombosis and pulmonary embolism with varying degrees of success.

Perineal versus radical retropubic prostatectomy

One of the advantages of the retropubic approach is that it allows simultaneous access to the prostate and pelvic lymph nodes. In the perineal approach access to pelvic lymph nodes requires a separate incision or laparoscopic approach. However, the majority of patients who are candidates for a radical prostatectomy have a low incidence of lymph node involvement. Advantages of the perineal approach are less blood loss and possibly less post-operative pain[18–20].

Many studies have compared positive margins and PSA recurrence between the retropubic approach and the perineal approach. Shalev et al. compared the retropubic versus the perineal approach in a group of men with similar Gleason scores and clinical stages[21]. In this study, the rate of positive surgical margins in the perineal approach was significantly lower (15.7% vs. 29.8%) and the rate of extracapsular disease with negative margins was significantly higher (15.7% vs. 7%) for the perineal approach.

Wahle et al. reviewed the surgical margin involvement in 64 patients that underwent radical prostatectomy (either a radical perineal, standard retropubic or nerve sparing retropubic prostatectomy) for clinical stage T1 or T2 prostate cancer[22]. They found that there was no significant difference between the standard retropubic and the nerve sparing retropubic approaches in terms of resection margin involvement (30% vs. 45%, respectively) but both retropubic approaches were significantly better than the perineal approach (78%).

Boccon-Gibod et al. also made a comparison between the retropubic and perineal approaches. They found in their series that the incidence of positive margins was 61% in the retropubic approach and 56% in the perineal group[10]. The biochemical disease-free survival was 67% each. However, surgically induced positive margins in patients with organ confined disease were significantly more frequent in the perineal than retropubic group (43% vs. 29%). In addition, capsular incisions exposing benign tissue were significantly more frequent in the perineal approach than in the retropubic approach (90% vs. 37%) irrespective of pathological stage. It was concluded that while there was no difference between the two approaches with respect to positive margins and biochemical failure rates, the perineal approach created a higher risk for capsular incision and surgically induced margins 'at risk' for biochemical failure.

Finally, Haab et al. retrospectively compared the efficacy of radical perineal prostatectomy and retropubic prostatectomy for patients with localized prostate cancer[11]. They found that both groups were identical as far as complications, hospital stay, operation time and pathology were concerned. Organ confined disease (55% in retropubic and 54% in perineal group) and positive margins (39% retropubic and 37% perineal group) were the same for both groups.

From these studies it is clear that there is no consensus about a 'right' approach and that the patient and surgeon must ultimately decide which one is correct for the situation. In the case of a patient at high risk for positive margins or nodal disease, the retropubic approach makes most sense in that lymphadenectomy may be accomplished easily at the same setting. The retropubic approach is also advantageous if urethra-sparing techniques are being utilized. The perineal approach allows close visualization of the apical dissection and might be advantageous in the obese patient.

Laparoscopic radical prostatectomy

The laparoscopic approach to prostatectomy (LRP) was initially tried with littel success but has recently gained popularity in certain European centers.[70] Guilloneau and Vallancien have recently reported their experience with 260 LRP's over a two year period.[71] The operation involves approaching the ampullae and seminal vesicles transperitoneally followed by bladder mobilization medial to the medial umbilical ligaments. After division of the urachal remnant, the retropubuc space is dissected in a similar fashion to the RRP. An antegrade dissection of the prostate from the bladder neck is then performed similar to that described for the open prostatectomy. Results from this approach are on par with the other RRP and RPP but the operative skill required makes it unlikely to be readily available to most patients in the short-term. The discussion which follows concentrates on the open surgical procedures.

Potential adverse events of the radical prostatectomy

There has been a marked increase in the number of radical prostatectomies performed as a result of recognizing the efficacy of this procedure and the ability to detect prostate 1cancer at an early stage through prostate cancer screening and increased community awareness. Over the last 10 years, advances in surgical technique based on a more detailed understanding of male pelvic anatomy and improved perioperative care have dramatically reduced the morbidity of the operation. Despite these advancements, the radical prostatectomy exposes patient to the immediate morbidity of blood loss and potentially the risks attendant with the transfusion of heterologous blood, post-operative thrombo-embolic events, and perioperative death (which is still <1%), (Table 15.3.2). Patients with compromised potency or continence will require subsequent medical or surgical treatment. Patients considering a radical prostatectomy require a discussion of the contemporary

Table 15.3.2   Complications of radical prostatectomy

Intra-operative	Early post-operative	Late
Blood loss	Incisional pain	Urinary incontinence
Rectal injury	Thromboembolic event	Impotence
Ureteral injury	Lymphocele	Bladder neck contracture
Obturator nerve injury		

estimate of these risks in order to provide an informed consent to the procedure.

Intraoperative complications: blood loss

The average blood loss during a radical retropubic prostatectomy is between 500 and 1500 cc[18,19]. If the surgeon is able to keep this loss below 1000 cc, a blood transfusion is usually not necessary in the patient with a normal preoperative hematocrit. The average blood loss encountered during a radical perineal prostatectomy is 600 cc[20]. The need for a blood transfusion has been decreased with recent advances in surgical technique as a result of a better understanding of the venous anatomy surrounding the prostate. The need to transfuse can be reduced significantly with careful control of the dorsal venous complex, accessory veins to the lateral pelvic side-wall and the veins draining to the lateral cavernosal neurovascular complex. In order to decrease further a patient's exposure to a heterogeneous blood transfusion, hemodilution or autologous blood banking should be available to the patient.

Erythropoietin alpha given subcutaneously preoperatively has been used to decrease the need for transfusions in patients who undergo radical prostatectomy. The best results are obtained when combined with normo-volemic hemodilution prior to radical prostatectomy. Erythropoietin alpha is still under study to determine the optimum dosage to be used for patients prior to radical prostatectomy[23].

Intraoperative complications: rectal injury

Rectal injury is reported to occur from 0.1% to 1.3% of cases of radical retropubic prostatectomy and in 1.5% of cases of radical perineal prostatectomy[18,19,24,25]. This injury generally occurs during the apical dissection when developing the plane between the rectum and Denonvillier's fascia and when dividing the rectourethralis muscle. If a rectal injury is identified the radical prostatectomy should be completed. Prior to placing the urethral sutures, the rectal injury should be repaired. This can be accomplished by first freshening the edges of the rectal injury then it can be closed in two layers. The inner

layer can be closed with a 2-0 or 3-0 chromic continuous suture. The outer layer can be closed with chromic Lembert sutures or 2-0 silk. An omental flap can be considered to prevent a rectourethral fistula. The pelvis is then copiously irrigated with antibiotic solution. After the rectal injury is repaired the vesicourethral anastomosis is performed. A pelvic drain is usually placed to the side of the repair and the anal sphincter dilated at the end of the procedure. The patient should be continued on postoperative intravenous antibiotics (aerobic and anaerobic coverage) for 5 to 6 days. If the patient has undergone radiation therapy or has a large rectal injury or if the rectal injury is detected post-operatively, it is prudent to consider a temporary diverting colostomy[18,25,26].

Intraoperative complications: ureteral injury

Ureteral injuries may occur as a result of significant 'J' hooking of the distal ureters combined with aggressive perivesical dissection. This uncommon complication is usually recognized at the time of surgery and repaired by ureteroneocystostomy or stenting if the injury is minor[18,19,24–26]. Discovery after closure of the abdomen may require temporary percutaneous nephrostomy placement on the affected side and later repair either endourologically or a second open procedure.

Intraoperative complications: obturator nerve injury

Obturator nerve injury is an uncommon complication of radical retropubic prostatectomy. It occurs in approximately 0.1% of cases[18]. Unilateral injury is often a symptomatic post-operatively. However, bilateral injury will result in significant gait disturbance. Careful attention to anatomic detail with clear identification of the structures in the obturator fossa when performing pelvic lymph node dissection can prevent this complication. If the obturator nerve is divided, an attempt should be made to re-anastomose the injured nerve with a fine non-absorbable suture or place a nerve graft[26].

Early post-operative complications: thromboembolic events

All pelvic surgery patients are at an elevated risk for perioperative deep venous thrombosis (DVT) and pulmonary embolism (PE). Deep venous thrombosis occurs in 0.8–2.3% of cases of radical prostatectomies (perineal and retropubic)[18,20,24]. Though the exact etiology of thrombosis is not well documented, the surgeon may be able to lower a patient's risk of such events.

The surgeon should avoid internal compression of the external iliac vein by excessive traction during the obturator lymph node dissection. Attention is also required to avoiding compression of the femoral vein during surgery by pressure on the patient's groin by the hand of an assistant or observer. Assisted lower extremity venous drainage by sequential compression devices with or without concurrent warfarin use is believed by many surgeons to lower the incidence of post-operative deep venous thromboses[27]. Several controlled trials do not support this belief, however[28].

The peri-operative use of anticoagulants is an established method to decrease the incidence of thrombotic complications for patients undergoing certain orthopedic and gynecologic procedures. Catalona et al. randomized post-radical retropubic prostatectomy patients to peri-operative subcutaneous heparin therapy. These patients did not have a significant difference in their incidence of deep venous thromboses but did have a significantly higher incidence of lymphoceles in comparison to patients not receiving peri-operative heparin[29]. Most surgeons, therefore, do not intentionally use an anticoagulant to lower the risk of a post-operative DVT unless the patient has had a previous DVT, PE or a strong family history of thromboembolism.

Early post-operative ambulation of the patient is the simplest and most agreed upon measure to decrease the risk of a DVT. With few exceptions, ambulation several times on the first post-operative day should be strongly encouraged. While not studied to date, it is interesting to speculate that the popular use of ketorolac may lower the risk of DVT and PE. In addition to inhibiting platelet aggregation, better post-operative pain control logically results in earlier and more frequent post-operative ambulation.

Early post-operative complications: post-operative pain

Most patients fear waking up after surgery more than the surgery itself due to their anticipation of the pain. These concerns are real and may contribute to the patient's perception of the overall success of the operation. To alleviate this problem, pre-emptive analgesia can be used to allow the patient to awaken with much less discomfort and allow earlier ambulation and use of incentive spirometry to prevent atelectasis. Though still somewhat controversial, some centers report excellent results. In the ideal situation, the analgesia should be induced prior to the incision with administration of local anesthetics and/or regional blockade (epidural or long-acting spinal block). If parenteral analgesia (PRN or patient-controlled analgesia – PCA) is to be administered only, it should be started prior to the patient awakening to minimize pain and the risk of valsalva induced bleeding. Non-steroidal medication such as ketorolac has been used with some success as have traditional opiates[30].

Grass et al. documented that patients receiving ketorolac report less pain from intestinal cramping and bladder spasms with ambulation than patients receiving opiate-based analgesia[31]. The routine use of 30 mg ketorolac IV at the time of incision closure, 15 mg IV every 6 hours for the first post-operative 24 hours, and 15 mg IV every 6 hours as needed for the remainder of the hospitalization is a popular and effective post-operative analgesic regimen. This regimen is not recommended for patients with compromised renal function or a history of peptic ulcer disease. Other pain control regimens are summarized in Table 15.3.3.

Early post-operative complications: lymphocele

Symptomatic lymphocele has been reported in most radical prostatectomy series at a rate between 0.4–2.3%[18,19,24]. This complication can be prevented with attention to carefully ligating or occluding the lymphatic channels at the moment of the pelvic lymph node dissection.

If a lymphocele is suspected a pelvic ultrasound or CT scan of the pelvis should be obtained. This condition can be treated with percutaneous drainage and catheter placement with radiological guidance. This catheter can be removed once the drain output becomes minimal. If there is persistence of drainage of fluid an attempt can be made to sclerose the cavity with tetracycline (500 mg in 50 ml of normal saline), alcohol, erythromycin or 10% povidine-iodine solution. Solutions are generally left in the cavity for 30 minutes and drained. Repeat treatments can be performed weekly until the cavity is ablated and the tube drainage is minimal. Sclerotherapy is effective in 90% of the time[32,33].

Table 15.3.3   Post-operative pain control regimens

Parental agent	Dosage	Route of administration
MSO$_4$	0.05 mg/kg/h	IV, IM
	0.05 mg/kg/cc @ 6 cc/h	Continuous epidural
Fentanyl	0.0002 mg/kg	IV
	0.005 mg/kg @ ~6 cc/h	Continuous epidural
Demerol	<0.2 mg/kg/2 h	IV, IM
Ketorolac	30 mg initial, then 15 mg/6 h	IV, IM
Oral		
Demerol	50–100 mg/3–4 h	PO
Codeine	32–65 mg/4–6 h	PO
Oxycodone	5–10 mg/4–6 h	PO
Ibuprofen	200–800 mg/8 h	PO
Acetomenophen	325–1000 mg/6 h	PO

Dosage are estimates for patients with normal hepatic and renal function and should be adjusted to meet the clinical situation.

In the cases where sclerotherapy is not successful, marsupialization of the lymphocele into the peritoneal cavity is usually curative. This is generally performed as an open procedure but recently has been performed laparoscopically[34].

Late post-operative complications: incontinence

The incidence and severity of post-prostatectomy incontinence associated with the perineal and retro-pubic approaches are equivalent. The likelihood of this complication based on the broad experience of major institutions depends on the degree of urine leakage that is considered to constitute incontinence. Weldon et al. reports 95% urinary continence in post-perineal prostatectomy patients after 10 months post-operatively[20]. Catalona et al. reports 94% urinary continence 18 months after radical retropubic prostatectomy[18].

The attention to several technical aspects of the prostatectomy are attributed to improved post-operative continence. Efforts to spare the functional sphincter created by the circular muscle fibers of the bladder neck have demonstrated a quicker return of post-operative continence but no significant difference in the overall incidence or degree of incontinence[35]. Most surgeons agree that a careful apical dissection which spares the maximal amount of urethral length proximal to the pelvic diaphragm minimizes trauma to the rhabdosphincter and preserves continence[36].

Most patients report return of continence within 3–6 months of catheter removal. However, those still complaining of leakage despite Kegel exercises and simple biofeedback maneuvers should be evaluated carefully. Though rare after an adequate mucosa to mucosa apposition, stricturing at the anastomosis may occur leading to overflow incontinence or overt urinary retention. A careful voiding history and check of post-void residual will usually suggest this diagnosis.

The management of non-obstructive post-prostat-ectomy incontinence should include studies (urodynamics and cystoscopy) to address sphincteric competence and bladder instability. Urodynamics are needed to assess the bladder-specific causes of incontinence. A small capacity bladder or hyper-reflexia may have been associated with bladder outlet obstruction pre-operatively and manifested post-prostatectomy as incontinence. Com-promised bladder contractility as a result of diabetes or previous radical pelvic surgery may result in overflow incontinence. Cystoscopy is performed to assess the sphincteric function and the bladder anastomosis. The sphincter typically does not contract fully if it has been damaged significantly by the previous prostatectomy.

Patients with severe incontinence can be offered condom catheters, urethral clamps, intraurethral injections of teflon or cross-linked collagen or an artificial urinary sphincter. While occasionally acceptable, the former two options are generally not chosen due to the limitations that they place on the patient's lifestyle and the problems that can occur due to erosion of the devices through the penile skin. Retrograde collagen injection for bulking the area around the membranous urethra after prostatectomy has been reported with some degree of short-term success[37]. Antegrade collagen injection procedures to add bulk to the bladder neck area have yielded mixed results and rarely result in complete durable continence[38]. The best results to date have been with the implantation of the AMS 800™ artificial urinary sphincter. It is reported up to 83% of patients are dry after placement of artificial urinary sphincter[39]. Alternatively, a sling of autologous or heterologous fascia may be placed intra-operatively to support the bladder neck if the urethral stump appears short or incompetent (S.P. Wan, personal communication). Though difficult and experimental at present, the sling procedure may be attempted post-operatively in the appropriately selected patient.

Late post-operative complications: impotence

Walsh et al. in 1982 described the innervation of the corpora cavernosa and recommended some modifications in the surgical technique of the radical retropubic prostatectomy[40]. With these modifications, the incidence of impotence after a radical prostatectomy was reduced considerably. Quinlan et al. reported a 68% potency rate among patients who underwent nerve sparing radical retropubic prostatectomy[41].

Catalona et al. have similar results. They report 30–75% potency rates for patients who underwent unilateral nerve sparing technique and 65–75% potency rates for patients who had bilateral nerve sparing radical retropubic prostatectomy for organ confined prostate cancer[18]. They also determined that bilateral nerve sparing is significantly more successful in preserving potency.

The reported experience of nerve sparing radical perineal prostatectomy is more limited. Weldon et al. reported 70% of potency in patients undergoing nerve sparing radical perineal prostatectomy[20].

Concern would exist with compromising surgical margins in the nerve sparing technique. Catalona et al. compared surgical margins of standard with nerve sparing radical retropubic prostatectomy[42]. They found that the incidence of positive margins was not significantly different between both groups. Eggleston et al. reviewed 100 cases of nerve sparing radical retropubic prostatectomy and determined that this technique does not compromise the surgical margins[43].

The ideal candidate for nerve sparing radical prostatectomy would be a young sexually active man with low volume, well differentiated, impalpable tumors with no perineural invasion on biopsy and a PSA less than 10 ng/ml. If it is obvious at the time of the prostatectomy that there is tumor extension to the neurovascular bundle, a nerve sparing procedure should be avoided[44,45].

Patients should be encouraged to resume sexual activity as soon as they are comfortable post-operatively. Erections may take 24 to 48 months to recover fully. In the interim, vacuum erection devices and vasoactive injection therapy (PGE1, papaverine, etc.) may be used[46].

Recently, interest in sildenafil citrate (Viagra™) has spawned its use for patients suffering impotence after a radical prostatectomy. An 80% response rate was obtained with this medication in patients who had bilateral nerve sparing. However, none of the unilateral nerve sparing patients or non-nerve sparing patients responded to sildenafil citrate[47,48].

Late postoperative complications: bladder neck contracture

Bladder neck contracture has been reported to occur in 1.3% to 22% of patients who had a radical prostatectomy[18,24,49,50,51]. Multiple etiologic factors have been identified including previous operations on the prostate, extravasation of urine, asymptomatic bacteriuria and excessive intraoperative blood loss[18,50,52]. A well vascularized, water-tight anastomosis is optimal for adequate healing. Meticulous mucosa-to-mucosa anastomosis over an adequately sized, non-reactive (e.g. 18 Fr silicone or silastic™) foley catheter should be performed.

Patients presenting with a bladder neck contracture can initially be managed with careful dilatation or urethrotomy. Half of patients fail initial dilatation and 62% of patients have been reported to fail incision with a cold knife. Steroid injection into the area at risk for scarring may obviate recurrence of the stricture[18,49].

Outcomes of radical prostatectomy

Biochemical evidence of cure vs. failure

Success or failure of the operation was difficult to assess in the short term until the development of the PSA assay. This test, originally approved for monitoring the outcome of surgery because it measures a protein not produced appreciably by any other organ, offers a sensitive and objective measure of efficacy. Serum PSA should be undetectable (< 0.2 ng/ml by the Hybritech assay) after a radical prostatectomy. Supersensitive assays may allow even earlier diagnosis of failure but their clinical relevance remains speculative.

Persistence of detectable PSA implies residual tumor, residual benign prostate tissue or metastatic disease. Differentiating among these is important in determining the next step in the patient's management. For instance, if the margins of resection were clear of tumor, but there is evidence on the specimen that the capsule of the prostate was violated, one might suspect residual 'at risk' but benign tissue. This patient might elect a close observation protocol. On the other hand, if the prostate specimen was intact and the margins negative, one has to assume an extraprostatic source of the PSA which would most likely be metastases. Hormone therapy may be the next best treatment for this patient.

The usual course after a radical prostatectomy (pT1, pT2, pN0 disease) is for the PSA to drop to undetectable quickly ($T_{1/2}$ ~2–3 days) and remain in this range indefinitely. However, in the case of margin positivity (documented or not) or local tumor implantation from surgery, a rising PSA generally will be detected 2–5 years prior to clinical recurrence[4,5]. The rate of margin involvement varies directly with Gleason score and tumor volume as reflected in the PSA level[6,9,17]. Margin negative patients, though theoretically 'cured' of the disease, are still at risk of recurrence in proportion to the amount of Gleason pattern 4 and 5 seen in the specimen. This may be an architectural indication of the development of the 'invasive potential' by the cancer cells. Many studies have documented the PSA progression rate after radical prostatectomy for clinically localized prostate cancer (Table 15.3.4).

Management of margin positive disease

Controversy exists to which is the most adequate treatment for positive surgical margins. Treatment options include

Table 15.3.4 Progression of PSA in men with clinically localized prostate cancer after radical prostatectomy

References	Patients	% pSA Progression free			
		5 years		10 years	
		Margin+	Margin−	Margin+	Margin−
Epstein et al.[53]	617	74	95	55	80
Paulson et al.[6]	441	–	–	40	70
Catalona et al.[54]	925	74	91	–	–
Ohori et al.[55]	478	64	83	–	–

external beam radiation (XRT), androgen ablation and observation. External beam radiation can be given either early or delayed. Indications reported for adjuvant XRT have been extracapsular tumor extension, high-grade tumor and positive surgical margins. Although sometimes useful, patients with a high post-operative PSA, pelvic lymph node metastasis or seminal vesicle invasion may gain little benefit from adjuvant XRT[5,56].

Gibbons et al. reported that there was a lower 5 year recurrence rate in those patients who received XRT when compared with patients who did not receive XRT for margin positive disease[57]. Unfortunately there was no statistical analysis in this report.

Paulson et al. reported a 5 year disease-free survival rate of 70% for patients who received adjuvant XRT and 50% in those who did receive XRT for positive surgical margins[6]. This difference was statistically significant. Meier et al also found that there was a statistically significant disease-free survival difference when comparing patients who received adjuvant XRT (91%) versus those who did not receive XRT (46%) for margin positive disease[58]. Neither of these studies showed an overall survival benefit. Local tumor control can also be achieved with delayed XRT but this does not improve disease-free or overall survival[59,60].

Androgen ablation has also been considered for the treatment of margin positive disease. Androgen ablation may delay the progression of the disease but no survival benefit has been proven. The literature is limited in studies regarding hormone therapy for locally advanced prostate cancer. Trials are underway to determine the efficacy of early and delayed hormone therapy for locally advanced disease[61].

Observation can also be considered since prostate cancer may not recur in some patients with surgical positive margins. This can be explained either because it was an artifact of preparation and handling or the remnant tumor was actually ablated during removal (e.g. with cautery). Observation would avoid unnecessary side effects in these patients. More studies and more information are required to determine if there truly exists a difference between early treatment and observation with delayed treatment.

Conclusions

Multiple modalities for the diagnosis and treatment of localized prostate cancer have emerged in the last decade. There continue to be studies on their way to improve the outcome in the treatment of prostate cancer. At the present time, there does not exist any treatment option that has successfully outperformed the results of radical prostatectomy for the treatment of localized prostate cancer. For this reason radical prostatectomy continues to be the gold standard of treatment for localized prostate cancer.

References

1. Landis S, Murray T, Bolden S, Wingo PA. Cancer statistics. *CA Cancer J Clin* 1999;**49**(1):8–31.
2. Mettlin C, Jones GW, Murphy GP. Trends in prostate cancer care in the United States, 1974–1990: observations from the patient care evaluation studies of the American College of Surgeons Commission on Cancer. *Ca*: 1993; **43**(2): 83–91.
3. Catalona WJ, Smith DS, Ratliff TL, Basler JW. Detection of organ-confined prostate cancer is increased through prostate-specific antigen-based screening [see comments]. *JAMA* 1993;**270**(8):948–954.
4. Lu-Yao GL, Yao SL. Population-based study of long-term survival in patients with clinically localized prostate cancer. *Lancet* 1997;**349**(9056):906–910.
5. Zincke H, Oesterling JE, Blute ML, Bergstralh EJ, Myers RP, Barrett DM. Long-term (15 years) results after radical prostatectomy for clinically localized (stage T2c or lower) prostate cancer. *J Urol* 1994;**152**(5 Pt 2):1850–1857.
6. Paulson DF, Moul JW, Robertson JE, Walther PJ. Postoperative radiotherapy of the prostate for patients undergoing radical prostatectomy with positive margins, seminal vesicle involvement and/or penetration through the capsule. *J Urol* 1990;**143**(6):1178–1182.
7. Lepor H, Walsh PC. Long-term results of radical prostatectomy in clinically localized prostate cancer: experience at the Johns Hopkins Hospital. *NCI Monographs* 1988;**7**(7):117–122.
8. Morton RA, Steiner MS, Walsh PC. Cancer control following anatomical radical prostatectomy: an interim report. *J Urol* 1991;**145**(6):1197–1200.
9. Partin AW, Lee BR, Carmichael M, Walsh PC, Epstein JI. Radical prostatectomy for high grade disease: a reevaluation 1994. *J Urol* 1994;**151**(6):1583–1586.
10. Boccon-Gibod L, Ravery V, Vordos D, Toublanc M, Delmas V, Boccon-Gibod L. Radical prostatectomy for prostate cancer: the perineal approach increases the risk of surgically induced positive margins and capsular incisions. *J Urol* 1998;**160**(4):1383–1385.
11. Haab F, Boccon-Gibod L, Delmas V, Boccon-Gibod L, Toublanc M. Perineal versus retropubic radical prostatectomy for T1, T2 prostate cancer. *Br J Urol* 1994;**74**(5):626–629.
12. Fleming C, Wasson JH, Albertsen PC, Barry MJ, Wennberg JE. A decision analysis of alternative treatment strategies for clinically localized prostate cancer. Prostate Patient Outcomes Research Team. *JAMA* 1993;**269**(20): 2650–2658.
13. Brasso K, Friis S, Juel K, Jorgensen T, Iversen P. Mortality of patients with clinically localized prostate cancer treated with observation for 10 years or longer: a population based registry study. *J Urol* 1999;**161**(2):524–528.
14. Lew EA, Garfinkel L. Mortality at ages 75 and older in the Cancer Prevention Study (CPS I). *Ca* 1990;**40**(4):210–224.
15. Johansson JE, Adami HO, Andersson SO, Bergstrom R, Holmberg L, Krusemo UB. High 10-year survival rate in patients with early, untreated prostatic cancer. *JAMA* 1992;**267**(16):2191–2196.
16. Mettlin C, Jones GW, Murphy GP. Trends in prostate cancer care in the United States, 1974–1990: observations from the patient care evaluation studies of the American College of Surgeons Commission on Cancer. *Ca* 1993;**43**(2): 83–91.
17. Partin AW, Kattan MW, Subong EN, Walsh PC, Wojno KJ, Oesterling JE, Scardino PT, Pearson JD. Combination of prostate-specific antigen, clinical stage, and Gleason score to predict pathological stage of localized prostate cancer. A multi-institutional update [published erratum appears in *JAMA* 1997;**278**(2):118]. *JAMA* 1997;**277**(18):1445–1451.
18. Keetch DW, Andriole GL, Catalona WJ. *Complications of radical retropubic prostatectomy.* AUA Update Series, Volume XIII, lesson 6, 1994.

19. Leandri P, Rossignol G, Gautier JR, Ramon J. Radical retropubic prostatectomy: morbidity and quality of life. Experience with 620 consecutive cases. *J Urol* 1992;**147**(3 Pt 2):883–887.

20. Weldon VE, Tavel FR, Neuwirth H. Continence, potency and morbidity after radical perineal prostatectomy [see comments]. *J Urol* 1997;**158**(4): 1470–1475.

21. Shalev M, Tykochinsky G, Richter S, Kessler OJ, Nissenkorn I. Does the narrow operating field in perineal radical prostatectomy lead to more positive surgical margins? *Euro J Surg Oncol* 1998;**24**(4):313–315.

22. Wahle S, Reznicek M, Fallon B, Platz C, Williams R. Incidence of surgical margin involvement in various forms of radical prostatectomy. *Urology* 1990;**36**(1):23–26.

23. Monk T. Improving the outcome of acute normovolemic hemodilution with epoetin alfa. *Sem Hematol* 1997;**33**(2 suppl 2):48; discussion 49–50.

24. Igel TC, Barrett DM, Segura JW, Benson RC Jr, Rife CC. Perioperative and postoperative complications from bilateral pelvic lymphadenectomy and radical retropubic prostatectomy. *J Urol* 1987;**137**(6):1189–1191.

25. Weldon VE. Radical perineal prostatectomy, In: Crawford DE, Sakti D (eds) *Current Genitourinary Cancer Surgery*. Williams & Wilkins, Baltimore 1997, pp. 258–287.

26. Eatham JA, Scardino PT. Radical prostatectomy., In Walsh PC, Retik AB, Vaughan ED, Wein AJ (eds). *Campbell's urology*. WB Saunders Co, Philadelphia, 1998, pp. 2547–2564.

27. Kibel AS, Creager MA, Goldhaber SZ, Richie JP, Loughlin KR. Late venous thromboembolic disease after radical prostatectomy: effect of risk factors, warfarin and early discharge. *J Urol* 1997;**158**(6):2211–2215.

28. Cisek LJ, Walsh PC. Thromboembolic complications following radical retropubic prostatectomy. Influence of external sequential pneumatic compression devices. *Urology* 1993;**42**(4):406–408.

29. Bigg SW, Catalona WJ. Prophylactic mini-dose heparin in patients undergoing radical retropubic prostatectomy. A prospective trial. *Urology* 1992;**39**(4):309–313.

30. Hinman F. Postoperative management. In: Hinman F (Ed.) *Atlas of urologic surgery*. W. B. Saunders Company, Philadelphia, 1998, pp. 16–18.

31. Grass JA, Sakima NT, Valley M, Fischer K, Jackson C, Walsh P, Bourke DL. Assessment of ketorolac as an adjuvant to fentanyl patient-controlled epidural analgesia after radical retropubic prostatectomy. *Anesthesiology* 1993;**78**(4):642–648; discussion 21A.

32. McDowell GC II, Babaian RJ, Johnson DE. Management of symptomatic lymphocele via percutaneous drainage and sclerotherapy with tetracycline. *Urology* 1991;**37**(3):237–239.

33. Gilliland JD, Spies JB, Brown SB, Yrizarry JM, Greenwood LH. Lymphoceles: percutaneous treatment with povidone-iodine sclerosis. *Radiology* 1989;**171**(1):227–229.

34. Clayman RV. Laparoscopic lymphocelectomy. In: Clayman RV, McDougall EM (eds) Laparoscopic urology St. Louis, Quality Medical Publishing, Inc., 1993, pp. 309–321.

35. Basler J, Figenshau R, Bullock A, McCarthy J, Arcangeli C. Does bladder neck sparing radical prostatectomy improve continence or compromise margins of resection? *J Urol* 1994;**151**(5):255A.

36. Walsh PC, Quinlan DM, Morton RA, Steiner MS. Radical retropubic prostatectomy. Improved anastomosis and urinary continence. *Urol Clin N Am* 1990;**17**(3):679–684.

37. Smith DN, Appell RA, Rackley RR, Winters JC. Collagen injection therapy for post-prostatectomy incontinence. *J Urol* 1998;**160**(2):364–367.

38. Klutke JJ, Subir C, Andriole G, Klutke CG. Long-term results after antegrade collagen injection for stress urinary incontinence following radical retropubic prostatectomy. *Urology* 1999;**53**(5):974–977.

39. Gundian JC, Barrett DM, Parulkar BG. Mayo Clinic experience with use of the AMS800 artificial urinary sphincter for urinary incontinence following radical prostatectomy. *J Urol* 1989;**142**(6):1459–1461.

40. Walsh PC, Donker PJ. Impotence following radical prostatectomy: insight into etiology and prevention. *J Urol* 1982;**128**(3):492–497.

41. Quinlan DM, Epstein JI, Carter BS, Walsh PC. Sexual function following radical prostatectomy: influence of preservation of neurovascular bundles. *J Urol* 1991;**145**(5):998–1002.

42. Catalona WJ, Dresner SM. Nerve-sparing radical prostatectomy: extraprostatic tumor extension and preservation of erectile function. *J Urol* 1985;**134**(6):1149–1151.

43. Eggleston JC, Walsh PC. Radical prostatectomy with preservation of sexual function: pathological findings in the first 100 cases. *J Urol* 1985;**134**(6):1146–1148.

44. Steiner MS. Current results and patient selection for nerve-sparing radical retropubic prostatectomy. *Sem Urol Oncol* 1995;**13**(3):204–214.

45. Andriole GL. Nerve sparing radical retropubic prostatectomy, patient selection and technique. *AUA Update Series*, Volume XII, lesson 13, 1993.

46. Walsh PC, Worthington JF. Treating prostate cancer: radical prostatectomy. In: *The Prostate: A guide for men and the women who love them.* Johns Hopkins University Press, Baltimore, 1995, pp. 92–119.

47. Marks LS, Duda C, Dorey FJ, Macairan ML, Santos PB. Treatment of erectile dysfunction with sildenafil. *Urology* 1999;**53**(1):19–24.

48. Zippe CD, Kedia AW, Kedia K, Nelson DR, Agarwal A. Treatment of erectile dysfunction after radical prostatectomy with sildenafil citrate (Viagra). *Urology* 1998;**52**(6):963–966.

49. Surya BV, Provet J, Johanson KE, Brown J. Anastomotic strictures following radical prostatectomy: risk factors and management. *J Urol* 1990;**143**(4):755–758.

50. Tomschi W, Suster G, Holtl W. Bladder neck strictures after radical retropubic prostatectomy: still an unsolved problem. *Br J Urol* 1998;**81**(6):823–826.

51. Popken G, Sommerkamp H, Schultze-Seemann W, Wetterauer U, Katzenwadel A. Anastomotic stricture after radical prostatectomy. Incidence, findings and treatment. *Euro Urol* 1998;**33**(4):382–386.

52. Hedican SP, Walsh PC. Postoperative bleeding following radical retropubic prostatectomy. *J Urol* 1994;**152**(4):1181–1183.

53. Epstein JI, Partin AW, Sauvageot J, Walsh PC. Prediction of progression following radical prostatectomy. A multivariate analysis of 721 men with long-term follow-up. *Am J Surg Pathol* 1996;**20**(3):286–292.

54. Catalona WJ, Smith DS. 5-year tumor recurrence rates after anatomical radical retropubic prostatectomy for prostate cancer. *J Urol* 1994;**152**(5 Pt 2):1837–1842.

55. Ohori M, Wheeler TM, Kattan MW, Goto Y, Scardino PT. Prognostic significance of positive surgical margins in radical prostatectomy specimens. *J Urol* 1995;**154**(5):1818–1824.

56. Coetzee LJ, Hars V, Paulson DF. Postoperative prostate-specific antigen as a prognostic indicator in patients with margin-positive prostate cancer, undergoing adjuvant radiotherapy after radical prostatectomy. *Urology* 1996;**47**(2):232–235.

57. Gibbons RP, Cole BS, Richardson RG, Correa RJ Jr, Brannen GE, Mason JT, Taylor WJ, Hafermann MD. Adjuvant radiotherapy following radical prostatectomy: results and complications. *J Urol* 1986;**135**(1):65–68.

58. Meier R, Mark R, St Royal L, Tran L, Colburn G, Parker R. Postoperative radiation therapy after radical prostatectomy for prostate carcinoma. *Cancer* 1992;**70**(7):1960–1966.

59. Forman JD, Wharam MD, Lee DJ, Zinreich ES, Order SE. Definitive radiotherapy following prostatectomy: results and complications. *Int J Rad Oncol Biol Phys* 1986;**12**(2):185–189.

60. Rosen EM, Cassady Jr, Connolly J, Chaffey JT. Radiotherapy for localized prostate carcinoma. *Int J Rad Oncol Biol Phys* 1984;**10**(12):2201–2210.

61. Mayer FJ, Crawford ED. The role of endocrine therapy in the management of local and distant recurrence of prostate cancer following radical prostatectomy or radiation therapy. *Urol Clin N Am* Nov. 1994;**21**(4):707–715.

62. Zerbib M, Methods and results of radical prostatectomy for localized cancer of the prostate. *Cancer Radiother* 2000 Nov; **4** Suppl 1: 109s–112s;

63. Hoznek A, Salomon L, Rabii R, Ben Slama MR, Cicco A, Antiphon P, Abbou CC, Vesicourethral anastomosis during laparoscopic radical prostatectomy: the running suture method. *J Endourol* 2000 Nov; **14**(9): 749–53;

64. Abbou CC, Hoznek A, Salomon L, Lobontiu A, Saint F, Cicco A, Antiphon P, Chopin D, Remote laparoscopic radical prostatectomy carried out with a robot. Report of a case. *Prog Urol* 2000 Sep; **10**(4): 520–3;

65. Thuroff JW, Laparoscopic radical prostatectomy: feasibility studies or the future standard technique? *Curr Opin Urol* 2000 Sep; **10**(5): 363–4;

66. Schulam PG, Link RE Laparoscopic radical prostatectomy. *World J Urol* 2000 Sep; **18**(4): 278–82.

67. Guillonneau B, Vallancien GJ Laparoscopic radical prostatectomy: the Montsouris technique. *Urol* 2000 Jun; **163**(6): 1643–9;

68. Abbou CC, Salomon L, Hoznek A, Antiphon P, Cicco A, Saint F, Alame W, Bellot J, Chopin DK Laparoscopic radical prostatectomy: preliminary results. *Urology* 2000 May; **55**(5): 630–4;

69. Jacob F, Salomon L, Hoznek A, Bellot J, Antiphon P, Chopin DK, Abbou CC, Laparoscopic radical prostatectomy; preliminary results. *Eur Urol* 2000 May; **37**(5): 615–20;

70. Abbou C, Hoznek A, Salomon 1, et al. Laparoscopic radical prostatectomy. *J Urol Suppl* 1999; **161**: abstract V4.

71. Guillonneau B, Vallancien G. Laparoscopic Radical Prostatectomy: The Montsouris Technique. *J Urol* 2000; **163**: 1643–1649.

15.4 Radiotherapy for organ confined prostate cancer

J T Roberts

Introduction

Two modalities of radiation are used for the treatment of prostate cancer. External beam therapy is usually delivered as high energy photons produced by a linear accelerator although particle beam irradiation, using protons or neutrons, has been used for locally advanced disease; it has limited availability. Interstitial radioisotopes may be implanted, using permanently placed iodine-125 (^{125}I) or, less commonly, palladium-103 (^{103}Pd) seeds. Temporary implants of Iridium-192 (^{192}Ir) may also be used, introduced via perineal needles. The largest body of data is available on the results of external beam irradiation.

Radiotherapy techniques

External beam irradiation

The choice of treatment volume is controversial. No randomized trial has established a benefit for the routine use of prophylactic pelvic lymph node irradiation and policy varies from institution to institution. Indeed, two randomized trials, in which patients were staged by lymphadenectomy[1] and either lymphangiogram, CT or lymphadenectomy[2], respectively, showed no significant difference in survival, disease-free survival, local control or distant metastasis rate when pelvic lymph nodes were electively irradiated in 'node negative' patients. Data from surgically staged series have been used to derive estimates of risk of nodal involvement, using Gleason score, clinical stage and PSA[3] and the suggestion made that elective nodal irradiation be applied when there is a 20% or greater risk of nodal involvement[4].

There is similar controversy surrounding the use of seminal vesicle irradiation; again PSA, tumour stage and Gleason score can also be used to predict the likelihood of seminal vesicle involvement[3] and a decision made to omit seminal vesicle irradiation in those in whom the risk of involvement is low. The aim of radical external beam irradiation is to deliver the maximum dose to the tumour, while sparing as much normal tissue as possible. The use of three, four or more radiation fields and of computerized, three-dimensional CT-based treatment planning techniques, allows conformal radiotherapy. Individualized patient immobilization devices, precisely aligned, carefully contoured, 'conformal' radiation fields, defined either by individually shaped metal blocks or by means of multileaf collimators, reduce the volume of normal tissue irradiated and hence reduce the morbidity of radiotherapy and allow escalation of the dose delivered to the tumour. Doses of 64–66 Gy, given in 32–33 fractions over $6\frac{1}{2}$ weeks are typically given with conventional, non-conformal radiotherapy techniques. Dose escalation beyond 70 Gy with conventional radiotherapy techniques is associated with a doubling of the severe morbidity rate, while patients have been treated with doses in excess of 80 Gy, using conformal techniques, with acceptable levels of morbidity[5].

Interstitial brachytherapy

Interstitial brachytherapy can be delivered either by means of permanent source placement or by temporary insertion of ^{192}Ir inside hollow, flexible catheters. There is currently more interest in the use of permanent implants, the prime advantage of which is that they can be performed on an outpatient basis, whereas ^{192}Ir temporary implants require an overnight stay. The major practical benefit of interstitial brachytherapy, however delivered, is the rapid fall-off of dose with distance from the radioactive source. This means that high doses can be delivered to the tumour volume, while careful placement allows the sparing of normal tissues. ^{125}I is the most commonly used isotope for permanent implants. It emits radiation of low average energy (30 keV) and therefore requires minimum shielding and protection arrangements. Its long half-life (60 days) allows several weeks storage prior to use. Its low dose rate is a theoretical disadvantage and has been cited as a reason for the high local failure rate observed with high-grade tumors[6,7]. For this reason ^{103}Pd has been used for the treatment of higher grade tumors. ^{103}Pd is also a low-energy emitter (21 keV) but has a shorter half-life (approximately 17 days) and therefore a greater initial dose rate, approximately three times greater than with an equivalent ^{125}I implant. Permanent implants are suitable only for those patients with disease confined within the capsule. For patients with extracapsular extension of disease either external beam therapy alone or combined with a boost dose achieved with brachytherapy, or a temporary iridium implant to a larger volume may be appropriate.

Treatment planning

In planning a radioactive prostate implant, digitized information either from CT or ultrasound images of the prostate are used to produce a three-dimensional reconstruction of the prostate which is then used to calculate a plan for seed placement and an isodose distribution for each cross-section. CT may produce less distortion of the prostatic contour but ultrasound provides sharper definition of the prostatic margin. At this stage adjustments to seed position can be made to adjust the dose delivered to prostate, urethra and rectum. The dose is prescribed at the periphery of the prostate and is intended as the minimum dose to the prostate. The dose delivered to the center of the prostatic volume is usually higher as a result of a cumulative contribution from multiple sources. As a result the urethral dose is invariably higher than the dose at the periphery of the gland and careful seed placement, with preferential peripheral placement of seeds, is used to keep urethral dose within tolerance. Minimum prostatic doses of 140–160 Gy are typically given with ^{125}I, which will give doses of around 250 Gy to the prostatic urethra.

Implant procedure

The lower bowel is cleared before the procedure and prophylactic antibiotics given. The patient is placed in the lithotomy position and either a general or spinal anaesthetic administered. A foley catheter helps identify the base of the prostate. A needle-guide template is placed against the perineum and needles inserted to steady the template, after which further needles are inserted, under ultrasound or fluoroscopic control and the seeds placed. Preoperative transrectal ultrasound allows control of seed placement and correction for the unavoidable difference in patient positioning from the planning scan and for prostate movement during the insertion of needles. When the implant is complete a CT scan is performed to evaluate the quality of the implant and to provide information on the precise position of the sources, thus allowing calculation of the dose and dose distribution provided by that implant.

Results

The largest body of published data on radiotherapy for early prostate cancer is from series treated with conventional external beam irradiation. High rates of local control may be obtained[8,9]. Conformal radiotherapy offers the opportunity of significant dose escalation compared with conventional external beam irradiation: this may lead to further improvements in control with acceptable morbidity. However, long-term follow up is lacking. For patients with disease confined within the capsule of the gland, PSA relapse-free survival rates equivalent to those obtained by radical prostatectomy are reported[10–14]. Morbidity appears acceptable with less than 1% of patients who have not previously been subjected to TURP experiencing incontinence and impotence occurring in less than 20% of those aged less than 70[15–17].

Conclusions

Excellent results, expressed in terms of freedom from PSA relapse, may be obtained, in appropriately selected patients, with modern radiotherapy; either external beam or brachytherapy. The influence of the mode of therapy, rather than the selection process, on outcome can only be determined by randomized comparisons of similar patient populations. In the absence of such studies and given the difficulty in obtaining informed consent to random selection of radical treatment procedures it is incumbent on all treating localized prostate cancer radically to agree common criteria for describing patients and disease and for assessing outcome, including morbidities.

References

1. Spaas PG, Bagshaw MA, Cox RS. The value of extended field irradiation in surgically staged carcinoma of the prostate. *Int J Radiat Oncol Biol Phys* 1988;**15**(suppl 1): 133–134.

2. Absell SO, Krall JM, Pilepich M-VAC *et al*. Elective pelvic irradiation in stage A2, B carcinoma of the prostate: analysis of RTOG-77-06. *Int J Radiat Oncol Biol Phys* 1988;**15**:1307–1316.

3. Partin AW, Yoo J, Cater HB *et al*. The use of prostate-specific antigen, clinical stage and Gleason score to predict pathological stage in men with localised prostate cancer. *J Urol* 1993;**15**:110–114.

4. Epstein BE, Hanks GE. Radiation therapy techniques and dose selection in the treatment of prostate cancer. *Semin Radiat Oncol* 1993;**3**:179–186.

5. Liebel SA, Heimann R, Kutcher GJ *et al*. Three-dimensional conformal radiation therapy in locally advanced carcinoma of the prostate: preliminary results of a phase I dose-escalation study. *Int J Radiat Oncol Biol Phys* 1994;**28**:55–65.

6. Ling CC. Permanent implants using Au-198, Pd-103 and I-125: radiobiological considerations based on the linear quadratic model. *Int J Radiat Oncol Biol Phys* 1992;**23**:81–87.

7. Orton CG, Webber BM. Time-dose factor (TDF) analysis of dose rate effects in permanent implant dosimetry. *Int J Radiat Oncol Biol Phys* 1977;**2**:55–60.

8. Perez C A, Hanks GE, Liebel SA *et al*. Localised carcinoma of the prostate (Stages T1B, T1C, T2 and T3): review of management with external beam radiation therapy. *Cancer* 1993;**72**:3156–3173.

9. Kaplan ID, Cox RS, Bagshaw MA. Prostate specific antigen after external beam radiotherapy for prostate cancer: follow up. *J Urol* 1993;**149**:519–522.

10. Priestley JB, Beyer DC. Guided brachytherapy for treatment of confined prostate cancer. *Urology* 1992;**40**:127–132.

11. Wallner K, Roy J, Harrison L. Tumour control and morbidity following transperineal iodine 125 implantation for stage T1/T2 prostatic carcinoma. *J Clin Oncol* 1996;**14**:449–53.

12. Kaye KW, Olsen DJ, Payne JT. Detailed preliminary analysis of iodine 125 implantation for localised prostate cancer using percutaneous approach. *J Urol* 1995;**153**:1020–1025.

13. Wallner K, Roy J, Zelefsky M *et al.* Short term freedom from disease progression after iodine 125 prostate implantation. *Int J Radiat Oncol Biol Phys* 1994;**30**:405–409.

14. Blasco JC, Wallner K, Grimm PD, Ragde H. Prostate specific antigen based disease control following ultrasound guided iodine 125

15. Blasco JC, Ragde H, Grimm PD. Transperineal ultrasound guided implantation of the prostate; morbidity and complications. *Scand J Urol Nephrol* 1991;**137**(suppl):113–118.

16. Stock RG, Stone NN, Iannuzzi C. Sexual potency following interactive ultrasound guided brachytherapy for prostate cancer. *Int J Radiat Oncol Biol Phys* 1996;**35**:267–272.

17. Arterbery VE, Wallner K, Roy J, Fuks Z. Short term morbidity from CT planned transperineal iodine 125 prostate implants. *Int J Radiat Oncol Biol Phys* 1993;**25**:661–667.

implantation for stage T1/T2 prostatic carcinoma. *J Urol* 1995;**154**:1096–1099.

16 Treatment of locally advanced disease

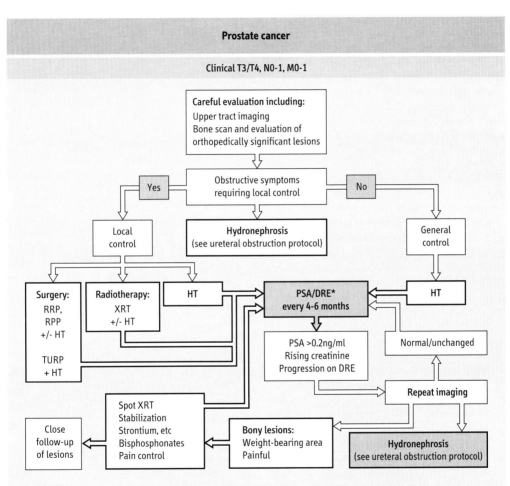

Prostate cancer

Clinical T3/T4, N0-1, M0-1

Careful evaluation including:
Upper tract imaging
Bone scan and evaluation of orthopedically significant lesions

Obstructive symptoms requiring local control

Yes — No

Local control

Hydronephrosis (see ureteral obstruction protocol)

General control

Surgery:
RRP,
RPP
+/- HT

TURP
+ HT

Radiotherapy:
XRT
+/- HT

HT

PSA/DRE* every 4-6 months

HT

PSA >0.2ng/ml
Rising creatinine
Progression on DRE

Normal/unchanged

Repeat imaging

Close follow-up of lesions

Spot XRT
Stabilization
Strontium, etc
Bisphosphonates
Pain control

Bony lesions:
Weight-bearing area
Painful

Hydronephrosis (see ureteral obstruction protocol)

*(add alkaline Phosphatase, Creatinine, periodic upper tract imaging)

179

16.1   Hormonal downstaging: myth or reality?

M Perrotti, B R Kava, N Stroumbakis and W R Fair

Introduction

Despite the increased public awareness of the importance of annual digital rectal examination and the widespread use of PSA by the medical community, only 37–58% of patients undergoing radical prostatectomy for presumed clinically localized prostate cancer will have pathologically organ confined cancer[1–6]. Tumors detected through prostate cancer screening programs[7], and by PSA elevation alone (i.e. clinical T1c), demonstrate extraprostatic extension approximately 25–30% of the time on examination of the pathologic specimen[8–10].

Although not all patients with disease beyond the prostatic capsule will eventually develop metastatic disease, the impact of extracapsular extension is associated with an increased risk of early biochemical relapse following prostatectomy. At a median follow up of 34 months, Stein et al.[11] reported PSA relapse rates of 15% in patients with pathologically organ confined prostate cancer, which was contrasted with a 29% PSA recurrence rate for those patients with extracapsular disease or positive surgical margins, and 39% in those patients with seminal vesical involvement. Similarly, Morton et al.[12] reported that the actuarial 5 year combined biochemical and clinical failure rate in those patients with organ confined disease at radical prostatectomy (n = 337) was 6%. This increased to 26% for patients with extraprostatic extension and negative surgical margins (n = 122) and 79% for those patients with either seminal vesical involvement, extracapsular extension and positive surgical margins, or lymph node metastases (n = 127).

The presence of cancer positive surgical margins as an independent risk factor for biochemical failure was demonstrated by Frazier et al.[13], who found that at a median follow up of 23 months, PSA recurrence in patients with extracapsular disease and cancer-free surgical margins was 39%, compared with 66% in many positive patients. These rates of PSA failure are comparable to the rates of local and radiological recurrences seen in another group of patients from the same institute at a period of 10 years following radical prostatectomy[13,14]. These data provide compelling evidence that tumor extension beyond the prostate at the time of radical prostatectomy is associated with an increased risk of early biochemical relapse which may eventually translate into clinical evidence of disease progression.

The rationale for the administration of neoadjuvant androgen deprivation therapy (ADT) prior to radical prostatectomy is to attempt medically to downsize the primary tumor, as well as the entire prostate gland, in order to improve the chances of complete tumor extirpation. This chapter will review the experimental and clinical basis for the use of neoadjuvant androgen deprivation prior to radical prostatectomy. It will review our experiences with neoadjuvant androgen ablation in patients with locally advanced (>T3) prostate cancer, as well as in those patients with clinically organ confined (T1, T2) disease.

Rationale for the use of neoadjuvant androgen deprivation therapy

How can neoadjuvant hormonal deprivation work? It is clear that tumor cells outside the prostate will not 'jump back' into the prostate. However, tumor extending beyond the confines of the prostatic capsule may regress following androgen ablation, and there is no evidence to suggest that extraprostatic cells are necessarily hormone-resistant. It is not inconceivable that some early (non-metastatic) prostate cancers may be composed entirely of hormonally sensitive cells. Studies in men undergoing ADT prior to radical prostatectomy have shown prostate cancer cells to exhibit active cellular degeneration in response to androgen deprivation[15]. The observed ADT effect consists of cytoplasmic vacuolization, nuclear pyknosis, nuclear fragmentation and cellular lysis. Morphologically, these effects are remarkably similar to the biological process of apoptosis[16], and may further explain the complete absence of tumor cells noted in some radical prostatectomy specimens following neoadjuvant ADT[17–21].

Experimental basis for neoadjuvant ADT

In the Dunning R-3327-H tumor, Isaacs et al.[22] noted a marked difference in the growth of inoculated tumor cells, which depended upon the temporal proximity to androgen deprivation. Maximum inhibition of tumor growth occurred when castration was performed at the time of tumor inoculation. When castration was performed 200 days following inoculation, little or no effect on tumor growth was observed. This suggests that sensitivity to androgen deprivation decreases markedly with increasing tumor size, and may be related to the differentiation status of the tumor.

Bruchovsky et al.[23] measured the relative stem cell concentration at various points of tumor growth in the Shionogi androgen sensitive mammary tumor. Though tumor volumes initially declined by 90% following castration, tumor regrowth led to a return to the original tumor volume within 1 month. Cell samples from the precastrate, castrate (at the point of maximal tumor regression) and recurrent tumors were injected into male and female nude mice. Table 16.1.1 illustrates that 1) not every injected cell produced a tumor, 2) the 'hormone-resistant' cells showed differential growth depending upon whether a male or female nude mouse was inoculated, indicating that the hormonal resistance following castration was a relative and not an absolute situation, 3) the recurrent tumor contained the highest percentage of stem cells, and 4) the lowest stem cell concentration was at the time of maximal castration effect. This final observation suggests that the ideal combination therapy may be an initial period of hormone deprivation to minimize the stem cell population, followed by definitive surgical excision to remove any remaining tumor cells that were not killed by ADT.

Clinical trials investigating neoadjuvant ADT

The use of neoadjuvant ADT in locally advanced prostate cancer (>clinical T3)

Patients with locally advanced prostate cancer have a 40–80% risk of lymph node metastases[24,25] and are at high risk for local and systemic recurrence following radical prostatectomy alone[26–28]. The high rates of cancer-positive post-irradiation biopsies[29,30] as well as high systemic failure rates following radiation therapy[31–34] make these modalities, too, less than optimal for the management of patients in the setting of locally advanced disease.

Early clinical experiences attested to the improved resectability of locally advanced tumors treated pre-operatively with ADT[35–39]. In 1964 Scott[40] reported on the use of pre-operative ADT in 21 patients with locally advanced disease, and in a follow up report, Scott and Boyd[41] confirmed the utility of pre-operative androgen deprivation in 44 patients. Most patients received surgical castration plus daily oestrogen for a period of at least 6 months prior to radical prostatectomy. Of those patients followed for 10 years (n = 33), 51.5% were alive without evidence of disease, 9.1% were alive with disease, 18.2% had died without evidence of recurrence, and 21.2% were dead as a

result of prostate cancer. Of 31 patients followed for 15 years or more (n = 31), 29% were alive without evidence of disease and 38.7% had died without evidence of disease. Thirty-two per cent of patients died from prostate cancer.

The advent of several potent, well tolerated pharmaceutical agents for induction of a reversible biochemically castrate state catalyzed a renewed interest in neoadjuvant ADT prior to radical prostatectomy in the late 1980s. In a pilot study at Memorial Sloan Kettering Cancer Center, Aprikian et al.[42] reported on 55 patients with locally advanced prostate cancer who were believed to be poorly amenable to surgical resection at the time of initial presentation. There were 18 patients with clinical stage T2b/c, 27 patients with clinical T3, and 10 patients with stage D0 (persistently elevated serum acid phosphatase levels) prostate cancer. Patients were treated with oral diethylstilbestrol (DES) at a dosage of 3 mg per day. At a median pre-treatment duration of 12 weeks (range 5–32 weeks), a marked reduction of serum PSA levels occurred, with 98% of patients achieving normal levels (<4.0 ng/ml) and 49% of patients achieving undetectable levels. In 15 patients who were evaluated with transrectal ultrasonography prior to and following androgen deprivation therapy there was a median reduction in calculated TRUS prostatic volume of 35%. Forty-seven patients underwent radical prostatectomy after five were found to have pelvic lymph node metastases on frozen section, and an additional three patients were believed to be unresectable as a result of pelvic sidewall fixation. Of the patients undergoing radical prostatectomy: 18 patients (38%) had pathologically organ confined prostate cancer and 30 patients (64%) were pathologically specimen confined. Ten patients (21%) had extracapsular extension with positive surgical margins, and seven patients (15%) had microscopic pelvic lymph node metastases. These patients had undergone prostatectomy after the initial frozen section analysis was reported as negative.

Figure 16.1.1 illustrates the results of 5 year interim follow up of the 47 patients undergoing radical prostatectomy in this series[43]. The actuarial 5 year freedom from PSA relapse rate approaches 45% in those patients with clinical T2b/c and T3 disease. This is similar to freedom from PSA rates observed in patients undergoing radical prostatectomy alone for clinical T2b and T2c prostate cancer in other series[44], and superior to results seen in radiation therapy with or without neoadjuvant androgen deprivation therapy[45]. The recurrence of detectable PSA in all of the patients with clinical D0 prostate cancer confirms that regardless of whether normalization occurs as a result of ADT, acid phosphatase elevation portends a poor prognosis. The fact that detectable PSA recurred within the first year in seven of nine patients (77%) with acid phosphatase elevation, even in the presence of cancer-free surgical margins and a negative pelvic lym-

Table 16.1.1 Stem cell assay (adapted from Bruchovsky et al.[23])

Cell sample injected	Stem cells: total cells	
	Male mice	Female mice
Precastrate	1:4000	1:370 000
Castrate	1:70 000	1:2 200 000
Recurrent	1:200	1:800

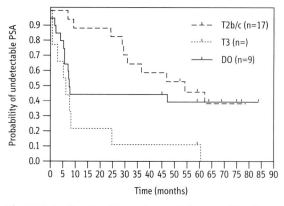

Fig. 16.1.1   Results of 5 year interin follow up of the 47 patients undergoing radical prostatectomy[43].

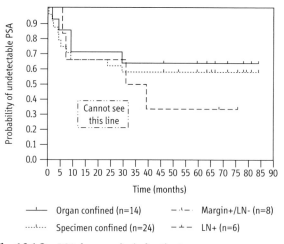

Fig. 16.1.2   PSA-free survival of patients.

phadenectomy, suggests that these patients probably harbored occult distant metastases that would not be expected to derive benefit from the improved local control afforded with ADT. Finally, it should be noted that all but two patients with lymph node metastases have developed PSA recurrence. These two patients were administered DES for several months post-operatively and are currently without detectable PSA after having discontinued DES for approximately 4 years each.

Figure 16.1.2 demonstrates the PSA-free survival for those patients with organ confined, specimen confined, margin-positive and lymph node-positive disease following neoadjuvant DES, excluding the patients with D0 prostate cancer. In this subset of patients, nine of 14 patients (64%) with pathologically organ-confined disease following ADT and 14 of 24 patients (58%) with specimen confined disease are currently without biochemical recurrence at a median follow up of 66.5 months (range 46.09–83.91 months). The durability of this response at 5 years, suggests that the declining incidence of cancer-positive surgical margins seen in patients treated with neoadjuvant ADT is a real occurrence, and not merely an artifact resulting from an inability to assess surgical margins accurately following androgen deprivation. If these patients had surgical margins that were mistakenly interpreted as negative as a result of ADT, we would expect a higher rate of PSA recurrence, that was comparable to the true margin-positive patients in this study.

Other contemporary studies have confirmed that neoadjuvant ADT consistently results in: 1) a dramatic reduction of serum PSA by 89–99%[46–55]; 2) acid phosphatase normalization[42]; and 3) a mean reduction in overall prostatic volume by 35–50% as measured by transrectal ultrasonography[42,46–56]. Several investigators[21,49] have noted that downsizing the prostate with neoadjuvant ther-

apy facilitated surgery, allowing for a reduction in operative time and blood loss. These observations have been disputed by others[47]. In several recent controlled trials[48,50] neoadjuvant ADT has had minimal effect on the technical aspects of radical prostatectomy, and post-operative complications were comparable between patients undergoing neoadjuvant therapy followed by surgery or surgery alone. Our surgical experience with several hundred patients who have been treated with neoadjuvant androgen deprivation concurs with these latter findings.

Table 16.1.2 summarizes the pathologic findings in several contemporary investigations utilizing neoadjuvant androgen deprivation therapy for patients with locally advanced prostate cancer. Attempts to derive significant meaning from these studies must be tempered, due to the fact that the majority of studies lacked control groups. Specifically with regard to the incidence of downstaging, studies evaluating the role of surgical monotherapy for clinical stage T3 prostate cancer[41,58] have shown that 18–24% of patients thought to have clinical stage C disease are found to have organ confined tumors on final pathological evaluation. Therefore, we must question whether patients with clinical stage T3 prostate cancer that have organ confined disease following neoadjuvant androgen deprivation therapy are actually overstaged initially, rather than downstaged following therapy. The only way truly to validate any potential downstaging effect of ADT is to incorporate randomized control groups in these studies. As indicated above, control groups in this setting would be at high risk for lymph node metastases and ultimate biochemical and clinical failure.

In a retrospective analysis of 22 patients who had undergone neoadjuvant ADT followed by radical prostatectomy, Oesterling et al.[52] used historical controls, that

Table 16.1.2 Influence of neoadjuvant androgen deprivation therapy on rates of organ confined and specimen confined disease in locally advanced (>T3) prostate cancer

Investigators	Patient number	Organ confined	Specimen confined
Aprikian et al. (1994)[42]	27	7 (26%)	15 (71%)
Kennedy et al. (1992)[51]	7	2 (29%)	–
MacFarlane et al. (1993)[47]	14	5 (36%)	–
Andros et al. (1993)[46]	16	3 (18%)	9 (56%)
Solomon et al. (1993)[56]	16	–	12 (75%)
Soloway et al. (1994)[48]	22	–	13 (59%)
Gomella et al. (1996)[57]	21	5 (24%)	12 (57%)
Schulman and Sassine (1993)[49]	15	4 (27%)	–
Labrie et al. (1993)[59]	12	9 (75%)*	8 (67%)†
Van Poppel et al. (1995)[53]	29	17 (59%)‡	–

* Compared with 2 patients (16.7%) in the control group (n=12).
† Compared with 4 patients (33%) in control group (n=12).
‡ Compared with 14 patients (56%) in the control group (n=25).

were matched for baseline PSA, pre-operative clinical stage, and pre-treatment tumor grade and underwent radical prostatectomy alone for clinical stages B2 and C prostate cancer. There were no significant differences with regard to maximal tumor dimensions, final pathological stage, and deoxyribonucleic acid ploidy status that were found between the treatment group and the controls. However, the use of both a retrospective cohort, along with matched historical controls, injects selection bias that precludes any definitive conclusions regarding the incidence of downstaging and margin positivity from this study.

In two randomized controlled studies, Labrie et al.[59] and Van Poppel et al.[53] evaluated the effects of neoadjuvant ADT prior to radical prostatectomy in patients with both clinically organ confined and locally advanced prostate cancer. In the former study, evaluation of the 24 patients with clinical stage T3 prostate cancer revealed that 75% of patients had pathologically organ confined cancer following neoadjuvant therapy versus 16% in the control group. In addition, controls had a dramatically higher rate of upstaging to D1 disease (42% versus 16%) and a higher rate of positive surgical margins (67.5% versus 17.5%). VanPoppel et al.[53], however, found no benefit from pretreatment with estramustine phosphate followed by radical prostatectomy versus radical prostatectomy alone among the 56 T3 patients who were evaluated. The authors speculated that the relatively short, 6 week duration of ADT may not have been sufficient for an optimal effect in large, predominantly poorly differentiated T3 tumors. They also postulated that the inflammatory effects of estramustine phosphate may have been responsible for fibrosis and adhesions, making the achievement of negative surgical margins more difficult.

While many of the trials investigating neoadjuvant androgen deprivation in the setting of locally advanced (>T3) prostate cancer have demonstrated potentially promising results, particularly with regard to decreasing the percentage of positive surgical margins, longer follow up in these controlled trials will be required to determine whether the perceived pathological responses will translate into decreased rates of PSA failure, and ultimately into improved clinical outcomes. Cher et al.[54] have recently reported that 63% of men with specimen confined disease following neoadjuvant androgen ablation developed clinical or PSA recurrence within a mean follow up of 32.7 months. This contrasts with the more favorable results seen in our interim follow up of patients treated with neoadjuvant DES (above), and once again, there were no control groups incorporated in this study.

Neoadjuvant ADT in clinically organ confined prostate cancer (< clinical T2)

Table 16.1.3 summarizes the pathologic outcome of controlled trials that have addressed the question of whether androgen deprivation can decrease the rate of unsuspected capsular penetration in patients with clinically localized (T1,T2) disease. Labrie et al.[59] randomized 118 patients with clinically localized prostate cancer either to radical prostatectomy alone (n = 53) or radical prostatectomy following 3 months of leuprolide and flutamide (n = 65). The incidence of positive surgical margins in patients with clinical stage B1 and B2 disease decreased from 15% to 9% and 35% to 15% in the control and treatment arms, respectively.

In a non-randomized prospective, controlled study, Fair et al.[55] examined the effect of 3 months of combination therapy with goserelin acetate and flutamide on the

183

Table 16.1.3   Influence of neoadjuvant androgen deprivation therapy on rates of organ confined and margin positive disease in clinically localized (T1,T2) prostate cancer

Investigators	Patient no.	Organ confined		Margin positive	
		Control	Neoadjuvant	Control	Neoadjuvant
Labrie et al. (1993)[59]	118	–	–	15–35%	9–15%
Fair et al. (1993)[55]	141	48%	74%	33%	10%
Soloway et al. (1995)[60]	287	22%	53%	48%	18%
Van Poppel et al. (1995)[53]	73	68%	82%	–	–
Goldenberg et al. (1996)[50]	192	19.8%	41.6%	64.8%	27.7%

final pathologic outcome in 141 patients with clinically localized disease. Seventy-two patients received neoadjuvant therapy, of whom 74% had pathologically organ confined disease. This was compared with the 48% of 69 patients undergoing radical prostatectomy alone. With respect to surgical margins, 10% of the hormonally pretreated patients had positive surgical margins, compared with 33% in the control group. Finally, 4% of the treatment group had no residual carcinoma in the prostatectomy specimen, following ADT.

In a prospective randomized trial evaluating 287 patients, Soloway et al.[60] examined the effect of 3 months of ADT in patients with clinical T2 tumors and a serum PSA < 50 ng/ml. No significant differences between the two groups with respect to operating time, blood loss, or morbidity was noted. Patients who received neoadjuvant androgen deprivation therapy had a significantly lower rate of capsular penetration (47% versus 78%) and cancer positive surgical margins (18% versus 48%).

Van Poppel et al.[53] randomized 37 patients with clinically localized prostate cancer to radical prostatectomy alone. The remaining 36 patients received 6 weeks of estramustine phosphate (560 mg/ day). The rate of organ confined cancer in the treatment arm was 82.3% versus 67.6% in the controls. There were no significant differences with regard to operative time or blood loss between the two groups. At 9 months following surgery, 100% (12/12) of the estramustine treated patients had undetectable PSA levels, compared with 93% (13/14) in the control group.

Finally, Goldenberg et al.[50] have published their randomized controlled trial utilizing 12 weeks of pre-treatment with the progestational agent, cyproterone acetate. Organ confined cancer was found in 18 of 91 control patients (19.8%), compared with 42 of 101 patients (41.6%) randomized to receive ADT. One or more positive surgical margins was found in 59 of 91 control patients (64.8%) compared with 28 of 101 patients (27.7%) in the neoadjuvant treatment arm. There was no difference noted with respect to the incidence of intraoperative or perioperative complications in either the control group or the pre-treated patients. Operative parameters such as transfusion requirements and the degree of surgical difficulty were also comparable between the two arms.

The results of these studies indicate that in patients with clinically localized prostate cancer, neoadjuvant androgen deprivation therapy decreases the incidence of unsuspected extracapsular tumor extension and positive surgical margins compared to control patients undergoing surgery alone. Analysis of the existing data also raises the possibility that longer periods of ADT may be more effective than the 1–3 months of treatment used in most studies. Solomon et al.[56] observed that three of eight patients receiving 3 months of ADT had positive surgical margins, compared with only one of six patients in a group of patients pre-treated for 6 months. Gleave et al. (61) demonstrated that neoadjuvant therapy administered for 8 months could increase the percentage of those patients achieving undetectable levels, which ultimately translated into improvement in pathological outcome in these patients. This latter study suggests that with a longer period of pre-treatment, perhaps to a PSA nadir, further benefit can be derived from ADT with regard to both increasing the rate of organ confined tumors, and decreasing the incidence of cancer-positive surgical margins.

Ongoing investigations to address the optimal pre-treatment duration of ADT are currently underway. We have recently evaluated the influence of neoadjuvant ADT on the incidence of circulating cancer cells in patients with prostate cancer. Using the highly sensitive, reverse transcriptase-polymerase chain reaction assay (RT-PCR) with prostate specific membrane antigen (PSM) primers, there was a decrease in the incidence of circulating tumor cells in patients pre-treated with an LHRH agonist and flutamide (17%) versus controls (38%). The significance of this effect is at the present time unknown. Correlation of this data with final pathological outcome, as well as the rate of clinical and biochemical failure in these patients, is currently being investigated.

Conclusions

The available data indicate that in the setting of locally advanced (>T3) prostate cancer, neoadjuvant androgen deprivation therapy prior to radical prostatectomy may result in a modest improvement in the rate of pathologically organ confined tumors with a more profound decrease in the rate of cancer-positive surgical margins. Randomized controlled studies need to investigate whether these effects are real, or a result of staging inaccuracies. Interim follow up of high risk, locally advanced (T2b/c,T3) patients in our pilot study, utilizing neoadjuvant DES, demonstrates that patients with organ confined disease following neoadjuvant ADT do as well as patients with clinically localized prostate cancer from other series, who have organ confined disease after surgery alone. Furthermore, these patients demonstrate lower rates of PSA failure than patients treated with external beam radiotherapy. The lack of control groups in these investigations, however, preclude any definitive statements defining the role of neoadjuvant ADT in the setting of locally advanced prostate cancer at the present time.

In patients with clinically localized prostate cancer, several randomized prospective series have demonstrated that there is a potential for neoadjuvant therapy to reduce the rate of unsuspected extracapsular disease, and improve the rate of specimen confined tumors. Whether this translates into decreased rates of biochemical failure, clinical progression, and survival will require longer follow up.

References

1. Walsh PC, Partin AW, Epstein JI. Cancer control and quality of life following anatomical radical retropubic prostatectomy: results at 10 years. *J Urol* 1994;**152**:1831–1836.
2. Rosen MA, Goldstone L, Lapin S, Wheeler T, Scardino PT. Frequency and location of extracapsular extension and positive surgical margins in radical prostatectomy specimens. *J Urol* 1992;**148**:331–337.
3. Zincke H, Oesterling JE, Blute ML, Bergstralh EJ, Myers RP, Barrett DM. Long-term (15 years) results after radical prostatectomy for clinically localized (stage T2c or lower) prostate cancer. *J Urol* 1994;**152**:1850–1857.
4. Murphy GP, Mettin C, Mek H, Winchester DP, Davidson AM. National patterns of prostate cancer treatment by radical prostatectomy: results of a survey by the American College of Surgeons Commission on Cancer. *J Urol* 1994;**152**:1817–1819.
5. Bostwick DG, Myers RP, Oesterling JE. Staging of prostate cancer. *Sem Surg Oncol* 1994;**10**:60–72.
6. Paulson DF. Impact of radical prostatectomy in the management of clinically localized disease: *J Urol* 1994;**152**:1826–1830.
7. Humphrey PA, Keetch DW, Smith DS, Shepherd DL, Catalona WJ. Prospective characterization of pathological features of prostate carcinomas detected via serum prostate specific antigen based screening. *J Urol* 1996;**155**:816–820.
8. Epstein JI, Walsh PC, Brendler CB. Radical prostatectomy for impalpable prostate cancer: the Johns Hopkins experience with tumors found on transurethral resection (stages T1a and T1b) and on needle biopsy (stage T1c). *J Urol* 1994;**152**:1721–1729.
9. Lerner SE, Seay TM, Blute ML, Bergstralh EJ, Barrett D, Zincke H. Prostate specific antigen detected prostate cancer (clinical stage T1c): an interim analysis. *J Urol* 1996;**155**:821–826.
10. Cookson MS, Fleshner N, Fair WR. Personal data, 1996.
11. Stein A, DeKernion JB, Smith RB, Dorey F, Patel H. Prostate specific antigen levels after radical prostatectomy in patients with organ confined and locally advanced prostate cancer. *J Urol* 1992;**147**:942–946.
12. Morton RM, Steiner PL, Walsh PC. Cancer control following anatomical radical prostatectomy: an interim report. *J Urol* 1991;**145**:1197–1200.
13. Frazier HA, Robertson JE, Humphrey PA, Paulson DF. Is prostate specific antigen of clinical importance in evaluating outcome after radical prostatectomy? *J Urol* 1993;**149**:516–518.
14. Paulson DF, Moul JW, Walther PJ. Radical prostatectomy for clinical stage T1-2N0M0 prostatic adenocarcinoma: long-term results. *J Urol* 1990;**144**:1180–1184.
15. Armas OA, Aprikian AG, Melamed J, Cordon-Cardo C, Cohen DW, Erlandson R, Fair WR, Reuter VE. Clinical and pathobiological effects of neoadjuvant total androgen ablation therapy on clinically localized prostatic adenocarcinoma. *Am J Surg Pathol* 1994;**18**:979–991.
16. Kyprianou N, English HF, Isaacs JT. Programmed cell death during regression of PC-82 human prostate cancer following androgen ablation. *Cancer Res* 1990;**50**:3748–3753.
17. Pinault S, Tetu B, Gagnon J, Monfette G, Dupont A, Labrie F. Transrectal ultrasound evaluation of local prostate cancer in patients treated with LHRH agonist in combination with flutamide. *Urology* 1992;**39**:254–261.
18. Tetu B, Srigley JR, Boivin JC *et al.* Effect of combination endocrine therapy (LHRH agonist and flutamide) on normal prostate and prostatic adenocarcinoma: a histopathologic and immunohistochemical study. *Am J Surg Pathol* 1991;**15**:111–120.
19. Labrie F. Endocrine therapy of prostate cancer. *Endocinol Metab Clin N Am* 1991;**20**:845.
20. Fair WR, Aprikian A, Sogani P, Reuter VE, Whitmore WF. The role of neoadjuvant hormonal manipulation in localized prostate cancer. *Cancer* (suppl) 1993;**71**:1031–1038.
21. Monfette G, Dupont A, Labrie F. Temporary combination therapy with flutamide and tryptex as adjuvant to radical prostatectomy for the treatment of early stage prostate cancer. In: Labrie F, Dupont A (eds) *Early stage prostate cancer: diagnosis and choice of therapy*. Excerpta Medica, New York, 1989, pp. 41–51.
22. Isaacs JT, Coffey DS. Adaptation versus selection as the mechanism responsible for the relapse of prostate cancer to androgen ablation therapy as studied in the Dunning R-3327-H adenocarcinoma. *Cancer Res* 1981;**41**:5070–5075.
23. Bruchovsky N, Rennie PS, Coldman AJ, Goldenberg SL, To M, Lawson D. Effects of androgen withdrawal on the stem cell composition of the Shionogi carcinoma. *Cancer Res* 1990;**50**:2275–2282.
24. van den Ouden D, Davidson PJT, Hop W, Schroder FH. Radical prostatectomy as a monotherapy for locally advanced (stage T3) prostate cancer. *J Urol* 1994;**151**:646–651.
25. Greskovich FJ III, Johnson DE, Tenney DM, Stephenson RA. Prostate specific antigen in patients with clinical stage C prostate cancer: relationship to lymph node status and grade. *J Urol* 1991;**145**:798–801.
26. Boxer RJ, Kaufman JJ, Goodwin WE. Radical prostatectomy for carcinoma of the prostate (1951–1976): a review of 329 cases. *J Urol* 1977;**117**:208–213.
27. Tomlinson RL, Currie DP, Boyce WH. Radical prostatectomy: palliation for stage C carcinoma of the prostate. *J Urol* 1977;**117**:85–87.
28. Lerner SE, Blute ML, Zincke H. Extended experience with radical prostatectomy for clinical stage T3 prostate cancer: outcome and contemporary morbidity. *J Urol* 1995;**154**:1447–1452.
29. Bagshaw MA, Cox RS, Ray GR. Status of radiation treatment of prostate cancer at Stanford University. *Natl Cancer Inst Monogr* 1988;**7**:47–60.
30. Kabalin JN, Hodge KK, McNeal JE, Freiha FS, Stamey TA. Identification of residual cancer in the prostate following radiation therapy: role of transrectal ultrasound-guided biopsy and prostate specific antigen. *J Urol* 1989;**142**:326–331.

31. Hanks GE, Diamond JJ, Krall JM. A ten year followup of 682 patients treated for prostate cancer with radiation therapy in the United States. *Int J Rad Oncol Biol Phys* 1987;**13**:499–504.

32. Zagars GK, vonEschenbach AC, Johnson DE, Oswald MJ. Stage C adenocarcinoma of the prostate: an analysis of 551 patients treated with external beam radiation. *Cancer* 1987;**60**:1489–1499.

33. Whitmore WF Jr, Hilaris B, Sogani P, Herr H, Batata M, Fair WR. Interstitial irradiation using I-125 seeds. *Prog Clin Biol Res* 1987;**243**B:177–195.

34. Kuban DA, El-Mahdi AM, Schellhammer PF.[125] I interstitial implantation for prostate cancer: what have we learned 10 years later? *Cancer* 1989;**63**:2415–2420.

35. Vallett BS. Radical perineal prostatectomy subsequent to bilateral orchiectomy. *Del Med J* 1944;**16**:19–23.

36. Parlow AL. Advanced cancer of the prostate: a consideration of the value of radical prostatectomy in selected cases. *NY J Med* 1945;**45**:383–387.

37. Colston JA, Brendler H. Endocrine therapy in carcinoma of the prostate: preparation of patients for radical perineal prostatectomy. *JAMA* 1947;**134**:848–853.

38. Parlow AL, Scott WW. Hormone control therapy as a preparation for radical perineal prostatectomy in advanced carcinoma of the prostate. *NY J Med* 1949;**49**:629–634.

39. Guttierez R. New horizons in the surgical management of carcinoma of the prostate. *Am J Surg* 1949;**78**:147–169.

40. Scott WW. An evaluation of endocrine therapy plus radical perineal prostatectomy in the treatment of advanced carcinoma of the prostate. *J Urol* 1964;**91**:97–102.

41. Scott WW, Boyd HL. Combined hormone control therapy and radical prostatectomy in the treatment of selected cases of advanced carcinoma of the prostate: a retrospective study based upon 25 years of experience. *J Urol* 1969;**101**:86–92.

42. Aprikian AG, Fair WR, Reuter VE, Sogani P, Herr H, Russo P, Sheinfeld J. Experience with neoadjuvant diethylstilboestrol and radical prostatectomy in patients with locally advanced prostate cancer. *Br J Urol* 1994;**74**:630–636.

43. Kava BR, Fair WR: (unpublished data).

44. Partin AW, Piantadosi S, Sanda M, Epstein JI, Marshall FF, Mohler JL, Brendler CB *et al.* Selection of men at high risk for disease recurrence for experimental adjuvant therapy following radical prostatectomy. *Urology* 1995;**45**(5):831–838.

45. Pilepich MV, Krall JM, Al-Sarraf M *et al.* Androgen deprivation with radiation therapy compared with radiation therapy alone for locally advanced prostatic carcinoma: a randomized comparative trial of the radiation therapy oncology group. *Urology* 1995;**45**(4):616–623.

46. Andros EA, Danesghari F, Crawford ED. Neoadjuvant hormonal therapy in stage C adenocarcinoma of the prostate. *Clin Invest Med* 1993;**16**(6):510–515.

47. MacFarlane M, Abi-Aad A, Stein A, Danella J, Belldegrun A, DeKernion JB. Neoadjuvant hormonal deprivation in patients with locally advanced prostate cancer. *J Urol* 1993;**150**:132–134.

48. Soloway MS, Hachiya T, Civantos F, Murphy WM, Gomez CC, Ruiz HE. Androgen deprivation prior to radical prostatectomy for T2b and T3 prostate cancer. *Urology* (suppl) 1994;**43**(2):52–56.

49. Schulman CC, Sassine AM. Neoadjuvant hormonal deprivation before radical prostatectomy. *Clin Invest Med* 1993;**16**(6):523–531.

50. Goldenberg SL, Klotz LH, Srigley J *et al.* Randomized, prospective, controlled study comparing radical prostatectomy alone and neoadjuvant androgen withdrawal in the treatment of localized prostate cancer. *J Urol* 1996;**156**:873–877.

51. Kennedy TJ, Sonneland AM, Marlett M, Troup R. Lutenizing hormone-releasing hormone downstaging of clinical stage C prostate cancer. *J Urol* 1992;**147**:891–893.

52. Oesterling JE, Andrews PE, Suman VJ, Zincke H, Myers RP. Preoperative androgen deprivation therapy: artificial lowering of serum prostate specific antigen without downstaging the tumor. *J Urol* 1993;**149**:779–782.

53. van Poppel H, Ridder DD, Elgamal AA, van de Voorde W, Werbrouck P, Ackaert K, Oyen R, Pittomvils G, Baert L. Neoadjuvant hormonal therapy

54. Cher ML, Shinohara K, Breslin S, Vapnek J, Carroll PR. High failure rate associated with long-term follow-up of neoadjuvant androgen deprivation followed by radical prostatectomy for stage C prostate cancer. *Br J Urol* 1995;**75**:771–777.

55. Fair WR, Aprikian AG, Cohen DW, Sogani P, Reuter VE. Use of neoadjuvant androgen deprivation therapy in clinically localized prostate cancer. *Clin Invest Med* 1993;**16**:516–522.

56. Solomon MH, McHugh TA, Dorr RP, Lee F, Siders DB. Hormone ablation therapy as neoadjuvant treatment to radical prostatectomy. *Clin Inv Med* 1993;**16**(6):532–538.

57. Gomella LG, Liberman SN, Mulholland SG, Petersen RO, Hyslop T, Corn BW. Induction androgen deprivation plus prostatectomy for stage T3 disease: failure to achieve prostate-specific antigen-based freedom from disease status in a phase II trial. *Urology* 1996;**47**(6):870–876.

58. Bosch RJLH, Kurth KH, Schroeder FH. Surgical treatment of locally advanced (T3) prostatic carcinoma: early results. *J Urol* 1987;**138**:816–821.

59. Labrie F, Dupont A, Cusan L, Gomez J, Diamond P, Koutsilieris M, Suburu R *et al.* Downstaging of localized prostate cancer by neoadjuvant therapy with flutamide and lupron: the first controlled and randomized trial. *Clin Invest Med* 1993;**16**(6):499–509.

60. Soloway MS, Roohollah S, Wajsman Z, McLeod D, Wood DP, Puras-Baez A. Randomized prospective study comparing radical prostatectomy alone versus radical prostatectomy preceded by androgen blockade in clinical stage B2 (T2bNxMO) prostate cancer. *J Urol* 1995;**154**:424–428.

61. Gleave ME, Goldenberg SL, Jones EC, Bruchovsky N, Sullivan LD. Biochemical and pathological effects of 8 months of neoadjuvant androgen withdrawal therapy before radical prostatectomy in patients with clinically confined prostate cancer. *J Urol* 1996;**155**:213–219.

before radical prostatectomy decreases the number of positive surgical margins in stage T2 prostate cancer: interim results of a prospective randomized trial. *J Urol* 1995;**154**:429–434.

16.2   Surgery: Is there a rationale?

D van den Ouden and F H Schröder

Staging

Over/understaging

Locally advanced disease (clinical stage T3 or C) is present in 12 to 40% of all newly diagnosed prostate cancer patients[1–3]. Despite the development of new techniques (MRI, PSA) and the improvement of existing techniques (TRUS, CT-scanning), it remains difficult to differentiate between locally confined and locally advanced disease. This is reflected not only in the understaging of T2 disease, which in 43–75% turns out to be histological pT3 disease[4–6], but also in the overstaging of T3 disease, which varies from 17–30%[7–9] This means that in 17–30% of the clinical T3 patients, the disease is locally confined, and that they are candidates for radical surgery according to generally accepted standards. This treatment may be denied because of staging errors. Understaging in clinical T3 disease occurs in 4%[8], which is pathologically pT4. These patients will suffer local recurrence and disease progression, despite surgery, and are therefore not candidates for radical prostatectomy. In cases of doubt, T4 can be diagnosed performing a cystoscopy and bimanual examination under anesthesia.

Lymph node metastases in clinical T3 carcinoma

Lymph node metastases (LNM) are frequently found in patients with clinical T3 carcinoma of the prostate; percentages of 33–56% are reported[7,8,10,12]. Once the pelvic lymph nodes are involved, the disease is no longer localized but systemic, and local radical therapy can not control the disease[13].

CT-scanning is of limited value in detecting LNM: Bosch described a sensitivity of only 35% for the detection of LNM, a positive predictive value (PPV) of 75% and a negative predictive value (NPV) of 59%[12]. MRI performs even worse, with a sensitivity for detecting LNM of 25%[14]. Wolf states that the probability of LNM should be 45% to make imaging beneficial. Partin developed nomograms which indicate a 50% risk for LNM when the Gleason score is 8–10 and the PSA is over 25 ng/ml[15]. Bluestein found LNM in 43% of patients with a PSA over 20 ng/ml and a primary Gleason grade 4 or 5[16]. If any doubt exists about the presence of LNM, a staging laparoscopic lymph node dissection should be performed, or frozen sections of the lymph node must be investigated intra-operatively prior to the radical prostatectomy.

Influence of high-grade disease on prognosis in T3 carcinoma

High-grade disease (poorly differentiated carcinoma) is associated with high mortality due to prostate cancer (10 times higher than well or moderately differentiated carcinoma), and a high morbidity due to a high metastatic rate. (74% at 10 years post-diagnosis even in locally confined disease in conservatively managed prostatic carcinoma)[17]. Therefore effective therapy is urgently needed for this group of biologically aggressive carcinomas. This aggressiveness is expressed in a high percentage of T3 disease (55–92%),[18,19] and a high percentage of aneuploidy, measured by DNA flow cytometry[26]. Nativ showed, however, that ploidy had no significant influence on progression once the tumor is poorly differentiated[21].

Ohori found progression in 0% of the organ confined and in 80% of the non-organ confined tumors with Gleason sum >8[18]. Partin showed that 24% of the specimen confined tumors with Gleason >8 progressed after 3 years, compared with 82% of the non-specimen confined tumors[19]. Both concluded that radical prostatectomy for high-grade disease is to be limited to locally confined tumors.

Van den Ouden reported on a group of 100 patients with clinical T3 carcinoma, which contained 15 patients with T3pT3G3 carcinomas, treated by radical prostatectomy without adjuvant therapy. Of these patients 14 (93%) progressed within 2 years post-surgery[8], whereas patients with T3pT3G1 and 2 had similar progression rates as T2 disease.

Lerner performed radical prostatectomy in 501 patients with T3 Gleason >7: 48% of the patients received adjuvant hormonal therapy. The actuarial cause specific survival rate at 5, 10 and 15 years was ± 80%, ± 70% and ± 50%[7], which may indicate a good response on the administration of adjuvant therapy in this high-risk group, despite the general known fact that adjuvant hormonal therapy does not influence survival.

In conclusion, patients with high-grade tumors and stage T3 are not good candidates for radical prostatectomy. If radical prostatectomy is performed in selected cases (for example in young patients) for T3G3 carcinoma, adjuvant therapy is desirable.

Results of radical surgery in clinically locally advanced disease (Stage T3/C)

Overall survival

Table 16.2.1 shows the results for overall survival and cancer-specific survival for patients with clinically advanced (stage T3/C) prostate cancer, treated by radical prostatectomy. There are many more reports in the literature concerning pathological stage T3/C, but this classification is only known after radical prostatectomy, when the major treatment decision has already been made; therefore these reports are not listed here.

Overall survival depends, besides tumor control, on age (for all series the median age is about 65 years) and general health. This can make comparison to other treatments difficult, because patients fit to undergo radical surgery are generally in a better condition than their age-matched controls, who are treated with radiotherapy or conservative (hormonal) treatment. Overall survival ranged from 64–95% at 5 years, from 12.5–72% at 10 years and from 20–51% at 15 years post-treatment. These differences can be explained by the difference in time (Jewett, 1958 vs Lerner, 1995)[7,22]; nowadays better post-operative care and better techniques of surgery are available. Many studies from early data do not evaluate LNM, since the prostatectomy is performed perineally. Therefore many patients with LNM may have early progression and death. Cancer-specific survival is not reported in most studies before

1980. Zincke[23] reported 5 and 10 years survival of 80 and 65%; this was not significantly different from the survival in a group of men of the same age in the general population. This finding indicates excellent chances for patients with T3 carcinoma treated by radical prostatectomy. However these patients represent a selection of otherwise very healthy persons, because they are fit to undergo major surgery. Furthermore, many underwent hormonal therapy which has impact on short- and long-term results.

Cancer-specific survival (CSS)

CSS is the best parameter to evaluate the results of treatment for prostate cancer for survival, since intercurrent death by other diseases are excluded and the parameter relates more to the disease under study. CSS at 5, 10 and 15 years post-treatment ranges from 85–92%, 79–82%, and 68–70% respectively. These ranges are remarkably narrow, considering the fact that a 25 years time difference lies between the first[24] and the last report[7]. Unfortunately this means also that little progress is made in the treatment of T3 carcinoma. Most studies administer either hormonal or adjuvant radiation treatment to a part of their patient populations. This, however, does not affect survival significantly[7].

Clinical progression

Clinical progression, local recurrence and biochemical progression are listed in Table 16.2.2. Clinical progression means (biopsy proven) local recurrence, and/or the occur-rence of distant metastasis as detected by bone scans, ultra sonography or CT-scans. Biochemical progression mean a rise in PSA over a certain value; this value differ between the different reported series.

The clinical progression rates vary from 12–45% at 5 years, 39–49% at 10 years and 50–71% at 15 years post treatment. The progression rates for patients who did no have adjuvant treatment[8,11] were not very different from those who did[23–25]. The other studies contain too few patients to be reliable in this matter. This is surprising since adjuvant hormonal therapy is known to prolong the interval to progression[7,26]; this effect does not seem to las longer than 5 years.

Local recurrence

Local recurrence is expected when there is residual disease because of a positive margin of resection. The limited amount of peri-prostatic tissue and the presence of extra capsular extension (ECE) leads to a higher percentage o positive margins with increasing stage[27]. In T3 disease 47–81% have positive surgical margins[27,28]. Many surgeons hesitate therefore to save the neurovascular bundles in T3 disease. Partin showed positive margins after radical prostatectomy for ECE positive disease in 55% when the bundle was saved, versus 42% when it was sacrificed. Margin positive patients had a decreased time to disease recurrence (not significant), but after 3 years both groups showed biochemical progression in 70%. This may be due to occult metastasis in ECE patients at the time of surgery.

Table 16.2.1   Overall survival and cancer-specific survival for patients with clinically diagnosed T3 or stage C prostate cancer

Reference	N	Therapy	Adjuvant therapy	Overall survival (%)			Cancer specific survival (%)		
				5	10 (years)	15	5	10 (years)	15
Jewett[22]	48	RP	–	–	12.5	–	–	–	–
Scott[24]	39	RP	HT (all)	74	61	29	83	79	68
Flocks[33]	69	RP	A 198	74	67	28	–	–	–
Tomlinson[34]	24	RP	HT (33%)	82	–	–	–	–	–
Schröder[35]	213	RP + PLND	HT (50%)	64	36	20	–	–	70*
Zincke[23]	49	RP + PLND	HT\RT(39%)	65	–	–	–	–	–
von Flamm[36]	20	RP	HT (90%)	46	–	–	–	–	–
Morgan[25]	232	RP + PLND	HT (54%)	84	72	–	89	82	–
Yamada[37]	25	RP + PLND	RT/HT	84	–	–	92	–	–
van den Ouden[27]	59	RP + PLND	–	83	–	–	90	–	–
Lerner[7]	812	RP + PLND	HT/RT (60%)	86	70	51	90	80	69

* During the observation period.
RP = radical prostatectomy.
PLND = pelvic lymph node dissection.
HT = Hormonal therapy.
RT = radiation therapy.
Au 198 = interstitial radioactive gold seeds implantation.
– = not reported.

Table 16.2.2   Clinical progression, local recurrence and biochemical progression in patients with clinically diagnosed T3 or stage C prostate cancer

Reference	N	Clinical progression (%)			Local recurrence (%)			Biochemical progression (%)	
		5	10	15	5	10	15	5	10
Scott[27]	39	38	49	71	–	–	–	–	–
Flocks[25]	69	–	–	–	–	–	4	–	–
Tomlinson[34]	24	–	–	–	9	–	–	–	–
Schröder[35]	213	–	–	–	–	–	13*	–	–
Zincke[23]	49	45	–	–	18	–	–	–	–
Morgan[25]	232	31	44	–	10	18	–	49	62
Yamada[37]	25	12	–	–	–	–	–	48	–
van den Ouden[27]	59	36	–	–	–	–	–	63	–
Lerner[7]	812	–	39	50	–	20	29	42	59
Olsson[38]	7	14	–	–	–	–	–	–	–
Bosch[39]	15	36	–	–	–	–	–	–	–

* During the observation period.
– = not reported.

and suggests that fate is not determined by the margins but by the extent of the tumor[29]. Epstein investigated secondary resection of the bundle (during the same operation) after initially saving it in patients in whom a positive margin was expected. In 40% no tumor was found in the resected bundle[30]. This indicates the inefficiency of decision-making intra-operatively. Despite the high percentage of positive margins, the local recurrence rate is low indicating that radical prostatectomy for T3 disease leads to an excellent local control (Table 16.2.2).

Biochemical progression

Data on biochemical progression are only available in four studies in this review. These were published after 1986, when PSA became available for routine use. As can be seen in Table 16.3.2 there are but little differences between the progression rates for the different groups, with the exception of the group who received no adjuvant therapy, which showed a 5 year progression of 63%. All other groups administered hormonal and/or radiation adjuvant therapy in a considerable percentage of their patients (54–100%). The biochemical progression rates are higher than the clinical progression rates in all groups. The knowledge that biochemical progression proceeds clinical progression by 3–5 years[31], and that all biochemical progressed patients will suffer clinical progression, reveals a gloomy scenario for these patients.

Complications

The mortality rate of surgery in T3 disease is 0.4–1.5%[7,32]. The overall complication rate is 43%[32]. Stenosis of the anastomosis requiring dilatation was present in 9–32%; incontinence in 14–23%, and impotence in 69%[7,32]. Davidson compared the complication rates of clinical stage T3 and T <3, and found no significant differences.

Conclusions

Radical prostatectomy for locally advanced (clinical stage T3 or C) disease is possible with acceptable mortality and morbidity, and is especially beneficial in patients who are downstaged to pT2 (17–30%) and in those with well or moderately differentiated disease. Surgery for poorly differentiated disease seems only advisable in combination with adjuvant treatment. Patients with lymph node metastasis should not undergo radical prostatectomy, but should be treated for systemic disease.

References

1. Murphy GP, Natarayan N, Pontes JE, Schmitz RL, Smart CR, Schmidt JD, Mettlin C. The national survey of prostate cancer in the United States by the American College of Surgeons. J Urol 1982;**17**:928.
2. Stamey TA, McNeal JE. Adenocarcinoma of the prostate. In: *Campbells urology* (6th edn), Philadelphia, WB Saunders, 1992, vol.2, ch. 29, pp. 1159–1221.
3. Whitmore WF. The natural history of prostatic cancer. Cancer 1973;**32**:1104.
4. Catalona WJ, Bigg SW. Nerve sparing radical prostatectomy: evaluation of results after 250 patients. J Urol 1990;**143**:538–544.
5. Elder JC, Jewett HJ, Walsh PC. Radical perineal prostatectomy for clinical stage B2 carcinoma of the prostate. J Urol 1982;**127**:704–706.
6. Hering F, Rist M, Roth J, Mihatsch M, Rütishauser G. Does microinvasion of the capsule and/or micro metastases in regional lymph nodes influence disease-free survival after radical prostatectomy? Br J Urol 1990;**66**: 177–181.

189

7. Lerner SE, Blute ML, Zincke H. Extended experience with radical prostatectomy for clinical stage T3 prostate cancer: outcome and contemporary morbidity. *J Urol* 1995;**154**:1447–1452.

8. van den Ouden D, Davidson PJT, Hop W, Schröder FH. Radical prostatectomy as a monotherapy for locally advanced (stage T3) prostate cancer. *J Urol* 1994;**151**:646–651.

9. Rannikko S, Salo JO. Radical prostatectomy as treatment of localized prostatic cancer. *Scand J Urol Nephrol* 1990;**24**:103–107.

10. Hanks G, Krall JM, Pilepich MV, Asbell SO, Perez CA, Rubin P. Comparison of pathologic and clinical evaluation of lymph nodes in prostate cancer: implications of RTOG data for patient management and trial design and stratification. *Int J Rad Oncol Biol Phys* 1992;**23**:293–298.

11. Andriole GL, Coplen DE, Mikkelsen DJ, Catalona WJ. Sonografic and pathological staging of patients with clinically localized prostate cancer. *J Urol* 1989;**142**:1259–1261.

12. Bosch RJLH, Schröder FH. Current problems in staging and grading prostatic carcinoma with special reference to T3 carcinoma of the prostate. *World J Urol* 1986;**4**:141–146.

13. Gervasi LA, Mata J, Easley JD, Wilbanks JH, Seale-Hawkins C, Carlton CE, Scardino PT. Prognostic significance of lymph nodal metastases in prostate cancer. *J Urol* 1989;**142**:332–336.

14. Wolf JS, Cher M, Dall'era M, Presti JC, Hricak H, Caroll PR. The use and accuracy of cross-sectional imaging and fine needle aspiration cytology for detection of pelvic lymph node metastases before radical prostatectomy. *J Urol* 1995;**153**:993–999.

15. Partin AW, Yoo J, Carter HB, Pearson JD, Chan DW, Epstein JI, Walsh PC. The use of prostate specific antigen, clinical stage and Gleason score to predict pathological stage in men with localized prostate cancer. *J Urol* 1993;**150**:110.

16. Bluestein DL, Bostwick DG, Bergstrahl EJ, Oesterling JE. Eliminating the need for bilateral pelvic lymphadenectomy in select patients with prostate cancer. *J Urol* 1994;**151**:1315.

17. Chodak GW, Thisted RA, Gerber GS, Johansson JE, Adolfsson J, Jones GW, Chisholm GD, Moskovitz CBEB, Livne PM, Warner J. Results of conservative management of clinically localized prostate cancer. *N Engl J Med* 1994;**330**:242–248.

18. Ohori M, Goad JR, Wheeler TM, Eastham JA, Thompson TC, Scardino PT. Can radical prostatectomy alter the progression of poorly differentiated prostate cancer? *J Urol* 1994;**152**:1843–1849.

19. Partin AW, Lee BR, Carmichael M, Walsh PC, Epstein JI. Radical prostatectomy for high grade disease: A reevaluation 1994. *J Urol* 1994;**151**:1583–1586.

20. Rönström L, Tribukait B, Esposti P. DNA pattern and cytological findings in fine-needle aspirates of untreated prostatic tumors. A flow-cytofluorometric study. *The Prostate*, 1980;**2**:79–88.

21. Nativ O, Winkler HZ, Raz Y, Therneau TM, Farrow GM, Myers RP, Zincke H, Lieber MM. Stage C prostatic adenocarcinoma. Flow cytometric nuclear DNA ploidy analysis. *Mayo Clin Proc* 1989;**64**:911–919.

22. Jewett HJ. Significance of the palpable prostatic nodule. *Bull NY Acad Med* 1958;**34**:26.

23. Zincke H, Utz DC, Taylor WF. Bilateral pelvic lymphadenectomy and radical prostatectomy for clinical stage C prostatic cancer: role of adjuvant treatment for residual cancer and in disease progression. *J Urol* 1986;**135**:1199–1205.

24. Scott WW, Boyd HL. Combined hormone control, therapy and radical prostatectomy in the treatment of selected cases of advanced carcinoma of the prostate: a retrospective study based upon 25 years of experience. *J Urol* 1969;**101**:86–92.

25. Morgan WR, Bergstralh EJ, Zincke H. Long-term evaluation of radical prostatectomy as treatment for clinical stage C (T3) prostate cancer. *Urology* 1993;**41**:113–120.

26. Veterans Administration Cooperative Urological Research Group. Estrogen treatment for cancer of the prostate: early results with three doses of diethylstilboestrol and placebo. *Cancer* 1970;**26**:257–261.

27. van den Ouden D, Bentvelsen FM, Boevé ER, Schröder FH. Positive margins after radical prostatectomy: correlation with local recurrence and distant progression. *Br J Urol* 1993;**72**:489–494.

28. Zietman AL, Edelstein RA, Coen JJ, Babayan RK, Krane RJ. Radical prostatectomy for adenocarcinoma of the prostate: The influence of preoperative and pathologic findings on biochemical disease free outcome. *Urology* 1994;**43**:828–833.

29. Partin AW, Borland RN, Epstein JE, Brendler CB. Influence of wide excision of the neurovascular bundle(s) on prognosis in men with clinically localized prostate cancer with established capsular penetration. *J Urol* 1993;**150**:142–148.

30. Epstein JE. Evaluation of radical prostatectomy capsular margins of resection: the significance of margins designated as negative, closely approaching and positive. *Am J Surg Pathol* 1990;**14**:626–632.

31. Paulson DF. Impact of radical prostatectomy in the management of clinically localized disease. *J Urol* 1994;**152**:1826–1830.

32. Davidson PJT, van den Ouden D, Schröder FH. Radical prostatectomy: prospective assessment of mortality and morbidity. *Eur Urol* 1996;**29**:168–173.

33. Flocks RH. The treatment of stage C prostatic cancer with special reference to combined surgical and radiation therapy. *J Urol* 1973;**109**:461–463.

34. Tomlinson RL, Currie DP, Boyce WH. Radical prostatectomy: Palliation for stage C carcinoma of the prostate. *J Urol* 1977;**117**:85–87.

35. Schröder FH, Belt E. Carcinoma of the prostate: a study of 213 patients with stage C tumors treated by total perineal prostatectomy. *J Urol* 1975;**114**:257–260.

36. von Flamm J, Kiesswetter H. Die radicale prostatektomie beim prostatakarzinom stadium C. *Z Urol Nephrol* 1987;**80**:185.

37. Yamada AH, Lieskovsky G, Petrovich Z, Chen S, Groshen S, Skinner DG. Results of radical prostatectomy and adjuvant therapy in the management of locally advanced clinical stage TC, prostate cancer. *Am J Clin Oncol* 1994;**17**:277–285.

38. Olsson CA, Babayan R, DeVere White R. Surgical management of stage B or C prostatic carcinoma: Radical surgery vs radiotherapy. *Urology* 1985;**25**:30–35.

39. Bosch RJLH, Kurth KH, Schröder FH. Surgical treatment of locally advanced (T3) prostatic carcinoma: Early results. *J Urol* 1987;**138**:816–822.

16.3   Radiation therapy

C A Perez

Optimal treatment for patients with localized carcinoma of the prostate is controversial. Radiation therapy is an established modality in the management of these patients and is the preferred treatment in patients with locally advanced tumors, frequently in combination with hormonal therapy.[1,2] Recently efficacy of therapy for carcinoma of the prostate is being evaluated in light of post-treatment prostate-specific antigen (PSA) determinations.[3–7] Effectiveness of any therapy in localized carcinoma of the prostate is always scrutinized against the background of what many describe as a fairly indolent clinical course of the disease. Whitmore[8] pointed out that the end results of treatment in these patients may be a combined consequence of host factors, tumor natural history and behavior, and therapy efficacy. Watchful waiting (expectant treatment) issues are discussed in Chapter 15.2.

Definitive external-beam irradiation

In most institutions external-beam irradiation is used as definitive therapy in the majority of patients with stage C or more locally extensive tumors. Tumor doses have ranged from 66 to 72 Gy for stage T3 (C) and T4 tumors.

Several retrospective studies indicate that dose has a strong impact on local tumor control; Perez et al.[9,10] noted improved local tumor control with doses greater than 65 Gy and, in patients with stage C tumors, Hanks et al.[11] reported 5 year local recurrence rates of 36% with doses below 64.9 Gy, 29% for 65 to 69.9 Gy, and 19% for those receiving 70 Gy or more.

The impact of elective pelvic lymph node irradiation on survival is controversial. McGowan[12] reported better survival and fewer pelvic failures in patients with stage B2 or C tumors treated with larger fields encompassing the pelvic lymph nodes compared with patients with treatment to the prostate and periprostatic tissues only. Ploysongsang et al.[13] described, in patients treated to the prostate and whole pelvis, a 5 year survival rate of 72% in stage C patients compared with 40% in patients irradiated to the prostatic area only. In 434 patients receiving definitive irradiation at our institution, for clinical stage C, the pelvic tumor control rate was 72% when the pelvic lymph nodes were treated with 50 Gy or higher dose in contrast to 60% with lower doses (P <0.01) (Figure 16.3.1); however, no correlation between irradiated volume and survival was demonstrated[14].

The importance of adequate radiation therapy techniques to achieve optimal tumor control in the pelvis has been emphasized[1]. Furthermore, a lower incidence of distant metastases and improved survival have been reported by Kaplan et al.[15] and Perez et al.[9] in patients with locoregional tumor control compared with patients developing pelvic failure in patients treated with external-beam irradiation (Figure 16.3.2) and by Kuban et al.[16,17] in patients treated with either external-beam or interstitial irradiation.

Results of treatment with external-beam irradiation

Survival

In 963 patients treated with definitive irradiation for localized carcinoma of the prostate at our institution between January 1967 and December 1992, 10 year disease-free survival rates were similar to those of other published series (Figure 16.3.3). In 434 patients with clinical stage T3 (C) disease, the actuarial disease-free survival rate was 45% at 10 years and 40% at 15 years.

Table 16.3.1 summarizes reported survival results in several reports[31].

Prognostic factors

Important prognostic factors in both univariate and multivariate analyses are clinical and pathologic stage, histologic degree of differentiation, elevation of prostatic acid phosphatase level, and, in more recent years, pretreatment PSA level[30,32–38]. In some studies age and race have been found to be significant prognostic factors, particularly for survival, although this is not a consistent finding[39–41].

In our experience race had no statistically significant impact on disease-free survival rates in patients with stage C (T3) tumors (55% for 364 white and 40% for 70 black patients) (P = 0.3). Age at diagnosis had a negative impact in patients with clinical stage C2 (T3b) disease (involvement of the seminal vesicles); those younger than 60 years of age exhibited a 10 year disease-free survival rate of 25% compared with 40% to 55% in older patients (P ≤ 0.01).

At our institution, in patients with clinical stage C (T3) tumors, histologic differentiation of the tumor had a

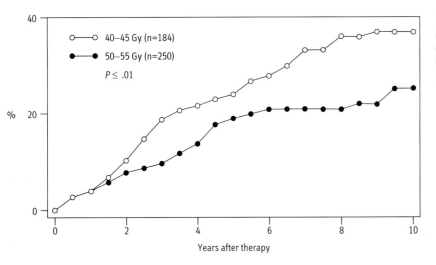

Fig. 16.3.1 Pelvic failure rate correlated with pelvic lymph node dose for 434 patients with stage C (T3) carcinoma of the prostate treated at Washington University.

profound effect on disease-free survival; the 10 year disease-free survival rates were 65%, 40% and 24%, respectively, for well, moderately, or poorly differentiated tumors (Figure 16.3.4).

Performance of a transurethral resection of the prostate (TURP) has also been reported to be an important prognostic factor only in stage C tumors with moderate or poor differentiation[35,42]. Stage C (T3) patients diagnosed with needle biopsy had a 48% 10 year survival rate compared with 30% if diagnosed by TURP ($P \leq 0.01$) (Figure 16.3.5).

Multivariate analysis of 963 patients treated at our institution showed that clinical stage, histological grade of the tumor, age younger than 60 years, and performance of TURP (in patients with stage C tumors) strongly correlated with disease-free survival. A separate analysis of the subpopulation of 301 patients for whom pre-treatment PSA levels were available documented a strong correlation of this parameter with disease-free survival (Table 16.3.2). Similar observations were reported by Zagars et al.[30] in 874 patients.

Patterns of failure after irradiation

Table 16.3.3 shows the overall incidence of pelvic failures, distant metastases, or combination of both in 963 patients treated at our institution (minimal follow up, 2 years; median, 6 years).

Pelvic failures

The majority of pelvic failures are in the prostate gland, but in some patients periprostatic extension is detected.

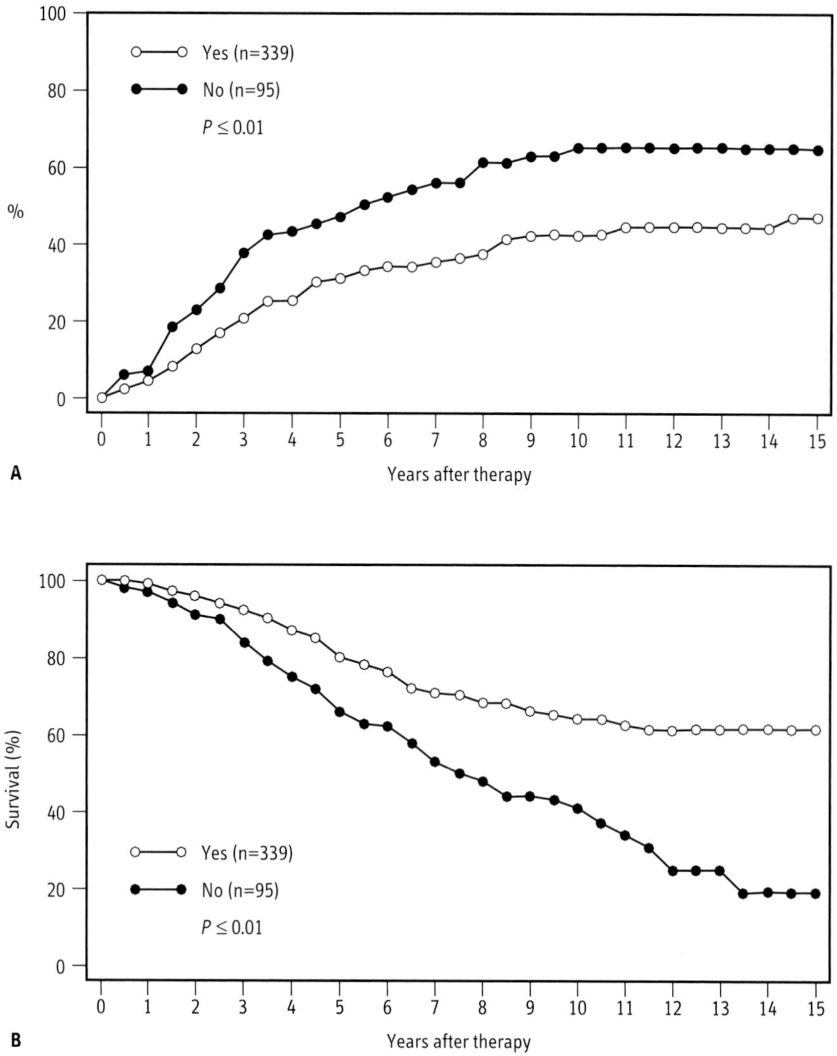

Fig. 16.3.2 Incidence of distant metastases (A) and cause-specific survival (B) correlated with pelvic tumor control in patients with stage C (T3) carcinoma of the prostate treated at Washington University.

Table 16.3.1 Survival with external beam irradiation: stage C (T3) carcinoma of the prostate

Study	No. of patients	Survival (%)		
		5 year	10 year	15 year
Aristizabal et al.[18]	82	60	–	–
Bagshaw et al.[19]	385	68 (70)	38 (50)	20 (35)
del Regato et al.[20]	372	66 (77)	38 (63)	17 (50)
Forman et al.[21]	125	(45)	–	–
Hanks[22]	296	56 (38)	32 (26)	23 (17)
	228	65	–	
Hanks[22]	197	66 (45)	33 (14)	
Hanks et al.[23]	503	70	38	
Harisiasdis et al.[24]	112	58	35	–
Neglia et al.[25]	97 (C1)	72	–	–
	53 (C2)	59	–	–
Perez et al.[9]	412	65 (58)	40 (44)	24 (40)
Rangala et al.[26]	93	78 (69)	–	–
Rosen et al.[27]	88	61 (53)	35 (35)	–
Rounsaville et al.[28]	140 (C1)	63 (67)	42 (44)	
	12 (C2)	32 (0)	11 (0)	
van der Werf-Messing et al.[29]	247	62 (52)	61 (25)	
Zagars et al.[30]	602	72 (59)	47 (44)	27 (30)

Open numbers = overall survival; numbers in parentheses = disease-free survival.
Modified from Perez CA: Prostate. In: Perez CA, Brady LW (eds) *Principles and practice of radiation oncology* (2nd edn) 1992[31].

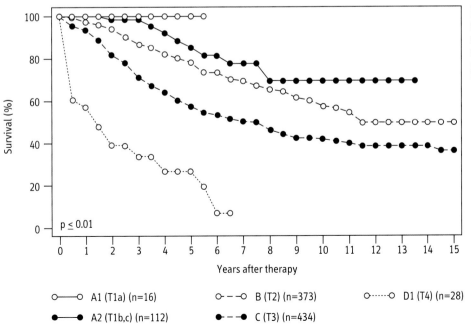

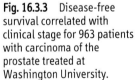

Fig. 16.3.3 Disease-free survival correlated with clinical stage for 963 patients with carcinoma of the prostate treated at Washington University.

Actuarial analyses are a more accurate method to report post-treatment failures, based on the number of patients at risk for any specific period of time. The 5 year pelvic failure rates in our patients are 12% for patients with stage B2 (T2c), 24% with C (T3) and 30% with clinical D1 (T4) tumors. The corresponding 10 year actuarial pelvic failure rates are 22% for B2 and 32% for C, and at 7 years 58% for D1 tumors.

No significant correlation of pelvic failures with pre-treatment PSA levels by clinical stage was observed, although patients with PSA higher than 20 ng/ml had a greater incidence of local recurrences ($P = 0.2$ to 0.37).

In 89 patients with stage C (T3), the pelvic failure rates were 42% in those younger than 60 years of age, about 30% in the group of patients 61 to 75 years of age, and 16% in patients older than 75 ($P = 0.01$). These differences may be related to the different life expectancy rates as a function of age at diagnosis.

Distant metastases

There is an increasing incidence of distant metastases with more advanced clinical stages. Also, the greatest incidence of distant metastases occurs in patients with poorly differentiated carcinoma (Gleason score 8 to 10). A greater incidence of distant metastases was noted in patients with stage C tumors diagnosed with TURP (57% at 10 years) compared with patients diagnosed with needle biopsy (44% at 10 years) ($P = 0.03$).

There was good correlation between the incidence of distant metastases and pre-treatment PSA in patients

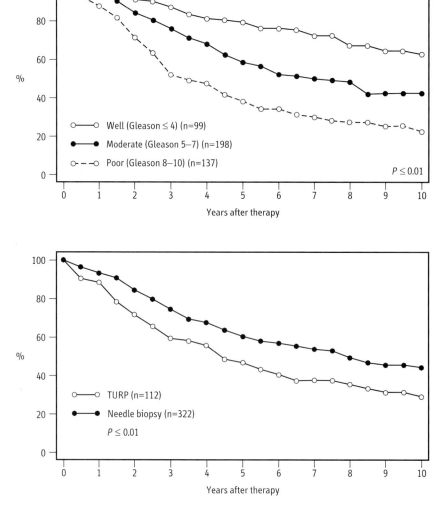

Fig. 16.3.4   Disease-free survival correlated with histologic grade for patients with stage C (T3) carcinoma of the prostate treated at Washington University.

Fig. 16.3.5   Disease-free survival correlated with method of diagnosis in patients with stage C (T3) carcinoma of the prostate treated at Washington University.

Table 16.3.2 Carcinoma of the prostate: multivariate analysis of chemical disease-free survival

Variable	Total patient population (n = 963)			Patient with pre-irradiation PSA (n = 301)		
	P-value	Final model regression coefficient (±SE)	Exponent of the regression coefficient	P-value	Final model regression coefficient (±SE)	Exponent of the regression coefficient
Clinical stage	0.001	0.2768+0.0413	1.3190	0.231	0.1354+0.1207	1.1450
Transurethral resection of prostate	0.045	−0.2284+0.1236	0.7958			
Lymph node status	0.078	−0.001+0.001	0.9999	0.017	−0.0002+0.001	0.9998
Histologic grade	0.001	0.2286+0.0335	1.2569	0.016	0.1655+0.0570	1.1800
Pelvic node dose	0.326	0.4664+0.2248	1.5942			
Central axis dose	0.111	−0.0002+0.0001	0.9998	0.861	0.0001+0.0003	1.0001
Initial prostate-specific antigen value				0.011	0.0068+0.0024	1.0069

Table 16.3.3 Carcinoma of the prostate: patterns of failure correlated with stage

Stage	No. of patients	Patterns of clinical failure		
		Pelvic	Pelvic and distant metastases	Distant metastases only
A1 (T1a)	16	0	0	0
A2 (T1b,c)	112	1 (9%)	3 (3%)	5 (4%)
B (T2)	373	30 (8%)	19 (5%)	45 (12%)
C (T3)	434	41 (9%)	54 (12%)	113 (26%)
D (T4)	28	4 (14%)	5 (18%)	12 (43%)

with clinical stage B (T2) and C (T3) tumors. With median follow up of 5 years patients with PSA of ≤ 20 ng/ml have significantly lower incidence of metastatic disease (20% or less) than those with higher PSA levels (30%) ($P = 0.12$).

Distant metastases developed in 60% of patients younger than 60 years of age with stage C tumors compared with 43% to 50% in the older patients ($P \leq 0.01$).

The reported incidence of distant metastases is approximately 20% in patients with stage T2 tumors in contrast with 40% in patients with T3 lesions. The incidence of local or pelvic recurrence and distant metastasis in patients with clinical stage C (T3) described in the literature is summarized in Table 16.3.4.

Impact of pre-treatment prostate-specific antigen on therapy results

Several authors have shown a close correlation between PSA levels, clinical and pathologic tumor stage, and, in conjunction with Gleason score, a predictable correlation with incidence of lymph node metastasis[36,37,41,45].

Worse outcome after external irradiation in patients with higher pre-treatment PSA has been reported. In patients with clinical stage C disease with a median follow up of up to 30 months and PSA below 10 ng/ml (Tandem R Hybritech), the probability of a chemical failure was 20%, whereas with initial PSA greater than 10 ng/ml, it ranged from 20% to 90%, depending on the pre-treatment PSA level[46–50].

'Gold standard' PSA values after irradiation have not been established[51]. Because the prostate gland remains in place and it is possible that some non-clonogenic cells may continue to produce PSA, it is not expected that values will decline to post-prostatectomy levels (less than 0.2 ng/ml) in many patients. The 'normal' post-irradiation PSA may be defined as that value associated with long-term disease-free survival[51]. Zagars et al.[49] observed a median of 1.2 ng/ml (normal 0 to 4 ng/ml), and Ritter et al.[52] a mean value of 1.1 ng/ml (normal 0 to 3.2 ng/ml).

Table 16.3.4   Incidence of locoregional recurrence, distant metastases, and intercurrent disease in patients with stage T3 treated with external radiation therapy

Study	Number of patients	Locoregional recurrence (%)	Distant metastases (%)	Intercurrent disease (%)
Aristizabel et al.[18]	82	12	33	23[a]
Bagshaw et al.[19]	385	38[b]		
del Regato et al.[20]				25[c]
Hanks[22]	296	30[c]		
Hanks[22]	197	42[d]		
Kurup et al.[43]	74	12	39	6
Perez et al.[9]	434	32[b]	42	
Rosen et al.[27]	88	30[b]		
Rounsaville et al.[28]	152	23	39	12
Sagerman et al.[44]	63	23	29	
Zagars et al.[30]	602	24[b]	45[b]	

[a] Total in all stages.
[b] 10 year actuarial.
[c] At 10 years.
[d] At 15 years.
Perez CA, Hanks GE, Leibel SA, Zietman AL, Fuks Z, Lee WR. Localized carcinoma of the prostate (stages T1B, T1C, and T3): Review of management with external beam radiation therapy. *Cancer* 1993;**72**:3156–3173[1].

Chemical failure precedes clinical recurrence by several years; even in patients with initial PSA of 4 to 30 ng/ml, 80% were clinically tumor-free 4 years after treatment. Others have reported shorter lead time from rising PSA to clinical evidence of relapse (from 6 months to 3 years on the average).[52–54]

Chemical disease-free survival (PSA below 2 ng/ml) in 68 patients with clinical stage C treated at Washington University (minimum follow up of 18 months and mean of 2.3 years) is shown in Figure 16.3.6A. With pre-treatment PSA levels of ≤ 10 ng/ml, the 5 year survival was 75% to 80%, and with higher PSA levels, about 40%. Patients are considered chemically free of disease if the post-treatment PSA level is less than 2 ng/ml in any of the post-treatment determinations. This value may be somewhat higher than that reported by Willett et al.[55] in 36 patients treated for pelvic malignancies without carcinoma of the prostate, in whom the median PSA level was 0.65 ng/ml (Tandem R, Hybretech assay).

As reported by Kavadi et al.[56] in 427 patients with localized carcinoma of the prostate treated with external irradiation (30 month median follow up), post-treatment PSA nadir values closely correlated with subsequent failure. In our experience, patients with nPSA of ≤ 1 ng/ml had only a 10% (eight of 83) probability of developing a chemical relapse compared with 16.7% (19 of 114) with nPSA of 1.1 to 2 ng/ml and 28% (28 of 99) with nPSA 2.1 to 3 ng/ml (Figure 16.3.6B).

Positive biopsy of the prostate after definitive radiation therapy

These data should be interpreted in the light of radiobiologic data indicating that cell death after radiation exposure is a post-mitotic event; cells that harbor lethal damage but have not had an opportunity morphologically to express it may be histologically misinterpreted as viable cells. Cox and Stoffel[57] noted that there was a decreasing incidence of positive biopsies as a function of time after irradiation (from 70% at 6 months to 20% after 24 months). Scardino[58] confirmed this observation, reporting that 32% of his patients with a positive biopsy at 12 months had a negative pathologic specimen at 24 months.

The rate of positive specimens is related to the initial clinical stage of the tumor; Scardino[58] noted a positivity of 28% for B1, 41% for B2 and 62% for stage C lesions. Freiha and Bagshaw[59] reported no positive biopsies in patients with stages A2 and B1, but rates of 38%, 59% and 74% for small stage B2, large B2, and stage C tumors, respectively.

In an analysis by Kuban and El-Mahdi[60], of 94 patients with clinically negative digital examination of the prostate who did not receive hormonal therapy until documented evidence of recurrence and on whom routine biopsies of the prostate were performed 18 months or longer after irradiation, the incidence of positive biopsies was one in 10 (10%) for stage A2, 10 in 55 (18%) for stage B,

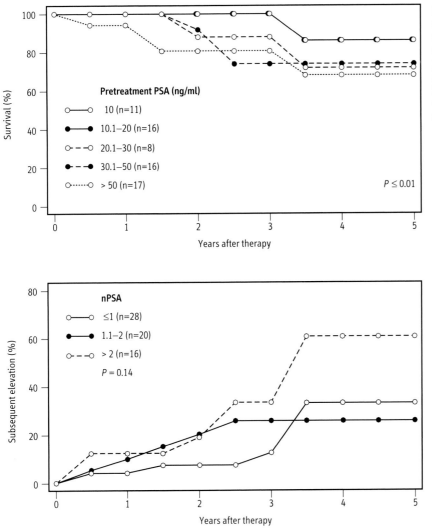

Fig. 16.3.6 (A) Chemical disease-free survival correlated with initial PSA value and (B) chemical failure correlated with nadir of postirradiation PSA for patients with stage C (T3) carcinoma of the prostate treated at Washington University (post treatment PSA below 2 ng/ml at any time).

and six in 29 (21%) for stage C lesions. By 10 years, 75% of patients with positive biopsies developed clinical local failure. Disease-free survival was 20% compared with 30% and 60%, respectively, in patients with negative biopsies.

Morbidity of external irradiation

As reported by Lawton et al.[61] and Perez et al.[62] the incidence of fatal complications in localized carcinoma of the prostate treated with external irradiation is about 0.2%, demonstrating the low risk of this therapy. The overall incidence of severe urinary or rectosigmoid sequelae is approximately 3% and moderate sequelae, 7% to 12%[19, 61–66]. The most frequent urinary sequelae are ure-

thral stricture and cystitis with intermittent hematuria (3% to 6%). Bladder fistula, hemorrhagic cystitis, or ureteral stricture occurs in fewer than 0.5% of patients. A higher incidence of urethral stricture (about 5%) has been described in patients irradiated after TURP compared with patients without such a history (3%). Some degree of urinary incontinence, in some cases related to stress, is noted in about 2% of patients, more frequently after TURP. The incidence of severe anal or rectal injury requiring colostomy is less than 1%; Perez et al.[62] reported one rectovesical and one vesicosigmoid fistula in 738 patients (0.27%), and Lawton et al.[61] recorded 11 (1%) grade 4 and 5 rectal injuries in 1020 patients. The incidence of proctitis or rectal ulcer causing bleeding is approximately 5%; occasionally a perianal abscess or anal stricture is noted.

197

Leg, scrotal, or penile edema is extremely rare in patients treated with irradiation alone (less than 1%), but its incidence ranges from 10% to 30% in patients undergoing lymph node dissection, depending on the extent of this procedure[64]. Erectile dysfunction, a significant treatment sequela affecting quality of life, particularly in younger men, has been described in 14% to 50% of patients, depending on patient age and techniques of irradiation. However, prospective, well documented quantitative assessment of this sequela is lacking[67].

Morbidity in 963 patients treated at Washington University is shown in Table 16.3.5.

Three-dimensional treatment planning and conformal therapy

With the advent of three-dimensional (3-D) treatment planning and conformal radiation therapy, it is feasible to deliver higher tumor doses to selected (conformed) target volumes while relatively sparing adjacent normal tissues, thus improving tumor control probability without increasing treatment morbidity. Improved dose distribution and smaller volumes of rectum and bladder receiving higher doses have been observed with conformal irradiation compared with conventional techniques in the treatment of prostate cancer (Figure 16.3.7)[68–72].

Hanks et al.[73] reported a 34% incidence of grade 2 morbidity in 247 patients treated with conformal therapy for prostate cancer in comparison with 57% in 162 patients treated with standard treatment. The 5 year chemical disease-free survival rates were 55% and 39%, respectively.

Acute toxicity during treatment has been quantitated weekly in 119 patients treated at Washington University with 3-D conformal irradiation and compared with that of 138 patients treated with conventional techniques (bilateral 120° arc rotation). Urinary symptoms (difficulty in urinating) were reported as moderate by 12% to 15% of patients with standard therapy in contrast to 3% to 8% in patients treated with conformal therapy. Proctitis or rectal bleeding, usually of no clinical significance, was recorded in 12% of patients in the standard therapy and 3% in the conformal group.

Leibel et al.[74] updated preliminary results in 324 patients with carcinoma of the prostate (135 with stage T2b,c and 102 with stage C) irradiated on a dose-escalation protocol (64.8 to 66.6 Gy in 70 patients, 70.2 Gy in 102, 75.6 Gy in 57, and 81 Gy in 25 patients). About 15% of patients had grade 2 or 3 rectal acute morbidity; only one patient (0.4%) has so far developed a severe grade 3 late complication. The overall 3 year actuarial PSA normalization rate was 86% with T2b tumors, 60% with stage T2c, and 43% with stage C tumors.

Table 16.3.5   Carcinoma of the prostate (1967–1992): sequelae correlated with irradiation

	Prostate and pelvis (n = 658)	Prostate only (n = 305)
Rectosigmoid and small bowel		
Moderate (Grade 2)		
Proctitis	39 (6%)	13 (4%)
Enteritis	9 (1%)	
Rectal fibrosis	2 (0.3%)	
Anal stricture	2 (0.3%)	
Rectal ulcer	1 (0.1%)	3 (1%)
Rectal stricture	1 (0.1%)	
Anal fissure	1 (0.1%)	
Perianal abscess	1 (0.1%)	
Anorectal telangiectasia	1 (0.1%)	
Severe (Grade 3)		
Perianal abscess	1 (0.1%)	1 (0.3%)
Proctitis	1 (0.1%)	
Small bowel obstruction	3 (0.5%)	
Urinary		
Moderate (Grade 2)		
Urethral stricture	22 (3%)	4 (1%)
Hematuria	4 (0.6%)	1 (0.3%)
Cystitis	7 (1%)	4 (1%)
Urinary incontinence	4 (0.6%)	1 (0.3%)
Ureteral stricture	1 (0.1%)	
Severe (Grade 3)		
Vesicosigmoid fistula[a]	1 (0.1%)	
Rectovesical fistula	1 (0.1%)	
Cystitis	1 (0.1%)	
Ureteral stricture	2 (0.3%)	1 (0.3%)
Other		
Moderate (Grade 2)		
Subcutaneous fibrosis	2 (0.3%)	
Leg, scrotal, penile edema	9 (1%)	
Impotence[b]	79 (12%)	19 (6%)
Severe (Grade 3)		
Pubic bone necrosis	1 (0.1%)	
Pelvic soft tissue necrosis	1 (0.1%)	
Fatal (Grade 4)		
Radiation-induced ileitis[c]	1 (0.1%)	

[a] Sigmoid diverticulitis.
[b] Only patients who were potent at the time of radiation therapy were included.
[c] History of aortic aneurysm and aorta-iliac graft.
Perez CA, Michalski J, Brown KC, Lockett MA. Nonrandomized evaluation of pelvic lymph node irradiation in localized carcinoma of the prostate. *Int J Radiat Oncol Biol Phys* (in press).[14]

New directions and future clinical trials

Three areas currently under investigation are dose-escalation, particle therapy, and radiation therapy combined with androgen suppression.

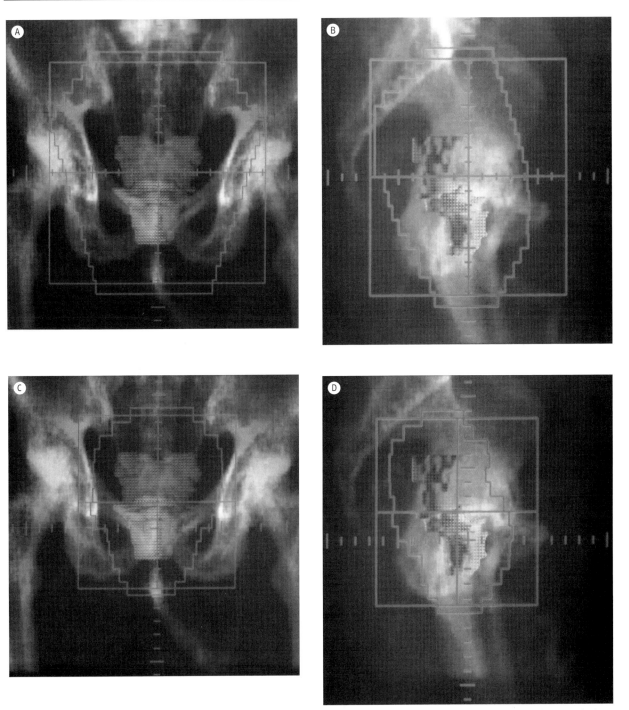

Fig. 16.3.7   Anteroposterior (A) and lateral (B) 3-D conformal irradiation portals used for treating patients with clinical stage C (T3) carcinoma of the prostate. (C) Anteroposterior and (D) lateral reduced portals, which in addition to 4 oblique fields are used for the diversional abnormal irradiation.

Dose-escalation studies

The benefit of 3-D conformal therapy hypothetically could be linked to improved local tumor control because of better coverage of the target volume with a specific dose of irradiation, less acute and late morbidity, possibility of carrying out dose-escalation studies if morbidity is held to acceptable levels, and improved survival. Several institutions[71,73,75–77], the Radiation Therapy Oncology Group (RTOG), and 10 institutions under cooperative agreement with the National Cancer Institute are conducting phase I/II dose-escalation studies. Depending on the results, the cost benefit of 3-D conformal irradiation must be further evaluated in a larger, multi-institutional protocol, comparing it with standard techniques in order to justify its initial increased cost.

Special particles

Special particles, such as protons and heavy ions, provide better dose distributions and some biologic advantages over photons; in preliminary studies they have been reported to yield a high probability of tumor control with sparing of normal tissues[78–81].

Laramore et al.[82] published the final report of an RTOG clinical trial of 91 patients with stage C or D1 carcinoma of the prostate randomized to receive either conventional photon irradiation (65 Gy) or equivalent doses with mixed photon and neutron beams. Ten year analysis showed local tumor control rates of 70% in the patients treated with mixed beams and 58% in the photon group ($P = 0.03$). The survival rates were 46% and 29%, respectively ($P = 0.04$). A total of seven mixed-beam and five photon-treated patients suffered significant sequelae from therapy (no statistical difference).

In the Neutron Therapy Collaborative Working Group Trial, 182 T3 or T4 or pelvic node-positive patients were treated with a pelvic field (50.4 Gy in the photon arm at 1.8 Gy per fraction and 13.6 nGy at 1.7 nGy per fraction in the neutron arm). The prostate was boosted with 20 Gy and 6.8 nGy, respectively. Five-year results show significantly better pathologic local tumor control with neutrons (82% versus 60%), but as yet no difference in disease-free or overall survival has been observed.[83] In this trial there was significant morbidity in the neutron arm; 10 of 87 patients had grade 4 morbidity (six requiring colostomy) compared with only one of 85 treated with photons.

Shipley et al.[84] reported on a phase I/II study of T3 and T4 prostate cancer in which, after 50.4 Gy to the pelvis delivered through four fields, 103 patients were randomized to receive a perineal conformal field proton (160 MV) boost of 25.2 CGE (cobalt Gray equivalent) or in 99 patients a 16.8 Gy boost with photons. Median follow up was 60 months. Among the patients completing randomization, the local relapse-free survival at 7 years was 80% for the proton and 66% for the photon group ($P = 0.14$). However, the local relapse-free survival at 7 years for 58 patients with poorly differentiated tumors was 85% with protons and 37% with photons ($P = 0.001$). The incidence of grade 1 and 2 rectal bleeding (32% versus 12%) and urethral stricture (19% versus 8%) was higher in the proton-treated patients compared with the photon-treated group.

External irradiation and endocrine therapy

Endocrine therapy in conjunction with radiation therapy has been explored as adjuvant therapy following irradiation for patients at high risk for occult metastatic disease or as neoadjuvant cytoreductive therapy in patients with bulky primary tumors to enhance the likelihood of local tumor control and disease-free survival.

RTOG protocol 8531 evaluated adjuvant goserelin acetate (Zoladex) (3.6 mg subcutaneously every 28 days indefinitely) combined with irradiation in T3 and T4 and node-positive patients or administered on relapse after identical irradiation alone. This study accrued 977 patients (479 in the adjuvant hormone arm and 471 in the observation arm); preliminary results showed higher pelvic tumor control (83% versus 68%) and disease-free survival (59% versus 40%) in the adjuvant hormone group compared with the control group, but no difference in overall survival (76% and 71%, respectively)[85].

Results were recently reported for RTOG protocol 8610[2] in 456 evaluable patients with large stage T2b,c (B2, B3, B4, C, D1) disease treated with either irradiation alone (45 Gy to pelvic lymph nodes and additional 20 to 25 Gy to the prostatic area) or a combination of the same radiation therapy and adjuvant hormonal therapy consisting of Zoladex (3.6 mg subcutaneously every 4 weeks) and Eulexin (250 mg po tid); both drugs started 2 months before initiation of irradiation and continued throughout the entire course of radiation therapy. With a median observation period of 3.3 years, the 4.5 year actuarial local failure rate was 46% in the study arm and 71% in the control arm ($P \leq 0.01$). A decreasing incidence of distant metastasis was also noted in patients receiving hormonal therapy (34% versus 41%) ($P = 0.09$). The actuarial clinical disease-free survival was 38% for the study arm and 16% for the control arm ($P < 0.001$). The corresponding chemical-free (PSA < 4 ng/ml) survival rates were 36% for the study arm and 15% for the control arm ($P < 0.001$). Overall survival differences are not statistically significant at this time.

The value of elective pelvic irradiation and neoadjuvant hormone therapy will be better assessed in a recently activated RTOG protocol (94-13) in which patients with clinical stage T2 and T3 carcinoma of the prostate are randomized to four arms: neoadjuvant total androgen suppression (Zoladex and flutamide) or not 2 months before and during irradiation or radiation therapy to the whole pelvis (50.4 Gy, 1.8 Gy fractions) and prostate (19.8 Gy boost) or to prostate volume only 70.2 Gy).

In summary, radiation therapy plays a major role in the management of patients with stage T3 (C) and T4 carcinoma of the prostate. Innovative approaches under investigation may enhance the efficacy of this therapeutic modality.

References

1. Perez CA, Hanks GE, Leibel SA, Zietman AL, Fuks Z, Lee WR. Localized carcinoma of the prostate (stages T1B, T1C, T2, and T3): Review of management with external beam radiation therapy. *Cancer* 1993;**72**:3156–3173.
2. Pilepich MV, Sause WT, Shipley WU *et al.* Androgen deprivation with radiation therapy compared with radiation therapy alone for locally advanced prostatic carcinoma: A randomized comparative trial of the Radiation Therapy Oncology Group. *Urology* 1995;**45**:616–623.
3. Benson MC, Whang IS, Olsson CA, McMahan DJ, Conner WH. The use of prostate specific antigen density to enhance the predictive value of intermediate levels of serum prostate specific antigen. *J Urol* 1992;**147**:817–821.
4. Catalona WJ, Smith DS, Ratliff TL *et al.* Measurement of prostate-specific antigen in serum as a screening test for prostate cancer. *N Engl J Med* 1991;**324**:1156–1161.
5. Oesterling JE. Prostate-specific antigen: A critical assessment of the most useful tumor marker for adenocarcinoma of the prostate. *J Urol* 1991;**145**:907–923.
6. Oesterling JE, Chan DW, Epstein JL *et al.* Prostate specific antigen in the preoperative and postoperative evaluation of localized prostatic cancer treated with radical prostatectomy. *J Urol* 1988;**139**:766–772.
7. Pisansky TM, Cha SS, Earle JD *et al.* Prostate-specific antigen as a pretherapy prognostic factor in patients treated with radiation therapy for clinically localized prostate cancer. *J Clin Oncol* 1993;**11**:2158–2166.
8. Whitmore WF. Overview: Historical and contemporary. *NCI Monogr* 1988;**7**:7–11.
9. Perez CA, Lee HK, Georgiou A, Logsdon MD, Lai PP, Lockett MA. Technical and tumor-related factors affecting outcome of definitive irradiation for localized carcinoma of the prostate. *Int J Radiat Oncol Biol Phys* 1993;**26**:581–591.
10. Perez CA, Pilepich MV, Zivnuska F. Tumor control in definitive irradiation of localized carcinoma of the prostate. *Int J Radiat Oncol Biol Phys* 1986;**12**:523–531.
11. Hanks GE, Martz KL, Diamond JJ. The effect of dose on local control of prostate cancer. *Int J Radiat Oncol Biol Phys* 1988;**15**:1299–1305.
12. McGowan DG. The value of extended field radiation therapy in carcinoma of the prostate. *Int J Radiat Oncol Biol Phys* 1981;**7**:1333–1339.
13. Ploysongsang SS, Aron BS, Shehata WM. Radiation therapy in prostate cancer: whole pelvis with prostate boost or small field to prostate? *Urology* 1992;**40**:18–26.
14. Perez CA, Michalski J, Brown KC, Lockett MA. Nonrandomized evaluation of pelvic lymph node irradiation in localized carcinoma of the prostate. *Int J Radiat Oncol Biol Phys*, 1996; **36**:573–84.
15. Kaplan ID, Prestidge BR, Bagshaw MA, Cox RS. The importance of local control in the treatment of prostatic cancer. *J Urol* 1992;**147**: 917–921.
16. Kuban DA, El-Mahdi AM, Schellhammer PF. Effect of local tumor control on distant metastasis and survival in prostatic adenocarcinoma. *Urology* 1987;**30**:420–426.
17. Kuban DA, El-Mahdi AM, Schellhammer PF. Potential benefit of improved local tumor control in patients with prostate carcinoma. *Cancer* 1995;**75**:2373–2382.
18. Aristizabal SA, Steinbronn D, Heusinkveld RS. External beam radiotherapy in cancer of the prostate: The University of Arizona experience. *Radiother Oncol* 1984;**1**:309–315.
19. Bagshaw MA, Cox RS, Ramback JE. Radiation therapy for localized prostate cancer: Justification by long-term follow-up. *Urol Clin North Am* 1990;**17**:787–802.
20. del Regato JA, Trailins AH, Pittman DD. Twenty years follow-up of patients with inoperable cancer of the prostate (stage C) treated by radiotherapy: Report of a national cooperative study. *Int J Radiat Oncol Biol Phys* 1993;**26**:197–201.
21. Forman JD, Wharam MD, Lee DJ, Zinreich ES, Order SE. Definitive radiotherapy following prostatectomy: Results and complications. *Int J Radiat Oncol Biol Phys* 1986;**12**:185–189.
22. Hanks GE. Treatment of early stage prostate cancer: Radiotherapy. In: Hellman S, De Vita V, Rosenberg S, Freeman S (eds). *Important advances in oncology*. JB Lippincott, Philadelphia, PA, 1993.
23. Hanks GE, Krall JM, Martz KL, Diamond JJ, Kramer S. The outcome of treatment of 313 patients with T-1 (UICC) prostate cancer treated with external beam irradiation. *Int J Radiat Oncol Biol Phys* 1988;**14**:243–248.
24. Harisiasdis L, Veenema RJ, Senyszyn JJ *et al.* Carcinoma of the prostate: treatment with external radiotherapy. *Cancer* 1978;**41**:2131–2142.
25. Neglia WJ, Hussey DH, Johnson DE. Megavoltage radiation therapy for carcinoma of the prostate. *Int J Radiat Oncol Biol Phys* 1977;**2**:873–882.
26. Rangala N, Cox JD, Byhardt RW, Wilson JF, Greenberg M, Lopes da Conceicao A. Local control and survival after external irradiation for adenocarcinoma of the prostate. *Int J Radiat Oncol Biol Phys* 1982;**8**:1909–1914.
27. Rosen EM, Cassady JR, Connolly J, Chaffey JT. Radiotherapy for localized prostate carcinoma. *Int J Radiat Oncol Biol Phys* 1984;**10**:2201–2210.
28. Rounsaville MC, Green JP, Vaeth JM, Purdon RP, Heltzel MM. Prostatic carcinoma: limited field irradiation. *Int J Radiat Oncol Biol Phys* 1987;**13**:1013–1020.
29. van der Werf-Messing BHP, Menon RS, van Putten WLJ. Prostatic cancer treated by external irradiation at the Rotterdam Radiotherapy Institute. *Strahlentherapie* 1984;**160**:293–300.
30. Zagars GK, von Eschenbach AC, Ayala AG. Prognostic factors in prostate cancer: analysis of 874 patients treated with radiation therapy. *Cancer* 1993;**72**:1709–1725.
31. Perez CA. Prostate. In: Perez CA, Brady LW (eds) *Principles and practice of radiation oncology* (2nd edn). JB Lippincott, Philadelphia, PA, 1992, pp. 1067–1116.
32. Blute ML, Nativ O, Zinke H, Farrow GM, Therneau T, Lieber MM. Pattern of failure after radical retropubic prostatectomy for clinically and pathologically localized adenocarcinoma of the prostate: Influence of tumor deoxyribonucleic acid ploidy. *J Urol* 1989;**142**:1262–1265.
33. Gleason DF. Histologic grade, clinical stage, and patient age in prostate cancer. *NCI Monogr* 1988;**7**:15–18.
34. Perez CA, Garcia D, Simpson JR, Zivnuska F, Lockett MA. Factors influencing outcome of definitive radiotherapy for localized carcinoma of the prostate. *Radiother Oncol* 1989;**16**:1–21.
35. Pilepich MV, Krall JM. Sause WT *et al.* Prognostic factors in carcinoma of the prostate: Analysis of RTOG study 75-06. *Int J Radiat Oncol Biol Phys* 1987;**13**:339–349.
36. Bluestein DL, Bostwick DG, Bergstralh EJ, Oesterling JE. Eliminating the need for bilateral pelvic lymphadenectomy in select patients with prostate cancer. *J Urol* 1994;**151**:1315–1320.
37. Partin AW, Lee BR, Chan DW, Epstein AW, Walsh PC. The use of prostate specific antigen (PSA) and Gleason score to predict pathologic stage in men with localized prostate cancer. *J Urol* 1993;**150**:110–114.
38. Sands ME, Zagars GK, Pollack A, von Eschenbach AC. Serum prostate-specific antigen, clinical stage, pathologic grade, and the incidence of nodal metastases in prostate cancer. *Urology* 1994;**44**:215–220.

39. Brawn P, Johnson E, Kuhl DL *et al.* Stage at presentation and survival of white and black patients with prostate carcinoma. *Cancer* 1993;**71**:2569–2573.

40. Kim JA, Kuban DA, El-Mahdi AM, Schellhammer PE. Carcinoma of the prostate: race as a prognostic indicator in definitive radiation therapy. *Radiology* 1995;**194**:545–549.

41. Roach M III, Krall J, Keller JW *et al.* The prognostic significance of race and survival from prostate cancer based on patients irradiated on Radiation Therapy Oncology Group protocols (1976–1985). *Int J Radiat Oncol Biol Phys* 1992;**24**:441–449.

42. McGowan DG. The effect of transurethral resection on prognosis in carcinoma of the prostate: real or imaginary? *Int J Radiat Oncol Biol Phys* 1988;**15**:1057–1064.

43. Kurup P, Kramer TS, Lee MS, Philips R. External beam irradiation of prostate cancer: Experience in 163 patients. *Cancer* 1984;**53**:37–43.

44. Sagerman RH, Chun HC, King GA, Chung CT, Dalal PS. External beam radiotherapy for carcinoma of the prostate. *Cancer* 1989;**63**:2468–2474.

45. Stamey TA, Yang N, Hay AR, McNeal JE, Freiha FS, Redwine E. Prostate-specific antigen as a serum marker for adenocarcinoma of the prostate. *N Engl J Med* 1987;**317**:909–916.

46. Fijuth J, Chauvet B, Vincent P, Felix-Faure C, Reboul F. Serum prostatic-specific antigen in monitoring the response of carcinoma of the prostate to radiation therapy. *Radiother Oncol* 1992;**23**:236–240.

47. Landmann C, Hunig R. Prostatic specific antigen as an indicator of response to radiotherapy in prostate cancer. *Int J Radiat Oncol Biol Phys* 1989;**17**:1073–1076.

48. Russell KJ, Dunatov C, Hafermann MD et al. Prostate specific antigen in the management of patients with localized adenocarcinoma of the prostate treated with primary radiation therapy. *J Urol* 1991;**146**:1046–1052.

49. Zagars GK, Sherman NE, Babaian RJ. Prostatic-specific antigen and external beam radiation therapy in prostatic cancer. *Cancer* 1991;**67**:412–420.

50. Zentner PG, Pao LK, Benson MC, Schiff PB. PSA density: A new prognostic factor for the prediction of outcome in patients with prostate cancer. *Int J Radiat Oncol Biol Phys* 1992;**24**(suppl 1): 150.

51. Russell KJ, Boileau MA. Current status of prostate-specific antigen in the radiotherapeutic management of prostatic cancer. *Semin Radiat Oncol* 1993;**3**:154–168.

52. Ritter MA, Messing EM, Shanahan TG *et al.* Prostate-specific antigen as a predictor of radiotherapy response and patterns of failure in localized prostate cancer. *J Clin Oncol* 1992;**10**:1208–1217.

53. Kaplan ID, Cox RS, Bagshaw MA. Prostate specific antigen after external beam radiotherapy for prostatic cancer: follow-up. *J Urol* 1993;**149**:519–522.

54. Kaplan ID, Prestidge BR, Cox RS, Bagshaw MA. Prostate specific antigen after irradiation for prostatic carcinoma. *J Urol* 1990;**144**:1172–1175.

55. Willett CG, Zietman AL, Shipley WU, Coen JJ. The effect of pelvic radiation therapy on serum levels of prostate specific antigen. *J Urol* 1994;**151**:1579–1581.

56. Kavadi VS, Zagars GK, Pollack A. Serum prostate-specific antigen after radiation therapy for clinically localized prostate cancer: prognostic implications. *Int J Radiat Oncol Biol Phys* 1994;**30**:279–287.

57. Cox JD, Stoffel TJ. The significance of needle biopsy after irradiation for stage C adenocarcinoma of the prostate. *Cancer* 1977;**40**:156–160.

58. Scardino PT. The prognostic significance of biopsies after radiotherapy for prostatic cancer. *Semin Urol* 1983;**1**:243–252.

59. Freiha FS, Bagshaw MA. Carcinoma of the prostate: results of post-irradiation biopsy. *Prostate* 1984;**5**:19–25.

60. Kuban DA, El-Mahdi AM. Prognostic significance of post-irradiation prostate biopsies. *Oncology* 1993;**7**(2):29–38.

61. Lawton CA, Won M, Pilepich MV *et al.* Long-term treatment sequelae following external beam irradiation for adenocarcinoma of the prostate: analysis of RTOG studies 7506 and 7706. *Int J Radiat Oncol Biol Phys* 1991;**21**:935–939.

62. Perez CA, Lee HK, Georgiou A, Lockett MA. Technical factors affecting morbidity in definitive irradiation for localized carcinoma of the prostate. *Int J Radiat Oncol Biol Phys* 1994;**28**:811–819.

63. Hanks GE, Leibel SA, Krall JM, Kramer S. Patterns of care studies: dose-response observations for local control of adenocarcinoma of the prostate. *Int J Radiat Oncol Biol Phys* 1985;**11**:153–157.

64. Pilepich MV, Asbell SO, Krall JM *et al.* Correlation of radiotherapeutic parameters and treatment related morbidity: analysis of RTOG study 77-06. *Int J Radiat Oncol Biol Phys* 1987;**13**:1007–1013.

65. Shipley WU, Prout GR Jr, Coachman NM *et al.* Radiation therapy for localized prostate carcinoma: experience at the Massachusetts General Hospital (1973–1981). *NCI Monogr* 1988;**7**:67–73.

66. Pilepich MV, Krall JM, Sause WT *et al.* Correlation of radiotherapeutic parameters and treatment related morbidity in carcinoma of the prostate: analysis of RTOG study 75-06. *Int J Radiat Oncol Biol Phys* 1987;**13**:351–357.

67. Zinreich ES, Derogatis LR, Herpst J, Auvil G, Piantadosi S, Order SE. Pre and post-treatment evaluation of sexual function in patients with adenocarcinoma of the prostate. *Int J Radiat Oncol Biol Phys* 1990;**19**:729–732.

68. Leibel SA, Ling CC, Kutcher GJ, Mohan R, Cordon-Cordo C, Fuks Z. The biological basis for conformal three-dimensional radiation therapy. *Int J Radiat Oncol Biol Phys* 1991;**21**:805–811.

69. Lichter AS. Three-dimensional conformal radiation therapy: a testable hypothesis. *Int J Radiat Oncol Biol Phys* 1991;**21**:853–855.

70. Perez CA, Purdy JA, Harms W *et al.* Three-dimensional treatment planning and conformal radiation therapy: Preliminary evaluation. *Radiother Oncol* 1995;**36**:32–43.

71. Sandler HM, Perez-Tamayo C, Ten Haken RK, Lichter AS. Dose escalation for stage C (T3) prostate cancer: Minimal rectal toxicity observed using conformal therapy. *Radiother Oncol* 1992;**23**:53–54.

72. Soffen EM, Hanks GE, Hwang CC, Chu JCH. Conformal static field therapy for low volume low grade prostate cancer with rigid immobilization. *Int J Radiat Oncol Biol Phys* 1991;**20**:141–146.

73. Hanks GE, Schultheiss TE, Hunt MA, Epstein B. Factors influencing incidence of acute grade 2 morbidity in conformal and standard radiation treatment of prostate cancer. *Int J Radiat Oncol Biol Phys* 1995;**31**:25–29.

74. Leibel SA, Zeletsky MJ, Kutcher GJ, Burman CM, Kelson S, Fuks Z. Three-dimensional conformal radiation therapy in localized carcinoma of the prostate: Interim report of a phase I dose escalation study. *J Urol* 1994;**152**:1792–1798.

75. Martinez A, Gonzalez J, Stromberg J *et al.* Conformal prostate brachytherapy: Initial experience of a phase I/II dose-escalating trial. *Int J Radiat Oncol Biol Phys* 1995;**33**:1019–1027.

76. Leibel SA, Heimann P, Kutcher GJ *et al.* Three-dimensional conformal radiation therapy in locally advanced carcinoma of the prostate: preliminary results of a phase I dose-escalation study. *Int J Radiat Oncol Biol Phys* 1994;**28**:55–65.

77. Wallner K. Iodine 125 brachytherapy for early stage prostate cancer: New techniques may achieve better results. *Oncology* 1991;**5**:115–122.

78. Castro JR, Collier JM Petti PL *et al.* Charged particle radiotherapy for lesions encircling the brain stem or spinal cord. *Int J Radiat Oncol Biol Phys* 1989;**17**:477–484.

79. Griffin TW, Pajak TF, Maor MH *et al.* Mixed neutron/photon irradiation of unresectable squamous cell carcinomas of the head and neck: The final report of a randomized cooperative trial. *Int J Radiat Oncol Biol Phys* 1989;**17**:959–965.

80. Suit HD, Urie M. Proton beams in radiation therapy. *J Natl Cancer Inst* 1992;**84**:155–164.

81. Munzenrider JE, Verhey IJ, Gargouda ES *et al.* Conservative treatment of uveal melanoma: Local recurrence after photon beam therapy. *Int J Radiat Oncol Biol Phys* 1989;**17**:493–498.

82. Laramore GE, Krall JM, Thomas FJ. Fast neutron radiotherapy for locally advanced prostate cancer: final report of a Radiation Therapy Oncology Group randomized clinical trial. *Am J Clin Oncol (CCT)* 1993;**16**:164–167.

83. Russell KJ, Krall JM, Laramore GE *et al.* Photon versus fast neutron external beam radiotherapy in the treatment of locally advanced prostate cancer: preliminary results of a randomized prospective trial of the Neutron Therapy Collaborative Working Group. *Int J Radiat Oncol Biol Phys* 1994; **28**: 47–54.

84. Shipley WU, Verhey LJ, Munzenrider JE *et al.* Advanced prostate cancer: The results of a randomized trial of high dose irradiation boosting with conformal protons compared with conventional dose irradiation using photons alone. *Int J Radiat Oncol Biol Phys* 1995;**32**:3–12.

85. Pilepich MV, Caplan R, Byhardt RW *et al.* Phase III trial of adjuvant androgen suppression using goserelin in patients with carcinoma of the prostate treated with definitive radiotherapy (Results of RTOG 85-31) (abstract). *Int J Radiat Oncol Biol Phys* 1995;**32**(suppl 1):188.

16.4 Locally advanced prostate cancer – hormonal treatment

T H Lynch and J M Fitzpatrick

Introduction

The widespread use of prostatic specific antigen (PSA) has enabled us to diagnose a greater proportion of prostate cancers when they are localized or locally advanced but the treatment remains controversial. The identification of a neoplastic focus within a surgically resected specimen from a TURP now has greater significance than heretofore in that it immediately raises the controversial issue of possible further treatment. The incidence of foci of carcinoma in resected specimens varies from 15% to 25% depending on the enthusiasm of the pathologist involved. Resected specimens come from the central and transitional zones, whereas the majority of residual tumor would be expected in the peripheral zone. What was thought to be localized may in fact be shown to be locally advanced on TRUS and biopsy. Traditionally, over half the patients labeled as having localized disease really have either low volume locally advanced disease or low volume disease with micrometastases.

Locally extensive prostate cancer may be fixed to or invade neighboring organs but there are no distant metastases (stage T3-4, N0, M0, according to the TNM system of classification as discussed in Chapter 14).

We have known for many years that there is wide variation in the rates of progression of invasive prostate cancer. Many low-grade lesions remain latent for several years and often go unrecognized and these patients clearly do not need any treatment. A minority of cases progress, invading surrounding tissues and metastasing, usually to bone.

The choice of treatment for locally advanced disease is influenced mainly by stage, grade, age and general health of the patient. Should one adopt a wait and see policy or commence hormonal treatment? If hormonal treatment is insti-

tuted should it be medical or surgical castration, should it be monotherapy or maximum androgen blockade? Should the patient have intermittent hormonal manipulation or should hormonal deprivation be combined with radiotherapy?

There is a consensus however that patients with locally advanced prostate cancer do not do well with any therapy. Whether newly diagnosed at an advanced stage or having progressed after diagnosis, it is generally accepted that the treatment of locally advanced disease is no longer curative. For years we have known that androgen ablation therapy alleviates symptoms of local and metastatic disease, shrinks tumors and delays disease progression but does not eliminate micrometastases.

The aims of treatment are to slow progression of the cancer and to palliate symptoms with quality of life being a high priority. The types of management include hormone deprivation, radiotherapy and palliative treatments including TURP.

Hormonal manipulation

Androgens are essential for the normal development of the prostate and their elimination is an effective treatment for prostate cancer. They originate either in the testicles (95%) or the adrenal glands (5%) (Figure 16.4.1). Adrenal androgens are transformed into testosterone in target cells such

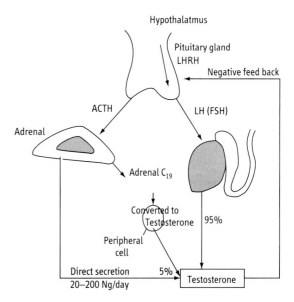

Fig. 16.4.1 Origin of plasma testosterone
Testosterone, the principal circulating androgen, is derived from the Leydig cells of the testicle and the peripheral conversion of C19 steroids from the adrenal glands.

LHRH   Lutenizing hormone releasing hormone
LH   Lutenizing hormone
ACTH   Adrenocorticotrophic hormone

as the prostate and adipose tissue. It is only the free unbound fraction of testosterone (2%) which is physiologically active because testosterone, when it is bound to plasma proteins, is unable to cross the cell membrane. Testosterone can only act at the cellular level having been transformed into dihydrotestosterone (DHT) by 5 alpha reductase.

Hormone treatment, even without any overt side effects, may leave a patient feeling under par thus it is unkind to submit a patient to hormone treatment unless an ultimate benefit can be proven. The financial implications of such treatment should also be borne in mind. Relapse after hormone treatment is usually fatal within a matter of months[1].

Hormonal deprivation can be achieved by removing the principal source of androgen by orchiectomy, administering LHRH analogues or blocking the peripheral effects of testosterone using antiandrogens (Table 16.4.1). It can be employed at first diagnosis or when the patient develops symptoms. About 70% to 80% of patients will respond to hormonal deprivation and the duration of their response ranges from a few months to several years.

Early or delayed hormonal ablation

One of the arguments against early treatment of any cancer, which leads to a prolonged survival, is simply a reflection of intervention at an earlier stage in the natural history of the patient's disease. We may only be affecting the lead time to progression rather than affecting the overall disease process. Advanced prostate cancer is treated at diagnosis in the hope of delaying the onset of symptoms and it may well prolong survival, although this is contentious. An elderly man may die from an unrelated cause before he develops symptoms requiring treatment, thus unless early treatment can be shown to have definite advantages, deferment until a definite indication arises might be preferable.

Table 16.4.1   Types of hormonal manipulation

Androgen withdrawal
Estrogens
   Diethylstilbestrol
   Estramustine phosphate
Bilateral orchiectomy
Luteinizing hormone releasing hormone agonists (LHRH)
   Goserelin
   Leuprolide
   Buserelin
   Triptoralin
Antiandrogens
   Steroid: cyproterone acetate
   Pure: flutamide, bicalutamide, nilutamide
Combination treatment
Castration (medical/surgical) and pure antiandrogens

This controversy over timing of treatment dates back to The Veterans Administration Co-operative Research Group (VACURG) study in the 1960s which demonstrated no survival advantage of early treatment in men with T3 disease[2]. This study included randomized control groups treated initially with a placebo but in whom active treatment was allowed on progression[3]. Many patients in this study died from cardiovascular complications associated with estrogen therapy and only 41% died from prostate cancer. This study concluded that treatment should be delayed until the onset of symptoms and showed no clear disadvantage in terms of survival in the treated group. However, later analysis of the results found that younger patients with poorly differentiated tumors might gain from immediate endocrine therapy[4].

This study formed the scientific basis for many years for withholding therapy and adopting a wait and see policy. The arguments against deferring such treatment have been: the risk of the loss of hormone sensitivity of the tumor, recurrent bladder outflow obstruction, obstructive uremia and development of spinal cord compression. Several uncontrolled and non-randomized studies have shown an advantage from early treatment[5].

In the MRC study[6] 938 men were recruited between 1985 and 1993. The study was designed to assess the impact of hormonal treatment commenced at the time of diagnosis on the course of the disease, compared with delay in treatment until clinical progression occurred. The need for treatment arose after a median of 9 months in men presenting with metastatic disease and few escape treatment before they die. Thus, the avoidance of side effects of hormonal treatment for a mean of 9 months has to be balanced against the risk of important complications.

Progression of disease will be arrested or slowed in patients treated immediately. This was shown by a more rapid onset of metastatic disease and local complications in the deferred group. Twice the number of patients in the deferred group developed spinal cord compression. A worrying aspect of this study is that 5% of patients died from prostate cancer before they received therapy and this may be due to the relatively infrequent follow up.

Although the survival data in this study are still relatively immature as only 64% of patients have died, the evidence from the study indicates that there is an advantage in terms of survival with early treatment, particularly in the younger patient.

This trial demonstrates that early therapy causes few complications and that at least for locally advanced disease it may improve survival. Those most likely to benefit from deferred treatment were elderly men with non-metastatic disease but the younger man with a good performance status should be given immediate hormonal treatment. These results have prompted urologists to commence treatment with androgen blockade after rising PSA levels indicate failure of local treatment.

Radiotherapy and androgen blockade

Although external beam radiotherapy is discussed elsewhere in this book the combination of androgen ablation and radiotherapy needs to be addressed. There is no modern study comparing external beam radiotherapy, brachytherapy and hormonal manipulation and patients are often confused by conflicting data and differing opinions, which may be strongly expressed.

Some studies have shown no benefit of androgen ablation combined with radiotherapy[4,8]. Other studies of neoadjuvant androgen ablation combined with external beam radiotherapy seem to show some benefit in terms of disease-free interval but no difference in overall survival[4,9]. Androgen ablation, whether used in combination or alone, significantly delayed metastases as compared with radiotherapy alone[10] and it often prolongs the suppression of the primary tumor following radiotherapy[11].

In the trial reported by Zietman[9] 471 men were randomly assigned to radiotherapy with or without androgen ablation for 16 weeks starting 8 weeks prior to radiation therapy. Despite this short exposure to androgen blockade, at 5 years the combined group had better local control (54% vs. 29%) and was more likely to be free of disease (36% vs. 15%). No difference in overall survival was observed.

The trial by Bolla and colleagues[12] had similar findings. They treated 415 men with radiotherapy and those randomized to receive goserelin were given this for a total of 3 years. The men given the combined treatment had better local control (97% vs. 76%), freedom from disease (85% vs. 48%), and, in a finding unique to this study, overall survival (79% vs. 62%). The main difference between this study and earlier trials is that other studies have compared short-term hormonal therapy, thus explaining the differences in results. Other reasons are the eligibility criteria and definition of local control in addition to a difference in the results of the radiotherapy treatment arm.

The main question here is whether the addition of androgen ablation to external beam radiotherapy is a true advance or just a rearrangement of existing approaches. The effect of androgen ablation on local control, disease-free survival and overall survival is well documented and this treatment alone without radiotherapy may be just as efficacious.

Conclusions

The many recent changes in the therapeutic approach to the management of locally advanced prostate cancer are challenging and exciting for the urologist but they can be bewildering for our patients. This chapter does not attempt to be a comprehensive review of hormonal treatment but rather an overview.

The evaluation of new treatment modalities poses a big problem because long-term follow up is required during which time clinical practice has often changed. The unpredictable course of the disease, classification of response and the need to include a large number of patients to attain a statistical significant difference also leads to difficulties.

Until the results of some of the ongoing trials are available we are unable to advise our patients as to which is the best form of treatment. Many men with prostate cancer are now well informed and it seems sensible to share the controversies with them as it is difficult to advise a patient categorically that he will not benefit from early treatment or MAB as clinical trials may well hide a few patients for whom the benefit is substantial. The approach to androgen deprivation may be to select a regimen which balances maximum quality of life against the side effects of androgen deprivation. Studies are underway on immunotherapy, growth factors and chemotherapy as an adjuvant to hormonal therapy and we await these with interest.

References

1. Beynon LL, Chisholm GD. The stable state is not an objective response in hormone-escaped carcinoma of the prostate. *BJU* 1984;**56**:702–705.
2. Veterans Administration Cooperative Urological Research Group. Treatment and survival of patients with cancer of the prostate. *Surg Gynecol Obstet* 1967;**124**:1011–1011.
3. Byar DP. The Veterans Administration Cooperative Research Group's studies of cancer of the prostate. *Cancer* 1973;**32**:1126–1130.
4. Sarosdy MF. Do we have a rational treatment plan for stage D-1 carcinoma of the prostate? *World J Urol* 1990;**8**:27–33.
5. Garrick MB. Hormonal therapy in the management of prostate cancer: from Huggins to the present. *Urology* 1997;**49**(suppl 3A):5–15.
6. The Medical Research Council Prostate Cancer Working Party Investigators Group. Immediate versus deferred treatment for advanced prostatic cancer: initial results of the Medical Research Council Trial. *BJU* 1997;**79**:235–246.
7. Neglia WJ, Hussey DH, Johnson DE. Megavoltage radiation therapy for carcinoma of the prostate. *Int J Radiat Oncol Biol Phys* 1977;**2**:873–883.
8. Taylor WJ, Richardson RG, Beynon LL. Radiation therapy for localised prostate cancer. *Cancer* 1988;**43**:1123–1127.
9. Zietmann AL, Prince EA, Nakfoor BM, Shipley WU. Neoadjuvant androgen suppression with radiation in the management of locally advanced adenocarcinoma of the prostate: experimental and clinical results. *Urology* 1997;**49**(suppl 3A):74–83.
10. Fellows GJ, Clark PB, Beynon LL *et al.* Treatment of advanced localised prostate cancer by orchiectomy, radiotherapy or combined treatment: a Medical Research Council study. *BJU* 1992;**70**:304–309.
11. Schroder FH. What is new in endocrine therapy of prostatic cancer? In:Newling DWW, Jones WG (eds). *EORTS Genitourinary Group monograph 7. Prostate cancer and testicular cancer.* Wiley-Liss, New York, 1990, pp. 45–52.
12. Bolla M, Gonzalez D, Warde P. Improved survival in patients with locally advanced prostate cancer treated with radiotherapy and goserelin. *N Engl J Med* 1997;**337**:295–300.

17 Treatment of metastatic prostate cancer

Algorithm

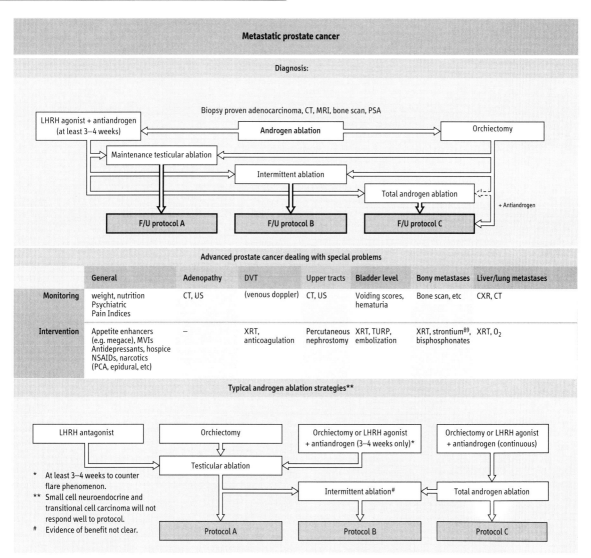

Metastatic prostate cancer

Diagnosis:

Biopsy proven adenocarcinoma, CT, MRI, bone scan, PSA

LHRH agonist + antiandrogen (at least 3–4 weeks)	Androgen ablation	Orchiectomy

Maintenance testicular ablation

Intermittent ablation

Total androgen ablation

+ Antiandrogen

F/U protocol A | F/U protocol B | F/U protocol C

Advanced prostate cancer dealing with special problems

	General	Adenopathy	DVT	Upper tracts	Bladder level	Bony metastases	Liver/lung metastases
Monitoring	weight, nutrition Psychiatric Pain Indices	CT, US	(venous doppler)	CT, US	Voiding scores, hematuria	Bone scan, etc	CXR, CT
Intervention	Appetite enhancers (e.g. megace), MVIs Antidepressants, hospice NSAIDs, narcotics (PCA, epidural, etc)	–	XRT, anticoagulation	Percutaneous nephrostomy	XRT, TURP, embolization	XRT, strontium^{89}, bisphosphonates	XRT, O$_2$

Typical androgen ablation strategies**

LHRH antagonist	Orchiectomy	Orchiectomy or LHRH agonist + antiandrogen (3–4 weeks only)*	Orchiectomy or LHRH agonist + antiandrogen (continuous)

Testicular ablation

Intermittent ablation#

Total androgen ablation

Protocol A | Protocol B | Protocol C

*   At least 3–4 weeks to counter flare phenomenon.
** Small cell neuroendocrine and transitional cell carcinoma will not respond well to protocol.
\# Evidence of benefit not clear.

Metastatic prostate cancer contd.

Follow up protocol A

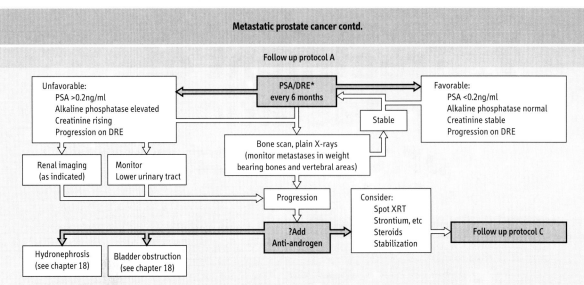

*   Add alkaline phosphatase, creatinine, periodic upper tract imaging.
    Due to the long-term risk of osteoporosis, bone density measurements should be obtained prior to initiation of androgen ablation and periodically throughout treatment. Supplementation with bisphosphonates may be appropriate.

Follow up protocol B – intermittent ablation

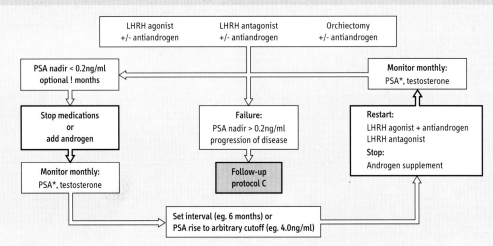

*Add alkaline phosphatase, creatinine, periodic upper tract imaging.
 Due to the long-term risk of osteoporosis, bone density measurements should be obtained prior to initiation of androgen ablation and periodically throughout treatment. Supplementation with bisphosphonates may be appropriate.

Metastatic prostate cancer contd.

Follow up protocol C – total androgen ablation

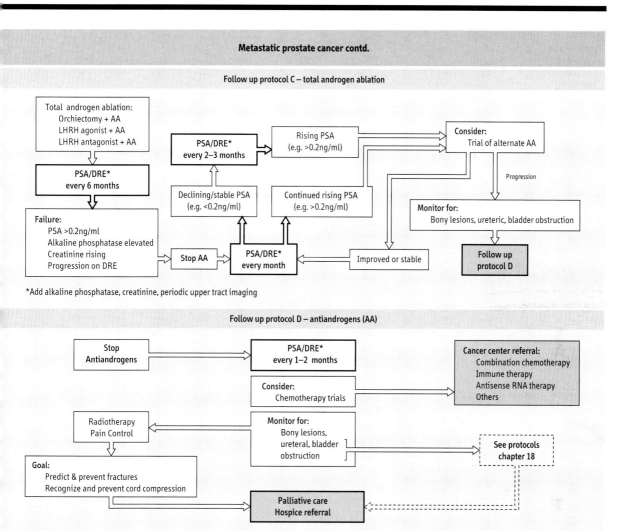

*Add alkaline phosphatase, creatinine, periodic upper tract imaging

Follow up protocol D – antiandrogens (AA)

*Add alkaline phosphatase, creatinine, periodic upper tract imaging

17.1 Endocrine therapy

F Rabbani and M E Gleave

Introduction

Androgens and the prostate gland

The male sex hormones are collectively known as androgens, which is derived from the Greek andros (man) and gennan (to produce). For millennia, Man has been aware of the more obvious effects of removing the testes from animals, including his own species. Reference to castration is found in mythology and certain religions, used as an instrument of punishment and revenge in many societies[1]. Castration of young boys up to the end of 19th century in Europe preserved the voice of popular male sopranos (castratos)[2], and served to guarantee the supply of eunuchs for guard duty in harems and the Forbidden City up to the beginning of the 20th century[2,3]. Aristotle was the first to make castration the subject of enquiry, describing its effect in considerable detail and recognizing that the testes were essential for the virility and fertility of an animal[2]. The first experimental demonstration that the testes contributed an endocrine factor to the bloodstream was made by John Hunter in 1794 when he showed that the spur of a hen would undergo masculine development if transplanted into the leg of a cock[4]. The actual isolation and characterization of naturally occurring androgens in the 1930s was therefore the crowning point of a process of observation and discovery which started at an early time in history[5]. The cellular and molecular actions of androgens have been further clarified over the past two decades.

Testosterone is the principal circulating androgen in man, and its presence is necessary for normal development of the penis, scrotum, testicles and male secondary sex characteristics at puberty. Testicular androgens are critical for prostate gland formation in the embryo and for normal function throughout adulthood. Furthermore, the ability of normal or cancerous prostate cells to produce prostate-specific antigen (PSA) is regulated by androgens. Testosterone has long been implicated as a possible promoter of prostatic cancer growth and, along with aging, is one of the most significant etiologic factors associated with the development of prostate cancer. Prostate cancer does not develop in eunuchs or other men castrated prior to puberty[3], and latent prostate cancer is less frequent among men with cirrhosis who have lower testosterone levels. Furthermore, differences in testosterone levels have been noted between low risk (Orientals, Nigerian blacks) and high risk (African American blacks) groups, paralleling the marked racial differences in prostate cancer incidence, with a 44-fold increased risk in black American males compared with oriental men living in Japan[6].

The ablation of testicular function for the palliative treatment of prostate cancer was first attempted in the 1930s with radio-orchiectomy[7]. This proved less effective than surgical orchiectomy, introduced about a decade later by Huggins and Hodges[8], which was subsequently to become the 'gold standard'. There is no other treatment that equals or surpasses androgen ablation in checking the growth of prostate cancer and reducing tumor volume in 80% of patients. However, for reasons that remain incompletely defined, the cell death process induced by androgen ablation fails to eliminate the entire malignant cell population. The result is inevitable progression to a state of androgen-independent (AI) tumor growth.

Over the past two decades, numerous alternatives to surgical castration have been developed. Drugs affecting the hypothalamic production of luteinizing hormone-releasing hormone (LHRH agonists) and those blocking the peripheral effects of androgens (steroidal and non-steroidal antiandrogens) have been used either alone or in various combinations to achieve medical castration. Many questions remain regarding their differing efficacies, toxicities and costs and, indeed, whether or not we have yet attained a new 'gold standard'. This chapter will discuss the issues of tumor regulation, androgen independence and androgen deprivation strategies. We will also review newer strategies of hormonal therapy aimed at improving quality of life.

Androgen-mediated tumor regulation

Mechanism of androgen action

Testosterone is the principal male sex hormone secreted by the testes, and circulates in association with two major plasma proteins, sex-hormone binding globulin (SHBG) and albumin[9]. Only 2% of the testosterone is unbound and available for diffusion into the target cell where it is converted to dihydrotestosterone (DHT) by the enzyme 5α reductase[10]. Two isoforms of the enzyme have been identified, type 1 which is found in skin, prostatic epithelium and to a lesser extent in stroma, and type 2 which predominates in prostatic stromal tissue[11,12]. Dihydrotestosterone binds with high affinity and specificity to an androgen-receptor protein in the cytoplasm causing its dissociation from heat-shock proteins (transformation) and subsequent translocation into the target cell nucleus.

The androgen receptor is a ligand-dependent transcription factor structurally organized into three major functional domains: a carboxyl (C)-terminal steroid binding domain, an amino (N)-terminal region involved in the activation of transcription, and an intermediate DNA-binding domain[13,14]. The latter contains two zinc-finger motifs, each containing a molecule of zinc. The first zinc-finger specifies the particular androgen response element located in genomic DNA adjacent to target genes to which the androgen receptor binds. The second zinc-finger contains a receptor dimerization region. Specific gene activation by androgens depends upon the binding of a homodimer of two androgen receptor molecules to two asymmetrical nucleotide sequences of 6 basepairs separated by a 3 basepair spacer, termed androgen responsive elements. Carried to completion, this complex receptor-DNA binding reaction triggers a cascade of transcriptional events underlying a given biological response. (Figure. 17.1.1.)

Until recently, the mechanisms of steroid receptor action appeared relatively straightforward, initiated by binding of DHT to the steroid binding domain of the AR, with subsequent binding of the activated receptor to the ARE of specific genes to regulate transcription. Unfortunately, it is becoming increasingly apparent that the process of steroid receptor-regulated transcription is much more complicated and is also affected by protein–protein interactions involving numerous co-regulators[15]. Steroid (and other nuclear) receptors can inhibit or enhance transcription by interacting with an

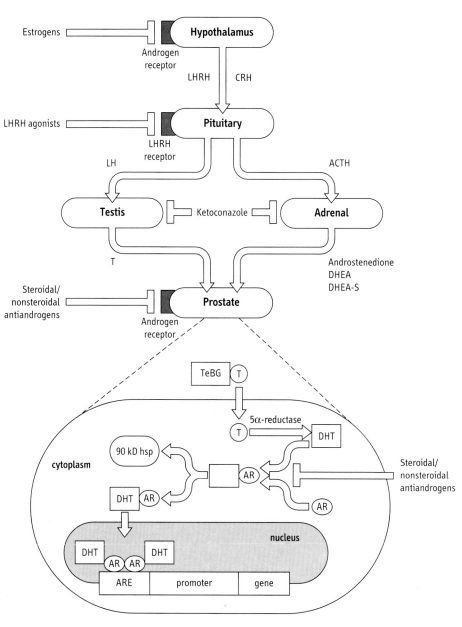

Fig. 17.1.1 Pathways of endocrine control of gonadal function. (LHRH = luteinizing hormone releasing hormone; CRH = corticotropin releasing hormone; LH = luteinizing hormone; ACTH = adrenocorticotropic hormone; T = testosterone; DHEA = dehydroepiandrosterone; DHEA-S = dehydro-epiandrosterone-sulfate; TeBG = testosterone binding globulin; DHT = dihydrotestosterone; AR = androgen receptor; hsp = heat shock protein; ARE = androgen response element)

array of putative co-activators or co-repressors, some of which may play a role in loss of androgen regulated gene expression that occurs with progression to androgen independence.

Biological effects

Androgenic regulation of target tissues is characterized by three broadly defined responses: a positive initiation phase, a negative feedback response phase and apoptosis[16]. In the presence of androgen, undifferentiated or involuted cells initiate new rounds of DNA synthesis and cell proliferation (i.e. androgen sensitivity), an example of positive gene regulation by androgens. When the tissue becomes normal in size, an inhibitory mechanism comes into play, which shuts down DNA synthesis and cell proliferation, a consequence of negative-gene regulation by androgens. Withdrawal of androgen induces apoptosis, a form of programmed cell death, in normal, benign hyperplastic, and malignant prostatic epithelial cells. Castration-induced apoptosis is a manifestation of androgen dependence[17–19].

Apoptotic cell death is distinctly different from necrotic cell death and involves a sequence of distinct events characterized morphologically by shrunken cells with condensed and fragmented nuclei (apoptotic bodies) and biochemically by preferential intranucleosomal DNA digestion resulting in 'DNA laddering' patterns[17]. Most interestingly, apoptosis is a 'genetic suicide' process that requires activation of a series of androgen-repressed genes along with Ca^{2+}-dependent endonucleases. These genes include c-fos and c-myc proto-oncogenes, TGF-β, and glutathione transferase. One particular gene, testosterone-repressed prostatic message (TRPM-2), is upregulated dramatically post-castration in a temporal pattern reflecting the period of maximal apoptosis, and may indeed represent an adaptive or protective mechanism by a dying cell to help abort apoptosis[18]. Another gene upregulated post-castration is BCL-2, a proto-oncogene believed to inhibit apoptosis and progression to androgen independence[19]. McDonnell et al.[19] demonstrated that BCL-2 expression is absent in most androgen dependent prostate cancers, but is present in virtually all androgen independent cancers. Other genes, like the tumor suppressor gene p53, may help promote apoptosis in cells that have sustained DNA damage[17]. Improved understanding of the molecular basis of apoptosis and progression to androgen independence will provide future therapeutic targets aimed at maximizing apoptotic cell death with androgen ablation.

Androgen independent progression

Data from animal studies[20] and observations of Chinese eunuchs[3] illustrate that normal prostatic epithelial cells undergo apoptotic regression and do not develop the ability to regenerate and grow in an androgen-depleted environment. In contrast, progression to androgen independence nearly always occurs following androgen ablation therapy for patients with prostatic carcinoma. A detailed discussion of the hypotheses proposed to define androgen independent progression is beyond the scope of this chapter, and reviewed in more detail elsewhere[20,21]. The clonal selection theory emphasizes tumor heterogeneity with a spectrum of androgen sensitivity; following castration, androgen dependent cells undergo apoptosis, while androgen independent cells survive and ultimately progress. The adaptation theory assumes the presence of androgen regulated stem cells with a capacity for adaptation and self-renewal in an androgen depleted environment. A third hypothesis emphasizes the importance of small amounts of residual androgens that selectively stimulates clones of androgen-sensitive cells. However, animal data[20,21] and clinical studies (see below, combined androgen blockade) do not support this hypothesis since blockage of adrenal androgens is ineffective in preventing progression, which suggests that non-androgen growth regulatory factors are more important. A fourth possibility involves production of mutant constitutively active androgen receptors capable of DNA binding and gene activation in the absence of androgen binding of their steroid binding region.

Progression to androgen-independence is a complex process that likely involves both selection and outgrowth of pre-existing clones of androgen independent cells (clonal selection) as well as adaptive up-regulation of genes that help the cancer cells survive and grow after androgen ablation (adaptation). These two mechanisms share an important characteristic – that prostate cancers are heterogenous tumors composed of various subpopulations of cells that respond differently to androgen withdrawal therapy. Indeed, this tumor heterogeneity may reflect either multifocal origin, adaptation to environmental stimuli, and/or genetic instability of the initial cancer; this heterogeneity, in turn, provides the basic requirements for androgen independent progression to occur because of clonal expansion or adaptive mechanisms in subpopulations of cells.

Androgen withdrawal therapy

Since the Nobel Prize winning reports by Dr Charles Huggins[8] in 1941, castration has remained the cornerstone of management for advanced prostate cancer. No other treatment exists that equals or surpasses androgen ablation in controlling the growth of prostate cancer. Until recently, androgen withdrawal therapy was restricted to a choice between bilateral orchiectomy and diethylstilbestrol. When these measures failed, adrenalectomy was occasionally tried, seldom yielding an objective response[22]. The advent of antiandrogens and luteinizing hormone releasing hormone (LHRH) agonists increased the options available for suppressing the influence of androgens on the growth of prostate cancer (Table 17.1.1).

The normal pathways of the endocrine control of gonadal function are summarized in Figure 17.1.1. Testicular synthesis of testosterone accounts for 90% or more of the dihydrotestosterone formed in the prostate, the remainder being derived from the weak adrenal androgens androstenedione and dehydroepiandrosterone, and dietary sources[23]. Testosterone provides a negative feedback signal to the hypothalamus regulating the secretion of LHRH and thereby of luteinizing hormone (LH). Negative feedback regulation of the hypothalamus by testosterone also involves the release of endogenous opioid peptides that act as inhibitory factors to suppress the intra-hypothalamic release of catecholamines[24].

Surgical castration

Bilateral orchiectomy has been the gold standard of hormonal therapy of metastatic prostate cancer with a response rate of 60–80%. Advantages include low cost, guaranteed compliance, rapidity of action in producing castrate levels of testosterone, and low morbidity. Lin and associates[25] found that the serum testosterone reaches castrate levels in 3 to 12 hours with a mean of 8.6 hours. Disadvantages include psychological trauma, irreversibility, low risk of infection and hematoma, and the general side effects of castration, including hot flushes in 40%, loss of libido and potency, and bone and muscle loss over time. Hot flushes result from loss of negative feedback regulation of the hypothalamus with a decrease in intra-hypothalamic testosterone-dependent opioid peptide and an increase in catecholamines[24]. Psychological trauma can be minimized by subcapsular orchiectomy[26].

Medical castration

Several types of agents are capable of inducing castrate levels of testosterone, usually through suppression of LH release from the pituitary gland.

Estrogens

Diethylstilbestrol (DES) results in castrate testosterone levels through negative feedback inhibition of hypothalamic androgen receptors with suppression of LHRH and LH. DES also has a peripheral action, increasing testosterone-binding globulin (TeBG) with a resultant decrease in free serum testosterone. DES is the least expensive of the synthetic oestrogens and castrate testosterone levels are achieved at doses of 1 mg daily[27]. The second Veterans Administration Cooperative Urological Research Group (VACURG) trial demonstrated that 1.0 mg daily was equivalent to 5 mg daily in delaying progression and was

associated with less cardiovascular toxicity[27]. Advantages of DES include its low cost, reduced psychological trauma, and hot flushes compared with orchiectomy. Disadvantages of DES include thromboembolic (6.9%) and cardiovascular (5.0%) complications, edema (15.8%), nausea and vomiting (15.8%), gynecomastia (48.5%), and loss of libido and potency, requiring withdrawal of treatment in 12% at a dose of 3 mg daily[28,29]. The cardiovascular side effects, which are significant at doses of 3 mg or greater daily, are due to fluid retention, changes in plasma lipids, and hypercoagulability due to increased platelet aggregation and decreased levels of plasma antithrombin III[30].

LHRH agonists

LHRH is a decapeptide produced by the hypothalamus that stimulates the secretion of LH by binding to LHRH receptors on the cell membrane of the anterior pituitary. LHRH agonists are produced by substitution of various amino acids for the glycine in the 6 position. This substitution increases the stability and binding affinity, thereby increasing potency 50 to 100-fold. The pituitary is normally stimulated by the pulsatile release of LHRH from the hypothalamus; when this periodicity is effaced by continuous administration of exogenous LHRH agonist, the pituitary becomes refractory to hypothalamic regulation. Continuous administration of LHRH agonist produces a biphasic response with an initial rise in LH and testosterone, termed the 'flare phenomenon', followed in 1 to 2 weeks by a fall in LH and testosterone[29,31]. Decreases in LH and testosterone result from the down-regulation and decrease in number of LHRH receptors as a result of the receptors being continuously occupied. The serum testosterone is suppressed into the castrate range within 3–4 weeks. The reported incidence of flare has ranged from 4–33%, with no distinction between clinical flare, consisting of precipitation of acute urinary retention, hydronephrosis or spinal cord compression, or biochemical flare[32]. The flare reaction is prevented by the initiation of therapy with cyproterone acetate or DES 1 week prior to the LHRH agonist, or blocked by non-steroidal antiandrogens prior to or concurrently with the LHRH agonist[32]. Although LHRH agonists appear equivalent to DES[29] and orchiectomy[33,34], the presence of the flare and 'acute on chronic' reactions (see below) questions the efficacy of LHRH agonist monotherapy.

Available LHRH agonists include buserelin acetate, triptorelin, leuprolide acetate, and goserelin acetate. The latter two agents are available as depot formulations: leuprolide 3.75 mg or 7.5 mg IM every 4 weeks and goserelin 3.6 mg SC every 4 weeks. Three month (10.8 mg goserelin[35] or 22.5 mg leuprolide[36]) and 4 month (30 mg leuprolide[37]) depot formulations are now available. Advantages of LHRH agonists include less psychological

Table 17.1.1   Agents used for androgen deprivation

Agent	Mechanism of action	Advantages	Disadvantages
Surgical therapy Bilateral orchiectomy	Removal of testicular production of T (which is source of > 90% of DHT formed in prostate)	Low cost Compliance Rapid onset of action Low morbidity	Psychological trauma Irreversible Hot flushes (40%) Side effects of castration (loss of libido, potency, bone and muscle loss with time)
Medical therapy **Medical castration** Estrogen/diethylstilbestrol	Negative feedback inhibition of hypothalamic androgen receptors (suppression of LHRH and LH production) Increases TeBG ($\therefore \downarrow$ free serum T)	Reversible Low cost Reduced hot flushes vs. orchiectomy Less psychologic trauma vs. orchiectomy	Side effects thromboembolic/cardiovascular complications edema nausea, vomiting gynecomastia loss of libido, potency Withdrawal of therapy in 12% at 3 mg daily
LHRH agonists leuprolide acetate goserelin acetate buserelin acetate triptorelin	Down-regulation of and decrease in number of LHRH receptors ($\therefore \downarrow$ LH $\Rightarrow \downarrow$ T synthesis)	Reversible Available in depot formulations Less psychologic trauma vs. orchiectomy Lack cardiovascular complications	Transient 'flare phenomenon' Frequent hot flushes (63%) High cost 'Acute-on-chronic' phenomenon
Ketoconazole	Inhibits testicular and adrenal P-450 enzymes	Rapid onset of action (castrate T in <24 h) Useful for impending spinal cord compression)	Toxicity Adrenal suppression Hepatotoxicity
Antiandrogens **Nonsteroidal** Flutamide Nilutamide Bicalutamide	Competitive inhibition of androgen receptors on peripheral target cells	Reversible Preservation of potency in 70–80% when used as monotherapy Once daily dosing with nilutamide and bicalutamide	Decreased survival with monotherapy Gynecomastia GI upset (diarrhea, nausea, vomiting with flutamide) Idiopathic hepatocellular toxicity $\downarrow$ adaptation to darkness (nilutamide) Alcohol intolerance (nilutamide) Interstitial pneumonitis (nilutamide) Hematuria (bicalutamide)
Steroidal Cyproterone acetate Megestrol acetate	Competitive inhibition of androgen receptors on peripheral target cells Progestational activity with inhibition of gonadotropin secretion (weakened effect after 6–9 months)	Reversible Suppression of hot flushes Intermediate expense	Requires addition of DES 0.1 mg daily for continued inhibition of gonadotropin secretion Loss of libido, potency Fatigue, mood changes Slightly $\uparrow$ risk of thrombosis

T = testosterone; DHT = dihydrotestosterone; TeBG = testosterone-binding globulin; LH = luteinizing hormone; LHRH = luteinizing hormone releasing hormone

trauma than orchiectomy, good tolerance with lack of cardiovascular complications, and reversibility. Disadvantages include the flare reaction, loss of libido and potency, frequent hot flushes (63%) and high cost[33,34]. A recently recognized disadvantage, termed acute-on-chronic, refers to a biochemical and clinical phenomenon in patients who sustained surges in testosterone and LH after each injection of LHRH agonist, perhaps due to repeated mini-flare reactions[38,39].

Sarosdy *et al.* reported no difference in efficacy between the goserelin plus an antiandrogen and leuprolide and an antiandrogen in a randomized, multicenter trial that was open-labeled for LHRH analogu and double-blind for antiandrogen[40]. In this study, 813 patients were allocated 2 : 1 to goserelin 3.6 mg every 28 days or leuprolide 7.5 mg every 28 days and 1 : 1 to bicalutamide 50 mg daily or flutamide 250 mg tid. Similar rates of progression (70.9% vs. 73.3%) and death (54.3% vs. 56.8%) were reported for goserelin plus antiandrogen and leuprolide plus antiandrogen. The corresponding hazard ratios for goserelin plus antiandrogen : leuprolide plus antiandrogen were 0.99 (95% CI: 0.84–1.18, $P = 0.92$) and 0.91 (95% CI: 0.75–1.11, $P = 0.34$) for time to progression and survival, respectively. However, exploratory analysis revealed an inferior outcome with leuprolide plus flutamide compared with the other three therapies.

LHRH antagonists (e.g. cetrorelix (SB-75) and teverelix (Antarelix)) are being evaluated in pre-clinical and phase I/II studies[41–44]. LHRH antagonists will have the advantage of absence of the flare phenomenon[45]. Chronic administration results in a marked down-regulation of pituitary LHRH receptors[46,47]. While side effects, such as edema and anaphylactoid reactions secondary to histamine release[48] as well as poor solubility[49], precluded clinical use of earlier compounds, newer agents have improved water solubility, improved activity and decreased histamine release[50]. Cetrorelix, at a dose of 300 µg SC, has been shown to decrease mean serum luteinizing hormone (LH) and the follicle stimulating hormone (FSH) after 1 hour, with nadir levels at 14 hours (69% decrease) and 24 hours (54% decrease), respectively[41]. Nadir serum total and free testosterone levels were attained at 6 hours (56% decrease) and 8 hours (60% decrease), respectively. Significant symptomatic improvement in bone pain and bladder outlet obstruction with normalization of acid and alkaline phosphatase has been reported after a 6 week course of cetrorelix 500 µg SC bid in men with locally advanced or metastatic prostate cancer[42]. Another study in five stage D2 prostate cancer patients with paraplegia secondary to spinal cord compression reported regression of their neurological symptoms in all five men and resolution of cord compression in one[43]. Suppression of gonadotropins and testosterone was maintained for the duration of therapy[43]. While further study of efficacy is needed with phase III studies, these agents may be useful in treatment of prostate cancer patients in whom the flare phenomenon should be avoided.

Antiandrogens

Antiandrogens competitively inhibit the effect of androgens peripherally by binding to androgen receptor (AR) binding sites in target cells. Receptor translocation to the nucleus or DNA binding is prevented with resultant inhibition of androgen regulated gene transcription and protein synthesis.

Non-steroidal antiandrogens. The non-steroidal, or pure, antiandrogens, which include flutamide, nilutamide and bicalutamide, act only at peripheral target tissues and have no direct gonadotrophic or progestational effects. However, competitive inhibition of androgen receptors in the hypothalamus leads to inhibition of the negative feedback by androgens on LH release with rising LH and testosterone levels and Leydig cell hyperplasia. Increased peripheral aromatization of testosterone leads to increased plasma oestradiol, which causes painful gynecomastia. Due to the competitive nature of the inhibition peripherally, the increased serum testosterone can partially negate the antiandrogenic effect, which permits preservation of potency in 70–80% of patients[51,52].

The gradual rise in serum testosterone raises concern regarding the efficacy of pure antiandrogens as monotherapy[53]. This point, however, is controversial as one study of 20 patients receiving flutamide revealed a rise in serum testosterone to 1.5 times normal within 3–6 months, which then reverted to normal within 9–12 months[54]. Flutamide has been found to have similar efficacy to DES in some prospective randomized trials[54,55]. More recently, Chang *et al.* reported on an Eastern Cooperative Oncology Group (ECOG) double-blind, randomized study in which 48 patients with stage D2 prostate cancer received DES 1 mg tid and 44 received flutamide 250 mg tid[56]. The overall response rate was similar (DES, 62% and flutamide, 50%). However, time to treatment failure and survival were longer with DES compared with flutamide [26.4 vs. 9.7 months ($P = 0.016$) and 43.2 vs. 28.5 months ($P = 0.040$), respectively].

While bicalutamide (Casodex, ICI 176,334) has peripheral selectivity in rats, this is not the case in human studies. Indeed, two of three randomized phase III studies comparing bicalutamide 50 mg daily to castration revealed it to be inferior to castration with respect to time to treatment failure and time to progression[57]. Higher doses of bicalutamide have been studied and a greater decline of PSA has been noted with doses of up to 200 mg daily with a slightly higher response rate[58]. Further responses have been seen with 200 mg daily used following failure of flutamide in combination with castration and following a flutamide withdrawal response. Further benefit is unlikely beyond doses of 200 mg daily. Data on the use of nilutamide as monotherapy is very limited[59]. In view of these findings non-steroidal anti-androgens should not be used as monotherapy but only in conjunction with surgical or medical castration.

Because of its short half-life of 5–6 hours, flutamide requires tid dosing (250 mg tid) which can reduce compliance. The longer half-life of nilutamide (Anandron, 45 h), and bicalutamide (Casodex, 5 days) permits once daily dosing which improves compliance. Side effects of flutamide and its active metabolite, hydroxyflutamide, include gynecomastia in 61%, diarrhea in 5–26%, and nausea and vomiting[51,52]. Idiosyncratic hepatocellular toxicity resulting in death may occur. Side effects of nilutamide include decreased adaptation to darkness in 33%, nausea in 25%, alcohol intolerance in 20% and case reports of interstitial pneumonitis[59]. Bicalutamide is better tolerated than flutamide with low toxicity including breast tenderness in approximately 32–36%, gynecomastia in 25%, hot flushes in 9%, and nausea, vomiting and diarrhea in 2–5%[60]. Recently, the flutamide withdrawal syndrome has been described, with a 50% decrease in serum PSA in 28% of patients, with median duration of 13 weeks[61,62]. This syndrome is not limited to flutamide and has been reported with both steroidal and non-steroidal anti-androgens, raising the possibility of a role for AR mutations and antiandrogens in tumor progression.

Comparison of non-steroidal antiandrogens has revealed similar efficacy when combined with an LHRH agonist, but different toxicity profiles. Recently, Shellhammer et al. reported on a randomized, double-blind, multicenter trial with a two-by-two factorial design where 813 patients were randomized 1 : 1 to bicalutamide 50 mg daily and flutamide 250 mg tid and 2 : 1 to goserelin acetate 3.6 mg every 28 days and leuprolide 7.5 mg every 28 days[63]. There was no difference in median time to progression and death (97 and 180 weeks for bicalutamide and LHRH agonist vs. 77 and 148 weeks for flutamide and LHRH agonist, respectively). The hazard ratios (bicalutamide plus LHRH agonist flutamide plus LHRH agonist) for time to progression was 0.93 (95% CI: 0.79–1.10, $P = 0.41$) and that for survival time was 0.87 (95% CI: 0.72–1.05, $P = 0.15$). Patients receiving bicalutamide and LHRH agonist had a higher incidence of hematuria compared with those receiving flutamide and LHRH agonist (12% vs. 6%, $P = 0.007$), while patients receiving flutamide and LHRH agonist had a higher incidence of diarrhoea compared with those receiving bicalutamide in LHRH agonist (26% vs. 12%, $P = 0.001$).

Steroidal antiandrogens. In addition to their anti-androgenic activity at peripheral receptors, steroidal anti-androgens possess progestational activity and inhibit gonadotropin secretion, thereby reducing serum testosterone levels[64]. The predominant mechanism of action is competitive inhibition of androgen receptors at the level of the target cells. Due to the weak progestational activity, monotherapy will suppress gonadotropin release only partially with weakening of the anti-gonadotropic effect after 6 to 9 months[64]. The two principal steroidal antiandrogens are cyproterone acetate and megestrol acetate with the former found to be more effective[65].

The combination of low-dose cyproterone acetate (50 mg bid) and mini-dose DES (0.1 mg daily) achieves potent androgen ablation, reducing whole tissue DHT, nuclear DHT and nuclear androgen receptor by 90–96% at one-third the cost of LHRH analogs[64–66]. Serum testosterone decreases to castrate levels within 48 h and the addition of mini-dose DES avoids the risk of 'progestational escape' associated with cyproterone acetate monotherapy. In a randomized study comparing DES 3 mg daily and megestrol acetate 120 mg/d plus mini-dose DES 0.1 mg/d, Venner reported no difference in response rate and survival[67]. However, DES 3 mg daily was less well tolerated with 20/54 patients withdrawing compared with 1/56 treated with megestrol acetate plus mini-dose DES; cardiovascular toxicity was higher in the DES arm (33% vs. 7%, $P = 0.001$).

Advantages of steroidal antiandrogens include reversibility and suppression of hot flushes, and intermediate expense. Side effects include uniform loss of libido and potency, fatigue, and mood changes with depression. There is a relatively low risk of cardiovascular toxicity due to the increased level of anti-thrombin III and increased fibrinolytic activity[64].

Prognostic markers of response to androgen withdrawal therapy

The discussion of prognostic factors is important to 1) determine factors which alter outcome; 2) to give more intensive therapy to those with a better prognosis while limiting toxicity in those with a poor prognosis; 3) to design properly randomized controlled trials to minimize bias between two different treatment arms.

Serum PSA

Serum PSA is very useful as a predictor of response to therapy[68]. Pre-treatment serum PSA levels correlate with extent of disease on bone scan[69] and has been shown to be a predictor of response to androgen deprivation[70]. Killian et al.[71] found that the PSA correlated with tumor recurrence rate and inversely with time to progression. Stamey et al.[72] found that almost all treated patients had an initial response with a rapid decrease in serum PSA in the first 6 months, into the normal range in 31% and undetectable in 9%. Furthermore, serum PSA at 6 months post-treatment is indicative of which patients will have a prolonged response. Serum PSA nadir between 24 and 32 weeks after androgen withdrawal therapy stratifies patients into good and poor prognostic groups[73,74]. Bruchovsky and associates[73] found that the PSA nadir was attained at 32 weeks with PSA falling below 4 μg/l in 70% of patients with advanced prostate cancer. Serum PSA levels > 4 μg/l between 24–32 weeks of therapy was associated with a median survival of 18 months compared with 40 months with a serum PSA below 4 μg/l. A similar difference in median survival (42 vs. 10 months) has been reported by other investigators with nadir PSA less than or greater than 4 μg/l[74]. In the EORTC trial 30853, a rise in PSA was the earliest and most common (45%) sign of progression[75]. Other investigators have also found that in almost all patients with tumor progression, serum PSA elevation pre-dates clinical recurrence by a lead-time of 6 to 12 months[71,74,75]. Thus it is clinically useful to monitor serial PSA levels in patients treated with androgen ablation. The pattern of response can distinguish patients with favourable from unfavourable outcomes.

Nature and burden of metastatic disease

Although there is little doubt that progressive multistep genetic changes, with either deletion of tumor suppressor genes or overexpression of oncogenes, contribute to malignant transformation[76], it is equally clear that the stromal microenvironment may either inhibit or accelerate the emergence and rate of progression of established carcinomas[77,78]. Prostate cancer selectively spreads to the cancellous bones of the axial skeleton, where it is the only malignancy consistently to produce osteoblastic lesions. Interaction between prostate cancer cells and stroma of various organs influences the patterns of dissemination seen in patients with advanced prostate cancer. Bidirectional stimulatory paracrine pathways between prostate cancer and bone stromal cells lead to selective spread of prostate cancer to bone with production of osteoblastic reactions[79].

Androgen withdrawal therapy is more effective in inducing regression of primary prostatic tumors and soft tissue metastases than the more lethal, skeletal component of the disease. In a series of 51 patients treated with cyproterone acetate plus low-dose DES, 41 of 49 patients (84%) with evaluable soft tissue disease (local and metastatic) responded with reduction in tumor volume[66]. In contrast, significant improvement occurred in only 13 (27%) of the 48 initially abnormal bone scans. This difference illustrates the relative resistance of skeletal metastases to androgen withdrawal therapy, as has also been noted by other investigators[80,81].

Patients with fewer than six metastatic deposits on their bone scan have a significantly better 2 year survival than those with more extensive disease[82]. Both the NCI Intergroup study[83] and the EORTC 30853 trial[84] showed that the number and location of bone metastases has a strong effect on treatment outcome. The good prognosis group, those with five or fewer metastases confined to the axial skeleton, and patients with good performance status, tended to derive the most benefit from treatment.

Other prognostic factors

The grade and ploidy of the primary tumor are important predictors of cancer behavior[85]. A low pre-treatment serum testosterone level (< 300 ng/dl)[82], the presence of anemia (hemoglobin < 85 g/l) and an elevated alkaline phosphatase (>1.25 times the upper limit of normal) are all considered important negative prognostic indicators[81,86]. Age and performance status have been identified in some studies as significant clinical parameters. Wilson et al.[87] found that the prognosis was worse for patients younger than 60 or older than 80 than in the 60–80-year-old age range. However, a number of other studies including the EORTC trials have not confirmed this[69,88]. Chodak and associates[89] identified performance status as a significant prognosticator of survival; however, the EORTC trials[88] identified this as the most important predictor of survival in advanced, non-metastatic disease but not in metastatic disease.

Controversial issues surrounding hormonal therapy in advanced prostate cancer

Up to 80% of patients with stage D_2 disease have objective responses following surgical or medical castration, with median progression-free survival of 12 to 33 months and median overall survival of 23 to 37 months[90,91]. However, for reasons that remain poorly defined, the cell death process induced by androgen ablation fails to eliminate the entire malignant cell population and accelerates the rate of progression of prostate cancer to an androgen-independent state[92]. Over the past 20 years, most efforts have focused on maximizing the degree of androgen ablation through combined androgen blockade (CAB) to inhibit or block both testicular and adrenal androgens. Another important issue surrounds timing of therapy, and whether immediate therapy prolongs survival compared with delaying hormonal therapy until the patient becomes symptomatic. More recently, investigators are focusing on the impact of treatment on quality of life issues to identify treatments that alter quality of life less without compromising efficacy.

217

Is combined androgen blockade superior to castration alone?

While the concept of combined androgen blockade (CAB) dates back to a report by Huggins in 1945[93], it remains a controversial topic even after 15 years of randomized controlled trials. The concept is supported by data showing that patients, following castration, can have significant amounts of residual DHT in prostate tissue, implicating the adrenals as a source of DHT[94]. Geller *et al.*[95] quantified prostate DHT concentrations in castrated patients and those treated with CAB, and reported that tissue DHT levels were 0.32 ng/g lower with CAB, a difference that is statistically significant.

Randomized clinical trials

Following the initial report by Labrie *et al.*[96], numerous randomized trials have been conducted with mixed results. Difficulty in synthesizing the results of these trials arises from heterogeneity in type of castration (medical vs. surgical) and type of antiandrogen (steroidal vs. nonsteroidal), as well as possible differences in study design, randomization procedures, assessment of treatment outcome, statistical evaluation and data maturity[97]. Confusion has also arisen from misinterpretation of negative studies, which have insufficient power to refute the positive trials and from early reports of interim analyses, which revealed no statistical significance[98].

The NCI Intergroup 0036 study[83] randomized 603 patients with previously untreated stage D2 prostate cancer to treatment with leuprolide in combination with either placebo or flutamide. The CAB arm had a longer progression-free survival (16.5 vs. 13.9 months; $P = 0.039$) and an increase in median length of survival (35.6 vs. 28.3 months; $P = 0.035$). In patients with good performance status and minimal disease, the median survival in the CAB arm was longer (51.9 vs. 39.6 months)[99]; the number of patients in this subgroup was too small, however, for these differences to reach statistical significance. Criticisms of this study correctly point out that daily leuprolide may be inferior to orchiectomy because of compliance, that the inferior results with the leuprolide only arm may be due to disease flare, and that the effect of CAB may be limited to patients with good performance status and minimal disease. Earlier studies had, however, found LHRH agonists to be equivalent to DES[29] and orchiectomy[33,34]. While the possibility of disease flare could not be ruled out, the EORTC 30853 trial[84] comparing goserelin acetate and flutamide vs. orchiectomy also showed a significant increase in time to subjective progression (87 vs. 52 weeks), objective progression (133 vs. 85 weeks) and duration of survival (34.4 vs. 27.1 months) with CAB. Again, the benefit was most prominent in those with WHO performance status 0 (death hazard ratio 0.67) and <5 bone metastases (death hazard ratio 0.60).

Ongoing debate regarding the superiority of CAB prompted the largest trial to date for advanced prostate cancer, randomizing 1387 patients to orchiectomy and either flutamide or placebo, which recently reported no differences in survival in any subgroup[100]. One explanation for the differences between this study and the earlier NCI Intergroup study[83] is that untreated flare with LHRH agonist monotherapy has an adverse effect on overall survival. One possible reason for the negative results of this SWOG study despite positive results of NCI Intergroup study[83,99] is that LHRH agonist monotherapy is inferior to orchiectomy and CAB in studies with sufficient power because of the flare[33,34] and/or acute-on-chronic[38,39] phenomena described earlier.

Meta-analyses

A meta-analysis is a quantitative review of all randomized trials assessing an intervention, which quantifies results of individual studies and combines results across studies. While not a substitute for a properly performed randomized trial, a meta-analysis will permit analysis of a larger group of patients. It should include all studies, whether published or not. The difference in outcome is measured separately for each study and the weighted average over all studies is calculated. The advantage of a meta-analysis is that the results of individual studies are graphically shown to determine consistency between studies and to identify outliers. These outliers may provide information regarding certain subgroups with a better prognosis. Also, the large sample size with a meta-analysis allows identification of a small difference in outcome and subgroup analysis. Potential pitfalls of a meta-analysis include heterogeneity between trials in dosing, interventions, compliance, follow up and reliability of data. Because of this heterogeneity, average results may not be representative of the results of individual trials, and treatment effects may be masked in certain subgroups. Finally, the results of a meta-analysis may be inconclusive due to lack of data or follow up.

Seven randomized double-blind trials involving 1191 stage D prostate cancer patients (1056 eligible patients) randomized to orchiectomy and placebo or nilutamide were included in a meta-analysis by Bertagna *et al.*[101]. In the CAB arm there was a greater degree of complete or partial regression (50% vs. 33%; $P < 0.001$), more frequent resolution of bone pain and normalization of prostatic acid phosphatase and alkaline phosphatase, and the odds of disease progression were significantly reduced (odds ratio 0.84; $P = 0.05$). Odds of death were reduced (odds ratio 0.90), but this did not attain statistical significance. The number of deaths/patients in the two arms are 321/506 and 333/550 for the placebo and nilutamide arms, respectively, suggesting that further follow up may be necessary. In a meta-analysis of 22 randomized trials evaluating CAB by the Prostate Cancer Trialists' Collaborative Group, 90% of randomized data from studies starting before December 1989 were included[102]. Median follow up was 40 months during which 3283/5710 patients (57%) died. Life-table analysis revealed no significant improvement in 5 year survival (22.8% for castration vs. 26.2% for CAB). Logrank time-to-death analyses found no significant heterogeneity among subgroups according to type of castration (orchiectomy vs. LHRH agonist) or type of anti-androgen (nilutamide vs. flutamide vs. cyproterone acetate).

The issue of CAB has been most definitively addressed by the Intergroup Study 0105, designed to compare overall survival and, secondarily, progression-free survival, in patients with stage D2 prostate cancer treated with bilateral orchiectomy with or without flutamide[100]. Surgical castration was used to avoid possible confounding due to disease flare with the use of LHRH agonists alone. This study had a target accrual of 1248 eligible patients with the assumptions of one-sided testing, a power of 90%, an α error of 0.05, a mean survival of 28.3 months in the placebo group, and a hazard ratio of 0.80 for death for the flutamide group vs. the placebo group. Of 1387 patients enrolled, 700 were randomized to the flutamide group and 687 to the placebo group, with stratification according to extent of disease and performance status. Median follow up was 49.2 months in the placebo group and 50.1 months in the flutamide group. There was no difference in overall survival (29.9 months [95% CI: 28.5–32.1 months] for the placebo group vs. 33.5 months [95% CI: 28.9–38.1 months] for the flutamide group; $P = 0.24$) or progression-free survival (18.6 months [95% CI: 17.2–21.0 months] for the placebo group vs. 20.4 months [95% CI: 18.2–22.7 months] for the flutamide group; $P = 0.21$). Furthermore, there was no benefit with flutamide with respect to overall or progression-free survival for patients with minimal disease.

Discussion

At the present time, data do not convincingly show a benefit of CAB over castration alone for patients with clinical stage D2 prostate cancer, implying that the role for adrenal androgens in progression after castration is insignificant. The large SWOG study comparing orchiectomy plus placebo to orchiectomy plus flutamide clearly demonstrates no benefits of CAB over orchiectomy alone. In view of these negative results, along with lack of significant differences in most meta-analyses, the role for adrenal androgens in progression after castration appears insignificant. Thus, bilateral orchiectomy remains the gold standard for the initial treatment of advanced prostate cancer. Antiandrogens should be reserved for patients on LHRH agonists to prevent flare reactions, including acute-on-chronic mini-fluctuations in serum testosterone, and for patients who progress after orchiectomy.

Timing of androgen withdrawal therapy

The question of when to initiate androgen ablation remains controversial and is discussed in Chapter 17.2. Increasing and evolving evidence suggests that treatment should commence at the time of diagnosis of locally advanced or metastatic disease. While the first VACURG study[28] found delayed endocrine therapy equivalent to immediate endocrine therapy, evidence from animal models of prostate cancer indicates that early androgen ablation is more effective[92,103]. The Goldie-Coldman[104] hypothesis of increasing somatic genomic alterations and tumor heterogeneity over time provides additional theoretical evidence supporting initiation of therapy as early as possible. Furthermore, the benefit to CAB in the good performance status, minimal disease subgroup observed in the NCI Intergroup 0036 study[83,99] and the EORTC 30853 study[84] may suggest a benefit to early therapy when the burden of disease is less. Finally, a randomized study in patients with locally advanced disease compared radiation therapy plus 3 years adjuvant hormone therapy to radiation therapy alone with hormone therapy initiated at the time of disease recurrence, demonstrated a significant difference in 5 year overall survival (78% vs. 56%)[105]. The EORTC protocol 30846 was designed to compare early vs. delayed endocrine therapy in patients with node-positive prostate cancer without distant metastases[106]. An interim analysis revealed a highly significant difference in time to progression favoring early therapy, but no differences in survival.

The Medical Research Council Prostate Cancer Working Party Investigators Group randomized 938 patients with locally advanced or asymptomatic metastatic prostate cancer to immediate therapy with orchiectomy or LHRH agonist or to deferred treatment, with stratification for age, clinical stage and metastatic status[107]. Patients in the deferred treatment group had a higher incidence of requiring transurethral prostate resection (30% vs. 14%, $P < 0.001$), pathological fracture (4.5% vs. 2.3%), spinal cord compression (4.9% vs. 1.9%), ureteral obstruction (12% vs. 7%), extraskeletal metastases (12% vs. 7.9%), and pain from metastases (45% vs. 26%, $P < 0.001$). In patients with M0 disease, fewer patients in the immediate therapy group had distant progression or death due to prostate cancer (96/256), compared with patients with deferred therapy (144/244) ($P < 0.001$). Overall and disease-specific survival rates were significantly different in the M0 group ($P = 0.002$ and $P < 0.001$, respectively), but not in the group of patients with M1 or MX disease.

Recently, Messing et al. reported on the phase III ECOG trial in which 98 men with node positive prostate cancer who had undergone radical prostatectomy and pelvic lymphadenectomy were randomized to early hormonal therapy or to observation until metastasis or symptomatic local recurrence occurred[108]. At a median follow up of 7.1 years, 7/47 (14.9%) and 18/51 (35.3%) died in the early and delayed hormonal therapy arms, respectively (P < 0.02), with 3 (6.4%) and 16 (31.4%) of the deaths due to prostate cancer, respectively. Recurrence or progression was noted in 11/47 (23.4%) and 42/51 (82.4%) patients in the early and delayed hormonal therapy arms, respectively (P < 0.001). Together, these studies suggest a benefit to immediate hormonal therapy.

Quality of life issues

Over the past 20 years, most efforts have focused on maximizing the degree of androgen suppression therapy by combining agents that inhibit or block both testicular and adrenal androgens. Although data from randomized trials suggest that quality of life may be improved by CAB[109,110], it is also evident that CAB increases treatment-related side effects and expense without significantly prolonging tumor progression or survival[91,100]. Quality of life assessments are important in clinical trials, given the discrepancy between the physician's and patient's evaluation of potency and pain[111,112]. Use of validated self-administered quality of life questionnaires in a study of 47 patients undergoing either early or delayed treatment for T1-3N1-3M0 prostate cancer revealed that patients receiving early therapy had more psychological distress, hot flushes, loss of potency and decreased sexual enjoyment[113].

Several factors are increasing the awareness of the potential adverse effects of long-term continuous androgen ablation. First, use of PSA in the early detection of prostate cancer has resulted in a stage migration and a 50% decrease in the incidence of stage D2 disease in recent years[114]. Because the median survival in D2 disease is only 2–3 years, the long-term effects of androgen ablation do not become apparent and are therefore not clinically relevant. However, use of PSA and stage migration has resulted in earlier diagnosis at younger ages and earlier stages of disease, with the prospect of much longer therapy and risk of chronic complications. Furthermore, the use of serum PSA to detect biochemical recurrences following radical prostatectomy or radiotherapy identifies men destined to recur who may benefit from early adjuvant therapy[106,107] but who have life expectancies exceeding 10 years. Hence, combinations of stage migration, PSA recurrences, longer life expectancies, and trend towards earlier therapy mean that clinicians will have to balance the potential benefits of early adjuvant therapy with risks of development of metabolic complications associated with long-term continuous androgen withdrawal therapy. These metabolic complications include loss of bone mass (osteoporosis)[115] and fractures[116], loss of mus-

cle mass with easy fatigue and decreased energy levels[117], changes in lipid profile with increased risk of cardiovascular complications, glucose intolerance[117], and depressive and/or irritable personality changes[112,113,117–119].

New approaches or combinations of reversible medical castration are being investigated to reduce the negative impact of androgen ablation on quality of life, with the realization that androgen withdrawal therapy is rarely curative, that CAB is not superior to orchiectomy, and that progression to androgen-independence is initiated and accelerated by androgen withdrawal[92]. Foulds[120] and Noble[121] both demonstrated that tumor cells are responsive to changes in their environment, and that efforts to kill cells by androgen withdrawal results in the induction of progressive autonomy, either immediately or after a delay. Restoring the environment to its normal state of hormonal balance may offer a pathway to reverse cellular mechanisms and aberrant metabolic pathways upregulated by androgen withdrawal. Our treatment goals should change from attempts to kill all cancer cells by maximizing androgen ablation to attempts to regain biological control of the tumor cells' growth and response to subsequent androgen ablation[122].

Intermittent androgen suppression (IAS)

IAS is based on the hypothesis that if tumor cells, which survive androgen withdrawal, are pressured along a normal pathway of differentiation by androgen replacement, then apoptotic potential may be restored and progression to androgen independence delayed. It follows that if androgens are replaced soon after regression of tumor, it should be possible to bring about repeated cycles of androgen-stimulated growth, differentiation and androgen withdrawal regression of tumor. Experimental animal data in the Shionogi[123] and LNCaP[124] tumor model systems support this hypothesis and demonstrate that progression to androgen independence can be delayed but not prevented by IAS. Klotz et al.[125] first tested IAS in a small cohort of patients with advanced prostate cancer prior to the PSA era. Goldenberg et al.[126] reported on 47 patients treated with IAS using changes in serum PSA as trigger points; this study was more recently updated by Gleave et al.[127] to include 60 patients with locally recurrent or metastatic disease. Mean initial serum PSA was 128 µg/l. Treatment was initiated with CAB and continued for an average of 9 months. Because prognosis is poor in patients who do not achieve normal PSA levels after androgen ablation, only patients with PSA nadir levels below 4 µg/l were eligible for the IAS protocol. After 9 months, medications were discontinued until serum PSA increased to 10–20 µg/l. This cycle of treatment and no-treatment was repeated until the regulation of PSA became androgen independent (Figure 17.1.2). The mean time to PSA nadir during the first three cycles was

5 months, and serum testosterone returned to the normal range within 8 weeks of stopping treatment. The first two cycles averaged 18 months in length with 45% of the time off therapy, while the third cycle averaged 15.5 months. The off-treatment period in all cycles was associated with an improvement in sense of well-being, and recovery of libido and potency in the men who reported normal or near-normal sexual function before the start of therapy. Median time to progression and survival in patients with D2 disease was similar to the expected results with continuous androgen ablation.

Observations from this preliminary study suggest that IAS does not have a negative impact on time to progression or survival, both of which are similar to continuous combined therapy. However, phase III randomized studies are required accurately to assess the effects of intermittent treatment on these critical parameters. IAS improves quality of life by permitting recovery of libido and potency, increasing energy levels and enhancing sense of well-being during off-treatment periods. The animal and preliminary clinical studies have helped identify groups of patients who are most likely to benefit from IAS, to determine optimal duration of treatment, and to suggest trigger points on when to re-start therapy again. The therapeutic strategy and trigger points in each situation are guided by serum PSA. IAS may offer a 'way out' of the immediate vs. delayed treatment controversy, balancing the benefits of immediate androgen ablation with reduced treatment-related side effects and expense. More information will become available from prospective randomized clinical trials of IAS which have been initiated in Canada, the USA, and Europe. Until survival data is available, IAS should be considered an investigational form of therapy.

Sequential androgen blockade

Another approach to reducing the side effects of therapy is the concept of sequential androgen blockade proposed by Fleshner and Trachtenberg[128,129]. By inhibiting conversion of testosterone to DHT, the relative potency of flutamide as an androgen receptor antagonist is increased, and the usual side effects of androgen ablation are avoided because testosterone levels are not reduced. Twenty-two sexually active men with stages C and D1 prostate cancer were treated with finasteride 5 mg daily and flutamide 125–250 mg tid. Mean serum PSA decreased from 42.9 ng/ml to 3.6 ng/ml and 2.9 ng/ml at 3 and 6 months, respectively, and the response was durable to 24 months. Potency was preserved in 86% of patients. Similar results were reported in 17 patients by Fleshner and Fair[130] with durable results in four patients treated for 2 years. In another study, when finasteride 5 mg was added after a nadir PSA was obtained in 20 men with advanced prostate cancer treated with flutamide 250 mg tid, a further 7% mean decline in PSA was obtained[131]. Others have reported a mean of 91% reduction in serum PSA (46% undetectable PSA) when flutamide 250 mg tid was added to finasteride 5 mg monotherapy[132]. Side effects with this approach of sequential androgen blockade include: gynecomastia in 23/72 (32%), elevated liver enzymes in 7/59 (12%) and, diarrhea in 13/72 (18%)[129–132]. Further follow up and comparative studies are necessary to

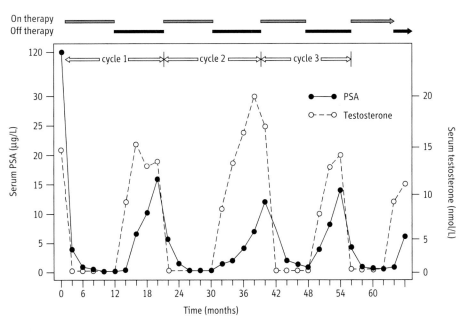

Fig. 17.1.2 Average serum PSA and testosterone in patients treated with intermittent androgen suppression with alternating cycles of treatment with combined androgen blockade (average 9 months duration) and time off treatment (average 9 months duration).

determine whether time to progression or survival is adversely affected.

Treatment of emergency conditions

Urinary retention is a common presentation of patients with locally advanced prostate cancer, which can be rapidly relieved by catheterization and subsequent transurethral resection. Procedures resulting in a rapid decline of serum testosterone may also be used to bring about regression of the obstructing lesion, particularly in the high-risk surgical patient or the individual with extensive local disease[133]. Orchiectomy and the use of cyproterone acetate or ketoconazole are recommended for this purpose.

Impending spinal cord compression should be treated urgently with dexamethasone and either cyproterone acetate or ketoconazole, with external beam radiotherapy where feasible. The use of an LHRH agonist is not advised since an acute elevation in the concentration of serum testosterone may stimulate tumor growth and exacerbate the condition.

Coagulation disorders complicating prostatic cancer have been well recognized entities for some time, but remain rare. The DIC syndrome that occurs is most likely due to a slow, continuous release of thromboplastic material from tumor cells, with fibrinolysis occurring secondarily. Prompt treatment of the cancer is required to correct the underlying pathophysiological defect, in addition to appropriate replacement of blood, platelets and clotting factors. This has been carried out successfully with high-dose intravenous diethylstilbestrol diphosphate (Honvol)[134], cyproterone acetate[64] or ketoconazole[135].

Treatment of hot flushes

The normal neuroendocrine mechanism for control of thermoregulation is centered within the hypothalamus[136]. When orchiectomy or LHRH agonist therapy leads to a peripheral androgen deficit, inhibitory factors, presumably opioid peptides, which are normally stimulated in the presence of sex steroids are no longer released from the hypothalamus. This results in increased central adrenergic activity, with release of norepinephrine and inappropriate stimulation of thermoregulatory centers; body heat is lost through peripheral vasodilation and manifests as hot flushes.

This effect can be blocked by the administration of central antiadrenergic medication (clonidine)[137] or steroids with central inhibitory action such as exogenous testosterone (contraindicated in prostate cancer), estrogens[138] (relatively contraindicated because of side effects) or progestogens[139]. Low-dose megestrol acetate[140] or cyproterone acetate 100 mg/day has been successful in significantly suppressing hot flushes with a minimum of side effects[64,141]. Hot flushes cannot be reduced by non-steroidal antiandrogens (e.g. flutamide) because of lack of central antigonadotrophic effects.

Conclusions

It is generally believed by most urologists today that hormonal therapy should be started at the time of diagnosis of metastatic prostate cancer, except in those asymptomatic patients who wish to remain sexually active. The choice of androgen ablation therapy for advanced prostate cancer depends on the philosophy of the physician and on patient preferences. Orchiectomy is the most cost-effective form of androgen withdrawal therapy for metastatic prostate cancer and has not been displaced as the 'gold standard' by newer forms of medical castration and combined androgen blockade. However, reversible androgen withdrawal therapies based on the use of antiandrogens and LHRH agonists are as efficacious as orchiectomy and have found a number of applications in the treatment of prostate cancer at different stages and offer flexibility and many new potential approaches. Intermittent therapy with reversible modalities based on antiandrogens and LHRH agonists offer potential for long-term control of prostate cancer while minimizing side effects, especially suppression of libido and potency, in the younger male patient. The main obstacle to improving survival and quality of life in patients with advanced prostate cancer is progression to androgen independence. The prospect of improving the results of androgen ablation can only be achieved by further research to identify new therapeutic strategies aimed at prolonging time to androgen independence.

References

1. Burrows H. *Biological actions of sex hormones* (2nd edn) Cambridge University Press; Cambridge, 1949, pp. 176–203.
2. Setchel BP. Introduction. In: Setchel BP (Ed.) *Male reproduction*. Van Nostrand Reinhold, New York, 1984, p. 1.
3. Wu CP, Gu FL. The prostate in eunuchs. *Prog Clin Biol Res* 1991;370: 249–255.
4. Berthold AA. Uber die Transplantation der Hoden. In: Setchel BP (Ed.) *Male reproduction*. Van Nostrand Reinhold, New York, 1984, p. 225.
5. Dorfman RI, Shipley RA. *Androgens: biochemistry, physiology, and clinical significance*. John Wiley & Sons Inc, New York, 1956, pp. 5–9.
6. Carter BS, Carter HB, Isaacs JT. Epidemiologic evidence regarding predisposing factors to prostate cancer. *Prostate* 1990;**16**:187–197.
7. Sharifi R, Kiefer J. History of endocrine manipulation in the treatment of carcinoma of the prostate – who was first? [abstract] *J Endocrinol Invest* 1987;**10**(suppl 2):91.

8. Huggins C, Hodges CV. Studies on prostatic cancer: I. The effect of castration, of estrogen and of androgen injection on serum phosphatases in metastatic carcinoma of the prostate. *Cancer Res* 1941;**1**:293–297.

9. Dunn JF, Nisula BC, Rodbard D. Transport of steroid hormones: binding of 21 endogenous steroids to both testosterone-binding globulin and corticosteroid-binding globulin in human plasma. *J Clin Endocrinol Metab* 1981;**53**:58–68.

10. Bruchovsky N, Wilson JD. The conversion of testosterone to 5α-androstan-17β-ol-3-one by rat prostate in vivo and in vitro. *J Biol Chem* 1968;**243**:2012–2021.

11. Andersson S, Bishop RW, Russell DW. Expression cloning and regulation of steroid 5α-reductase, an enzyme essential for male sexual differentiation. *J Biol Chem* 1989;**264**:16249–16255.

12. Normington K, Russell DW. Tissue distribution and kinetic characteristics of rat steroid 5α-reductase isoenzymes. Evidence for distinct physiological functions. *J Biol Chem* 1992;**267**:19548–19554.

13. Carson-Jurica MA, Schrader WT, O'Malley BW. Steroid receptor family: structure and functions. *Endocr Rev* 1990;**11**:201–220.

14. Beato M. Gene regulation by steroid hormones. *Cell* 1989;**56**:335–344.

15. Horwitz KB, Jackson TA, Bain DL, Richer JK, Takimoto GS, Tung L. Nuclear receptor coactivators and corepressors. *Mol Endocrinol* 1996;**10**:1167–1176.

16. Bruchovsky N, Goldie JH. Basis for the use of drug and hormone combinations in the treatment of endocrine-related cancer. In: Bruchovsky N, Goldie JH (eds) *Drug and hormone resistance in neoplasia, volume II, Clinical concepts.* CRC Press, Boca Raton 1983, p. 129.

17. Kerr JFR, Winterford CM, Harmon BV. Apoptosis: its significance in cancer and cancer therapy. *Cancer* 1994;**73**:2013–2026.

18. Rennie PS, Bruchovsky N, Buttyan R, Benson M, Cheng H. Gene expression during the early phases of regression of the androgen-dependent Shionogi mouse mammary carcinoma. *Cancer Res* 1988;**48**:6309–6312.

19. McDonnell TJ, Troncoso P, Brisbay SM, et al. Expression of the protooncogene bcl-2 in the prostate and its association with emergence of androgen-independent prostate cancer. *Cancer Res* 1992;**52**:6940–6944.

20. Gleave ME, Hsieh JT. Animal models in prostate cancer. In: Raghavan D, Scher HI, Leibel SA, and Lange P (eds) *Principles and practice of genitourinary oncology.* Lippincott-Raven, Philadelphia, 1997, pp. 367–378.

21. van Weerden WM. Animal models in the study of progression of prostate and breast cancers to endocrine independency. In: Berns PMJJ, Romijn JC, Schröder FH (eds) *Mechanisms of progression to hormone-independent growth of breast and prostate cancer.* Parthenon Publishers, New Jersey, 1991, pp. 55–70.

22. Grayhack JT. Adrenalectomy and hypophysectomy for carcinoma of the prostate. *JAMA* 1969;**210**:1075–1076.

23. Bruchovsky N. Comparison of the metabolites formed in rat prostate following the in vivo administration of seven natural androgens. *Endocrinology* 1971;**89**:1212–1222.

24. Radlmier A, Bormacher K, Neumann F. Hot flushes: mechanism and prevention. *Prog Clin Biol Res* 1990;**359**:131–140.

25. Lin BJT, Chen K-K, Chen M-T, Chang LS. The time for serum testosterone to reach castrate level after bilateral orchiectomy or oral estrogen in the management of metastatic prostate cancer. *Urology* 1994;**43**:834–837.

26. O'Connor VJ, Chiang SP, Grayhack JT. Is subcapsular orchiectomy a definitive procedure? Studies of hormone excretion before and after orchiectomy. *J Urol* 1963;**89**:236–240.

27. Byar DP. Proceedings: The Veterans Administration Cooperative Urological Research Group's studies of cancer of the prostate. *Cancer* 1973;**32**:1126–1130.

28. Mellinger GT. Carcinoma of the prostate: a continuing co-operative study. Veterans Administration Co-operative Urological Research Group. *J Urol* 1964;**91**:590–594.

29. The Leuprolide Study Group. Leuprolide versus diethylstilbestrol for metastatic prostate cancer. *N Engl J Med* 1984;**311**:1281–1286.

30. Cox RL, Crawford ED. Estrogens in the treatment of prostate cancer. *J Urol* 1995;**154**:1991–1998.

31. Waxman J, Man A, Hendry WF et al. Importance of early tumor exacerbation in patients treated with long acting analogues of gonadotrophin releasing hormone for advanced prostatic cancer. *BMJ* 1985;**291**:1387–1388.

32. Mahler C. Is disease flare a problem? *Cancer* 1993;**72**:3799–3802.

33. Kaisary AV, Tyrrell CJ, Peeling WB, Griffiths K. Comparison of LHRH analogue (Zoladex) with orchiectomy in patients with metastatic prostate cancer. *Br J Urol* 1991;**67**:502–508.

34. Soloway MS, Chodak G, Vogelzang NJ et al. for Zoladex Prostate Study Group. Zoladex versus orchiectomy in treatment of advanced prostate cancer: a randomized trial. *Urology* 1991;**37**:46–51.

35. Dijkman GA, Debruyne FMJ, Fernandez del Moral P et al. on behalf of the Dutch South East Cooperative Urological Group. A phase III randomized trial comparing the efficacy and safety of the 3-monthly 10.8-mg depot of Zoladex with the monthly 3.6-mg depot in patients with advanced prostate cancer. *Eur Urol* 1994;**26**(suppl 1):1–2.

36. Sharifi R, Bruskewitz RC, Gittleman MC, Graham SD Jr, Hudson PB, and Stein B. Leuprolide acetate 22.5 mg 12-week depot formulation in the treatment of patients with advanced prostate cancer. *Clin Ther* 1996;**18**:647–657.

37. Lupron depot – 4 month 30 mg. Deerfield, Ill.: Tap Pharmaceticals. In: *Physicians' desk reference* (53rd edn). Montvale: Medical Economics Company Inc, 1999, pp. 3147–3148.

38. Kerle D, Williams G, Ware H, Bloom SR. Failure of long-term luteinising hormone treatment for prostatic cancer to suppress serum luteinising hormone and testosterone. *BMJ* 1984;**289**:468–469.

39. Garnick MB. Hormonal treatment of prostate cancer [letter]. *N Engl J Med* 1999;**340**:812–813.

40. Sarosdy MF, Schellhammer PF, Sharifi R et al. Comparison of goserelin and leuprolide in combined androgen blockade therapy. *Urology* 1998;**52**:82–88.

41. Gonzalez-Barcena D, Vadillo Buenfil M, Garcia Procel E et al. Inhibition of luteinizing hormone, follicle-stimulating hormone and sex-steroid levels in men and women with a potent antagonist analog of luteinizing hormone-releasing hormone, Cetrorelix (SB-75). *Eur J Endocrinol* 1994;**131**:286–292.

42. Gonzalez-Barcena D, Vadillo-Buenfil M, Gomez-Orta F et al. Responses to the antagonistic analog of LH-RH (SB-75, Cetrorelix) in patients with benign prostatic hyperplasia and prostatic cancer. *Prostate* 1994;**24**:84–92.

43. Gonzalez-Barcena D, Vadillo-Buenfil M, Cortez-Morales A et al. Luteinizing hormone-releasing hormone antagonist cetrorelix as primary single therapy in patients with advanced prostatic cancer and paraplegia due to metastatic invasion of spinal cord. *Urology* 1995;**45**:275–281.

44. Sorenson S, Rondeau JJ, Lenaerts V et al. Radioimmunoassay of Antarelix, a luteinizing hormone releasing-hormone antagonist, in plasma and its application for pharmacokinetic study in dogs. *J Immunoassay* 1996;**17**:205–226.

45. Reissmann T, Felberbaum R, Diedrich K, Engel J, Comaru-Schally AM, Schally AV. Development and applications of luteinizing hormone-releasing hormone antagonists in the treatment of infertility: an overview. *Hum Reprod* 1995;**10**:1974–1981.

46. Pinski J, Lamharzi N, Halmos G et al. Chronic administration of the luteinizing hormone-releasing hormone (LHRH) antagonist cetrorelix decreases gonadotrope responsiveness and pituitary LHRH receptor messenger ribonucleic acid levels in rats. *Endocrinology* 1996;**137**:3430–3436.

47. Halmos G, Schally AV, Pinski J, Vadillo-Buenfil M, Groot K. Down-regulation of pituitary receptors for luteinizing hormone-releasing hormone (LH-RH) in rats by LH-RH antagonist Cetrorelix. *Proc Natl Acad Sci USA* 1996;**93**:2398–2402.

48. Hahn DW, McGuire JL, Vale WW, Rivier J. Reproductive/endocrine and anaphylactoid properties of an LHRH antagonist (ORF-18260). *Life Sci* 1985;**37**:505–514.

49. Rivier JE. Novel antagonists of GnRH: a compendium of their physicochemical properties, activities, relative potencies and efficacy in humans. In: Lunenfeld B, Insler V (eds) *GnRH analogues – The State of the Art.* Parthenon Publishing Group, London, 1993, pp. 13.

50. Janecka A, Janecki T, Bowers CY, Folkers K. New, highly active antagonists of LHRH with acylated lysine and p-aminophenylalanine in positions 5 and 6. *Int J Pept Protein Res* 1994;**44**:19–23.

51. Prout GR Jr, Keating MA, Griffin PP, Schiff SF. Long-term experience with flutamide in patients with prostatic carcinoma. *Urology* 1989;**34**(4 suppl):37–45.

52. Sogani PC, Vagaiwala MR, Whitmore WF Jr. Experience with flutamide in patients with advanced prostate cancer without prior endocrine therapy. *Cancer* 1984;**54**:744–750.

53. Schroeder FH. Pure antiandrogens as monotherapy in prospective studies of prostatic carcinoma. *Prog Clin Biol Res* 1990; **359**:93–103.

54. Lund F, Rasmussen F. Flutamide versus stilboestrol in the management of advanced prostatic cancer. *Br J Urol* 1988;**61**:140–142.

55. Jacobo E, Schmidt JD, Weinstein SH, Flocks RH. Comparison of flutamide (SCH-13521) and diethylstilbestrol in untreated advanced prostatic cancer. *Urology* 1976;**8**:231–234.

56. Chang A, Yeap B, Davis T et al. Double-blind, randomized study of primary hormonal treatment of stage D2 prostate carcinoma: flutamide versus diethylstilbestrol. *J Clin Oncol* 1996;**14**:2250–2257.

57. Iversen P on behalf of the International Casodex Investigators. Update of monotherapy trials with the new anti-androgen, Casodex (ICI 176,334). *Eur Urol* 1994;**26**(suppl 1):5–9.

58. Blackledge GR. High-dose bicalutamide monotherapy for the treatment of prostate cancer. *Urology* 1996;**47**(1A suppl):44–47.

59. Decensi AU, Boccardo F, Guarneri D et al. Monotherapy with nilutamide, a pure nonsteroidal anti-androgen in untreated patients with metastatic carcinoma of the prostate. The Italian Prostatic Cancer Project. *J Urol* 1991;**146**:377–381.

60. Schellhammer PF, Sharifi R, Block NL et al. for the CASODEX Combination Study Group. A controlled trial of bicalutamide vs flutamide, each in combination with luteinizing hormone-releasing hormone analogue therapy, in patients with advanced prostate carcinoma. *Cancer* 1996;**78**:2164–2169.

61. Kelly WK, Scher HI. Prostate specific antigen decline after antiandrogen withdrawal: the flutamide withdrawal syndrome. *J Urol* 1993; **149**:607–609.

62. Herrada J, Dieringer P, Logothetis CJ. Characterization of patients with androgen-independent prostatic carcinoma whose serum prostate specific antigen decreased following flutamide withdrawal. *J Urol* 1996;**155**:620–623.

63. Schellhammer PF, Sharifi R, Block NL et al. for the Casodex Combination Study Group. Clinical benefits of bicalutamide compared with flutamide in combined androgen blockade for patients with advanced prostatic carcinoma: final report of a double-blind, randomized, multicenter trial. *Urology* 1997;**50**:330–336.

64. Goldenberg SL, Bruchovsky N. Use of cyproterone acetate in prostate cancer. *Urol Clin North Am* 1991;**18**:111–122.

65. Rennie PS, Bruchovsky N, Goldenberg SL, Lawson D, Fletcher T, Foekens JA. Relative effectiveness of alternative androgen withdrawal therapies in initiating regression of rat prostate. *J Urol* 1988;**139**: 1337–1342.

66. Goldenberg SL, Bruchovsky N, Gleave ME, Sullivan LD. Low-dose cyproterone acetate plus mini-dose doethylstilbestrol – a protocol for reversible medical castration. *Urology* 1996;**47**:882–884.

67. Venner PM. Therapeutic options in treatment of advanced carcinoma of the prostate. *Semin Oncol* 1990;**17**(suppl 9):73–77.

68. Gleave ME, Goldenberg SL, Bruchovsky N. Prostate specific antigen as a prognostic predictor for prostate cancer. In: Pasqualini JR, Katzenellenbogen BS (eds) *Hormone-dependent cancer*. Marcel Dekker, New York, 1996, pp. 425–452.

69. Ernst DS, Hanson J, Venner PM, Uro-oncology Group of Northern Alberta. Analysis of prognostic factors in men with metastatic prostate cancer. *J Urol* 1991;**146**:372–376.

70. Kuriyama M, Wang MC, Lee CI et al. Use of human prostate-specific antigen in monitoring prostate cancer. *Cancer Res* 1981;**41**:3874–3876.

71. Killian CS, Yang N, Emrich LJ et al. Prognostic importance of prostate specific antigen for monitoring patients with stages B2 to D1 prostate cancer. *Cancer Res* 1985;**45**:886–891.

72. Stamey TA, Kabalin JN, Ferrari M, Yang N. Prostate specific antigen in the diagnosis and treatment of adenocarcinoma of the prostate: IV. Anti-androgen treated patients. *J Urol* 1989;**141**:1088–1090.

73. Bruchovsky N, Goldenberg SL, Akakura K, Rennie PS. Luteinizing hormone-releasing hormone agonists in prostate cancer: elimination of flare reaction by pretreatment with cyproterone acetate and low-dose diethylstilbestrol. *Cancer* 1993;**72**:1685–1691.

74. Miller JI, Ahmann FR, Drach GW, Emerson SS, Bottaccini MR. The clinical usefulness of serum prostate specific antigen after hormonal therapy of metastatic prostate cancer. *J Urol* 1992;**147**:956–961.

75. Newling DWW, Denis L, Vermeylen K for the European Organization for Research on Treatment of Cancer – Genitourinary Group. Orchiectomy versus goserelin and flutamide in the treatment of newly diagnosed metastatic prostate cancer: analysis of the criteria of evaluation used in the European Organization for Research on Treatment of Cancer – Genitourinary Group Study 30853. *Cancer* 1993;**72**:3793–3798.

76. Fearon ER, Vogelstein B. A genetic model for colorectal tumorigenesis. *Cell* 1990;**61**:759–767.

77. DeCosse JJ, Gossens CL, Kuzma JF, Unsworth BR. Breast cancer: induction of differentiation by embryonic tissue. *Science* 1973;**181**:1057–1058.

78. Gleave ME, Chung LWK. Stomal–epithelial interaction affecting prostate tumor-growth and hormonal responsiveness. *Endocr-Relat Cancer* 1995;**2**:243–265.

79. Gleave M, Hsieh JT, Gao CA, von Eschenbach AC, Chung LWK. Acceleration of human prostate cancer growth in vivo by factors produced by prostate and bone fibroblasts. *Cancer Res* 1991;**51**:3753–3761.

80. Sayer J, Ramirez EI, von Eschenbach AC. Retrospective review of prostate cancer patients with lymph node metastases [abstract]. *J Urol* 1992;**147**:52A.

81. Fossa SD, Heilo A, Lindegaard M, Skinningrud A, Ous S. Clinical significance of routine follow-up examinations in patients with metastatic cancer of the prostate under hormone treatment. *Eur Urol* 1983;**9**:262–266.

82. Matzkin H, Perito PE, Soloway MS. Prognostic factors in metastatic prostate cancer. *Cancer* 1993;**72**:3788–3792.

83. Crawford ED, Eisenberger MA, McLeod DG et al. A controlled trial of leuprolide with and without flutamide in prostatic carcinoma. *N Engl J Med* 1989;**321**:419–424.

84. Denis LJ, Carneiro De Moura JL, Bono A et al. Goserelin acetate and flutamide versus bilateral orchiectomy. *Urology* 1993;**42**:119–129.

85. Soloway MS. The importance of prognostic factors in advanced prostate cancer. *Cancer* 1990;**66**:1017–1021.

86. Mulders PFA, Dijkman GA, Fernandez del Moral P, Theeuwes AGM, Debruyne FM, members of the Dutch Southeastern Urological Cooperative Group. Analysis of prognostic factors in disseminated prostatic cancer. *Cancer* 1990;**65**:2758–2761.

87. Wilson JM, Kemp IW, Stein GJ. Cancer of the prostate: do younger men have a poorer survival rate? *Br J Urol* 1984;**56**:391–396.

88. de Voogt HJ, Suciu S, Sylvester R, Pavone-Macaluso M, Smith PH, de Pauw M. Prognostic factor analysis from EORTC trials in advanced prostatic cancer. *Prog Clin Biol Res* 1990;**357**:69–72.

89. Chodak GW, Vogelzang NJ, Caplan RJ, Soloway M, Smith JA for the Zoladex Study Group. Independent prognostic factors in patients with metastatic (stage D2) prostate cancer. *JAMA* 1991;**265**:618–621.

90. Bruchovsky N. Androgens and antiandrogens. In: Holland J, Frei E III, Bast R Jr, Kufe D, Morton D, Weichselbaum (eds) *Cancer Medicine* (3rd edn), Lea & Febiger, Philadelphia 1993, pp. 884–896.

91. Denis L, Murphy GP. Overview of phase III trials on combined androgen treatment in patients with metastatic prostate cancer. *Cancer* 1993;**72**:3888–3895.

92. Bruchovsky N, Rennie PS, Coldman AJ, Goldenberg SL, To M, Lawson D. Effects of androgen withdrawal on the stem cell composition of the Shionogi carcinoma. *Cancer Res* 1990;**50**:2275–2282.

93. Huggins C, Scott WW. Bilateral adrenalectomy in prostate cancer. *Ann Surg* 1945;**122**:1031–1041.

94. Geller J, Albert J, Vik A. Advantages of total androgen blockade in the treatment of advanced prostate cancer. *Semin Oncol* 1988;**15**(suppl 1): 53–61.

95. Geller J, Albert JD, Nachtsheim DA, Loza D. Comparison of prostate cancer tissue dihydrotestosterone levels at the time of relapse following orchitectomy or estrogen therapy. *J Urol* 1984;**132**:693–696.

96. Labrie F, Dupont A, Bélanger A. Complete androgen blockade for the treatment of prostate cancer. In: de Vita VT, Hellman S, Rosenberg SA (eds) *Important advances in oncology*. JB Lippincott, Philadelphia, 1985, pp. 193–217.

97. Suciu S, Sylvester R, Iversen P, Christensen I, Denis L. Comparability of prostate trials. *Cancer* 1993;**72**:3841–3846.

98. Blumenstein BA. Some statistical considerations for the interpretation of trials of combined androgen therapy. *Cancer* 1993;**72**:3834–3840.

99. Crawford ED, Allen JA. Treatment of newly diagnosed stage D2 prostate cancer with leuprolide and flutamide or leuprolide alone, phase III, intergroup study 0036. *J Steroid Biochem Mol Biol* 1990;**37**:961–963.

100. Eisenberger MA, Blumenstein BA, Crawford ED et al. Bilateral orchiectomy with or without flutamide for metastatic prostate cancer. *N Engl J Med* 1998;**339**:1036–1042.

101. Bertagna C, de Géry A, Hucher M, François JP, Zanirato J. Efficacy of the combination of nilutamide plus orchidectomy in patients with metastatic prostatic cancer: a meta-analysis of seven randomized double-blind trials (1056 patients). *Br J Urol* 1994;**73**:396–402.

102. Prostate Cancer Trialists' Collaborative Group. Maximum androgen blockade in advanced prostate cancer: an overview of 22 randomised trials with 3283 deaths in 5710 patients. *Lancet* 1995; **346**:265–269.

103. Isaacs JT. The timing of androgen ablation therapy and/or chemotherapy in the treatment of prostatic cancer. *Prostate* 1984;**5**:1–17.

104. Goldie JH, Coldman AJ. A mathematic model for relating the drug sensitivity of tumors to the spontaneous mutation rate. *Cancer Treat Rep* 1979;**63**:1727–1733.

105. Bolla M, Gonzalez MD, Warde P et al. Improved survival in patients with locally advanced prostate cancer treated with radiotherapy and goserelin. *N Engl J Med* 1997;**337**:295–300.

106. van den Ouden D, Tribukait B, Blom JHM et al. Deoxyribonucleic acid ploidy of core biopsies and metastatic lymph nodes of prostate cancer patients: impact on time to progression. The European Organization for Research and Treatment of Cancer Genitourinary Group. *J Urol* 1993;**150**:400–406.

107. The Medical Research Council Prostate Cancer Working Party Investigators Group. Immediate versus deferred treatment for advanced prostatic cancer: initial results of the Medical Research Council trial. *Br J Urol* 1997;**79**:235–246.

108. Messing E, Manola J, Sarosdy M, Wilding G, Crawford ED, Trump D. Immediate hormonal therapy compared with observation after radical prostatectomy and pelvic lymphadenectomy in men with node-positive prostate cancer. N Engl J Med 1999;**341**:1781–1788.

109. Dijkman GA, Fernandez del Moral P, Debruyne FM, Janknegt RA on behalf of the International Anandron Study Group. Improved subjective responses to orchiectomy plus nilutamide (Anandron) in comparison to orchiectomy plus placebo in metastatic prostate cancer. *Eur Urol* 1995;**27**:196–201.

110. Di Silverio F, Serio M, D'Eramo G, Sciarra F. Zoladex vs. Zoladex plus cyproterone acetate in the treatment of advanced prostatic cancer: a multicenter Italian study. *Eur Urol* 1990;**18**(suppl 3):54–61.

111. Calais da Silva F. Quality of life in prostatic cancer patients. *Cancer* 1993;**72**:3803–3806.

112. Calais da Silva F, Reis E, Costa T, Denis L, and the members of the Quality of Life Committee of the EORTC Genitourinary Group. Quality of life in patients with prostatic cancer. *Cancer* 1993;**71**:1138–1142.

113. van Andel G, Kurth KH, de Haas H. Quality of life assessment in patients with prostatic carcinoma category T1-3N1-3M0, receiving or not receiving hormonal treatment. In: *Recent advances in prostate cancer and BPH* (Proceedings of the Fourth Symposium of Progress and Controversies in Oncological Urology). Rotterdam, 1996, p. P50.

114. Newcomer LM, Stanford JL, Blumenstein BA, Brawer MK. Temporal trends in rates of prostate cancer: declining incidence of advanced stage disease, 1974 to 1994. *J Urol* 1997;**158**:1427–1430.

115. Daniell HW. Osteoporosis after orchiectomy for prostate cancer. *J Urol* 1997;**157**:439–444.

116. Townsend MF, Sanders WH, Northway RO, Graham SD Jr. Bone fractures associated with luteinizing hormone-releasing hormone agonists used in the treatment of prostate carcinoma. *Cancer* 1997;**79**:545–550.

117. Higano CS, Ellis W, Russell K, Lange PH. Intermittent androgen suppression with leuprolide and flutamide for prostate cancer: a pilot study. *Urology* 1996;**48**:800–804.

118. Roth AJ, Kornblith AB, Batel-Copel L, Peabody E, Scher HI, Holland JC. Rapid screening for psychologic distress in men with prostate carcinoma: a pilot study. *Cancer* 1998;**82**:1904–1908.

119. Moinpour CM, Savage MJ, Troxel A et al. Quality of life in advanced prostate cancer: results of a randomized therapeutic trial. *J Natl Cancer Inst* 1998;**90**:1537–1544.

120. Foulds L. *Neoplastic development*. Vol. 1. Academic Press Inc, New York, 1969, pp. 69–76.

121. Noble RL. Hormonal control of growth and progression in tumors of Nb rats and a theory of action. *Cancer Res* 1977;**37**:82–94.

122. Schipper H, Goh CR, Lim Wang T. Rethinking cancer: should we control rather than kill? Part 2. *Can J Oncol* 1993;**3**:220.

123. Akakura K, Bruchovsky N, Goldenberg SL, Rennie PS, Buckley AR, Sullivan LD. Effects of intermittent androgen suppression on androgen-dependent tumors: apoptosis and serum prostate specific antigen. *Cancer* 1993;**71**:2782–2790.

124. Sato N, Gleave ME, Bruchovsky N et al. Intermittent androgen suppression delays progression to androgen-independent regulation of prostate specific antigen gene in the LNCaP prostate tumor model. *J Steroid Biochem Mol Biol* 1996;**58**:139–146.

125. Klotz LH, Herr HW, Morse MJ, Whitmore WF Jr. Intermittent endocrine therapy for advanced prostate cancer. *Cancer* 1986;**58**:2546–2550.

126. Goldenberg SL, Bruchovsky N, Gleave ME, Sullivan LD, Akakura K. Intermittent androgen suppression in the treatment of prostate cancer: a preliminary report. *Urology* 1995;**45**:839–844.

127. Gleave ME, Bruchovsky N, Goldenberg, SL, Rennie P. Intermittent androgen suppression: rationale and clinical experience. In: Schroeder FH (Ed.) *Recent advances in prostate cancer and BPH*. Parthenon Publishing, London, 1997, pp. 109–121.

128. Fleshner NE, Trachtenberg J. Sequential androgen blockade: a biological study in the inhibition of prostatic growth. *J Urol* 1992;**148**:1928–1931.

129. Fleshner NE, Trachtenberg J. Combination finasteride and flutamide in advanced carcinoma of the prostate: effective therapy with minimal side effects. *J Urol* 1995;**154**:1642–1646.

130. Fleshner NE, Fair WR. Anti-androgenic effects of combination finasteride plus flutamide in patients with prostatic carcinoma. *Br J Urol* 1996;**78**:907–910.

131. Brufsky A, Fontaine-Rothe P, Berlane K et al. Finasteride and flutamide as potency-sparing androgen-ablative therapy for advanced adenocarcinoma of the prostate. *Urology* 1997;**49**:913–920.

132. Ornstein DK, Rao GS, Johnson B, Charlton ET, Andriole GL. Combined finasteride and flutamide therapy in men with advanced prostate cancer. *Urology* 1996;**48**:901–905.

133. Fleischmann JD, Catalona WJ. Endocrine therapy for bladder outlet obstruction from carcinoma of the prostate. *J Urol* 1985; **134**:498–500.

134. Goldenberg SL, Fenster HN, Perler Z, McLoughlin MG. Disseminated intravascular coagulation in carcinoma of prostate: role of estrogen therapy. *Urology* 1983;**22**:130–132.

135. Lowe FC, Somers WJ. The use of ketoconazole in the emergency management of disseminated intravascular coagulation due to metastatic prostatic cancer. *J Urol* 1987;**137**:1000–1002.

136. Neumann F, el Etreby MF, Habenicht UF, Radlmaier A, Bormacher K. Pharmacological basis of androgen deprivation by various antiandrogens and their combination with LHRH agonists. In: Klosterhalfen H (Ed.) *Endocrine management of prostatic cancer*. de Gruyter, Berlin,1988, p. 57.

137. Parra RO, Gregory JG. Treatment of post-orchiectomy hot flashes with transdermal administration of clonidine. *J Urol* 1990;**143**:753–754.

138. Steinfeld AD, Rheinhardt C. Male climacteric after orchiectomy in patient with prostatic cancer. *Urology* 1980;**16**:620–622.
139. Charig CR, Rundle JS. Flushing: long term side effect of orchiectomy in treatment of prostatic carcinoma. *Urology* 1989;**33**:175–178.
140. Loprinzi CL, Michalak JC, Quella SK et al. Megestrol acetate for the prevention of hot flashes. *N Engl J Med* 1994;**331**:347–352.
141. Eaton AC, McGuire N. Cyproterone acetate in the treatment of post-orchiectomy hot flushes: double-blind cross-over trial. *Lancet* 1983;1336–1337.

17.2 Immediate versus deferred hormonal treatment

D Kirk

Introduction

Over the half century since the hormonal dependence of prostatic cancer was first recognized,[1] androgen deprivation continues to be the main treatment for advanced prostate cancer, especially metastatic disease[2]. Although some response is seen in most patients, it will be temporary and relapse will occur, usually within 2 years in patients with metastases. While radiotherapy and other palliative measures may then be helpful in relieving symptoms, relapse after hormone therapy is usually fatal within a matter of months[3].

The concept of deferred treatment

A man with metastatic prostate cancer presenting with bone pain or other symptoms almost always needs hormonal therapy commenced as soon as possible. It is in the asymptomatic patient that the possibility of deferring treatment arises. Although treatment at diagnosis should prolong survival, this has been disputed[4]. Treatment left until symptoms occur should be followed by a further asymptomatic period and possibly a similar survival[5].

The Veterans Administration studies

It was the Veterans Administration Cooperative Research Group (VACURG) studies[6], which included randomized control groups treated initially with a placebo but started on active treatment on progression, which led to the acceptance of deferred treatment. It should be noted that it was for men with locally advanced non-metastatic disease that deferring treatment until metastases occurred appeared not to be detrimental for survival. Deferring treatment in patients who already have metastatic disease until they develop pain is an extension of this principle. In any case,

Byar in his review in 1973[6], could only state that 'These data support the concept that treatment can be delayed'. In metastatic disease the same potential advantages of deferring treatment arise – any side effects resulting from treatment will occur for a shorter period of time, and in elderly patients, death from an unrelated cause might occur before the patient develops symptoms requiring treatment. In the VACURG studies, even in those with metastatic disease, only 50% of patients dying did so from prostate cancer[6] and thus many patients might not need treatment in their lifetime. Unless early treatment can be shown to have advantages, deferment until an indication arises might be preferable[7].

Immediate or deferred treatment

Although deferred treatment became a fairly widespread practice following the VACURG studies, recently there has been more doubt about the justification for delaying hormonal therapy. The arguments are as follows[5,7]:

- Treatment while tumor bulk is smaller should be more effective;
- The evidence that deferring treatment has no effect on survival is not conclusive;
- Prostate cancer may become less hormone-sensitive as it progresses,
- Local progression in the absence of treatment increases the number of patients requiring TURP for recurrent outflow obstruction;
- Catastrophic events such as spinal cord compression and pathologic fractures may occur in untreated patients;
- The absence of specific symptoms might mask a general malaise associated with uncontrolled cancer – the patient might simply feel better if he were treated.

These possible benefits of immediate treatment must be balanced against the side effects of hormone treatment. It has been argued that new developments such as LH RH analogs have reduced the disadvantages of hormone therapy and swing the balance back towards early treatment[8]. On the other hand, since these new treatments are expensive, they have added an economic component to the argument. However, impotence remains a problem for many patients, not least the younger man for whom, paradoxically, deferring treatment is probably least appropriate. Into this debate came the suggestion by Crawford and his colleagues[9] that any benefit from maximal androgen blockade appeared most marked in those with least disease, reviving an old argument about loss of hormone sensitivity as prostate cancer progresses, used by Nesbit and Baum in 1950[10] at the time of the first debate on timing of treatment.

The need for a controlled trial

This discussion was based for many years on the results of the VACURG studies, which were rapidly becoming obsolete, which involved a rather elderly selected group of patients (mainly World War I survivors) and were never actually designed to answer this question. Retrospective reviews of anecdotal series gave conflicting results[11,12]. What was needed was hard evidence from a prospective controlled study designed specifically to answer the question 'In asymptomatic advanced prostate cancer, should hormone therapy be commenced on diagnosis or can it be deferred until clinically significant progression occurs?' Such a study has been sponsored by the British Medical Research Council[13]. Recruitment into the study ended in 1993. The first results were published in 1997[14] some of which have been updated here to April 1999 with unpublished data.

Medical Research Council study

Protocol design

The study was designed to assess the impact of hormonal treatment commenced at the time of diagnosis on the course of the disease compared with delaying treatment until clinical progression occurred. Participants were encouraged to manage patients according to their clinical practice. Entry and follow up were simplified as much as possible, and only data considered relevant to the main issue were collected. Eligibility was largely governed by Peto's uncertainty principle: if the clinician had genuine uncertainty as to whether the patient would benefit from immediate hormone treatment, and no clear reason to defer treatment, and provided this concurred with the informed view of the patient, he was eligible for entry. Similarly, indications for treatment in deferred patients were at the discretion of the participant.

Metastatic status of patients

After the trial had commenced, it was discovered that many British urologists did not have ready access to nuclear medicine facilities and that some patients entered as 'non-metastatic' had not had this confirmed by a bone scan. In classifying patients' metastatic status, these patients were categorized as 'Mx' (Table 17.2.1).

Trial follow up

The absence of stringent trial follow up schedules in the protocol has been criticized. However, it should be noted that although data collection was carried out annually,

patients were actually followed up more frequently, but according to the practice of the participant.

Results

Timing of treatment

Fifty per cent of patients with metastases (M1) randomized to deferred treatment had been treated 9 months after randomization compared with 27 months in those with non-metastatic disease. Approximately 10% died from other causes before treatment was indicated, mostly patients over the age of 70 and mainly with non-metastatic disease at presentation (Table 17.2.2). At the time of the initial report of the study, it was considered that some 29 patients had died from other causes before treatment was commenced. A subsequent review of these cases[15] has been performed. In fact, there are 15 men who do seem to have died from prostate cancer. This was due to a variety of reasons, including in three refusal of treatment by the patient or his relatives. In 11 there is considerable doubt as to the exact cause of death. These were mainly elderly patients with considerable comorbidity, emphasizing the difficulty in management in this age group and, paradoxically, most had M0 disease at presentation.

Table 17.2.1   MRC immediate vs. deferred treatment study – patients with follow up information available (total numbers recruited are shown in brackets)

	Immediate	Deferred
M0	256 (256)	244 (247)
Mx*	83 (83)	90 (91)
M1	130 (130)	131 (131)
Total	469 (469)	465 (469)

* Patients who did not undergo bone scan, but with no other evidence of metastatic disease.

Table 17.2.2   MRC immediate vs. deferred treatment study – death from other causes before treatment (deferred patients)

Age at randomization	No. randomized	No. of deaths
<60	10	1
60–64	41	0
65–69	80	4
70–74	116	10
75–79	136	20
80 +	82	16
M stage		
M0	247	29
Mx	91	16
M1	131	6

Progression

As would be expected, progression from M0 to M1 disease was significantly more rapid in patients with deferred treatment, and in those with M1 disease at randomization, bone pain occurred earlier. The philosophy of deferred treatment accepts this, progression being the indication for treatment. However, local progression also was more rapid[16], and almost twice the number of patients in the deferred arm needed a TURP (149 vs. 79). In M1 patients, 31 patients have required TURP in the deferred group, compared with 12 in those treated immediately. The significance of local progression is emphasized by the fact that 48 patients required more than one TURP (in addition to any TURP carried out at diagnosis), and 10% of patients, whether immediately treated or not, required TURP within 1 year of dying. Since 246 (120 immediate, 126 deferred) of the original 261 patients with M1 disease have now died, it is unlikely that the discrepancy in the number of TURPs will change, a comment which applies also to the differences in complication rates reported in the next section.

Complications

A major concern with deferred treatment is leaving the patient exposed to serious complications. As demonstrated in Table 17.2.3 the incidence of spinal cord compression, pathologic fracture, ureteric obstruction and extraskeletal metastases is more frequent in deferred patients. Although true statistical significance generally only applies to the overall differences, it seems clear that it is the patient who has metastatic disease at presentation who is most at risk. It should be noted that of 23 patients in the original report[14] who developed spinal cord compression in the deferred group, in 18, treatment had already been commenced for another reason (in 17, more than 6 months before the onset of the spinal cord compression). Thus the risk of this complication may be irrevocably increased when treatment is deferred, and its prevention is not simply a matter of vigilance in commencing treatment[17].

Survival

There is overall a clear difference in the numbers and rate of death in those randomized to deferred treatment (Figure 17.2.1). However, two important qualifications must be made. First, although overall survival from all causes of death (Figure 17.2.1a) is just statistically significant, the difference is clearly much greater when only prostate cancer deaths (Figure 17.2.1b) are considered. Does this mean that early treatment merely makes it likely that the patient will die from something else but still die at about the same time? Alternatively, since the trial was not double blind, there may have been a bias in ascribing

Table 17.2.3 MRC immediate vs. deferred treatment study – major complications

	Immediate (n=467)	Deferred (n=465)
Pathologic fracture		
M0	6	8
Mx	1	4
M1	7	11
Total	14	23
Cord compression		
M0	4	3
Mx	1	6
M1*	5	14
Total**	10	23
Ureteric obstruction a		
M0	30	31
Mx***	1	12
M1	11	15
Total**	42	58
Extra skeletal metastases		
M0	19	29
Mx	8	9
M1	14	21
Total*	41	59

A denominator excludes seven patients receiving local radiotherapy to the prostate
*2P<0.05, **2P<0.025, ***2P<0.005, otherwise statistically non-significant.

cause of death in patients randomized to deferred treatment. However, from the statistician's viewpoint (Peto, personal communication) it is more correct to consider prostate cancer deaths not as part of the overall deaths, but to compare them with non-cancer deaths as independent events (Figure 17.2.2). Due to the small numbers, the excess of non-cancer deaths in the immediate arm is not significant, and indeed as data has matured this discrepancy has become less marked.

The second issue arises when the mortality is considered in relation to metastatic status. For those with M0 disease, confirmed by a negative bone scan, both overall and prostate cancer survival was clearly better in the immediate treatment group (Figure 17.2.3) while, in those with metastatic disease, no difference in survival can be identified (Figure 17.2.4). Thus as far as survival is concerned, the man with metastatic disease may not benefit from immediate treatment.

Cause of death

Of all the patients who died during the study, 65% did so from prostate cancer, a proportion rising to 78% in those with M1 disease on entry. The relevant figures in the VAC-URG studies were 41% and 50% respectively. Clearly improvements in life expectation now make prostate

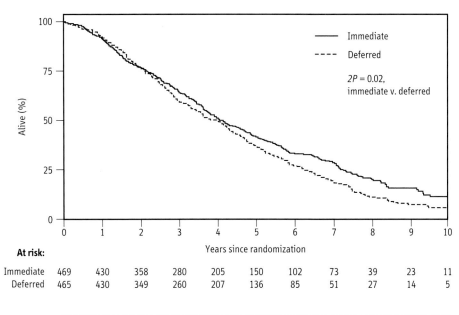

Fig.17.2.1a MRC immediate vs. deferred treatment study – survival curves, death from all causes. All patients, immediate versus deferred treatment.

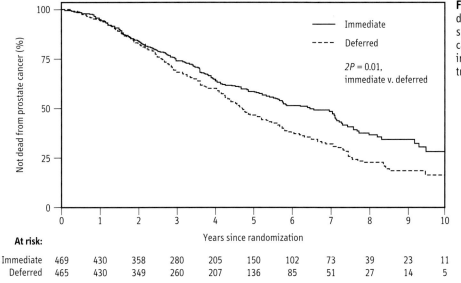

Fig.17.2.1b MRC immediate vs. deferred treatment study – survival curves for prostate cancer deaths. All patients, immediate versus deferred treatment.

cancer a more potent cause of death, and reduce the chance of a man avoiding the need for treatment, as reflected in the fact that few men entered under the age of 70 died from other causes before treatment was started (Table 17.2.2).

Interpretation of MRC trial data

Although 85% of patients entered into the study have now died, some aspects of the data will always remain open to debate. Superficially they support immediate treatment. However, two irrevocable deficiencies will remain. The

absence of PSA data during the study will be discussed in a later section. At the time the study was commenced, there were no acceptable quality of life questionnaires available, and indeed, the level of recruitment achieved, in a study largely performed by busy district general hospital urologists without significant financial support, would have been jeopardized by such an addition. It is, therefore, not possible to assess the adverse effects of treatment on those in the immediate arm. A case against deferred treatment will depend on its deficiencies being so great that they will clearly mitigate any treatment-induced loss of

229

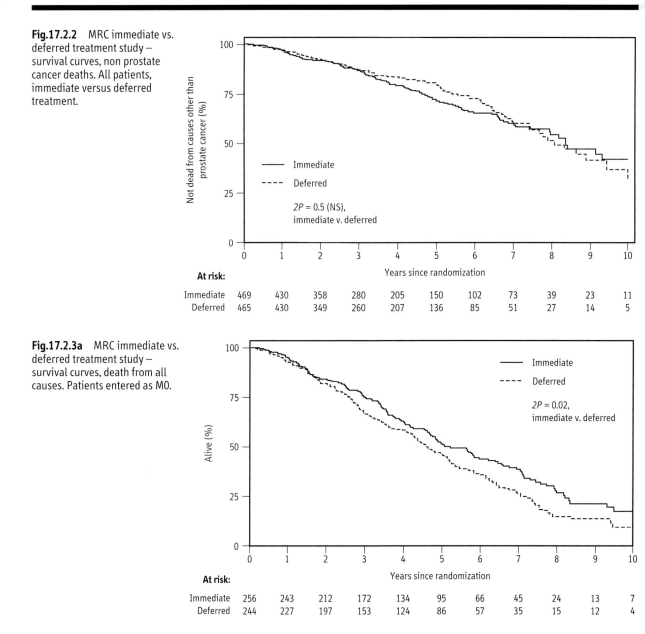

Fig.17.2.2 MRC immediate vs. deferred treatment study – survival curves, non prostate cancer deaths. All patients, immediate versus deferred treatment.

Fig.17.2.3a MRC immediate vs. deferred treatment study – survival curves, death from all causes. Patients entered as M0.

quality of life. For those with metastatic disease, the real subject of this chapter, the majority are not going to escape treatment, and on these grounds it seems reasonable to recommend that deferred treatment is not considered for men under 70. For the majority, treatment will be necessary within 1 year. Although no clear adverse effect on survival is apparent, there will be an increased chance that during his relatively short survival, he will require a further TURP[16] as discussed in an earlier section. The chances of sustaining spinal cord compression or other complications seem greater[14,18]. Since 246 of 261 patients with metastatic disease have already died it is likely that

the overall incidence of these complications will remain higher in the deferred group.

Complications of hormone treatment

The tendency towards earlier hormone treatment has occurred at a time when the complications of androgen deprivation are coming to be more appreciated. The possibility that improved cause-specific survival from early treatment is not reflected in overall survival rates has raised the possibility of treatment related mortality from

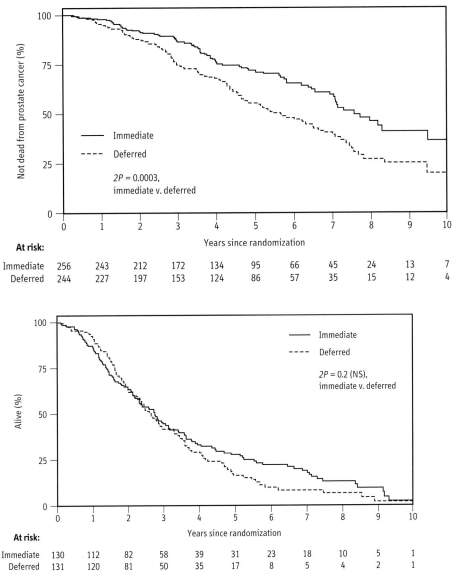

Fig.17.2.3b MRC Immediate vs. deferred treatment study – survival curves for prostate cancer deaths. Patients entered as M0.

At risk:

Immediate	256	243	212	172	134	95	66	45	24	13	7
Deferred	244	227	197	153	124	86	57	35	15	12	4

Fig.17.2.4a MRC Immediate vs. deferred treatment study – survival curves, death from all causes. Patients entered as M1.

At risk:

Immediate	130	112	82	58	39	31	23	18	10	5	1
Deferred	131	120	81	50	35	17	8	5	4	2	1

hormone therapies other than estrogens. Loss of bone density has also been recognized[18]. However, these problems are less likely to be significant within the short life expectation of those with metastatic disease.

The role of prostate-specific antigen

As the routine use of PSA in monitoring prostate cancer is comparatively recent, the MRC study has not, unfortunately, provided information on PSA levels on diagnosis or follow up, although as the use of PSA has become more widespread, 'rising tumor markers' has become a more common indication for abandoning deferred treatment. A high PSA correlates with tumor progression19. The use

of PSA in assessing and monitoring patients can reduce some of the concern about missing tumor progression in deferred treatment patients. In patients who are keen to avoid treatment, a short period monitoring PSA, with the advice that a rapid rise should be taken as an indication for treatment, seems a reasonable compromise.

Immediate or deferred treatment – the current position

In patients with metastatic disease, the timing of treatment may not have a dramatic effect on survival. However, the other problems considered to arise from deferred treatment listed in an earlier section seem to have been con-

231

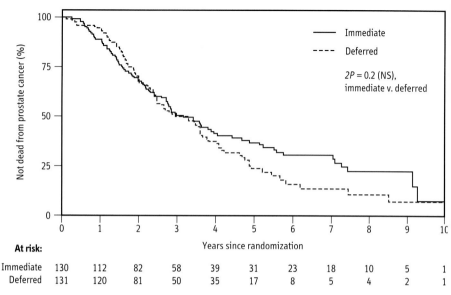

Fig.17.2.4b MRC Immediate vs. deferred treatment study – survival curves for prostate cancer deaths. Patients entered as M1.

At risk:	0	1	2	3	4	5	6	7	8	9	10
Immediate	130	112	82	58	39	31	23	18	10	5	1
Deferred	131	120	81	50	35	17	8	5	4	2	1

firmed by the MRC study. Completely avoiding treatment is likely only in men over the age of 70 – and it should be noted of those dying from other causes before treatment, 27 had confirmed M0 disease and only seven were men with definite metastases[14]. It must be concluded that there is an increased risk of complications or catastrophes such as spinal cord compression if treatment is deferred. Although careful assessment in selecting patients for deferred treatment and by subsequent close follow up may reduce their incidence, clearly these risks are significant. There is a substantially increased chance of needing a further TURP and it is difficult to see how careful assessment and closer follow up could prevent this.

Is deferred treatment still acceptable?

Hot flushes and loss of potency may still be significant problems for some men. The author has a policy of discussing management issues with the patient, and even after introducing the results of the MRC study into such conversations, some men are still reluctant to start treatment when they have no appreciable symptoms. In such cases, my practice is to advise regular monitoring of PSA. If this suggests rapid tumor progression treatment is then started. Otherwise, accepting that a stable PSA is not entirely reliable[20] careful follow up is mandatory. It is essential if treatment is deferred that the patient and his GP are fully aware of the situation. However, it is the author's impression that the climate was already swinging away from deferred treatment, certainly in patients with metastatic disease, and that the results of the MRC study may be taken as confirmation of this.

References

1. Huggins C, Hodges CV. Studies in prostate cancer. 1. The effect of castration of oestrogen and of androgen injection on serum phosphatase in metastatic carcinoma of the prostate. *Cancer Res* 1941;**1**:293–297.
2. Jacobi GH. Hormonal treatment of metastatic carcinoma of the prostate. In: Fitzpatrick JM, Krane RJ (eds) *The Prostate*. Churchill Livingstone, Edinburgh, 1989, pp. 389–399.
3. Beynon LL, Chisholm GD. The stable state is not an objective response in hormone-escaped carcinoma of the prostate. *Br J Urol* 1984;**56**:702–705.
4. Lepor H, Ross A, Walsh PC. The influence of hormonal therapy on survival of men with advanced prostatic cancer. *J Urol* 1982;**128**:335–340.
5. Kirk D. Deferred treatment for advanced prostatic cancer. In: Waxman J, Williams G (eds) *Urological oncology*. Edward Arnold, Sevenoaks, 1991, pp. 117–125.
6. Byar DP. The Veterans Administration Cooperative Research Group's studies of cancer of the prostate. *Cancer* 1973;**32**:1126–1130.
7. Kirk D. Trials and tribulations in prostatic cancer. *Br J Urol* 1987;**59**:375–379.
8. Kozlowski JM, Ellis WJ, Grayhack JT. Advanced prostatic carcinoma. Early versus late endocrine therapy. *Urol Clin N Am* 1991;**15**:15–24.
9. Crawford ED, Eisenberger MA, McLeod DG *et al*. A controlled trial of leuprolide with and without flutamide in prostatic carcinoma. *N Eng J Med* 1989;**321**:419–424.
10. Nesbit RM, Baum WC. Endocrine control of prostatic cancer. Clinical survey of 1818 cases. *JAMA* 1950;**143**:1317–1320.
11. Parker MC, Cook A, Riddle PR, Fryatt I, O'Sullivan J, Shearer RJ. Is delayed treatment justified in carcinoma of the prostate? *Br J Urol* 1985;**57**:724–728.
12. Carr TW, Handley RC, Travis D, Powell PH, Hall RR. Deferred treatment of prostate cancer. *Br J Urol* 1988;**62**:249–253.
13. Kirk D. Prostatic carcinoma. *Br Med J* 1985;**290**:875–876.
14. Medical Research Council Prostate Cancer Working Party Investigators Group. Immediate versus deferred treatment for advanced prostatic cancer: initial results of the Medical Research Council Trial. *Br J Urol* 1997;**79**:235–246.
15. Kirk D and Medical Research Council Prostate Cancer Working Party Investigators Group. MRC immediate versus deferred treatment study: patients dying without treatment (abstract). *Br J Urol* 1998; **81**(suppl 4):31.

16. Kirk D and Medical Research Council Prostate Cancer Working Party Investigators Group. MRC immediate versus deferred treatment study: how important is local progression in advanced prostate cancer (abstract) *Br J Urol* 1998;**81**(suppl 4):30.

17. Kirk D and Medical Research Council Prostate Cancer Working Party Investigators Group. Complications in advanced prostate cancer: results from the Medical Research Council immediate vs deferred treatment study. *Br J Urol* 1997;**79**(suppl 4):27.

18. Carlstrom K, Stege R, Henriksson P, Grande M, Gunnarsson PO, Pousette A. Possible bone-preserving capacity of high dose intramuscular depot estrogen as compared to orchiectomy in the treatment of patients with prostate cancer. *The Prostate* 1997;**31**:193–197.

19. Armitage TG, Cooper EH, Newling DWW, Robinson MRG, Appleyard I. The value of measurements of serum prostate specific antigen in patients with benign prostatic hyperplasia and untreated prostate cancer. *Br J Urol* 1988;**62**:584–589.

20. Josefsen D, Waehre H, Paus E, Fossa SD. Increase in serum prostate specific antigen and clinical progression in pN+ M0 prostate cancer. *Br J Urol* 1995;**75**:502–506.

17.3 Radiation therapy

C A Perez

Several reports document the value of external or interstitial irradiation in the management of post-radical prostatectomy local recurrences and interstitial irradiation for local failure after external irradiation. Furthermore, irradiation is widely used to relieve symptoms caused by locally extensive or metastatic carcinoma of the prostate in many anatomic sites. The techniques and results reported for various indications of radiation therapy are reviewed in this chapter.

Treatment of locally recurrent carcinoma of the prostate

Some patients who fail locally after radical prostatectomy may be later treated with irradiation. Selection of the appropriate method depends on 1) extent of the tumor (prostatic or pelvic); 2) general condition of the patient (including metastatic dissemination); 3) age of patient; 4) sexual potency preservation, if present; 5) initial treatment modality; and 6) time span between initial therapy and retreatment[1].

Post-radical prostatectomy elevation of prostate-specific antigen

Several authors[2,3] have reported a significant decrease in prostate-specific antigen (PSA) levels after pelvic irradiation in 60% to 70% of patients with persistent or increasing PSA levels after radical prostatectomy. Usually the prostatic bed is treated with 62 to 65 Gy using 10×12 cm

or 12×12 cm portals and 120-degree bilateral arc rotation or three-dimensional (3-D) conformal irradiation with high-energy photons.

Initially, Hudson and Catalona[4] reported on 21 patients, and McCarthy et al.[5] later noted that 62% of patients with elevated PSA had steadily decreasing or undetectable PSA levels after pelvic irradiation. In an update of their experience, McCarthy et al.[6] reported that, of 43 men irradiated for post-prostatectomy delayed PSA elevation, 27 (63%) were disease-free with a median follow up of 72 months. Less than 50% of patients with persistently detectable PSA (eight of 20) remained disease-free (median follow up, 52 months). Link et al.[3] reported on 25 patients receiving post-radical prostatectomy pelvic irradiation for elevated PSA levels. In 15 patients (60%) PSA levels decreased to less than 0.3 ng/ml. At the time of the report, eight patients had no detectable PSA levels with median follow up of 18 months. Only one of 12 patients with detectable PSA levels immediately after radical prostatectomy had a sustained response after pelvic irradiation as opposed to seven of 13 patients with delayed elevated PSA levels. Link et al.[3] noted that the number of patients showing decrease of PSA levels to less than 0.3 ng/ml was greater in patients receiving 50 Gy to the whole pelvis (six of six, 100%) than in those treated to the prostatic bed only (five of 11, 45%).

Irradiation for local failure after radical prostatectomy

The majority of patients who have clinically palpable post-prostatectomy recurrent lesions are believed to have a high propensity for pelvic lymph node metastases. The pelvis is usually treated with anterior/posterior (AP) and lateral portals (Figure 17.3.1) to doses of 45 to 50 Gy in 1.8 Gy fractions per day, five fractions per week; the prostatic bed receives an additional dose for a total of 65 to 70 Gy with reduced portals depending on tumor volume (Figure 17.3.2), in 2 Gy daily fractions[7]. The isodose curve for this plan of therapy is shown in Figure 17.3.3.

In 23 patients with isolated post-prostatectomy local recurrence treated at our institution, 17 (74%) had local tumor control, 45% survived relapse-free for 5 years and 17% at 10 years after irradiation of the recurrence; six of these patients later developed distant metastases. Seven additional patients (30%) later developed metastatic disease without local recurrence for an overall distant metastatic rate of 56%[8]. The disease-free survival from the time of prostatectomy was 70% at 5 years and 54% at 10 years; results are similar to those observed in patients with clinical or surgical stage C (T3) disease[9]. Dose of irradiation had an impact on survival; none of four patients receiving less than 50 Gy showed local control or long-term survival, as opposed to four of four (100%) treated

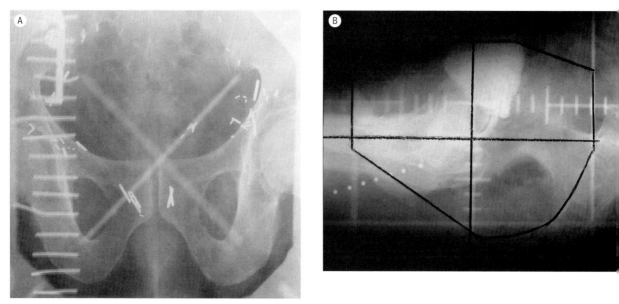

Fig. 17.3.1   (A) AP and (B) lateral simulation films illustrating portals used to treat the pelvic lymph nodes and prostate bed in patients with recurrent prostatic carcinoma.

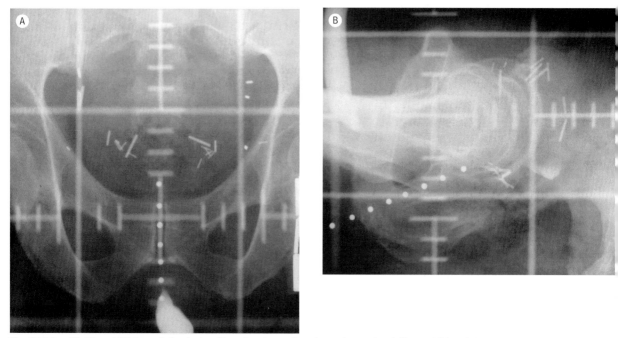

Fig. 17.3.2   (A) AP and (B) lateral simulation films showing reduced portals used to deliver additional dose to the prostate bed. In some patients only the reduced fields are used.

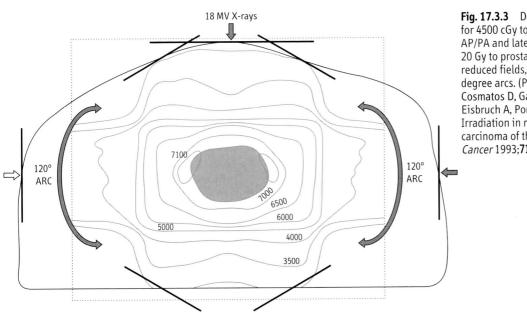

18 MV X-rays

120°
ARC

120°
ARC

7100

7000
6500
6000
5000
4000
3500

Fig. 17.3.3 Dose distribution for 4500 cGy to the pelvis with AP/PA and lateral fields and 20 Gy to prostate bed with reduced fields, bilateral 120-degree arcs. (Perez CA, Cosmatos D, Garcia DM, Eisbruch A, Poulter CA. Irradiation in relapsing carcinoma of the prostate. *Cancer* 1993;**71**:1110–1112[7].)

with 60 to 65 Gy and 13 of 15 patients (87%) receiving 55.01 to 70 Gy. Irradiated volume had no significant influence on local tumor control (71% to 75%). However, in the patients treated with a prostatic field only, 21% survived disease-free for 5 years as opposed to 54% of the group treated to the whole pelvis and the prostatic bed (P=0.65).

Minor sequelae were noted in seven of 23 patients (30%): three cases of scrotal/penile edema (17.6%), two of moderate cystitis with occasional hematuria, one small bowel obstruction, one urinary incontinence, and one partial small bowel obstruction treated conservatively.

In other reports the local tumor control rate with irradiation for pelvic recurrence after radical prostatectomy ranges from 58% to 100%[10–13]. When compared with hormonal treatment in a similar group of patients, pelvic irradiation conferred better local tumor control and disease-free survival, although no advantage in overall survival was reported by Anscher and Prosnitz[14] in a retrospective series.

Irradiation for pelvic recurrence after initial irradiation

Interstitial irradiation

Implantation with ^{125}I seeds has been carried out in patients with limited-volume (under 75 cc) recurrent prostatic carcinoma following external irradiation (60 to 70 Gy in 6 to 7 weeks).

Goffinet *et al.*[15] reported their experience with 14 patients with histologically proven, locally recurrent tumor 16 to 51 months after completion of radiation therapy. Cystoscopy and proctosigmoidoscopy were performed to rule out bladder or rectal tumor extension; a suprapubic extraperitoneal approach was used for selective lymph node biopsies of suspicious nodes or for lymphadenectomy. The prostate was isolated, and the ^{125}I seeds were implanted. The dose administered ranged from 40 to 225 Gy (average, 120 Gy). Clinical local tumor control was noted in 11 of 14 patients (79%) with a follow up of 6 to 36 months after implantation, and eight patients (57%) were disease-free at the time of the report. Complications occurred in four patients (two cystoproctitis, one abscess with urinary incontinence, and one vesicorectal fistula).

Martinez *et al.*[16] used interstitial ^{192}Ir irradiation to treat six patients with recurrent prostatic tumor. Therapy was well tolerated. Follow up was too short to allow tumor control assessment.

External irradiation

In patients initially treated with interstitial irradiation alone, it may be possible to retreat with external irradiation to the prostatic bed or limited volumes of the pelvis, depending on tumor extent. A significant difficulty is the inability to protect the bladder or the anterior rectal wall without compromising tumor coverage. Therefore, to diminish the probability of major sequelae, it is advisable to limit the re-treatment dose to 45 to 50 Gy (1.8 Gy daily, 5 weekly fractions) using small volumes and 3-D conformal therapy to decrease the dose to the bladder and the rectosigmoid.

Palliative radiation therapy for symptomatic locally extensive prostatic carcinoma

Irradiation at doses of 60 to 65 Gy may be quite effective in the treatment of massive pelvic carcinoma of the prostate or extensive lymph node involvement, which may produce pelvic or perineal pain, hematuria, urethral or ureteral obstruction, or leg edema because of lymphatic obstruction. Tissue swelling during the initial phase of irradiation may cause increased urinary difficulty in patients with partial urethral obstruction. An indwelling catheter may avert a complete blockage, but ideally it should not be used for more than 2 or 3 weeks because of irritation and the danger of superimposed infection. After a urine culture is obtained, antibiotics may be electively administered. A transurethral resection may be required if there is no improvement of the obstruction during the initial course of irradiation; an interval of 3 to 4 weeks would be allowed before resuming radiation therapy to decrease the probability of urinary incontinence or urethral fibrosis.

At Washington University, we irradiated the pelvis of 26 patients with various symptoms or signs secondary to locally advanced prostatic carcinoma, usually recurrent after initial hormonal therapy. All patients with pelvic or perineal pain or hematuria had relief of symptoms, usually complete; six of eight showed decreased urinary outlet obstruction, whereas only 50% had significant decrease in the size of the tumor or relief of ureteral obstruction. Carlton et al.[17] noted relief of bladder neck obstruction in 20 of 40 patients (50%) who failed to respond to estrogen therapy, improvement of hydronephrosis in eight of 11 patients (73%), and disappearance of intractable hematuria in seven patients (100%). Kraus et al.[18] also described satisfactory palliation in 27 patients with locally advanced prostatic cancer with doses of 40 to 50 Gy. Twenty-two of these patients had previous hormonal therapy, and 19 had undergone one or more transurethral resections. Marked improvement of rectal symptoms (pain, constipation and tenesmus) occurred in five patients (100%), and severe rectal bleeding caused by tumor invasion was controlled in one patient. Gross hematuria disappeared in 13 patients (100%), and there was definitive decrease in the size and induration of the gland in 19 of 23 patients (82%). Symptoms of lower urinary tract obstruction improved after irradiation in 14 patients; four of five patients treated for ureteral obstruction had a favorable response. Severe edema of the lower extremities improved in two patients, and perineal and inguinal pain were relieved in three patients.

Kynaston et al.[19] reported symptomatic improvement in 15 of 17 patients treated with irradiation. Ten of 13 patients with indwelling bladder catheters did not require further catheterization after irradiation; 50% of patients with obstructive symptoms maintained symptomatic improvement with follow up ranging from 5 to 24 months (median, 11 months). Eleven of 13 patients with hematuria showed disappearance of this distressing symptom. Approximately 50% of patients stopped bleeding after the first fraction of 8 Gy.

Lankford et al.[20] reported on 29 patients with regionally localized hormone refractory carcinoma of the prostate treated with irradiation (36 Gy in 12 fractions to 66 Gy in 33 Gy fractions). Actuarial local failure rate at 4 years was 39%; 80% of patients had disease progression or rising PSA. Doses above 60 Gy to the prostate were associated with symptom-free local tumor control in 90% of patients at 3 years.

Table 17.3.1 summarizes the palliative results reported by various authors.

Palliation of metastases

Bone metastases

External local irradiation

Irradiation is frequently used in the treatment of bony metastases from carcinoma of the prostate. Marked symptomatic relief is noted in about 80% of patients treated with doses of 30 to 35 Gy in 2 to 3 weeks. Large portals to include the entire bone, such as in the extremities or the pelvis, yield better palliative results.

Table 17.3.1   Radiation therapy for local palliation of extensive pelvic prostatic carcinoma

| | Relief of symptoms/signs | | | | |
	Kraus et al.[18]	Carlton et al.[17]	Kynaston et al.[19]	Perez et al. (present study)	Total (%)
Hematuria	13/13	7/7	11/13	5/5	36/38 (95)
Outlet obstruction	14/15	20/24	10/12	6/8	52/75 (69)
Ureteral obstruction	4/5	8/11		2/4	14/20 (70)
Pelvic/perineal pain				5/5 (3 CR, 2 PR)	8/8 (100)
Rectal symptoms	6/6				6/6 (100)
Lower extremity edema	2/2				2/2 (100)
Decreased large pelvis tumor	19/23			2/4	21/27 (78)

Perez CA, Cosmatos D, Garcia DM, Eisbruch A, Poulter CA. *Cancer* 1993;**71**:1110–1122.[7]

The Radiation Therapy Oncology Group (RTOG) conducted several trials with different fractionation and dose schedules to determine the most effective irradiation in patients with osseous metastases from various primary tumors. Fifty-four per cent of the patients experienced complete and 36% partial relief of pain[21]. The lesions treated with 40.5 Gy had an 18% incidence of fracture compared with 8% to 9% for those treated with 25 to 30 Gy and only 5% for those receiving 15 to 20 Gy. Blitzer[22], in a re-analysis of the above data after longer follow up, concluded that for all endpoints two high-dose programs ($2.7 \times 15 = 40.5$ Gy and $3.0 \times 10 = 30$ Gy) had the best results (absence of pain and cessation of use of narcotics) when compared with the short course, lower-dose schedules (Figure 17.3.4A). In patients with solitary metastasis, the retreatment rate was 11% (eight of 74) with 40.5 Gy in 15 fractions versus 24% (17 of 72) treated with 20 Gy in five fractions. In the multiple metastases group, the re-treatment rate was 12% (20 of 167) in patients receiving 30 Gy in 10 fractions versus 16% to 23% with lower doses ($P = 0.02$). When the score for use of narcotics is combined with the pain score, the patients receiving the higher doses and larger number of fractions showed better therapeutic results than those treated with lower doses (Figure 17.3.4B) ($P = 0.0003$). The higher rate of pathologic fractures in the high-dose protracted arm of the solitary metastasis

group may have been the result of increased bone healing or perhaps secondary to pain relief and subsequent weight-bearing[22].

Hemibody irradiation

Hemibody irradiation has yielded good palliation of disseminated bone metastases in a large proportion of patients. Kuban et al.[23], in 31 patients treated with half-body irradiation (doses of 4 to 10 Gy) for palliation of multiple symptomatic osseous metastases, noted that 67% of patients treated to the lower and 82% of those treated to the upper half of the body achieved good pain relief until death with median intervals of 4 to 6 months.

Zelefsky et al.[24] administered 29 hemibody irradiation courses in 26 patients with hormone refractory metastatic adenocarcinoma of the prostate; 15 courses were given in fractionated regimens (25 to 30 Gy in nine or 10 fractions over 3 weeks), and 14 courses used a single dose of 8 Gy for the lower hemiskeleton and 6 Gy for the upper hemiskeleton. They reported that 11 of 14 patients (78%) treated with single-dose and 13 of 15 (86%) treated with fractionated hemibody irradiation showed complete pain relief. The median time to relapse in the single-dose group was 2.8 months in contrast to 6 and 11 months in the fractionated schedule group.

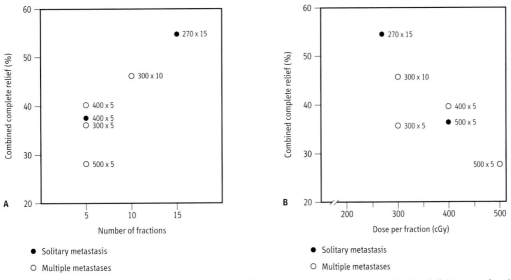

Fig. 17.3.4 Local irradiation for bone metastases. (A) Number of fractions versus complete combined relief. Percent of patients achieving complete combined relief (both narcotic score and pain score falling to zero) is plotted versus the number of fractions of irradiation for the solitary and multiple metastases groups ($P = 0.0003$). Next to each point is the dose per fraction (in cGy) times the total number of fractions. (B) Dose per fraction correlated with complete combined relief. Percent of patients achieving complete combined relief is plotted versus the dose per fraction of irradiation for the solitary and multiple metastases groups ($P > 0.10$). (Blitzer PH. Reanalysis of the RTOG study of the palliation of symptomatic osseous metastasis. *Cancer* 1985;**55**:1468–1472[22].)

In an RTOG phase III randomized study of patients with painful bony metastases from various malignant tumors, symptomatic bone metastases were treated with 30 Gy in 10 fractions over 14 days; patients were randomized to receive or not a single dose of hemibody irradiation (8 Gy) with lung correction and thin lung shields in upper hemibody[25]. Analysis of 146 patients with primary carcinoma of the prostate showed that 1 year after treatment, 78% of 69 patients treated with local irradiation alone and 54% of 77 patients treated with local and hemibody irradiation required further treatment in the treated hemibody (Figure 17.3.5) ($P = 0.001$). Although the difference was not statistically significant ($P = 0.16$), there was better survival for patients receiving hemibody irradiation, particularly at 1 year (44% versus 33%). The main acute and subsequent sequelae of hemibody treatment were nausea and vomiting, diarrhea, anemia, leukopenia and thrombocytopenia in 1% to 5% of patients.

Strontium[89]

[89]Sr is a calcium analog, beta-article emitter with a maximum energy of 1.43 MeV and physical half-life of 50.5 days, decaying to Yttrium-89.[89]Sr has been administered intravenously (40 µCi/kg, total dose about 3 to 4 mCi) for diffuse bone metastases with relief of pain in 60% to 80% of patients[26–29].

Buchali et al.[27] in a randomized study of 49 patients with skeletal metastases of prostatic carcinoma treated with either three doses of [89]Sr (75 MBq) or saline as placebo, observed no significant difference in pain relief between the two groups. However, the 2 year survival rate

was 46% in 25 patients receiving the ^{89}Sr as opposed to 4% in 24 patients treated with placebo.

Efficacy data from RTOG 88-21 demonstrated that patients treated on the 4 mCi dose arm had a 50% decrease in pain scores on average, while those treated on the 6.5 mCi dose arm reported a 22% to 46% decrease in pain scores.

Porter et al.[30] reported on a multicenter Canadian study in which 126 patients with painful metastasis from carcinoma of the prostate refractory to hormone therapy were treated with local-field radiation therapy and either [89]Sr (single dose of 10.8 mCi in 11 ml of isotonic solution) or a placebo. In the ^{89}Sr-treated group, 17.1% of patients stopped taking analgesics as compared with 2.4% in the placebo group. At 3 months, 58.7% of the ^{89}Sr group were free of new painful metastases, in comparison with 34% in the placebo group ($P < 0.002$). The median time to further radiation therapy was 35.3 weeks in the study group compared with 20.3 weeks in the placebo group ($P = 0.006$). Quality of life, pain relief, and improvement in physical activity were statistically superior in the patients treated with [89]Sr ($P < 0.05$). In the ^{89}Sr-treated patients grade 3 and 4 toxicity was 10.4% and 1.49% for the white blood cells and 22.4% and 10.4%, respectively, for platelet count.

A United Kingdom study[31,32] compared pain relief after ^{89}Sr or external-beam irradiation. A total of 305 patients were randomized and 284 treated according to protocol. Median survival after ^{89}Sr was 33 weeks compared with 28 weeks after external irradiation. Patients receiving ^{89}Sr developed fewer new sites of pain and required additional therapy less often than those treated with external irradiation.

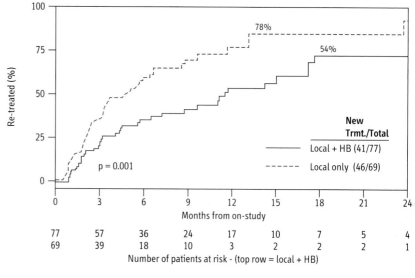

Fig. 17.3.5   Time to additional treatment for patients with osseous metastases from prostatic carcinoma treated with local irradiation alone or combined with hemibody radiation therapy. (Perez CA, Cosmatos D, Garcia DM, Eisbruch A, Poulter CA. Irradiation in relapsing carcinoma of the prostate. *Cancer* 1993;**71**:1110–1122[7].)

Laing et al.[33] reported on 83 patients with metastatic prostatic carcinoma treated with [89]Sr. At 3 months, 17% of patients had dramatic, 33% had substantial and 25% had some improvement of pain. Relief of pain was maintained for 4 to 15 months (mean, 6 months). The main toxicity was decreased white blood cell and platelet counts, which was dose dependent.

Pain relief as reported by various authors is summarized in Table 17.3.2.

A flushing sensation, particularly facial, after injection of ^{89}Sr has been noted in some patients but is self-limiting. The side effects of ^{89}Sr therapy appear to be limited to hematologic toxicity and an occasional transient increase in bone pain. The latter effect 'pain flare' seems to occur a few days after ^{89}Sr administration. Most patients show a decreased platelet count (24% to 70% from baseline) from pre-treatment levels with doses of 3 mCi to 4 mCi. The platelet nadir occurs between 4 to 8 weeks after the injection. Recovery is gradual and often complete.

Some practical aspects of ^{89}Sr use are presented in a later chapter.

Systemic [32]P

Radioactive phosphorus (^{32}P) has been administered systemically after priming with testosterone[35,36] or parathormone[37,38]. Testosterone cyprinate (100 mg) is given intramuscularly each day for 7 to 15 days. After the first 5 or 6 days,[32]P is administered either orally or intravenously (1.5 mCi for 6 or 7 days). Some advocate administration of a single dose of 5 to 7 mCi. Edland[39] reported good-to-excellent relief of pain in 86% of 42 patients treated with this method. Glaser et al.[40] noted complete pain relief in four of 24 patients after administration of four doses of 3 mCi ^{32}P intervenously on alternate days. Aziz et al.[41] described palliation of pain in 12 of 15 patients (80%) with

diffuse bony metastases from carcinoma of the prostate treated with intravenous sodium [32]P (10 to 12 mCi in single or divided doses over 1 week), preceded by daily intramuscular injections of testosterone propionate (100 mg) for 5 days. In seven patients (47%) relief was complete, and analgesics were no longer required. Pinck and Alexander[42] treated 32 patients with parathormone before ^{32}P administration and noted acute pain relief in 22 (69%); 14 of the patients maintained pain relief for 1 year or longer. The results reported by other investigators are summarized in Table 17.3.3. The authors pointed out that because of the rather delayed response to ^{32}P therapy, it has fallen out of favour.

Rhenium-186

Use of [186]Re was reported by Maxon et al.[47] in 20 patients, nine of whom had skeletal metastases from carcinoma of the prostate. Average activity administered by intravenous injection was 34 mCi (1258 MBq). The average overall decline in the pain index was about 40%, while there was essentially no change following a placebo. The main toxicity following administration of [186]Re(Sn) was a moderate decrease in white blood cell and platelet counts.

Yttrium-90 hypophysectomy

Straffon et al.[48] reported use of ^{90}Y hypophysectomy in the palliative treatment of patients with painful widespread bony metastases from prostate carcinoma. About half of 13 patients had good response, including a group of seven who had not responded to orchiectomy or estrogen therapy.

Brain metastases

Although brain metastases are very rare in patients with prostatic carcinoma, irradiation has been shown to be an effective palliative therapy when this situation occurs. In

Table 17.3.2   Selected clinical trials of ^{89}Sr in patients with bone metastases secondary to prostate or breast cancer

Investigator	No. of patients	[89]Sr dose range	Overall response rate	No. of pain-free patients
Robinson et al.[28]	137[*†]	30–40 µCi/kg	80%	10/100 (10%) prostate 5/28 (18%), breast
McEwan et al.[33]	26[‡]	40 µCi/kg	77%	27% (7/26)
Laing et al.[32]	83[‡]	40–80 µCi/kg	75%	22% (18/83)
Dusing et al.[34]	70[§]	40 µCi/kg	81%	–
Porter et al.[29]	62	10.8 mCi	58.7%	40%
Bolger et al.[30]	305	5.4 mCi	73%	66% (201/305)

*Patients who survived more than 3 months post-treatment.
†Patients with prostate or breast cancer.
‡Patients with prostate cancer.
§Patients with breast cancer.

Table 17.3.3   Relief of bone pain with ^{32}P therapy in metastatic prostatic carcinoma

Author	No. of patients	Total response (%)	Complete response (%)	Average duration of response (months)
Maxfield et al.[43]	21	76	47	–
Vermooten et al.[44]	27	75	–	–
Joshi et al.[35]	13	92	60	–
Smart[36]	9	95	33	5.0
Donati et al.[45]	12	91	50	6.3
Corwin et al.[46]	20	70	45	3.3
Glaser et al.[40]	24	58	17	5.0
Aziz et al.[41]	15	80	47	6.0

Aziz B, Choi K, Sohn C, Yaes R, Rotman M. Am J Clin Oncol 1986;9:264–268[41].

a randomized study the RTOG demonstrated that several dose schedules (20 Gy in five fractions in 1 week, 30 Gy in 10 fractions in 2 weeks, or 40 Gy in 15 fractions in 3 weeks) were equally effective in inducing relief of symptoms and improvement of neurologic function in 60% to 75% of patients. Complete relief of headaches ranged from 52% to 69%, whereas motor and coordination functions, impaired mentation and cranial nerve functions showed a complete response of 34% to 52%. Stereotactic irradiation has been used for the treatment of small solitary brain metastasis, with reported local tumor control of 85% to 96%[49].

Patchell et al.[50] described results in a randomized study of 48 patients with cerebral metastases from several types of primary tumors treated with irradiation alone (36 Gy in 12 fractions) or combined with surgical resection of single brain metastasis. Recurrence at the original metastatic site was less frequent in the combined-therapy group (5 of 25, 20%) than in the irradiation-alone group (12 of 23, 52%) (P < 0.02).

Mediastinal metastases

Occasionally, patients with prostatic carcinoma may develop metastases to mediastinal lymph nodes, which can be effectively palliated with doses of 35 to 40 Gy in 3 to 4 weeks.

Liver metastases

When patients with prostatic carcinoma develop symptomatic liver metastases, palliative relief may be accomplished with hepatic irradiation to doses of 27 to 30 Gy in fractions of 2.5 to 3 Gy, five fractions per week.

Leibel et al.[51] reported on 187 patients with liver metastases treated with 21 Gy in seven fractions, alone or combined with misonidazole (1.5 g/m² PO, 4 to 6 h before irradiation). Relief of pain was observed in 87% of patients treated with radiation therapy plus misonidazole compared with 74% with radiation therapy alone (P = 0.08). At these doses radiation hepatitis has not been observed, although in children this complication has been described when moderate doses of irradiation (25 Gy) are combined with cytotoxic agents[52]. Localized portions of the liver can be treated with higher doses (50 to 60 Gy)[53].

Spinal cord compression secondary to metastatic prostatic carcinoma

Although rare, patients with advanced prostate carcinoma may present with acute spinal cord compression. In a review by Flynn and Shipley[54], prostatic carcinoma metastasis accounted for 9% of 735 patients with spinal cord compression reported in the literature. Kuban et al.[55]

described a 6.8% incidence of spinal cord compression in patients with prostatic carcinoma, the greatest incidence being noted in patients with metastatic disease (27 of 157, 17.2%) or with poorly differentiated tumors (28 of 229, 12.2%). The most common signs and symptoms of cord compression are pain, usually radicular, progressive weakness of the lower extremities, and sensory loss. Autonomic dysfunction may be seen in approximately 50% of patients at diagnosis; related symptoms include difficulty in emptying the bladder, followed by retention and overflowing incontinence. Although the patient may be able to urinate, there is residual urine volume after voiding greater than 150 ml. Constipation may occur; a relaxed anal sphincter is noted on physical examination.

Besides physical examination, prompt magnetic resonance or computed tomography scan imaging usually confirms the diagnosis and localizes the cord compression level. Bony abnormalities associated with cord compression may be noted, such as erosion or collapse of vertebral bodies, paravertebral soft tissue masses, or osteoblastic metastasis.

The most common sites of cord compression are the thoracic (56.2% to 72.5% of patients), lumbar (18% to 36.5%) and cervical spine (2.9% to 14%), as reported by Flynn and Shipley.[54]

Spinal cord compression is a medical emergency that must be promptly treated. Preservation or restoration of ambulation and bladder function are measures of successful treatment, although pain relief is also an important goal. Corticosteroids at high doses as soon as the diagnosis is made may be of value in reducing neurologic deficiencies[54]. Some authors recommend doses as high as 100 mg of intravenous dexamethasone administered initially, followed by similar oral doses that are tapered every few days. However, in a report by Greenberg et al.[56] no difference was seen in neurologic outcome after this type of therapy in comparison with historic controls from the same institution.

Irradiation alone or following surgical decompression has been the standard method of treatment. The doses of irradiation range from 30 to 45 Gy, 2.5 to 3 Gy daily, four or five fractions per week, depending on the general condition and prognosis of the patient. The target volume should be generous, usually three vertebral bodies above and below the limits of the cord compression noted on radiographic studies. Based on experimental studies, Rubin et al.[57] recommended doses of 3 to 4 Gy for the first 3 days to induce greater tumor regression that would offset the initial cord edema induced by the irradiation.

Shoskes and Perrin[58] reported that 15 ambulatory patients remained ambulatory and eight of 13 (62%) bedridden patients became ambulatory after surgical laminectomy and radiation therapy for prostatic carcinona. Of the 20 patients who could walk after laminectomy, 15 remained ambulatory until death. In a group of 34 patients, decompression relieved pain in 26 (77%). Flynn and Shipley[54] reported a 36% ambulatory rate in 11 bedridden patients treated with surgery alone, 53% in 15 patients treated with irradiation alone, and 44% in 18 patients treated with surgery plus radiation therapy for cord compression from prostate carcinoma.

The best results with irradiation alone are seen in patients who are ambulatory and have minimal to moderate paraparesis, rather than in patients who are paraplegic, for whom the probability of motor function recovery is small. Barcena et al.[59] reported 100% post-treatment ambulation in nine ambulatory patients with minimal paresis compared with 52% in 25 with paraparesis and only 38% in 21 who were paraplegic. Flynn and Shipley[54] noted that patients treated within 24 h of initiation of motor dysfunction had significantly better recovery than those treated later. Median survival in patients with spinal cord compression secondary to prostatic carcinoma ranges from 6 to 13 months, with 50% of patients surviving for 1 year and 30% surviving for 2 years[54,60]. Functional palliation depends on early treatment, and survival depends primarily on the progress of systemic disease and response to hormonal therapy.

References

1. Perez CA, Eisbruch A. Role of postradical prostatectomy irradiation in carcinoma of the prostate. *Semin Radiat Oncol* 1993;**3**:198–209.

2. Keisch MK, Perez CA, Grigsby PW, Bauer WC, Catalona WJ. Preliminary report on 10 patients treated by irradiation after radical prostatectomy for isolated elevated prostate specific antigen. *Int J Radiat Oncol Biol Phys* 1990;**19**:1503–1506.

3. Link P, Freiha FS, Stamey TA. Adjuvant radiation therapy in patients with detectable prostate specific antigen following radical prostatectomy. *J Urol* 1991;**145**:532–534.

4. Hudson MA, Catalona WJ. Effect of adjuvant radiation therapy on prostate specific antigen following radical prostatectomy. *J Urol* 1990;**143**:1174–1177.

5. McCarthy JF, Catalona WJ, Hudson MA. Effect of radiation therapy on detectable serum prostate specific antigen levels following radical prostatectomy: Early versus delayed treatment. *J Urol* 1994;**151**:1575–1578.

6. McCarthy JF, Hudson MA, Catalona WJ. Radiation therapy after radical prostatectomy: Long-term followup (abstract). *J Urol* 1996;**155**(suppl):608A.

7. Perez CA, Cosmatos D, Garcia DM, Eisbruch A, Poulter CA. Irradiation in relapsing carcinoma of the prostate. *Cancer* 1993;**71**:1110–1122.

8. Eisbruch A, Perez CA, Roessler EH, Lockett MA. Adjuvant irradiation after prostatectomy for carcinoma of the prostate with positive surgical margins. *Cancer* 1994;**73**:884–887.

9. Forman JA, Wharam MD, Lee DJ, Zinreich ES, Order SE. Definitive radiotherapy following prostatectomy: Results and complications. *Int J Radiat Oncol Biol Phys* 1986;**12**:185–189.

10. Hanks GE, Dawson AK. The role of external beam radiation therapy after prostatectomy for prostate cancer. *Cancer* 1986;**58**:2406–2410.

11. Jacobson GM, Smith JA, Stewart JR. Postoperative radiation therapy for pathologic stage C prostate cancer. *Int J Radiat Oncol Biol Phys* 1987;**13**:1021–1024.

12. Ray GR, Bagshaw MA, Freiha F. External beam radiation salvage for residual or recurrent local tumor following radical prostatectomy. *J Urol* 1984;**132**:926–930.

13. Perez CA, Pilepich MV, Garcia D, Simpson Zivnuska F Jr, Hederman MA. Definitive radiation therapy in carcinoma of the prostate localized to the pelvis: experience at the Mallinckrodt Institute of Radiology. *NCI Monogr* 1988;**8**:85–94.

14. Anscher MA, Prosnitz LR. Radiotherapy versus hormonal therapy for the management of locally recurrent prostate cancer following radical prostatectomy. *Int J Radiat Oncol Biol Phys* 1989;**17**:963–958.

15. Goffinet DR, Martinez A, Freiha F et al. 125 Iodine prostate implants for recurrent carcinomas after external beam irradiation: Preliminary results. *Cancer* 1980;**45**:2717–2724.

16. Martinez M, Edmundson GD, Cox RS, Gunderson LL, Howes AE. Combination of external beam irradiation and multiple-site perineal applicator (MUPIT) for treatment of locally advanced or recurrent prostatic, anorectal, and gynecologic malignancies. *Int J Radiat Oncol Biol Phys* 1985;**11**:391–398.

17. Carlton CE Jr, Dawoud F, Hudgins P, Scott R Jr. Irradiation treatment of carcinoma of the prostate: a preliminary report based on 8 years of experience. *J Urol* 1972;**18**:924–927.

18. Kraus PA, Lutton B, Weiss RM, Prosnitz LR. Radiation therapy for local palliative treatment of prostatic cancer. *J Urol* 1972;**108**:612–614.

19. Kynaston HG, Keen CW, Matthews PH. Radiotherapy for palliation of locally advanced prostatic carcinoma. *Br J Urol* 1990;**66**:515–517.

20. Lankford SP, Pollack A, Zagars GK. Radiotherapy for regionally localized hormone refractory prostate cancer. *Int J Radiat Oncol Biol Phys* 1995;**33**:907–912.

21. Tong D, Gillick L, Hendrickson FR. The palliation of symptomatic osseous metastases: Final results of the study by the Radiation Therapy Oncology Group. *Cancer* 1982;**50**:893–899.

22. Blitzer PH. Reanalysis of the RTOG study of the palliation of symptomatic osseous metastasis. *Cancer* 1985;**55**:1468–1472.

23. Kuban DA, Delbridge T, El-Mahdi AM, Schellhammer PF. Half-body irradiation for treatment of widely metastatic adenocarcinoma of the prostate. *J Urol* 1989;**141**:572–574.

24. Zelefsky MJ, Scher HI, Forman JD, Linares LA, Curley T, Fuks Z. Palliative hemiskeletal irradiation for widespread metastatic prostate cancer: a comparison of single dose and fractionated regimens. *Int J Radiat Oncol Biol Phys* 1989;**17**:1281–1285.

25. Poulter CA, Cosmatos D, Rubin P et al. A report of RTOG 8206: A phase III study of whether the addition of single dose hemibody irradiation to standard fractionated local field irradiation is more effective than local field irradiation alone in the treatment of symptomatic osseous metastases. *Int J Radiat Oncol Biol Phys* 1992;**23**:207–214.

26. Blake GM, Wood JF, Wood PJ, Zivanovic MA, Lewington VJ. [89]Sr therapy: Strontium plasma clearance in disseminated prostatic carcinoma. *Eur J Nucl Med* 1989;**15**:49–54.

27. Buchali K, Correns H-J, Schuerer M, Schnorr D, Lips H, Sydown K. Results of a double blind study of 89-strontium therapy of skeletal metastases of prostatic carcinoma. *Eur J Nucl Med* 1988;**14**:349–351.

28. Robinson RG, Blake GM, Preston DF et al. Strontium-89: Treatment results and kinetics in patients with painful metastatic prostate and breast cancer in bone. *Radiographics* 1989;**9**:271–281.

29. Dusing RW et al. Strontium-89 chloride for pain palliation in the skeletal metastases of breast cancer. Clin Nucl Med (abstract) (in press)

30. Porter AT, McEwan AJB, Powe JR et al. Results of a randomized phase III trial to evaluate the efficacy of strontium-89 adjuvant to local field external beam irradiation in the management of endocrine resistant metastatic prostate cancer. *Int J Radiat Oncol Biol Phys* 1993;**25**:805–813.

31. Bolger JJ, Dearnaley DP, Kirk D et al. Strontium-89 (Metastron) versus external beam radiotherapy in patients with painful bone metastases secondary to prostatic cancer: Preliminary report of a multicenter trial. UK Metastron Investigators Group. *Semin Oncol* 1993;**20**:32–33.

32. Quilty PM, Kirk D, Bolger JJ et al. A comparison of the palliative effects of strontium-89 and external beam radiotherapy in metastatic prostate cancer. Radiother Oncol 1994;**31**:33–40.

33. Laing AH, Ackery DM, Bauly RJ et al. Strontium-89 chloride for pain palliation in prostatic skeletal malignancy. Br J Radiol 1991; **64**:816–822.

34. McEwan AJ, Porter AT, Venner PM, Amyotte G. An evaluation of the safety and efficacy of treatment with strontium-89 in patients who have previously received wide field radiotherapy. Antibodies Immunoconjugates Radiopharm 1990;**3**:91–98.

35. Joshi DP, Seery WH, Goldberg LG, Goldman L. Evaluation phosphorus-32 for intractable pain secondary to prostatic carcinoma metastases. JAMA 1965;**193**:621–623.

36. Smart JF. The use of P32 in the treatment of severe pain from bone metastases of carcinoma of the prostate. Br J Urol 1965;**37**:139–147.

37. Rubenfeld S. Treatment of bone metastases from carcinoma of the prostate with parathyroid hormone and radioactive phosphorus. Urology 1973;**1**:268–269.

38. Tong ECK, Finkelstein P. The treatment of prostatic radiophosphorus therapy in prostatic carcinoma. Urology 1973;**1**:71–75.

39. Edland RW. Testosterone potentiated radiophosphorus therapy of osseous metastases in prostatic cancer. Am J Roentgenol 1974;**120**: 678–683.

40. Glaser MG, Howard N, Waterfall N. Carcinoma of the prostate: the treatment of bone metastases by radiophosphorus. Clin Radiol 1981;**32**:695–697.

41. Aziz H, Choi K, Sohn C, Yaes R, Rotman M. Comparison of ^{32}P therapy and sequential hemibody irradiation (HBI) for bony metastases as methods of whole body irradiation. Am J Clin Oncol 1986;**9**:264–268.

42. Pinck BD, Alexander S. Parathormone potentiated radiophosphorus therapy in prostatic carcinoma. Urology 1972;**1**:201–204.

43. Maxfield JR, Maxfield JJG, Maxfield WS. The use of radioactive phosphorus and testosterone in metastatic bone lesions from breast and prostate. South Med J 1958;**51**:320–328.

44. Vermooten V, Maxfield JR, Maxfield JGS. The use of radioactive phosphorus in the management of advanced carcinoma of the prostate. West J Surg 1959;**67**:245–249.

45. Donati RM, Ellis H, Gallahar NI. Testosterone potentiated ^{32}P therapy in prostate cancinoma. Cancer 1966;**19**:1088–1090.

46. Corwin SH, Maxwell M, Small M et al. Experiences with ^{32}P in advanced carcinoma of prostate. J Urol 1970;**104**:745–748.

47. Maxon HR III, Schroder LE, Hertzberg VS et al. Rhenium-186(Sn)HEDP for treatment of painful osseous metastases: Results of a doubleblind crossover comparison with placebo. J Nucl Med 1991;**32**:1877–1881.

48. Straffon RA, Kiser WS, Robitalle M, Dohn DF. Yttrium hypophysectomy in the management of metastatic carcinoma of the prostate gland in 13 patients. J Urol 1968;**99**:102–105.

49. Loeffler JS, Alexander E III, Kooy H, Wen RY, Fine HA, Black PM. Radiosurgery for brain metastases. PPO Updates 1991;**5**:1–12.

50. Patchell RA, Tibbs PA, Walsh JW et al. A randomized trial of surgery in the treatment of single metastases to the brain. N Engl J Med 1990;**322**:494–500.

51. Leibel SA, Pajak TF, Massullo V et al. A comparison of misonidazole sensitized to radiation therapy alone for the palliation of hepatic metastases: Results of a Radiation Therapy Oncology Group randomized prospective trial. Int J Radiat Oncol Biol Phys 1987;**13**:1057–1064.

52. Tefft M, Mitus A, Das I et al. Irradiation of the liver in children: Review of experience in the acute and chronic phases, and in the intact normal and partially resected. Am J Roentgenol 1970;**108**:365–385.

53. Lawrence TS, Tesser RJ, Ten Haken RK. An application of dose volume histograms to the treatment of intrahepatic malignancies with radiation therapy. Int J Radiat Oncol Biol Phys 1990;**19**:1041–1047.

54. Flynn DF, Shipley WU. Management of spinal cord compression secondary to metastatic prostatic carcinoma. Urol Clin North Am 1991;**18**(1):145–152.

55. Kuban DA, El-Mahdi AM, Sigfred SV et al. Characteristics of spinal cord compression in adenocarcinoma of prostate. Urology 1986;**28**: 364–369.

56. Greenberg HS, Kim JH, Posner JB. Epidural spinal cord compression from metastatic tumor: Results with a new treatment protocol. Ann Neurol 1980;**8**:361–366.

57. Rubin H, Lome LG, Presman D. Neurological manifestation of metastatic prostatic carcinoma. J Urol 1974;**111**:799–802.

58. Shoskes DA, Perrin RG. The role of surgical management for symptomatic spinal cord compression patients with metastatic prostate cancer. J Urol 1989;**142**:337–339.

59. Barcena A, Lobato RD, Rivas JJ et al. Spinal metastatic disease: An analysis of factors determining functional prognosis and the choice of treatment. Neurosurgery 1984;**15**:820–827.

60. Liskow A, Chang CC, DeSanctis P et al. Epidural cord compression in association with genitourinary neoplasms. Cancer 1986;**58**:949–954.

17.4 Strontium[89] in metastatic disease

J Bolger

Introduction

Strontium[89] is an alkaline earth element found adjacent to calcium in the periodic table. Strontium[89] should be distinguished from strontium[90]. Strontium[90] is a hazardous gamma ray emitting isotope with a very prolonged half-life produced by nuclear explosions. Strontium[89] has a relatively short half-life and is essentially a beta-emitter (Table 17.4.1). It is used to treat bone metastases but is of no help in the palliation of soft tissue disease[1].

Physiology

After intravenous injection strontium[89] follows the biochemical pathways of calcium in the body. It is taken up in the mineral matrix of the bone and is eliminated primarily by the kidneys, the remainder by biliary excretion. It is selectively taken up at sites of high bone turnover and so is concentrated in sites of metastatic disease. Only small amounts are taken up by healthy bone and elimination from healthy bone is rapid. Consequently the radiation dose to healthy bone and marrow is approximately one-fifth to one-tenth that of metastatic sites. Retention of iso-

Table 17.4.1 Physical characteristics of strontium[89]

Physical half-life	= 50.5 days
Beta energy (Mev)	= 1.5
Penetration of beta rays	= 8 mm
Gamma ray emission	= negligible

tope is dependent upon the number of sites of metastatic disease, the greater the number of sites the greater the retention[2].

Administration

Strontium[89] is administered by intravenous injection in a dose of 150 MBq over a few minutes. It should only be given by those experienced in the use of radio-isotopes who are suitably licensed. Such injections should only be given in a designated department of nuclear medicine or radiotherapy. All the usual precautions concerned with the administration of unsealed isotopes should be taken with appropriate facilities for dealing with isotope spillage and disposal.

Radiation protection

Radiation protection regulations vary from country to country. In the United Kingdom a patient who has received a therapeutic dose of strontium[89] is not considered to be a hazard to those in proximity to the patient, as strontium[89] is a beta-emitter with only a short range in tissue. Strontium[89] can be given as an outpatient without risk to the general population. Low concentrations of strontium[89] are present in the patient's urine for 1 to 2 weeks after treatment. It is recommended that incontinent patients are not treated or are catheterized prior to therapy.

After passing urine the patient should 'double flush' the lavatory and dispose of any spillage in the same way. Burial or cremation of a cadaver previously treated with strontium[89] does not require any special precautions[3].

Efficacy

Uncontrolled studies have shown that strontium[89] produces significant pain relief from bone metastases in approximately 75% to 80% of patients. A randomized trial comparing strontium[89] with conventional external beam radiotherapy (local and hemibody) confirm this level of pain relief and also show strontium[89] to be as effective as conventional radiotherapy[4,5]. In addition it significantly decreases the number of new sites of symptomatic bone pain developing. Further studies using strontium[89] as an adjuvant to external beam radiotherapy have also demonstrated this effect of decreasing new sites of symptomatic pain[6]. Symptomatic response to strontium[89] begins approximately 2 to 3 weeks following therapy and reaches a maximum at approximately 6 weeks. The use of strontium[89] as an adjuvant to radical primary therapy or for treatment of asymptomatic patients with a biochemical relapse has not yet been explored. The use of strontium[89]

rather than conventional radiotherapy does not appear to confer any survival benefit.

Toxicity

The principal toxicity of strontium[89] is hematologic. White blood count and platelet depression to approximately two-thirds of baseline values occurs around 4 to 8 weeks post-treatment. The blood parameters gradually return towards normal over subsequent months. If the patient has a suitable white cell and platelet count pre-treatment (white count 3×10^9/l; platelets 100×10^9/l) with normal renal function such depression will not be clinically significant. Occasionally patients have a brief exacerbation of their pain but only rarely is this serious and settles spontaneously after suitable temporary increase in analgesia.

Re-treatment

If a patient has been treated successfully on one occasion with strontium[89] repeat administration is possible if the peripheral blood count is satisfactory and renal function normal. If a patient has responded to initial therapy and then had a symptomatic relapse prospects for a second response are good. Repeat administration after initial failure is very unlikely to be helpful. A repeat dose of strontium[89] should not be given for a minimum period of 3 months after first treatment. A significant number of patients have received several doses of strontium[89] over a period of years and this ability to repeat treatment highlights an advantage over conventional external beam radiotherapy.

Cost

The absolute cost of strontium[89] is high. Its economic viability as a therapy is dependent upon the health care system in which it is used. The cost may be offset against such expenses as inpatient care, conventional radiotherapy facilities and the cost of support medication to treat side effects of other treatments. The fact that strontium[89] significantly reduces the number of new sites requiring treatment must also be taken into account. There is no doubt that in terms of patient convenience and upset the cost is justified as strontium[89] therapy is an outpatient procedure with a minimum of side effects. For the majority of patients therapy is no more demanding than a single venepuncture.

Conclusion

Strontium[89] is a simple, single visit, outpatient medication giving relief of pain in the majority of patients. It is as effective as conventional radiotherapy with a minimum of side effects. Toxicity is predominantly hematologic but is seldom a problem if pre-treatment peripheral blood count and renal function are satisfactory. An additional benefit is the delay in the development of new sites of pain. It is effective for bone metastases but is not suitable for soft tissue disease. If the patient's peripheral blood count and renal function allow, the treatment may be repeated on a number of occasions.

References

1. Bolger JJ. Strontium[89] for treatment of prostate cancer. *Cope* 1995;**11**: 20–21.
2. Ackery D, Yardley J, Radionuclide-targeted therapy for the management of metastatic bone pain. *Semin Oncol* 1993 (June)**20**:27–31.
3. Cooper JR, Walmsley A, Charles D. Individual and collective doses from the release of SR[89] into the environment following medicine administration. National Radiological Protection Board contract report 1989; NRPB-M193.
4. Bolger JJ, Dearnley DP, Kirk D *et al.* Strontium[89] (Metastron) versus external beam radiotherapy in patients with painful bone metastases secondary to prostatic cancer: preliminary report of a multicenter trial. *Semin Oncol* 1993; (June)**20**:32–33.
5. Quilty PM, Kirk D, Bolger JJ *et al.* A comparison of the palliative effects of Strontium[89] and external beam radiotherapy in metastatic prostate cancer. *Radiother Oncol* 1994;**31**:33–40.
6. Porter AT, McEwan AJB, Powe JE *et al.* Results of a randomised phase III trial to evaluate the efficacy of SR[89] adjuvant to local field external beam irradiation in the management of endocrine resistant metastatic prostate cancer. *Int J Rad Oncol Biol Phys* 1993;**25**:805–813.

17.5 The use of biophosphonates in prostate carcinoma metastatic to the skeleton

N A T Hamdy

Bisphosphonates

Bisphosphonates are potent inhibitors of osteoclast-mediated bone resorption which are established as the treatment of choice in disorders associated with increased bone resorption such as Paget's disease of bone and malignancy-associated hypercalcaemia. Over the last decade, these agents have also been increasingly used at lower dose regimens in the management of osteoporosis[1,2]. The exact cellular and molecular mechanism by which bisphosphonates inhibit all aspects of normal and stimulated bone resorption has been recently elucidated. Nonnitrogen-containing bisphosphonates such as etidronate, clodronate and tiludronate are metabolized intracellularly to substances toxic to osteoclasts[3,4]. Nitrogen-containing bisphosphonates such as pamidronate, olpadronate, alendronate, risedronate, ibandronate and zoledronate interfere with specific enzymes of the mevalonate pathway, resulting in early osteoclast apoptosis by disrupting cytoskeletal integrity and intracellular signalling of these cells[5–9].

All bisphosphonates are poorly absorbed from the gastrointestinal tract. Absorption is indeed in the order of 1–5% of an orally administered dose, further decreased if ingested with food, particularly if calcium-containing, which would bind to the agent and diminish its absorption further. Pharmacokinetics data on these agents are scarce. About 50% of an absorbed dose is believed to be rapidly taken up by the skeleton where it remains for years, probably in a biologically inert form with no effect on bone remodelling, and the remainder is rapidly excreted in the urine. More of the drug has thus to be presented more frequently to bone to be effective in conditions of ongoing stimulation of bone remodeling such as in malignancy-induced events. The potency of bisphosphonates to inhibit bone resorption varies from compound to compound and this can be quantitated by measuring changes in biochemical parameters of bone turnover, which are also used to evaluate biological responses[1,2].

The use of bisphosphonates in the clinic is associated with very few side effects. Gastro intestinal intolerance may occur specially with the use of nitrogen-containing bisphosphonates such as pamidronate and alendronate, particularly when large doses are given. An acute phase reaction is also described when these agents are used for the first time. Etidronate, has a narrow therapeutic window so that caution must be exerted with its continuous long-term use in high doses as the doses that effectively inhibit bone resorption are close to those which inhibit bone mineralization. Finally, large doses of bisphosphonates infused rapidly may result in acute renal failure due to their capacity to chelate calcium with precipitation of the insoluble complexes in the renal tubules. Slow intravenous delivery is recommended for all bisphosphonates in current use although the use of bolus administrations is being explored for the more potent newer bisphosphonates[1,2].

Bisphosphonates in metastatic prostate carcinoma

Bone metastases in prostate carcinoma

Pathophysiology

The metastatic potential of tumor cells to 'seed' skeletal sites, the 'soil' to which they must attach to grow, is critically determined by their adhesion properties which are modulated at least in part by the bony microenvironment[10–14]. Once implanted, prostate carcinoma cells secrete soluble factors with selective mitogenic properties for osteoblasts, thereby stimulating their proliferation[15,16]. Increased bone resorption at metastatic and non-metastatic sites is likely to be due to the production of cytokines by tumor cells. This increase in osteoclast-mediated bone resorption further releases growth regulatory factors, large stores of which are found in the bone matrix. A number of these factors such as transforming growth factor ß (TGFß), fibroblast growth factors, insulin growth factors I and II, proteases, particularly the plasminogen activator uPA, bone morphogenetic proteins and endothelin 1, modulate tumor growth and activity, and act as chemoattractants for further tumor cells, thereby amplifying the metastatic process[17–19].

Morbidity

Prostate carcinoma metastasizes frequently to the skeleton and some two-thirds of patients with this malignancy would have evidence for bone metastases at the time of diagnosis. Skeletal metastases are associated with significant morbidity, mostly due to severe bone pain, worse at night, soon progressing to become intractable despite maximum use of analgesics and opiates. Other complications include pathological fractures, nerve compression syndromes, spinal cord compression and bone marrow compromise due to widespread invasion and replacement of the marrow space by tumor cells[20].

Rationale for use of bisphosphonates in prostate carcinoma

The mechanism responsible for osteolytic bone metastases is the stimulation of osteoclast–mediated bone resorption by tumor cells or their products and bisphosphonates are highly efficient in inhibiting this process[21]. Prostate carcinoma is, however, typically associated with osteoblastic metastases so that the rationale for using bisphosphonates in this malignancy appears to be much less impeccable. Notwithstanding, an increase in bone resorption has been consistently demonstrated in bone biopsies from metastatic as well as tumor-free skeletal sites[22–24]. Urinary excretion of hydroxyproline, a marker of bone resorption also correlates significantly with that of serum alkaline phosphatase activity: a marker of bone formation[23], suggesting an overall concommitant increase in bone resorption. In addition to their stimulatory effect on osteoblasts, prostate carcinoma cell lines (PC III) were also found to induce osteoclast-mediated bone resorption in animal models[25]. Finally, there is increasing evidence that in patients with metastatic bone disease, pain is associated with an increased rate of bone resorption and that suppression of bone resorption results in a decrease in bone pain[26].

Pretreatment of PC3 and PmCIII cells (a highly metastatic PCIII subline) for 24 h in vitro with ibandronate, risedronate, pamidronate or clodronate, was shown to dose- dependently inhibit tumor cell attachment to mineralized and unmineralized extracellular bone matrix[27]. No effect was observed on tumor cell attachment when only the bone matrix was pretreated suggesting a direct effect of bisphosphonates on tumor cells. The inhibitory activity of bisphosphonates on in vitro tumor cell attachment correlated with their known in vivo relative potencies. Pretreatment with clodronate or pamidronate has been shown to retard in vivo the process of spinal tumor invasion in male Copenhagen rats intravenously injected with prostatic carcinoma cells[28]. These findings are in keeping with similar data on the attachment of breast carcinoma cells to bone matrix after pretreatment with bisphosphonates[29]. In prostate cancer, bisphosphonates may also directly affect the metastatic process by inhibiting the invasion of bone matrices by tumor cells[30] as well as by inhibiting their growth[31]. These findings hold promise for a potential beneficial effect of bisphosphonates in modulating the metastatic process in this malignancy.

Clinical studies

Several problems are encountered in the evaluation of treatment modalities in metastatic bone disease. In prostate carcinoma, bone metastases are often multiple and diffuse and are notoriously difficult to monitor. The main measure of response is symptomatic improvement in pain, but this is essentially subjective and uniform criteria for assessment of pain are lacking so that assessment of efficacy and comparison between different treatment modalities is difficult. Compliance to oral medication is also less than optimal in patients in the late stages of their malignancy and bisphosphonates may be poorly tolerated at the large doses required. Three of the commercially available bisphosphonates: etidronate, clodronate and pamidronate have been tested in the palliation of pain in patients with metastatic carcinoma of the prostate.

Etidronate

An open study conducted in a small number of patients originally showed promise[32], but these results could not be reproduced in a large double-blind placebo controlled trial[33]. Etidronate appears to be ineffective in the palliation of metastatic bone pain at least at the mode of administration used and dose tested. The narrow therapeutic window of this bisphosphonate and the need for long-term treatment in prostate carcinoma precluded the design of further studies using larger doses for prolonged periods of time.

Clodronate

The use of clodronate in the palliation of painful bone metastases has been more extensively addressed. Seventeen patients treated with intravenous clodronate at a dose of 300 mg/day for 14 days followed by 3.2 g po or 100 mg i.m/day for 4 to 11 weeks demonstrated a significant improvement in pain and a decrease in the daily consumption of analgesics within 2 weeks of treatment, with symptoms recurring 4–8 weeks after discontinuation[34]. A dramatic improvement in pain is further reported in 80 of 92 patients treated with 300 mg i.v./day for 10 days with maintenance of the beneficial effect with oral clodronate. The intramuscular and oral routes were found to be much less effective in controlling symptoms[35]. A similar decrease in pain symptoms is demonstrated in a different study in 29 of 41 patients (71%) within 3–5 days of iv clodronate 300 mg/d for 8 days followed by oral maintenance therapy 1.6 g/day[36].

The only double-blind placebo controlled trials using clodronate come from the finnish group of Elomaa et al. The first study compares the use of oral clodronate at a dose of 3.2 g/d for 1 month followed by 1.6 g/day for 5 month to placebo, in a group of 75 patients with hormone-resistant prostate carcinoma[37]. An only marginal benefit was observed in the actively treated group compared to controls, but these results are confounded by simultaneously starting anti-tumor treatment with estramustine and clodronate at the beginning of the study. Using the same study design, but additionally examining bone histology, 57 patients were further treated with iv clodronate at a dose of 300 mg/day for 5 days followed by 1.6 g/day for 3 months. Features of osteomalacia were rather surprisingly observed in both groups of patients treated with either clodronate or placebo in addition to estramustinea possible role for a relative deficiency of calcium and phosphate was suggested[38]. Although double-blind placebo-controlled, the confounding role of concommitant antitumour treatment renders the evaluation of the outcome of both these studies rather difficult. The Newcastle group studied 27 patients with progressive hormone-resistant prostatic carcinoma in an open multicentre trial comparing clodronate given at a dose of 300 mg/d i.v. for 10 days followed by 1.6 g/d p.o. for 4 to 12 weeks to placebo. An effective response was reported in only 10 of the 27 patients and long-term response was poor, sustained in only three of the patients on continuous oral maintenance therapy[39]. Lastly, a significant palliative response was observed in 75% of patients treated with daily intravenous infusions of 300 mg clodronate for 8 days followed by maintenance oral therapy at a dose of 1600 mg/day. The response was relatively short-lived: mean duration nine weeks[40]. Taken overall these data suggest that using clodronate, the intravenous route of administration is necessary for an adequate symptomatic response, and that long-term oral therapy, at the dose tested, is inadequate in maintaining this response.

Pamidronate

Symptomatic relief of metastatic bone pain was also reported with the use of intravenous pamidronate, but the response was short-lived requiring repeat infusions at regular 2 weekly intervals[41]. A significant relationship between biochemical and clinical response was additionally demonstrated in a separate study of seven patients with hormone-resistant metastatic prostatic carcinoma treated with 15 mg pamidronate intravenously daily for 7 days[42]. Similar responses were obtained in 25 patients treated with intravenous pamidronate at a dose of 30 mg once a week for 4 weeks and every 2 weeks thereafter for 5 months[43]. In this study, the authors document the discrepancy between the consistent decreases in urinary calcium after treatment with bisphosphonates and the more variable changes in urinary hydroxyproline excretion suggesting an additional tumor source for the hydroxyproline measured. Bone biopsies obtained before and 6 months after intravenous pamidronate in 27 patients, and at baseline and after 6 months on no treatment in 9 more patients, confirmed increased bone resorption in metastatic (7 biopsies through metastases) and non-metastatic sites, the mechanism of which could not be further elucidated[44].

No significant dose–response relationship could be shown in 58 patients given intravenous pamidronate 30 mg every 2 weeks, 60 mg every 4 weeks, 60 mg every 2 weeks or 90 mg every 4 weeks in which all groups demonstrated improvement in symptoms[45].

Other bisphosphonates

In metastatic prostate carcinoma, similar to other malignancies, bone resorption is likely to continuously stimulated by local and systemic factors so that the response to any administered bisphosphonate is expected to be short-lived with a reversal of beneficial effects within 2–4 weeks of discontinuing therapy. Oral doses are poorly absorbed and large doses are therefore required to achieve adequate suppression of bone resorption. The relatively narrow therapeutic window of etidronate precludes its long-term use in high doses due to the risk of impairing mineralisation. The large doses of oral pamidronate required to effectively control symptoms are also likely to be associated with gastrointestinal side-effects. The delivery to the skeleton of adequate doses of a bisphosphonate which would be well tolerated and would also be safe and efficacious is in practice better achieved with the use of the more potent bisphosphonates which are currently in development. An example of such a bisphosphonate is olpadronate, a bisphosphonate obtained by the dimethylation of the nitrogen molecule of pamidronate which results in a 5 to 10–fold increase in anti-resorptive potency and has the distinct advantage of being very well tolerated in its oral form. Our group has demonstrated a beneficial clinical response in 75% of patients with hormone-resistant prostate carcinoma treated with intravenous olpadronate at a dose of 4 mg/day for 5 days. This response could be maintained with continuous oral olpadronate at a dose of 200 mg/day[26]. This bisphosphonate has also been shown to reduce the incidence of spinal cord compression in hormone-refractory prostate cancer metastatic to the skeleton[46]. Other experimental bisphosphonates such as ibandronate[47] and zoledronate[48] have also been tested in the management of metastatic prostate carcinoma and a number of studies are currently in progress to establish the beneficial effects of different agents in this malignancy.

Conclusions

Metastatic hormone-resistant prostatic carcinoma is incurable so the main goal of treatment is essentially palliative, aiming at decreasing morbidity by controlling pain[49–51]. Available evidence strongly suggests a role for bisphosphonates in the palliative management of metastatic prostate carcinoma. For successful responses, initial high doses of potent agents should be followed by maintenance treatments at doses sufficient to keep bone resorption suppressed. Bisphosphonates hold an advantage over the widely used bone-seeking radionuclides in that they do not result in bone marrow suppression. The trend has been to use these agents at a late stage in the natural history of prostate cancer, and the question arises whether bisphosphonates may not hold further therapeutic potential were they to be used earlier in the course of this ubiquitous malignancy. The inhibition of tumor cell attachment to bone matrix by bisphosphonates and their ability to effectively suppress bone resorption which enhances metastatic spread suggest that these agents may hold promise in the disruption of the metastatic process, thereby opening exciting new avenues for their potential use in the prevention of bone metastases. Further studies are certainly warranted to address this issue.

References

1. H Fleisch. Bisphosphonates in bone disease: From the laboratory to the patients. The Parthenon Publishing Group, New York; London, 1995, p.31–66.
2. Bijvoet OLM, Fleisch HA, Canfield RE, Russell RGG (eds) *Bisphosphonates on Bones.* Elsevier, Amsterdam 1995.
3. Frith JC, Monkkonen J, Blackburn GM, Russell RG, Rogers MJ. Clodronate and liposome-encapsulated clodronate are metabolized to a toxic ATP analog, adenosine 5'-(beta, gamma- dichloromethylene) triphosphate, by mammalian cells in vitro. *J Bone Miner Res* 1997;**12(9)**:1358–67.
4. Russell RGG, Rogers MJ, Frith JC, et al. The pharmacology of bisphosphonates and new insights into their mechanism of action. *J Bone Miner Res* 1999;**14(Supp)**:56–65.
5. Rogers MJ, Frith JC, Luckman SP, et al. Molecular mechanism of action of bisphosphonates. *Bone* 1999;**24**:73S–79S.
6. Luckman SP, Hughes DE, Coxon FP, et al. Nitrogen- containing bisphosphonates inhibit the mevalonate pathway and prevent post-translational prenylation of GTP-binding proteins including Ras. *J Bone Miner Res* 1998;**13**:581–589.
7. Van Beek E, Löwik C, van der Pluijm G, et al. The role of geranylgeranylation in bone resorption and its suppression by bisphosphonates in fetal bone explants in vitro: a clue to the mechanism of action of nitrogen-containing bisphosphonates. *J Bone Miner Res* 1999;**14**:722–729.
8. Fisher JE, Rogers MJ, Halasy JM, et al. Mechanism of action of alendronate: geranylgeraniol, an intermediate of the mevalonate pathway, prevents inhibition of osteoclast formation, bone resorption and kinase activity in vitro. *Proc Natl Acad Sci USA* 1999;**96**:133–138.
9. Van Beek E, Pieterman E, Cohen L, et al. Nitrogen- containing bisphosphonates inhibit isopentyl pyrophosphate isomerase/farnesyl pyrophosphate synthetase activity with relative potencies corresponding to their antiresorptive potencies in vitro and in vivo. *Biochem Biophys Res Commun* 1999;**255**:491–494.
10. Guise T, Mundy G. Cancer and bone. *Endocr Rev* 1998;**19**:18–54.
11. Mundy GR. Mechanisms of bone metastases. *Cancer* 1997;**80**:1546–1556.
12. Goltzman D. Mechanisms of the development of osteoblastic metastases. *Cancer* 1997;**80(8 Suppl)**:1581–7. Review.
13. Miyasaka M. Cancer metastasis and adhesion molecules. *Clin Orthop Rel Res* 1995;**312**:10–18.
14. Bussemakers MJG, Schalken JA. The role of cell adhesion molecules and proteases in tumor invasion and metastasis. *World J Urol* 1996;**14**:151–156.
15. Jacobs SC, Pikna D, Lawson RK. Prostatic osteoblastic factor. *Invest Urol* 1979;**17**:195–198.
16. Koutsilieris M, Rabbani SA, Bennett HPJ, Goltzman D. Characteristics of prostate-derived growth factors for cells of the osteoblast phenotype. 1987;**80**:941–946.
17. Orr FW, Varani J, Gondek MD, Ward PA, Mundy GR. Chemotactic responses of tumor cells to products of resorbing bone. *Science* 1979;**203**:176–179.
18. Kostenuik PJ, Singh G, Suyama KL, Orr FW. Stimulation of bone resorption results in a selective increase in growth rate of spontaneously metastatic Walker 256 cancer cells in bone. *Clin Exp Metastasis* 1992;**10**:411–418.
19. Manishen WJ, Sivananthan K, Orr FW. Resorbing bone stimulates tumor cell growth. A role for the host microenvironment in bone metastasis. *Am J Pathol* 1996;**123**:39–45.
20. Body JJ. Metastatic bone disease: Clinical and therapeutic aspects. *Bone* 1992;**13**:S57–S62.
21. Scher HI, Yagoda A. Bone metastases: Pathogenesis, treatment and rationale for use of resorption inhibitors. *Am J Med* 1987;**82**:6–28.
22. Urwin GH, Percival RC, Haris S, Beneton MNC, Williams JL, Kanis JA.Generalized increase in bone resorption in carcinoma of the prostate. *Br J Urol* 1985;**57**:721–723.
23. Percival RC, Urwin GH, Yates AJP, Williams JL, Beneton M, Kanis JA. Biochemical and histological evidence that carcinoma of the prostate is associated with increased bone resorption. *Eur J Surgical Oncology* 1987;**13**:41–49.
24. Clarke NW, McClure J, George JR. Morphometric evidence for bone resorption and replacement in prostate cancer. *Br J Urol* 1991;**68**:74–80.
25. Pollard M, Luckert PH. Effects of dichloromethylene diphosphonate on the osteolytic and osteoplastic effects of rat prostate adenocarcinoma cells. *J Natl Cancer Inst* 1985;**75**:949–951.
26. Pelger RC, Hamdy NA, Zwinderman AH, Lycklama a Nijeholt AA, Papapoulos SE. Effects of the bisphosphonate olpadronate in patients with carcinoma of the prostate metastatic to the skeleton. *Bone* 1998;**22(4)**:403–8.
27. Boissier S, Magnetto S, Frappart L, et al: Bisphosphonates inhibit prostate and breast carcinoma cell adhesion to unmineralized and mineralized bone extracellular matrices. *Cancer Res* 1997;**57**:3890–3894.
28. Yu-Cheng S, Geldof AA, Newling DWW, Rao R. Progression delay of prostate tumor skeletal metastasis effects by bisphosphonates. *J Urol* 1992;**148**:1270–1273.
29. van der Pluijm G, Vloedgraven H, van Beek E, van der Wee-Pals L, Lowik C, Papapoulos S. Bisphosphonates inhibit the adhesion of breast cancer cells to bone matrices in vivo. *J Clin Invest* 1996;**98**:1–8.
30. Boissier S, Ferreras M, Peyruchaud O, et al. Bisphosphonates inhibit breast and prostate carcinoma cell invasion, an early event in the formation of bone metastases. *Cancer Res* 2000;**60**:2949–2954.
31. Lee MV, Fong EM, Singer FR, Guenette RS. Bisphosphonate treatment inhibits the growth of prostate cancer cells. *Cancer Res* 2001;**61**:2602–2608.
32. Carey PO, Lippert MC. Treatment of painful prostatic bone metastases with oral etidronate disodium. *Urology* 1988;**22**:403–407.
33. Smith JA. Paliation of painful bone metastases from prostate cancer using sodium etidronate: Results of a randomized, prospective, double-blind, placebo-controlled study. *J Urol* 1989;**141**:85–87.
34. Adami S, Salvagno G, Guarrera G, Bianchi G, Dorizzi R, Rosini S, Mobilio G, Lo Cascio V. *J Urol* 1985;**134**:1152–1154.

35. Adami S, Mian M. Clodronate therapy of metastatic bone disease in patients with prostatic carcinoma. *Recent Results Cancer Res* 1989;**116**:67–72.
36. Vorreuther R. Bisphosphonates as an adjunct to palliative therapy of bone metastases from prostatic carcinoma. A pilot study on clodronate. *Br J Urol* 1993;**72**:792–795.
37. Elomaa I, Kylmala T, Tammela T, et al. . Effect of oral clodronate on bone pain. A controlled study in patients with metastatic prostatic carcinoma. *Int Urol Nephrol* 1992;**24**:159–166.
38. Taube T, Kylmala T, Lamberg-Allardt C, Tammela TLJ, Elomaa I. The effect of Clodronate on bone in metastatic prostate cancer. Histomorphometric report of a double-blind randomized placebo-controlled study. *Eur J Cancer* 1994;**30A**:751–758.
39. Cresswell SM, English PJ, Hall RR, Roberts JT, Marsh MM. Pain relief and quality of life assessment following intravenous and oral clodronate in hormone-escaped metastatic prostate cancer. *Br J Urol* 1995;**76**:360–365.
40. Heidenreich A, Hofmann R, Engelmann UD. The use of bisphosphonate for the palliative treatment of painful bone metastasis due to refractory prostate cancer. *J Urol* 2001;**165**:136–140.
41. Masud T, Slevin ML. Pamidronate to reduce bone pain in normocalcaemic patient with disseminated prostatic carcinoma. *Lancet* 1989;**ii**:1021–1022.
42. Pelger RCM, Lycklama a Nijeholt AAB, Papapoulos SE. Short-term metabolic effects of pamidronate in patients with prostatic carcinoma and bone metastases. *Lancet* 1989;**ii**:865.
43. Clarke NW, Holbrook IB, McClure J, George NJR. Osteoclast inhibition by pamidronate in metastatic prostate cancer: a preliminary study. *Br J Cancer* 1991;**63**:420–423.
44. Clarke NW, McClure J, George NJR. Disodium pamidronate identifies differential osteoclastic bone resorption in metastatic prostate cancer. *Br J Urol* 1992;**69**:64–70.
45. Lipton A, Glover D, Harvey H, Grabelsky S, Zelenakas K, Macerata R, Seaman J. Pamidronate in the treatment of bone metastases: Results of 2 dose-ranging trials in patients with breast or prostate cancer. Ann Oncol 1994;**5**:S31–S35.
46. Soerdjbalie-Maikoe V, Pelger RCM, Lycklama à Nijeholt AAB, Arndt J-W, Zwinderman AH, Papapoulos SE, Hamdy NAT. Strontium–89 (Metastron®) and the bisphosphonate olpadronate reduce the incidence of spinal cord compression in patients with hormone-refractory prostate cancer metastatic to the skeleton. *Eur J Nucl Med* 2002 (in press)
47. Coleman RE, Purohit OP, Black C, et al. Double-blind, randomized, placebo-controlled, dose-finding study of oral ibandronate in patients with metastatic bone disease. Ann Oncol 1999;**10**:311–316.
48. Coleman RE, Seaman JJ. The role of zoledronic acid in cancer: clinical studies in the treatment and prevention of bone metastases. *Semin Oncol* 2001;**28**:11–16.
49. Papapoulos SE, Hamdy NAT, van der Pluijm. Bisphosphonates in the management of prostate carcinoma metastatic to the skeleton. *Cancer* 2000;**88**:3047–3053.
50. Pelger RCM, Soerdjbalie-Maikoe V, Hamdy NAT. Strategies for management of prostate cancer related bone pain. *Drugs Aging* 2002 (in press).
51. Hamdy NAT, Papapoulos SE. The palliative management of skeletal metastases in prostate cancer: use of bone-seeking radionuclides and bisphosphonates. *Semin Nucl Med* 2001;**31**:62–68.

17.6   The role of monoclonal antibody imaging in the management of prostate cancer

D Khan, J C Austin and R D Williams

Introduction

Managing prostate cancer continues to be enigmatic, related in part to the inability accurately to stage patients prior to treatment. Currently, the serum level of PSA combined with the histologic differentiation (Gleason sum) of the tumor provides more predictable clinical staging than any imaging modality. In an attempt to improve upon the inability of conventional imaging to detect metastatic prostate cancer in lymph nodes or other soft tissue sites, monoclonal antibody imaging using radioimmunoconjugates specific to prostate antigens has been developed. In this chapter we will review the concept of monoclonal antibody imaging, the history of its use in prostate cancer imaging, and current data with respect to the use of ^{111}In-capromab pendetide (ProstaScint®).

Radioimmunoconjugates

Antibodies are distinct proteins, which are produced in response to an immune reaction, and are specific to the antigen, which elicited the response. In the case of anti-cancer antibodies, a tumor-associated antigen is typically used to generate the antibody. To be used in radioimmunoscintigraphy (RIS), the antibody must first be radiolabeled. Most whole, anticancer antibodies used for RIS (including those used for patients with prostate cancer) are labeled with either [131]I (half-life 8 days) or [111]In (half-life 2.8 days). [99m]Tc (half-life 6 h) can be used with whole antibodies, but poses special problems in terms of the chemical labeling procedure. Protein labeling with ^{131}I is relatively simple using techniques such as the cholamine-T or iodogenic methods. The principal disadvantages of RIS with ^{131}I-labeled antibodies are the dehalogenation which occurs and the lower dose of ^{131}I that must be used for safety concerns (both of which degrade image quality). Compared with iodinated antibodies, ^{111}In-labeled immunoconjugates offer the advantage of quality images (single-photon emission computerized tomography or SPECT) when between 3 and 6 mCi is administered, substantially more stable binding of the radioatom to the protein, and a physical half-life which is approximately equal to the biologic serum half-life of many murine whole monoclonal antibodies. The main drawbacks of ^{111}In are that considerably more complex chemistry procedures are required for antibody labeling, and, unlike radioiodinated antibodies, a significantly higher fraction of the injected dose normally accumulates in the liver and bone marrow. This accumulation of activity degrades the lesion-to-background ratio such that tumor metastases in the bone and liver are often not detectable.

Imaging technique

Following intravenous injection most ^{131}I or ^{111}In-radiolabeled whole antibodies have blood clearance half-times in excess of 24 h; imaging therefore is typically delayed for

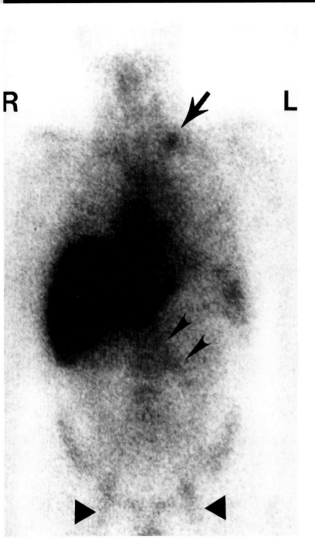

Fig. 17.6.1 Whole-body planar image obtained 5 days after injection of ^{111}In-capromab pendetide in a 74-year-old man with a PSA of 6.8 4 years following radical prostatectomy. A lesion is seen in the left supraclavicular region (arrow) and subtly in the upper abdomen to the left of the spine (arrowheads). Normal accumulation of the radioimmunoconjugate is seen in the liver, spleen, bone marrow (e.g. spine and pelvis) and in the blood pool within the femoral vessels (triangles). R = right; L = left.

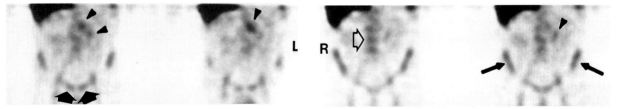

Fig. 17.6.2 Four abdominal coronal images (moving posterior to anterior, left to right) of the same patient seen in Figure 17.7.1. The lesions (small arrowheads) in the abdomen are now clearly seen anterior off the left of the spine (open arrowhead) in the periaortic and left perirenal locations. Normal bone marrow activity is seen in the pubic rami (large arrowheads) and in the pelvis (arrows). Normal activity in the liver is seen in the upper right of each image. R = right; L = left.

at least 48 h following injection. Imaging of patients receiving [99mTc]-labeled proteins is often started by 1 to 6 h and completed by 18 to 24 h. In either case, the principal reason for the delay between the time of injection and scanning is to permit the activity in the blood (and therefore in the body tissues) to decline so that antibody preferentially attached to the target site (e.g. tumor) can be detected.

Imaging is carried out using conventional nuclear medicine gamma cameras. Typically a planar, whole-body set of images is obtained so as to evaluate the entire body for sites of disease. The patient will have multiplanar tomography performed of the regions of the body which are most likely to have disease present. SPECT is more accurate than planar imaging when studying patients with cancer, and must be performed in all cases. Current gamma-camera technology has advanced to the point that larger field-of-view cameras, which are multi-headed and can have their camera head's orbit programmed to match a particular patient's body habitus, are most effective.

Imaging antiprostate cancer radioimmunoconjugates in humans

Over 20 years ago Kohler and Milstein first reported producing a monoclonal antibody through the use of their hybridoma system[1]. Until their method of producing 'pure' murine antibodies became available, polyclonal antibodies had been used in clinical practice since about 1948, when Pressman and Keighley reported on their investigations of the murine kidney in vivo[2]. In the late 1970s, a number of studies were performed using radioiodinated polyclonal antibodies directed against a variety of tissues, including the pioneering work of Goldenberg et al.[3] and Mach et al.[4] in tumors. The first report of RIS in patients with prostate cancer was published in 1983 by Goldenberg and DeLand using prostatic acid phosphatase (PAP) antibodies[5]. They later expanded their work in a larger group of patients with prostate cancer using the same polyclonal antibodies[6].

Prostate cancer lesions were successfully imaged with these radioimmunoconjugates, and the authors concluded that RIS with this agent was safe and reasonably effective (Table 17.6.1). Notably, bone lesions were not detected with this radioimmunoconjugate.

Monoclonal radioimmunoconjugates: anti-PSA and anti-PAP antibodies

Vihko and co-workers employed [111In]- or [99mTc]-labeled monoclonal antibodies of murine origin or fragments against PAP[7]. They injected varying doses of protein and radionuclide in four patients with prostate cancer. All sites of tumor, including the prostate, were seen with these immunoconjugates. They also reported five patients who, prior to scheduled prostatectomy and lymphadenectomy, had 1 mg of [99mTc]-labeled F(ab)$_2$' directed against PAP injected percutaneously into the periprostatic space[8]. In one patient, abnormal activity was detected in multiple lymph nodes including periaortic nodes. Histopathologic examination of multiple nodes in the obturator, iliac and periaortic regions confirmed the scan findings in the single scan-positive patient, and confirmed the negative scan in the other four patients. The authors concluded from their preliminary data that lymphoscintigraphy may accurately determine the extent of regional spread of prostate cancer before prostatectomy.

Dillman and co-workers studied nine patients with an anti-PSA monoclonal antibody: four with [111In]-labeled PSA-399 and five with an anti-prostatic acid phosphatase antibody, [111In]-labeled PAY-276[9]. With all doses administered, the fraction of tumor sites detected was 55% and 16% for the [111In]-labeled PSA-399 and the [111In]-labeled PAY-276, respectively. The results of this limited trial led the authors to conclude that antibodies directed against PSA were more promising than those against PAP. This same group confirmed their experience with anti-PAP radioimmunoscintigraphy in 10 patients following [111In]-labeled PAY-276 infusion[10].

Table 17.6.1   MAbs used for imaging prostate cancer

Author	n	Antigen	Isotope-mAb	Results
Goldenberg et al.	9	PAP	[131I] (polyclonal)	Imaged primary tumor, lymph nodes, and lung metastases; no imaging of bone metastases
Vihko et al.	9	PAP	[111In]/[99mTc]	Primary tumor imaged; lymphoscintigraphy detected metastases to pelvic lymph nodes
Dillman et al.	4	PSA	[111In]-PSA-399	Detected 55% of tumor sites with PSA-399; detected 16%
	5	PAP	[111In]-Pay276	of tumor sites with Pay-276
Babaian et al.	25	PAP	[111In]-Pay276	Detected bone metastases but not lymph node metastases
Maguire	217	PSMA	[111In]-CYT-356	Detected soft tissue metastases in nodes and prostate fossa; less accurate in bone
Feneley et al.	22	PSMA	[99Tc] CYT-351	Detected 20% of bone metastases and high percentage of soft tissue metastases

Babaian and co-workers, using the same anti-PAP monoclonal antibody (^{111}In-labeled PAY-276), studied a larger series of patients (n = 25) with escalating doses of unlabeled antibody and 1 mg of the radioimmunoconjugate[11]. All patients had metastatic disease. They reported a high incidence of human anti-mouse-antibody (HAMA) formation in eight of 16 tested, but no other adverse reactions. Both lesion- and patient-sensitivity in the bone improved markedly in those patients who received the higher doses (between 20 and 80 mg) of unlabeled antibody (patient sensitivity increased from 40% to 100%, lesion sensitivity increased from 23% to 75%). The enhanced lesion sensitivity in this report, compared with the series reported by Halpern et al.[10], is possibly explained by the dose of unlabeled antibody. In many of Babaian's patients the dose was considerably higher than the dose used by Halpern. Notably, however, lymph node metastases were not detected with this agent.

Monoclonal antibody 7E11-C5.3

The murine monoclonal antibody 7E11-C5.3 is an IgG1 protein. It is produced from a hybridoma using the human prostate cancer cell line LNCaP originally described by Horoszewicz et al. in 1987[12]. This antibody recognizes a transmembrane (intracellular domain) prostate-specific membrane glycoprotein that is only expressed by prostatic epithelial cells (benign and malignant) and whose DNA coding sequence has significant homology to that of the human transferrin receptor[13]. The monoclonal antibody 7E11-C5.3 underwent site-specific conjugation with the linker-chelator glycyl-tyrosyl-(N, e-diethylenetriaminepentaacetic acid)-lysine (GYK-DTPA) using the procedure developed by Rodwell and co-workers[14]. The resulting immunoconjugate, 7E11-C5.3-GYK-DTPA labeled with [111]In (^{111}In-CYT-356 or ^{111}In-capromab pendetide) and a very similar immunoconjugate [99m]Tc (^{99m}Tc-CYT-351), has been investigated in patients with prostate cancer prior to or following radical prostatectomy.

[111]In-capromab pendetide studies in patients with prostate cancer

A phase I/II trial using ^{111}In-capromab pendetide (Table 17.6.2) in patients with prostate cancer was reported by Abdel-Nabi et al.[15]. Two types of patients were scanned:

a group of men with no detectable metastatic disease prior to staging pelvic lymphadenectomy (n = 28) and a group of patients with known metastatic prostate cancer (n = 40). There were no significant adverse effects. Serum HAMA measurements were available in 44 patients, and were measured 8 weeks after antibody infusion. Only three developed evidence of a significant HAMA response. Results of RIS demonstrated that two of four surgically proven pelvic lymph node metastases were detected with the scan. The scan was correctly negative in 25 of 27 histologically confirmed negative lymph nodes. Sixteen of the 27 prostates with confirmed cancer were detected by the scan. In those patients with metastatic disease, 38 of 40 had bony lesions, which had been documented using conventional radiographic modalities. The antibody scan detected lesions in 55% of these patients, but in only a minority of the patients were all bony lesions detected. Biopsies of bone lesions, particularly those that were discordant with the scan, were not obtained. The scan was also positive in four of six patients with extraprostatic soft tissue lesions. Overall, ^{111}In-capromab pendetide appeared to be safe, able to detect soft tissue lesions, but had only modest sensitivity for bone lesions.

Babaian and co-workers assessed the diagnostic accuracy of ^{111}In-capromab pendetide for the detection of prostate cancer in the pelvic lymph nodes prior to bilateral pelvic lymph node dissection[16]. Whole-body scanning and SPECT were performed in 19 men twice between 48 and 120 h after ^{111}In-capromab pendetide administration. HAMA titers were not detected in any of the men during follow up. Results of the scan were compared with the histopathologic findings and the conventional radiographic appearance of the pelvic lymph nodes. Eight of the 19 patients had pathologic evidence of metastatic disease to the pelvic lymph nodes, with the scan detecting four of these cases. CT and MR imaging detected abnormalities in only one of the eight patients. The scan was normal in nine of 11 patients who did not have metastatic cancer to the pelvic nodes.

Feneley et al. investigated the ^{99m}Tc-labeled form of 7E11 (^{99m}Tc-CYT-351) in 22 patients prior to and after prostatectomy[17]. Their patients included a mixture of those with incidental carcinoma following prostatectomy for apparently benign disease as well as patients with metastatic cancer. Based on results from small subgroups of these patients, the authors concluded that this agent is able to detect cancer in the prostate fossa and in lymph node

Table 17.6.2 Detection of pelvic lymph node metastases by ^{111}In-capromab pendetide

Author	n	Pathologic + nodes	Scan sensitivity	Scan specificity
Abdel-Nabi et al.	28	4	2/4 (50%)	25/27 (92%)
Babaian et al.	19	8	4/8 (50%)	9/11 (81%)
Maguire	217	85	51/85 (60%)	105/132 (80%)

regions. However, only one of the five men with bone metastases documented by bone scan showed abnormal accumulation of this agent. While the data using ^{99m}Tc-CYT-351 is sparse, the ^{99m}Tc-labeled antibody offers potential advantages over the ^{111}In-labeled form, including study completion time (1 day vs. 3–5 days for ^{111}In-capromab pendetide) and possible improved image quality. Further investigations with this agent seems warranted.

[111]In-capromab pendetide studies at the University of Iowa and the Iowa City Veterans Affairs Medical Center

As part of the multicenter phase II and phase III trials, we have studied patients following bilateral pelvic lymph node dissections and radical prostatectomy with curative intent. All of the patients had evidence of residual or recurrent cancer as evidenced by abnormally elevated PSA (defined as 'occult prostate cancer recurrence'). The patient's physical examination and all other tests, such as bone scans, CT or MR imaging, or trans-rectal ultrasound (TRUS) were negative for evidence of recurrent prostate cancer.

We reported data from our institution and the Lahey Clinic Medical Center (Burlington, MA) obtained during the phase II trial of the first 27 subjects with occult prostate cancer recurrence[18]. In this series, we studied 27 men with 5 mCi of ^{111}In-capromab pendetide from 9 to 141 months (range) following radical prostatectomy. We did not detect a significant correlation between the serum PSA and the likelihood of detecting scan abnormalities. However, the initial pathologic grade of the tumor was related to the probability of an abnormal scan: those with disease confined to the prostate were statistically less likely to have disease seen on scan compared with those with unconfined disease (64% vs. 94%). Based on scan findings from the initial infusion data, 22 of the 27 subjects had abnormalities seen in the prostatic fossa and/or extrafossa sites. In 11 of 22 patients, some of the abnormalities were confirmed by CT or MR imaging or by fossa biopsy. Included in this group were subjects with abnormalities seen in the prostate fossa (biopsy confirmed n = 8), mediastinum (radiographically confirmed n = 2), abdominal lymph nodes (unconfirmed n = 5) and lumbar spine (radiographically confirmed n = 1). None of the subjects have developed detectable HAMA titers during at least 8 weeks of follow up. This preliminary data, like the data from the phase I/II trials described above, suggested that ^{111}In-capromab pendetide imaging was able to detect prostatic fossa cancer recurrence and that extrafossa sites of soft tissue disease were also being seen.

Following the phase II trial, our medical center participated in and published the results of a multicenter phase III trial where 0.5 mg of ^{111}In-capromab pendetide was administered to patients with occult prostate cancer recurrence as defined above[19]. The phase III trial had the same entrance criteria as did the phase II trial described above except that all men had a TRUS-guided needle biopsy of the prostatic fossa within 8 weeks after the scan. Of 183 patients, 181 had interpretable scans, of which 158 (87%) underwent a prostatic fossa biopsy. Scan abnormalities were seen in 108 of 181 (60%) men, 18%, 17% and 25% seen respectively in the fossa only, the fossa plus extraprostatic fossa sites and extraprostatic sites only. Using the fossa biopsy as the standard, the sensitivity of ^{111}In-capromab pendetide (with 95% confidence intervals) was 49% (41–57%) and the specificity was 71% (63–78%). CT or MRI examinations were performed in 48 of the 76 (63%) men with scan evidence of extrafossa abnormalities. In only seven men were these scan abnormalities confirmed. We concluded that the relatively low accuracy of the scan was undoubtedly in part due to the diagnostic inaccuracy of a single fossa biopsy[20–22]. Abnormalities seen outside the prostatic fossa region, as in the phase II trial reported above, remain largely unconfirmed. While proof of accuracy is lacking, from our data it appears that, in patients who were treated with radical prostatectomy with curative intent, ^{111}In-capromab pendetide is able to detect prostate fossa recurrences with reasonable accuracy. The scan was certainly superior to reports of conventional techniques such as CT scanning, which has been shown to be relatively inaccurate[23].

Clinical follow up continues in patients who have occult cancer and underwent scanning. We are particularly interested in the outcome of the subgroup of patients who undergo salvage radiotherapy with curative intent. We therefore investigated and reported our findings on whether clinical outcome is related to scan findings, i.e. whether patients with abnormally elevated PSAs and scan abnormalities limited to their prostate fossa show complete responses (PSA 0.3 ng/ml) to radiation therapy whereas those with extrafossa scan abnormalities do not[24].

To answer this question, we retrospectively reviewed the records of 32 men scanned with ^{111}In-capromab pendetide after failed radical prostatectomy (by PSA criteria). All of these men underwent salvage radiotherapy to the prostatic fossa and pelvis (a treatment decision made independent of the scan results) with curative intent. These men had PSA follow up for a median of 13 months. In 16 of 23 (70%) patients with a normal scan outside the prostate fossa, the PSA declined to ≤0.3 ng/ml and remained at or below this level for at least 6 months and at last follow up (defined as a durable complete response). However, in men with scan evidence of disease outside the region of the prostatic fossa only two of nine (22%) had a durable complete response (difference significant, P = 0.0225). No other clinical variables were found to be prelictive of a durable complete response, including tumor stage and grade, or time interval between initial surgery and radiation. While our findings are preliminary, the scan appears to detect extraprostatic sites of disease and to predict the success or failure of salvage pelvic radiotherapy using PSA criteria. We are currently preparing to launch a prospective, multicenter trial to confirm our results in a large group of similar patients.

Conclusions

The clinical utility of monoclonal antibody imaging in the management of prostate cancer remains controversial due to the limited histologic evidence that positive scans for soft-tissue lesions are true positives and not false positives. The data available, however, indicates that correlation between scan findings and pathology is 70% accurate. Our retrospective radiation treatment data also suggests similar accuracy.

In our view the current ^{111}In-capromab pendetide scans are useful in two clinical situations. First, during pre treatment evaluation in patients with a serum PSA greater than 20, a Gleason sum greater than 7, and/or a palpable T_3 cancer, the scan will be more accurate than MRI or CT for detecting positive lymph nodes in the pelvis or abdomen. We base management on scan results, i.e. a positive scan in nodal areas outside the prostate would eliminate definitive local therapy as an option although histologic nodal evaluation should be considered. The ^{111}In-capromab pendetide scan is not useful to evaluate bone lesions. The scan can also be useful if a second local treatment with curative intent is contemplated after failure of primary definitive treatment. We use the scan for patients who previously had primary definitive treatment of localized prostate cancer (pelvic X-ray therapy, brachytherapy or radical prostatectomy) but subsequently have evidence of recurrence (newly palpable nodule on digital rectal examination or a persistently rising PSA) without distant metastases (negative bone scan) Management in these patients is based on scan results as well. A positive scan in nodal areas outside of the prostate fossa would preclude pelvic X-ray therapy in the post-radical prostatectomy patient or radical prostatectomy in the postradiation therapy patient. Thus, radioimmunoscanning for prostate cancer has utility in selected patients suspected of having initial metastatic or recurrent disease but is not applicable otherwise at present.

We anticipate that improvements can and will be made in monoclonal antibody imaging of prostate cancer. The use of ^{99m}Tc can decrease the scan time and may improve scan quality. A monoclonal antibody against the extracellular domain of prostate-specific membrane antigen rather than that against the intracellular portion of the antigen is used currently for ^{111}In-capromab pendetide scans could improve scan accuracy. Humanized antibodies to these and other prostate-specific antigens may decrease HAMA formation and allow use of serial scan and eventually radioimmunotherapy. While monoclonal antibody imaging of prostate cancer has limited indications today, we believe future innovations will substantially improve the efficacy of the technique.

References

1. Kohler G, Milstein C. Continuous cultures of fused cells secreting antibody of predefined specificity. *Nature* 1975;**256**:495–497.
2. Pressman D, Keighley G. The zone of activity of antibodies as determined by the use of radioactive tracers: the zone of activity of nephrotoxic antikidney serum. *J Immunol* 1948;**59**:141–146.
3. Goldenberg DM, DeLand F, Kim E *et al.* Use of radiolabeled antibodies to carcinoembryonic antigen for the detection and localization of diverse cancers by external photoscanning. *N Engl J Med* 1978;**298**:1384–1386.
4. Mach JP, Carrel S, Forni M *et al.* Tumor localization of radiolabeled antibodies against carcinoembryonic antigen in patients with carcinoma. *N Engl J Med* 1980;**305**:5–10.
5. Goldenberg DM, DeLand FH, Bennett SJ *et al.* Radioimmunodetection of prostate cancer. In vivo use of radioactive antibodies against prostatic acid phosphatase for diagnosis and detection of prostatic cancer by nuclear imaging. *JAMA* 1983;**250**:630–635.
6. Goldenberg DM, DeLand FH. Clinical studies of prostatic cancer imaging with radiolabeled antibodies against prostatic acid phosphatase. *Urol Clin North Am* 1984;**11**:277–281.
7. Vihko P, Kontturi M, Lukkarinem O *et al.* Radioimaging of prostate and metastases of prostate carcinoma with Tc 99m-labeled prostatic acid phosphatase-specific antibodies and their Fab fragments. *Am Clin Res* 1984;**16**:51–52.
8. Vihko P, Kontturi M, Lukkarinen O *et al.* Immunoscintigraphic evaluation of lymph node involvement in prostate carcinoma. *Prostate* 1987;**11**:51–57.
9. Dillman RO, Beauregard J, Ryan KP *et al.* Radioimmunodetection of cancer with the use of indium-111-labeled monoclonal antibodies. *NCI Monogr* 1987;**3**:33–36.
10. Halpern SE, Haindl W, Beauregard J *et al.* Scintigraphy with indium-labeled monoclonal antibodies: kinetics, biodistribution, and tumor detection. *Radiology* 1988;**168**:529–536.
11. Babaian RJ, Murray JL, Lamki LM *et al.* Radioimmunological imaging of metastatic prostatic cancer with [111]Indium-labeled monoclonal antibody PAY-276. *J Urol* 1987;**137**:439–443.
12. Horoszewicz JS, Kawinski E, Murphy GP. Monoclonal antibodies to a new antigenic marker in epithelial prostatic cells and serum of prostatic cancer patients. *Anticancer Res* 1987;**7**:927–936.
13. Israeli RS, Powel CT, Fair WR, Heston WDW. Molecular cloning of a complementary DNA encoding a prostate-specific membrane antigen. *Cancer Res* 1993;**53**:227–230.
14. Rodwell JD, Alvarez VL, Lee C *et al.* Site-specific covalent modification of monoclonal antibodies: in vitro and in vivo evaluations. *Proc Natl Acad Sci USA* 1986;**83**:2632–2636.
15. Abdel-Nabi H, Wright GL, Gulfo JV *et al.* Monoclonal antibodies and radioimmunoconjugates in the diagnosis and treatment of prostate cancer. *Semin Urol* 1992;**10**:45–54.
16. Babaian RJ, Sayer J, Podoloff DA, Steelhammer LC, Bhadkamkar VA, Gulfo JV. Radioimmunoscintigraphy of pelvic lymph nodes with In-111-labeled monoclonal antibody CYT-356. *J Urol* 1994;**152**:1952–1955.
17. Feneley MR, Chengazi VU, Kirby RS *et al.* Prostatic radioimmunoscintigraphy: preliminary results using technetium-labeled monoclonal antibody, CYT-351. *Br J Urol* 1996;**77**:373–381.

18. Kahn D, Williams RD, Seldin DW *et al.* Radioimmunoscintigraphy with [111]Indium labeled CTY-356 for the detection of occult prostate cancer recurrence. *J Urol* 1994;**152**:1490–1495.

19. Kahn D, Williams RD, Manyak MJ *et al.* In-111 capromab pendetide in the evaluation of patients with residual or recurrent prostate after radical prostatectomy. *J Urol* 1998;**159**:2041–2047.

20. Abi-Aad AS, MacFarlane MT, Stein A, deKernion JB. Detection of local recurrence after radical prostatectomy by prostate specific antigen and transrectal ultrasound. *J Urol* 1992;**147**:952.

21. Lightner DJ, Lange PH, Reddy PK, Moore L. Prostate specific antigen and local recurrence after radical prostatectomy. *J Urol* 1990;**144**:921.

22. Foster LS, Jajodia P, Fournier G *et al.* The value of prostate specific antigen and transrectal ultrasound guided biopsy in detecting prostatic fossa recurrences following radical prostatectomy. *J Urol* 1993;**149**:1024.

23. Platt JF, Bree RL, Schwab RE. The accuracy of CT in the staging of carcinoma of the prostate. *AJR* 1987;**149**:315–318.

24. Kahn D, Williams RD, Haseman MK *et al.* Radioimmunoscintigraphy with ^{111}In-capromab pendetide predicts prostate cancer response to salvage after failed radical prostatectomy. *J Clin Oncol* 1998;**16**:284–289.

17.7 Chemotherapy in patients with androgen independent prostate cancer

P M Swanson, E M O' Reilly and W K Kelly

In the past, chemotherapy has had a limited role in androgen independent prostate cancer. A retrospective analysis found that only 8% of 1683 patients treated with chemotherapy achieved a complete or partial remission[1]. Currently, there is no standard therapy for these patients, but more contemporary clinical trials using post-therapy declines in PSA and instruments which can detect improvement in quality of life and pain have identified several chemotherapeutic agents (Table 17.7.1) which have shown clinical benefit.

Clinical trials using post-therapy declines in PSA

Part of the problem in new drug development for prostate cancer has been the lack of relevant surrogate endpoints to follow the disease status in patients being treated. Recently, clinical investigators have tried to adapt the prostate-specific antigen test (PSA) as a way to monitor disease status. The clinical significance of using post-therapy declines in PSA as a measure of outcome is debated, but multiple studies in patients have shown that changes in PSA do correlate with disease progression or regression. For instance, Scher *et al.* showed that a 50% rise from the nadir value correlates with measurable disease progression[2] while Sella *et al.* reported that a 50% decline in the PSA was representative of measurable disease regression[3].

Retrospective multivariate analysis in 110 patients with androgen independent prostate cancer has found that a 50% post-therapy decline in PSA, defined as three consecutive declines of PSA greater than 50%, each measurement taken at least 2 weeks apart, is the strongest predictor of overall survival. In this study, patients who met the 50% decline in PSA criteria had an overall median survival of 20.1 months, versus 8.6 months for non responders. This model was verified independently on data from the Norwegian Radium Hospital[4], and subsequently several other series have reported similar outcomes. This would suggest that an agent that can produce a sustained post-therapy decline in PSA does have anti tumor activity and should be further tested. Using PSA as a screening modality, several studies have identified agents which have produced PSA declines, and these agents have gone on to be tested in randomized trials.

Estramustine-based regimens

Estramustine phosphate is a nor-nitrogen mustard carbamate derivative of estradiol-17-β-phosphate which binds to the microtubule associated proteins, resulting in microtubular depolymerization[5,6]. Combining estramustine phosphate with other antimicrotubule agents such as vinblastine, etoposide or paclitaxel has shown both in vitro synergy and significant clinical activity. Seidman *et al.* treated 24 patients with the combination of estramustine and vinblastine and 13 (54%, 95% CI 34–74%) patients with a rising PSA prior to therapy had a 50% or more decline in PSA post-therapy[7]. In five patient with bi-dimensional measurable disease, two (40%) patients had a partial regression of the tumor mass. The overall median duration of response was 7 months and the therapy was well tolerated with peripheral edema and nausea being the most common adverse affects. These preliminary findings were confirmed by two additional centers[8,9] and the combined results from all three clinical trials showed that a significant decline in PSA can be achieved in over 50% of the patients (56%, 46 out of 82) and that one third of the cases with measurable disease will have a partial or complete regression of the tumor mass.

A recent phase III trial comparing estramustine and vinblastine versus vinblastine alone confirmed that the progression free survival was superior for the combination of estramustine and vinblastine but overall survival was not significantly greater than the single agent alone[10]. Additional phase III studies are currently ongoing.

Other investigators have taken advantage of the in vitro synergy of estramustine and etoposide[11]. Pienta *et al.* treated 42 patients with androgen independent prostate cancer with estramustine and etoposide and found significant clinical activity. Fifty-two per cent of the patients had a greater than 50% decline in PSA while half of the patients had regression of their measurable disease[12]. The most

Table 17.7.1   Selected chemotherapy regimens

Author	Dose and schedule	Major toxicities	Response proportion	Endpoint
Seidman[7]	Estramustine, 10 mg/kg/day in three divided doses for 6 weeks	leukopenia, mild nausea, peripheral neuropathy, edema	54%	PSA decline
	Vinblastine, 4 mg/m^2 Q week for 6 weeks on, 2 weeks off		40%	Measurable disease Regression
Pienta[12]	Estramustine, 15 mg/kg/day in four divided doses for 3 weeks, 1 week off	Alopecia, leukopenia, anemia, edema	52%	PSA decline
	Etoposide, 50 mg/m^2/day in two divided doses for 3 weeks, 1 week off		50%	Measurable disease regression
Hudes[15]	Estramustine, 600 mg/m^2/day	Leukopenia, mucositis, edema	69%	PAS decline
	Paclitaxel, 120 mg/m^2 Q 21 days			
Petrylak[16]	Estramustine, 280 mg PO TID for 5 days	Fluid retention, transaminitis, granulocytopenia	62%	PSA decline
	Docetaxel, 60 mg/m^2 Q 21 days			
Reese[17]	Estramustine, 140 mg TID days 1–14	Nausea, febrile neutropenia	50%	PSA decline
	Vinorelbine, 25 mg/m^2 days 1 and 8, recycle Q 21 days			
Sella[3]	Doxorubicin, 20 mg/m^2 weekly (400 mg/m^2 total dose)	Acraylerythema, mucositis, neutropenia	55%	PSA decline
	Ketoconazole, 400 mg PO TID		58%	Measurable disease regression
Tannock[28]	Mitoxantrone, 12 mg/m^2 Q 21 days	Leukopenia, cardiac toxicity	29%	Palliation of symptoms
	Prednisone, 5 mg BID			

common toxicities encountered were alopecia (100%), leukopenia (57%), anemia (56%), edema (48%) and venous thrombosis (10%). A similar trial at Memorial Sloan Kettering Cancer Center utilized estramustine and etoposide with cisplatin or carboplatin in patients with a very aggressive phenotype of prostate cancer classified as 'anaplastic' carcinoma of the prostate. These patients typically present with locally aggressive tumors with soft tissue metastasis, a low PSA relative to the tumor burden and a short response to primary hormonal therapy. In 18 patients, 11 (61%) had a complete or partial response to the three drug regimen with the duration of response over a year in some patients[13]. While the toxicities were modest, patients did have significant palliative benefit from the therapy.

Combinations of estramustine with other agents have also shown some promise. Roth *et al.* investigated paclitaxel as a single agent and showed only one partial response out of 23 patients[14]. However, combining paclitaxel using a 96 h continuous infusion with estramustine, Hudes and colleagues reported 69% (95% CI 41–89%) of the patients had a 50% or more post-treatment decline in PSA[15]. In seven patients with measurable disease, three had a partial or complete response. While significant hematologic toxicities were initially reported with the prolonged administration of paclitaxel, shorter infusions have been well tolerated with the preliminary results showing similar efficacy. Both docetaxel[16] and vinorelbine[17] have also been combined with estramustine and the initial results are consistent with other reported estramustine regimens.

Suramin

Suramin is a polysulfonated naphthylurea initially used to treat trypanosomiasis, which has been shown to inhibit multiple polypeptide growth factors, alter protein kinases, induce differentiation and effect several other intracellular and extracellular enzymes[18]. Initial reports by Myers *et al.* showed that 21 out of 38 (42%) patients had a greater than 50% post-therapy decline in PSA with measurable disease regression in six out 17 (35%) patients[19]. Similar reports from the University of Maryland confirmed the activity with over 70% of the patients having a significant decline in PSA and half of the patients with measurable disease obtaining a complete or partial response[20]. Reports from Memorial Sloan Kettering Cancer Center had less dramatic results, and further evaluation showed that the initial trials did not control for the antiandrogen withdrawal effect[21], nor the effects of hydrocortisone which is given concomitantly with suramin[22]. Two prospective phase II clinical trials which controlled for the effects of antiandrogen withdrawal and hydrocortisone prior to the administration of suramin demonstrated a greater than 50% decline in PSA in 18% and 19% of the patients, respectively[23,24]. These results showed that suramin had modest activity in this disease. Further testing of suramin

255

using contemporary dosing schemes with improved toxicity profiles are ongoing in randomized clinical trials.

Anthracycline-based regimens

Others have re-evaluated the efficacy of more conventional chemotherapy agents or combinations such as doxorubicin or doxorubicin plus ketoconazole using post-therapy declines in PSA. Doxorubicin at low doses, e.g. 20 mg/ m^2/week, has modest activity and is generally well tolerated. Torti *et al.* reported that a third of the patients with measurable disease had complete or partial response to low-dose weekly doxorubicin[25]. The combination of doxorubicin and ketoconazole has also been studied in a phase II setting and 21 out of 55 patients (55%) had a greater than 50% decline in baseline PSA with measurable disease regression documented in seven out of 12 (58%) patients[3].

Clinical trials using quality of life endpoints

There has been an increased interest in the development of new outcome measures to assess response to a therapeutic modality which may improve the quality of a patient's life. Instruments which reproducibly quantify improvements in patient's symptoms such as fatigue, overall well-being, physical activity, appetite, mood or pain have been developed. Initial studies by Tannock *et al.* evaluated the effects of prednisone on pain and found that a third of the patients had significant improvement in pain at one month[26]. Moore and colleagues expanded this experience and studied the benefits of the combination of mitoxantrone and prednisone on the patient's pain and overall quality of life. A palliative response was defined as a decrease in analgesic score by at least 50% without an increase in pain intensity, or a decrease in pain intensity with no increase in analgesic consumption over a course of at least two cycles (6 weeks). In this study, nine out of 25 patients (36%, 95% CI 18–57%) had significant and durable palliative response[27].

With these encouraging results, Tannock *et al.* conducted a randomized trial between mitoxantrone plus prednisone versus prednisone using reduction in pain as the primary endpoint[28]. There was a significant difference in the palliative effect in favour of the combination arm (29% vs. 12%, $P = 0.1$) which was maintained for an average of 43 weeks versus 12 weeks for prednisone alone. The reduction in analgesics consumption was also greater in the combination arm which was similar to other palliative therapies such as strontium-89[29].

In a similar study from the Cancer and Leukemia Group B, patients with androgen independent prostate cancer were randomized to receive hydrocortisone plus mitoxantrone or hydrocortisone alone evaluating survival and quality of life as the major endpoints. There was no difference in overall survival but patients treated with mitoxantrone and hydrocortisone had better pain palliation compared with the control arm[30].

Future treatment approaches

Over the last decade, there has been an increased understanding in the events leading to the development and progression of malignant diseases. This has led to the discovery of novel agents which target specific steps in the malignant process. Novel treatment strategies currently under investigation include the use of drugs which influence tumor differentiation, inhibit neovascularization of tumors or inhibit basement membrane erosion and metastasis. Others are developing strategies to modulate the immune system by using vaccines which target glycoproteins on prostate cell surface, or specific monoclonal antibodies which target growth factor receptors such as the epidermal growth factor (EGF). These new technologies are under intensive research and many of these agents are now being evaluated in patients with prostate cancer.

References

1. Eisenberger MA, Simon R, O'Dwyer PJ, Wittes RE, Friedman MA. A reevaluation of nonhormonal cytotoxic chemotherapy in the treatment of prostatic carcinoma. *J Clin Oncol* 1985;**3**:827–841.
2. Scher HI, Curley T, Geller N, Engstrom C, Dershaw DD, Lin SY et al. Trimetrexate in prostatic cancer: preliminary observations on the use of prostate-specific antigen and acid phosphatase as a marker in measurable hormone-refractory disease. *J Clin Oncol* 1990;**8**:1830–1838.
3. Sella A, Kilbourn R, Amato R, Bui S, Zukiwski A, Ellerhorst J et al. A phase II study of ketoconazole (KC) combined with weekly doxorubicin (DOX) in patients (PTS) with hormone refractory prostate cancer (PC). *Proc Am Soc Clin Oncol* 1992;**11**:219.
4. Kelly WK, Scher HI, Mazumdar M, Vlamis V, Schwartz M, Fossa SD. Prostate specific antigen as a measure of disease outcome in hormone-refractory prostatic cancer. *J Clin Oncol* 1993;**11**:607–615.
5. Perry CM, McTavish D. Estramustine phosphate sodium. A review of its pharmacodynamic and pharmacokinetic properties, and therapeutic efficacy in prostate cancer. *Drugs Aging* 1995;**7**:49–74.
6. Gunnarsson PO, Forshell GP, Fritjofsson A, Norlen BJ. Plasma concentrations of estramustine phosphate and its major metabolites in patients with prostatic carcinoma treated with different doses of estramustine phosphate (estracyt). *Scand J Urol Nephrol* 1981;**15**:201–206.
7. Seidman AD, Scher HI, Petrylak D, Dershaw D, Curley T. Estramustine and vinblastine: Use of prostate specific antigen as a clinical trial endpoint for hormone-refractory prostatic cancer. *J Urol* 1992;**147**:931–934.
8. Hudes GR, Greenberg R, Krigel R. Phase II study of estramustine and vinblastine, two microtubule inhibitors, in hormone-refractory prostate cancer. *Journal of Clinical Oncology* 1992;**10**:1754–1761.
9. Amato RJ, Ellerhorst J, Bui C, Logothetis CJ. Estramustine and vinblastine for patients with progressive androgen-independent adenocarcinoma of the prostate. *Urol Oncol* 1995;**1**:168–172.

10. Hudes G, Roth B, Loehrer P, Ramsey H, Sprandio J, Entmacher M *et al.* Phase III trial of vinblastine versus vinblastine plus estramustine phosphate for metastatic hormone refractory prostate cancer. *Proc Am Soc Clin Oncol* 1997;**16**:1127.

11. Pienta KJ, Lehr JE. Inhibition of prostate cancer growth by Estramustine and etoposide: evidence for interaction at the nuclear matrix. *J Urol* 1993;**149**:1622–1625.

12. Pienta KJ, Redman B, Hussain M, Cummings G, Esper PS, Appel C *et al.* Phase II evaluation of oral estramustine and oral etoposide in hormone-refractory adenocarcinoma of the prostate. *J Clin Oncol* 1994; **12**:2005–2012.

13. Frank SJ, Amsterdam A, Kelly WK, Netto G, Liebertz C, Reuter V *et al.* Platinum-based chemotherapy for patients with poorly differentiated hormone-refractory prostate cancers (HRPC) response and pathologic correlations. *Proc Am Soc Clin Oncol* 1995;**14**:.

14. Roth B, Yeap B, Wilding G, Kasimis B, McLeod D, Loehrer P. Taxol (NSC 125973) in advanced, hormone-refractory prostate cancer: An ECOG phase II trial. *Proc Am Soc Clin Oncol* 1992;**11**:196.

15. Hudes GR, Nathan FE, Khater C, Greenberg R, Gomella L, Stern C *et al.* Paclitaxel plus estramustine in metastatic hormone-refractory prostate cancer. *Sem Onc* 1995;**22**(suppl 12):41–45. (abstract).

16. Petrylak DP, Shelton G, Judge T, O'Connor J, MacArthur RB. Phase I trial of docetaxel + estramustine in androgen-insensitive prostate cancer. *Proc Am Soc Clin Oncol* 1997;**16**:1103.

17. Reese D, Burris H, Belledgrun A, White L, O'Rourke T, Yates B *et al.* A phase I/II study of Navelbine (vinorelbine) and estramustine in the treatment of hormone refractory prostate cancer (HRPC). *Proc Am Soc Clin Oncol* 1996;**15**:673 (abstract).

18. Scher HI, Kelly WK. Suramin. Defining the role in the clinic. *Principles and Practice of Oncology. PPO Updates* 1993;**9**:1–16.

19. Myers CE, La Rocca R, Stein C, Cooper M, Dawson N, Choyke P *et al.* Treatment of hormonally refractory prostate cancer with suramin. *Proc Am Soc Clin Oncol* 1990;**9**:133 (abstract).

20. Eisenberger MA, Sinibaldi VJ, Reyno LM, Sridhara R, Jodrell DI, Zuhowski EG *et al.* Phase I clinical evaluation of a pharmacologically guided regimen of suramin in patients with hormone-refractory prostate cancer. *J Clin Oncol* 1995;**13**:2174–2186.

21. Scher HI, Kelly WK. The flutamide withdrawal syndrome: its impact on clinical trials in hormone-refractory prostatic cancer. *J Clin Oncol* 1993;**11**:1566–1572.

22. Kelly WK, Scher HI, Mazumdar M, Pfister D, Curley T, Leibertz C *et al.* Suramin and hydrocortisone: determining drug efficacy in androgen-independent prostate cancer. *J Clin Oncol* 1995;**13**:2214–2222.

23. Kelly WK, Curley T, Leibertz C, Dnistrian A, Schwartz M, Scher HI. Prospective evaluation of hydrocortisone and suramin. *J Clin Oncol* 1995;**13**:2208–2213.

24. Dawson NA, Cooper MR, Figg WD, Headlee DJ, Thibault A, Bergan RC *et al.* Antitumor activity of suramin in hormone-refractory prostate cancer controlling for hydrocortisone treatment and flutamide withdrawal as potentially confounding variables. *Cancer* 1996;**76**:453–462.

25. Torti FM, Aston D, Lum B *et al.* Weekly doxorubicin in endocrine-refractory carcinoma of the prostate. *J Clin Oncol* 1983;**1**:477–482.

26. Tannock I, Gospodarowicz M, Meakin W, Panzarella T, Stewart L, Rider W. Treatment of metastatic prostatic cancer with low-dose prednisone: evaluation of pain and quality of life as pragmatic indices of response. *J Clin Oncol* 1989;**7**:590–597.

27. Moore MJ, Tannock IF, Osoba D, Armitage G, Neville P, Murphy K. Mitoxantrone (M) + prednisone (P) in patients (PTS) with hormonally resistant prostate cancer. Use of a quality of life endpoint. *Proc Am Soc Clin Oncol* 1992;**11**:215.

28. Tannock IF, Osoba D, Stockler MR, Ernst S, Neville AJ, Moore MJ *et al.* Chemotherapy with mitoxantrone plus prednisone or prednisone alone for symptomatic hormone-resistant prostate cancer: a Canadian randomized trial with palliative end points. *J Clin Oncol* 1996;**14**:1756–1764.

29. Quilty PM, Kirk D, Bolger JJ, Dearnaley DP, Lewington VJ, Mason MD *et al.* A comparison of the palliative effects of strontium-89 and external beam radiotherapy in metastatic prostate cancer. *Radiother Oncol* 1994;**31**:33–40.

30. Kantoff PW, Conaway M, Winer E, Picus J, Vogelzang NJ. Hydrocortisone (HC) with or without mitoxantrone (M) in patients (pts) with hormone refractory prostate cancer (HRPC): preliminary results from a prospective randomized Cancer and Leukemia Group B Study (9182) comparing chemotherapy to best supportive care. *Proc Am Soc Clin Oncol* 1996; **14**:1748.

18 Management of sequelae, voiding dysfunction and renal failure

J W Basler and J Werschman

Algorithm

Prostate cancer

Bladder outflow obstruction algorithm

High PSA
Elevated creatinine, decrease urine output
Edema, congestive heart failure
Irritative/obstructive symptoms
Hematuria

→ Renal ultrasound
IVP → Hydronephrosis → See Ureteric obstruction algorithm

↓

Cystoscopy ± urodynamic studies

Non-obstructive ← Obstruction
Bleeding → Transurethral resection
Urethral stent
Radiotherapy
Hormone therapy

Pressure | Urodynamics: | **Residual**

Low — Low
Normal — Low → Follow up

Low — High
Normal — High → CISC*, urethral/suprapubic catheter

Not improved ← — Improved

Continue to monitor:
PSA
IPSS
Upper tracts

*CISC, clean intermittent self-catheterization

Ureteric obstruction algorithm

Newly diagnosed cancer — High PSA
Elevated creatinine*, decrease urine output
Edema, congestive heart failure
Irritative/obstructive symptoms — **Known cancer**

Hydronephrosis ← Renal ultrasound → **Hydronephrosis**

Hormone naïve ← Aggressive
management ← Patient and family
Counseling

Unilateral | Bilateral **Previous HT**

HT | HT and high dose
Dexamethasone 3–4wk | Diversion†
PCN, stent#
Ureteroneocystostomy | Expectant
management
(recommended)

Close monitoring ← Urgent diversion†
PCN, stent# | Consider ↓ | **Hospice**
Pain control
Supportive care

Deteriorating function | Pelvic XRT
? Chemotherapy trial

Dialysis → Await response to HT ← Poor/none

Improved function → PSA/DRE##
every 3 months → Deteriorating function

Antegrade; retrograde cannulation is usually very difficult
add alkaline phosphatase, creatinine, periodic upper tract imaging
* May be only minimally elevated.

† Unilateral to best kidney for palliation, bilateral for aggressive management but may be necessary for palliation as well.

Introduction

The advent of the prostate-specific antigen (PSA) blood test and a raised awareness of the need for routine cancer screening have led to many more cancers being discovered in the early, and curable, stages. However, a small but significant percentage of men will still present with or progress to a metastatic and terminal stage of the disease. After attempts to control the cancer with surgery, radiation or hormonal therapy, the urologist must also know how to treat complications related to the progression of incurable cancer. Most commonly, these complications are: bone pain and pathologic fractures related to bone metastases, urethral and ureteral obstruction with progression to renal failure, and disseminated intravascular coagulation. Long-term complications of the previous attempts at controlling the cancer through hormone therapy (weight loss, muscle wasting, weakness, hot flushes, impotency, osteoporosis, gynecomastia, etc.), radiation therapy (hemorrhagic cystitis, proctitis, etc.) and surgery (impotency, incontinence, bladder neck contractures, etc.) must also be addressed in providing care for these men. Because there is no known treatment capable of curing patients who are refractory to hormone therapy, treatment is aimed at preventing or minimizing the symptoms from these complications and prolonging survival where possible and desirable.

Managing the complications of the cancer

Parts of these sections will briefly summarize important management issues which may have been elaborated upon in previous sections concerning hormone therapy and radiotherapy.

Bony destruction and bone pain

Bone pain, an indication of bony destruction mediated by tumor cells, is a common symptom in patients with metastatic prostate cancer. The axial skeleton, specifically the vertebrae, pelvis, ribs, femur, skull and humerus, are commonly involved and cause pain that may be constant or intermittent from different sites at variable times[1]. Less frequently, patients may present with a pathologic fracture of the femur or vertebrae with or without neurologic deficit. If not already started, hormonal therapy is the first-line treatment of choice, providing relief in up to 80% of patients[2]. The most rapid method of achieving castrate levels of serum testosterone is by surgical orchiectomy, which is effective within 12 hours[3]. The fastest non-surgical method of androgen suppression is ketoconazole given in oral dosages of 400 mg every 8 hours, which will lower testosterone to castrate levels within 24 hours[4]. Decadron

(and other corticosteroids) have been used to treat acute spinal compression due to tumor in doses of 1 mg/kg/24 hours and higher. Oral estrogens such as diethylstilbestrol (1–5 mg daily or higher) elicit an effect in 3 to 4 days but may be complicated by cardiovascular side effects. Finally, luteinizing hormone releasing hormone (LHRH) agonists (Leuprolide, Gosereilin, others) take 3 to 4 weeks to reach a maximal effect but are expensive and cause a 'flare response' in which there is an initial increase in testosterone production and therefore potential exacerbation of symptoms. The flare response must be suppressed by using an antiandrogen (flutamide 250 mg orally three times daily, nilutamide 150 mg/day, bicalutamide 50–150 mg/day, cyproterone acetate 150 mg/day or others) for the first 3 to 4 weeks. Pure LHRH antagonists (e.g. cetrorelix) will soon be available more readily and may eliminate the need for the antiandrogen.

Radiation delivered by external beam to either specific sites or up to whole body treatment can also relieve severe bone pain. External beam irradiation to a specific site (usually administered in daily increments of 200 to 300 cGy up to a total of 2000 to 3000 cGy) may be effective in 75% of patients for up to 7 months[5]. For patients with multiple metastatic sites, half-body irradiation of 600 cGy to the upper body or 800 cGy to the lower body can be given in a single dose. If full-body irradiation needs to be given, each half of the body should be irradiated with a temporal separation of 1 month. Pain relief is prompt in 75–80% of patients but often of short duration[6]. Patients should be monitored for complications of radiation, such as nausea and vomiting, and less commonly pancytopenia and pneumonitis.

Another method of delivering radiation to the bone involves the use of ^{32}P and the administration of an activated form of parathyroid hormone. When given intravenously for several days, the bone becomes deplete of phosphorus. When the treatment is stopped, radioactive phosphorus is given and becomes deposited in the bone. Success rates are about equal to external beam radiation[7]. More recently, strontium-89 (^{89}Sr) has been used intravenously with mean response rates of 68%. Strontium-89 has a relative selectivity for bone and causes less myelotoxicity than other agents[6]. These agents should be considered adjuvants to external beam irradiation because their effect is best with osteoblastic but not osteolytic lesions, which are most likely responsible for compression fractures leading to neurologic damage[8]. Other agents having a measurable effect on bone pain including estramustine phosphate have been discussed in the section on chemotherapy.

Glucocorticoids may decrease bone pain. The usual dosage is prednisone 20 mg/day and though its effect is usually short-lived, it can be helpful for temporary relief. Although the mechanism of action is uncertain, it has been suggested that steroids prevent the release of prostaglandins, and because prostaglandins lower the pain threshold by sensitizing nerve endings, pain tolerance will be enhanced. In addition, as edema around the tumor is reduced there will be less pressure on the nerves and subsequently less pain[2].

Oral analgesics are a vital part of controlling metastatic bone pain. Most often, non-steroidal antiinflammatory drugs (NSAIDs) are used. Similar to the steroids, they inhibit the production of prostaglandins, and therefore, the pain threshold increases. The side effects of NSAIDs are gastrointestinal distress and bleeding and less commonly renal failure and sodium and water retention. For severe pain not controlled by NSAIDs or other methods, narcotics are often effective. Intravenous (PCA) or intrathecal (continuous spinal or epidural) narcotic therapy with demerol, morphine, fentanyl and others can alleviate severe pain but should be an adjunct to other attempts at tumor control. The main side effects of narcotics are nausea, vomiting, constipation and respiratory distress (although this is rarely seen with controlled oral dosages). Though often feared by patients, there is no evidence that use of narcotics for pain relief, in this setting, leads to addiction. Short-term nerve blocks with local anesthetic agents, permanent nerve blocks using alcohol and freezing, and epidural or spinal blocks are all viable options as well.

Surgical intervention is a final attempt at pain control from bone metastasis. Cordotomy through the cervical or thoracic anterior-lateral spinothalamic tract is able to relieve pain immediately in the lower half of the body. However, the effect usually lasts only up to 6 months in 60% of patients. Potential side effects include transient urinary retention and ipsilateral paralysis[9]. Hypophysectomy also can have excellent results in as many as 75% of patients and last up to 20 weeks[10,11]. No clear etiology for this effect is known. Because of the morbidity, expense and variable results of these ablative pain control methods, surgery is rarely used as palliative treatment.

Pathologic fractures

As prostate cancer metastasizes to the bones, particularly the long weight-bearing bones, the tumor-invested bone will become weaker. Subsequently, pathologic fractures may result. Prostate cancer bone metastases, unlike many other types of bone metastases, are classically osteoblastic so that when a pathologic fracture does occur, the healing rate is almost that of normal bone. If at least 50% of the cortical bone has been replaced by metastatic disease, lesions will appear on plain films or CT scans heralding an impending fracture. Nuclear bone scan will usually detect tumor spread earlier than other radiologic tests although MRI may be better able to ascertain marrow replacement. Treatment of a pathologic fracture consists of appropriate analgesia, stabilization and radiation as described for bone pain. Because of the rapid healing of these bone lesions, surgical stabilization may only be absolutely necessary in about a quarter of these fractures[12]. However, many feel that early fixation will allow earlier ambulation and improvement in quality of life. External beam irradiation can be given in combination with a surgical repair, provided that at least 1 or 2 weeks have passed prior to radiation.

It should also be mentioned that some fractures in elderly men can be osteoporotic in nature especially if hormonal therapy has been instituted for a long period of time (see below). These should be differentiated from those caused by pathologic invasion of the bone by tumor cells since the treatments are different.

Spinal cord compression

Spinal cord compression resulting from vertebral fracture is a medical emergency. Vertebral fracture occurs in up to 12% of patients with bone metastases and is due either to direct invasion of the vertebral body or extradural tumor tissue[13]. The most common site of vertebral invasion is thoracic (46–68%), but it can occur anywhere along the spine including the lumbar (18–48%) and cervical (5–14%) vertebrae[14]. The most common clinical manifestations of spinal cord compression are back pain (75–100%) or pain along a specific nerve root distribution. Very often, pain precedes an actual fracture by several weeks. Motor weakness may develop with the potential quickly to progress to paraparesis or paraplegia. Sensory deficits (68%) and autonomic dysfunction such as neurogenic bladder and fecal incontinence (40%) occur less frequently[15]. In the past, the diagnosis has been made by myelogram or CT scan, but MRI has since become the best diagnostic tool due to the detail of the spinal cord and nearby structures it provides. When evaluating one specific area of the spine, there is a 15% chance of discovering another, clinically silent, vertebral lesion using MRI[16]. Most patients who have been diagnosed with prostate cancer spinal metastases will have already been started on therapy to prevent the acute onset of cord compression. However, this devastating complication may be seen in those who have neglected follow up or those in whom cancer has not previously been diagnosed.

Immediate treatment of spinal cord compression is essential. Steroids should be given to decrease the surrounding edema and lessen the compression on the spinal cord. Conventionally, dexamethasone (Decadron) 10 mg IV bolus followed by 4 mg IV every 6 h has been the suggested regimen[2,17]. A steroid taper can begin after 2 days, ultimately converting to oral steroids such as prednisone which may be further tapered as the effects of androgen ablative therapy progress. Ketoconazole should also be given immediately, specifically 400 mg IV every 8 hours to lower testosterone to castrate levels within 24 hours. Alternatively, bilateral orchiectomy in the patient stable for surgery is effective in 12 hours. Unfortunately, patients who have already failed hormonal therapy will have less of a response to these treatments than those presenting primarily. Median survival for patients who have not had hormonal therapy is approximately 16 months as opposed to 6 months for those who have had previous hormonal therapy[18]. The next treatment option can be either radiation plus surgical decompression or radiation alone. There have been no conclusive studies that show one option to be more effective than the other. Each may result in improvement of the neurologic symptoms for over 50% of treated patients. Usually, radiation and steroid therapy are the initial choices because the combination is as effective but less invasive than surgical therapy[19]. However, patients who have developed bladder dysfunction or rapidly progressive paraplegia (i.e. neurologic instability) have a poorer prognosis for recovery with radiation and immediate surgery may be more beneficial.

Surgical options are laminectomy for posterior vertebral lesions and anterior decompression for extensive vertebral body involvement. Surgery is followed 3 to 5 days later by 3000 to 4000 cGy of radiation, divided over a 2 week period. Daily doses of 500 cGy for 3 days followed by a 4 day rest period, followed by 300 cGy daily for 5 days have been advocated by Young[20]. Rapid pain relief is seen in about 66% of patients and another 20% will improve over the course of several months. It is recommended that the radiation ports be two vertebral bodies above and two below the lesion in order to decrease the chance of local recurrence, as approximately 15% of such patients will have a local recurrence[21,22]. For patients who maintain neuromuscular function through the event, ambulatory function is usually always preserved but in patients who have developed paraplegia, only one-third will regain ambulatory ability[23,24].

Bladder outlet obstruction

In the absence of efforts to control the local tumor burden within the prostate, from 18–72% of cancer patients will progress to significant bladder outlet obstruction[25,26]. Associated problems may include suprapubic pain, urinary tract infections, hematuria and renal failure. Therapy involves relieving the obstruction in a way that will maintain the highest quality of life for the individual patient. In a motivated and facile patient with an easily traversed urethra, intermittent self-catheterization (SIC) is an option. For those not able or unwilling to perform SIC, the simplest therapy may be placement of an indwelling urethral catheter although placement may be difficult or impossible depending on the degree of tumor obstruction. Alternatively, a suprapubic catheter can be placed in the event of an acute obstruction or for long-term

management in the terminal patient. Partial transurethral ablation of the prostate simply to open a urethral channel through the rigid tumor tissue (e.g. 'channel' TURP, contact laser ablation, electrovaporization (Vaportrode™), and other means of ablation) is effective in allowing patients to void more freely and may eliminate the discomfort of catheterization. Side effects include urinary incontinence (up to 8%), bleeding and the development of urethral strictures. There has been controversy regarding the possibility of seeding tumor cells while performing the resection, but several studies have not substantiated this fear[27–29].

If not already instituted, hormonal therapy is usually the first line of treatment for non-acute bladder outlet obstruction. Bilateral orchiectomy provides improvement at an average of 2.7 months compared with standard doses of estrogens or antiandrogens (3.4 months). Six months after initiation of any type of hormonal therapy, about two-thirds will be voiding without the need for catheterization. This improvement may last for another 6 months[30]. Practically speaking, for those patients who fail to void after 2 months of hormonal therapy, TURP is a reasonable option.

External beam radiation to the prostate is not often used to treat outlet obstruction. If it is attempted no more than a total of 2000 cGy should be used in order to avoid the development of complete urinary retention as a side effect of transient edema. Between 80–90% of patients have improved voiding that persists for up to 1 year. However, in almost 50% significant side effects of radiation (impotence (50–70%), urethral strictures (8%), cystitis and proctitis (<5%)) occur as well. These problems have led to radiation being reserved for those who refuse hormone treatment or are not surgical candidates[31,32].

A new treatment option for patients who fail standard hormonal therapy or who need a less invasive and more immediate treatment is placement of a prostatic stent (UroLume Wallstent™). The stents are cylindrical wire mesh made of corrosion-resistant super-alloy which are placed cystoscopically under local anesthesia with IV sedation. Stents have been available in lengths between 2 to 4 cm, fitting effectively in prostatic urethra from 2.5 to 4.5 cm long. In a study by Guazzoni, 11 of 11 patients could void spontaneously immediately after stent placement and none of 10 patients had recurrent obstruction at 1 year as determined by urodynamic studies[33]. Interestingly, all stents had become completely covered with epithelium and there were no serious side effects such as incontinence or fistulae, although tumor growth through the mesh did become apparent in some patients at longer follow up.

A self-expanding ProstaCoil™ urethral stent can be inserted at 17°F and expanded to a maximum size of

30°F. It can be placed in uninfected patients using viscous lidocaine urethral anesthesia on an outpatient basis. In a study by Yachia[34], 24 of 27 patients could void spontaneously immediately after stent insertion while three developed clot retention. Over a mean follow up time of about 24 months, all patients, except one patient who was incontinent prior to stent insertion, who had stents in place were able to void well and remained continent. No stent became occluded by tumor mass. This stent is most effective as a temporary alternative to an indwelling catheter during hormonal therapy attempts to shrink the prostate cancer mass.

Ureteral obstruction

Ureteral obstruction can occur due to local progression of prostate cancer into the bladder base in and around the trigone. The tumor progresses superiorly via the ureteral sheath causing obstruction due to direct compression if not frank invasion of the ureter. The obstruction is almost always unilateral initially and may be heralded by few if any signs (slight elevation of creatinine, haematuria) or symptoms (urinary frequency, mild flank pain) unless accompanied by bladder outlet obstruction, gross hematuria or concurrent UTI. Early detection requires a high index of suspicion since there is no easy way to make the diagnosis without imaging tests that are not routine when following prostate cancer patients. Patients with palpably extensive disease (cT2c, cT3, cT4) or those progressing to (or presenting with) metastatic disease should have upper tract imaging with ultrasound or CT to rule out obstruction. Confirmatory renal scan with furosemide wash-out may be ordered as indicated.

Before beginning extensive evaluation and treatment of this complication, the patient and physician should realize that this is one of the later sequelae of prostate cancer and relieving obstruction could mean eliminating one of the more humane mechanisms of death from this disease. Even with adequate preservation of renal function, survival outlook is especially dismal if the patient has already failed hormonal intervention[35]. However, if the patient is presenting primarily, has a high quality of life and desires to expend all options for survival, monitoring and treatment should be as aggressive as necessary. One approach to follow up of patients at risk for obstruction is outlined in the algorithms for locally advanced disease.

As with bladder outlet obstruction, if the patient is presenting without the prior diagnosis of prostate cancer, immediate treatment with hormone ablation is most appropriate[36,37]. Additionally, high-dose dexamethasone[38] and/or ketoconazole can be administered until the effects of standard therapy (e.g. LHRH agonists) take hold and the diagnosis is confirmed.

When unilateral obstruction is identified, the degree of function and obstruction of the involved renal unit should be assessed with a renal scan (^{99m}Tc-DTPA). If the function is <10% and the patient is asymptomatic, no intervention is usually indicated. When treatment is indicated, several options are available and their use should be tailored to the individual patient's situation.

Experience with radiotherapy for ureteral obstruction has been reviewed recently[39,40]. However, a review of these reports suggest that surgical intervention may be more effective as a specific treatment.

Surgical methods including the following have all been described with varying degrees of success: percutaneous nephrostomy[41–45]; percutaneous antegrade stenting of the ureter (nephrostent, universal stent, etc.); retrograde stenting (often difficult or impossible in the presence of infiltration of the trigone)[42,46]; ureteral endoprosthesis placement (similar to the prostatic stents)[47,48]; retrograde transurethral resection or unroofing of the ureter (works best with short length of ureteral obstruction in un-irradiated areas)[49]; uretero-neocystostomy[50]; percutaneous nephrosto-neocystostomy (with subcutaneous tunneling of the tubing)[51]; or laparoscopic cutaneous ureterostomy[52].

Bilateral obstruction is often seen as progressive anuria with azotemia in the emergency setting. A quick assessment of the kidneys with ultrasound can identify the renal unit which most likely has the best function by measuring the amount of remaining cortex. Percutaneous nephrostomy is the treatment of choice in this setting. This is one situation where a true post-obstructive diuresis may be seen so careful monitoring is essential. Generally, the treatment of post-obstructive diuresis is to replace half of the excess urine output with half normal saline and monitor electrolytes frequently. After the uremia subsides and electrolyte abnormalities are controlled, antegrade studies can be performed to assess the degree and level of obstruction. Generally the same treatment options as for unilateral obstruction apply except that if operative ureteral reimplantation is contemplated, unilateral rather than bilateral procedures are usually indicated. The option for internal stenting or drainage of any variety is limited by the degree of bladder outlet obstruction. Indeed, channel TUR or other prostatic ablative therapy in conjunction with stenting is often necessary. Foley catheterization or suprapubic tube placement may also be used to provide adequate low-pressure bladder drainage.

Disseminated intravascular coagulation

Disseminated intravascular coagulation (DIC) is an uncommon but difficult complication of metastatic prostate cancer. Chronic rather than acute DIC is more common in prostate cancer, seen in approximately 13% of patients, presenting as low-grade bleeding intermittently over months and may be associated with venous thrombosis[53]. Laboratory tests for the diagnosis of DIC include platelet count, fibrinogen and fibrin split product levels, Factors V and VIII levels, and prothrombin and partial thromboplastin times. In acute DIC, more often caused by septicemia, burns and trauma, the platelet and fibrinogen and Factors V and VIII levels are expected to be low and the PT, PTT, and fibrin split products high. Laboratory diagnosis of chronic DIC is not simple. The laboratory values vary from deficiencies due to depletion of factors to elevations due to overcompensation.

Initial treatment is aimed at the underlying cause, i.e. the prostate cancer. If the diagnosis of prostate cancer has been made but hormone therapy has not been initiated, it should be. For patients in whom the diagnosis has not been made prior to this presentation, but the clinical findings are highly suspicious (suspicious DRE, grossly elevated PSA, characteristic bone scan, etc.) treatment can be initiated pending confirmatory biopsy. Ketoconazole, 400 mg orally every 8 hours, should be administered and followed with standard hormone therapy as the diagnosis is confirmed[53]. The urologist should be aware that this treatment is not without potential complications including acute adrenal insufficiency[54]. While orchiectomy provides the most rapid decrease of testosterone to castrate levels, this may not be feasible in an individual with DIC due to risk of significant hemorrhage.

Unfortunately, if the patient has already failed hormonal therapy, the clinician must attempt to treat the coagulopathy. Intravenous heparin has been recommended[55] but should be used with caution as its use may occasionally lead to fatal hemorrhage. Epilson-aminocaproic acid given intravenously can be beneficial in patients with fibrinolysis because it inhibits the fibrinolytic pathway[56]. However, it may also cause fatal bleeding or thrombosis and should be given with low-dose heparin. Transfusion of blood products such as platelets, packed red blood cells, fresh frozen plasma and cryoprecipitate should be instituted based on the serum levels of the various blood components. Unfortunately, DIC is often difficult to control, and active therapy lies in prompt treatment of the prostate cancer.

Treating the side effects of cancer management

Some of the most troubling problems that patients are faced with involve dealing with iatrogenic complications from attempts to eradicate or control the prostate cancer. This section outlines several of the most commonly seen problems and attempts to provide a rational approach to management.

Side effects of hormone manipulation

Hormone therapy side effects depend on the agents or procedures being used and can often be pre-empted with some forethought. The most common adverse consequences of the various medications used in hormonal manipulation are listed in Table 18.1. Surgical or medical castration results in an early symptom complex of hot flushes, loss of libido and impotency. Management of hot flushes has recently been reviewed[57]. Hot flushes are expected in >50%[58] and are controllable to an extent with the addition of low doses of medications with estrogenic effects (DES, 0.25–1.0 mg daily, megestrol acetate 10–20 mg q12–24 h)[59] and possibly with phyto-estrogenic dietary supplements[60]. Less of an effect is seen with vasopressive agents (e.g. clonidine 0.1–0.3 mg patch daily)[61].

Loss of libido is most likely secondary to direct loss of brain stimulation by testosterone but impotency per se is not an absolute consequence of castration. Indeed, a significant number of newly castrate men retain the ability to obtain and maintain erections with appropriate stimulation[62]. In many cases, supportive measures (PGE-1 suppositories, PGE-1 injection, papavarine injection, vacuum erection devices, Viagra™, etc.) and reassurance may allow continued sexual activity. Loss of libido will ultimately limit these efforts. Some patients have expressed a desire to improve this with over the counter supplements of DHEA (dihydroepiandrosterone) which is marketed as a male rejuvenating substance. This weak adrenal androgen has unproven bioavailability when taken orally but could be converted to DHT in prostate tissue. Caution should be recommended for those who choose this remedy and monitoring serum DHT levels might be in order. The possibility of development of super-selective testosterone analogs that are capable of stimulating sexual behavior and maintaining muscle mass and bone density but not be convertible to DHT, has been raised by a recent study by Morali et al.[63]. Such drugs, if not stimulatory to cancer cells, could prove to be a major step forward in maintaining quality of life for men in need of hormonal therapy.

Osteoporotic changes as a result of androgen ablation appear as early as 12 months after initiation of therapy[64]. These have been associated with a high incidence of pathologic fractures and have led some to recommend that baseline bone mineral density studies be performed at the onset of treatment and annually thereafter[65,66]. Studies are underway to determine if bisphosphonates and/or low doses of estrogens may eliminate this potentially troublesome iatrogenic complication[67,68].

Gynecomastia and mastodynia have been associated with all efforts at hormone manipulation to varying degrees. The most common drugs associated with this problem are the antiandrogens and oral estrogens, though it has even been reported after orchiectomy and

Table 18.1 Common short- and long-term side effects of hormonal therapies

Agent/Action	Early onset side effect	Treatment	Long-term side effect	Treatment
Orchiectomy	Hot flushes Impotency	DES, Megace, Clonidine Viagra, PGE1, VED, prosthesis	Loss of muscle mass Osteoporosis	Creatine supp., MVI Calcium supp., bisphosphonates transdermal estrogens
	Loss of libido	?DHEA*		
Estrogens DES	(see Orchiectomy) Gynecomastia Cardiovascular	(see Orchiectomy) Breast irradiation Lower dose (1 mg) ?Thrombolytics	(see Orchiectomy) Cardiovascular	(see Orchiectomy) Lower dose (1 mg) ?Thrombolytics
LHRH agonists Gosereilin Luprolide	(see Orchiectomy) Flare	(see Orchiectomy) Antiandrogens (1 month) or CAB†	(see Orchiectomy)	(see Orchiectomy)
Antiandrogens Steroidal Cyproterone Acetate	(see Orchiectomy) Gynecomastia	(see Orchiectomy) Breast irradiation	(see Orchiectomy) Hepatic toxicity	(see Orchiectomy) Monitor, Reduce dosage, stop
Antiandrogens Non-steroidals ‡ Flutamide	Less impotency GI upset	Supportive care	Gynecomastia, diarrhea, nausea, hepatic toxicity	Breast irradiation Supportive care Reduce dosage, stop
Nilutamide	Vision problems	Avoid low light	Milder GI Sxs Pneumonitis	Supportive care Reduce dosage, stop Periodic exam, CXRs,
Bicalutamide	Less impotency Fewest GI Sxs	Supportive care		

* Since this medication could be converted to DHT via 5-alpha reductase, and its effects on prostate cancer cell growth in vivo are uncertain, patients should be cautioned about this commonly available over the counter medication. †CAB = continuous androgen ablation. ‡ in decreasing order of frequency of side effects.

LHRH agonist therapy[69]. Treatment is with pre-emptive radiotherapy (200 cGy each side) prior to the initiation of hormone therapy. After therapy has begun, some relief may be obtained with tamoxifen 10 mg po BID[69,70].

Side effects of radiotherapy

Adverse consequences of radiation therapy including hemorrhagic cystitis, proctitis, urgency incontinence and impotence are well described[71–73]. The worst short-term side effects seem to abate for most patients within a few weeks after completion of external beam treatments. Urinary urgency and obstructive symptoms can still be significant problems with brachytherapy. Prolonged urinary frequency and rectal urgency can be seen in 25–30% of

patients and potency problems may be noted in 30–60% at 2 years follow up[74,75].

Treatment of the immediate rectal effects include antidiarrheals (imodium, etc.) and in some cases short-term discontinuation of radiotherapy pending resolution of symptoms. Fewer immediate rectal problems are noted with brachytherapy.

Urinary frequency and urgency incontinence must be thoroughly evaluated to assure that the patient has not developed retention. For patients without significant post-void residual urine, anticholinergics (e.g. oxybutinin 5 mg TID, hyoscyamine sulfate 0.125–0.375 mg TID, etc.) and alpha-antagonists (terazosin 1–5 mg QD, doxazosin 1–4 mg QD, tamsulosin 0.4 mg QD) may be helpful. For those with significant obstruction (either pre-existing or as a result of radiotherapy induced swelling) the alpha antagonists may be of value but intermittent self-catheterization or a suprapubic cystostomy tube are often necessary. Indwelling foley catheters during radiotherapy may be problematic and should be avoided due to the chronic inflammatory changes around them and subsequent risk of strictures. Occasionally, a patient will remain in retention after radiotherapy and require further intervention. TUR procedures should be delayed for a sufficient time to allow the inflammation to resolve. Hormone therapy in this interval may eliminate the need for the surgical procedure and its consequent risk of incontinence and strictures. The long-term management of urinary frequency in the absence of obstruction should include anticholinergics, alpha-blockade as tolerated and urinary analgesics (methylene blue, phenazopyridine HCl, etc.) as needed.

Chronic hemorrhagic cystitis and proctitis is seen in 1–2% of patients after standard radiotherapy but can be minimized theoretically with conformal and brachytherapy techniques. Proctitis is generally managed conservatively with steroid-containing cream products followed by laser therapy when these fail but may ultimately require diverting colostomy and proctectomy.

The management of hemorrhagic cystitis begins initially with an evaluation of the underlying cause of the bleeding, hydration and catheterization with wash-out of all clot material. Coagulation studies and urine culture are sent and broad spectrum antibiotics are started. Any infection discovered on the urine culture should be treated aggressively by adjusting the antibiotic therapy according to sensitivities. Coagulation parameters are brought back into the normal ranges as indicated with fresh frozen plasma (FFP) and / or platelets as indicated.

If the urine is sterile and clears with gentle irrigation, an initial imaging of the upper tracts is completed with ultrasound, CT or IVP, if not already done in the pre-treatment evaluation for prostate cancer. Follow up cystoscopy is performed to remove remaining clots and confirm the absence of vesicle malignancy. The patient can then be observed. If the hematuria does not respond, continuous bladder irrigation with normal saline can be instituted to prevent further clotting while coagulation studies are being completed. Irrigation with 1% alum[76], silver nitrate, prostaglandins[77] and 1–4% formalin (under anesthesia)[78] have been reported to decrease the bleeding. Alternatively, hyperbaric oxygen therapy, if available, may improve bleeding in some patients[79]. Temporary or permanent urinary diversion may be necessary to control hemorrhage[80]. Interestingly, cystectomy is usually not required since the bleeding seems to stop when urine is diverted, possibly as a result of decreasing urokinase contact with the irradiated epithelium[80]. Unfortunately, successful management of one episode of hemorrhagic cystitis does not preclude future events so close monitoring is recommended.

Impotency after radiotherapy is generally gradual in onset but in many cases responsive to the same measures that are offered to the non-irradiated patients. The etiology of the erectile problems is uncertain but probably arises as a result of progressive vasculitis of the small vessels around the cavernosal nerves and fibrosis of the penile arteries. Since significant beam scattering can occur, if the testes are not adequately shielded, a drop in testosterone may also occur. Initial evaluation includes a testosterone level and management begins with a trial of Viagra™ or intraurethral PGE-1 (MUSE™). Intracavernosal PGE-1 (Caverject™, etc.) can be used but the risk of cavernosal fibrosis is unknown. Vacuum erection devices are a reasonable option as well but implants should be reserved for those failing less invasive therapies and a suitable amount of time should pass between the radiotherapy and surgical implantation.

Side effects of surgery

Long-term complications of surgical intervention including impotency, incontinence, bladder neck contractures are becoming more uncommon with the development of better surgical techniques.

Incontinence and bladder neck contracture after radical prostatectomy can largely be prevented by observing careful technique. Meticulous dissection of the distal circular urethral muscle fibers and eversion of the mucosa at the site of anastomosis are key aspects of the retropubic prostatectomy that allow this dramatic improvement. These are discussed in the section on surgery for localized disease above (Chapter 15). In situations where optimal dissection is not possible or advisable (e.g. wider dissection necessary for tumor advancing from the apex distally), there are some maneuvers which may improve control post-operatively. These include: tubularization of the bladder neck (largely abandoned due to a higher than normal stricture and rate of urinary retention); bladder neck-sparing (which may preserve the circular fibers distal to the trigone and possibly improve control); and placement of a pubo-urethral sling (similar to that performed for female urethral incompetence). Post-operative incontinence should be evaluated with cystoscopy to evaluate for recurrent disease and bladder neck contracture. If the urethra coapts well and no stricture is seen, urodynamics with documentation of the vesicle and valsalva leak point pressures can be helpful in tailoring further therapy. Kegel exercises or collagen injection (Contigen™) around the urethra can sometimes be successful for cases of mild stress incontinence. However, the artificial urinary sphincter (AMS-800™) may be the best option for severe cases.

Radical prostatectomy without cavernosal nerve-sparing will result in nearly universal erectile dysfunction.

267

Indeed, transient erectile dysfunction is seen after most nerve-sparing radical prostatectomies. Return of erectile function is age-related to a large extent as evidenced by the fact that younger patients (in their fifties) who functioned normally prior to surgery, will have >90% chance of normal erections post-operatively whereas this percentage drops significantly with each successive decade for the same operation and tumor stages[81]. Treatment options are the same as outlined above for radiotherapy. However, Viagra™ would not be expected to work well if both nerve bundles have been sacrificed.

References

1. Pollen II, Schmidt JD. Bone pain in metastatic cancer of the prostate. *Urology* 1979;**8**:129–134.
2. Labasky RF, Smith JA. Management of pain and other symptoms of advanced prostatic cancer. *Seminars in Urology*, 1988;**4**(4):311–321.
3. Robinson MRG, Thomas BS. Effect of hormonal therapy on plasma estosterone levels I prostatic carcinoma. *Dr Mcd Journal* 1997;**4**:391–394.
4. Trachtenberg J. Ketoconazole therapy in advanced prostatic cancer. *J Urology* 1984;**132**:61–63.
5. Benson RC, Hasan SM, Jones AC et al. External beam radiotherapy for palliation of pain from metastatic carcinoma of the prostate. *J Urol* 1982;**127**:69–71.
6. Nielson O, Munro AJ, Tannock IF. Bone metastases: pathophysiology and management policy. *J Clin Oncology* 1991;**9**:509–524.
7. Tong ECK. Parathormone and P-32 therapy in prostatic cancer with bone metastases. *Radiology* 1971;**98**:343–351.
8. De Ruysscher D, Spaas P, Specenier P. The treatment of osseous metastases of hormone-refractory prostate cancer with external beam radiotherapy and Strontium-89. *Acta Urol Belg* 1996;**64**(3):13–19.
9. Payne R. Pain management in the patient with prostate cancer. *Cancer supplement* 1993;**71**(3):1131–1137.
10. Tindall GT, Payne NS, Nixon DW. Transphenoidal hypophysectomy for disseminated carcinoma of the prostate gland. *J Neurosurgery* 1979;**50**:275–282.
11. Waldman SD, Feldstein LS, Allen ML. Neuroadenolysis of the pituitary: description of a modified technique. *J Pain Symptom Management* 1987;**2**(1):45–49.
12. Coyler RA. Surgical stabilization of pathological neoplastic fractures. *Curr Prob Cancer* 1986;**10**:121–168.
13. Rubin H, Lome LG, Presman D. Neurological manifestation of metastatic prostatic carcinoma. *J Radiol* 1974;**111**:799–802.
14. Osborn JL, Getzenberg RH, Trump DL. Spinal cord compression in prostate cancer. *J Neuro-Oncology* 1995;**23**:135–147.
15. Shoskes DA, Perrin RG. The role of surgical management for symptomatic spinal cord compression in patients with metastatic prostate cancer. *J Urol* 1989;**142**:337–339.
16. Payne R. Pain management in the patient with prostate cancer. *Cancer Suppl* 1993;**71**(3):1131–1137.
17. Osborn JL, Getzenberg RH, Trump DL. Spinal cord compression in prostate cancer. *J Neurooncol* 1995;**23**:135–147.
18. Flynn DF, Shipley WU. Management of spinal cord compression secondary to metastatic prostate carcinoma. *Urol Clin N Amer* 1989;**18**:145–152.
19. Perez CA, Cosmatos D, Garcia DM, Eisbruch A, Poulter CA. Irradiation in relapsing carcinoma of the prostate. *Cancer* 1993;**71**(3 suppl):1110–1122.
20. Young RF, Post EM, King GA. Treatment of spinal epidural metastases. *J Neurosurgery* 1980;**53**:741–748.
21. Smith EM, Hampel N, Ruff R et al. Spinal cord compression secondary to prostate carcinoma: treatment and prognosis. *J Urol* 1993;**149**:330–333.
22. Kaminski HJ, Diwan VG, Ruff RL. Second occurrence of spinal epidural metastasis. *Neurology* 1991;**41**:744–746.
23. Constans JP, de Divitiis E, Donzelli R et al. Spinal metastases with neurological manifestations. *J Neurosurgery* 1983;**59**:111–118.
24. Smith EM, Hampel N, Ruff R et al. Spinal cord compression secondary to prostate carcinoma: treatment and prognosis. *J Urol* 1993;**149**:330–333.
25. Forman JD, Orderr SE, Zinreich BS et al. The correlation of pretreatment transurethral resection of prostatic cancer with tumor dissemination and disease-free survival. A univariate and multivariate analysis. *Cancer* 1986;**58**:1770.
26. Varenhorst E, Alund G. Urethral obstruction secondary to carcinoma of the prostate: response to endocrine treatment. *Urology* 1985;**25**:354.
27. Meacham RB, Scardino PT, Hoffman GS et al. The risk of distant metastases after transurethral resection of the prostate versus needle biopsy in patients with localized prostate cancer. *J Urol* 1989;**142**:320.
28. Lloyd-Davies RW, Collins CD, Swan AV. Carcinoma of the prostate treated by radical external beam radiotherapy using hypofractionation. Twenty-two years' experience. *Urology* 1990;**36**:107.
29. Nativ O, Bergstralh EJ, Boyle ET et al. Transurethral resection versus needle biopsy prior to radical prostatectomy for stage C prostate cancer. Influence on progression and survival. *Urology* 1991;**37**:22.
30. Schmid HP. The problem of obstruction in prostate cancer. *Urol Res* 1991;**19**:323–326.
31. Kynston HG, Keen CW, Matthews PN. Radiotherapy for palliation of locally advanced prostatic carcinoma. *Br J Urol* 1990;**66**:515.
32. Gibbons RP, Mason JT, Correa RJ et al. Carcinoma of the prostate: local control with external beam radiation therapy. *J Urol* 1979;**121**:310.
33. Guazzoni G, Montorsi F, Bergamaschi F et al. Prostatic urolume wallstent for urinary retention due to advanced prostate cancer: a 1-year follow up study. *J Urol* 1994;**152**:1530–1532.
34. Yachia D, Aridogan IA. The use of a removable stent in patients with prostate cancer and obstruction. *J Urol* 1996;**155**:1956–1958.
35. Paul AB, Love C, Chisholm GD. The management of bilateral ureteric obstruction and renal failure in advanced prostate cancer. *Br J Urol* 1994;**74**(5):642–645.
36. Honnens de Lichtenberg M, Miskowiak J, Rolff H. Hormonal treatment of obstructed kidneys in patients with prostatic cancer. *Br J Urol* 1993;**71**(3):313–316.
37. Briggs TP, Parker C, Green AN, Miller RA. Emergency orchiectomy under sedoanalgesia for uraemic ureteric obstruction secondary to prostatic carcinoma. An alternative to percutaneous and stenting procedures. *Br J Urol* 1993;**71**(1):111.
38. Hamdy FC, Williams JL. Use of dexamethasone for ureteric obstruction in advanced prostate cancer: percutaneous nephrostomies can be avoided. *Br J Urol* 1995;**75**(6):782–785.
39. Perez CA, Cosmatos D, Garcia DM, Eisbruch A, Poulter CA. Irradiation in relapsing carcinoma of the prostate. *Cancer* 1993;**71**(3 suppl):1110–1122.
40. Ampil FL. Radiation therapy palliation in malignancy-associated ureteral obstruction. *Radiat Med* 1989;**7**(6):282–286.
41. Demetriou D, Sebeikat D. Percutaneous nephrostomy in malignant ureteral obstruction. *Dtsch Med Wochenschr* 1996;**121**(49):1526–1530.
42. Desportes L, Blanchet P, Benoit G, Lecouturier S, Langloys J, Decaux A, Di Palma M, Richard C, Jardin A. Neoplastic ureteral obstruction: drainage by percutaneous nephrostomy or double J catheterization. *Presse Med* 1995;**24**(29):1332–1336.
43. Bordinazzo R, Benecchi L, Cazzaniga A, Vercesi A, Privitera O. Ureteral obstruction associated with prostate cancer: the outcome after ultrasonographic percutaneous nephrostomy. *Arch Ital Urol Androl* 1994;**66**(4 suppl):101–106.
44. Dowling RA, Carrasco CH, Babaian RJ. Percutaneous urinary diversion in patients with hormone-refractory prostate cancer. *Urology* 1991;**37**(2):89–91.
45. Chiou RK, Chang WY, Horan JJ. Ureteral obstruction associated with prostate cancer: the outcome after percutaneous nephrostomy. *J Urol* 1990;**143**(5):957–959.

46. Giannakopoulos X, Gartzios A, Giannakis D, Tsamboulas K, Kotoulas KJ. Internal urinary diversion in pelvic cancers and quality of life. Value of double 'J' endoprosthesis. Urol (Paris) 1995;**101**(5–6):221–227.

47. Pandian SS, Hussey JK, McClinton S. Metallic ureteric stents: early experience. Br J Urol 1998;**82**(6):791–797.

48. Lopez-Martinez RA, Singireddy S, Lang EK. The use of metallic stents to bypass ureteral strictures secondary to metastatic prostate cancer: experience with 8 patients. J Urol 1997;**158**(1):50–53.

49. Chefchaouni MC, Flam TA, Pacha K, Thiounn N, Zerbib M, Debre B. Endoscopic ureteroneocystostomy: palliative urinary diversion in advanced prostatic cancer. Tech Urol 1998;**4**(1):46–50.

50. Wawroschek F, Hamm M, Rathert P. Results of ureterocystoneostomy for inner urinary diversion in locally advanced prostate carcinoma. Urologe A 1998;**37**(4):372–376.

51. Di Lelio A. Circumvallate nephro-cystostomy. Arch Ital Urol Nefrol Androl 1992;**64**(suppl 2):45–49.

52. Puppo P, Ricciotti G, Bozzo W, Pezzica C, Geddo D, Perachino M. Videoendoscopic cutaneous ureterostomy for palliative urinary diversion in advanced pelvic cancer. Eur Urol 1995;**28**(4):328–333.

53. Lowe FC, Somers WJ. The use of ketoconazole in the emergency management of disseminated intravascular coagulation due to metastatic prostatic cancer. J Urol 1987;**137**:1000–1002.

54. Sarver RG, Dalkin BL, Ahmann FR. Ketoconazole-induced adrenal crisis in a patient with metastatic prostatic adenocarcinoma: case report and review of the literature. Urology 1997;**49**(5):781–785.

55. Cabane J, Etarian C, Louvet C, Robert A, Blum L, Wattiaux MJ, Imbert JC. Disseminated intravascular coagulation associated with prostatic cancer. Rev Med Interne 1995;**16**(3):219–224.

56. Cooper DL, Sandler AB, Wilson LD, Duffy TP. Disseminated intravascular coagulation and excessive fibrinolysis in a patient with metastatic prostate cancer. Response to epsilon-aminocaproic acid. Cancer 1992;**70**(3):656–658.

57. Aubert J, Vigouroux V, Dore B. Hot flushes in men after surgical or pharmacologic castration. Prog Urol 1995;**5**(4):507–509.

58. Iversen P. Orchidectomy and oestrogen therapy revisited. Eur Urol 1998;**34**(suppl 3):7–11.

59. Smith JA Jr. Management of hot flushes due to endocrine therapy for prostate carcinoma. Oncology (Huntingt) 1996;**10**(9):1319–1322; discussion 1324.

60. Adlercreutz H, Mazur W. Phyto-oestrogens and Western diseases. Ann Med 1997;**29**(2):95–120.

61. Smith JA Jr. A prospective comparison of treatments for symptomatic hot flushes following endocrine therapy for carcinoma of the prostate. J Urol 1994;**152**(1):132–134.

62. Greenstein A, Plymate SR, Katz P. Visually stimulated erection in castrated men. J Urol 1995;**153**(3 Pt 1):650–652.

63. Morali G, Lemus AE, Munguia R, Arteaga M, Perez-Palacios G, Sundaram K, Kumar N, Bardin CW. Induction of male sexual behavior in the rat by 7-alpha-methyl-19-nortestosterone, an androgen that does not undergo 5 alpha-reduction. Biol Reprod 1993;**49**(3):577–581.

64. Suzuki Y, Aikawa K, Oishi Y, Yamazaki H, Onishi , Suzuki M, Kobari T et al. A clinical study of decreased bone density in the patients treated with long term luteinizing hormone releasing hormone analogue (LHRH-a)—The risk of iatrogenic osteoporosis due to treatment of carcinoma of prostate. Nippon Hinyokika Gakkai Zasshi 1998;**89**(12):961–966.

65. Galus MA. Re: Osteoporosis after orchiectomy for prostate cancer. J Urol 1998;**159**(4):1314.

66. Daniell HW. Osteoporosis after orchiectomy for prostate cancer. J Urol 1997;**157**(2):439–444.

67. Levis S, Kim C, Roos B, Krongrad A. Dopestrogens protect against bone loss in men treated for prostate cancer? Proc 76th Annual Meeting of the Endocrine Society, p. 1565, 1994.

68. Eriksson S, Eriksson A, Stege R, Carlstrom K. Bone mineral density in patients with prostatic cancer treated with orchidectomy and with estrogens. Calc Tissue Int 1995;**57**:97.

69. Serels S, Melman A. Tamoxifen as a treatment for gynecomastia and mastodynia resulting from hormonal deprivation. J Urol 1998;**159**:1309.

70. Fentiman I, Caleffi M, Hamed H, Chaudary M. Studies of tamoxifen in women with mastalgia. Br J Clin Pract 1989;**68**(suppl):34.

71. Moreno JG, Ahlering TE. Late local complications after definitive radiotherapy for prostatic adenocarcinoma. J Urol 1992;**147**(3 Pt 2):926–928.

72. Talcott JA, Rieker P, Clark JA, Propert KJ, Weeks JC, Beard CJ, Wishnow KI et al. Patient-reported symptoms after primary therapy for early prostate cancer: results of a prospective cohort study. J Clin Oncol 1998;**16**(1):275–283.

73. Perez CA, Lee HK, Georgiou A, Lockett MA. Technical factors affecting morbidity in definitive irradiation for localized carcinoma of the prostate. Int J Radiat Oncol Biol Phys 1994;**28**(4):811–819.

74. Nguyen LN, Pollack A, Zagars GK. Late effects after radiotherapy for prostate cancer in a randomized dose-response study: results of a self-assessment questionnaire. Urology 1998;**51**(6):991–997.

75. Beard CJ, Lamb C, Buswell L, Schneider L, Propert KJ, Gladstone D, D'Amico A, Kaplan I. Radiation-associated morbidity in patients undergoing small-field external beam irradiation for prostate cancer. Int J Radiat Oncol Biol Phys 1998;**41**(2):257–262.

76 Goswami AK, Mahajan RK, Nath Rm, Sharma SK. How safe is 1% alum irrigation in controlling intractable vesical hemorrhage? Urology 1993;**149**(2): 264–267.

77. Yamamoto M, Hibi H, Ohmura M, Miyake K. Successful treatment of hemorrhagic cystitis secondary to cyclophosphamide chemotherapy with intravesical instillation of prostaglandin F2 alpha. Hinyokika Kiyo 1994;**40**(9):833–835.

78. Vicente J, Rios G, Caffaratti J. Intravesical formalin for the treatment of massive hemorrhagic cystitis: retrospective review of 25 cases. Eur Urol 1990;**18**(3):204–206.

79. Del Pizzo JJ, Chew BH, Jacobs SC, Sklar GN. Treatment of radiation induced hemorrhagic cystitis with hyperbaric oxygen: long-term followup. J Urol 1998;**160**(3 Pt 1):731–733.

80. Sneiders A, Pryor JL. Percutaneous nephrostomy drainage in the treatment of severe hemorrhagic cystitis. J Urol 1993;**150**(3):966–967.

81. Catalona WJ, Basler JW. Return of erections and urinary continence following nerve sparing radical retropubic prostatectomy. J Urol 1993;**150**(3):905–907.

PART THREE

Upper urinary tract, adrenal and retroperitoneal tumors

Chapter 19
Renal cell carcinoma: Incidence, etiology, epidemiology and genetics

Chapter 20
Pathology of renal tumors

Chapter 21
Renal cell carcinoma: Presentation, diagnosis and staging

Chapter 22
Surgical treatment of renal cell carcinoma

22.1   Radical nephrectomy

22.2   Surgery for neoplastic involvement of the renal vein and inferior vena cava

22.3   Partial radical nephrectomy

22.4   Von Hippel-Lindau disease

Chapter 23
Minimally invasive therapy

23.1   Focused ultrasound ablation

23.2   Focused microwave ablation and cryotherapy

23.3   Laparoscopic surgery

Chapter 24
Metastatic renal cancer

24.1   The role of surgery and tumor embolization

24.2   The role of immunotherapy

24.3   The role of chemotherapy

Chapter 25
Transitional cell carcinoma of the upper urinary tract: Incidence, etiology, epidemiology and genetics

Chapter 26
Transitional cell carcinoma of the upper urinary tract: Presentation, diagnosis and staging

Chapter 27
Transitional cell carcinoma of the upper urinary tract: Pathology

Chapter 28
Transitional cell carcinoma of the upper urinary tract: Surgical treatment

28.1   Nephro-ureterectomy and partial ureterectomy

28.2   Percutaneous, ureteroscopic resection and novel approaches

Chapter 29
Chemotherapy immunotherapy for upper urinary tract transitional cell carcinoma

Chapter 30
Rare renal tumors

Chapter 31
Adrenal tumors

Chapter 32
Retroperitoneal malignancies and processes

Chapter 33
Pathology of adrenal and retroperitoneal tumors

10 Renal cell carcinoma: Incidence, etiology, epidemiology and genetics

R B Nadler and J M Kozlowski

Incidence

World-wide incidence

There are an estimated 80 000 to 100 000 new cases of renal cell carcinoma diagnosed world-wide each year, representing approximately 1.5% of all cancers. There is a ten-fold range in incidence world-wide with the highest rates occurring in Europe and lowest rates in Asia, Africa and South America. The incidence of and mortality from renal cell carcinoma has been increasing over the past 50 years world-wide, especially in western Europe and Scandinavia[1]. The incidence of renal cell cancer is 8.4 per 100 000 among white men, 8.6 among black men, 3.7 among white women and 3.8 among black women with an average rise in incidence rates of 2% per year[2]. Recently, however, the mortality from renal cell carcinoma seems to be decelerating world-wide[1].

United States incidence

It is estimated that there will be 30 800 cases of renal and upper urinary tract cancer in the United States in 2001, resulting in 12 100 cancer deaths. The majority of these upper urinary tract cancers will be renal cell carcinoma (approximately 26 000)[3]. Renal cell carcinoma accounts for approximately 2% of all new cancer cases in the United States and has been reported in children as young as 6 months of age, although the majority of cases occur in patients in their 60s and 70s. The incidence and mortality from renal cell carcinoma is twice as high in the United States as compared with Central and South America and similar to that in western Europe. The male to female ratio is approximately 2 : 1, similar to that found in Europe[3,4].

Etiology

Immunohistochemical and ultrastructural analysis has demonstrated that the common histologic variants of the renal cell carcinoma (clear cell, granular cell, sarcomatoid) originate from proximal convoluted tubule cells[5–7]. In distinction, distal tubular origin has been proposed for renal oncocytomas[8], papillary renal cell carcinomas[9], chromophobe carcinomas[10], and collecting duct carcinomas of the kidney[11].

A variety of epigenetic (i.e. environmental) and genetic factors have been causally linked to the development of renal cell carcinoma[12,13]. Cigarette smoking has been implicated in the development of nearly 30% of these tumors in men and about one-quarter of those in women[14]. Recently, an international, multicenter, population-based, case-control study found statistically significant links between smoking and renal cell carcinoma. Furthermore, this risk of developing renal cell carcinoma increased for the number of cigarettes and duration (years) of smoking, and decreased with long-term cessation[15]. Obesity, particularly in women, may also constitute a risk factor for the development of renal cell carcinoma[16,17]. At-risk occupations include: refinery workers; petroleum products distribution workers; leather tanners; shoe workers; and individuals chronically exposed to asbestos[18–21]. Exposure to a variety of other agents has also been correlated with an increased risk of renal cell carcinoma, including cadmium[22], thorium dioxide[23], lead phosphate, dimethyl nitrosamine, aflatoxin B1, and streptozotocin[13,24]. Although analgesic abuse (particularly with phenacetin-containing compounds) has been primarily linked with an increased frequency of carcinomas of the renal pelvis, there is also an increased risk of renal parenchymal tumors[12,25]. There does not appear to be a human correlate to the observations implicating the prolonged administration of estrogen to male Syrian golden hamsters and the subsequent development of renal cell carcinoma[26].

Recent reports have suggested that the incidence of renal cell carcinoma in patients with end-stage renal disease is seven to 50 times greater than that identified in the general population[27]. This relationship appears to be linked to the acquisition of cystic disease of the kidney in patients with chronic renal failure. Approximately 8% of these patients have evidence of acquired cystic disease prior to the initiation of dialysis and its a subsequent development after 1–3 years, 3–5 years and 5–10 years of dialysis is reported to be 10–40%, 40–60% and greater than 90%, respectively[28,29]. However, the observation that approximately 6% of such patients develop renal cell carcinoma[30]. was not validated in a literature review of 1645 patients with end-stage renal disease (with and without dialysis) in which the occurrence rate of renal cell carcinoma was 1% and the incidence of metastases was 0.2 to 0.5%[28].

Epidemiology

Very little is known about the epidemiology of renal cell carcinoma because of its relatively infrequent presentation, hidden anatomic location, unpredictable clinical course and poor response to non-surgical treatment[31].

Most patients present over the age of 40 in industrialized countries (North America, Europe, Scandinavia). Several occupational exposures and risk factors such as tobacco use have been identified and already discussed. No link between socioeconomic status and renal cell carcinoma has been found[32,33], but a clear link between an urban versus rural environment and renal cell carcinoma has been established. Several studies in the United States and in Europe confirm that the incidence and mortality is higher in an urban environment[32,34,35].

A few studies have looked at the role of ethnicity and renal cell cancer. Several studies have shown a higher rate of renal cell carcinoma among native born Jewish inhabitants of New York City as compared with Catholics, Protestants, and Jewish people born outside of the United States[36,37].

The role of diet in the development of renal cell carcinoma is poorly understood. Several case control studies have shown the relationship between the high consumption of meat[16,38] and margarine and oils[39]. A recent study has shown fried meats to be associated with an increased renal cell cancer risk while vegetables and fruits particularly orange/dark green vegetables are associated with a

protective effect[38]. There has been no link between coffee and tea consumption with renal cell cancer[40]. Similarly no link between alcohol consumption and renal cell carcinoma exists[41,42].

Genetics/molecular biology

Renal cell carcinoma occurs in both inherited and sporadic (non-inherited) forms[43]. Hereditary cancers account for about 4% of renal cell cancers and are generally distinguished from their sporadic counterparts by a distinct predisposition to multifocality, bilaterality and occurrence at a younger age[44].

Three distinct forms of hereditary or familial renal cell carcinoma have been identified. The first is designated hereditary, non-papillary renal cell carcinoma. This variant is inherited with an autosomal dominant mode of penetrance and is typified by the production of clear cell renal carcinomas in approximately 50% of the at-risk cohort[44–46]. In each case, reciprocal translocations of a portion of the short arm of chromosome 3 to other chromosomes (8, 11, 6) have been identified.

Von Hippel-Lindau (VHL) disease constitutes the second form of hereditary renal cell carcinoma. This condition affects 1/36 000 live births and is also inherited as an autosomal dominant condition[12]. The following phenotypes have been associated with the full expression of VHL disease: pancreatic cysts; pancreatic islet cell tumors; retinal angiomas; hemangioblastomas of the central nervous system; pheochromocytomas; benign epididymal cysts and cystadenomas; and multiple, bilateral renal cystic tumors. With respect to the latter, clear cell type renal cell carcinomas occur in 40% of patients with VHL disease and constitute the cause of death in about 30% of such patients[47]. Examination of tumor tissues using cytogenetic techniques and restriction fragment length polymorphism have consistently demonstrated loss of a segment of the short arm of chromosome 3 (3p). This loss of heterozygosity has been correlated with rearrangements, deletions, and translocations involving this chromosomal segment which is thought to harbor a critical tumor suppressor gene[48]. More recent studies utilizing linkage analysis have permitted the localization of the VHL gene to a site between 3p25 and 3p26[49]. The human VHL gene encodes a protein of 213 amino acids with no significant homology to known proteins[50]. The functional target of the VHL protein appears to be a critical cellular transcription factor designated Elongin (S III). The VHL protein appears to bind tightly and specifically to Elongin B and C subunits and, consequently, to inhibit Elongin (S III) transcriptional activity. Hypermethylation, in addition to the standard mechanisms of VHL gene inactivation, may play a role in the abnormal expression of this critical transcriptional regulator[51].

Hereditary papillary renal cell carcinoma is the third familial variant of this disease. About 5–10% of renal cancers exhibit a papillary growth pattern[44]. As was the case with clear cell carcinomas, a sporadic variant of papillary renal carcinoma has also been identified. Unlike the hereditary clear cell carcinomas, loss of heterozygoty of chromosome 3p has not been detected in the tumor tissue or cell lines from patients with papillary kidney cancer[52]. The cytogenetic abnormalities which have been detected in these tumors include translocations involving chromosome 1 and trisomy of chromosomes 7, 16, or 17[46].

The molecular epidemiology of sporadic renal cell carcinomas appears to involve aberrations in growth control in addition to those that are obviously linked to abnormalities involving the short arm of chromosome 3. Indeed, the molecular analysis of sporadic renal cancers has demonstrated, with variable frequency, a loss of heterozygosity on chromosomes 3, 11p, 17p and 18q[53]. Perhaps most noteworthy are those tumors associated with chromosome 17p deletions and associated mutations of the p53 tumor suppressor gene. The wild-type (i.e. normal) variant of p53 is one of the major regulators of entry into the G_1 phase of the cell cycle. Deletions of this tumor suppressor gene or mutations in that gene are associated with uncontrolled proliferation. The presence of p53 mutations in renal cell carcinoma closely correlates with advanced stage and poor prognosis[54]. It is not surprising, therefore, that the vast majority of sarcomatoid renal cancers avidly express the mutated form of p53.

Finally, it should be emphasized that the majority of non-papillary renal tumors aberrantly overexpress the genes for the epidermal growth factor receptor (EGF-R) and its ligand, transforming growth factor-α (TGF-α). Amplified expression of this receptor–ligand combination has been associated with metastatic propensity and poor prognosis[55]. Of interest, papillary tumors have a significantly lower rate of EGF-R positivity than solid pattern renal cancers and this feature may be directly linked to the more favourable overall prognosis exhibited by papillary tumors[55].

References

1. Coleman MP, Esteve J, Damiecki P, Arslan A, Renard H. Kidney and other urinary organs. In: *Trends in cancer incidence and mortality*. Lyon: IARC Scientific Publications No. 121. International Agency for Research on Cancer, 1993, pp. 577–608.

2. Devesa SS, Silverman DT, McLaughlin JK, Brown CC, Connelly RR, Fraumeni JF Jr. Comparison of the descriptive epidemiology of urinary tract cancers. *Cancer Causes Control* 1990;**1**:133–141.

3. Greenlee RT, Hill-Harmon MB, Murrag T, Than M. Cancer Statistics 2001. *Cancer* 2001;**51**:15–37.

4. Jennings SB, Linehan WM. Renal, perirenel, and ureteral neoplasms. In: Gillenwater JY, Grayhack JT, Howards SS, Ducket JW (eds) *Adult and pediatric urology*. Mosby St Louis, 1996, pp. 643–694.

5. Golimbu M, Joshi P, Sperber A, Tessler A, Al-Askari S, Morles P. Renal cell carcinoma: survival and prognostic factors. *Urology* 1986;**27**:291–301.

6. Tannenbaum M. Ultrastructural pathology of human renal cell tumors. *Pathol Ann* 1971;**197**(6):249–277.

7. Cooper PH, Waisman J. Tubular differentiation and basement-membrane production in a renal adenoma: Ultrastructural features. *J Pathol* 1973 Feb; 109(2):113.

8. Morra MN, Das S. Renal oncocytoma: a review of histogenesis, histopathology, diagnosis and treatment. *J Urol* 1993;**150**:295–302.

9. Mancilla-Jimenez R, Stanley RJ, Blath RA. Papillary renal cell carcinoma. *Cancer* 1976;**38**:2469–2480.

10. Crotty TB, Farrow GM, Lieber MM. Chromophobe cell renal carcinoma: clinicopathological features of 50 cases. *J Urol* 1995;**154**:964–967.

11. Fleming S, Lewi HJE. Collecting duct carcinoma of the kidney. *Histopathology* 1986;**10**:1131–1141.

12. Linehan WM, Gnarra JR, Lerman MI, Latif F, Zbar B. Genetic basis of renal cell cancer. In: DeVita VT Jr, Hellman S, Rosenberg SA (eds) *Important advances in oncology 1993*, J.B. Lipincott Company, Philadelphia, 1993, pp. 47–70.

13. Richie JP. Renal cell carcinoma. In: Holland JF, Frei E III, Bast RC Jr *et al.* (eds), *Cancer medicine* (3rd edn) Philadelphia, Lea & Febiger, 1993, pp. 1529–1538.

14. Yu MC, Mack TM, Hanisch R, Cicioni C, Henderson BE. Cigarette smoking, obesity, diuretic use, and coffee consumption as risk factors for renal cell carcinoma. *JNCI* 1986;**77**:351–356.

15. McLaughlin JK, Lindblad P, Mellemgaard A *et al.* International renal-cell cancer study I. tobacco use. *Int J Cancer* 1995;**60**:194–198.

16. McLaughlin JK, Mandel JS, Blot WJ, Schuman LM, Mehl ES, Fraumeni JF. A population-based case control study of renal cell carcinoma. *JNCI* 1984;**72**:275–284.

17. Kantor AF. Current concepts in the epidemiology and etiology of primary renal cell carcinoma. *J Urol* 1977;**117**:415–417.

18. Malker HR, Malker BK, McLaughlin JK, Blot WJ. Kidney cancer among leather workers. *Lancet* 1984; Jan 7;**1**(8367):56.

19. Maclure M. Asbestos and renal adenocarcinoma: a case-control study. *Environ Res* 1987;**42**:353–361.

20. Ross RK, Pagannini-Hill A, Landolph J, Gerkins V, Henderson BE. Analgesics, cigarette smoking, and other risk factors for cancer of the renal pelvis and ureter. *Cancer Res* 1989;**49**:1045–1048.

21. Enterline PE, Viren J. Epidemiologic evidence for an association between gasoline and kidney cancer. *Environ Health Perspect* 1985;**62**:303–312.

22. DeKernion JB, Smith RB. The kidney and adrenal glands. In: Paulson DF (Ed.) *Genitourinary surgery*. Churchill Livingstone, New York, 1984, pp. 1–153.

23. Kauzlaric D, Barmeir E, Binek J, Ramelli F, Petrovic M. Renal carcinoma after retrograde pyelography with thorotrast. *AJR* 1987;**148**:897–898.

24. Mauer SM, Lee CS, Najarian JS, Brown DM. Induction of malignant kidney tumors in rats with streptozotocin. *Cancer Res* 1974 Jan;**34**(1):158.

25. Lornoy W, Becaus I, De Vleeschouwer M. Renal cell carcinoma, a new complication of analgesic nephropathy. *Lancet* 1986;**2**:1271–1272.

26. Harris DT. Hormonal therapy and chemotherapy of renal-cell carcinoma. *Semi Oncol* 1983 Dec;**10**(4):422.

27. Terasawa Y, Suzuki Y, Morita M, Kato M, Suzuki K, Sekino H. Ultrasonic diagnosis of renal cell carcinoma in hemodialysis patients. *J Urol* 1994;**152**:846–851.

28. Chandhoke PS, Torrence RJ, Clayman RV, Rothstein M. Acquired cystic disease of the kidney: a management dilemma. *J Urol* 1992;**147**:969–974.

29. Matson MA, Cohen EP. Acquired cystic kidney disease: occurrence, prevalence, and renal cancers. *Medicine* 1990;**69**:217.

30. Brennan JF, Stilmant MM, Babayan RK, Siroky MB. Acquired renal cystic disease: Implications for the urologist. *Br J Urol* 1991;**67**:342–348.

31. Dayal H, Kinman J. Epidemiology of kidney cancer. *Semin Oncol* 1983;**10**:366–377.

32. Kantor AFL, Meigs JW, Heston JF *et al.* Epidemiology of renal cell carcinoma in Connecticut, 1935–1973. *J Natl Cancer Inst* 1976;**57**:495–500.

33. Williams R, Stegens N, Goldsmith J. Associations of cancer site and type with occupation and industry from the Third National Cancer Survey Interview. *J Natl Cancer Inst* 1977;**59**:1147–1185.

34. Hoover R, Mason TJ, McKay FW *et al.* Geographic patterns of cancer mortality in the United States. In: Fraumeni JF Jr (Ed.) *Persons at high risk of cancer.* Academic Press, New York, 1975, pp. 343–360.

35. Case RAM. Mortality from cancer of the kidney in England and Wales. In: Riches E (Ed.) *Tumors of the kidney and ureter.* E. & S. Livingston, Edinburgh and London, 1964, pp. 3–38.

36. Newill V. Distribution of cancer mortality among ethnic subgroups of the white population of New York City, 1953–1958. *J Natl Cancer Inst* 1961;**26**:405–417.

37. Seidman H. Cancer death rates by site and sex for religions and socioeconomic groups in New York City. *Environ Res* 1970;**3**:234–250.

38. Wolk A, Gridley G, Niwa S *et al.* International renal cell cancer study. VII. role of diet. *Int J Cancer* 1996;**65**:67–73.

39. Maclure M, Willett W. A case-control study of diet and risk of renal adenocarcinoma. *Epidemiology* 1990;**1**:430–440.

40. Kreiger N, Marrett LD, Dodds L, Hilditch S, Darlington GA. Risk factors for renal cell carcinoma: results of a population-based case-control study. *Cancer Causes Control* 1993;**4**:101–110.

41. Breslow NE, Enstrom JE. Geographic correlations between cancer mortality rates and alcohol-tobacco consumption in the United States. *J Natl Cancer Inst* 1977;**53**:631–639.

42. Williams RR, Horm JV. Association of cancer sites with tobacco and alcohol consumption socioeconomic status of patients: Interview study for the Third National Cancer Society. *J Natl Cancer Inst* 1977;**58**: 525–547.

43. Walther MM, Jennings SB, Gnarra JR, Zbar B, Linehan WM. Molecular genetics of renal cell carcinoma. In: Vogelzang NJ, Scardino PT, Shipley WU, Coffey DS, (eds) *Comprehensive textbook of genitourinary oncology.* Williams & Wilkins, Baltimore, Md, 1996, pp. 160–170.

44. Linehan WM, Lerman MI, Zbar B. Identification of the von Hippel-Lindau (VHL) Gene. *JAMA* 1995;**273**(7):564–570.

45. Cohen AJ, Li FP, Berg S *et al.* Hereditary renal-cell carcinoma associated with a chromosomal translocation. *N Engl J Med* 1979;**301**:592–595.

46. Kovacs G, Fuzesi L, Emanual A, Kung HF. Cytogenetics of papillary renal cell tumors. *Genes Chromosom Cancer* 1991;**3**:249–255.

47. Glenn GM, Choyke PL, Zbar B, Linehan WM. Von Hippel-Lindau disease, clinical review and molecular genetics. *Problems in Urology* 1990;**4**(2):312–330.

48. Presti JC, Rao PH, Chen Q *et al.* Histopathological, cytogenic, and molecular characterization of renal cortical tumors. *Cancer Res* 1991;**51**:1544–1552.

49. Lerman MI, Latif F, Glenn GM, *et al.* Isolation and regional localization of a large collection (2,000) of single copy DNA fragments on human chromosome 3 for mapping and cloning tumor suppressor genes. *Hum Genet* 1991;**86**:567–577.

50. Duan DR, Pause A, Burgess WH, Aso T, Chen DYT, Garrett KP, Conaway RC, Conaway JW, Linehan WM, Klausner RD. Inhibition of transcription elongation by the VHL tumor suppressor protein. *Science* 1995;**269**:1402–1446.

51. Herman JG, Latif F, Weng Y *et al.* Silencing of the VHL tumor suppressor gene by DNA methylation in renal carcinoma. *Proc Natl Acad Sci USA* 1994;**91**:9700–9704.

52. Zbar B, Tory K, Merino M, Schmidt L, Glenn G, Choyke P, Walther MM, Lerman M, Linehan WM. Hereditary papillary renal cell carcinoma. *J Urol* 1994;**151**:561–566.

53. Presti JC, Reuter VE, Cordon-Cardo C, Mazumdar M, Fair WR, Jhanwar SC. Allelic deletions in renal tumors: histopathological correlations. *Cancer Res* 1993;**53**:5780–5783.

54. Uhlman DL, Nguyen PL, Manivel JC, *et al.* Association of immunohistochemical staining for p53 with metastatic progression and poor survival in patients with renal cell carcinoma. *J Natl Cancer Inst* 1994;**86**:1470–1475.

55. Uhlman DL, Nguyen P, Manivel JC, Zhang G, Hagen K, Fraley E, Aeppli D, Niehans GA. Epidermal growth factor receptor and transforming growth factor α expression in papillary and nonpapillary renal cell carcinoma: Correlation with metastatic behavior and prognosis. *Clin Cancer Res* 1995;**1**:913–920.

20 Pathology of renal tumors

D J M DiMaio

Tumors of the kidney

Tumors of the kidney can be divided into adult and pediatric tumors. While this division is a useful way to approach renal tumors, it is artificial. Many so-called adult tumors have been reported in children and pediatric tumors have been reported in adults. This chapter will focus mainly on the more common epithelial and non-epithelial, pediatric and adult, renal tumors (Table 20.1). Transitional cell carcinoma of the renal pelvis, while certainly not uncommon, will not be covered here because the histologic criteria used to evaluate transitional cell carcinoma is better discussed in the chapter concerning tumors of the bladder.

Malignant adult tumors of the kidney

Renal cell carcinoma accounts for only 3% of the cancers in the United States but 85% of all primary malignant renal tumors[1]. The tumor occurs in men two to three times more often than women and may occur with equal frequency in either kidney[2]. In patients with von Hippel-Lindau disease, 20–50% will develop renal cell carcinoma[3].

Table 20.1 Adult and pediatric renal tumors

Adult	Pediatric
Renal cell carcinoma	Nephroblastoma (Wilms' tumor)
Clear cell carcinoma	Cystic nephroma
Papillary carcinoma	Cystic partially differentiated nephroblastoma
Chromophobe carcinoma	Mesoblastic nephroma
Collecting duct carcinoma	Clear cell sarcoma of kidney
Oncocytoma	Malignant rhabdoid tumor of kidney
Papillary adenoma	
Metanephric adenoma	
Juxtaglomerular cell tumor	
Angiomyolipoma	

These patients develop renal cell carcinoma at an earlier age and have a greater incidence of bilateral renal cell carcinoma[4]. Approximately one-third of all patients with renal cell carcinoma have metastatic disease at the time of diagnosis[5]. Renal cell carcinoma is known for its ability to metastasize to almost any location in the body. The lungs, however, are the most common sites for metastatic disease[6]. The number of patients with advanced disease at time of diagnosis is gradually decreasing as the number of incidentally detected carcinomas is increasing. In 1976 only 4% of asymptomatic tumors were discovered. By 1991 the number had increased to 61%[7].

Although sometimes discussed as such, renal cell carcinoma is not a single disease. While the 'variants' of renal cell carcinoma do share some common features, they also have very distinct and important clinical, histologic and chromosomal differences. The following sections discuss the currently recognized types of renal cell carcinoma[8–9].

Clear cell renal carcinoma

Clear cell carcinoma (conventional renal cell carcinoma) is the most common type of renal cell carcinoma, representing 70–80% of all such tumors (Figure 20.1)[3,10]. The age of presentation is wide with a peak incidence in the sixth decade of life. The average diameter of the tumor is 8 cm. The cut surface is yellow to tan to red depending on the amount of lipid present. Hemorrhage, necrosis and cystic degeneration are common. The tumor may be multifocal in the same kidney (4.5%) or bilateral (0.5 to 1.5%)[1]. Microscopically, the tumor is composed of polygonal cells with clear to lightly eosinophilic granular cytoplasm. The cells may be arranged in a variety of non-papillary patterns such as sheets and tubules. High-grade neoplasm may appear sarcomatoid with sheets of spindle cells.

The most important histologic feature when evaluating any renal cell carcinoma is the nuclear grade as it is an

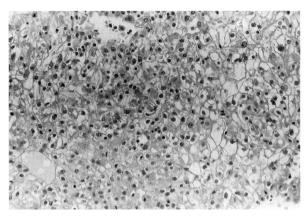

Fig. 20.1 Clear cell renal carcinoma consisting of cells with clear cytoplasm, moderate nuclear atypia and prominent nucleoli.

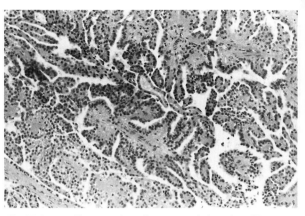

Fig. 20.2 Papillary renal carcinoma consisting of papillae lined by cells with eosinophilic cytoplasm and inconspicuous nucleoli.

independent predictor of survival[11]. Nuclear grade is evaluated using Fuhrman's nuclear grading (Table 20.2), a four-tier system based upon nuclear atypia and the presence or absence of nucleoli[11]. The architectural pattern or the characteristics of the cells cytoplasm are not independent predictors of survival[12]. The only exception to this is the sarcomatoid pattern which is associated with poor outcome independent of nuclear grade[12–13].

Unlike most epithelial neoplasms, renal cell carcinoma will stain with cytokeratin and vimentin antibodies[10]. Cytogenetically, 96% of clear cell renal carcinoma will show an abnormality of the short arm of chromosome 3[14]. Additional chromosomal abnormalities are usually present.

Papillary renal carcinoma

Papillary carcinoma (Figure 20.2) is the second most common type of renal cell carcinoma. It represents 10 to 15% of all renal cell carcinomas and is the most common carcinoma in tumors less then 3 cm[3,10]. Like clear cell carcinoma, it most commonly presents in the sixth decade of life having an average diameter of 8 cm. Papillary carcinoma was previously grouped with clear cell carcinoma but there are several important differences between the two tumors. Microscopically, papillary carcinoma is characterized by polygonal cell with eosinophilic granular cyto-

plasm lining fibrovascular stalks of the papillae. Some tubule formation may also be present. Calcifications (psammoma bodies) and areas of necrosis are common. The nuclei are usually low grade (grade 1 to 2) and the tumor is usually low stage[10]. It is common to have multiple smaller papillary tumors (less than 3 cm) in the same or contralateral kidney[15]. Cytogenetically, papillary carcinoma shows unique chromosomal abnormalities with loss of the Y chromosome and trisomy of chromosomes 7 and 17[16]. The more favorable prognosis associated with papillary carcinoma versus other types of renal cell carcinoma is most likely due to its association with a low nuclear grade After factoring in nuclear grade, the presence of a papillary pattern is of limited prognostic significance[11,12].

Chromophobe renal carcinoma

Chromophobe renal carcinoma (Figure 20.3) is the third most common type of renal cell carcinoma. It represents approximately 5% of all renal cell carcinomas[3,10]. Like clear cell carcinoma, they most often occur in the sixth decade of life (mean age 53 years)[17]. Grossly, they may resemble an ordinary renal cell carcinoma with the tumor having an average diameter of 8 cm (range 2 to 22 cm)[10,17]. The cut surface ranges from light brown to yellow to grey. Microscopically two variants exist: the typical variant and the eosinophilic variant. Both variants are composed of polygonal cells of varying sizes most often arranged in sheets. The cells contain abundant cytoplasm and centrally located nuclei. The nuclei may range from low to high grade. The difference in the two variants is based upon the cytoplasm. The cytoplasm of the typical variant (66% of cases) is pale and reticular with condensation along the periphery of the cell causing accentuation of the cell membrane. The cytoplasm of the eosinophilic variant is markedly eosinophilic with similar accentuation of cell

Table 20.2 Fuhrman system for assessing nuclear grade*

Grade 1	Small uniform nuclei with inconspicuous or absent nucleoli
Grade 2	Larger nuclei with some irregularities and small nucleoli
Grade 3	Large nuclei with prominent atypia and nucleoli
Grade 4	Grade 3 nuclei with bizarre multinucleated nuclei

* Based upon reference 11

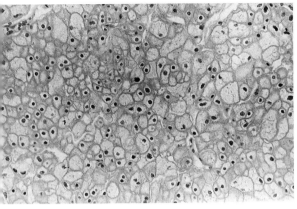

Fig. 20.3 Chromophobe renal carcinoma consisting of cells with pale to eosinophilic cytoplasm. Notice how the cytoplasm has a reticular appearance and the accentuation of the cell membrane.

membrane. The eosinophilic variant usually has some areas characteristic of the typical variant. The electron microscopic findings of these two variants are diagnostic. The cytoplasm of the typical variant is filled with microvesicles while the cytoplasm of the eosinophilic variant is filled with mitochondria[18]. Also characteristic of chromophobes is that they will stain weakly positive for periodic acid-Schiff (PAS) but strongly positive for Hale's acid iron colloid stain. Some studies have reported better survival in patients with chromophobe renal carcinoma versus typical renal cell carcinoma[18]. Larger series of cases are required before anything definitive can be said.

Collecting duct carcinoma

Collecting duct carcinoma (carcinoma of ducts of Bellini) is rare representing less than 1% of all renal cell carcinomas[3]. The mean age of presentation is 55 years[19]. Grossly, tumors may range from 2.5 to 12 cm with a mean diameter of 5 cm. They have poorly defined margins with a cut surface that is firm and gray to white in color. The tumor arises in the renal medulla and then may extend in to the cortex. Microscopically, the tumor is composed of irregular infiltrating tubules and papillae in a desmoplastic background. A prominent inflammatory component is present. The individual cells may have lightly eosinophilic to basophilic cytoplasm with high-grade nuclei. A prominent sarcomatoid component may be present. The presence of the desmoplastic stroma and the location of the tumor in the medulla help in differentiating collecting duct carcinoma from high-grade clear cell carcinoma. It is important to remember, however, that any of the renal cell carcinomas can occur in the medulla. Collecting duct carcinoma is the most aggressive type of renal cell carcinoma with 35 to 40% of patients with metastatic disease at time

of presentation. Approximately 66% of patients will die of disease within 2 years[19–20]. Common sites of metastatic disease include the lung, regional lymph nodes, bone, liver and skin[21].

Benign adult tumors of the kidney

Oncocytoma

Oncocytomas (Figure 20.4) are benign tumors that represent approximately 5% of all renal neoplasms[3]. They are most often discovered incidentally with a mean age of presentation of 57 years (range 26 to 87)[22]. Grossly, the tumor may range from 2 to 25 cm with a mean diameter of 5 to 8 cm[22]. They are well circumscribed with a cut surface that is mahogany in color. A central stellate scar may occasionally be seen. Areas of cysts or necrosis are rare. Although uncommon, cases of bilateral or multicentric oncocytomas have been reported[23]. Microscopically, the tumor is composed of nests or sheets of cells with abundant granular eosinophilic cytoplasm and low-grade nuclei (grade 1 to 2). No clear cells or mitotic figures are present. Electron microscopy shows the cytoplasm to be filled with numerous large mitochondria.

Papillary adenoma

The diagnosis of papillary adenoma is controversial. Many pathologists will not make the diagnosis except in autopsy cases. The reason for this reluctance is that microscopically there is no difference between papillary adenoma and low-grade papillary carcinoma. They even share similar cytogenetic abnormalities as papillary carcinoma[3]. The main criteria that is being used to separate the two entities is tumor size. Tumors that resemble low-grade papillary carcinoma but are less than 5 mm are classified as adenomas while tumors that are greater than

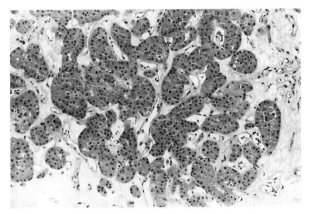

Fig. 20.4 Oncocytoma consisting of nests of cells with eosinophilic cytoplasm and minimal nuclear atypia.

5 mm are classified as carcinomas[3,24]. Papillary adenomas are typically located just beneath the renal capsule. They are well circumscribed and their cut surface is yellow to gray in color. Microscopically they resemble low-grade papillary carcinoma. In one study of 212 autopsy kidneys, 21% of the kidneys showed papillary adenomas[25]. Their frequency increased with patient age from 10% in patients 21 to 40 years old to 40% in patients 70 to 90 years old. There also appears to be an increased incidence of papillary adenomas in patients with arteriolonephrosclerosis[26]. The reason for choosing 5 mm as the size limit is that more than 90% of papillary lesions at autopsy are less than 5 mm[24]. Since these small papillary tumors have clinically behaved in a benign fashion (i.e. the patient did not die or develop metastatic disease from them), the chance of detecting a tumor less than 5 mm that is going to behave in a malignant fashion is remote.

Metanephric adenoma

Metanephric adenomas are rare tumors that appear to be benign[3]. As of yet, the number of reported cases is too small to make any definitive decision. They may occur in patients of any age but most often occur in the fifth to sixth decade. Grossly, they are well circumscribed tumors that typically are between 3 to 6 cm in diameter[24]. The cut surface is gray to tan in color. Areas of hemorrhage and necrosis are common. Microscopically they are composed of tightly compact tubules to the point that they may appear as a solid sheet of cells. The individual cells have minimal cytoplasm and small uniform nuclei. Occasional small cysts with papillary structures resembling immature glomeruli are present. Rare mitotic figures may be seen. A variant of metanephric adenoma is the metanephric adenofibroma. Adenofibromas are similar to metanephric adenomas except that adenofibromas have a cellular stroma. The stroma is composed of spindle fibroblast like cells with eosinophilic cytoplasm and benign appearing oval nuclei.

Juxtaglomerular cell tumor

Juxtaglomerular cell tumors are rare benign tumors that typically occur in young adults (mean 24 years) and always cause hypertension[27]. Grossly, they are well circumscribed tan to gray tumors typically located near the renal capsule and measuring 2 to 3 cm in diameter[22]. The microscopic appearance of juxtaglomerular cell tumors is variable and the diagnosis can be difficult to make without clinical information. One common pattern is sheets of small cells with eosinophilic granular cytoplasm and hypochromatic nuclei. Alternatively, the cells may become more spindled and begin to resemble smooth muscle. A prominent

lymphocytic infiltrate is frequently present. Nests of medium sized cells with pale cytoplasm and central nuclei are often present. These cells are referred to as Spiegelei cells and their presence can help in making the diagnosis.

Angiomyolipoma

Angiomyolipomas are the most common mesenchymal tumors of the kidney. They may occur either sporadically or in patients with tuberous sclerosis. They are four times more likely to occur sporadically. In patients with tuberous sclerosis, however, 47% develop angiomyolipomas. Of these patients, 71% had bilateral tumors and 87% had multiple tumors[28]. The presence of multiple angiomyolipomas in a patient of any age or a single angiomyolipoma in a child is almost diagnostic of tuberous sclerosis[29]. Patients without tuberous sclerosis present much later (mean 45 to 55 years) than those with tuberous sclerosis (mean 25 to 35 years)[29]. Typical angiomyolipomas are well circumscribed with a mean diameter of 9 cm[22]. Their color can range from yellow to gray depending on the amount of fat and muscle present. Microscopically they are composed of mature adipose cells, mature smooth muscle and thick walled vessels. The percentage of fat and smooth muscle present can vary greatly. Some nuclear pleomorphism and rare mitotic figures may be seen. Rarely, regional lymph nodes may contain tumor but this is felt to represent multifocal expression of the tumor and not true metastatic disease[22].

Epithelioid angiomyolipoma is a recently described variant that can recur locally, metastasize and cause death[29–30]. Microscopically, this tumor is composed of numerous polygonal cells with abundant eosinophilic cytoplasm and mild to prominent nuclear atypia. Occasional multinucleated cells and cells that resemble ganglia are present. Hemorrhage, necrosis and mitotic figures may be prominent. The amount of fat and thick-walled vessels present is minimal. Both the typical variant and the epithelioid variant stain positive with the HMB-45 antibody[31].

Pediatric tumors of the kidney

Nephroblastoma (Wilms' tumor)

Wilms' tumor (Figure 20.5) is the most common intra-abdominal malignant tumor of childhood. It accounts for 13 to 20% of all solid malignant tumors in children less than 15 years of age[22]. Approximately 80% of cases occur between 1 to 5 years of age with a peak incidence between 3 to 4 years[32]. It is rare for Wilms' tumor to occur after 10 years of age[22]. Bilateral Wilms' tumor occurs in 4 to 5% of cases[33]. Children with Wilms' tumor have an increased incidence of having a variety of congenital abnormalities or syndromes such as: aniridia (1%), musculoskeletal

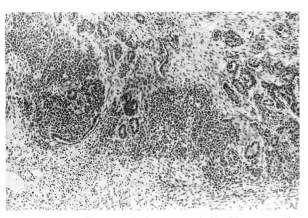

Fig. 20.5 Wilms' tumor. Tubules surrounded by blastema and immature stroma.

malformations (3%), Beckwith-Wiedemann syndrome (3%), and various 'hamartomatous disorders' (5–10%)[34]. Changes in the short arm of chromosome 11 are seen in 40 to 50% of cases of Wilms' tumor[35]. Familial cases are rare and are not associated with abnormalities of chromosome 11[36].

Grossly, these tumors are well demarcated with a mean diameter of 11.3 cm[37]. The cut surface is gray to light tan with areas of hemorrhage (25%), necrosis (20%), cysts (17%) and rarely calcifications (5%)[22]. The consistency of the tumor ranges from soft to firm. Microscopically, Wilms' tumors are triphasic composed of epithelial, mesenchymal and blastemal components. The epithelial component consists of tubules lined by columnar cells with hyperchromatic nuclei. Some of the tubules are dilated and have papillary invaginations giving the appearance of an immature glomeruli. The stromal component consists of undifferentiated spindle cells. Areas of muscle, fat or cartilage differentiation may be present. The blastemal component consists of medium sized undifferentiated cells with hyperchromatic nuclei, small nucleoli and sparse cytoplasm. The cells are arranged in sheets, cords or nodules. The ratio of the three components to each other can vary. By tradition, if one of the three components makes up more than two-thirds of the tumor then the tumor is designated by that component (e.g. blastemal predominant Wilms' tumor). Blastemal predominant tumors behave in a more aggressive fashion with early metastatic spread and more advanced disease at presentation[38]. In most cases (40.8%), none of the three elements predominates. In the remaining cases, blastemal predominant Wilms' tumor (39%) is more common than epithelial predominant (18.3%) or stromal predominant (1.4%)[36]. In patients treated with chemotherapy, however, the blastemal component may become a very minor element because it is the most sensitive to chemotherapy.

The most important histologic finding in determining a patient's outcome is the presence or absence of anaplasia. Anaplasia is defined by the presence of nuclei three times the diameter of nuclei of the same cell type and the presence of bizarre mitotic figures. Approximately 5% of Wilms' tumor have areas of anaplasia[38]. Anaplasia is subdivided into focal and diffuse. In the past, focal and diffuse anaplasia were defined by the percentage of anaplastic changes in the tumor. Less than 10% was considered focal and greater than 10% was considered diffuse. This definition was recently changed so that now focal anaplasia is defined as anaplastic change confined to one or a few discrete foci within the primary tumor and with no anaplasia or marked nuclear atypia elsewhere. Diffuse anaplasia is now defined as possessing at least one of four attributes: 1) non-localized anaplastic change within the tumor; 2) localized anaplastic change but with the presence of marked nuclear atypia elsewhere; 3) anaplastic change extending outside the tumor capsule or in metastases; or 4) anaplastic change in a random biopsy[38]. The reason for the change in the definition was to help predict more accurately the clinical behavior of the tumor and identify those children requiring more aggressive therapy. Under the new definition, patients with focal anaplasia have outcomes comparable to patients with non-anaplastic Wilms' tumor. In addition, the presence or absence of anaplasia does not appear to affect the prognosis of stage I tumors[38].

Nephrogenic rests

Nephrogenic rests are foci of immature nephrogenic tissue present in the kidney after 36 weeks gestation. Microscopically, they may resemble Wilms' tumor. It can be very difficult to distinguish between the two entities. Nephrogenic rests are thought to be precursor lesions for Wilms' tumor. They have been found in 25% of kidneys with Wilms' tumor[39]. The vast majority of nephrogenic rests, however, undergo spontaneous regression since they are also present in 1% of random neonatal autopsies and 40 to 50% of patients with trisomies 13 and 18[34].

Nephrogenic rests have been subdivided into perilobar (75% of cases) and intralobar (25%) rests based upon their location in the kidney Microscopically, other differences exist between the two types of rests Perilobar rests are well demarcated nodules composed predominantly of blastemal or epithelial cells. Intralobar rests are poorly demarcated, infiltrating into the surrounding parenchyma. They are composed predominantly of undifferentiated stromal cells.

Instead of regressing, nephrogenic rests may undergo hyperplastic change and enlarge. Differentiating between a hyperplastic nephrogenic rest and a nephrogenic rest that has become neoplastic (i.e. Wilms' tumor) can be difficult. Imaging studies can be more helpful than biopsies,

281

since, histologically, both entities may look the same. Wilms' tumors are believed to arise from a single point source. Tumor cell division, therefore, should result in uniform spherical growth early on. Hyperplastic growth, on the other hand, occurs at multiple sites and therefore should result in an irregularly shaped mass[36].

Cystic nephroma and cystic partially differentiated nephroblastoma

Cystic nephroma and cystic partially differentiated nephroblastoma (CPDN) are both believed to be low-grade variants of Wilms' tumor. Cystic nephromas occur mainly in children less than 4 years of age. They are well demarcated, multilocular, cystic tumors that average 9 cm in diameter[40]. The tumor is completely cystic with no solid areas (except the septa). The cysts may contain a serous or hemorrhagic fluid. The septa are thin, typically less than 5 mm in thickness[41]. Microscopically, the cysts are lined by a flat to cuboidal epithelium. The stroma of the septa consists of fibrous tissue. No heterologous elements such as muscle or fat are present. No blastema is present either. Occasional tubules lined by benign appearing cuboidal cells are present.

Cystic partially differentiated nephroblastoma resemble cystic nephromas both clinically and grossly. Microscopically, however, the septa of CPDN contain all three of the elements seen in Wilms' tumor: blastema, immature stroma and epithelial elements. Heterologous elements are also commonly seen in the septa. If the cystic areas are accompanied by solid areas that show the histologic features of Wilms' tumor then the tumor should be regarded as a Wilms' tumor[35].

Mesoblastic nephroma

Mesoblastic nephroma is the most common renal tumor of the first year of life[42]. They range in size from 0.8 to 14 cm, with a mean diameter of 6.2 cm[22]. Approximately 60% are diagnosed in the first 3 months, and 90% during the first year of life[36]. Although rare, adult variants of the tumor have been reported in patients up to 78 years of age[43]. The cut surface is white to tan and may resemble a leiomyoma. Focal areas of hemorrhage, necrosis and cyst formation are occasionally present. Two histologic variants of mesoblastic nephromas exist: the classic (fibroleiomyomatous) type and the cellular type. Microscopically, the classic type resembles a leiomyoma. Interlacing fascicles of spindle cells with benign appearing nuclei and eosinophilic cytoplasm are seen. In the cellular variant, the tumor is hypercellular with the cells arranged in a more compact fashion; less well differentiated and the nuclei more hyperchromatic. Numerous mitotic figures are present. The majority of tumors show a mixture of both patterns. There is no difference in prognosis between the two

variants[44]. Although the tumor may grossly appear to be well circumscribed, microscopically the tumor has an infiltrating margin that may extend beyond the kidney into the peri-renal fat. Extension through the kidney has been seen in 25% to 30% of cases and may explain some of the reason for local recurrence[34]. The vast majority of recurrences occur within 1 year of resection[35]. Mesoblastic nephromas are considered benign tumors only requiring surgical removal but rare metastases have been reported[45].

Malignant rhabdoid tumor of the kidney

Malignant rhabdoid tumors of the kidney are rare but extremely lethal renal neoplasms of childhood. They account for 0.9% to 2.4% of all pediatric renal tumors[46]. Approximately 50% are diagnosed in patients before 1 year of age[37]. They rarely occur in patients greater than 5 years old. Rhabdoid tumors may range in size from 4 to 15 cm with a mean diameter of 9.6 cm. They have infiltrating poorly demarcated margins. The cut surface is soft and friable with areas of hemorrhage and necrosis. The color of the tumor ranges from gray to pink. Microscopically, the tumor may have multiple histologic patterns. The most common is sheets of loosely cohesive rhabdoid cells. The cells are polygonal in shape with eosinophilic cytoplasm; large nuclei, eccentrically located and prominent nucleoli[47]. Frequent mitotic figures are seen. Although the cells may look like rhabdomyoblasts, both immunohistochemistry and electron microscopy have failed to demonstrate myogenic origin[46]. Rhabdoid tumors behave in a very aggressive fashion. In one study, at time of diagnosis, 44% of patients had metastatic disease with another 38% eventually developing metastates[46]. The vast majority of patients will die within 1 year of diagnosis with a mean survival of 5.5 months[35]. Two interesting associations seen with this tumor are hypercalcemia (3.6 to 18% patients) and the development of a synchronous or metachronous primary brain tumor (4.5 to 13.5% of patients)[46,48]. The brain tumors are primitive neuroepithelial tumors of the cerebellar or pineal midline region[36].

Clear cell sarcoma of the kidney

Clear cell sarcoma of the kidney is a malignant neoplasm of the kidney that accounts for approximately 5% of all pediatric renal tumors[35]. The age of presentation is similar to Wilms' tumor with most patients presenting between 1 to 4 years of age. The gross appearance of the tumor also resembles Wilms' tumor with the cut surface being tan to gray in color with focal areas of hemorrhage, necrosis and cyst formation. Unlike Wilms' tumor it is almost never bilateral or multifocal[34]. Microscopically, the tumor is composed of a deceptively bland population of cells with pale cytoplasm, indistinct cell membranes and bland hypochromatic nuclei. The cells are often arranged in nest and sheets. Infiltrating between the cells is a characteristic fine network of branching vessels. Clear cell sarcoma of the kidney used to be called bone metastasizing renal tumor of childhood due to its frequency in metastasizing to the skeletal system (40% patients)[34]. New regimens of chemotherapy have dramatically improved long-term survival from 30% to 60–70%[49].

References

1. Bannayan GA, Lamm DL. Renal cell tumors. *Pathol Ann* 1980;**15**:271–308.
2. MacDonald EJ. The present incidence and survival picture in cancer and the promise of improved prognosis. *Bull Am Coll Surgeons* 1978;**33**:75.
3. Storkel S, Eble JN, Adlakha K *et al.* Classification of renal cell carcinoma, workgroup 1. *Cancer* 1997;**80**:987–989.
4. Seizinger BR, Rouleau GA, Ozelius LJ *et al.* Von Hippel-Lindau disease maps to the region of chromosome 3 associated with renal cell carcinoma. *Nature* 1988;**332**:268–269.
5. Sokoloff MH, deKernion JB, Figlin RA, Belldegrun A. Current management of renal cell carcinoma. *CA Cancer J Clin* 1996;**46**:284–302.
6. Parks CM, Kellett MJ. Staging renal cell carcinoma. *Clin Radiol* 1994;**29**:223–230.
7. Moll V, Becht E, Ziegler M. Kidney preserving surgery in renal cell tumors: Indications, technique and results in 152 patients. *J Urol* 1991;**150**:319–323.
8. Thoenes W, Storkel S, Rukmpelt H-J. Histopathology and classification of renal cell tumors (adenomas, oncocytomas and carcinomas) the basic cytological and histopathological elements and their use for diagnostics. *Pathol Res Pract* 1986;**181**:125–143.
9. Kovacs G. Molecular differential pathology of renal cell tumors. *Histopathology* 1993;**22**:1–8.
10. Weiss LM, Gelb AB, Medeiros LJ. Adult renal epithelial neoplasms. *Am J Clin Pathol* 1995;**103**:624–635.
11. Fuhrman SA, Lasky LC, Limas C. Prognostic significance of morphologic parameters in renal cell carcinoma. *Am J Surg Pathol* 1982;**6**:655–663.
12. Medeiros LJ, Gelb AB, Weiss LM. Renal cell carcinoma: prognostic significance of morphologic parameters in 121 cases. *Cancer* 1988;**61**:1639–1651.
13. Ro JY, Ayala AG, Sella A, Samuels ML, Swanson DA. Sarcomatoid renal cell carcinoma: clinicopathologic: a study of 42 cases. *Cancer* 1987;**59**:516–526.
14. Kovacs G, Frisch S. Clonal chromosome abnormalities in tumor cells from patients with sporadic renal cell carcinomas. *Cancer Res* 1989;**49**:651–659.
15. Kovacs G, Kovacs A. Parenchymal abnormalities associated with papillary renal tumors: a morphologic study. *J Urol Pathol* 1993;**1**:301–312.
16. Kovacs G, Fuzesi L, Emanuel A, Kung H. Cytogenetics of papillary renal cell tumors. *Genes Chromosom Cancer* 1991;**3**:249–255.
17. Renshaw AA, Henske EP, Loughlin KR, Shapiro C, Weinberg DS. Aggressive variants of chromophobe renal cell carcinoma. *Cancer* 1996;**78**:1756–1761.
18. Thoenes W, Storkel S, Rumpelt HJ *et al.* Chromophobe cell renal carcinoma and its variants: a report on 32 cases. *J Pathol* 1988;**155**:227–287.
19. Srigley JR, Eble JN. Collecting duct carcinoma of kidney. *Semin Diagn Pathol* 1998;**15**:54–67.
20. Matz LR, Latham BI, Fabian VA, Vivian JB. Collecting duct carcinoma of the kidney: a report of three cases and review of the literature. *Pathology* 1997;**29**:354–359.
21. Natsume O, Ozono S, Futami T, Ohta M. Bellini duct carcinoma: a case report. *Jpn J Clin Oncol* 1997;**27**:107–110.
22. Mostofi FK, Davis CJ Jr. Tumors and tumor-like lesions of the kidney. *Curr Probl Cancer* 1986;**10**:56–114.
23. Zhang G, Monda L, Wasserman NF, Fraley EE. Bilateral renal oncocytoma: report of 2 cases and literature review. *J Urol* 1985;**133**:84–86.
24. Grignon DJ, Eble JN. Papillary and metanephric adenomas of the kidney. *Semin Diagn Pathol* 1998;**15**:41–53.
25. Eble JN, Warfel K. Early human renal cortical epithelial neoplasia. *Mod Pathol* 1991;**4**:45A (abstract).
26. Budin RE, McDonnell PJ. Renal cell neoplasms: their relationship to arteriolonephrosclerosis. *Arch Pathol Lab Med* 1984;**108**:138–140.
27. Squires JP, Ulbright TM, Deschryver-Kecskemeti K, Engleman W. Juxtaglomerular cell tumor of the kidney. *Cancer* 1984;**53**:516–523.
28. Stillwell TJ, Gomez MR, Kelalis PP. Renal lesions in tuberous sclerosis. *J Urol* 1987;**138**:477–481.
29. Eble JN. Angiomyolipoma of the kidney. *Semin Diagn Pathol* 1998;**15**:21–40.
30. Mai KT, Perkins DG, Collins JP. Epithelioid variant of renal angiomyolipoma. *Histopathology* 1996;**28**:277–280.
31. Eble JN, Amin MB, Young RH. Epithelioid angiomyolipoma of the kidney: a report of five cases with a prominent and diagnostically confusing epithelioid smooth muscle component. *Am J Surg Pathol* 1997;**21**:1123–1130.
32. Breslow N, Beckwith JB, Ciol M, Sharples K. Age distribution of Wilms' tumor: report from the National Wilms' Tumor Study. *Cancer Res* 1988;**48**:1653–1657.
33. Blute ML, Kelalis PP, Offord KP, Breslow N, Beckwith JB, D'Angio GJ. Bilateral Wilm's tumor. *J Urol* 1987;**138**:968–973.
34. Kissane JM, Dehner LP. Renal tumors and tumor-like lesions in pediatric patients. *Pediatr Nephrol* 1992;**6**:3656–382.
35. Charles AK, Vujanic GM, Berry PJ. Renal tumors of childhood. *Histopathology* 1998;**32**:293–309.
36. Schmidt D, Beckwith JB. Histopathology of childhood renal tumors. *Hematol Oncol Clin North A* 1995;**9**:1179–1200.
37. Webber BL, Parham DM, Drake LG, Wilimas JA. Renal tumors in children. *Pathol Ann* 1992;**27**:191–232.
38. Faria P, Beckwith B, Mishra K *et al.* Focal versus diffuse anaplasia in Wilms' tumor – new definitions with prognostic significance: a report from the National Wilms Tumor Study Group. *Am J Surg Pathol* 1996;**20**:909–920.
39. Beckwith JB, Kiveat NB, Bonadio JF. Nephrogenic rests, nephroblastomatosis and the pathogenesis of Wilms' tumor. *Pediatr Pathol* 1990;**10**:1–36.
40. Madewell JE, Goldman SM, Davis CJ Jr *et al.* Multilocular cystic nephroma: A radiographic-pathologic correlation of 58 patients. *Radiology* 1984;**146**:309–321.
41. Eble JN, Bonsib SM. Extensively cystic renal neoplasms: cystic nephroma, cystic partially differentiated nephroblastoma, multilocular cystic renal cell carcinoma, and cystic hamartoma of renal pelvis. *Semin Diagn Pathol* 1998;**15**:2–20.
42. Chan HSL, Chen M-Y, Mancer K *et al.* Congenital mesoblastic nephroma: a clinicoradiologic study of 17 cases representing the pathologic spectrum of the disease. *J Pediatr* 1987;**111**:64–70.
43. Luan DT, Williams R, Ngo T *et al.* Adult mesoblastic nephroma: expansion of the morphologic spectrum and review of literature. *Am J Surg Pathol* 1998;**22**:827–839.
44. Pettinato G, Manivel JC, Wick MR, Dehner LP. Classical and cellular (atypical) congenital mesoblastic nephroma. A clinicopathologic, ultrastructural, immunohistochemical, and flow cytometric study. *Hum Pathol* 1998;**20**:682–690.
45. Heidelberger KP, Ritchey ML, Dauser RC, McKeever PE, Beckwith JB. Congenital mesoblastic nephroma metastatic to the brain. *Cancer* 1993;**72**:2499–2502.
46. Vujanic GM, Sandstedt B, Harms D, Boccon-Gibod L, Delemarre JFM. Rhabdoid tumor of the kidney: a clinicopathologic study of 22 patients from the International Society of Paediatric Oncology (SIOP) nephroblastoma file. *Histopathology* 1996;**28**:333–340.
47. Wick MR, Ritter JH, Dehner LP. Malignant rhabdoid tumors: a clinicopathologic review and conceptual discussion. *Semin Diagn Pathol* 1995;**12**:233–248.
48. Weeks DA, Beckwith JB, Mierau GW, Luckley DW. Rhabdoid tumor of kidney: a report of 111 cases from the National Wilms' Tumor Study Pathology Center. *Am J Surg Pathol* 1989;**13**:429–458.
49. Green DM, Breslow NE Beckwith JB, Moksness J, Finklestein JZ, D'Angio GJ. Treatment of children with clear-cell sarcoma of the kidney: a report from the National Wilms' Tumor Study Group. *J Clin Oncol* 1994;**12**:2132–2137.

21 Renal cell carcinoma: Presentation, diagnosis and staging

D K Ornstein and G L Andriole

Presentation

About 40 to 50% of patients with renal cell carcinoma are asymptomatic at the time of presentation and are diagnosed incidentally from an abdominal computed tomography scan or abdominal ultrasonography performed for unrelated symptoms[1,2]. Incidental tumors are more likely to be clinically localized and potentially curable than symptomatic tumors[3]. The widespread use of newer more sensitive imaging techniques (i.e. CT scanning and ultrasonography) have dramatically increased the number of renal masses detected and have led to a substantial downward stage migration for newly diagnosed renal cell carcinoma[4]. Currently, over 80% of patients have clinically localized disease[4] and up to 40% have tumors smaller than 3 cm at the time of diagnosis[5].

Localized symptoms from primary tumor mass

The most common symptom of renal cell carcinoma is hematuria, historically occurring in 40% to 60% of patients[6]. Flank pain occurs in 35% to 40%, and a palpable flank mass is present in 25% to 50% of cases[7,8,9]. The classic triad of flank pain, hematuria and flank mass occurs in less than 10% of cases[7,8]. Significant bleeding from the tumor can occasionally lead to clot formation in the ureter or bladder with temporary obstruction and ureteral colic. Even though the presence of hematuria (both gross and microscopic), flank mass, or flank pain are non-specific, these findings should alert the clinician to the possible diagnosis of renal cell carcinoma.

Renal cell carcinoma has the propensity to invade the renal vein and grow into and up the inferior vena cava extending as far as the right ventricle[10]. Tumor thrombus within the inferior vena cava usually does not cause symptoms since the development of caval obstruction is relatively slow; allowing time for the development of collateral channels[10,11]. When symptoms do occur they are secondary to caval obstruction and include dilated superficial collateral veins on the lower abdomen, lower extremity edema and pulmonary embolism[10,11]. The tumor thrombus can obstruct the testicular vein (particularly on the left side) leading to development of a fixed varicocele (present in 3% to 5% of patients with renal cell carcinoma). The development of a non-reducible left-sided varicocele in a man older than 40 years of age should alert the clinician to the potential for renal cell carcinoma[8].

Cachexia and chronic debilitation are present in approximately 30% of patients and can be seen with localized as well as metastatic disease[6]. Hypertension occurs about 30% of the time and can result from different factors such as hyperreninemia and renal artery compression[6]. Anemia is present in 20% to 40% of cases and results from persistent hematuria, decreased erythropoetin production and splenic red blood cell destruction[6]. Other paraneoplastic syndromes such as pyrexia, hepatic dysfunction without hepatic metastasis (Stauffer's syndrome), hypercalcemia, erthrocytosis and amyloidosis occur less commonly[6]. In general, patients with these symptoms have a poor prognosis but some have localized disease and are potentially curable.

Diagnosis

Radiologic imaging

Intravenous urogaphy (IVU)

The intravenous urogram (IVU) should be used as the initial test in the evaluation of gross and microscopic hematuria, since it is a relatively inexpensive test and may be useful in excluding a urothelial tumor. IVU findings demonstrating distortion or displacement of the renal collecting system as well as lack of homogeneity of the renal nephrogram is suggestive of a renal mass. The IVU is about 80% sensitive in diagnosing renal parenchymal tumors larger than 3 cm, but is less than 50% sensitive for tumors smaller than 3 cm[12]. The performance of nephrotomograms may enhance sensitivity.

The presence of calcification within the renal mass is suggestive of malignancy (peripheral curvilinear calcification is suggestive of a calcified benign cyst) but is found in less than 20% of renal cell carcinomas[13]. The IVU is poor at determining the nature of a renal mass, that is, distinguishing between solid and cystic lesions. Therefore, all IVU examinations that reveal a renal mass should be followed up with either a renal sonogram or CT scan. IVU is not helpful in staging renal cell carcinoma.

Administration of intravenous contrast is required for this test and is contraindicated in patients with a history of anaphylactic reaction to intravenous contrast[14]. Relative contraindications include chronic renal insufficiency (serum creatinine >2.0 mg/dl), multiple myeloma with associated proteinuria or hypercalcemia, and myasthenia gravis[14]. Patients with a history of non-anaphylactic reactions to intravenous contrast can be injected with contrast following pre-medication with steroids[14].

Computed tomography (CT)

Contrast-enhanced CT scanning is the most accurate test in detecting and diagnosing renal cell carcinoma[9,15,16]. Diagnostic accuracy has been reported to be as high as 95%[17]. Features on CT scans that are suspicious for renal cell carcinoma include attenuation that is equal to or lower than the surrounding parenchyma, irregular margins, displacement of collecting system or deformity of renal contour, enhancement after contrast injection (a rise in CT attenuation of more than 10 Houndsfield Units), and centrally located or thick peripherally located calcifications (Figure 21.1A)[9,17].

The sensitivity and accuracy of CT scanning is dependent on ideal radiographic technique[9]. Scans should be obtained on machines capable of obtaining thin sections (≤ 5 mm) and rapid sequence images (≤ 2–3s)[5]. Rapid helical and spiral CT scanners are now available and allow for complete renal images during a single breath thereby

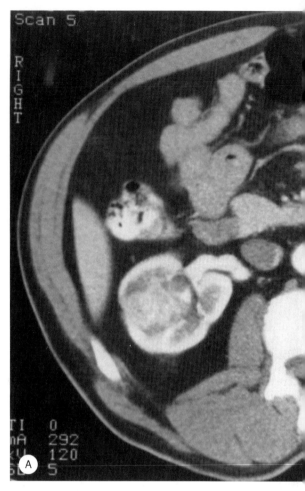

Fig. 21.1   Shows a 4 cm renal cell carcinoma imaged by CT, ultrasound and MRI. The CT scan (A) demonstrates hyperdense areas that enhance with contrast.

eliminating artefact associated with respiration. For all techniques, images should be obtained prior to administration of intravenous contrast. Contrast should be injected by power injection at a rate of at least 2 ml/s and images should be obtained during the nephrographic phase (that is 90 s after the start of mechanical injection of contrast)[5]. Oral contrast should be given at least 1 h prior to the examination in order to opacify bowel loops.

Since CT scanning requires injection of intravenous contrast the same contraindications for IVU, mentioned previously, apply to contrast-enhanced CT scanning.

Contrast-enhanced CT scanning should be performed on all patients (without contraindication to intravenous contrast) with renal masses that have not been proven to be simple cysts.

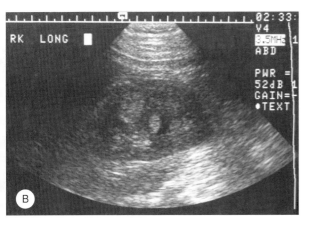

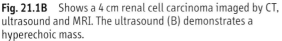

Fig. 21.1B Shows a 4 cm renal cell carcinoma imaged by CT, ultrasound and MRI. The ultrasound (B) demonstrates a hyperechoic mass.

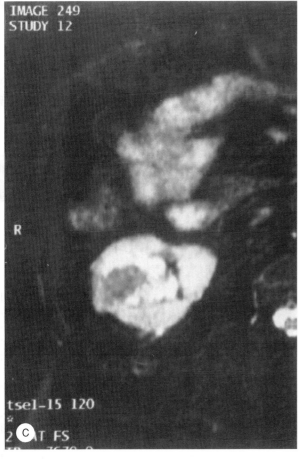

Fig. 21.1C Shows a 4 cm renal cell carcinoma imaged by CT, ultrasound and MRI. The MRI (C) demonstrates a heterogeneous mass on T1 weighted images that enhances after administration of intravenous gadolinium (as seen on a T2 weighted fat-saturation image).

Ultrasonography

Ultrasonography is a non-invasive test that is highly - accurate in distinguishing simple cysts from solid masses or more complex cysts. Sonographic criteria for the diagnoses of a simple cyst include good through and through transmission of echoes, absence of internal echoes and sharply marginated smooth walls. Like CT scanning, ultrasonography is almost 100% accurate in distinguishing solid from cystic masses for lesions larger than 2 cm, but may be indeterminate for smaller lesions. Ultrasonography detects virtually all masses larger than 3 cm[19], but may miss up to 40% of lesion detected by CT scanning that are smaller than 3 cm[12]. Renal cell carcinoma is typically isoechoic, but hypoechoic and hyperechoic tumors do exist and therefore echogenicity can not be reliably used to exclude malignancy (Figure 21.1B).

The usefulness of ultrasonography is dependent on the quality of the equipment and on the skill of the examiner. Masses in the left upper pole may be difficult to evaluate sonographically because of interference from overlying bone and a lack of a good acoustic window[18]. In addition it may be impossible to obtain adequate images in obese patients.

Ultrasonography can be used as the initial follow up test (instead of CT scanning) to evaluate patients with a renal mass/cyst discovered by IVU. Ultrasonography should be the first renal parenchymal imaging technique used in patients with intravenous contrast allergies and compromised renal function, and should be used to serially follow patients with small indeterminate cysts.

Magnetic resonance imaging

MRI is usually not the first-line imaging modality in the evaluation of renal masses, but may be useful as an adjunct to CT scanning and ultrasonography. With proper technique, MRI can be as accurate as CT scanning in the detection and characterization of renal masses. In general a mass is considered solid and suspicious for malignancy if it enhances after intravenous administration or gadolidium[20]. Variable signal intensities on pre-contrast images can be seen with renal cell carcinoma (Figure 21.1C).

Standard MRI protocols use a body coil to obtain both T1 and T2 weighted images. Since renal tumors tend to have similar signal intensity compared with surrounding parenchyma, non-enhanced scans can miss over 50% of masses smaller than 3 cm[17]. Calcifications are usually not appreciated with these MRI sequences[17].

Fat-saturation and fast scanning (i.e. spin or gradient echo) techniques in conjunction with intravenous administration of gadolinium enhances the sensitivity of MRI to equal that of CT scanning[20]. Gadolinium can be administered to patients with iodinated contrast allergies. Gadolinium enhanced MRI is also useful for patients

287

with compromised renal function. Gadolinium is not nephrotoxic and can be safely given to patients with serum creatinine levels as high as 5.0 mg/dl[21]. Hemodialysis may be required to clear gadolinium administered to patients with glomerular filtration rates lower than 20 cc/min[22].

Cost and availability are the major factors that limit the overall utility of MRI[9]. In addition, this imaging technique requires good patient cooperation for as long as 30 to 45 minutes. MRI scanning can not be safely performed in patients with cardiac pacemakers or cerebral aneurysm clips, and patients with compromised mental status or with clostrophobia may require sedation. MRI can safely be performed in patients with non-mobile metallic prosthesis such as artificial joints and hemostatic surgical clips.

MRI is indicated to evaluate sonographically indeterminate renal masses in patients with compromised renal function or severe allergies to iodinated intravenous contrast material.

Solid renal masses

Renal cell carcinoma accounts for 80% to 90% of all solid renal masses in adults[23]. Other possible malignant renal masses include transitional cell carcinoma of the urothelium, metastasis from other malignancies, lymphoblastoma, nephroblastoma, multilocular cystic nephroma, sarcoma and renal medullary carcinoma[23,24]. Benign lesions included in the differential diagnoses are angiomyolipoma, oncocytoma, adenoma, lipoma, fibroma and renin-secreting juxtaglomerular tumor[23,24] (Table 21.1).

Urothelial tumors account for only 6% to 7% of all malignant renal tumors[24], and distinguishing them from renal cell carcinoma pre-operatively is critical, since the surgical management for these tumors is different (nephroureterectomy is required for most upper tract transitional cell tumors). CT scanning and ultrasonography may be unable definitively to differentiate transitional cell carcinoma from renal cell carcinoma. It is therefore prudent to evaluate patients with centrally located tumors, filling defect in the collecting system, or thickening of the renal pelvis (i.e. tumors with characteristics suspicious for transitional cell carcinoma) with an intravenous or retrograde pyelogram (Figure 21.2). If transitional cell carcinoma can not be ruled out by radiographic imaging, ureteroscopy and biopsy should be performed.

The most common tumors to metastasize to the kidneys are lung, breast, uterine, malignant melanoma, colon, esophagus and testis[23]. Even though these tumors tend to be multifocal and hypovascular, differentiating them from primary renal cell carcinomas may not be possible from renal imaging alone[8]. It is therefore critical to obtain a detailed history and to perform a complete physical examination on all patients with a renal mass.

Lymphoma generally involves the kidney in an infiltrative pattern, but on rare occasions can cause a discrete

Table 21.1   Symptoms of renal cell carcinoma

Local	Systemic
Gross hematuria	Cachexia
Flank pain	Hypertension
Flank mass	Anemia
Varicocele	Pyrexia
Vena caval obstruction	Distant metastasis
lower abdominal varicocities	cough/pneumonia
lower extremity edema	bone pain
Ureteral colic	neurologic deficit
	Hepatic dysfunction (Stauffer's
	syndrome)
	Hypercalcemia
	Erythrocytosis
	Amyloidosis

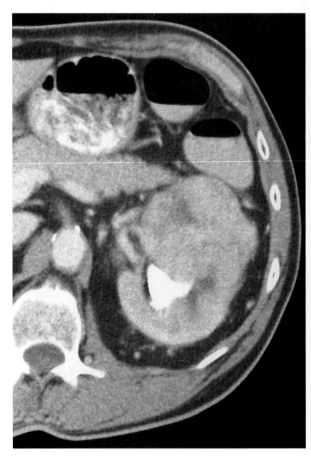

Fig. 21.2   (A) CT scan showing a large heterogenous renal mass in the anterior lateral aspect of the kidney with an associated filling defect in the renal pelvis.

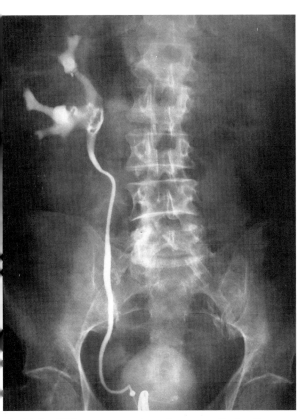

Fig. 21.2 (B) Prone retrograde pyelogram confirming the filling defect in the renal pelvis. Pathology revealed a transitional cell carcinoma.

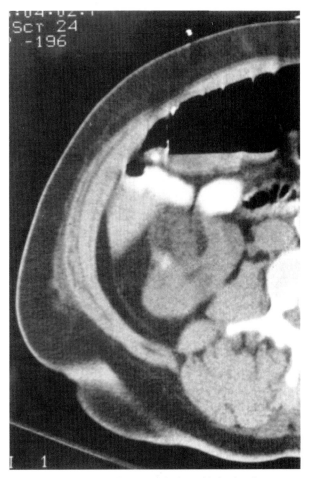

Fig. 21.3 Is a CT showing a 3 cm lesion with fat density characteristic of an angiomyolipoma.

mass[25]. However, renal involvement usually occurs late in the disease and is rarely the presenting sign[25].

Nephroblastoma (Wilms' tumor), multi-locular cystic nephroma, and sarcomas are all extremely rare renal tumors in adults[26]. These tumors are usually not distinguished from renal cell carcinoma pre-operatively and their diagnosis is made by pathologic examination of the surgical specimen[26].

Renal medullary carcinoma is a very rare tumor that occurs most commonly in young black teenagers and adults with sickle-cell trait[27,28]. These tumors tend to be very aggressive and carry a poor prognosis[27,28]. This diagnosis is usually made pathologically but some characteristic features on CT scan have been reported (i.e. tumors located deep within the renal parenchyma demonstrating an infiltrative pattern)[27].

A definitive diagnoses of angiomyolipoma can often be made by CT scan if characteristic fat density (−20 to−80Houndsfield units) is present (Figure 21.3)[9,24]. These lesions appear hyper-intense on T1 weighted pre-contrast MRI images. Fat saturation images are usually required to differentiate the angiomyolipoma from hemorrhage

into a renal cell carcinoma. Ultrasonography is, usually not helpful in distinguishing angiomyolipoma from renal cell carcinoma.

Even though oncocytomas (which account for about 5% to 7% of renal tumors) can have a characteristic central stellite scar they can not be reliably distinguished from malignant tumors radiographically, and pathologic examination is required for definitive diagnosis[29]. Some studies have suggested that MRI may be helpful but this has not been proven definitively[30]. It is these facts that limit the conservative (watchful waiting) management of these potentially benign renal lesions.

Adenomas are another potentially benign lesion that can not be reliably distinguished from renal cell carcinoma[8,29]. In addition, there has been extensive debate regarding the malignant potential of these 'benign' tumors. Because of these two reasons, renal adenomas should be managed as renal cell carcinoma.

Cystic renal masses

The vast majority of renal cysts are harmless benign lesions. However, renal cell carcinoma can be cystic, and differentiating benign from malignant cysts is critical. Bosniak has devised a classification system based on various CT findings in order to help determine the likelihood that a given cyst is malignant (Table 21.2)[31,32]. In select cases, MRI may provide unique information in the evaluation of patients with indeterminate renal masses by CT scan criteria[14]. Ultrasonography does not add unique information to CT scanning in terms of detection or classification of renal masses, and is not indicated if a contrast-enhanced CT scan has already been obtained[14].

Diagnostic cyst aspiration is less accurate than CT or MRI and is generally not recommended[33].

Cysts that are unquestionably benign and do not need further evaluation do not enhance with contrast, are well marginated with imperceptibly thin walls, and have homogeneously low attenuation (that is Hounsfield units 0–20).

Minimally complicated cysts that do not require follow up are defined by the presence of either one thin septations or thin border calcifications.

Minimally complicated cysts that require follow up are characterized by one or more thin septations or irregular border-forming calcification. This category also includes small (< 3 cm) non-enhancing hyper-dense (Hounsfield units 40–90) cysts. These cysts have a very low likelihood of malignancy and can be followed with repeat imaging at 3 months, 6 months and 1 year[32].

Indeterminate cysts with up to a 50% chance of malignancy should be surgically removed by either a radical nephrectomy or partial nephrectomy[31,32]. These are cysts that have either a thick wall, numerous thin septations, one or more thick septations, an enhancing septation, or large and non-border forming calcifications[31,32].

Malignant cysts should be treated as renal cell carcinoma. These are cysts that have definite solid features or have at least three suspicious features shown in Table 21.3 (Figure 21.4).

Table 21.2   Solid renal masses

Malignant	Benign lesions
Renal cell carcinoma	Angiomyolipoma (renal hamartoma)
Transitional cell carcinoma	Oncocytoma
Metastasis from other malignancies	Adenoma
Lymphoblastoma	Fibroma
Nephroblastoma (adult Wilms' tumor)	Lipoma
Multilocular cystic nephroma	Renin-secreting juxtaglomerular
Sarcoma	tumor
Renal medullary carcinoma	

Table 21.3   CT characteristics of benign and cystic renal masses

Benign characteristics	Malignant characteristics
No enhancement with contrast	Enhancement with contrast
Small border-forming calcifications	Large or non-border forming
Low attenuation	calcifications
Thin septations	High attenuation
Imperceptible wall	Thick septations
	Thick wall

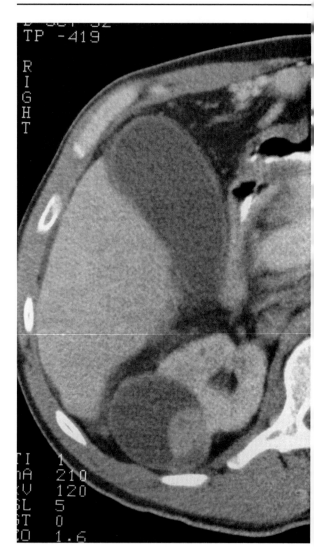

Fig. 21.4   CT scan showing an enhancing mass in the wall of acyst.

Staging

Radiologic imaging

CT scanning is the imaging modality most widely used for staging renal cell carcinoma. As mentioned previously the diagnostic accuracy of CT scanning is dependent on the administration of intravenous contrast and the use of proper scanning techniques. MRI can be used accurately to stage the patient with iodinated contrast allergies and impaired renal function. MRI should also be used to evaluate patients with vena caval tumor thrombus that appears to extend beyond 1 cm of the renal vein ostia. The role of ultrasonography in staging is limited to evaluating the renal vein and vena cava for tumor thrombus.

All patients with suspected renal cell carcinoma should be evaluated for distant metastasis with a chest X-ray and laboratory tests (blood count, chemistry and liver enzymes). Patients with suspicious findings on chest X-ray should be evaluated with a chest CT scan (a routine chest CT is not necessary)[9]. Patients with large tumors (> 5 cm), with an abnormal renal vein or vena cava, bone pain, or an elevated alkaline phosphatase should be evaluated with a radionuclide bone scan (a routine bone scan is not necessary)[34].

Staging systems

The stage of the disease (i.e. the anatomical extent of the tumor) is the most important factor determining the prognosis for patients with renal cell carcinoma[35]. The modified Robson and TNM systems are currently the most commonly used staging systems. The TNM system is more specific but the Robson system is less cumbersome and therefore more practical. Both systems are shown in Table 21.4, and estimated survival for each stage is provided[8,36].

Prognosis based on stage

Although larger tumors (i.e. > 4 cm) tend to be associated with more advanced disease, the size of the primary tumor does not independently impact prognosis[35]. On the other hand the presence of perinephric tumor involvement sub-

stantially reduces long-term survival; that is, the 5 year survival for Robson stage II is 50% to 60% compared with 80% to 90% for stage I[8,36]. In general both CT and MRI are poor at differentiating between stage I (T1/T2) and stage II (T3a)[37].

The ipsilateral adrenal is involved with tumor in less than 5% of patients undergoing radical nephrectomy for clinically localized renal cell carcinoma[38,39]. The prognosis from patients with ipsilateral adrenal involvement is about the same as the prognosis for patients with perinephric tumor invasions (i.e. both are stage T3a)[36]. CT scanning is very accurate in predicting adrenal metastasis, and a normal appearing adrenal gland on CT scan virtually guarantees the presence of a pathologically normal adrenal gland (less than 2% have micrometastasis)[40].

Tumor thrombus is found within the vena cava in 5% to 10% of all cases of renal cell carcinoma[41]. The prognosis for patients with isolated vena cava tumor thrombus (Robson stage IIIa) is the same as for patients with perinephric involvement (Robson stage II)[41]. With proper technique (as previously described) CT scanning is very sensitive (85–100%) in detecting renal vein and vena caval tumor thrombus[9,37]. Both ultrasonography and MRI can provide unique information with regard to the presence of a tumor thrombus; they can accurately assess the extent of tumor thrombus and define its relationship to the hepatic veins, superior vena cava and right atrium. MRI has the particular advantage of differentiating tumor and bland thrombus and is more accurate at detecting invasion of the vena cava wall than either CT or ultrasonography (Figure 21.5)[37]. Several different MRI scanning sequences are available that can be used accurately to determine the extent of the thrombus[20].

The presence or absence of lymph node metastasis is the single most important prognostic indicator for patients with renal cell carcinoma; that is, the 5 year survival for patients with lymph node metastasis is 30% compared with about 60% for patients without[35,36]. Approximately 10% to 25% of patients undergoing radical nephrectomy for renal cell carcinoma will have nodal metastasis[41–43]. CT and MRI are equally accurate at detecting enlarged lymph nodes and are both relatively poor at differentiating malignant from benign reactive lymph nodes[27]. Most investigators have advocated using a size of 1.0 cm or greater as criteria for determining disease[9,35]. However, up to 60% of enlarged (> 1 cm) lymph nodes contain inflammation rather than malignancy[45] and up to 50% of lymph node metastasis are microscopic and undetectable[42].

A majority of patients with metastatic renal cell carcinoma will have multiple sites of involvement. The most common sites of metastasis are the lungs (76%), retroperitoneal lymph nodes (64%), bone (43%), liver (41%), contralateral kidney (25%), contralateral adrenal gland

Table 21.4   Robson staging systems and 5 year survival stratified by stage

Robson stage	Tumor extent	5 year survival
I	Confined to kidney	80–90%
	< 2.5 cm	
	> 2.5 cm	
II	Invades perinephric fat/adrenal gland	50–60%
IIIA	Invades vena cava above diaphram	40–60%
		30–40%
IIIB	Involves regional lymph nodes	25–40%
IIIC	Lymph nodes and vena cava	20%
IVA	Involves contiguous organs	10–20%
IVB	Distant metastasis	5–20%

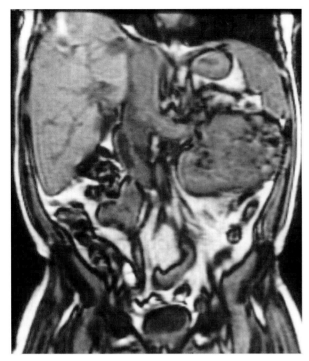

Fig. 21.5   MRI showing a large left renal mass with extension of the caval tumor thrombus to the level of the diaphragm.

(12%) and brain (11%)[46,47]. This group of patients has a particularly dismal prognosis, with a 5 year survival of 5–7%[48,49]. Patients with a solitary metastasis however should be considered separately, as the 5 year survival following nephrectomy and resection of the metastatic lesion can be as high as 25% in select patients[48,49]. Both CT and MRI have equivalent accuracy in predicting the presence of adjacent organ involvement.[37] CT scanning is more accurate at detecting pulmonary metastasis than CXR, but as previously mentioned should not be used routinely. The role of MRI in the detection of pulmonary metastasis has yet to be determined. MRI is the most useful imaging modality to evaluate for spinal cord or nerve root compression in patients with vertebral metastasis.

References

1. Mevorach RA, Segal AJ, Tesegno ME *et al.* Renal cell carcinoma: incidental diagnoses and natural history. *Urology* 1992;**39**:519.
2. Lanctin HP, Futter NG. Renal cell carcinoma: incidental detection. *Can J Surg* 1990;**33**:488–490.
3. Smith SJ, Bosniak MA, Megibow AJ, Hulnick DH, Horii SC, Raghavendra BN. Renal cell carcinoma: earlier discovery and increased detection. *Radiology* 1989;**170**:699–703.
4. Silverman SG, Bloom DA, Seltzer SE. The radiological evaluation of renal masses: approach, analysis, and new technologies. *AUA Update Series* 1994;**13**(1).

Table 21.5   Results of 2, 5 and 10-year disease specific survival depicted by stage in the 1987 and 1997 TNM classifications

	% 2 Years	% 5 Years	% 10 Years
1987 Stage I	100	96	96
1997 Stage I	98	95	95
1987 Stage II	97	94	92
1997 Stage II	95	88	81
1987 Stage III	74	59	43
1997 Stage III	74	59	43
1987 Stage IV	23	20	14
1997 Stage IV	23	20	14

TNM 1997 Classification - renal cancer

T–Primary tumor	
Tx	Primary tumor cannot be assessed
T0	No evidence of primary tumour
T1	Tumor 7 cm or less in greatest dimension, limited to kidney
T2	Tumor more than 7 cm in greatest dimension, limited to the kidney
T3	Tumor extends into major veins or invades adrenal gland or perinephric tissues but not beyond Gerota's fascia
T3a	Tumor invades adrenal gland or perinephric tissues but not beyond Gerota's fascia
T3b	Tumor grossly extends into renal vein(s) or vena cava below diaphragm
T3c	Tumor grossly extends into vena cava above diaphragm
T4	Tumor invades beyond Gerota's fascia
N–Regional lymph nodes	
Nx	Regional lymph nodes cannot be assessed
N0	No regional lymph node metastasis
N1	Metastasis in a single regional lymph node
N2	Metastasis in more than one regional lymph node
M–Distant metastasis	
M0	No distant metastasis
M1	Distant metastasis

5. Curry NS. Small renal masses (lesions smaller than 3 cm): imaging evaluation and management. *Am J Radiology* 1995;**164**:355–362.
6. Jennings SB, Linehan WM. Renal, perirenal, and ureteral neoplasms. In: Gillenwater JY, Grayhack JT, Howards SS, Duckett JW (eds) *Adult and pediatric urology.* Mosby-Year Book, St Louis, MO 1996, pp. 654–694.
7. Waters WB, Richie JP. Aggressive surgical approach to renal cell carcinoma: review of 130 cases. *J Urol* 1979;**122**:306–309.
8. Malkowicz BS. Clinical aspects of renal tumors. *Semin Roentgenol* 1995;**30**:102.
9. McClennan BL, Deyoe LA. The imaging evaluation of renal cell carcinoma: diagnoses and staging. *Radiol Clin North Am* 1994;**32**:55–69.
10. Blute ML, Zincke H. Surgical management of renal cell carcinoma with intracaval involvement. *AUA Update Series* 1994; Vol. 13, lesson 17.
11. Missal ME, Robinson JA, Tatum RW. Inferior vena cava obstruction. Clinical manifestation, diagnostic methods, and related problems. *Ann Intern Med* 1965;**62**:133–161.

12. Warshauer DM, McCarthy SM, Street L, Brookbinder MJ, Glickman MG, Richter J, Hammers L, Taylor C, Rosenfield AT. Detection of renal masses: sensitivities and specificities of excretory urography/linear tomography, US, and CT. *Radiology* 1988;**169**:363–365.

13. Daniel WW, Hartman GW, Witten DM, Farrow GM, Kelalis PP. Calcified renal masses. A review of ten years experience at the Mayo Clinic. *Radiology* 1972;**103**:503–508.

14. Leder RA, Walther PJ. Radiologic imaging of renal cell carcinoma: its role in diagnoses, staging, and management. In: Vogelzang NJ, Scardino PT, Shipley WU, Coffey DS (eds) *Comprehensive textbook of genitourinary oncology* (1st edn). Wilkins and Wilkins, Baltimore, MD 1996, pp. 187–206.

15. Holmberg G, Hietala SO, Ljungberg B. A comparison of radiologic methods in the diagnoses of renal mass lesions. *Scand J Urol Nephrol* 1988;**22**:187–196.

16. Dinney CPN, Awad SA, Gajewski JB, Belitsky P, Lannon SG, Mack FG, Millard OH. Analysis of imaging modalities, staging systems, and prognostic indicators for renal cell carcinoma. *Urology* 1992;**39**:122–129.

17. Levine E. Renal cell carcinoma: clinical aspects, imaging diagnosis, and staging. *Semin Roentgen* 1995;**30**:128–148.

18. Jamis-Dow CA, Choyke PL, Jennings SB, Linehan WM, Thakore KN, Walther MM. Small (< 3 cm) renal masses: Detection with CT versus US and pathologic correlation. *Radiology* 1996;**198**:785–788.

19. Einstein DM, Herts BR, Weaver R, Obuchowski N, Zepp R, Singer A. Evaluation of renal masses detected by excretory urography: cost-effectiveness of sonography versus CT. *Am J Radiology* 1995;**164**:371–375.

20. Choyke PL. Detection and staging of renal cancer. *MRI Clin N Am* 1997;**5**:29–47.

21. Haustein J, Niendorf HP, Krestin G, Gouton T. Renal tolerance of gadolinium DTPA/dimeglumine in patients with chronic renal failure. *Invest Radiol* 1992;**27**:153–156.

22. Haustein J, Schuhmann-Giampieri G. Elimination of Gd-DTPA by means of hemodialysis. *Eur J Radiol* 1990; 227–229.

23. Peterson RO. *Urologic pathology*, Philadelphia, PA: Lippincott, 1992.

24. Rodriguez R, Fishman EK, Marshall FF. Differential diagnoses and evaluation of the incidentally discovered renal mass. *Semin Urol Oncol* 1995;**13**:246–253.

25. deKernion JB, Belldegrun A. Renal tumors. In: Walsh PC, Retik AB, Stamey TA, Vaughan DE (eds) *Campbell's urology*. WB Saunders, Philadelphia, PA, 1992, pp. 1053–1093.

26. Newhouse JH. The radiographic evaluation of the patient with renal cancer. *Urol Clin North Am* 1993;**20**:231–246.

27. Avery RA, Harris JE, Davis CJ, Borgaonkar DS, Byrd JC, Weiss RB. Renal medullary carcinoma. Clinical and therapeutic aspects of a newly described tumor. *CA* 1996;**78**:128–132.

28. Davis CJ, Mostofi FK, Sesterhenn IA. Renal medullary carcinoma, the seventh sickle cell nephropathy. *Am J Surg Path* 1995;**19**:1–11.

29. Licht MR. Renal adenoma and oncocytoma. *Semin Urol Oncol* 1995;**13**:262–266.

30. Harmon WJ, King BF, Lieber MM. Renal oncocytoma: magnetic resonance imaging characteristics. *J Urol* 1996;**155**:863–867.

31. Bosniak MA. The current radiological approach to renal cysts. *Radiology* 1986;**158**:1.

32. Bosniak MA. Problems in the radiological diagnoses of renal parenchymal tumors. *Urol Clin North Am* 1993;**20**:217–230.

33. Herts BR, Baker ME. The current role of percutaneous biopsy in the evaluation of renal masses. *Semin Urol Oncol* 1995;**13**:254–261.

34. Linder A, Golman DG, deKernion JB. Cost effective analysis of prenephrectomy radioisotope scans in renal cell carcinoma. *Urology* 1983;**22**:127–129.

35. Parks CM, Kelett MJ. Review, staging renal cell carcinoma. *Clin Radiology* 1994;**49**:223–230.

36. Guinan P, Frank W, Saffrin R, Rubenstein M. Staging and survival of patients with renal cell carcinoma. *Semin Surg Oncol* 1994;**10**:47–50.

37. Zagoria RJ, Bechtold RE, Dyer RB. Staging of renal adenocarcinoma: role of various imaging procedures. *Am J Radiol* 1995;**164**:363–370.

38. Shalev M, Cipolla B, Guille F, Staerman F, Lobel B. Is ipsilateral adrenalectomy a necessary component of radical nephrectomy? *J Urol* 1995;**153**:1415–1417.

39. Sagalowsky AI, Kadesky KT, Ewalt DM, Kennedy TJ. Factors influencing adrenal metastasis in renal cell carcinoma. *J Urol* 1994;**151**:1131–1184.

40. Gill IS, McClennan BL, Kerbl K *et al.* Adrenal involvement from renal cell carcinoma: predictive value of computerized tomography. *J Urol* 1994;**152**:1082.

41. Kallman DA, King BF, Hattery RR, Charboneau WJ, Ehman RL, Guthman DA, Blute ML. Renal vein and inferior vena cava tumor thrombus in renal cell carcinoma: CT, US, MRI and venacavography. *J Comput Assist Tomogr* 1992;**16**:240–247.

42. Skinner DG, Colvin RB, Vermillion CD, Pfister RC, Leadbetter WF. Diagnoses and management of renal cell carcinoma, a clinical and pathologic study of 309 cases. *Cancer* 1971;**28**:1165–1176.

43. Herrlinger A, Schrott KM, Schott G, Sigel A. What are the benefits of extended dissection of the regional renal lymph nodes in the therapy of renal cell carcinoma? *J Urol* 1991;**146**:1224–1227.

44. Marshall FF, Powell KC. Lymphadenectomy for renal cell carcinoma: anatomical and therapeutic considerations. *J Urol* 1982;**128**:677–681.

45. Johnson CD, Dunnick NR, Cohan RH, Illescas FF. Renal adenocarcinoma: CT staging of 100 tumors. *Am J Radiol* 1987;**148**:59–63.

46. Studer UE, Scherz S, Scheidegger J, Kraft R, Sonntag R, Ackermann D, Zingg EJ. Enlargement of regional lymph nodes in renal cell carcinoma is often not due to metastases. *J Urol* 1990;**144**:243–245.

47. Saitoh H, Hida M, Nakayama K, Shimbo T, Shiramizu T, Satoh T. Metastatic processes and a potential indication of treatment from metastatic lesions of renal adenocarcinoma. *J Urol* 1982;**128**:916–918.

48. Saitoh H, Nakayama M, Nakamura K, Satoh T. Distant metastasis of renal adenocarcinoma in nephrectomized cases. *J Urol* 1982;**127**:1092–1095.

49. Giuliani L, Giberti C, Martorana G, Rovida S. Radical extensive surgery for renal cell carcinoma long-term results and prognostic factors. *J Urol* 1990;**143**:468–474.

50. Golimbu M, Joshi P, Sperber A, Tessler A, Al-Akari S, Morales P. Renal cell carcinoma: survival and prognostic factors. *Urology* 1986;**27**:291–301.

51. Dernevik L, Berggren H, Larsson S, Roberts D. Surgical removal of pulmonary metastases from renal cell carcinoma. *Scand J Urol Nephrol* 1985;**19**:133–137.

52. Tolia BM, Whitmore WF. Solitary metastases from renal cell carcinoma. *J Urol* 1975;**114**:836–838.

53. Nishimura K, Hida S, Okada K *et al.* Staging and differential diagnoses of renal cell carcinoma: a comparison of magnetic resonance imaging and computed tomography. *Acta Urol Jpn* 1988;**34**:1323–1331.

22 Surgical treatment of renal cell carcinoma

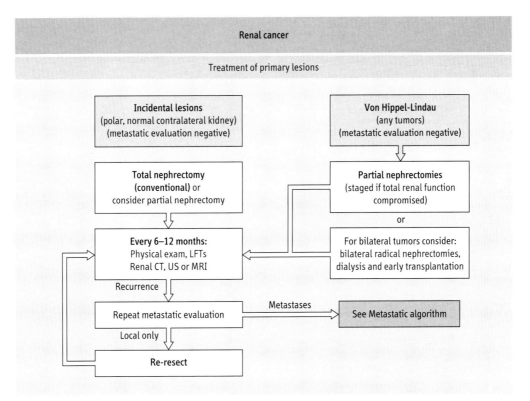

22.1   Radical nephrectomy

R J Krane

Indications

The primary indication for radical nephrectomy is a localized renal carcinoma without any evidence of metastatic disease. Radical nephrectomy was introduced in 1963 by Robson[1] and in contradistinction to simple nephrectomy, it involves removal of the adrenal gland and Gerota's fascia with a regional lymphadenectomy. The use of partial nephrectomy for a localized renal carcinoma has been commonly used for many years in solitary kidneys or when the contralateral kidney is poorly functioning. More recently, partial nephrectomy for localized carcinoma of the kidney, even in the presence of a normal contralateral kidney, has gained acceptance for smaller tumors (less than 4 cm) and will be discussed elsewhere in this text. Radical nephrectomy may also be performed in the presence of metastatic disease because of local symptoms such as pain and bleeding. It has also been shown that radical nephrectomy will improve survival and response rates to various immunotherapeutic strategies. In and of itself, however, radical nephrectomy in the presence of metastatic disease is really not a therapeutic endeavor.

The need for concomitant adrenalectomy has come into question recently. Several large series have shown that if the adrenal gland is normal on CT scan or MRI, the likelihood of localized metastasis to that organ is essentially nonexistent[2]. Therefore the vast majority of radical nephrectomies can now be performed without concomitant adrenalectomy. Lymph node metastases from renal cell carcinoma may go to regional lymph nodes, but may also metastasize to lymph nodes of the interaortocaval region or even to nodes surrounding the contralateral great vessel. A truly adequate lymph node dissection would encompass both great vessels and is rarely performed. Most lymph node dissections are local – regional dissections or the lateral and sometimes medial aspect of the ipsilateral great vessel. The need for a regional lymph node dissection does come into question as it is not unreasonable to assume that positive lymph nodes imply microscopic metastatic focal elsewhere in the body and therefore lymphadenectomy on its own would not offer a surgical cure, except possibly in a very small subset of patients. As more and more biological response modifiers are introduced, protocols for adjuvant immunotherapy have been developed which usually treat positive lymph nodes or T4 disease. In that context, it would seem appropriate to carry out a regional lymph node dissection. It should also be remembered that as more and more renal cell carcinomas are found incidentally, the percentage of patients with positive lymph nodes will decrease. In one large European series[3], only 5% of patients who underwent radical lymphadenectomy in conjunction with radical nephrectomy had positive lymph nodes.

On rare occasions it may be beneficial pre-operatively to infarct the kidney in the angiographic suite several hours prior to surgery. These instances usually involve significant tumor burden in the renal vein or obvious nodal disease close to the renal hilum (Figure 22.1.1). In both these situations infarction will allow for dissection of the more anterior renal vein prior to ligating the renal artery and may save considerable time as well as blood loss.

The pre-operative assessment and staging of the patient has been discussed already. The main pre-operative finding that will affect choice of surgery is the presence of a vena caval thrombus diagnosed on ultrasound or MRI. The removal of a caval thrombus in conjunction with radical nephrectomy will be discussed later. The mere extension of tumor into the renal vein will generally not alter the surgical plan except in the case of a large thrombus which may require pre-operative renal infarction as described above.

Operative approach

Incisions

The incision used to perform a radical nephrectomy may be either thoraco-abdominal, lumbar or transabdominal. In most abdominal cases the incision used is determined

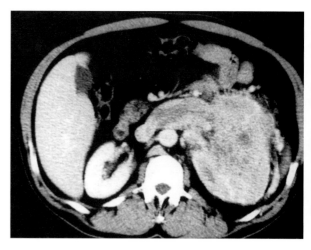

Fig. 22.1.1   An abdominal CT scan showing a 12 cm left renal carcinoma and a large tumor thrombus along the entire course of the left renal vein ending with a small thrombus in the vena cava. This patient underwent pre-operative angio-infarction of the left kidney which aided in the surgical dissection.

by the operator's preference. In cases involving large upper pole tumors, a thoraco-abdominal incision may be preferable. Obviously, transabdominal incisions allow for closer inspection of intra-abdominal organs when metastatic disease is in question. For most radical nephrectomies the author employs an 11th rib incision with the patient at about 30° from the horizontal and flexed at the point of the 11th rib. The incision is begun at approximately the distal half of the 11th rib and carried down over the abdomen towards the umbilicus (Figure 22.1.2). Usually there is no need to take any of the rectus abdominus muscle, although on occasion this may be divided. The advantage of this approach is that the surgery may be performed in an extraperitoneal manner. Although there are obvious limitations superiorly, the incision may be orientated inferiorly from the point of the lateral aspect of the rectus abdominus if more inferior exposure is necessary. If an extensive assessment of the intraperitoneal contents

is needed, a simple peritoneal incision could be made during the procedure through the same incision.

Other incisions

Supra 11th rib flank incision

A supra 11th rib flank or partial flank incision is similar to the 11th rib incision except the incision is made between the 10th and 11th ribs and carried down through intercostal muscles (Figure 22.1.3). At that point dissection through the diaphragm and the pleura inferiorly out of the field are carried out.

Thoraco-abdominal incisions

A thoraco-abdominal incision[4] is made through the 9th and 10th interspace (Figure 22.1.2), again dividing intercostal muscles and avoiding injury to the intercostal neurovascular bundle. Through this incision, a large amount of diaphragm is usually encountered and incised as a separate layer which later will be approximated during closure. A thoraco-abdominal incision is usually only reserved for large upper pole tumors or venal cava tumor thrombus extension.

Abdominal incisions

Chevron, subcostal, and mid-line incisions are all accomplished in the supine position. Abdominal incisions in general are more suited for thinner patients. The Chevron incision[5] is rarely necessary for a unilateral radical nephrectomy, but is certainly realistically utilized during bilateral renal explorations. A subcostal incision, which can include the ipsilateral or bilateral rectus abdominus muscles, may offer excellent exposure for radial nephrectomy. Lastly the midline incision is made from the xiphoid process to an infra-umbilical location. When access to the vena cava is required this is best achieved with a mid-line incision. As with other abdominal incisions the antero-posterial distance of the patient may impose some limitations to this incision, especially during the dissection of the renal hilum.

Operative procedure

An incision is first made over the distal half of the 11th rib and carried down medially over the abdomen toward the umbilicus, stopping at the approximately later aspect of the rectal abdominus. The distal 11th rib is removed in a subperiosteal manner and below this the small amount of underlying diaphragm is sharply incised and the pleura can be brought inferiorly out of the field by sharp and finger dissection. The three abdominal wall layers are incised and the retroperitoneum is entered. At this point a Finachetto retractor is placed so that the superior and inferior aspects of the wound are adequately separated. After

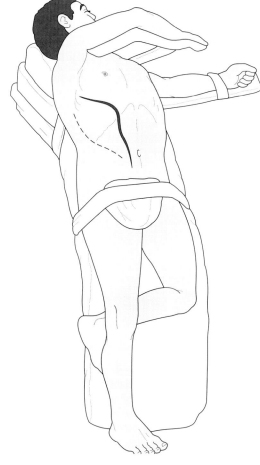

Fig. 22.1.2 Thoraco-abdominal (solid line) and 11th rib (dotted line) incisions performed with the patient's operative side at 30° to the horizontal.

Fig. 22.1.3   A supra 11th rib incision. After the intercostal muscles have been divided the costa-vertebral ligament must be cut to allow for proper retraction of the wound.

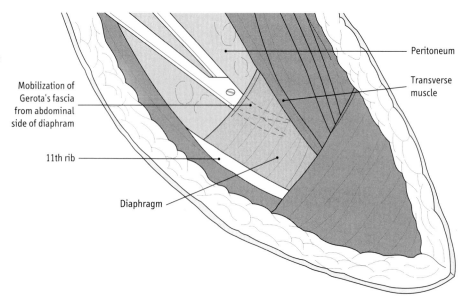

Peritoneum

Transverse muscle

Mobilization of Gerota's fascia from abdominal side of diaphram

11th rib

Diaphragm

the abdominal musculature has been divided, the plane between peritoneum and Gerota's fascia is found and the peritoneum is bluntly dissected medially. At this point Dever retractors are placed to retract the intraperitoneal contents. With this retraction the hilum is usually palpable and visible.

The initial dissection begins inferiorly with Gerota's fascia being dissected free of surrounding tissue until the ureter is identified medially. On the left side both the ureter and gonadal vein can be identified and ligated just below the lower pole of Gerota's. The area between the lower pole of Gerota's fascia and the renal hilum is usually easily dissected. One can then rotate the kidney medially and identify the renal artery or arteries and doubly ligate them with 0 silk sutures. On occasion it may be more practical and safer to ligate the right renal artery from its position between the vena cava and the aorta. (Figure 22.1.4) After renal artery ligation and division the kidney can be replaced in its normal position and the renal vein can then be ligated and cut in a similar manner. When the renal vein is dissected from its surrounding structures, it should be flat due to lack of arterial inflow into the kidney. If the vein is not flat at this point, it usually implies that there is another arterial vessel to the kidney that still requires ligation. On the left side the renal vein is longer than on the right and during left renal vein dissection the left gonadal vein and left inferior adrenal veins are ligated and cut. Dissection of the superior aspect of Gerota's fascia is then carried out using either sharp dissection, electrocautery or vascular clips. As mentioned above, it is usually not necessary to remove the adrenal which is easily spared during the superior dissection.

When there is a potential issue of an adrenal metastasis, the adrenal must be removed during the course of the radical nephrectomy. Especially on the right, care should be taken to use vascular clips surrounding the entire adrenal, as bleeding from adrenal veins, especially high up on the right side can cause difficulties.

Although in routine radical nephrectomies intra-abdominal organs are usually not at risk, care should be taken during right radical nephrectomy to avoid the retroperitoneal portion of the duodenum. When necessary, a Kocher maneuver should be made. Both the spleen and pancreas may be injured during a left radical nephrectomy. On rare occasions with large tumors, the overlying colon may be involved or at least unable to be dissected free from the tumor mass. A pre-operative indication of this is usually apparent from the CT scan and, in those cases, a pre-operative bowel preparation should be performed and a surgical approach which would allow for a localized bowel resection should be entertained.

Intra-operative complications

During the course of the procedure the pleura may inadvertently be entered. A repair should not be entertained at this point, and a sponge should be placed on the pleura to avoid undue bleeding into the pleural cavity during the procedure. At the end of the procedure, during the closure, we usually close the pleura with a continuous 3-0 absorbable suture over a small red rubber catheter which is brought out through the wound and clamped. After all layers of the wound are closed, the catheter is placed in a basin of water and unclamped during periods of inspira-

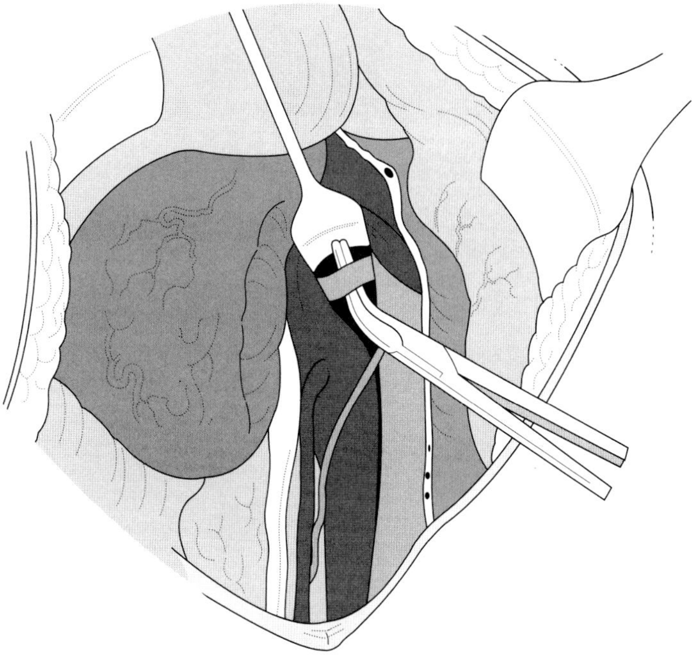

Fig. 22.1.4 When necessary the right renal artery may be identified, ligated and resected in its position between the vena cava and aorta.

tion only. When all air bubbles cease to be visible, the catheter is removed and a chest X-ray is obtained in the recovery room.

Intra-abdominal bleeding will usually result from a venous avulsion off the vena cava (right gonadal veins or small lumbar veins), an unexpected lumbar vein at the level of the renal vein or a large right adrenal vein as mentioned above. As with acute and profuse bleeding anywhere, the area should be compressed so that fluid and blood replacement if necessary should be undertaken prior to consideration of directly surgically controlling the bleeding. After this has been accomplished with continued compression the vena cava and renal veins should be dissected as best as possible. In cases of avulsions from the vena cava a small Satinsky or even an Allis clamp may be placed over the bleeding cava prior to surgical closure. Bleeding from an unsuspected lumbar vein just posterior to the renal vein can be annoying and will usually require continued compression of the vena cava above and below the area until the exact site of bleeding can be located and controlled. The lumbar vein may, if completely avulsed, retract into the underlying psoas muscle and may require a figure of eight suture through the muscle in the area of bleeding.

Intra-abdominal gastrointestinal injury may occur as mentioned above. The spleen and pancreas may be injured during the performance of a left radical nephrectomy. In the past most splenic injuries were treated with splenec-

tomy, however more and more at present are merely managed with Avitene and electrocautery, especially if the injury is small. An injury to the tail of the pancreas can cause considerable problems and usually will require an amputation of the tail. Despite this maneuver, a pancreatic fistula may result which requires a considerable length of time to heal. Usually the patient is placed on some form of hyperalimentation until healing occurs. In cases of an unrecognized pancreatic lesion which results in a pancreatic leak, percutaneous drainage may be necessary. A pancreaticocutaneous fistula will usually form and can be treated as discussed above.

Results

Radical nephrectomy remains the only reasonable and effective treatment for localized renal cell carcinoma. There is at present no role for pre- or post-operative radiation therapy. The pros and cons of radical nephrectomy in the metastatic setting when considering biological response modifiers will be discussed in another chapter.

The results of radical nephrectomy are best looked at in terms of the pathological stage of the tumor. In patients with T1 or T2 disease, the five year survival is excellent and at times approaches 90% for T1 and 70–80% for T2 disease[5,6]. Patients with T3 disease which implies extension

299

outside of the renal capsule or into major veins or the adrenal gland but not beyond Gerota's fascia, have a diminished 5 year survival of about 47–70%. This obviously may be modified depending on the renal vein and vena caval involvement. Patients with T4 disease implying extension beyond Gerota's fascia have a poor 5 year prognosis, in the range of 20–35%. As mentioned above, the performance of a regional or radical lymphadenectomy does not appear to be a therapeutic maneuver since at the time of positive nodes it would be expected that almost all patients would have microscopic metastatic disease elsewhere. The vast majority of these patients will in fact have visible metastatic disease within 18–24 months. The prognosis for patients undergoing radical nephrectomy with positive lymph node disease is probably in the 10–20% range. Clearly, patients with T4 or N-positive disease following radical nephrectomy would potentially benefit from adjuvant therapy if and when such therapy was proven beneficial.

References

1. Robson CJ. Radical nephrectomy for renal cell carcinoma. *J Urol* 1963;**89**:37.
2. Kletscher B, Qian J, Bostwick D, Zincke H, Blute M, Barrett D. Prospective analysis on the incidence of ipsilateral adrenal metastasis in renal cell carcinoma. *J Urol* 1995;**153**:143A.
3. Blom JHM, Schroder FH, Sylvester R, Hammond B, EORTC Genitourinary Group. The therapeutic value of lymphadenectomy in conjunction with radical nephrectomy in non-metastatic renal cancer – Results of an EORTC phase III study. *J Urol* 1992;**147**:422A.
4. Chute R, Soutter L, Kerr W. The value of thoraco-abdominal incisions in kidney tumors. *NEJM* 1949;**241**:951.
5. McNichols DW, Segura JW, de Weerd JH. Renal cell carcinoma: Long term survival and late recurrence. *J Urol* 1981;**127**:17.
6. Robson CJ, Churchill BM, Anderson W. The results of radical nephrectomy for renal cell carcinoma, *Trans Am Ass Genitourin Surg* 1968;**60**:122.

22.2   Surgery for neoplastic involvement of the renal vein and inferior vena cava

T J Polascik and F F Marshall

One characteristic of renal cell carcinoma is its tendency to form a tumor thrombus extending into the renal vein and the inferior vena cava (IVC). The extent of tumor thrombus involving the IVC can vary from extension just beyond the ostium of the renal vein to complete occlusion of the IVC with encroachment upon the heart (Figure 22.2.1)[1]. We have removed tumor from both renal veins, lumbar veins, hepatic veins, the right atrium and the right ventricle. Technical difficulties and complications (exces-

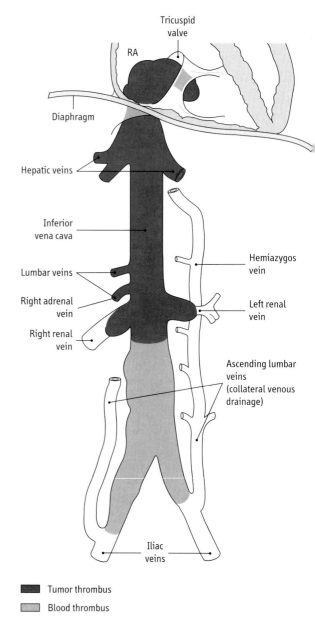

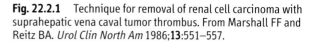

Tumor thrombus

Blood thrombus

Fig. 22.2.1   Technique for removal of renal cell carcinoma with suprahepatic vena caval tumor thrombus. From Marshall FF and Reitz BA. *Urol Clin North Am* 1986;**13**:551–557.

sive bleeding, coagulopathy and post-operative renal failure) can accompany these procedures, especially with extensive intra- or suprahepatic caval neoplastic extension. The tumor can also be adherent to the caval wall and tumor with extensive neovascularity can be difficult to remove surgically.

Pre-operative evaluation and management

Surgical candidates should have a thorough evaluation for metastatic disease including computerized tomography (CT) of the chest and abdomen and routine blood work. A bone scan should be performed if an elevated alkaline phosphatase or symptoms are present. If metastatic disease is identified, we do not typically recommend proceeding with surgery. Occasionally, nephrectomy is performed if a clinical protocol or adjuvant immunotherapy or chemotherapy are considered for metastatic disease. Non-invasive imaging of the renal vein and IVC is easily accomplished using magnetic resonance imaging (MRI). MRI can usually define the superior limit of the caval thrombus unless the thrombus is mobile thus limiting its accuracy. MRI is also effective when total caval occlusion is present. Venocavography can be used to define a caval tumor, however its invasive nature, its false positive and negative results, and a decreased ability to define the superior extent of the tumor limit its use. To delineate fully the extent of a large caval tumor, the combination of MRI and intraoperative transesophageal sonography provide the best results[2]. A thorough medical evaluation is required to optimally prepare the patient prior to surgery.

For most tumors, standard monitoring includes arterial pressure tracings, central venous pressure, urinary output and electrocardiography. For extensive vena caval tumors, pulmonary arterial wedge pressure, esophageal and rectal temperature monitoring, oxygen and carbon dioxide measurements and transesophageal sonography are utilized. Body temperature can be maintained with a hypothermic blanket. A cephalosporin usually provides adequate antibiotic coverage.

Operative technique

The extent of the tumor and the patient's body habitus govern the selection of the surgical approach. For renal tumors with minimal extension of neoplasm into the inferior venacava, a supra11th rib or standard thoracoabdominal approach with rib excision is ideal, especially in obese patients. Anterior incisions provide good exposure for more extensive caval tumors and left-sided tumors. When the intracaval neoplasm extends into or beyond the liver and cardiopulmonary bypass is considered, a median sternotomy extending into either a midline abdominal or a chevron incision (for patients with a wide abdominal girth) is recommended (Figure 22.2.2)[1]. Although the excellent exposure obtained with

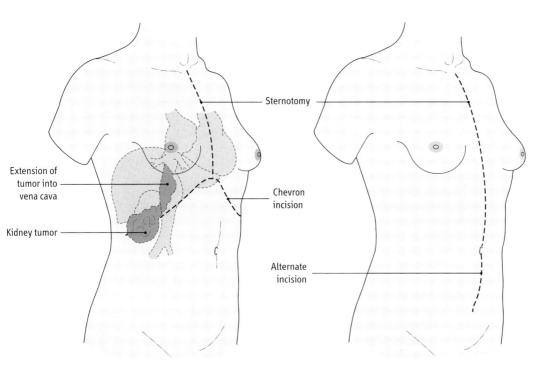

Fig. 22.2.2 Anterior incisions providing excellent exposure of extensive vena caval tumors. Median sternotomy with chevron incision (for patients with wide abdominal girth) or midline abdominal. From Marshall FF (ed.) *Operative Urology*. WB Saunders Co., Philadelphia, PA, ch 4, 1991, p. 27.

301

these extensive incisions allows for additional operations to be performed including coronary artery bypass grafting, we recommend limiting the procedure to nephrectomy and caval thrombectomy whenever possible.

To excise a right renal tumor with minimal neoplasm extending into the vena cava, a flank or thoracoabdominal approach is preferred as previously described. The Omni-Tract retractor (Minnesota Scientific Inc.) provides excellent superficial and deep exposure of the surgical field. The entire kidney including Gerota's fascia is mobilized. The kidney is first approached posterolaterally by developing the plane between the quadratus/psoas muscles and Gerota's fascia. On the anterolateral aspect of the kidney, the mesocolon is reflected medially from the anterior surface of Gerota's fascia until the vena cava is reached. A Kocher maneuver provides further exposure medially at the level of the vena cava. After mobilizing the kidney posteriorly, the renal artery is ligated. The adrenal vein is ligated and divided followed by dissection of the adrenal superiorly. The kidney is then mobilized inferiorly with ligation of the gonadal vein followed by ligation of the ureter. This leaves the entire specimen attached to the vena cava via the renal vein.

With right-sided renal tumors, the vena cava must be isolated in proportion to the extent of the intracaval tumor. Dissection should proceed on the vena cava using care to prevent potential dislodgment of caval tumor. If the intracaval tumor extends slightly beyond the ostium of the renal vein into the vena cava, a Satinsky vascular clamp can be placed on the caval sidewall beyond the tumor. This segment of caval wall can be excised with the nephrectomy specimen en bloc, and the cava can be oversewn.

With a more extensive infrahepatic intracaval tumor, a midline transperitoneal approach should be performed. Exposure to the right kidney is obtained by mobilizing the right colon medially after incising the line of Toldt from the cecum to the ligament of Treitz superiorly. The intestines can then be placed in a bowel bag and reflected medially. After the kidney is dissected free leaving only its renal vein attached, control of the IVC must be obtained below both renal veins. One or more posterior lumbar veins may require ligation to prevent unexpected bleeding. A Rummel tourniquet is placed loosely around a segment of the left renal vein in case control of this vessel becomes necessary. Superiorly, additional exposure to the vena cava can be gained by dividing the posterior attachments of the liver followed by rotation of the liver medially. Depending upon the superior extent of the thrombus, several venous branches draining the caudate lobe of the liver may need to be ligated and divided to mobilize the vena cava below the liver (Figure 22.2.3). The venous

drainage of the caudate lobe is quite variable. If these veins are short, they can be controlled with suture ligatures placed into the liver parenchyma. If a vascular clamp or Rummel tourniquet can be placed across the cava above the superior extent of the tumor, cardiopulmonary bypass can be avoided.

Once adequately mobilized, Satinsky clamps or Rummel tourniquets are placed on the superior and inferior extent of the vena cava defined by the intracaval tumor. An elliptical incision circumscribing the ostium of the involved renal vein is made and the tumor is extracted under direct vision. Additional tumor may be removed using a Fogarty or Foley catheter. Although direct vision usually suffices, we have used a dental mirror to inspect the hepatic veins and the flexible cystoscope to inspect the cava as necessary. If one is uncertain whether the superior

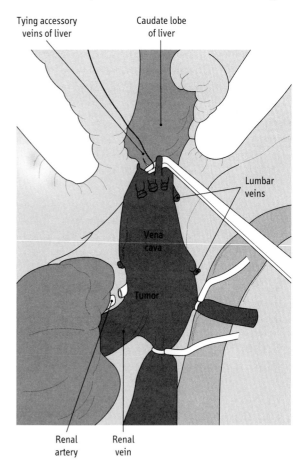

Fig. 22.2.3   Venous branches supplying caudate lobe are ligated and divided to allow vascular control of vena cava superior to the tumor. From Marshall FF *et al.* Surgical management of renal cell carcinoma with intracaval neoplastic extension above the hepatic veins. *J Urol* 1988;**139**:1169.

extent of the thrombus has been completely removed, transesophageal or direct sonography can be utilized intraoperatively[2]. Tumor in the vena cava below the renal veins is generally a blood thrombus without neoplastic cells. This blood thrombus can adhere to the caval wall, and in some instances the cava has been oversewn to prevent subsequent embolism. In cases in which the tumor is inseparable from the caval endothelium superior to the renal veins, the involved cava has been excised. Caval reconstruction can be accomplished using prosthetic grafts although we prefer using autologous material such as pericardium since it is less thrombogenic[3]. If caval excision reduces the vascular diameter by 50% or greater, reconstruction of the vena cava is recommended to prevent the risk of caval thrombosis (Figure 22.2.4). Venous drainage of the right kidney must always be preserved to prevent venous infarction. We reconstruct the cava with 4-0 or 5-0 cardiovascular polypropylene sutures.

A left-sided tumor with caval thrombus is often a more difficult procedure than a right-sided lesion since dissection on both sides of the abdomen must be performed to access the vena cava and the left kidney. Depending on the superior extent of the caval tumor, an anterior incision provides adequate exposure. The descending colon is first reflected medially by incising the line of Toldt. In a dissection similar to a right-sided tumor, the entire kidney within Gerota's fascia is mobilized until only the left renal vein remains. The ascending colon is then mobilized medially by incising the line of Toldt and the duodenum is reflected by the Kocher maneuver. Once adequate exposure to the vena cava is obtained, the remainder of the procedure is as previously described.

Cardiopulmonary bypass, hypothermia and temporary cardiac arrest greatly facilitates the resection of a suprahepatic caval thrombus[1]. It is best to dissect as much of the kidney and the vena cava as possible prior to cardiac bypass. To reduce the incidence of complications, circulatory arrest time is best limited to 45 minutes. Dissections of this nature are often difficult and are best performed in specialized centers.

References

1. Marshall FF, Dietrick DD, Baumgartner WA, Reitz BA. Surgical management of renal cell carcinoma with intracaval neoplastic extension above the hepatic veins. *J Urol* 1988;**139**:1166.
2. Treiger BFC, Humphrey LS, Peterson JCV, Oesterling JE, Mostwin JL, Reitz BA, Marshall FF. Transesophageal echocardiography in renal cell carcinoma: an accurate diagnostic technique for intracaval neoplastic extension. *J Urol* 1991;**145**:1138.
3. Marshall FF, Reitz BA. Supradiaphragmatic renal cell carcinoma tumor thrombus: indications for vena caval reconstruction with pericardium. *J Urol* 1985;**133**:266.

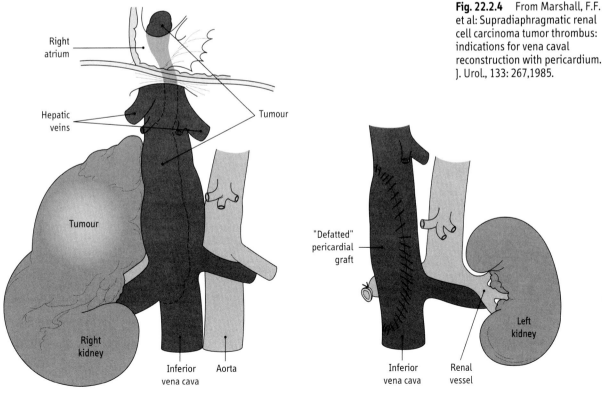

Fig. 22.2.4 From Marshall, F.F. et al: Supradiaphragmatic renal cell carcinoma tumor thrombus: indications for vena caval reconstruction with pericardium. J. Urol., 133: 267,1985.

22.3 Partial nephrectomy

T J Polascik and F F Marshall

Introduction and indications

In patients with limited functional renal parenchyma, such as those with a solitary kidney, bilateral renal cell carcinoma, or severe renal insufficiency, the benefits of nephron-sparing surgery for renal tumors are clear since this operation can potentially avoid hemodialysis or renal transplantation. Recent reports describe a growing acceptance to perform partial nephrectomy for patients with a normal contralateral kidney if the size and location of the tumor is favorable. Several contemporary series indicate the disease-free survival for patients undergoing partial nephrectomy for small stage T1 renal adenocarcinomas is comparable to radical nephrectomy[1–3]. The complication rate of partial nephrectomy has been diminished due to improvements in surgical technique and an increased incidence of smaller, serendipitously discovered tumors[1].

Our definition of partial nephrectomy is the surgical resection of the renal lesion accompanied by a margin of normal parenchyma. Partial 'radical' nephrectomy includes the excision of perinephric fat (with Gerota's fascia) directly above the tumor. We have identified capsular penetration in five of 27 renal cell carcinomas (18.5%) with a diameter of 3.5 cm or less, and demonstrated perinephric invasion in three of these five tumors[1]. This finding strongly suggests that aggressive surgical resection with adequate tumor-free parenchymal and perinephric margins is necessary even for small lesions.

One concern regarding partial nephrectomy is the possibility of incompletely excising the tumor. The technique of partial radical nephrectomy is designed for complete tumor excision including negative parenchymal and perinephric surgical margins. Multifocal tumors, ranging in frequency from 7–19.7%, can potentially account for local tumor recurrence if not excised[1,4–7]. Because many of these accessory tumors are small, current imaging modalities are often unable to consistently identify these lesions. However, the biologic potential of these satellite tumors contributing to local recurrence has been questioned and it is not clear that these are all clinically significant tumors[1]. In our experience, partial nephrectomy with intraoperative ultrasound can preserve renal parenchyma while providing good local control of renal cell carcinoma with minimal surgical morbidity[1,4].

Intraoperative sonography

We routinely utilize intraoperative sonography to delineate the extent of the tumor when planning the surgical limits of partial nephrectomy[4]. Sonography can assess the size, number, echo texture and location of renal lesions and define the spatial relationship of the tumor(s) to the collecting system, vasculature and renal capsule. Extrarenal structures can be evaluated for tumor involvement, such as the renal vein, inferior vena cava, adrenal gland and liver. Intraoperative ultrasound is particularly beneficial in defining pre-operative indeterminate renal lesions and some complex cysts. In select cases, it may identify the presence of a satellite tumor. Real-time Doppler imaging can be used to distinguish between renal arteries, renal veins and the collecting system. For these reasons, we rely upon intraoperative sonography for all partial nephrectomies since it provides greater assurance for the surgeon.

Pre-operative evaluation

Candidates for partial nephrectomy for renal malignancy should not have metastatic disease and be medically able to withstand the anesthetic and surgery. Pre-operative evaluation consists of an abdominal computerized tomography (CT) scan, chest roentgenogram, and standard blood work including liver and renal function tests. We recommend a chest CT to study those patients with suspicious lesions found on standard chest roentgenogram. Other studies including magnetic resonance imaging (MRI), inferior venocavography, angiography, radionuclide imaging, and bone scintigraphy are obtained as indicated. All patients undergo a thorough medical evaluation, and a nephrologist is consulted if a patient is at high risk for post-operative hemodialysis.

Operative technique

A thoracic epidural catheter is routinely placed at the start of the case and can later serve as patient-controlled analgesia (PCA) post-operatively. Following the induction of general anesthesia, an indwelling urethral catheter and oropharyngeal tube are placed. The patient is placed in a standard flank position and secured to the table. A cephalosporin is administered for antibiotic coverage.

The choice of incision depends on the side of the lesion, the location and the size of the tumor. Typically, we use an extraperitoneal flank incision unless the location or size of the tumor mandates a thoracoabdominal approach. The incision is deepened through the three abdominal muscle layers. The transversus abdominis muscle is sharply incised directly medial to the tip of the rib and the underlying peritoneum is bluntly swept away from the overlying musculature. After incising the remainder of the transversus abdominis, the Omni-Tract retractor (Minnesota Scientific Inc.) is placed, providing fixed superficial and deep exposure of the surgical field.

The kidney is approached posterolaterally, defining the plane between the quadratus and psoas muscles and Gerota's fascia to the level of the renal artery. Inferiorly, the ureter is identified and tagged with a vessel loop. Anteriorly, the mesocolon is reflected off Gerota's fascia in a medial direction until hilar vessels are reached. Minimal dissection around the hilar vessels is undertaken so that perivascular adipose tissue will act as a 'cushion' when subsequently clamping the renal hilum. Gerota's fascia is incised distal to the tumor and perirenal adipose tissue is removed from the capsular surface. However, Gerota's fascia and perinephric tissue are left adherent to the kidney overlying the tumor. If the tumor is located in the upper pole, we typically excise the adrenal gland with the specimen.

Intraoperative sonography (7.5 MHz probe most commonly used) is utilized initially to confirm the location and extent of the lesion. It can define tumors in relation to hilar anatomy and allow partial nephrectomy to be performed safely while avoiding hilar vessels and the collecting system. Additionally, intraoperative sonography can assess for possible inconspicuous satellite tumors and further evaluate pre-operatively indeterminate lesions. The renal vein and vena cava are sonographically studied for patency. After the initial sonographic evaluation of the kidney, intraoperative ultrasound is used to define the surgical limits of partial nephrectomy[4].

Intravenous mannitol is administered prior to manipulating the renal vasculature to ensure a brisk diuresis. The renal artery is carefully evaluated for the presence of plaques prior to clamping. The renal artery(s) and vein(s) are not skeletonized but rather are clamped as a single unit since venous back bleeding can occur, especially on the right side. The kidney is placed in an intestinal bag and, after occluding the vasculature, ice-slush is placed around the kidney for regional hypothermia (Figure 22.3.1). Intrarenal arterial branches are then appropriately divided if they clearly supply the renal segment with tumor. The renal capsule is sharply incised leaving a 0.5–1.0 cm margin of normal-appearing parenchyma beyond the visual limits of the tumor. A neurosurgical brain elevator is used bluntly to separate the lesion from the surrounding parenchyma. Segmental renal vessels encountered are individually ligated with 4-0 vicryl and disruptions in the collecting system are oversewn with 4-0 chromic suture (Figure 22.3.2). The specimen consists of the tumor circumscribed by a rim of normal-appearing parenchyma and abundant perinephric soft tissue overlying the lesion. Multiple frozen sections of the deep margins of the

remaining kidney are obtained to verify the absence of residual cancer at the surgical margin. The kidney is then sonographically studied to confirm that all suspicious lesions have been excised.

After temporarily occluding the ureter with a vessel loop, the collecting system is injected with a dilute solution of methylene blue dye (Figure 22.3.2). Small defects in the collecting system are repaired with 4-0 chromic suture. Argon beam coagulation is applied to the surface of the operative site to achieve hemostasis (Figure 22.3.3). Microfibrillar collagen hemostat is then placed on the cut surface of the kidney and 2-0 chromic sutures approximate the remaining renal parenchyma (Figure 22.3.4). Following removal of the vascular clamp, the kidney is manually compressed for 5 minutes. The kidney is fixed by reapproximating Gerota's fascia with absorbable suture. A closed drainage system is placed at the surgical site and the flank and abdominal musculature is closed in two layers. Ureteral stenting is not used and lymphadenectomy is not routinely performed.

During the extended post-operative period, patients are routinely evaluated with serum creatinine measurements, urinalysis and renal sonography. A CT scan is obtained if further anatomic detail is required.

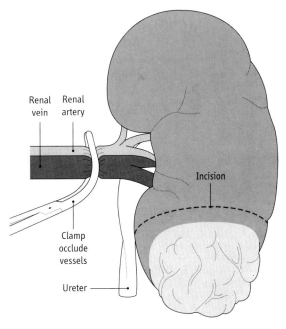

Fig. 22.3.1 Technique of partial incision of the tumor and a 0.5–1.0cm margin of normal parenchyma are marked. The hilar vessels are then clamped and the kidney is cooled with ice slush.

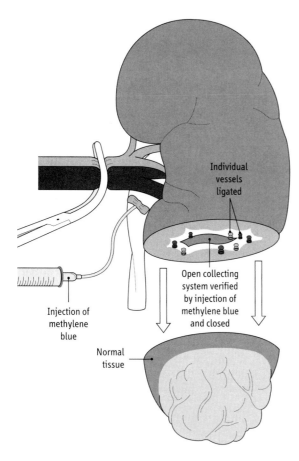

Fig. 22.3.2   Following excision of tumor with adequate margin of normal tissue, methylene blue is injected to verify absence of urinary leak. All rerts in collecting system are oversewn and hemostasis is confirmed. Frozen-section biopsies of remnant kidney ensure adequacy of surgical margins.

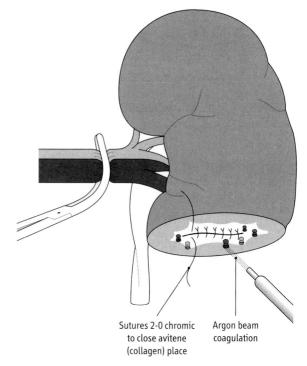

Fig. 22.3.3   Hemostasis is achieved by individual ligation of vessels and judicious application of the Argon beam coagulation. Avitene collagen is placed on the raw surface of the kidney for additional hemostasis.

References

1. Polascik TJ, Pound CR, Meng MV, Partin AW, Marshall FF. Partial nephrectomy: technique, complications and pathological findings. *J Urol* 1995;**154**:1312.
2. Steinbach F, Stockle M, Muller SC, Thuriff JW, Melchior SW, Stein R, Hohenfellner R. Conservative surgery of renal cell tumors in 140 patients: 21 years of experience. *J Urol* 1992;**148**:24.
3. Butler BP, Novick AC, Miller DP, Campbell SC, Light MR. Management of small unilateral renal cell carcinomas: radical versus nephron-sparing surgery. *Urology* 1995;**45**:34.
4. Polascik TJ, Meng MV, Epstein JI, Marshall FF. Intraoperative sonography for evaluation and management of renal tumors: experience with 100 patients. *J Urol* 1995;**154**:1676.
5. Amendola MA, Bree RL, Pollack HM, Francis IR, Glazer GM, Jafri SZ, Tomaszewski JE. Small renal cell carcinomas: resolving a diagnostic dilemma. *Radiology* 1988;**166**:637.
6. Cheng WS, Farrow GM, Zincke H. The incidence of multicentricity in renal cell carcinoma. *J Urol* 1991;**146**:1221.
7. Mukamel E, Konichezky M, Engelstein D, Servadio C. Incidental small renal tumors accompanying clinically overt renal cell carcinoma. *J Urol* 1988;**140**:22.

22.4   Von Hippel-Lindau disease

E R Maher

Von Hippel-Lindau (VHL) disease is a dominantly inherited familial cancer syndrome with a minimal incidence of 1 in 36 000[1]. Although rare, VHL disease is the commonest cause of familial renal cell carcinoma (RCC) and early diagnosis and recognition of VHL disease is important if morbidity and mortality is to be avoided.

Clinical features and natural history

The age at onset of VHL disease is variable. The first manifestations may be detected in childhood or not until old age. However most patients present in the second and third decades and penetrance is almost complete by 60 years of age. The relative frequencies and mean age at diagnosis of the major complications of VHL disease are shown in Table 22.4.1. The most frequent initial manifestations are retinal and cerebellar hemangioblastomas, but RCC is the presenting feature in ~10% of cases[2,3].

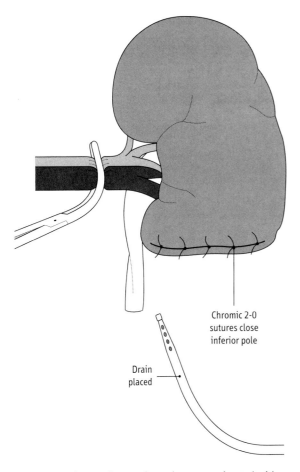

Fig. 22.3.4 The renal parenchyma is reapproximated with suture, the vascular clamp is released and a drain placed.

Chromic 2-0 sutures close inferior pole

Drain placed

Table 22.4.1   Major manifestations of VHL disease

Lesion	UK series (n = 152)	Literature review (n = 554)	Mean age of onset : (years) (Maher et al.[1])
Retinal angioma	89 (59%)	317 (57%)	25.4 ± 12.7
Cerebellar hemangioblastoma	89 (59%)	304 (55%)	29.0 ± 10.0
Spinal cord hemangioblastoma	20 (13%)	79 (14%)	33.9 ± 12.6
Renal cell carcinoma	43 (28%)	133 (24%)	44.0 ± 10.9
Pheochromocytoma	11 (7%)	106 (19%)	20.2 ± 7.6

Retinal angiomas occur in most VHL patients and are multiple in many cases. Histologically they are benign hemangioblastomas, but untreated they enlarge progressively and may produce retinal detachment and hemorrhage resulting in visual impairment. The early detection of these tumors enables treatment by laser- or cryotherapy and reduces the risk of visual loss.

Within the central nervous system, the cerebellum is the most frequent site of hemangioblastoma followed by the spinal cord and brain stem[4]. The incidence of supratentorial lesions is small. Approximately 30% of all patients with cerebellar hemangioblastoma have VHL disease and the mean age at diagnosis in those with VHL disease is considerably younger than in sporadic cases[5]. Hemangioblastomas are benign and the results of surgery for cerebellar lesions are often excellent. However, the treatment of multiple CNS hemangioblastomas and the management of brain stem and spinal tumors is often difficult. Hence CNS hemangioblastomas remains an important cause of morbidity and mortality for VHL patients.

The onset of RCC in VHL disease is usually later than that for retinal or cerebellar hemangioblastomas. As a result of advances in neurosurgery, an increasing number of VHL patients survive to an age when there is a significant risk of RCC. The lifetime risks (> age 60 years) of retinal and cerebellar hemangioblastomas and of RCC are in excess of 70%, and RCC has emerged as a leading cause of death in VHL disease[3]. Patients with VHL disease are not only at high risk of RCC, they also develop tumors at an early age (solid renal lesions have been reported as early as 16 years) (Table 22.4.1) and frequently have bilateral and multicentric tumors. Indeed microscopic examination of VHL kidneys has suggested that they may contain hundreds of small tumor foci[6].

Pheochromocytoma is an important complication of VHL disease[7], although it does not occur in most VHL families (Type I families). However in some families (Type II), pheochromocytoma is the most common manifestation of VHL disease. These interfamilial differences in pheochromocytoma susceptibility are caused by variations in the extent to which specific VHL mutations predispose to pheochromocytoma. Specific missense mutations may cause a very high risk of pheochromocytoma. Rarely, specific missense mutation may be associated with mutations[8–11]. The identification of a VHL gene mutation may not only allow reliable presymptomatic diagnosis, but may also provide a guide to the risk of pheochromocytoma. Generally the risk of pheochromocytoma is low in individuals with gene deletions or mutations predicted to cause a truncated pVHL whereas certain missense mutations (e.g. substitutions at codon 167) are associated with a high risk[12].

Familial cancer syndromes account for only a small proportion of all human cancers, but they can, as exemplified by retinoblastoma, provide important insights into the mechanism of tumorigenesis in both familial and sporadic cancers. Inactivating mutations in tumor suppressor genes causes many familial cancer syndromes, including familial retinoblastoma and VHL disease. The mechanism of tumorigenesis in VHL disease is similar to that in retinoblastoma such that inactivation of both alleles is required to initiate tumor development (two-hit model of tumorigenesis). In patients with VHL disease one allele is inactivated by a germline mutation and the remaining allele may be inactivated by loss of a large part of chromosome 3, a localized intragenic mutation or by hypermethylation and transcriptional silencing[13–15]. Importantly similar mechanisms of VHL inactivation occur in most sporadic clear cell RCC. In the majority of clear cell RCC both VHL alleles have been inactivated by somatic mutation events[16–19]. These findings suggest that VHL gene inactivation is an early and important event in the pathogenesis of sporadic clear cell RCC and the reintroduction of a function VHL tumor suppressor gene into RCC cell lines reduces in vivo tumorigenicity[20,21].

Management of VHL disease

Ascertainment and screening

VHL disease is a multisystem disorder and the effective management of VHL patients and families requires a multidisciplinary approach. Specific complications may require expert investigations and treatment from ophthalmologists and other organ based specialists. However, there is also a need for the overall coordination of family ascertainment and screening. Thus when an individual with VHL disease is identified strenuous efforts should be made to identify all at risk relatives and offer them information on the inheritance and clinical manifestations of VHL disease. Patients and relatives should also be offered systematic screening to detect subclinical disease as outlined in Table 22.4.2. For affected individuals and individuals at high risk by DNA testing, lifelong surveillance should be offered. In the absence of DNA testing, at risk individuals without clinical or subclinical evidence of VHL should be followed up until after 60 years of age[3]. Increasingly, however, it is possible to modify the risk of such relatives by DNA testing and then change the surveillance program as appropriate. Early detection and treatment of VHL associated neoplasms (particularly in the eye and kidney) reduces morbidity and mortality. A proactive approach to identifying VHL families by contacting those specialists likely to be involved (ophthalmologists, neurosurgeons, urologists, etc.) is most likely to result in a high level of ascertainment.

Individuals with VHL disease without a family history can only be identified clinically when they have developed two manifestations (see above). Hence the diagnosis of 'new mutation' cases is delayed compared with familial VHL disease. Molecular genetic studies provide a method by which an early diagnosis of VHL disease could be made in patients who do not satisfy the current clinically-based diagnostic criteria. Molecular genetic testing is of course complementary to documenting a detailed family history and investigations to detect subclinical manifestations of

Table 22.4.2 Example surveillance program for von Hippel-Lindau disease in affected patients and at risk relatives (adapted from Maher et al, 1990a)[3]

Affected patient

1. Annual physical examination and urine testing.
2. Annual direct and indirect ophthalmoscopy
3. MRI (or CT) brain scan every 3 years to age 50 and every 5 years thereafter.
4. Annual renal ultrasound scan, with CT or MRI scan every 3 years (more frequently if multiple renal cysts present).
5. Annual 24 hour urine collection for catecholamines.

At risk relative

1. Annual physical examination and urine testing.
2. Annual direct and indirect ophthalmoscopy from age 5. Annual fluoroscein angioscopy or angiography from age 10 (see text) until age 60.
3. MRI (or CT) brain scan every 3 years from age 15 to 40 years and then every 5 years until age 60 years.
4. Annual renal ultrasound scan, with abdominal CT scan every 3 years from age 16 to 65 years.
5. Annual 24 hour urine collection for catecholamines from age 11.

VHL disease. A diagnosis of VHL disease should be considered in all cases of retinal and central nervous system hemangioblastomas, but also patients with familial, multicentric or young onset pheochromocytoma and RCC. Molecular genetic testing has revealed that ~50% of patients with apparently isolated familial pheochromocytoma or bilateral pheochromocytoma have germline VHL gene mutations[22–24]. For patients with familial RCC, in addition to VHL disease, a diagnosis of familial papillary RCC and familial clear cell RCC which is not allelic with VHL disease should also be considered[25–26].

Management of renal lesions

The recognition that RCC is a frequent complication and a leading cause of death in VHL disease, provided a basis for recommending regular renal imaging in VHL patients and at risk relatives. As a result of this, renal lesions in VHL disease are increasingly being detected at an early asymptomatic stage. Consequently the management of renal lesions in VHL disease is changing with the emphasis no longer on how to operate on large symptomatic RCC, but on how to manage small asymptomatic tumors. The identification of renal cysts in VHL patients is a frequent and expected finding. As these do not usually compromise renal function no treatment is necessary. It is known, however, that the epithelium lining the cysts in VHL kidneys is frequently atypical and may contain carcinoma in situ. If renal imaging suggests only simple cysts are present then annual follow up is sufficient. However if complex cysts are detected these should be reviewed more frequently as they can develop into solid lesions[28]. Although CT scanning is the most accurate method for following renal lesions (particularly in the presence of renal cysts) MRI or ultrasound scanning avoids the potential adverse effects of a large cumulative radiation exposure in cancer-predisposed individuals and are preferred for regular follow up. The investigation of a specific lesion may, however, require multiple imaging modalities. Most small solid renal tumors enlarge slowly (mean < 2 cm/ year). Having established the growth rate of an individual lesion these can usually be followed by CT scanning every 6 months[28]. The risk of distant metastasis from a solid lesion < 3 cm appears to be very remote and a conservative approach is applied until a solid lesion reaches ~3 cm in size. It is very likely that individuals with VHL disease and RCC will ultimately develop further tumors in their remaining renal tissue as a result of new primary tumors. This observation has been used as a rationale for bilateral nephrectomy in VHL patients with bilateral RCC. Increasingly, however, a conservative nephron sparing approach is being applied for the management of RCC in VHL disease[29,30]. The objective of this strategy is to maintain adequate renal function for as long as possible by avoiding the removal of normal renal tissue. Thus wherever possible solid tumors are removed by a limited partial nephrectomy or by 'shelling out' small encapsulated lesions. When elective surgery is performed, it is helpful if, in addition to removing the primary lesion, other smaller lesions are also removed when accessible and when this is possible without damaging normal renal tissue. This approach should then delay the need for further surgery. Follow up of VHL patients managed by such a nephron-sparing approach suggests that although the risk of local recurrence (most likely from new primary tumors) is high the risk of distant metastasis is low[29]. As many VHL patients undergoing surgery for RCC are young, any delay in the requirement for renal replacement therapy is beneficial. Anephric VHL patients on dialysis may be more susceptible to fluid balance problems because of the lack of endogenous renal function. Renal transplantation is an option for a VHL patient in end stage renal failure and experience so far suggests that immunosuppression does not effect adversely the underlying course of VHL disease. It is customary to wait at least 2 years for performing a transplant in patients who have had a RCC removed, but this may be unnecessary in VHL patients who have had only small tumors (3 cm or less).

Conclusion

VHL disease is a multisystem disorder and the successful management of VHL disease requires a multidisciplinary team with a wide range of expertise. The management of RCC in VHL disease is challenging and the optimal approach is still evolving. The emphasis, however, is on pre-serving functioning renal tissue for as long as possible. The optimal management of VHL disease requires more than the successful treatment of specific complications such as RCC or retinal angioma. In addition, it is important that a coordinated system for ascertaining families and providing appropriate surveillance is available. This approach reduces morbidity and mortality from VHL disease.

References

1. Maher ER, Bentley E, Yates JRW, Latif F, Lerman M, Zbar B, Affara NA, Ferguson-Smith MA. Localization of the gene for von Hippel-Lindau disease to a small region of chromosome 3p by genetic linkage analysis. *Genomics* (1991);**10**:957–960.
2. Lamiell JM, Salazar FG, Hsia YE. von Hippel-Lindau disease affecting 43 members of a single kindred. *Medicine* 1989;**68**:1–29.
3. Maher ER, Yates JRW, Harries R, Benjamin C, Harris R, Ferguson-Smith MA. Clinical features and natural history of von Hippel-Lindau disease. *Q J Med* (1990a);**77**:1151–1163.
4. Fillery-Katz MR, Choyke PL, Oldfield E, Charnas L, Patronas NJ, Glenn GM, Gorin MB, Morgan JK, Linehan WM, Seizinger BR *et al.* Central nervous system involvement in Von Hippel-Lindau disease. *Neurology* (1991);**41**:41–46.
5. Maher ER, Yates JRW, Ferguson-Smith MA. Statistical analysis of the two stage mutation model in von Hippel-Lindau disease and in sporadic cerebellar haemangioblastoma and renal cell carcinoma. *J Med Gen* (1990b);**27**:311–314.
6. Walther MM, Choyke PL, Weiss G, Manolatos C, Long J, Reiter R, Alexander RB, Linehan WM (1995). Parenchymal sparing surgery in patients with hereditary renal cell carcinoma. *J Urol* 1995a;**153**:913–916.
7. Richard S, Chauveau D, Chretien Y, Beigelman C, Denys A, Fendler JP, Fromont G, Paraf F, *et al.* Renal lesions and pheochromocytoma in von Hippel-Lindau disease. *Adv Nephrol* 1994;**23**:1–27.
8. Richards FM, Maher ER, Latif F, Phipps ME, Tory K, Lush M, Crossey PA, Oostra B *et al.* Detailed genetic mapping of the von Hippel-Lindau disease tumor suppressor gene. *J Med Gen* (1993);**30**:104–107.
9. Crossey PA, Foster K, Richards FM, Phipps ME, Latif F, Tory K, Jones MH, Bentley E *et al.* Molecular genetic investigation of the mechanism of tumorigenesis in von Hippel-Lindau disease: Analysis of allele loss in VHL tumors. *Hum Gen* (1994);**93**:53–58.
10. Chen F, Kishida T, Duh FM, Renbaum P, Orcutt ML, Schmidt L, Zbar B. Suppression of growth of renal carcinoma cells by the von Hippel-Lindau tumor suppressor gene. *Cancer Res* (1995);**55**:4804–4807.
11. Zbar B, Kishida T, Chen F, Schmidt L, Maher ER, Richards FM, Crossey PA, Webster AR *et al.* Germline mutations in the von-Hippel-Lindau disease (VHL) gene in families from North-America, Europe, and Japan. *Hum Mut* (1996);**8**:348–357.
12. Maher ER, Webster AR, Richards FM, Green JS, Crossey PA, Payne SJ, Moore AT. Phenotypic expression in von Hippel-Lindau disease: correlations with germline VHL gene mutations. *J Med Gen* (1996);**33**(4):328–332.
13. Tory K, Brauch H, Linehan M, Barba D, Oldfield E, Filling-Katz M, Seizinger B, Nakamura Y *et al.* Specific genetic change in tumors associated with von Hippel-Lindau disease. *J Natl Cancer Inst* 1989;**81**:1097–1101.
14. Crossey PA, Richards FM, Foster K, Green JS, Prowse A, Latif F, Lerman MI, Zbar B *et al.* Identification of intragenic mutations in the von Hippel-Lindau disease tumor suppressor gene and correlation with disease phenotype. *Hum Mol Gen* (1994);**3**:1303–1308.
15. Prowse AH, Webster AR, Richards FM, Richard S, Olschwang S, Resche F, Affara NA, Maher ER. Somatic inactivation of the VHL gene in Von Hippel-Lindau disease tumors. *Am J Hum Gen* (1997);**60**:765–771.
16. Foster K, Prowse A, van den Berg A, Fleming S, Hulsbeek MMF, Crossey PA, Richards FM, Cairns P *et al.* Somatic mutations of the von Hippel-Lindau

disease tumor suppressor gene in nonfamilial clear cell renal carcinoma. *Hum Mol Gen* (1994);**3**:2169–2173.

17. Gnarra JR, Tory K, Weng Y, Schimdt L, Wei MH, Li H, Latif F, Liu S *et al.* Mutations of the VHL tumor suppressor gene in renal carcinoma. *Nat Gen* (1994);**7**:85–90.

18. Shuin T, Kondo K, Torigoe S, Kishida T, Kubota Y, Hosaka M, Nagashima Y, Kitamura H *et al.* Frequent somatic mutations and loss of heterozygosity of the von Hippel-Lindau tumor suppressor gene in primary human renal cell carcinomas. *Cancer Res* (1994);**54**:2852–2855.

19. Herman JG, Latif F, Weng Y, Lerman MI, Zbar B, Liu S, Samid D, Duan DSR *et al.* Silencing of the VHL tumor suppressor gene by DNA methylation in renal carcinomas. *Proc Natl Acad Sci USA* (1994);**91**:9700–9704.

20. Chen F, Kishida T, Yao M Hustad T, Glavac D, Dean D, Gnarra JR, Orcutt ML *et al.* Germline mutations in the von Hippel-Lindau disease tumor suppressor gene: correlations with phenotype. *Hum Mutat* (1995);**5**:66–75.

21. Iliopoulos O, Kibel A, Gray S, Kaelin WG Jr. Tumor suppression by the human von Hippel-Lindau gene product. *Nat Med* (1995);**1**:822–826.

22. Crossey PA, Eng C, Ginalska-Malinowska M, Lennard TW, Wheeler DC, Ponder BA, Maher ER. Molecular genetic diagnosis of von Hippel-Lindau disease in familial phaeochromocytoma. *J Med Gen* (1995); **32**:885–886.

23. Neumann HPH, Eng C, Mulligan L, Glavac D, Ponder BAJ, Crossey PA, Maher ER, Brauch H. Consequences of direct genetic testing for germline mutations in the clinical management of families with multiple endocrine neoplasia type 2. *JAMA* (1995);**274**:1149–1151.

24. Woodward ER, Eng C, McMahon R, Voutilainen R, Affara NA, Ponder BAJ, Maher ER. Genetic predisposition to phaeochromocytoma: Analysis of candidate genes GDNF, RET and VHL. *Hum Mol Gen* 1997;**6**:1051–6.

25. Zbar B, Glenn G, Lubensky I, Choyke P, Walther MM, Magnusson G, Bergerheim US, Pettersson S *et al.* Hereditary papillary renal cell carcinoma: clinical studies in 10 families. *J Urol* (1995);**153**:907–912.

26. Teh BT, Giraud S, Sari NF, Hii SI, Bergerat JP, Larsson C, Limacher JM, Nicol D. Familial non-VHL non-papillary clear-cell renal cancer. *Lancet* (1997);**349**:848–849.

28. Choyke PL, Glenn GM, Walther MM, Zbar B, Weiss GH, Alexander RB, Hayes WS, Long JP *et al.* The natural history of renal lesions in von Hippel-Lindau disease: A serial CT study in 28 patients. *Am J Radiol* (1992);**159**:1229–1234.

29. Steinbach F, Novick AC, Zincke H, Miller DP, Williams RD, Lund G, Skinner DG, Esrig D *et al.* Treatment of renal cell carcinoma in von Hippel-Lindau disease: a multicenter study. *J Urol* (1995);**153**:1812–1816.

30. Walther MM, Lubensky IA, Venzon D, Zbar B, Linehan WM. Prevalence of microscopic lesions in grossly normal renal parenchyma from patients with von Hippel-Lindau disease, sporadic renal cell carcinoma and no renal disease: clinical implications. *J Urol* (1995a);1995; **154**(6): 2010–2014.

23 Minimally invasive therapy

23.1 Focused ultrasound ablation

K U Köhrmann and P Alken

Introduction

For the treatment of kidney tumors, invasive surgery or systemic application of immuno-chemotherapy are first choice options. Minimal invasive procedures are not routinely performed. The common trend is currently towards new technologies for tissue ablation without the trauma of open surgery. The aim is the contactless destruction of defined parts of an organ by extracorporeally applied energy. This aim could be fulfilled by focused ultrasound targeted with high precision to the focus where it induces a well defined thermonecrosis.

Technical principle

Ultrasound waves are generated by piezo-electric elements and focused by spherical arrangement, acoustic lens or paraboloid reflectors. Due to physical laws the appropriate range to induce a small focus of a size around 10×1 mm the frequency and corresponding to that the wave length is restricted to 0.5 to 10 MHz and 3.0 to 0.25 mm respectively[1]. The ultrasound is coupled by degassed water between the source and the skin of the patient. Owing to the comparable acoustic properties of water and tissue the sound waves should penetrate the skin and further precursory tissue with only slight absorption and reflection. The power density of the converging ultrasound increases as it approaches the focal point (Figure 23.1.1). The interaction of acoustic energy and tissue causes thermonecrosis (Figs 23.1.2 and 23.1.3). To induce a clearly demarcated lesion the power density should be high enough and exceed 100 W/cm^2. This is sufficient to reach temperatures above 65°C within a pulse duration of less than 5 s. The size of the ablated tissue is around that of the physical focal zone but can be controlled within a limited range by power and duration of the ultrasound pulses. By scanning the target using multiple pulses, larger areas of tissue can be ablated. Diagnostic sonography by an additional integrated or adapted scanner is applied to position the focus within the target organ and to supervise the induced lesion.

Ablation of malignant tumors

The destruction of malignant tissue by focused ultrasound has been demonstrated by different sudies, but complete ablation is not achieved in all specimens[4]. The application of a new technique to such tumors with the risk of promoting metastasis must be discussed. Since ultrasound energy is not completely transferred to thermic and also to mechanical energy (cavitation effects), there is the possibility of cell mobilization causing them to enter the circulation. Until now, this hypothesis is controversely discussed in the literature. An early study revealed an increased metastasis rate of 17–44% after focused ultrasound application in contrast to control animals[5]. The rate of pulmonary metastasis after sonication of prostate cancer in rats was calculated to be 23% (3/13) and 15% (4/26) after sham treatment which was classified as comparable[6]. Further studies concluded that focused ultrasound does not increase metastatic spread of cancer significantly but may even reduce it[7–9]. A further positive effect was seen in the treatment induced alteration of the host response against cancer resulting in control of tumor not directly exposed to ultrasound[10–12].

Fig. 23.1.1   Principle of tissue ablation by focused ultrasound.

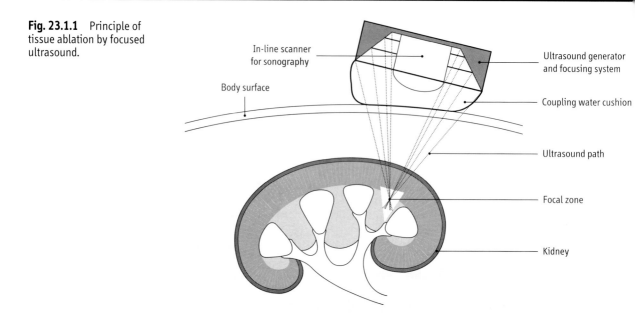

In-line scanner for sonography

Body surface

Ultrasound generator and focusing system

Coupling water cushion

Ultrasound path

Focal zone

Kidney

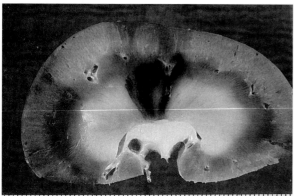

Fig. 23.1.2   Macroscopic aspect of the lesion in the in vivo canine kidney 10 days after ultrasound application.

Clinical application

The clinical application of focused ultrasound commenced in the early 1950s for neurosurgical indications in about 50 patients. After trepanation of the skull accurately positioned lesions were produced in the central nervous system[13]. A large series of 1117 sessions for treatment of glaucoma in 880 eyes was performed with a success rate of 79% after 1 year[14]. Up to now, six devices have proved suitable for clinical application. Four of them are primarily applied for urological disorders[15]. The Sonablate (Focal

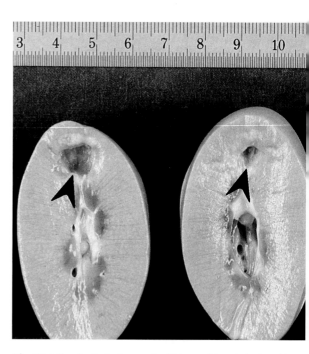

Fig. 23.1.3   Cavity in the ex vivo kidney of the pig induced by multiple pulses of focused ultrasound.

Surgary) generator with a focal depth up to 4.0 cm for transrectal application to the prostate could reach subjective and objective improvement in a phase II study including 50 patients with BPH[16]. The Ablatherm transrectal device (Technomed) was also focused to the prostate but aimed to control localized prostate cancer (see below). The Pyrothec (EDAP) generator with a diameter of 32 cm was used to destroy bladder, kidney and liver tissue by extracorporeal application[17].

Despite the discussion on promoting metastasis three study groups reported their clinical experience of ultrasound ablation in carcinomas. Recurrent superficial bladder tumors (12 patients) were treated using the Pyrothec generator. Marked alteration with intense congestion of the bladder mucosa and inflammatory changes of the underlying lamina propria were detected. In one patient, laceration and monocellular necrosis was observed in liver metastasis[17]. The transrectal treatment of prostate cancer using the Ablatherm achieved normalization of PSA and negative control biopsies reported in more than 200 patients treated so for[18,19].

Application to the kidney

In the experimental set-up ultrasound sources with a limited focal depth reached the kidneys of smaller animals, thus offering the possibility of sonablation in this organ. The 'transrectal' probe of the Sonablate can be used to ablate rabbit kidney tumors induced by injection of VX-2 tumor cell suspension in the renal segmental artery or into the lower pole parenchyma[20]. In phase 1 of this experi-

mental study, focused ultrasound was applied after eventration of the kidney under direct contact of the source to the kidney. Four hours after treatment, seven of nine insonated tumors showed macroscopical evidence of ablation. Histologically, in all nine rabbits, a well-defined area of renal and tumor tissue was damaged corresponding to the chosen regions. Tissue destruction was characterized by eosinophilic cytoplasm and separation of the cells. This was surrounded by hemorrhage. The area immediately adjacent to the targeted tissue was apparently normal. In phase 2, ultrasound was applied through the shaved skin of the flank. Thus, insufficient clarity of imaging the tumor was explained by indirect extracorporal application. One week later, four rabbits exhibited skin burns and only seven of nine kidneys showed gross or histologic tissue ablation. After this longer follow up time, nuclei were absent and the cytoplasm was pale pink in the damaged cells. Lymphocytes infiltrated from the border of the damaged area. Furthermore, coagulative necrosis, including mineralization and tubular atrophy, was described. Limited tumor localization by the 4 MHz diagnostic ultrasound and kidney movement due to ventilation were given as reasons for insufficient ablation by percutaneous ultrasound application. Using a power Doppler ultrasound and the Sonablate device targeting an area of 10 by 10 by 18 mm, a zone of tumor destruction was histologically demonstrated in all animals without severe side effects to

Table 23.1   Technical characterization of generators for clinical application of focused ultrasound

	Extracorporeal devices		Transrectal devices	
	Pyrothec	FOCUS	Sonablate	Ablatherm
	EDAP	STORZ Medical	Focus Surgery Inc.	Technomed
Generator				
Piezoelement	16 ceramics	1 cylindric ceramic	1 lead tilanate ceramic	1 ceramic
total size	ø 32 cm	ø10 cm	3 x 2.2 cm	ø 3.5 cm
power	-	≤ 400 Watt	≤ 25 Watt	-
frequency	1 MHz	1.07 MHz	4 MHz	2.25 Mhz
focusing system	spheric arrangement of multiple ceramics	cylindric ceramic + paraboloid reflector	spheric ceramic	spheric ceramic
Focus				
size	10 x 2 mm	10 x 1.5 mm	10 x 2 mm	8 x 1.5 mm
focal depth	320 mm	100 mm	25, 30, 35 or 40 mm	35 or 45 mm
power density	≤ 10,000 W/cm²	≤ 5,500 W/cm²	1260 - 2200 W/cm²	≤ 6300 W/cm²
Localization system	in-line sonography: 3.5 MHz, transrectal probe 7.5 MHz	in-line sonography: integrated 5 MHz	in-line sonography: central part of therapeutic probe ceramic 4 MHz	in-line sonography: 7.5 MHz probe
Application				
coupling	water cushion	water cushion	waterfilled condome	waterfilled condome
puls duration	0.015–60 s	0.1–10 s	4 s	1–10 s
repositioning	computer controled, motorized	free, manual controled	computer controled, motorized: longitudinal (45 mm), sector (40°) motion	computer controled, motorized

renal function[21]. In 124 rat and 16 canine kidneys localized coagulating necrosis or punched out cavities were induced by the 'transrectal' probe of the Ablatherm device. In 63% of canine kidneys this was achieved extracorporeally[22]. Using bowl-shaped transducers with a focal length of 10 and 15 cm respectively, it was shown that kidney tissue can be destroyed at depths of up to 10 cm in large animals (dogs, pigs) without damaging overlying structures[23,24].

In *clinical* practice, successful tissue ablation in the kidney demands a penetration depth of around 5 to 15 cm. This can only be provided by larger generators reaching higher power and longer focal depth. The Pyrothec[17] and two other sources[2,24] are recent constructions for this indication. Therefore, the number of patients treated by focused ulttrasound was limited. The Pyrothec was applied to kidney tissue to confirm experimental in vivo studies without therapeutic intention in eight patients: two cases of renal atrophy, one complex stone bearing kidney, five kidneys with cancer each requiring nephrectomy. Focused ultrasound was directed to renal parenchyma apart from tumor. Depth of the target tissue was 35 to 80 mm, treated volume 1 to 8 cm³. The applied dose was 110 to 314 shots with a pulse duration of 0.015 to 0.125 s each. Nephrectomy immediately (n = 5) or 2 to 3 days (n = 2) after application revealed moderate edema without hemorrhage of the perirenal fat (n = 2). In case of delayed operation, CT revealed a low-density zone and macroscopically blackish zone corresponding to the treated volume. Histologically, immediately after ultrasound application, intense congestion with severe hyperemia and marked alteration of the microcapillaries was observed. Two days later, additional early signs of limited subcapsular necrosis were demonstrated. A first and third grade skin burn are described as the only complications[17]. Figure 23.4 illustrates the ultrasound application to the kidney using an extracorporeal device (STORZ Medical). The patient in general anesthesia is positioned laterally as for nephrectomy. After primary evaluation of the best application route using an external diagnostic ultrasound probe, the therapeutic ultrasound source with its water cushion is coupled (Figure 23.1.4a). Contact is optimized by ultrasound gel. The inline diagnostic ultrasound scanner enables exact positioning of the focus within the kidney (Figure 23.1.4b). Focused ultrasound is applied with a dose of 10 pulses, each with a duration of 5 s and an interval of at least 20 s. During firing, ventilation of the patient is controlled by the anesthestist. The macroscopic aspect (Figure 23.1.4c) revealed distinct areas of tissue ablation within the treated area. Histologically the typical aspect of the thermolesion was found (Figure 23.1.4d).

As a perspective focused ultrasound will find many indications. With a curative intention it can be applied to small tumors which formerly were called adenomas.

Larger tumors with contraindicated surgical treatment or for suspected benign tumors (angiomyolipoma, oncocytoma) will be adequate fields of application. As a palliative procedure, this new technology will be a useful alternative to embolization.

Focused ultrasound is a promising but presently an experimental procedure. It will achieve access to clinical routine when technical problems concerning visualization of the target organ and lesion, protection from skin burns and precise control of lesion size have been solved.

Conclusions

Focused ultrasound induces thermal necrosis in the depth of the body without damaging skin and other precursory tissue. This is achieved by absorption of the high acoustic energy in the focus. Extracorporeally applied ultrasound generators are proved to destroy kidney tissue in

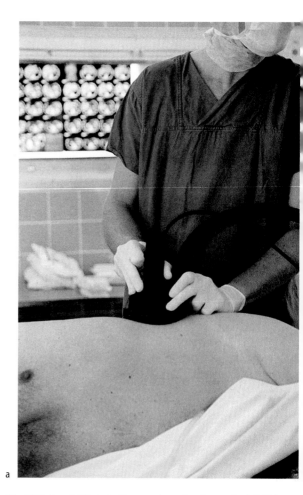

a

Fig. 23.1.4   a) Clinical ultrasound application to the left kidney (STORZ Medical device): a) coupling of the source.

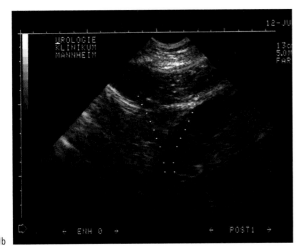

b) sonographic focus positioning;

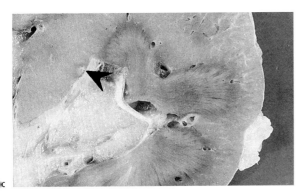

c) macroscopic aspect of the lesion in the humen kidney (Courtesy of W. Back, Institute of Pathology, Mannheim, Germany);

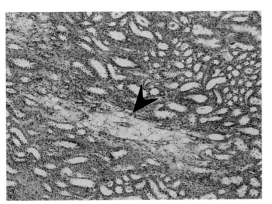

d) histologic aspect of the lesion (Courtesy of W. Back, Institute of Pathology, Mannheim, Germany)

the experimental clinical set-up. This is a promising technique for minimal invasive ablation of renal tissue in the treatment of benign and malignant diseases.

References

1. Fry FJ. Intense focused ultrasound in medicine. *Eur Urol* 1993;**23**:2–7.
2. ter Haar GR, Robertson G. Tissue destruction with focused ultrasound in vivo. *Eur Urol* 1993;**23**:8–11.
3. Susani M, Madersbacher S, Kratzik Ch, Vingers L, Marberger M. Morphology of tissue destruction induced by focused ultrasound. *Eur Urol* 1993;**23**:34–38.
4. Gelet A, Chapelon JY. Effects of high-intensity focused ultrasound on malignant cells and tissues. In Marberger M, Madersbacher S (eds) *Newer forms of energy in urology.* Isis Medical Media, Oxford, 1995.
5. Fry FJ, Johnson LK. Tumor iradiation with intense ultrasound. *Ultrasound Med Biol* 1978;**4**:377–341.
6. Oosterhof GON, Cornel EB, Smits GAHJ, Debruyne FMJ, Schalken JA. The influence of physical exposure on metastatic spread of prostate cancer. *J Urol* 1995;**153**(Abstract 613).
7. Yang R, Reilly DR, Rescorla FJ, Sanghvi NT, Fry FJ, Franklin TD, Grosfeld JL. High intensity focused ultrasound in the treatment of experimental liver cancer. *Arch Surg* 191;**126**:1002–1010.
8. Goss SA, Fry FJ. The effects of high intensity ultrasonic irradiation on tumor growth. *IEEE Trans Sonics Ultrasonics* 1984;**31**:491–496.
9. Chapelon JY, Margonary J, Vernier F Gorry F, Ecochard R. Gelet A. In vivo effects of high intensity ultrasound on prostatic adenocarcinoma Dunning R3327. *Cancer Res* 1992;**52**:6353–6357.
10. Dimitrieva NP. Resorption of not exposed metastases following the effect of ultrasound of high intensity on Brown-Pierce tumors in rabbits. *Biull Eksp Biol Med* 1957;**44**:81–85.
11. Kaketa K, Bagai , Mizuno S *et al.* Annual report (1971) Tokyo: Medical Ultrasonics Research Center Tokyo, Juntendo University School of Medicine 1971;
12. Yang R, Reilly CR, Rescorla F *et al.* Effects of high intensity focused ultrasound in the treatment of experimental neuroblastoma. *J Pediatr Surg* 1992;**27**:246–251.
13. Fry WJ, Barnard JW, Fry FJ, Krumins RF, Brennan JF. Ultrasonic lesions in the mammalian central nervous system. *Science* 1955;**122**:517–518.
14. Silverman RH, Vogelsang B, Rondeau MJ, Coleman J. Therapeutic ultrasound for the treatment of glaucoma. *Am J Ophthal* 1991;**111**:327–337.
15. Köhrmann KU, Michel MS, Rassweiler J, Alken P. Focused ultrasound. In: Smith AD, (ed) *Smith's textbook of endourology,* Quality Medical Publishing, St Louis, 1996.
16. Madersbacher S, Kratzik Ch, Susani M, Marberger M. Tissue ablation in benign prostatic hyperplasia with high intensity focused ultrasound. *J Urol* 1994;**152**:1956–1961.
17. Vallancien G, Harouni M, Veillon B, Mombet A, Prapotnich D, Brisset JM, Bougaran J. Focused extracorporeal pyrotherapy: Feasibility study in man. *J Endourol* 1992;**6**:173–181.
18. Gelet A, Chapelon JY, Bouvier R, Souchon R, Pangaud C, Abdelrahin AF, Cathignol D, Dubernard JM. Treatment of prostate cancer with transrectal focused ultrasound: early clinical experience. *Eur Urol* 1996;**29**:174–183.
19. Madersbacher S, Pedevilla M, Vingers L, Susani M, Marberger M. Effect of high-intensity focused ultrasound on human prostate cancer in vivo. *Cancer Res* 1995;**55**:3346–3351.
20. Adams JB, Moore RG, Anderson JH, Strandberg JD, Marshall FF, Kavoussi LR. High-intensity focused ultrasound ablation of rabbit kidney tumors. *J Endourol* 1996;**1**:71–75.
21. Averch TD, Adams JB, Anderson JH, Strandberg RD, Moore RG, Kavoussi LR, Marshall FF. Transcutaneous ablation of rabbit tumors utilizing high intensity focused ultrasound. *J Urol* 1996;**155**(Abstract 932).

22. Chapelon JY, Morgonary J, Theillere Y, Gorry F, Vernier F, Blanc E, Gelet A. Effects of high-energy focused ultrasound on kidney tissue in the rat and the dog. *Eur Urol* 1992;**22**:147–152.
23. ter Haar GR, Vaughan MG, Hill CR. In vivo destruction of porcine bladder and renal tissue using high intensity focussed ultrasound. *J Urol* 1992;**1148**:(Abstract 188).
24. Köhrmann U, Back W, Kahmann F, Michel MS, Rassweiler J, Alken P. Morphological aspect of tissue lesions induced by focused ultrasound on different organs. *J Urol* 1995;**153**(Abstract 1222).

23.2 Focused microwave ablation and cryotherapy

E Keahey and J W Basler

Microwave therapy

The microwave tissue coagulator, a proven method in solid vascular organs, has been applied in the setting of open partial nephrectomy. Traditional surgery, with clamping of the renal pedicle, results in renal ischemia, which increases the chance of acute tubular necrosis post-operatively. With the use of microwave tissue coagulation, there is no loss of blood flow to the unaffected parenchyma, and subsequently no increased risk of acute tubular necrosis[1]. The technique described involves isolating the kidney using techniques similar to a partial radical nephrectomy. Blunt dissection exposes the perirenal fat, being careful to leave the perirenal fat overlying the tumor as much as possible. Ultrasound can be used to check for satellite tumors and verify the region to be coagulated. Tissue coagulation was performed with 5 to 8 mm margins, at 5 to 8 mm intervals. The renal parenchyma could then be cut with scissors in the coagulated area. Pathologic evaluation of the resection margins can be performed intraoperatively by frozen section. Indigo carmine injected into the ureter allows for detection and suturing of ruptured areas of the collecting system. After repair, the cut surface of the kidney is covered with fibrin glue and surrounding fatty tissue replaced over the defect. The coagulation results in little or no blood loss at the operative site.

Combining a laparoscopic approach with a non-ischemia producing partial nephrectomy may be less traumatic overall to the patient and residual renal function. Indeed, Winfield *et al.* pursued this approach by combining laparoscopic partial nephrectomy, without renal pedicle clamping, and hemostasis via an argon beam coagulator[2]. Banya *et al.* took this one step further, describing the use of microwave tissue coagulation with laparoscopic partial nephrectomy in dogs[3]. As more experience is gained with the technique, laparoscopic partial nephrec-

tomy with use of the microwave tissue coagulator could become preferred for treatment of patients requiring nephron-sparing surgery.

Cryotherapy

While literature abounds on cryotherapy for hepatic, prostatic and other solid organ tumors, there is only one report in the general literature concerning its use in the kidney[4]. This feasibility study, performed on sheep, suggests that the procedure can be performed safely with preservation of renal function. Theoretically, cryotherapy, like microwave and ultrasound ablation, could be used to destroy solitary or multiple lesions in situations where nephrectomy may be less desirable. Obviously, more work needs to be done before any of these techniques come into the mainstream of urologic practice.

References

1. Kagebayashi Y, Hirao Y, Samma S, Fukui Y, Hirohashi R. In situ non-ischemic enucleation of multilocular cystic renal cell carcinoma using a microwave tissue coagulator. *Int J Urol* 1995;**2**(5):3399–3343.
2. Winfield HN, Donovan JF, Lund GO, Kreder KJ, Stanley KE, Brown BP, Loening SA, Clayman RV. Laparoscopic partial nephrectomy: initial experience and comparison to the open surgical approach. *J Urol* 1995;**153**(5):1409–1414.
3. Banya Y, Kajikawa T, Kanai H, Tamura T, Sugimura J, Hatafuku F, Kubo T. Laparoscopic partial nephrectomy in a canine model: application of microwave tissue coagulation technique. *J Microwave Surg*, 1996;**14**:7.
4. Cozzi PJ, Lynch WJ, Collins S, Vonthethoff L, Morris DL, Renal cryotherapy in a sheep model; a feasibility study. *Urology* 1997;**157**(2):710–712.

23.3 Laparoscopic surgery

R V Clayman, D Hoenig and E M McDougall

Introduction

Major changes are afoot in the realm of surgery. Progress in ablative surgery from a maximally invasive approach to minimally invasive procedures and eventually to non-invasive treatments is occurring in all surgical disciplines. These changes are best viewed in the recent alteration in the approach to surgical urolithiasis which has undergone two paradigm shifts in the last 20 years. First in the late 1970s and early 1980s came the transformation of a century old maximally invasive surgical approach to a minimally invasive percutaneous or ureteroscopic. Next, in the mid 1980s came the conversion from minimally invasive to non-invasive procedures in the form of extracorporeal shock wave lithotripsy. Similar changes are now afoot in he realm of renal ablative surgery, for benign and, most recently, malignant disease. Whether here too the minimally invasive approach will eventually be superseded by progress in even less invasive or non-invasive modalities is difficult to predict, however work in both areas has already begun[1-3].

Background

In 1869, Gustav Simon performed the initial nephrectomy in Heidelberg, Germany, thereby curing the ravages of a post-ovariectomy vesicoureteral fistula. In the subsequent 100 years, the success of ablative open renal surgery benefited greatly from advances in anesthesia, analgesia and antibiotics. Interestingly, aside from technical nuances with regard to approaching the diseased kidney, little change occurred in the basic surgical technique or instrumentation used for the nephrectomy procedure[4].

The first development of a minimally invasive technique occurred in June of 1990 when Clayman, Kavoussi and associates at Washington University performed a laparoscopic total nephrectomy in an 85-year-old woman with a 5 cm oncocytic tumor. Following this report laparoscopic techniques for simple nephrectomy rapidly proliferated. Both laparoscopic transperitoneal and soon thereafter December, 1990; Washington Unviersity) laparoscopic retroperitoneal simple nephrectomies were successfully accomplished at many urological institutions. To date, more than 500 of these procedures have been performed world-wide[5,6].

Laparoscopic simple nephrectomy for removal of the benign kidney has now been carefully compared with open surgical nephrectomy by many clinical investigators. In all series, the laparoscopic approach resulted in a significant decrease in blood loss, use of less parenteral analgesics, a shorter hospital stay and a more rapid convalescence. Complication rates for this approach have been similar or less. The only drawback to the technique has been the longer operative times needed and the higher cost. Both of these problems are gradually being overcome by increased operator experience and streamlining of the technique[7-9].

While laparoscopic simple nephrectomy for benign disease has become a widespread and well accepted procedure, the application of these same techniques to renal malignancy is as yet in its controversial infancy. To date, the anecdotal pioneering efforts of multiple investigators have been documented; each form of renal surgery for renal cancer has now been performed laparoscopically: renal biopsy, wedge excision, partial nephrectomy, total nephrectomy and radical nephrectomy. However, in no instance has any of these procedures become widespread. This acceptance awaits the development of larger series, longer follow up, and careful comparison with a contemporary series of like patients.

Current status

In discussing the application of laparoscopic techniques to renal malignancy, the first order of business is to separate the 'possible' from the 'reasonable'. Indeed as previously noted all currently available open surgical techniques for diagnosing and treating renal malignancy have already been accomplished laparoscopically. However, it is one thing to perform a procedure for the first time, and quite another to develop, critique, and compare it to a point whereby it gains widespread acceptance; the former is the realm of the pioneering surgeon whereas the latter belongs to the surgeon scientist.

At present all of the aforementioned procedures are 'possible', it is their 'reasonableness' that remains unsettled. In order to evaluate a procedure from the standpoint of its reasonableness, the laparoscopic approach must be carefully compared with the results of open surgical techniques in a contemporary group of similar patients. In this regard, both approaches need to be evaluated with respect to four areas: efficacy, efficiency, morbidity and cost. Efficacy, or 'getting the right job done', addresses specimen size, completeness of the surgical excision, and achieving proper pathological assessment of the disease. The efficiency of the procedure, 'getting the job done right', has to do with the operating room time and the hospital stay. With regard to morbidity, the complications of the procedure as well as the use of postoperative analgesics and length of convalescence are considered. Lastly with respect to costs, the tangible monetary expenditure for the procedure needs to be considered; ideally this should include costs for hospitalization, equipment, operative time and complications. Unfortunately, the intangible costs of time to return to work and time to full recovery are never included in this analysis.

Diagnosis

In the diagnosis of renal cell cancer, there really is little if any role for laparoscopic surgery. In today's world the diagnosis of renal tumor is made in the vast majority of patients via the combination of intravenous urography, computed tomography, renal ultrasonography and/or magnetic resonance imaging. In those few cases in which the nature of a renal mass is in doubt, percutaneous renal biopsy under computed tomographic control or ultrasonographic control almost invariably resolves the problem. Indeed, while laparoscopic renal biopsy has been reported on one occasion for diagnosis of underlying renal disease, there are no published reports on renal biopsy of a known renal mass for the sake of diagnosis[10].

317

Treatment of renal cell cancer

Wedge excision

Overall wedge excision is a relatively rarely performed procedure for dealing with renal cell cancer. As such, it is not surprising that the total reported experience with laparoscopic wedge excision of a renal mass consists of only case reports[11,12,13]. Both were performed using a retroperitoneal approach. An operating time of 2 hours was noted with blood loss of less than 100 cc. Hemostasis was achieved using the Argon beam coagulator and specially prepared 'plugs' of hemostatic material[11]. In one detailed case report the patient left the hospital on the third post-operative morning and required no post-operative analgesics. Regular activity was resumed within 1 week post-operatively. Final pathology showed a low-grade granular cell cancer; the margin was negative for tumor. While these early anecdotal reports are promising, many additional case reports are needed prior to even beginning to compare this approach with its open surgical counterpart.

Partial nephrectomy

Interest in nephron-sparing procedures for renal cell cancer has grown rapidly over the past 5 years. Presently there are multiple reports revealing that the nephron-sparing approach for tumors less than 5 cm in size achieves 5 year survival results similar to a radical nephrectomy. Although it is a more difficult procedure to perform than radical nephrectomy, the virtues of a nephron-sparing procedure lie in the decreased chance of renal insufficiency in later life should a contralateral tumor or other renal disease develop. The concern over multicentric lesions and recurrence of cancer in the renal remnant is the one major objection to this approach. Multicentricity is noted in upwards of 20–25% of radical nephrectomy specimens; however follow up at 5 years has failed to show clinically detectable lesions or decreased survival[14–17]. Nonetheless, careful surveillance with a CT scan every 6 months for recurrence of cancer in the renal remnant is currently recommended.

Laparoscopic partial nephrectomy has only been reported anecdotally. The largest series consists of only six cases reported by Winfield and colleagues[18]. In only one of the six cases was the procedure attempted for excision of a renal tumor; in this case, the procedure had to be converted from a laparoscopic to an open procedure. Of the remaining five cases, one of the patients was found on frozen section to have an unsuspected focus of renal cancer and thus was converted to an open procedure. As such, in the overall series a third of the patients had to be converted to an open procedure; in both instances these were patients with renal tumors. Of the remaining four patients, all with benign disease, the operative time averaged 6.1 h with an estimated blood loss of 525 cc.

It is of note that 52 mg of morphine sulfate analgesics were required and the hospital stay was 8.25 days with a 2.25 week convalescence. When these authors compared their laparoscopic experience with a contemporary group of patients undergoing open partial nephrectomy, the operative time was almost twice as long, however, the use of analgesics was half as much and the convalescence was decreased almost fourfold. However the hospital stay was unchanged at 8 days. Based on these results the authors concluded that even for benign disease laparoscopic partial nephrectomy was a 'technically intensive procedure fraught with difficulty' and it 'should not be considered routine or state of the art' at this point in time.

With regard to laparoscopic partial nephrectomy for malignant renal disease to date there are only two reported successful cases. In one case, an 80 year old gentleman with an incidentally discovered 2 cm left lower pole renal mass underwent a 7.3 h procedure with an estimated blood loss of 150 cc. The pathology specimen revealed an oncocytoma; the surgical margins were negative for tumor. The patient spent 9 days in the hospital. The case was complicated by a nephrocutaneous fistula that resolved with percutaneous drainage[19]. The other case report was found among a wide range of laparoscopic procedures and no details of the case were provided[13]. As with wedge excision of a renal lesion, the laparoscopic partial nephrectomy for renal malignancy remains investigational and anecdotal.

It is obvious that in order to improve the efficiency of these laparoscopic procedures newer instrumentation and increased operator experience are essential. With regard to the former, extensive research in pigs has been performed on the development of an electrosurgical cutting snare and the use of various ultrasound dissecting and resecting probes to excise renal tissue[20]. Unfortunately, to date, the ultrasonic forms of energy while capable of removing renal tissue are slow and associated with significant blood loss. In contrast, the electrosurgical snare had the greatest potential for the rapid removal and hemostasis of renal tissue; with this device a lower pole partial nephrectomy could be completed in under a minute. Of note was a minimal depth of injury of only 0.8 mm thereby sparing as much renal parenchyma as possible. This snare has subsequently been used twice clinically, however it performed poorly, perhaps due to the larger size of the human kidney. Obviously, further refinements are necessary, however, this is the beginning of perhaps additional instrumentation that could be brought to bear on the problem of performing a laparoscopic partial nephrectomy.

Radical nephrectomy

Presently, 68 cases of laparoscopic radical or total nephrectomy have been reported world-wide for suspected renal cell cancer. The average operative time has been 5.7 h with an estimated blood loss of 352 cc. The oral intake has usually begun within the first 24 h following surgery. Use of post-operative analgesia has been minimal with only 20 mg of morphine sulfate on average and the mean hospital stay has been 6.6 days. The average time to return to normal activity has been 3.5 weeks. While in most cases, tumors were less than 5 cm in size, it is of note that tumors as large as 10 cm as well as tumors invading the renal vein have been successfully removed laparoscopically[13,21–28].

There have been two publications in which the laparoscopic and open approaches were directly compared. In 1993, Kavoussi, Clayman and colleagues compared their initial experience with eight laparoscopic radical nephrectomies with 58 patients undergoing open radical nephrectomy; in all cases the renal tumors were less than 6 cm in size. The average age of the patients was similar as was their surgical risk. The laparoscopic procedure at that time, being quite new, required 7.5 h of surgery versus only 2.7 h for the open procedure. However, among the laparoscopic patients the estimated blood loss was less (295 cc versus 410 cc) as was the post-operative use of parenteral analgesics (15 mg of morphine sulfate equivalent versus 145 mg of morphine sulfate equivalent). Also in the laparoscopic group, the hospital stay was shorter (5.2 days versus 7.5 days) and return to normal activities was quicker (3 weeks versus 7.1 weeks)[22]. More recently McDougall, Clayman and Elashry compared 12 open with 12 laparoscopic radical nephrectomies performed during a similar period of time at Washington University School of Medicine. All patients had pT1 or pT2 tumors. The average operating time was 6.9 h in the laparoscopic group versus 2.2 h in the open group; the estimated blood loss was similar in the two groups. Post-operative complications of a major or minor nature were similar in both groups: 8% major and 18% minor complications. Of note, however, was a statistically significant decrease in the amount of post-operative pain medications used in the laparoscopic group (24 mg of morphine sulfate versus 40 mg of morphine sulfate plus ketoralac 15 mg), earlier oral intake (1 day versus 3 days), shorter hospital stay (4.5 days versus 8.4 days), decreased time to return to normal activity (3.5 weeks versus 5.1 weeks), and more rapid full recovery (5.8 weeks versus 39 weeks)[28].

In both studies, the efficacy of the procedure was found to be equivalent to open surgery with a marked decrease in the morbidity (i.e. analgesics and convalescence). However, the efficiency of the procedure was found to be lacking due to the prolonged operating time despite the markedly shortened hospital stay. With regard to cost, hospital charges for both groups were examined in the second study, and the operating room charges for open radical nephrectomy were only a third that of the laparoscopy group ($3309 versus $10 090). However, due to the prolonged hospital stay and other complicating factors in the open group, the overall charges for open radical nephrectomy were $16 620 compared with $18 470 for laparoscopic radical nephrectomy. In this regard, it needs to be stressed that with increased surgeon experience, the operative time for this procedure has slowly decreased from 7.5 h in the first study to 6.9 h in the second study. This trend has continued such that among the most recent six laparoscopic radical nephrectomies performed in 1995–1996, at Washington University, the operative time has dropped to 5.6 h; associated with this decreased operative time has also been a fall in hospital stay to only 2.4 days. These changes have decreased the charges another $1000 thus making the laparoscopic radical nephrectomy economically competitive with the open radical nephrectomy.

From the standpoint of the efficiency and cost of the procedure, this can be markedly improved if a laparoscopic assisted procedure is performed. The 7–10 cm incision used to retrieve the specimen is made at the outset of the procedure, allowing for manual dissection of the operative site throughout the procedure[23,24,26,27]. With this approach, operative times as brief as 2 to 3 h have been reported, which is no different from the time necessary to perform an open radical nephrectomy.

From the patient's standpoint, this is a step in the right direction as the decreased pain, improved cosmesis, shortened hospital stay and more rapid convalescence are all desirable features of the laparoscopic procedure. However, there are several as yet unsettled concerns with regard to the laparoscopic approach to malignant disease: adequacy of the specimen, the ability to stage and grade the disease, and concerns over seeding of the peritoneal cavity or port sites from the tumor specimen. With regard to adequacy of the specimen, the laparoscopic approach is certainly satisfactory. McDougall, Clayman and Elashry noted that in comparing patients with pT1 and pT2 renal cell cancer undergoing laparoscopic or open radical nephrectomy, the laparoscopic group had a 65% larger specimen then the open group (514 g versus 311 g)[28]. Part of the reason for this discrepancy is that the laparoscopic approach affords the surgeon a greater ability to visualize the hepatic ligaments on the right side and as such the nephrectomy specimen encompasses all the tissue from the supra-adrenal cava downward. Likewise, on the left side the surgeon is able to incise the lienocolic as well as the lienophrenic ligaments and again obtain a large specimen incorporating all of the perirenal and pararenal fat and Gerota's fascia.

With regard to staging and grading the tumor and the concerns about seeding, many surgeons have answered this problem by removing the free or entrapped laparoscopic surgical specimen intact. As such, the specimen is removed directly or placed in an impermeable entrapment sack and then delivered whole through a 7 to 10 cm incision.[23,24,26–28]. This provides an intact specimen for the pathologist while, in theory, reducing any chance of wound seeding since the specimen does not come into contact with the incision.

However, others have not chosen to answer the question of staging, grading and seeding with intact specimen removal. Instead, in an effort to decrease procedural morbidity, these surgeons have eschewed making a 7–10 cm incision and have championed in situ morcellation of the entrapped specimen in an impermeable entrapment sack (LapSac, Cook Urological Inc., Spencer, Indiana)[28]. Earlier animal laboratory studies by Urban and colleagues revealed that high-speed electrical tissue morcellation of the kidney in a specially designed entrapment sack was safe[29]. Following morcellation, testing of the integrity of the sack with cells, bacteria and indigo carmine revealed no leakage from the sack of any material into the surrounding dialysate. As such, based on these findings, Clayman and colleagues at Washington University as well as Kavoussi and colleagues at Johns Hopkins have continued to morcellate the entrapped tumor specimen in the sack. The morcellated tissue has been adequate for tumor grading but accurate staging cannot be obtained with this method. In the authors' opinion, until stage specific adjunctive chemotherapy is shown to be a beneficial treatment modality, the pathological staging will remain only of academic interest.

With the practice of morcellation, seeding remains a major concern. However, to date, with follow up to 5 years, there has been only one case of post-operative peritoneal or trocar site malignant implantation of renal cell cancer at any institution. Indeed, it would appear that seeding of the peritoneal cavity or of a port site with tumor cells requires direct contact with the malignant tissue. As such, most of the cases reported in the world's literature have to do with carcinoma of the ovary, gallbladder or colon in which direct peritoneal contact with the surface of the tumor has been made or in which the tumor was biopsied[30–32]. In the realm of urology to date there are only three other case reports of seeding after a laparoscopic procedure: one from prostate cancer and two associated with bladder cancer. In each case the bare tumor had been removed intact or piecemeal through a port site[33–35]. Of note, peritoneal seeding following any laparoscopic urological procedure has yet to be reported.

To settle the controversy of intact removal versus morcellation, two bits of data are needed. First, longer follow up in both groups is necessary; any sign of seeding in either group will be sufficient to condemn that specific approach. Secondly, the morcellated and intact removal groups need to be carefully compared with regard to post-operative (e.g. incisional pain, wound infection) and long-term (i.e. incisional hernia) morbidity. Indeed if the laparoscopic-assisted approach can be shown to have no significant increased morbidity versus the pure laparoscopic approach, then the savings in operating room time, reduced hospital costs, improved pathology assessment and reduced risk of seeding would make the laparoscopic-assisted approach the preferred method.

Surgical future

Minimally invasive surgery is moving like a vortex throughout the surgical realm. Currently we are only on the outer edge of the vortex, however, there are forces afoot that will carry us deeper into this exciting field. In the realm of ablative surgery, the time and energy required to 'excise' the specimen from the patient may soon be replaced with the philosophy of merely destroying the tumor tissue in situ. Already, laboratory studies have shown successful ablation of normal and malignant tissues using laparoscopically or fluoroscopically guided cryotherapy probes or microwave probes[2,3].

However, at the very center of this vortex lies the demise of minimally invasive surgery; indeed, as this force field implodes our energies will become concentrated in creating a new field: non-invasive ablative surgery. Laboratory and clinical ablative studies have already been completed with energy sources that can be directed from outside the body to focus upon and destroy diseased tissue deep within the body. High intensity focused ultrasound and piezoelectric energy have both been successfully used to treat benign and malignant prostatic tissue and bladder tumors [1, 36]. Given the current pace of progress, the two problems inherent in this approach, resolution and accurate energy delivery, should soon be solved. The day is truly not too far distant when the 'surgeon' treating a renal tumor will merely sit down at a high resolution MRI or CT screen and proceed to outline the lesion; with the press of a button, all designated tissue would then be systematically destroyed using an extracorporeal energy source.

If as physicians our goal is to relieve pain and suffering while prolonging life, then we must continue to seek out those advances that will provide our patients with the greatest good for the least harm. In this way we find ourselves in the unusual situation of realizing our goals by eliminating the very skills we have trained so long and hard to acquire. Primum non nocere!

References

1. Vallancien G, Harouni M, Veillon B, Mombet A, Prapotnich D, Brisset JM, Bougaran J. Focused extracorporeal pyrotherapy: Feasibility study in man. *J Endo* 1992;**6**:173–183.
2. Delworth MG, Pisters LL, Fornage BD, von Eschenback AC. Cryotherapy for renal cell carcinoma and angiomyolipoma. *J Urol* 1996;**155**: 252–255.

3. Seki T, Inoue K. Microwave coagulation therapy of hepatocellular carcinoma. *Nippon Naika Gakkai Zasshi* 1995;**84**:2024–2027.

4. Murphy L]T. The kidney. In: *The history of urology.* Charles C. Thomas 1972;**8**:191–271.

5. Clayman RV, Kavoussi LR, Soper NJ, Dierks SM, Meretyk S, Darcy MD, Roemer FD, Pingleton ED, *et al.* Laparoscopic nephrectomy: initial case report. *J Urol* 1991;**146**:278–282.

6. Gill IS, Clayman RV, McDougall EM. State of the art: Advances in urological laparoscopy. *J Urol* 1995;**154**:1275–1294.

7. Winfield HN, Rashid TM, Lund GO, Troxel SA, Donovan]F. Comparative financial analysis of laparoscopic versus open nephrectomy. *J Urol* 1994;**151**:342A.

8. Parra RO, Perez MG, Boullier JA, Cummings JM. Comparison between standard flank versus laparoscopic nephrectomy for benign renal disease. *J Urol* 1995;**153**:1171–1174.

9. Kerbl K, Clayman RV, McDougall EM, Gill IS, Wilson BS, Chandhoke PS, Albala DM, Kavoussi LR. Transperitoneal nephrectomy for benign disease of the kidney: A comparison between laparoscopic and open surgical techniques. *Urol* 1994;**43**:607–613.

10. Squadrito]F]r, Coletta AV. Laparoscopic renal exploration and biopsy. *J Lap Surg* 1991;**1**:235–239.

11. McDougall EM, Clayman RV, Anderson K. Laparoscopic wedge resection of a renal tumor: Initial experience. *J Lap Surg* 1994;**3**:577–583.

12. Luciani RC, Greiner M, Clement]C, Houot A, Didierlaurent]F. Laparoscopic enucleation of a renal cell carcinoma. *Surg Endosc* 1994;**8**:1329–1331.

13. Gasman D, Saint F, Barthelemy Y, Antiphon P, Chopin D, Abbou CC. Retroperitoneoscopy: A laparoscopic approach for adrenal and renal surgery. *Urology* 1996;**47**:801–806.

14. Mukamel E, Konichezky M, Engelstein D, Servadio C. Incidental small renal tumors accompanying clinical overt renal cell carcinoma. *J Urol* 1998;**140**:22–24.

15. Whang M, O'Toole, K, Bixon R, Brunetti], Ikeguchi E, Olsson CA, Sawczuk TS, Benson MC. The incidence of multifocal renal cell carcinoma in patients who are candidates for partial nephrectomy. *J Urol* 1995;**154**:968–971.

16. Licht MR, Novick AC, Goormastic M. Nephron sparing surgery in incidental versus suspected renal cell carcinoma. *J Urol* 1994;**152**:39–42.

17. Morgan WR, Zincke H. Progression and survival after renal-conservative surgery for renal cell carcinoma: experience in 104 patients and extended follow-up. *J Urol* 1990;**144**:852–858.

18. Winfield HN, Donovan]F, Lund GO, Kreder KJ, Stanley KE, Brown BP, Loening SA, Clayman RV. Laparoscopic partial nephrectomy: Initial experience and comparison to the open surgical approach. *J Urol* 1995;**153**:1409–1415.

19. Elashry OM, Wolf]r]S, McDougall EM, Clayman RV. Laparoscopic partial nephrectomy of a renal tumor using a new instrument. *J Lap Surg* 1996 (submitted)

20. Elashry OM, Wolf]r]S, Rayala HJ, McDougall EM, Clayman RV. Recent advances in laparoscopic partial nephrectomy: comparative study of electrosurgical snare electrode and ultrasound dissection. *J Urol* 1997;**11**:15–22

21. Matsuda, T Terachi T, Mikami O, Komatz Y, Yoshida O. Laparoscopic nephrectomy with lymphadenectomy for renal cell carcinoma: Initial two cases. *Min Invas Therapy* 1993;**2**:221–226.

22. Kavoussi LR, Kerbl K, Capelouto CC, McDougall EM, Clayman RV. Laparoscopic nephrectomy for renal neoplasms. *Urology* 1993;603–610.

23. Suzuki K, Ihara H, Kurita Y, Kageyman S, Masuda H, Ushiyama T, Ohtawara Y, Kawabe K. Laparoscopy-assisted radical nephrectomy without pneumoperitoneum. *Eur Urol* 1994;**25**:237–241.

24. Tierney]P, Oliver SR, Kusminsky RE, Tiley EH, Boland]P. Laparoscopic radical nephrectomy with intra-abdominal manipulation. *Min Invas Therapy* 1994;**3**:303–307.

25. Kinukawa T, Hattori R, Ono Y, Kato N, Hirabayashi S, Ohshima S, Matsuura O. Laparoscopic radical nephrectomy. Analysis of 10 cases and preliminary report of retroperitoneal approach. *Nippon Hinyokika Gakkai Zasshi* 1995;**86**:1625–1630.

26. Suzuki K, Masuda H, Ushiyama T, Hata M, Fujita K, Kawabe K. Gasless laparoscopy-assisted nephrectomy without tissue morcellation for renal carcinoma. *J Urol* 1995;**154**:1685–1687.

27. Nishiyama T, Terunuma M. Laparoscopy-assisted radical nephrectomy in combination with minilaparotomy: report of initial 7 cases. Int *J Urol* 1995;**2**:124–127.

28. McDougall EM, Clayman RV, Elashry OM. Laparoscopic radical nephrectomy for renal tumor. The Washington University experience. *J Urol* 1996;**155**:1180–1185.

29. Urban DA, Kerbl K, McDougall EM, Stone AM, Fadden PT, Clayman RV. Organ entrapment and renal morcellation: Permeability studies. *J Urol* 1993; **150**:1792–1795.

30. Clair DG, Lautz DB, Brooks DC. Rapid development of umbilical metastases after laparoscopic cholecystectomy for unsuspected gallbladder carcinoma. *Surg* 1993;**113**:355–358.

31. Gleeson NC, Nicosia SV, Mark]E, Hoffman MS, Cavanagh D. Abdominal wall metastases from ovarian cancer after laparoscopy. Am *J Obstet Gynecol* 1993;**169**:522–523.

32. Fodera M, Pello MJ, Atabek U, Spence RK, Alexander]B, Camishion RC. Trocar site tumor recurrence after laparoscopic-assisted colectomy. *J Lap Surg* 1995;**5**:259–263.

33. Andersen]R, Steven K. Implantation metastasis after laparoscopic biopsy of bladder cancer. *J Urol* 1995;**153**:1047–1048.

34. Stolla V, Rossi D, Bladou F, Rattier C, Ayuso D, Serment G. Subcutaneous metastases after coelioscopic lymphadenectomy for vesical urothelial carcinoma. *Eur Urol* 1994;**26**:342–3.

35. Bangma CH, Kirkels WJ, Chadha S, Schroeder FH. Cutaneous metastasis following laparoscopic pelvic lymphadenectomy for prostatic carcinoma. *J Urol* 1995;**153**:1635–1636.

36. Madersbacher S, Kratzik C, Susani M, Marberger M. Tissue ablation in benign prostatic hyperplasia with high intensity focused ultrasound. *J Urol* 1994;**152**:1956–1962.

24 Metastatic renal cancer

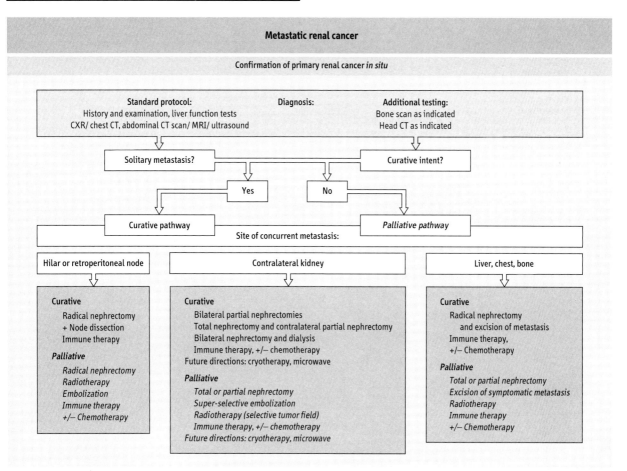

Metastatic renal cancer

Confirmation of primary renal cancer *in situ*

Standard protocol:	Diagnosis:	Additional testing:
History and examination, liver function tests CXR/ chest CT, abdominal CT scan/ MRI/ ultrasound		Bone scan as indicated Head CT as indicated

Solitary metastasis? — Curative intent?

Yes — No

Curative pathway — *Palliative pathway*

Site of concurrent metastasis:

Hilar or retroperitoneal node	Contralateral kidney	Liver, chest, bone
Curative Radical nephrectomy + Node dissection Immune therapy *Palliative* *Radical nephrectomy* *Radiotherapy* *Embolization* *Immune therapy* *+/– Chemotherapy*	**Curative** Bilateral partial nephrectomies Total nephrectomy and contralateral partial nephrectomy Bilateral nephrectomy and dialysis Immune therapy, +/– chemotherapy Future directions: cryotherapy, microwave *Palliative* *Total or partial nephrectomy* *Super-selective embolization* *Radiotherapy (selective tumor field)* *Immune therapy, +/– chemotherapy* *Future directions: cryotherapy, microwave*	**Curative** Radical nephrectomy and excision of metastasis Immune therapy, +/– Chemotherapy *Palliative* *Total or partial nephrectomy* *Excision of symptomatic metastasis* *Radiotherapy* *Immune therapy* *+/– Chemotherapy*

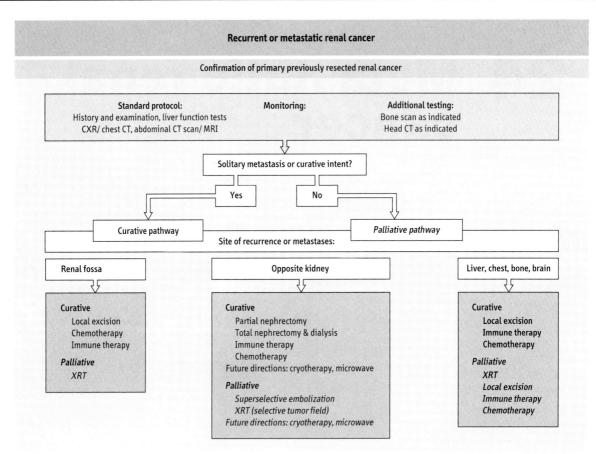

Recurrent or metastatic renal cancer

Confirmation of primary previously resected renal cancer

Standard protocol:	**Monitoring:**	**Additional testing:**
History and examination, liver function tests		Bone scan as indicated
CXR/ chest CT, abdominal CT scan/ MRI		Head CT as indicated

Solitary metastasis or curative intent?

Yes — No

Curative pathway — Palliative pathway

Site of recurrence or metastases:

Renal fossa

Curative
Local excision
Chemotherapy
Immune therapy

Palliative
XRT

Opposite kidney

Curative
Partial nephrectomy
Total nephrectomy & dialysis
Immune therapy
Chemotherapy
Future directions: cryotherapy, microwave

Palliative
Superselective embolization
XRT (selective tumor field)
Future directions: cryotherapy, microwave

Liver, chest, bone, brain

Curative
Local excision
Immune therapy
Chemotherapy

Palliative
XRT
Local excision
Immune therapy
Chemotherapy

24.1 The role of surgery and tumor embolization

A P Patel and J B deKernion

Introduction

The natural history of renal cell carcinoma (RCC) is such, that of all patients currently diagnosed with the disease, approximately one-third will already harbor clinically detectable metastases at the time of presentation while another third will manifest metastatic disease during follow up. Although metastasis from this tumor can be found in almost any body organ, the most commonly involved sites are the lungs (55%), lymph nodes (34%), bones (32%), liver (32%), adrenal gland (19%), contralateral kidney (11%), brain (5.7%) and heart (5%). It is undisputed that there is no effective management strategy for this tumor which is clearly better than surgical excision, for the tumor is both radio- and chemo-resistant and yet the median survival for those with metastases is dismally short (10 months). Modern treatment of those with unresectable metastases has sought to extend the indications for radical surgery, either as a prelude to, or as an adjunct to systemic therapy (immunotherapy), but the demonstration of a clear survival advantage in favor of this practice is lacking from any well designed prospective study. At the same time, reports of morbidity remain high in many centers and mortality often reaches double figures, for most patients are debilitated by the extent of their tumor burden.

Tumor embolization

Pre-operative

The practice of pre-operative occlusion or embolization in patients with advanced RCC serves primarily to reduce catastrophic blood loss and permit early control of the renal vein and vena cava, when both are occluded by tumor thrombus. In theory, pre-operative embolization may devascularize the venous tumor thrombus and facilitate its detachment into the pulmonary circulation before or during surgery. Such an event can be fatal immediately (large embolus) or later on from established lung metastases (small emboli). A better approach to this problem may be provided by the pre-operative placement of a balloon occlusion catheter on the day of surgery, which can be inflated to occlude the renal artery during nephrectomy. Others[1] have reported a twofold advantage in favor of delayed nephrectomy 22–44 days after ethanol infarction, suggesting that this may cause shrinkage of venous tumor thrombus to permit easier surgical resection and allow

time for an improvement in the clinical status of a malnourished or anemic patient. Unfortunately, ethanol infarction of the kidney can be associated with complications such as colonic and skin necrosis from reflux into mesenteric and lumbar arteries. Furthermore, the experience in this study was limited to only six patients and has not been validated in a larger series.

Some[2] have previously moved to popularize tumor angio-infarction prior to nephrectomy in the face of metastases on the basis that in situ tumor destruction may enhance the host immune response. Of the patients treated at M.D. Anderson in this study, objective responses were seen in only 24%, there was a bias in favor of patients with only lung metastases, the evidence for improved lymphocyte blastogenesis was scant and outcomes were confounded by the effects if any of adjuvant hormones. A later Southwest Oncology Group (SWOG) study of 30 patients treated by angio-infarction and delayed nephrectomy, reported by Gottesman and colleagues[3] with at least 1 year of follow up, also reported poor outcomes with only four responders (none with complete response) and a 7 month median survival that equated to a comparable series of untreated patients. Both this and an EORTC study[4] failed to show any advantage in favor of this practice and, consequently, it has not received widespread application by other specialist units.

Palliative embolization of the primary tumor

Angio-infarction of the entire kidney or tumor vessels has been used with success to treat intractable bleeding from a primary tumor site and to palliate symptoms. This is achieved by the accurate placement of occlusive material using the retrograde Seldinger technique, while steerable catheters allow sub-selective access into individual tumor branch vessels. A variety of particulate and fluid materials have been utilized including absorbable gelatin sponge, polyvinyl alcohol foam particles, stainless steel or platinum coils, ethanol and lipiodol. The advantages of particulate emboli are minimal necrosis of adjacent healthy tissue, when surgical intervention is planned as definitive treatment within 24 h for a tumor in a solitary kidney (or for selected metastases). The morbidity of this minimally invasive technique overall is small, and saves an occasional ill patient from the necessity of surgical nephrectomy with all its attendant hazards. It is also useful in the rare patient who develops cardiac failure from massive arteriovenous shunting through fistulae within the primary tumor.

Embolization of bone metastases

Osseous metastases from renal cell cancer are often lytic in nature and hypervascular as a rule. The main indications for surgical treatment of bony lesions are intractable pain, cortical destruction leading to impending pathological fracture, associated neurological deficit, rapid onset of paraplegia that fails to respond to high-dose steroid treatment and objective or symptomatic relapse after failed palliative radiation. Since RCC metastases are noted to be both chemo-resistant and relatively radio-resistant, surgery is often the treatment of first choice and has been shown to have worthwhile outcomes, in selected candidates with good performance status, solitary or metachronous metastasis, or those with co-existent low volume lung metastases.

RCC is the fourth most common tumor to metastasize to the spine after lung, breast and prostate. It accounts for less than 10% of all malignant metastases at this site and is the most likely to cause neurological deficit from cord compression or from pathological fracture. The poor response of mechanical instability of the spine to radiation makes prompt surgical curettage and internal fixation all the more important. Several centers have reported promising results from anterior or posterior spinal decompression, but the high attendant morbidity and mortality related to significant blood loss from a hyper-vascular tumor bed is not inconsequential. Recurrence rates may approach 50%. In one such study[5] survival did not correlate with the time elapsed since nephrectomy, but was related to the extent of neurological deficit as measured by the Frankel grading system. The better survival observed in those who tolerated multiple operations (15 months vs. 6 months) in this series can almost certainly be related to selection bias. A subsequent report by Olerund and colleagues[6] addressed the issue of intra-operative blood loss and the therapeutic role of pre-operative embolization. They found that mean blood loss was reduced from 6.4 to 2.2 l ($P < 0.02$) when a posterior approach was used in combination with pre-operative embolization while the difference was less dramatic for the more bloody anterior approach. Furthermore, there were no ischemic complications from the embolization in this series. Experience from other centers suggests that the anterior approach is best suited to those in whom the tumor is localized to less than two contiguous levels and is anterior to the dura, while the posterior approach is optimal in all other instances.

Nephrectomy and resection of lymph node metastases

The resurgence of extended retroperitoneal lymphadenectomy at the time of radical nephrectomy in the modern era has been driven largely through the improved survival reported (in retrospective studies) by some centers[7–9] and yet, the literature is replete with series that have demonstrated the dismal long-term survival in those with lymph node metastases from RCC[10–12]. Almost invariably,

this finding is indicative of the presence of undetected microscopic disease elsewhere. Although the hilum is the most common site for nodal involvement in the first instance, RCC has a marked propensity for a haphazard pattern of lymphatic dissemination in the retroperitoneum or pelvis, a feature which is compounded by tumor neovascularity. These observations on the natural history of metastatic RCC, combined with the extra morbidity of an extended retroperitoneal lymph node dissection, mitigate against early reports that such an aggressive dissection might impact positively on increasing survival. One might, however, expect better survival (and better staging) through a locally extended lymphadenectomy in the small cohort of patients with microscopic low volume hilar disease but, to date, no study has related survival quantitatively to the number and distribution of positive lymph nodes.

Resection of non-regional metastases

Surgical resection of RCC metastases has been reported on occasion to produce long-term survival, as exemplified by the case reported by Barney and Churchill in 1939[13] where the patient developed an isolated metastasis 5 years after nephrectomy and survived for another 18 years after its resection. All the more likely when an apparent solitary metastasis is present (1–3%), 5 year survival in such circumstances has varied from 34–62%[14,15], but even in these series, long-term cure is exceptional and the majority of patients will ultimately succumb to other manifestations of metastatic disease and suffer a disease related death. Furthermore, it is difficult to ascertain the true benefit of surgery in this instance, for most retrospective analyses of this nature are colored by an element of inherent bias towards the selection of patients with good performance status who can withstand an aggressive surgical approach. Golimbu and associates[16] have attempted to refine the issue of selection by the application of a prognostic index which incorporated tumor histology, size, local and regional pathological stage. They found the best prognosis in patients with tumors of low biological activity compatible with an extended life expectancy (50% at 5 years). The appearance of metachronous metastases after nephrectomy in this series was associated with only 25% survival at 5 years. In this latter group, the cohort with a long interval between the original nephrectomy and the subsequent development of metastases had the best outcome. The favorable prognosis in this subset is disputed by others[17] but is probably related to a combination of inherently indolent behavior of the metastatic tumor cell line and intrinsic host-tumor immunity. Furthermore, it persisted even when second and third generation metastases occurred provided these were treated aggressively. Investigations of tumor biology through DNA flow cytometry, even in early stage disease, has suggested that prognosis and rates of tumor progression both show a correlation with a non-diploid pattern in the primary tumor.[18,19]

The best outcomes after surgical resection of metastatic disease are undoubtedly seen in the case of solitary or low volume unilateral deposits in the lungs and for solitary adrenal metastasis[20]. Several series, including one from our own institution, have reported 5 year survival of 34 to 42% in patients with lung deposits. Although the majority of these patients will later succumb to disease relapse or recurrence, occasional long-term survivors undoubtedly reap the benefits of an aggressive surgical curative attempt, especially if the metastases appear two years or more after the original nephrectomy and the patient has good performance status.

Of many common sites for RCC metastases, the brain often represents a daunting challenge to both treatment philosophy and aggressive surgical intent. Fortunately, most metastases in this location are relatively firm and well circumscribed making them technically suitable for complete en-bloc resection. To counterbalance this, the incidence of intra-tumoral hemorrhage and the need for emergent surgical intervention is high (45%). There are few good reported series, but Wronski and associates[21] have recently reported on an updated group of 50 such patients from the Memorial Sloan Kettering Cancer Center. The laudable survival (median of 31.4 months after resection of the primary tumor and 12.1 months after diagnosis of brain metastases) in this series once again emphasizes the influence of selection bias, for there was a preponderance of patients (47) who had undergone prior nephrectomy and had presented with metachronous secondaries at a median interval of 17 months. Other factors that contributed to the favorable outcome in this series included the presence of a single metastasis (41/50), lung involvement (37/50) and male gender (38/50). Nevertheless, peri-operative mortality was 10% after craniotomy and these patients were excluded from the calculation of median survival, while 31% suffered significant surgical complications and recurrence was seen in 49% (20% local and 29% at distant sites). Survival was worse when metastases were infra-tentorial (cerebellar) and, curiously, also for the group with right-sided primary tumors (a possible reflection of overall tumor burden and lower Karnofsky performance status). These results once again confirm the paramount importance of patient selection when palliation is the primary goal of the surgeon. The outcomes are most rewarding in the patient who begins with good performance status and has delayed presentation of low volume metastatic lesions, for longevity is a serendipitous bonus in the majority.

Clearly, a curative surgical intent for metastatic disease may be fulfilled in a rational manner with the least unnecessary morbidity, when the natural biology of the individual tumor is comprehensively understood. Only the prospective application of biological selection criteria in randomized studies will provide further clarification on this issue.

Palliative nephrectomy and unresectable metastatic disease

The most common indications for palliative nephrectomy, without altering survival in the presence of metastatic disease, are symptoms related to the local tumor. These include intractable bleeding with anemia (requiring repeated hospitalization for blood transfusion) or clot colic, flank pain from local invasion of adjacent parietes or viscera uncontrolled by opiates and tumor related toxic systemic reactions such as fever, hypertension and Stauffers' syndrome. Symptoms from endocrine effects such as hypercalcemia and erythrocytosis are rarely amenable to cure by nephrectomy, for these para-neoplastic syndromes are often perpetuated by the metastases that remain. The practice that palliative nephrectomy can invoke the regression of metastases has largely fallen into disrepute, for observations of this phenomenon have been anecdotal at best and subject to certain selection biases. In the two largest reported series[22,23], there was a large preponderance of males with lung metastases (both favorable prognostic indicators). In these series, histological confirmation was not obtained for the majority of metastatic lesions, some patients showed regression prior to nephrectomy and in the majority, the regression observed was short lived and did not translate to long-term cure.

Initial nephrectomy

The debate on the indications for cytoreductive nephrectomy as an initial procedure for patients treated with systemic combination immunotherapy protocols has re-emerged as better treatment success has been observed than was seen earlier with interferon monotherapy. The rationale in favor of nephrectomy prior to immunotherapy lies in the recognition that interactions between the RCC tumor cells and the host immune system causes an impairment of several facets of the host defense mechanism. These include decreased delayed-type hypersensitivity reactions, decreased lymphocyte cytolytic function and lymphocyte proliferation response to presented tumor antigens. Although nephrectomy in this instance should theoretically facilitate patient responses to multi-modality systemic treatments and eliminate the small risk of metachronous metastases, there is little data to support this contention convincingly.

327

The higher responses seen after treatment with interferon α (IFNα) in patients who had undergone previous nephrectomy were not subjected to univariate analysis, with the exception of the report from Umeda and colleagues[24], but were probably consequent upon the often observed selection bias in favor of including patients with good performance status (Karnofsky) and lungs as the sole site of metastases. Furthermore, the data presented by Umeda et al. may be criticized on the basis that they were summaries of different clinical trials using varying doses, schedules and types of interferon, and therefore not amenable to meaningful statistical analysis. In a retrospective study of patients with metastatic RCC from UCLA treated with human leukocyte IFNα, a group of 33 patients who had undergone immunotherapy within a year of nephrectomy was compared with a smaller group of 12 patients who underwent immunotherapy within 1 year of presenting with metastases with the primary tumor still in place[25]. The two groups were well matched for mean Karnofsky score and the percentage with lung metastases alone. Therapeutic response rates were better in the group who had undergone prior nephrectomy (24.3% vs. 8.3%), but these differences did not reach statistical significance (possibly due to under-powering of the size of the no-nephrectomy group) and differences in disease bulk were not taken into account. With the advent of newer immunotherapy protocols, pre-treatment nephrectomy is undoubtedly a requisite for those entered into an adoptive TIL treatment protocol, with or without cytokines.

We would conclude that if significant morbidity from nephrectomy is to be avoided in patients with extensive metastatic disease, it should be reserved only for those considered for entry into a TIL protocol until there is firm evidence from a prospective randomized study to support the contention that initial nephrectomy improves outcomes when used in combination with immunotherapy. In this respect, the results of an intergroup cooperative study comparing nephrectomy followed by interferon treatment, to interferon alone (with the primary tumor in situ) should prove to be illuminating. Finally, adjunctive nephrectomy may be justifiable in the occasional patient whose distant metastases have completely regressed after immunotherapy (by CT criteria) but the primary tumor is large or undiminished in size.

The recent report by Bennett and colleagues[26] has suggested a high peri-operative mortality rate (17%) and a high failure to treat with adjuvant immunotherapy (77%) due to accelerated disease progression and surgical morbidity. This perverse rapid progression after nephrectomy has also been noted by some others and may be explained by an observation made in a murine model, that suggests elaboration of an angiogenesis inhibitor, 'angiostatin', from the primary tumor which partially suppresses the growth of metastases. Removal of the primary tumor in

this case can permit rapid growth at metastatic sites. Our own experience at UCLA with respect to surgical morbidity in a series of 63 patients who underwent nephrectomy as part of a planned immunotherapy program (IFNα, IL2 + IFNα, pTIL + IL2 + IFNα) does not match that reported from other institutions. Surgical mortality in this series was absent and only seven patients have failed to receive immunotherapy subsequently. It is therefore clear from this discrepancy that many factors related to patient selection contribute to the rate of patient morbidity.

Adjunctive nephrectomy in patients with unresectable metastases

The place of nephrectomy in patients with unresectable metastatic disease is small indeed and does not seem to impact on survival[16]. It has no place in clinical practice outside of the strict confines of investigational controlled protocols seeking new combinations of immune modulators to enhance anti-tumor activity. On the other hand, nephrectomy and resection of metastases may be technically possible in some patients with objective partial responses greater than 50% after adoptive immunotherapy. Here, surgery can be used to achieve a complete response by removing low volume residual disease which can be submitted for histological evaluation of residual tumor or scar tissue. Surgery is also appropriate in those who have shown durable response to planned multi-modality immunotherapy in all metastatic sites (complete remission or partial remission) and have a low surgical risk with locally resectable stable disease. Our recent experience with the investigational use of positron emission tomography (PET) scan imaging as it correlates to findings on CT scans, has been encouraging in the subset of patients that has shown objective response to an immunotherapy regimen and, provided the cost of such imaging is acceptable, it may be of use in selecting the best surgical candidates for salvage surgery in the future.

Some investigators have reported benefit from adjunctive nephrectomy in patients with skeletal metastases[27] while others[28] have suggested that benefit only accrued to those with solitary rather than multiple metastatic sites irrespective of bony involvement.

Nephrectomy and spontaneous regression of metastases

Spontaneous regression of metastatic renal cell cancer was first described by Bumpus in 1928[29]. Unfortunately, this phenomenon is too infrequent (1 in 250 at best) after nephrectomy and rarely durable enough to make it worthwhile. The hypothesis that nephrectomy aids this process has been based on two possibilities:

1. That surgical manipulations of the tumor releases a shower of tumor cells into the circulation (vascular and lymphatic) resulting in a large tumor antigen load which stimulates a strong host immune response.
2. That the antigen load of the primary tumor is too great and overwhelms the host anti-tumor response until nephrectomy is performed.

In practical terms, nephrectomy alone is seldom curative, but exceptions may arise in the rare patient with good performance status, a diploid tumor and a solitary or few metastatic sites not suitable for surgical excision but amenable to palliative embolization or radiation.

In conclusion, the true fraction of patients with metastases from RCC whose longevity will be increased as a result of complete surgical resection of detectable disease is small. Surgical intervention is most worthwhile in the selected subset with good performance status who have the most to gain from a prolonged disease-free interval and in those considered for treatment in experimental immunotherapy protocols.

References

1. Craven WM, Redmond PL, Kumpe DA, Durham JD, Wettlaufer JN. Planned delayed nephrectomy after ethanol embolization of renal carcinoma. *J Urol* 1991;**146**:704–708.
2. Swanson DA, Wallace S, Johnson DE. The role of embolization and nephrectomy in the treatment of metastatic renal cell carcinoma. *Urol Clin N Am* 1980;**7**:719–730.
3. Gottesman JE, Crawford ED, Grossman HB, Scardino P, McCracken JD Infarction-nephrectomy for metastatic renal carcinoma. Southwest oncology group study. *Urology* 1985;**25**(3):248–250.
4. Kurth KH, Cinqualbre J, Oliver RTD, Schulman CC. Embolization and subsequent nephrectomy in metastatic renal cell carcinoma. *Prog Clin Biol Res* 1984;**153**:423–436.
5. King GJ, Kostuik JP, McBroom RJ, Richardson W. Surgical management of metastatic renal carcinoma of the spine. *Spine* 1991;**16**(3):265–271.
6. Olerund C, Jonsson H, Lofberg AM, Lorelius LE, Sjostrom L. Embolization of spinal metastases reduces peroperative blood loss. *Acta Ortho Scand* 1993;**64**(1):9–12.
7. Robson CJ, Churchill BM, Anderson W. The results of radical nephrectomy for renal cell carcinoma. *J Urol* 1969;**101**:297–301.
8. Pizzocaro G, Piva L. Pros and cons of retroperitoneal lymphadenectomy in operable renal cell carcinoma *Eur Urol* 1990;**18**:22–23.
9. Giuliani L, Giberti C, Martorana G, Rovida S. Radical extensive surgery for renal cell carcinoma: long term results and prognostic factors. *J Urol* 1990;**143**:468–474.
10. Skinner DG, Vermillion CD, Colsin RB. The surgical management of renal cell carcinoma. *J Urol* 1972;**107**:705–710.
11. Hultén L, Rosencrantz M, Seeman T, Wahlqvist L and Achren Ch. Occurrence and localization of lymph node metastases in renal cell carcinoma. *Scand J Urol Nephrol* 1969;**3**:129–133.
12. Bassil B, Dosoretz DE, Prout GR Jr. Validation of the tumor, nodes and metastases classification of renal cell carcinoma. *J Urol* 1985;**134**:450–454.
13. Barney JD, Churchill EJ. Adenocarcinoma of the kidney with metastasis to the lung. *J Urol* 1939;**42**:269–276.
14. Middleton RG. Surgery for metastatic renal cell carcinoma. *J Urol* 1967;**97**:973–977.
15. Watanabe M, Kitamura Y, Komatsubara S, Sakata Y. The evaluation of surgical management for metastatic lesions of renal cell carcinoma. *Hinyokika Kiyo Acta Urologica Japonica* 1995;**41**(11):847–853.
16. Golimbu M, Joshi P, Sperber A, Tessler A, Al-Askari S, Morales P. Renal cell carcinoma: survival and prognostic factors. *Urology* 1986;**27**:291–301.
17. Dineen MK, Pastore RD, Emrich LJ, Huben RP. Results of surgical treatment of renal cell carcinoma with solitary metastasis. *J Urol* 1988;**140**(2):277–279.
18. DeKernion JB, Mukamel E, Ritchie AWS, Blyth B, Hannah J, Bohman R. Prognostic significance of the DNA content of renal carcinoma. *Cancer* 1989;**64**(8):1669–1673.
19. Grignon DJ, el-Naggar A, Green LK, Ayala AG, Ro JY, Swanson DA, Troncoso P et al. DNA flow cytometry as a predictor of outcome of stage 1 renal cell carcinoma. *Cancer* 1989;**63**(6):1161–1165.
20. Kinouchi T, Kotake T. Management of advanced renal cell carcinoma: Surgical treatment of metastasis. *Hinyokika Kiyo Acta Urologica Japonica* 1994;**40**(10):919–924.
21. Wronski M, Arbit E, Russo P, Galichich JH. Surgical resection of brain metastases from renal cell carcinoma in 50 patients. *Urology* 1996;**47**(2):187–193.
22. Bloom HJG. Hormone induced and spontaneous regression of metastatic renal cancer. *Cancer* 1973;**32**:1066–1071.
23. Freed SZ, Halperin JP, Gordon M. Idiopathic regression of metastases from renal cell carcinoma. *J Urol* 1977;**118**:538–542.
24. Umeda T, Aso Y, Niijima T. Treatment of advanced renal cell carcinoma with alpha interferon: summary of three collaborative trials. In: deKernion (ed.) *Immunotherapy of urological tumors.* International Society of Urology Monograms, London, Churchill Livingstone, 1988, pp. 219–222.
25. Belldegrun A, Koo AS, Bochner B, Figlin R, deKernion JB Immunotherapy for advanced renal cell cancer: the role of radical nephrectomy. *Euro Urol* 1990;**18**(suppl 2):42–45.
26. Bennett RT, Lerner SE, Taub HC, Dutcher JP, Fleischmann J. Cytoreductive surgery for stage IV renal cell carcinoma. *J Urol* 1995;**154**(1):32–34.
27. Montie JE, Stewart BH, Straffon RA, Banowsky LHW, Hewitt CB, Montague DK. The role of adjunctive nephrectomy in patients with metastatic renal cell carcinoma. *J Urol* 1977;**117**(3):272–275.
28. Swanson DA, Orovan WL, Johnson DE, Giacco G. Osseous metastases secondary to renal cell carcinoma. *Urology* 1981;**18**(6):556–561.
29. Bumpus HC Jr. The apparent disappearance of pulmonary metastases in a case of hypernophroma following nephrectomy. *T. Am A Genito Urin Surgeons* 1928;**21**:19–25.

24.2   The role of immunotherapy

C A Kim and R K Babayan

Introduction

Of all renal cancers, 13–48% will present with metastatic disease[1–5]. The median survival for this group is 6–12 months[1,4,5] with the majority of the patients dying within 1 year[1,4,5]. Unlike other solid tumors, renal cell cancer is relatively resistant to traditional systemic therapies such as radiation therapy, hormonal therapy and chemotherapy[6–9]. Interest in immunotherapy arose from observations on the variable natural history of renal cell cancer. The recognition that renal cell carcinoma may remain stable for long intervals or even spontaneously regress, as well as disease recurrence noted 10–30 years later, suggest a host response to the tumor[2,10]. These observations along with the necessity for more effective therapeutic strategies led to clinical trials employing immunotherapy for treatment of metastatic renal cell carcinoma (mRCC).

Interferons (IFN)

Interferons were one of the first biological agents to demonstrate activity against mRCC. Interferons are glycoproteins that share anti-viral, tumoristatic, or immunoregulatory activities. They were initially identified as substances secreted by virally infected cells which prevented or 'interfered' with infection of uninfected cells[11]. In 1983, deKernion and Quesada both reported positive results using partially purified human leukocyte IFNα in the treatment of mRCC[12,13]. They noted response rates of 16% and 26% respectively. However, subsequent phase II trials proved disappointing. While objective response rates to alpha-interferon remain in the 10–20% range, the mean duration of response is only 6 to 10 months with little impact on survival. Table 24.2.1 summarizes the results of several clinical trials which employed IFNα in the treatment of mRCC.

Responses to IFN therapy tend to be correlated with good performance status, nephrectomy prior to therapy, and an interval of 1–2 years from the time of diagnosis to the time of treatment[6,14–17]. Adverse effects of IFN therapy occur more frequently at higher doses and include a flu-like syndrome characterized by fever, fatigue, chills and myalgias. Hematological and hepatic toxicity are usually reversible on cessation of the therapy[14,15,18].

Alpha, beta, and gamma-IFNs have all been used for the treatment of mRCC. While there are significant differences between IFNα and IFNβ in the immunoregulatory and anti-proliferative actions, reported response rates between the two are similar[19]. However, response rates for IFNγ are conflicting, varying from 0–30%[19,20]. In a recent phase III trial designed to investigate the possible benefit of adding IFNγ to IFNα therapy in mRCC, the authors found no benefit. In fact, the issue of a possible detrimental effect with its addition was raised[20]. Further studies are needed to determine the therapeutic efficacy of IFNγ in the treatment of mRCC.

Interleukin-2

Interleukin-2 (IL-2), originally referred to as T-cell growth factor, was isolated in 1976 as a factor that allowed human T-cells to grow in vitro[21]. IL-2 is produced by activated helper T cells. It has been shown to increase the production of other cytokines, enhance natural killer (NK) cell activity, and stimulate the production of cytotoxic lymphocytes and lymphokine activated killer (LAK) cells.

High-dose intravenous IL-2 is the only biological agent approved by the Food and Drug Administration (FDA) for the treatment of mRCC. FDA approval came in May 1992, after reviewing the data from seven phase II studies on 255 patients[22]. The overall response rate was 14% (5% CR). However, unlike interleukin therapy, these responses proved durable, with a median duration of response of 20.3 months. For the CRs, the median duration of response has not yet been reached, with eight of the 12 responses still ongoing, and two of these for a period over 5 years. In analyzing the data on those who responded, the only statistically signifi-

Table 24.2.1   Clinical trials of IFN- α in renal cell carcinoma

Source	Dose regimen ($\times 10^6$ IU)	No. Pts	CR	PR	RR (%)
Human leukocyte IFN-α					
deKernion et al. (1983)[12]	3, daily, 5 x weekly, IM	43	1	6	7 (16)
Quesada et al. (1983)[13]	3, daily, IM	19	0	5	5 (26)
Kirkwood et al. (1985)[18]	1, daily, IM	14	0	0	0 (0)
	10, daily, IM	16	1	2	3 (19)
Recombinant IFN-α					
Quesada et al. (1985)[72]	20/m², daily, IM	41	1	11	12 (29)
	2/m², daily, IM	15	0	0	0 (0)
Umeda and Niijma (1986)[14]	3 to 36 daily, IM	108	2	13	15 (14)
	6 to 10, 3–5 weekly, IM	45	1	7	8 (18)
Creagan et al. (1991)[73]	20/m², 3 x weekly, IM	87	1	6	7 (8)
Minasian et al. (1993)[15]	50/m², 3 x weekly, IM	39	0	7	7 (18)
	3 to 36, daily, SC	59	2	5	7 (12)
Tsavaris et al. (1993)[74]	5 to 15, 3 x weekly, IM	41	0	6	6 (13)
DeMulder et al. (1995)[20]	20/m², daily, IM	53	2	5	7 (13)

CR = Complete response; PR = Partial response; RR = Response rate; IM = Intramuscular; SC = Subcutaneous

cant predictor of response was a good performance status. Unlike prior immunotherapy trials, responses were not limited to small tumor burdens or microscopic disease. In fact, responses were seen in patients with large tumor burdens, intact primary tumors, and in those with bone metastases. However, the toxicity of IL-2 was significant with a combined mortality rate of 4% for the seven studies.

IL-2 toxicity causes fevers, chills, malaise, nausea and diarrhea. More importantly, IL-2 causes a capillary leak syndrome[23,24]. This may result in hypotension, pre-renal azotemia, oliguria, pulmonary edema, acute respiratory distress, cardiac ischemia and arrhythmias. With careful screening for cardiac and pulmonary disease, newer studies report a much improved morbidity and mortality rate, but this also limits the group of people eligible for treatment.

In an effort to decrease the toxicity of high-dose IL-2 and allow the treatment of patients with poorer performance status, several alternative dose treatment regimens were developed. High-dose regimens deliver 600 000 to 720 000 IU/kg IV every 8 h for a total of 14 doses or as tolerated. After a 5 to 9 day rest period, the cycle is repeated. In Europe, high-dose 24 h continuous IV infusion protocols are used which deliver up to 18×10^6 IU/m^2/day of IL-2. The rationale is that the more constant serum levels would decrease the toxicity. In practice, the infusion rates often need to be decreased due to hemodynamic instability.

Support for low-dose regimens came from animal studies in which low-dose IL-2 demonstrated immunologic activity and produced objective regressions in metastatic lesions[25,26]. Low-dose intravenous (IV) and subcutaneous (SC) therapy have both been utilized. Table 24.2.2 summarizes the data from several clinical trials using both high and low-dose IL-2.

While initial clinical trials using low-dose IL-2 show favorable response rates, the long-term durability of these responses as compared with high-dose IL-2 regimens is not known. The National Cancer Institute (NCI) conducted a randomized, prospective study objectively to compare the effectiveness and the toxicity between high- and low-dose IL-2 regimens. The final report is not yet in press. However, on interim analysis of the data, the response rates between high- and low-dose IL-2 were similar (20% for high-dose vs. 15% for low-dose), while the toxicity was markedly reduced with the low-dose therapy[27].

Combination therapy

The concept of combining agents with different mechanisms of action is a natural development in the effort to discover more effective therapy. Experimental data using animal models demonstrated a synergistic response with the combination of IL-2 and IFNα against established RCC metastases than either agent alone[28,29]. After animal models demonstrated synergy between IL-2 and IFNα, clinical trials using this combination were performed. An initial, non-randomized trial by Rosenberg and colleagues resulted in an objective response rate of 31% (4 CR; 7 PR)[30]. They used an escalating IV dose combination of IL-2 and IFNα in 35 patients and found the highest response rates (38%) in the patients who received the highest dose schedules. Aside from elevations in transaminases (AST and

Table 24.2.2 Clinical trials of IL-2 in renal cell carcinoma

Source	Dose regimen	No. Pts	CR	PR	RR (%)
High-dose IV bolus					
Rosenberg et al. (1989)[42]	720 000 IU/kg q8h	54	4	8	12 (22)
Atkins et al. (1993)[32]	600 000 IU/kg q8h	71	4	8	12 (17)
Yang et al. (1994)[27]	720 000 IU/kg q8h	65	2	11	13 (20)
Rosenberg et al. (1989)[75]	720 000 IU/kg q8h	149	10	20	30 (20)
Fyfe et al. (1995)[22]	60–72 x 10^4 IU/kg q8h	255	12	24	36 (14)
Continuous infusion IL-2					
Negrier (1989)[76]	18×10^6 IU/m^2/d	32	2	4	6 (19)
von der Maase (1991)[77]	18×10^6 IU/m^2/d	51	2	6	8 (16)
Geertsen (1992)[78]	18×10^6 IU/m^2/d	30	2	4	6 (20)
Low dose IV bolus IL-2					
Yang (1994)[27]	72 000 IU/kg q8h	60	4	5	9 (15)
Subcutaneous IL-2					
Stein (1991)[79]	0.6 MU, 5 d/wk x 8 wks	9	0	2	2 (22)
Lissoni (1992)[80]	9 MU/m^2 bid x 2 d then 1.8 MU/m^2 bid x 5d/wk x 6 wks	13	0	4	4 (31)
Sleijfer (1992)[81]	18 MU/d x 5 d then 9 MU/d x 2 d then 18 MU/d x 3 d/wk x 6 wks	26	2	4	6 (23)

CR = Complete response; PR = Partial response; RR = Response rate; IM = Intramuscular; SC = Subcutaneous

ALT) and a greater incidence of confusion, increased toxicity with combination therapy was not noted.

In an extended, long-term follow up of this study by the NCI, higher response rates continued to be associated with the group given the highest dose of IFN. However, markedly increased toxicity was associated with this dosing regimen, with no overall survival benefit[31]. Atkins and colleagues conducted a randomized trial comparing high-dose IL-2 alone or in combination with IFNα, response rates were 17% (4 CR; 8 PR) and 11% (0 CR; 3 PR) respectively[32]. Median survival was similar for both groups, 15.5 months for IL-2 alone versus 16 months for combination therapy, while more patients on combination therapy experienced neutropenia, myocarditis and ischemic events. Based on this data, combination therapy with high-dose IL-2 and IFNα is not felt to be synergistic, with increased toxicity seen with higher doses of both IL-2 and IFN.

In an attempt to reduce toxicity while maintaining or improving response rates of low-dose IL-2 therapy, clinical trials began using subcutaneous or intramuscular delivery of IFNα with an outpatient regimen of IL-2[33–37]. Dosing regimens varied, but reported objective response rates ranged from 8% to 36%. A summary of these clinical trials is listed in Table 24.2.3.

Atzpodien and colleagues recently reported the results of a European phase II, multi-institutional, outpatient trial using combination subcutaneous IL-2 and IFNα. One hundred and fifty-two patients were treated with an overall response rate of 25% (9 CR, 29 PR). Median duration of responses were 16+ months for CRs and 9 months for PRs. Systemic toxicity was noted to be markedly reduced. A prospective, randomized study is needed to compare this combination to single agent SC IL-2. Both efficacy with

regard to actual survival benefit as well as treatment toxicity need to be addressed.

Other forms of combination therapy include the use of 5-fluorouracil (5-FU), vinblastine, 13-cis-retinoic acid with IFNα, IL-2, or both. In these phase I/II clinical trials, response rates of 38–48% have been reported with acceptable toxicity[38,39]. Again, larger numbers of randomized trials are necessary fully to evaluate the long-term effectiveness of combination IL-2 and IFNα with or without the addition of other agents.

Cellular therapy (LAK cells, TILs and ALTs)

Cellular therapy for mRCC has largely been adoptive or passive immunotherapy. Cells are removed from the patient, stimulated and activated in vitro, and then reinfused into the patient. Lymphokine-activated killer (LAK) cells result from in vitro activation of peripheral blood lymphocytes with IL-2. LAK cells are non-major histocompatibility (MHC) restricted killer cells, cytolytic against a wide range of neoplastic cells. In 1984, Rosenberg and colleagues performed an initial clinical trial employing LAK cells in conjunction with high dose IL-2 to treat patients with metastatic disease[40]. This study was extended and an additional 33 patients with mRCC were treated with high-dose IL-2 and LAK cells[41]. A 33% response rate was noted in 36 patients with four CRs and eight PRs. In a separate, larger trial by Rosenberg and colleagues, 72 patients were treated with combination IL-2/LAK cell therapy[42]. Again, a 35% objective response rate resulted with eight CRs and 17 PRs. Schoof also reported high response rates of 50% with IL-2/LAK cell therapy, but duration of response

Table 24.2.3   Clinical trials of low-dose IL-2 and IFN-α in renal cell carcinoma

Source	Dose regimen	No. Pts	CR	PR	RR (%)
Budd et al. (1989)[82]	IL-2: 0.1–2 x U/m² IV 3x/wk x 4 wks IFN-α: 0–10 x 10⁶ U/m² SC 3x/wk x 4 wks	12	0	1	1 (8)
Atzpodien et al. (1990)[33]	IL-2: 9 x 10⁶ IU SC bid x 2 d then 18 x 10⁶ IU SC bid 5x/wk x 6 wks IFN-α: 5 x 10⁶ U/m² SC 3x/wk	17	2	3	5 (36)
Mittelman et al. (1991)[34]	IL-2: 9 x 10⁶ IU CIV 4d/wk x 4 wks IFN-α: 5 x 10⁶ U/m² IM d1–4/wk/ x 4 wks	15	2	2	4 (27)
Figlin et al. (1992)[35]	IL-2: 6 x 10⁶ IU CIV/SC d1–4/wk x 4 wks IFN-α: 6 x 10⁶ U/m² SC d1–4/wk x 4 wks	52	4	9	13 (25)
Vogelzang et al. (1993)[83]	IL-2: 4 x 10⁶ U/m2 SC d1–4/wk x 4 wks IFN-α: 9 x 10⁶ U/m² SC d1, d4/wk x 4 wks	42	2	3	5 (12)
Atzpodien et al. (1995)[37]	IL-2: 20 x 10⁶ IU/m² SC 3x/wk, wks 1,4 IL-2: 5 x 10⁶ IU/m² SC 3x/wk, wks 2,3,5,6 IFN-α: 6 x 10⁶ U/m² SC 1x/wk, wks 1,4 IFN-α: 6 x 10⁶ U/m² SC 3x/wk, wks 2,3,5,6	152	9	29	38 (25)

CR = Complete response; PR = Partial response; RR = Response rate; IM = Intramuscular; SC = Subcutaneous; CIV = Continuous IV infusion.

was short (3–4+ months), and there was no survival advantage[43].

In order to determine whether the addition of LAK cells to high-dose IL-2 therapy truly resulted in improved therapeutic efficacy, the NCI conducted a prospective, randomized trial comparing IL-2 to IL-2 plus LAK[44]. A total of 97 patients with mRCC were randomized. No statistical difference in either response rates between IL-2 or IL-2/LAK (24% vs. 33%) or in survival at 48 months (25% vs. 29%) was found. Treatment toxicity was related to the dose of IL-2 administered. Based on this data, it is generally believed that LAK cells provide no additional benefit to IL-2 therapy alone.

The two forms of cellular therapy currently being investigated are tumor infiltrating lymphocytes (TIL) and autolymphocyte therapy (ALT). The TIL approach is conceptually based on the knowledge that renal tumors are populated with lymphocytes presumed to be capable of recognizing tumor antigens[45,46]. By incubating lymphocytes harvested from the tumor with IL-2, TILs are created. These cells are theoretically tumor specific with markedly enhanced tumoricidal capability[45,47]. These TILs are then reinfused into the patient along with IL-2.

More recently, an improved technique referred to as cytokine priming was developed to improve the CD8+ (cytolytic) fraction of TIL[48,49]. A radical nephrectomy is performed and the primary tumor is mechanically then enzymatically digested into a single cell suspension. The cells are then incubated with low-dose IL-2 and expanded over 8 to 12 days. During this time, the tumor cells die and the remaining TILs are further expanded in the presence of IL-2. With further purification, the CD8+ only portion of TIL can be isolated. Figlin and colleagues reported a 33% objective response rate in a clinical trial of 48 patients, 15 of whom were treated with purified CD8+ TILs plus low-dose IL-2 and the remaining 33 with bulk TILs plus low-dose IL-2[49]. A response rate of 33% was noted for the group with an objective response rate of 40% for the purified TILs vs. 30% for the bulk TILs. Eight patients (17%) experienced complete responses with a median duration of 24+ months. A phase III trial is currently in progress comparing treatment with combination TIL/IL-2 to IL-2 alone in patients with mRCC.

Autolymphocyte therapy (ALT) is a form of passive immunotherapy utilizing autologous memory T-cells activated ex vivo[50]. Lymphocytes are removed by leukophoresis and are cultured in the presence of an antibody directed against the CD3 portion of the T-cell receptor (i.e. OKT-3). These in vitro conditions activate the T-cells and cause them to secrete a variety of cytokines. The supernatant of this culture, containing OKT-3 and a variety of autologously generated cytokines, is removed and frozen. The patient undergoes leukophoresis monthly, and his/her white cells are cultured with an aliquot of the above cytokine rich supernatant (polyclonal activation). These cells, which have been shown phenotypically to be activated T-cells capable of producing IFN-γ, tumor necrosis factor (TNF) beta and granulocyte macrophage colony stimulating factor (GM-CSF) in response to stimulation, are reinfused into the patient. Cimetidine is also infused to decrease suppressor cell activity.

In a non-randomized study of 36 patients with mRCC treated with ALT, median survival was 15 months, with 36% alive at 24 months and minimal side effects from the treatment[51]. A phase III study of 90 patients treated with ALT plus cimetidine versus cimetidine alone revealed a 21% PR rate for the ALT group versus a 5% PR rate for the cimetidine only group[52]. Median survival had not yet been reached in the ALT group, but was only 265 days for the cimetidine only group. The projected survival advantage was 2.5 times greater in the ALT group. Again, toxicity was mild and treatment was delivered entirely on an outpatient basis. A multicenter, randomized phase III study between ALT and IFNα is underway in the USA and Canada.

Gene therapy

Recent advances in molecular biology and gene transfer have led to the possibility of treating tumors by inserting new genetic material into either the tumor cells from the patient and/or their normal tissue[53–57]. This form of therapy, termed gene therapy, is in its infancy. However, there are a number of early phase trials in progress. This section will review some of the methods and strategies for gene therapy.

There are three key elements to successful gene therapy: 1) transfer of the DNA to cells by a vector, 2) expression of the gene following its introduction into cells, 3) persistence of gene expression in the target cell. Vectors are the vehicles used to transfer the therapeutic gene into the target cells. They are pieces of deoxyribonucleic acid (DNA) or ribonucleic acid (RNA) that have been engineered to express the gene of interest. The most popular vectors at present are based on viruses, such as retroviruses or adenoviruses. These viruses have been altered to make them non-replicating and for adenoviruses, less immunogenic. An alternative to viral transfer methods is direct transfer of the DNA into the target cell. Although this method is less efficient than viral transfer, direct transfer of DNA into the cell has the advantage of lower immunogenicity and improved safety[58]. At present, all of these vectors are non-specific in that they allow gene transfer to most cells. Methods to allow transfer to specific cell types, such as renal cells, are currently being developed.

Following transfer of the gene into the target cell, successful gene therapy requires expression of the gene. In most cases, this results in protein production, however, strategies have been described whereby expression of the vector DNA results in expression of anti-sense mRNAs or dominant-negative peptides that block expression of a gene[59,60]. Gene expression results from the placement of the DNA sequences adjacent to promoter and enhancer elements. In most cases, these regulatory elements are in the vector. Examples of commonly used enhancers/promoters are from cytomegalovirus and Moloney murine leukemia virus. Both of these enhancer/promoter combinations result in sustained, high level expression of the introduced gene. There have been a number of reports of promoters/enhancers that confer cell type specificity to a gene, i.e. that limit the expression of a gene to certain cells such as renal cells or hepatic cells. Incorporation of these elements into vectors may allow cell type specificity of the introduced genetic material. In addition, some promoters/enhancers may be induced by manipulating the proteins that control gene expression. As a result, it may be possible both to turn on and turn off expression of a gene within a cell. Use of these elements may allow further control of gene expression within target cells. In addition, methods are being developed that may allow insertion of the introduced genetic material into specific sites in the genome. This offers the possibility of expressing the genetic material from the endogenous control elements. For example, replacement of a damaged P53 gene with its 'healthy' counterpart by homologous recombination would cause the introduced gene to be expressed from the P53 control elements.

Stability of gene transfer refers to the ability of genes to be transferred to cells in either a stable or transient fashion. Methods such as adenoviral gene transfer and plasmid transfer do not cause integration of the gene into the cell's DNA. Thus, as the cells replicate, the sequences are lost. This has the advantage of not disrupting the genome, which in rare cases may in itself be transforming. Potential application of this technique may be for cytokine gene therapy where only a short period of expression of the specific cytokine is required.

In stable gene transfer, the DNA integrates into the chromosome and the integrated DNA is maintained as chromosomal DNA. Thus, as the cells replicate, the sequences replicate, and there is potential for long-term expression of the gene of interest. Vectors such as retroviruses or adeno-associated viruses produce stable gene transfer. Situations where stable gene transfer is desirable include corrective gene therapy where replacement of a missing gene, such as P53, would correct the neoplastic transformation.

The most promising methods for gene therapy seek to modulate the immune system similar to the strategies described above for IL-2 and other cytokine-based therapies. This approach is based on the premise that current gene therapy methods are insufficient directly to treat the large number of cells that comprise a tumor (usually greater than 10^8). Instead, these methods seek to stimulate the immune system with the hope that this stimulation will cause the immune system to render a cure. One strategy currently in clinical trials is to introduce an immunostimulatory cytokine, such as IL-2, directly into the tumor cells ex vivo, and subsequently inject them into the patient as a tumor vaccine. In practice the tumor cells are removed from the patient and the cytokine gene is introduced into these cells in vitro by an engineered retrovirus or similar methodology. The cells are then assayed for expression, irradiated to prevent neoplastic growth and reintroduced into the patient. The goal is to achieve sufficient secretion of IL-2 by these transduced tumor cells to activate the surrounding T-cells, NK cells, and other immune mediator cells which can then elicit a cytotoxic response without significant toxicity to the patient and confer anti-tumor memory. In comparison to the methods described earlier in this chapter, it is hoped that direct injection of the stimulatory cytokines into the tumor cells will achieve a sufficiently high local concentration of these factors to elicit a significant clinical response. Similar approaches are in clinical trials with a number of different cytokines including GM-CSF and IL-4[61–63].

An alternative method to immune stimulation is specifically to alter the tumor cells either by inserting genes that will express proteins leading to cell death or genes that will correct the specific genetic defects that lead to cellular transformation. 'Suicide' genes encode an enzyme that can activate a non-toxic, pro-drug into its potent cytotoxic form[64]. An example of this is the insertion of the herpes simplex virus type 1 kinase gene into the tumor followed by the administration of systemic gancyclovir. This results not only in the cell death of the transformed cells, but also the surrounding cells by a 'bystander effect'. Another method involves the insertion of genes that induce apoptosis or programmed cell death, such as members of the fas pathway. Other strategies involve correcting a mutant gene, with the hope that this will prevent the malignant growth of the tumor cells. For example, restoring the normal copy of the tumor suppressor gene, P53, into tumor cells that do not express normal copies of this protein, results in cessation of abnormal growth in tissue culture experiments. One problem with these non-immune therapies is that the genetic material must be transferred to the great majority of the tumor cells. As discussed above, the present methods of gene therapy will not allow this. Nevertheless, treatment of cancer by gene therapy is currently an extremely active area of research and it is anticipated that successes in this area will lead to many of the future innovations in treatment.

Surgery

The role of surgery in IL-2 based immunotherapy remains controversial with no randomized studies comparing the benefits of immunotherapy alone or after cytoreductive surgery. While nephrectomy alone does not generally confer a survival advantage in patients with mRCC, in select cases, nephrectomy combined with the resection of a solitary pulmonary metastasis has been associated with extended survival[65,66]. In addition, many studies report improved response rates in patients who had a nephrectomy prior to immunotherapy[1,67,68].

The controversy arises from reports documenting significant morbidity and mortality associated with the surgery itself, often resulting in inability to treat with immunotherapy. Significant perioperative complications have been reported in 13–50% of patients treated with nephrectomy prior to systemic immunotherapy[68–70]. This surgical morbidity and mortality along with disease progression resulted in a failure to treat rate of up to 77%[69]. However, in another study where nephrectomy was performed prior to definitive treatment with TIL therapy, only 1 (9%) failed to be treated with IL-2 therapy[71]. The issue is whether the retained intact primary tumor affects responses of the metastatic deposits to immunotherapy. To help answer this question, an ongoing Southwestern Oncology Group phase III trial is currently randomizing patients prospectively to receive systemic interferon therapy either after nephrectomy or without nephrectomy.

Conclusion

There are a number of potentially new approaches to treating mRCC. Some are in phase III trials while others are still in their inception with technical obstacles that must be surmounted. It is hoped that in the future more immunotherapy trials will be controlled and survival data rather than just response rate will be reported. Although response rates are important they may ultimately not translate to prolonged survival in immunotherapy as in cytotoxic chemotherapy. In addition, many studies have reported late or delayed responses and long-term survival has between seen in non-responders. The concept of long-term immunotherapy that produces tumor stability rather than tumor regression remains an intriguing one. If this proves to be the case, then therapies which are effective with less toxicity and less expense will become more widely used. The treatment of cancer by gene therapy is an exciting and extremely active area of research. Successes in this area will lead to many new innovations in the treatment and potential cure of metastatic renal cell carcinoma.

References

1. deKernion JB, Ramming KP, Smith RB. The natural history of metastatic renal cell carcinoma: a computer analysis. *J Urol* 1978;**120**:148–152.
2. Hellsten S, Berge T, Wehlin L. Unrecognized renal cell carcinoma: clinical and pathological aspects. *Scand J Urol Nephrol* 1981;**15**:273–278.
3. Hermanek P, Schrott KM. Evaluation of the new tumor, nodes and metastases classification of renal cell carcinoma. *J Urol* 1990;**144**:238–242.
4. Katz SA, Davis JE. Renal adenocarcinoma: prognostics and treatment reflected by survival. *Urology* 1977;**10**(1):10–11.
5. Ritchie AWS, Chisholm GD. The natural history of renal carcinoma. *Semin Oncol* 1983;**40**(4):390–400.
6. deKernion JB. Treatment of advanced renal cell carcinoma – traditional methods and innovative approaches. *J Urol* 1983;**130**:2–7.
7. Harris DT. Hormonal therapy and chemotherapy of renal-cell carcinoma. *Sem Onc* 1983;**10**:422–430.
8. Finney R. An evaluation of postoperative radiotherapy in hypernephroma treatment – a clinical trial. *Cancer* 1973;**32**:1332–1340.
9. Yagoda A, Bassam A, Petrylak D. Chemotherapy for advanced renal-cell carcinoma: 1983–1993. *J Clin Oncol* 1995;**22**(1):42–60.
10. Oliver RTD, Nethersell ABW, Bottomeley JM. Unexplained spontaneous regression and alpha-interferon as treatment for metastatic renal carcinoma. *Br J Urol* 1989;**63**:128–131.
11. Friedman PM. Antiviral activity of interferons. *Bacteriol Rev* 1977;**41**:543–567.
12. deKernion JB, Sarna G, Figlin R, Lindner A, Smith RB. The treatment of renal cell carcinoma with human leukocyte alpha-interferon. *J Urol* 1983;**130**:1063–1066.
13. Quesada JR, Swanson DA, Trindade A, Gutterman JU. Renal cell carcinoma: antitumor effects of leukocyte interferon. *Cancer Res* 1983;**43**:940–947.
14. Umeda T, Niijima T. Phase II study of alpha interferon on renal cell carcinoma. Summary of three collaborative trials. *Cancer* 1986;**58**:1231–1235.
15. Minasian LM, Motzer RJ, Gluck L, Mazumdar M, Vlamis V, Krown SE. Interferon Alfa-2a in advanced renal cell carcinoma: treatment results and survival in 159 patients with long-term follow-up. *J Clin Oncol* 1993;**11**(7):1368–1375.
16. Fossa SD, Martinelli G, Otto U *et al*. Recombinant interferon alfa-2a with or without vinblastine in metastatic renal cell carcinoma: results of a European multi-center phase III study. *Annals Oncol* 1992;**3**(4):301–305.
17. Fossa S, Jones M, Johnson P *et al*. Interferon-alpha and survival in renal cell cancer. *Br J Urol* 1995;**76**(3):286–290.
18. Kirkwood JM, Harris JE, Vera R *et al*. A randomized study of low and high doses of leukocyte alpha-interferon in metastatic renal cell carcinoma: The American Cancer Society Collaborative Trial. *Cancer Res* 1985;**45**:863–871.
19. Wirth MP. Immunotherapy for metastatic renal cell carcinoma. *Urol Clin N Am* 1993;**20**(2):283–295.
20. De Mulder PH, Oosterhof G, Bouffioux C, van Oosterom AT, Vermeylen K, Sylvester R. EORTC (30885) randomised phase III study with recombinant interferon alpha and recombinant interferon alpha and gamma in patients with advanced renal cell carcinoma. The EORTC Genitourinary Group. *Br J Cancer* 1995;**71**(2):371–375.
21. Morgan DA, Ruscetti FW, Gallo R. Selective in vitro growth of T lymphocytes from normal human bone marrows. *Science* 1976;**193**:1007–1008.
22. Fyfe G, Fisher RI, Rosenberg SA, Sznol M, Parkinson DR, Louie AC. Results of treatment of 255 patients with metastatic renal cell carcinoma who received high-dose recombinant interleukin-2 therapy. *J Clin Oncol* 1995;**13**(3):688–696.
23. Taneja SS, Pierce W, Figlin R, Belldegrun A. Immunotherapy for renal cell carcinoma: the era of interleukin-2 based treatment. *Urology* 1995;**45**(6):911–924.
24. Siegel JP, Puri RK. Interleukin-2 toxicity. *J Clin Oncol* 1991;**9**:694–704.
25. Donohue JH, Rosenstein M, Chang AE *et al*. The systemic administration of purified interleukin-2 enhances the ability of sensitized murine lymphocytes

335

to cure a disseminated syngeneic lymphoma. *J Immunol* 1984;**132**:2123–2128.

26. Ettinghausen SE, Rosenberg SA. Immunotherapy of murine sarcomas using lymphokine activated killer cells: Optimization of the schedule and route of administration of recombinant interleukin-2. *Cancer Res* 1986;**46**:2784–2792.

27. Yang JC, Topalian SL, Parkinson D et al. Randomized comparison of high-dose and low-dose intravenous interleukin-2 for the therapy of metastatic renal cell carcinoma: an interim report. *J Clin Oncol* 1994;**12**(8):1572–1576.

28. Brunda MJ, Bellantoni D, Sulich V. In vivo antitumor activity of combinations of interferon-alpha and interleukin-2 in a murine model. Correlation of efficacy with the induction of cytotoxic cells resembling natural killer cells. *Int J Cancer* 1987;**40**:365–371.

29. Cameron RB, McIntosh JK, Rosenberg SA. Synergistic antitumor effects of combination immunotherapy with recombinant interleukin-2 and a recombinant hybrid alpha-interferon in the treatment of established murine hepatic metastases. *Cancer Res* 1988;**48**:5810–5817.

30. Rosenberg SA, Lotze MT, Yang JC et al. Combination therapy with interleukin-2 and alpha-interferon for the treatment of patients with advanced cancer. *J Clin Oncol* 1989;**7**(12):1863–1874.

31. Marincola FM, White DE, Wise AP, Rosenberg SA. Combination therapy with intereferon alfa-2a and interleukin-2 for the treatment of metastatic cancer. *J Clin Oncol* 1995;**13**(5):1110–1122.

32. Atkins MB, Sparano J, Fisher RI et al. Randomized phase II trial of high-dose interleukin-2 either alone or in combination with interferon alfa-2b in advanced renal cell carcinoma. *J Clin Oncol* 1993;**11**(4):661–670.

33. Atzpodien J, Korfer A, Franks CR, Poliwoda H, Kirchner H. Home therapy with recombinant interleukin-2 and interferon-α2b in advanced human malignancies. *Lancet* 1990;**335**:1509–1512.

34. Mittelman A, Puccio C, Ahmed T, Zeffren J, Choudhury A, Arlin Z. A phase II trial of interleukin-2 by continuous infusion and interferon by intramuscular injection in patients with renal cell carcinoma. *Cancer* 1991;**68**:1699–1702.

35. Figlin RA, Belldegrun A, Moldawer N, Zeffren J, deKernion J. Concomitant administration of recombinant human interleukin-2 and recombinant interferon alpha-2A: an active outpatient regimen in metastatic renal cell carcinoma. *J Clin Oncol* 1992;**10**:414–421.

36. Lipton A, Harvey H, Givant E et al. Interleukin-2 and interferon alpha-2 alpha outpatient therapy for metastatic renal cell carcinoma. *J Immunother* 1993;**13**:122–129.

37. Atzpodien J, Hanninen EL, Kirchner H et al. Multiinstitutional home-therapy trial of recombinant human interleukin-2 and interferon alfa-2 in progressive metastatic renal cell carcinoma. *J Clin Oncol* 1995;**13**(2):497–501.

38. Hofmockel G, Langer W, Theiss M, Gruss A, Frohmuller HGW. Immunochemotherapy for metastatic renal cell carcinoma using a regimen of interleukin-2, interferon-α and 5-fluorouracil. *J Urol* 1996;**156**:18–21.

39. Atzpodien J, Kirchner H, Hanninen EL, Deckert M, Fenner M, Poliwoda H. Interleukin-2 in combination with interferon-α and 5-fluorouracil for metastatic renal cell cancer. *Eur J Cancer* 1993;**29A**(suppl 5): S6–S8.

40. Rosenberg SA, Lotze MT, Muul LM et al. Observations on the systemic administration of autologous lymphokine-activated killer cells and recombinant interleukin-2 to patients with metastatic cancer. *New Eng J Med* 1985;**313**(23):1485–1492.

41. Rosenberg SA, Lotze MT, Muul LM et al. A progress report on the treatment of 157 patients with advanced cancer using lymphokine-activated killer cells and interleukin-2 or high-dose interleukin-2 alone. *N Eng J Med* 1987;**316**(15):889–897.

42. Rosenberg SA, Lotze MT, Yang JC et al. Experience with the use of high-dose interleukin-2 in the treatment of 652 cancer patients. *Ann Surg* 1989;**210**:484–485.

43. Schoof DD, Gramolini BA, Davidson DL, Massaro AF, Wilson RE, Eberlein T. Adoptive immunotherapy of human cancer using low-dose recombinant interleukin-2 and lymphokine-activated killer cells. *Cancer Res* 1988;**48**:5007–5010.

44. Rosenberg SA, Lotze MT, Yang JC et al. Prospective randomized trial of high-dose interleukin-2 alone or in conjunction with lymphokine-activated killer

cells for the treatment of patients with advanced cancer. *J Natl Cancer Inst* 1993;**85**(8):622–632.

45. Rosenberg SA, Spiess PRL. A new approach to the adoptive immunotherapy of cancer with tumor infiltrating lymphocytes. *Science* 1986;**233**: 1318–1321.

46. Belldegrun A, Muul LM, Rosenberg SA. Interleukin 2 expanded tumor-infiltrating lymphocytes in human renal cell cancer: isolation, characterization, and antitumor activity. *Cancer Res* 1988;**48**:206–214.

47. Choudhary A, Davodeau F, Moreau A, Peyrat MA, Bonneville M, Jotereau F. Selective lysis of autologous tumor cells by recurrent gamma delta tumor-infiltrating lymphocytes from renal carcinoma. *J Immunol* 1995;**154**:3932–3940.

48. Figlin RA. Cancer immunotherapy using tumor-infiltrating lymphocytes. *Semin Hematol* 1992;**29**(2 suppl 1): 33s–35s.

49. Pierce WC, Belldegrun A, Figlin RA. Cellular therapy: scientific rationale and clinical results in the treatment of metastatic renal cell carcinoma. *Semin Oncol* 1995;**22**(1):74–80.

50. Sawczuk IS. Autolymphocyte therapy in the treatment of metastatic renal cell carcinoma. *Urol Clin N Am* 1993;**20**(2):297–301.

51. Krane RJ, Carpinito GA, Ross SD, Lavin PT, Osband ME. Treatment of metastatic renal cell carcinoma with autolymphocyte therapy. *Urology* 1990;**35**(5):417–422.

52. Osband ME, Lavin PT, Babayan RK et al. Effect of autolymphocyte therapy on survival and quality of life in patients with metastatic renal-cell carcinoma. *Lancet* 1990;**335**:994–998.

53. Mulligan RC. The basic science of gene therapy. *Science* 1993;**260**(5110):926–932.

54. Jaffee EM, Pardoll DM. Gene therapy: its potential applications in the treatment of renal-cell carcinoma. *Sem Oncol* 1995;**22**(1):81–91.

55. Foa R, Guarini A, Gansbacher B. IL2 treatment for cancer: from biology to gene therapy. *Br J Cancer* 1992;**66**:992–998.

56. Mickisch GH. Gene therapy on renal-cell carcinoma: magic bullet or tragic insanity? *World J Urol* 1995;**13**:178–185.

57. Mastrangelo MJ, Berd D, Nathan FE, Lattime EC. Gene therapy for human cancer: an essay for clinicians. *Sem Onc* 1996;**23**(1):4–21.

58. Nabel EG, Plautz G, Nabel GJ. Site-specific gene expression in vivo by direct gene transfer into the arterial wall. *Science* 1990;**249**:1285–1288.

59. Gudkov AV, Zelnick CR, Kazarov AR et al. Isolation of genetic suppressor elements, inducing resistance to topoisomerase II-interactive cytotoxic drugs, from human topoisomerase II cDNA. *Proc Natl Acad Sci USA* 1993;**90**(8):3231–3235.

60. Gudkov AV, Kazarov AR, Thimmapaya R, Axenovich SA, Mazo IA, Roninson IB. Cloning mammalian genes by expression selection of genetic suppressor elements: association of kinesin with drug resistance and cell immortalization. *Proc Natl Acad Sci USA* 1994;**91**(9):3744–3748.

61. Golumbek PT, Lazenby AJ, Levitsky HI et al. Treatment of established renal cell cancer by tumor cells engineered to secrete interleukin-4. *Science* 1991;**254**:713–716.

62. Gansbacher B, Motzer R, Houghton A, Bander S. A pilot study of immunization with interleukin-2 secreting allogenic HLA-A2 matched renal cell carcinoma cells in patients with advanced renal cell carcinoma. *Hum Gene Ther* 1992;**3**:691–703.

63. Dranoff G, Jaffee E, Lazenby A et al. Vaccination with irradiated tumor cells engineered to secrete murine granulocyte-macrophage colony-stimulating factor stimulates potent, specific, and long-lasting anti-tumor immunity. *Proc Natl Acad Sci USA* 1993;**90**(8):3539–3543.

64. Freeman SM, Whartenby KA, Freeman JL, Abboud CN, Marrogi AJ. In situ use of suicide genes for cancer therapy. *Sem Oncol* 1996;**23**(1):31–45.

65. Morrow CE, Vassilopoulos PP, Grage TB. Surgical resection for metastatic neoplasms of the lung: experience at the University of Minnesota Hospitals. *Cancer* 1980;**45**:2981–2985.

66. Johnson DE, Kaesler KE, Samuels ML. Is nephrectomy justified in patients with metastatic renal carcinoma. *J Urol* 1975;**114**:24–29.

67. Marcus SG, Choyke PL, Reiter R et al. Regression of metastatic renal cell carcinoma after cytoreductive nephrectomy. *J Urol* 1993;**150**: 463–466.

8. Walther MM, Alexander RB, Weiss GH et al. Cytoreductive surgery prior to interleukin-2 based therapy in patients with metastatic renal cell carcinoma. Urology 1993;42(3):250–258.

9. Bennett RT, Lerner SE, Taub HC, Dutcher JP, Fleischmann J. Cytoreductive surgery for stage IV renal cell carcinoma. J Urol 1995;154:32–34.

70. Rackley R, Novick A, Klein E, Bukowski R, McLain D, Goldfarb D. The impact of adjuvant nephrectomy on multimodality treatment of metastatic renal cell carcinoma. J Urol 1994;152:1399–1403.

71. Belldegrun A, Pierce W, Kaboo R et al. Interferon-α primed tumor-infiltrating lymphocytes combined with interleukin-2 and interferon-α as therapy for metastatic renal cell carcinoma. J Urol 1993;150:1384–1390.

72. Quesada JR, Rios A, Swanson D et al. Antitumor activity of recombinant-derived interferon alpha in metastatic renal cell carcinoma. J Clin Oncol 1985;3:1522–1528.

73. Creagan ET, Twito DI, Johansson SL et al. A randomized prospective assessment of recombinant leukocyte α human interferon with or without aspirin in advanced renal adenocarcinoma. J Clin Oncol 1991;9:2104–2109.

74. Tsavaris N, Mylonakis N, Bacoyiannis C, Tsoutsos H, Karabelis A, Kosmidis P. Treatment of renal cell carcinoma with escalating doses of alpha-interferon. Chemotherapy 1993;39(5):361–366.

75. Rosenberg SA, Yang JC, Topalian SL et al. Treatment of 283 consecutive patients with metastatic melanoma or renal cell cancer using high-dose bolus interleukin 2. JAMA 1994;271:907–913.

76. Negrier S, Philip T, Stoter G et al. Interleukin-2 with or without LAK cells in metastatic renal cell carcinoma: A report of a European multicentre study. Eur J Cancer Clin Oncol 1989;25:S21.

77. von der Maase H, Geertsen P, Thatcher N et al. Recombinant interleukin-2 in metastatic renal cell carcinoma – a European multicentre phase II study. Eur J Cancer 1991;27:1583–1589.

78. Geertsen PF, Hermann GG, von der Maase H, Steven K. Treatment of metastatic renal cell carcinoma by continuous intravenous infusion of recombinant interleukin-2: a single-center phase II study. J Clin Oncol 1992;10(5):753–759.

79. Stein RC, Malkovska V, Morgan S et al. The clinical effects of prolonged treatment of patients with advanced cancer with low-dose subcutaneous interleukin-2. Br J Cancer 1991;63:275–278.

80. Lissoni P, Barni S, Ardizzoia A et al. Second line therapy with low-dose subcutaneous interleukin-2 alone in advanced renal cancer patients resistant to interferon-alpha. Eur J Cancer 1992;28(1):92–96.

81. Sleijfer DT, Janssen RAJ, Butler J et al. Phase II study of subcutaneous interleukin-2 in unselected patients with advanced renal cell cancer on an outpatient basis. J Clin Oncol 1992;10:1119–1123.

82. Budd GT, Osgood B, Barna B et al. Phase I clinical trial of interleukin 2 and α-interferon: toxicity and immunologic effects. Cancer Res 1989;49:6432–6436.

83. Vogelzang NJ, Lipton A, Figlin RA. Subcutaneous interleukin-2 plus interferon alfa-2a in metastatic renal cancer: an outpatient multicenter trial. J Clin Oncol 1993;11(9):1809–1816.

24.3   The role of chemotherapy

G Velikova and P J Selby

Introduction

Cancer of the kidney accounts for 1.6% of all cancers in the UK and for 1.8% of cancer deaths[1]. Thirty per cent of the patients with renal cancer have metastatic disease at initial presentation and 25% have locally advanced disease[2–4]. Thirty per cent of patients with localized

tumors relapse after radical nephrectomy with median time before relapse of 15 to 18 months and with 85% of the relapses occurring within 3 years[5]. Even patients who are free of disease 10 years after diagnosis have a 10% risk of developing late recurrence[6]. Overall only about one-third of the patients with renal cell cancer (RCC) are cured from their disease by surgery. The prognosis of patients with advanced RCC is poor. The expected 5 year survival for patients with recurrent and metastatic disease is between 0 and 10%[2,7]. Median survival duration following diagnosis of metastatic renal cancer is 6–16 months[5,6].

Many types of systemic therapy have been studied to assess their effects against metastatic RCC. The main approaches include hormonotherapy, chemotherapy and more recently biologic therapy. In this chapter we will review the results of the studies assessing the efficacy of hormonal and chemotherapeutic agents and discuss the few studies where chemotherapy has been used in combination with immunotherapy.

Hormonal therapy

The treatment of metastatic RCC with hormonal agents developed from encouraging results obtained in animal models showing that renal cancer may be hormone-dependent and hormone-sensitive[8–10]. Epidemiological and clinical observations suggest that hormones affect the growth of RCC in humans. RCC shows a predominance in male patients, with a male/female ratio of about 3 : 1 with increased incidence in females after the menopause suggesting that ovarian activity might protect women against RCC. The more aggressive course of renal cancer in men has been related to hormonal factors[11]. Receptors for estradiol and progesterone were found both in normal human kidney and in human renal cell carcinoma[12,13]. However, further studies suggested that the number of patients whose tumors expressed significant amounts of hormone receptors is very small and there is no correlation of steroid receptors with response to hormones[14,15].

Attempts have been made to treat renal cancer using progesterones, androgens or anti-estrogens. In a review of the clinical literature between 1967 and 1971, Bloom found a total of 173 cases (including 80 of his own) that had been treated with progesterone or androgen with a response rate from 7% to 25%. The overall objective response rate for the whole series was 16%[16]. Subsequent studies reported response rates varying between 5% and 10%, but these responses were usually partial, short and only for patients with lung metastases. Further review of hormonal therapy of RCC in 1977 suggested that if stricter criteria were applied to the earlier studies, the response rate declined to below 2%. However, at least in some series the response rate to hormonal treatment appeared to be greater than the rate of spontaneous regression[17]. A randomized trial of adjuvant medroxyprogesterone acetate following radical nephrectomy failed to show reduction in recurrence rate or prolongation of disease-free survival in the hormonotherapy arm[18]. More recent clinical studies assessed the effectiveness of anti-estrogens, mainly Tamoxifen, but failed to demonstrate any superior results. The overall results from hormonal therapy in advanced RCC are summarized in Table 24.3.1.

Taking the results of these hormonal studies as a group it seems reasonable to conclude that hormonotherapy has a minimal effect against human RCC with infrequent and incomplete responses, which are short-lived and do not appear to improve survival. Despite these data, hormonal therapy is still often used in advanced RCC because of its ease of administration, lack of toxicity and some positive symptomatic effects (e.g. increased appetite and weight gain), which can improve patients' quality of life. With the recent development of biological treatment achieving higher response rates, the hormonal treatment is usually considered only as a second/third line treatment for metastatic RCC or for elderly patients with poor performance status unlikely to tolerate biological therapy. However, evidence for improved long-term survival after biologic therapy compared with hormonal therapy remains scanty.

Chemotherapy

Many chemotherapeutic agents have been studied to assess their effect against metastatic RCC (Table 24.3.2). The most extensively studied are vinblastine, fluo-rodeoxyuridine (FUDR) and 5-fluorouracil (5-FU) Vinblastine 0.1–0.3 mg/kg/week has been considered until recently, the conventional chemotherapeutic regimen for metastatic RCC. Earlier studies of this drug reviewed by Hrushesky and Murphy[17] yielded a median response rate of 17.5%. However, more recent trials failed to demonstrate significant anti-tumor activity for vinblastine Efforts to improve the efficacy of vinblastine by administering it by continuous infusion have been largely unsuccessful.

5-FU administered as a continuous infusion or 5-day boluses with leukovorin has shown some limited activity in advanced RCC.

An innovative approach to the use of chemotherapy for metastatic RCC has been developed by Hrushesky[19] based on chronobiological cytokinetic and pharmacological administration of FUDR. It is based upon the theory that tumors with low growth fractions may respond better if there is long-term sustained concentration of a cytotoxic agent. They also noted variability of susceptibility of tumor and host cells as a result of an interaction of cytokinetic, pharmacokinetic, endocrine and immunological circadian rhythms. They designed circadian infusion pattern with a maximal flow rate in the afternoon which showed a higher dose intensity, better therapeutic index and lower gastrointestinal toxicity than constant FUDR infusion. A 21% remission rate was initially reported, but the overall remission rate in further trials was only 14%.

Alkylating agents and nitrosoureas have been investigated in the past with negligible therapeutic activity. Newer agents such as carboplatin, ifosfamide, amsacrine, paclitaxel, suramin, gemcitabine, topotecan, docetaxel all underwent phase II trials testing as potential agents against metastatic RCC but failed to show any activity superior to that of vinblastine, FUDR and 5FU (Table 24.3.2).

A recent extensive review of the results of 65 agents evaluated in phase II trials involving 4542 patients (of them 4093 adequately treated) revealed an objective response rate of 6% and usually of short duration[20]. The only cytotoxic agents that showed modest antitumor activity against metastatic RCC were FUDR and 5FU. No chemotherapeutic agent produced responses in proportions that would justify its use as single-agent therapy. However the use of combination chemotherapy did not yield better results than single agents, despite an increase in toxicity. A few examples of phase II studies of combination chemotherapy in advanced RCC are provided in Table 24.3.3.

This intrinsic resistance of RCC to multiple chemotherapeutic agents has been explained by expression of multiple drug resistance (MDR) associated P-170 glycoprotein by renal carcinomas. P-170 glycoprotein is encoded by the MDR1 gene and functions as an energy dependent transmembrane efflux pump which actively

Table 24.3.1 Clinical activity of hormonal therapy in advanced RCC

Agents	No. studies	No. patients	No. responders	Response rate (%)	Response rate (%) Range
Progestins					
Medroxyprogesterone acetate [16,52–61]	12	317	29	9	0–20
Others	4	47	3	6.3	0–12
Androgens					
Testosterone propionate [54,56,57,62]	4	61	8	13	0–29
Others [58,60,61]	3	54	1	1.8	0–5
Antioestrogens					
Tamoxifen-high dose* [63–66]	4	146	10	6.8	1.7–12
Tamoxifen-low dose** [67–70]	4	118	7	5.9	0–13

* Tamoxifen between 150 mg/m^2/day and 400 mg/m^2/day.
** Tamoxifen between 20 mg/day and 80 mg/day.

Table 24.3.2 Clinical activity of single-agent chemotherapy in advanced RCC

Agents	No. studies	No. patients	No. responders	Response rate (%)	Response rate (%) Range
Alkylating agents					
Chlorambucil[71]	1	133	19	14.2	13–17
Lomustine (CCNU)[72]	1	302	32	10.6	0–20
Ifosfamide[73–75]	3	43	1	2.3	0–9
Diaziquone[76–78]	4	132	2	1.5	0–4
Plant alkaloids					
Vinblastine (early studies)[17]	15	626	110	17.5	0–31
Vinblastine[79–84]	6	152	18	11.8	0–16
Vindesine[85–88]	3	69	0	0	0
Navelbine[89]	1	14	0	0	–
VM-26[90–92]	3	106	4	3.7	0–9
Antimetabolites					
5-FU[93, 94]	4	142	9	6.3	0–11
FUDR (cont. infusion)[95–98]	4	102	13	12.7	0–28
FUDR (Circadian infusion)[19, 99–108]	11	307	44	14.3	0–43
Gemcitabine[109–111]	3	93	7	7.5	6–10
Trimetrexate[112, 113]	2	54	1	1.8	0–3
Fludarabine[114, 115]	2	54	0	0	–
Antitumor antibiotics					
Doxorubicin[116]	1	14	0	0	0
Epirubicin[117,118]	2	41	0	0	0
Idarubicin[119]	1	21	0	0	0
Mitoxantrone[120–123]	4	177	0	0	0
Miscellaneous					
Amsacrine[124–127]	4	145	4	2.7	0–2
Bisantrene[128–132]	5	140	5	3.5	0–10
Carboplatin[133, 134]	2	42	0	0	0
Elliptinium[135–137]	3	70	7	10	0–21
Mitoguazone[138–142]	5	212	11	5.2	0–16
Rhizoxin[143]	1	18	0	0	–
Suramin[144,145]	2	38	1	2.6	0–4
Taxol[146,147]	2	35	0	0	0
Taxotere[148]	1	33	2	6	–
Topotecan[149]	1	15	0	0	–

Table 24.3.3 Clinical activity of combination chemotherapy for advanced RCC – examples

Agents	No. patients	No. responders	Response rate (%)
Dacarbasine + Cyclophosphamide + Cisplatin + Doxorubicin + Vindesine[150]	18	1	6.25
Mitoguazone + Melphalan[151]	16	0	0
FUDR + Vinblastine[152]	14	3	21
Vinblastine + Adriamycin[153]	11	2	18

The understanding of MDR has led to intensive investigation of many compounds that appear to inhibit or interfere with the function of P-glycoprotein. Several classes of reversing agents have been studied (e.g. calcium channel blockers, calmodulin antagonists: neuroleptics and antidepressants, steroid agonists/antagonists, immunosuppressants, anti-arrhythmics). These agents inhibit the binding of cytostatic agents to P-glycoprotein, thus allowing the anticancer drugs to accumulate in the cells. Dexverapamil, tamoxifen and trifluoperazine have been demonstrated in vitro to reverse the resistance of renal cancer cell lines to vinblastine and doxorubicin[29–33]. Unfortunately many of the chemosensitizing agents, although active in vitro, are not clinically effective or the required doses to overcome drug resistance are associated with unacceptable clinical toxicity, limiting their use. A few clinical trials using different chemosensitizing agents together with chemotherapy for advanced RCC have been largely unsuccessful (Table 24.3.4). Current research on reversal of MDR has focused on two approaches: 1) development of non-toxic reversing agents; 2) development of cytotoxic analogs of chemotherapeutic agents with lower affinity to P-glycoprotein; and both approaches hold some promise[21].

Biological therapy combined with chemotherapy

Late relapses of RCC after nephrectomy, prolonged stabilization of disease in the absence of systemic treatment and rare spontaneous regressions of metastases following nephrectomy or embolization, suggest that host immune mechanisms are important in regulating tumor growth and led to the initial studies of immunotherapy in metastatic RCC[35]. Indeed biologic therapy has altered the prospects for the treatment of RCC substantially. Used alone, interferons (IFN) and interleukin-2 (IL-2), with or without lymphocyte activated killer cells (LAK-cells), obtained responses in 10–15% [34] and 15–35%[35] of patients. Responses to IFN occur predominantly in patients with good performance status, prior nephrectomy

transports various chemotherapeutic agents out of the cell thus decreasing their intracellular concentration and their cytotoxicity. The group of drugs comprises a broad spectrum of structurally and functionally unrelated, naturally occurring, large hydrophobic compounds which share the property of binding to P-glycoprotein[21]. A series of studies confirmed strong MDR1 expression in most renal cell adenocarcinomas[22–27] although other mechanisms (e.g. glutathione and related enzymes) were also suggested[28].

Table 24.3.4   Phase I/II trials of combinations of chemotherapeutic drugs with chemosensitizing agents in advanced RCC

Agents	No. patients	No. responders	Response rate (%)	Toxicity
Vinblastine + Dipyridamole[154]	15	0	0	Leukopenia
Vinblastine + Nifedipine[155]	14	0	0	–
Vinblastine + Quinidine[156]	23	1	4	Leukopenia
Vinblastine + Verapanmil[157]	7	0	0	–
Vinblastine + Dexverapamil[158]	23	0	0	Hypotension, bradycardia, heart failure
Vinblastine + Dexverapamil*[159]	9	1	–	–
Vinblastine + Cyclosporin A[160]	15	0	0	–
Vinblastine + Cyclosporin A[161]	16	0	0	Leukopenia, vomiting, constipation, malaise
Vinblastine + Acrivastine[162]	17	0	0	Vomiting, leukopenia
Vinblastine and Adriamycin + Cepharanthine[163]	6	2	33	–
Lomustine + Amphotericin B[164]	5	0	0	–
Teniposide + Cyclosporin A[165]	5	0	0	Leukopenia

* Ongoing.

and limited metastatic disease, particularly when confined to the lungs [36,37]. Patients responding to IL-2 have a prolonged disease-free survival, good performance status and a limited number of disease sites[38]. It is possible that IFNs and IL-2 may offer a survival advantage to those patients who respond[36,38,39]. In combination IFN and IL-2 achieve response rates of 7–42% and with similar progression free intervals as monotherapy[40]. A major disadvantage of biologic therapy is toxicity which can be life-threatening in the case of intravenous IL-2.

The combination of IFN with chemotherapeutic agents is supported by substantial pre-clinical data showing synergistic effect in vitro between IFN and a number of cytotoxic drugs, including doxorubicin, cyclophosphamide, 5-FU and vinblastine[41]. The phase II studies assessing the clinical activity of combination of biologic therapy with chemotherapy are summarized in Table 24.3.5.

Most extensively studied in phase II trials is the combination of IFN and vinblastine, probably because vinblastine is regarded as the most effective cytotoxic drug. The results of the individual studies remain contradictory with response rate between 0 and 43% (Table 24.3.5). Overall the response rate seems comparable with that achieved with IFN alone. One randomized trial including 160 patients compared vinblastine and IFN with vinblastine alone and showed higher objective response and prolonged survival in the patient group receiving the combination treatment (response rate 16% vs. 2.5% and survival 15.8 vs. 8.8 months, respectively[42]. Whether the addition of vinblastine to IFN results in improvement in response rate and survival in metastatic RCC remains unclear. Two randomized trials addressed this question.

The European study involved 178 patients randomized to receive IFNα with or without vinblastine. The response rate was 11% for patients on monotherapy and 24% for combination therapy. There was no difference in survival, with 5 year survival of 9% for both arms[43]. However no significant difference in response rate emerged from a large American study where patients were randomized to receive human lymphoblastoid IFN alone or in combination with vinblastine (response rate 17% and 15% respectively[44]. In all studies the combination IFN and vinblastine produced increased toxicity, mainly myelosuppression. The two studies assessing the combination of IL-2 and vinblastine did not show any increased effectiveness (Table 24.3.5). Therefore the significance of adding vinblastine to biologic therapy is uncertain. It may increase slightly the response rate but has no influence on survival and certainly leads to increased toxicity.

The combination of IFN with FUDR has been clinically evaluated in three phase II studies. Two of them using continuous infusion of FUDR, reported response rate of 33%, but no remission were observed in the third one (using boluses of FUDR and folinic acid). One small study employing IFN in combination with 5-FU showed objective response of 23% of the patients, but in other studies the response rate was low. No significant increase over the activity of IFN alone was observed with its combinations with various other cytotoxic agents (Table 24.3.5).

A combination regimen including 5-FU, IFN and IL-2 has been developed based on pre-clinical models suggesting that: 1) IFN may augment IL-2 induced cell killing through activation of cytotoxic lymphocytes and via enhanced expres-

Table 24.3.5   Results achieved with combination of biologic therapy with chemotherapy

Agents	No. studies	No. patients	No. responders	Response rate (%)	Response rate (%) range
IFN and chemotherapy					
IFN + Vinblastine[42,43,166–183]	18	505	105	18.5	0–43
IFN + 5-FU[184–187]	4	86	12	14	0–25
IFN + FUDR (cont. infusion)[188,189]	2	55	18	33	–
IFN + FUDR + Leukovorin	1	20	0	0	–
IFN + Vinblastine + Doxorubicin[153]	1	11	2	18	–
IFN + Epirubicin + Vinblastine + MPA[190]	1	35	9	26	–
IFN + 5-FU + Mitomycin-C[191]	1	49	17	35	–
IFN + Cyclophosphamide[192]	1	25	1	4	–
IFN + Vindesine + Ifosfamide[193]	1	29	7	24	–
IL-2 and chemotherapy					
IL-2 + Vinblastine[194,195]	2	23	2	9	6–12
IFN, IL-2 and chemotherapy					
IFN, IL-2,5-FU[46–49,196]	5	265	88	38	9–48
IFN, IL-2,5-FU, Vinblastine and Retinoic acid[51]	1	45	20	44	–
IFN + IL-2 + Retinoic acid[197]	1	34	6	22	–
IFN + IL-2 + cyclophosphamide[198]	1	16	2	12	–

Cyclophosphamide[198].

sion of major histocompatibility complex-I antigens on tumor cells; 2) synergistic anti-neoplastic activity of IFN, IL-2 and 5-FU[41,43]. The initial results of this outpatient regimen showed overall response rate of 48.6% suggesting that the regimen may represent a genuine advance in the management of metastatis RCC[46]. Further studies from the same group of investigators confirmed high response rate around 38–39% with mild to moderate toxicity[47,48].

We treated 55 patients with advanced RCC in a phase II study using the same combination of IFN, IL-2 and 5-FU. Thirty-eight patients were evaluable for response and there were nine partial remissions, representing a response rate of 24% (95% CI 10–38%) of evaluable patients and 16% of all patients. The median survival for patients with stable disease or partial remission exceeded 22 months. Outcome and survival were related to performance status, number of sites of metastatic disease and prior nephrectomy. Among 25 evaluable patients who previously had nephrectomy, the response rate was 32% (95% CI 14–50%) where as there was only one response amongst 22 patients who had not undergone nephrectomy. All responses were seen in patients with metastases in the lungs, regional nodes and with good performance status. The toxicity of the regimen was considerable with 44% of patients experiencing at least one grade III toxicity and only 14% reported less than grade II toxicities. The main side effects associated with this regimen were fatigue, nausea, pyrexia, mucositis, diarrhoea and renal impairment. Assessment of quality of life of the patients showed significant deterioration in the Rotterdam Symptom Checklist measurements of activity and symptoms 4 weeks after commencement of treatment.

Our results confirm that the combination of IFN, IL-2 and 5-FU is an active regimen in metastatic and recurrent RCC but the patients who are likely to benefit are limited to those with good performance status, limited sites of disease and who have undergone nephrectomy[49].

Recently this regimen was further extended by adding 13-cis-retinoic acid with initial response rate of 42–44%. Further more the combination of 13-cis-retinoic acid and IFN achieved objective response in four out of 19 patients with disease resistant to IFN, IL-2 and 5-FU[50,51].

Overall the combination of biologic therapy with chemotherapy seems to achieve a moderate response rate in a selected group of patients with good prognosis but it needs further assessment in randomized trials.

Conclusions

The current results of systemic treatment of advanced RCC are largely unsatisfactory. Most of the studies of hormonal and cytotoxic agents are 10–20 years older than those of biologic therapy. Therefore stage migration, quality of care and improvement in defining response may influence the response to a drug and contribute to the higher response rate seen in the more recent studies. Also IFN and IL-2 are considered better than hormones and cytotoxics mainly from comparison of results from phase II studies. There is a remarkable lack of randomized phase III trials in the treatment of metastatic RCC. Never the less IFN and IL-2 (with or without chemotherapy) appear to have an encouraging antitumor activity in patients with favorable prognostic characteristics and may also have a positive impact on survival. However further studies are needed in this subgroup of patients to identify the treatment of choice and the best sequence and combination of drugs. Use of chemobiological treatments may be considered as adjuvant therapy in patients at high risk of relapse after nephrectomy but this should only happen in prospective randomized trials.

For patients with unfavorable prognostic factors biologic therapy and chemotherapy do not show satisfactory activity while the toxicity is even higher. Hormonotherapy, especially with progestins, may offer useful palliation and improvement in quality of life for these patients. They also should be encouraged to enter controlled clinical trials aimed to evaluate investigational drugs and new therapeutic approaches.

In view of the resistance of RCC to systemic therapy two aspects of patients care should be emphasized: 1) asymptomatic patients could be offered the option of initial close surveillance with systemic therapy delayed (and toxicity thus avoided) until symptoms appear or there is evidence of progression; 2) systemic therapy can not be relied on to palliate symptoms (e.g. pain) or treat complications (e.g. spinal cord compression, hypercalcemia) and these must be managed with active supportive care.

New drugs are urgently required and as soon as they are described, they should be rapidly tested in RCC. This should continue for both chemotherapy and biological therapy. While some progress may come from a better understanding of patients selection and new schedules for existing agents, the best hope for patients with advanced renal cancer lies in the development of effective new agents.

References

1. Doll R, Peto R, Weatherall DJ, Ledingham JGG, Warrell DA (eds). Epidemiology of cancer. In: *Oxford textbook of medicine* (3rd edn) Oxford University Press, Oxford, New York; 1996, pp. 197–222.
2. Couillard DR, deVere White RW. Surgery of renal cell carcinoma. *Urol Clin N Am* 1993; **20**:263–275.
3. Kidney cancer: a report by 97 Illinois hospitals on cases diagnosed in 1975–85. Report no.12 of results in treating cancer. American Cancer Society, Chicago, 1989.
4. Ritchie AWS, Chisholm GD. The natural history of renal carcinoma. *Semin Oncol* 1983; 10:390–400.
5. Rabinovitch RA, Zelefsky MJ, Gaynor JJ, Fuks Z. Patterns of failure following surgical resection of renal cell carcinoma: implications for adjuvant local and systemic therapy. *J Clin Oncol* 1994; **12**(1):206–212.
6. McNichols DW, Segura JW, DeWeerd JH. Renal cell carcinoma: long-term survival and late recurrence. *J Urol* 1981; **126**(1):17–23.
7. Motzer RJ, Bander NH, Nanus DM. Renal-cell carcinoma. *N Engl J Med* 1996; **335**(12):865–875.
8. Kirkman H, Bacon RL. Estrogen-induced tumors of the kidney. I. Incidence of renal tumors in intact and gonadectomized male golden hamsters treated with diethylstilbestrol. *J Natl Cancer Inst* 1952; **13**: 745–756.

9. Kirkman H, Bacon RL. Estrogen-induced tumors of the kidney. II Effect of dose, administration, type of estrogen and age on the induction of renal tumors in intact male golden hamsters. *J Natl Cancer Inst* 1952; **13**:757–764.
10. Horning ES. Observations on hormone-dependent renal tumors in the golden hamster. *Br J Cancer* 1956; **10**:678–682.
11. Bloom HJ. Proceedings: Hormone-induced and spontaneous regression of metastatic renal cancer. *Cancer* 1973; **32**(5):1066–1071.
12. Concolino G, Marocchi A, Conti C, Tenaglia R, Di Silverio F, Bracci U. Human renal cell carcinoma as a hormone-dependent tumor. *Cancer Res* 1978; **38**(11:Pt 2)4340–4344.
13. Concolino G, Marocchi A, Tenaglia R, Di Silverio F, Sparano F. Specific progesterone receptor in human renal cancer. *J Ster Biochem* 1978; **9**(5):399–402.
14. Pearson J, Friedman MA, Hoffman PG Jr. Hormone receptors in renal cell carcinoma. Their utility as predictors of response to endocrine therapy. *Cancer Chemother Pharmacol* 1981; **6**(2):151–154.
15. Karr JP, Pontes JE, Schneider S, Sandberg AA, Murphy GP. Clinical aspects of steroid hormone receptors in human renal cell carcinoma. *J Surg Oncol* 1983; **23**(2):117–124.
16. Bloom HJ. Medroxyprogesterone acetate (Provera) in the treatment of metastatic renal cancer. *Br J Cancer* 1971; **25**(2):250–265.
17. Hrushesky WJ, Murphy GP. Current status of the therapy of advanced renal carcinoma. [Review]. *J Surg Oncol* 1977; **9**(3):277–288.
18. Pizzocaro G, Piva L, Di Fronzo G, Giongo A, Cozzoli A, Dormia E, Minervini S, Zanollo A, Fontanella U, Longo G et al. Adjuvant medroxyprogesterone acetate to radical nephrectomy in renal cancer: 5-year results of a prospective randomized study. *J Urol* 1987; **138**(6):1379–1381.
19. Hrushesky WJ, Von Roemeling R, Fraley EE, Rabatin JT. Circadian-based infusional chrono-chemotherapy controls progressive metastatic renal cell carcinoma. *Semin Surg Oncol* 1988; **4**(2):110–115.
20. Yagoda A, Abi-Rached B, Petrylak D. Chemotherapy for advanced renal-cell carcinoma: 1983–1993. [Review]. *Semin Oncol* 1995; **22**(1):42–60.
21. Chapman AE, Goldstein LJ. Multiple drug resistance: biologic basis and clinical significance in renal-cell carcinoma. [Review]. *Semin Oncol* 1995; **22**(1):17–28.
22. Fojo AT, Shen D, Mickley LA et al. Intrinsic drug resistance in human kidney cancer is associated with expression of a human multidrug-resistance gene. *J Clin Oncol* 1987; **5**:1922–1927.
23. Kakehi Y, Kanamaru H, Yoshida O, et al. Measurement of multidrug-resistance messenger RNA in urogenital cancers: Elevated expression in renal carcinomais associated with intrinsic drug resistance. *J Urol* 1988; **139**:862–865.
24. Goldstein LJ, Galski H, Fojo A. Expression of the multidrug resistance gene in human cancers. *J Natl Cancer Inst* 1989; **81**:116–124.
25. Nishiyama K, Shirahama T, Yoshimura A et al. Expression of the multidrug transport P-glycoprotein in renal and transitional cell carcinoma. *Cancer* 1993; **71**:3611–3619.
26. Bak M Jr, Efferth T, Mickisch G, Mattern J, Volm M. Detection of drug resistance and P-glycoprotein in human renal cell carcinomas. *Eur Urol* 1990; **17**(1):72–75.
27. Tobe SW, Noble-Topham SE, Andrulis IL, Warren R, Hartwick J, Skorecki KL, Warner E. Expression of the multiple drug resistance gene in human renal cell carcinoma depends on tumor histology, grade, and stage. *Clin Cancer Res* 1995; **1**(2):1611–1615.
28. Naito S, Sakamoto N, Kotoh S, Goto K, Matsumoto T, Kumazawa J. Expression of P-glycoprotein and multidrug resistance in renal cell carcinoma. *Eur Urol* 1993; **24**(1):156–160.
29. Mickisch GH, Kossig J, Tschada RK, Keilhauer G, Schlick E, Alken PM. Circumvention of multidrug resistance mediated by P-170 glycoprotein using calcium antagonists in primary human renal cell carcinoma. *Urol Int* 1991; **47**(3):118–125.
30. Mickisch GH, Merlino GT, Aiken PM, Gottesman MM, Pastan I. New potent verapamil derivatives that reverse multidrug resistance in human renal carcinoma cells and in transgenic mice expressing the human MDR1 gene. *J Urol* 1991; **146**(2):447–453.

31. Lai T, Collins CM, Hall P, Morgan AP, Smith PJ, Stonebridge BR, Symes MO. Verapamil enhances doxorubicin activity in cultured human renal carcinoma cells. *Eur J Cancer* 1993; **29A**(3):378–383.

32. Volm M, Pommerenke EW, Efferth T, Lohrke H, Mattern J. Circumvention of multi-drug resistance in human kidney and kidney carcinoma in vitro. *Cancer* 1991; **67**(10):2484–2489.

33. Fine RL, Williams A, Jett M *et al*. Tamoxifen (TAM) potentiates the antitumour effect of vinblastine against intrinsically multidrug resistant (mdr) human renal cell carcinoma lines. [Abstract] *Proc AACR* 1990; **31**:359.

34. Pittman K, Selby P. The management of renal cell carcinoma. [Review]. *Crit Rev Oncol Hematol* 1994; **16**(3):181–200.

35. Whittington R, Faulds D. Interleukin-2: A review of its pharmacological properties and therapeutic use in patients with cancer. *Drugs* 1993; **46**:446–514.

36. Fossa SD, Kramar A, Droz JP. Prognostic factors and survival in patients with metastatic renal cell carcinoma treated with chemotherapy or interferon-alpha. *Eur J Cancer* 1994; **30A**(9):1310–1314.

37. Minasian LM, Motzer RJ, Gluck L, Mazumdar M, Vlamis V, Krown SE. Interferon alfa-2a in advanced renal cell carcinoma: treatment results and survival in 159 patients with long-term follow-up. *J Clin Oncol* 1993; **11**(7):1368–1375.

38. Jones M, Philip T, Palmer P, von der Maase H, Vinke J, Elson P, Franks CR, Selby P. The impact of interleukin-2 on survival in renal cancer: a multivariate analysis. *Cancer Biother* 1993; **8**(4):275–288.

39. Fossa SD, Jones M, Johnson P, Joffe J, Holdener E, Elson P, Ritchie A, Selby P. Interferon-alpha and survival in renal cell cancer. *Br J Urol* 1995; **76**:286–290.

40. Negrier S, Escudier B, Lasset C, Savary J, Douillard JY, Chevreau C, Ravaud A, Peny J, Mousseau M. The FNCLCC Crecy trial: interleukin 2 (IL2) + interferon (IFN) is the optimal treatment to induce responses in metastatic renal cell carcinoma (MRCC) (Meeting abstract). *Proc Am Soc Clin Oncol* 1996; **15**:A629.

41. Wadler S, Schwartz EL. Antineoplastic activity of the combination of interferon and cytotoxic agents against experimental and human malignancies: a review. *Cancer Res* 1990; **50**:3473–3486.

42. Pyrhonen S, Salminen E, Lehtonen T, Nurmi M, Tammela T, Juusela H, Ruutu M, Kellokumpu-Lehtinen P. Recombinant interferon alfa-2a with vinblastine vs vinblastine alone in advanced renal cell carcinoma: a phase III study (Meeting abstract). *Proc Am Soc Clin Oncol* 1996; **15**:A614.

43. Fossa SD, Martinelli G, Otto U, Schneider G, Wander H, Oberling F, Bauer HW, Achtnicht U, Holdener EE. Recombinant interferon alfa-2a with or without vinblastine in metastatic renal cell carcinoma: results of a European multi-center phase III study. *Ann Oncol* 1992; **3**(4):301–305.

44. Neinhart JA, Anderson SA, Harris JE *et al*. Vinblastine fails to improve response of renal cancer to interferon alpha-n1: high response rate in patients with pulmonary metastases. *J Clin Oncol* 1991; **9**: 832–840.

45. Reiter Z, Ozes ON, Blatt LM, Taylor MW. A dual anti-tumor effect of a combination of interferon-alpha and 5-fluorouracil on natural killer cell-mediated toxicity. *Clin Immunol Immunopath* 1992; **62**:103–111.

46. Atzpodien J, Kirchner H, Hanninen EL, Deckert M, Fenner M, Poliwoda H. Interleukin-2 in combination with interferon-alpha and 5-fluorouracil for metastatic renal cell cancer. *Eur J Cancer* 1993; **29A**(suppl 5):S6–8.

47. Hofmockel G, Langer W, Theiss M, Gruss A, Frohmuller HG. Immunochemotherapy for metastatic renal cell carcinoma using a regimen of interleukin-2, interferon-alpha and 5-fluorouracil [see comments]. *J Urol* 1996; **156**(1):18–21.

48. Lopez Hanninen E, Kirchner H, Atzpodien J. Interleukin-2 based home therapy of metastatic renal cell carcinoma: risks and benefits in 215 consecutive single institution patients. *J Urol* 1996; **155**(1):19–25.

49. Joffe JK, Banks RE, Forbes MA, Hallam S, Jenkins A, Patel PM, Hall GD, Velikova G *et al*. A phase II study of interferon-alpha, interleukin-2 and 5-fluorouracil in advanced renal carcinoma: clinical data and laboratory evidence of protease activation. *Br J Urol* 1996; **77**(5):638–649.

50. Atzpodien J, Kirchner H, Duensing S, Lopez Hanninen E, Franzke A, Buer J, Probst M *et al*. Biochemotherapy of advanced metastatic renal-cell carcinoma: results of the combination of interleukin-2, alpha-interferon, 5-fluorouracil, vinblastine, and 13-cis-retinoic acid. *World J Urol* 1995; **13**(3):174–177.

51. Atzpodien J, Buer J, Probst M, Duensing S, Kirchner H, Ganser A. Clinical and pre-clinical role of 13-cis-retinoic acid in renal cell carcinoma: Hannover experience (Meeting abstract). *Proc Am Soc Clin Oncol* 1996; **15**:A625.

52. Steineck G, Strander H, Carbin BE, Borgstrom E, Wallin L, Achtnich U, Arvidsson A *et al*. Recombinant leukocyte interferon alpha-2a and medroxyprogesterone in advanced renal cell carcinoma. A randomized trial. *Acta Oncol* 1990; **29**(2):155–162.

53. Paine CH, Wright FW, Ellis F. The use of progestogen in the treatment of metastatic carcinoma of the kidney and uterine body. *Br J Cancer* 1970; **24**(2):277–282.

54. Papac RJ, Ross SA, Levy A. Renal cell carcinoma: analysis of 31 cases with assessment of endocrine therapy. *Am J Med Sci* 1977; **274**(3):281–290.

55. Stolbach LL, Begg CB, Hall T, Horton J. Treatment of renal carcinoma: a phase III randomized trial of oral medroxyprogesterone (Provera), hydroxyurea, and nafoxidine. *Cancer Treat Rep* 1981; **65**(7–8):689–692.

56. Werf-Messing B van der, Gilse HA van. Hormonal treatment of metastases of renal carcinoma. *Br J Cancer* 1971; **25**(3):423–427.

57. Wagle DG, Murphy GP. Hormonal therapy in advanced renal cell carcinoma. *Cancer* 1971; **28**(2):318–321.

58. Talley RW, Moorhead EL II, Tucker WG, San Diego EL, Brennan MJ. Treatment of metastatic hypernephroma. *JAMA* 1969; **207**(2):322–328.

59. Samuels ML, Sullivan P, Howe CD. Medroxyprogesterone acetate in the treatment of renal carcinoma (hypernephroma). *Cancer* 1968; **22**(3):525–532.

60. Morales A, Kiruluta G, Lott S. Hormones in the treatment of metastatic renal cancer. *J Urol* 1975; **114**(5):692–693.

61. Alberto P, Senn HJ. Hormonal therapy of renal carcinoma alone and in association with cytostatic drugs. *Cancer* 1974; **33**(5):1226–1229.

62. Jenkin RDT. Androgens in metastatic renal adenocarcinoma. *BMJ* 1967; 1:361.

63. Schomburg A, Kirchner H, Fenner M, Menzel T, Poliwoda H, Atzpodien J. Lack of therapeutic efficacy of tamoxifen in advanced renal cell carcinoma. *Eur J Cancer* 1993; **29A**(5):737–740.

64. Papac RJ, Keohane MF. Hormonal therapy for metastatic renal cell carcinoma combined androgen and provera followed by high dose tamoxifen. *Eur J Cancer* 1993; **29A**(7):997–999.

65. Stahl M, Wilke H, Schmoll HJ, Schober C, Diedrich H, Casper J, Freund M, Poliwoda H. A phase II study of high dose tamoxifen in progressive, metastatic renal cell carcinoma. *Ann Oncol* 1992; **3**(2):167–168.

66. Stahl M, Schmoll E, Becker H, Schlichter A, Hoffmann L, Wagner H, Possinger K *et al*. Lonidamine versus high-dose tamoxifen in progressive, advanced renal cell carcinoma: results of an ongoing randomized phase II study. *Semin Oncol* 1991; **18**(2:suppl 4):33–37.

67. Glick JH, Wein A, Torri S, Alavi J, Harris D, Brodovsky H. Phase II study of tamoxifen in patients with advanced renal cell carcinoma. *Cancer Treat Rep* 1980; **64**(2–3):343–344.

68. al-Sarraf M, Eyre H, Bonnet J, Saiki J, Gagliano R, Pugh R, Lehane D *et al*. Study of tamoxifen in metastatic renal cell carcinoma and the influence of certain prognostic factors: a Southwest Oncology Group Study. *Cancer Treat Rep* 1981; **65**(5–6):447–451.

69. Weiselberg L, Budman D, Vinciguerra V, Schulman P, Degnan TJ. Tamoxifen in unresectable hypernephroma. A phase II trial and review of the literature. *Cancer Clin Trials* 1981; **4**(2):195–198.

70. Lanteri VJ, Dragone N, Choudhury M *et al*. High-dose tamoxifen in metastatic renal cell carcinoma. *Urology* 1982; **19**:623.

71. Moore GE, Brass DJ, Ansman R. *et al*. Effects of chlorambucil (NSC-3088) in 374 patients with advanced cancer. *Cancer Chemother Rep* 1968; **52**:641–653.

72. Mittelmann A, Albert DJ, Murphy GP. Lomustine treatment of metastatic renal cell carcinoma. *JAMA* 1973; **225**:32–35.

73. DeForges A, Droz JP, Ghosn M et al. Phase II trial of ifosfamide and mesna in metastatic adult renal carcinoma. Cancer Treat Rep 1987; 71:1103.

74. Fossa SD, Talle K. Treatment of metastatic renal cell carcinoma with ifosfamide and mesnum with and without irradiation. Cancer Treat Rep 1980; 64:1103–1108.

75. Bodrogi I, Baki M, Sinkovics I, Eckhardt S. Ifosfamide chemotherapy of metastatic renal cell cancer. Semin Surg Oncol 1988; 4(2):95–96.

76. Nichols WC, Kvols LK, Richardson RLE. A phase II trial of azirinylbenzoquinone (AZQ) in advanced genitourinary (GU) cancer. [Abstract] Proc Am Soc Clin Oncol 1982; 1:117.

77. Hansen M, Gallmeier WM, Vermorken J et al. Phase II trial of diaziquone in advanced renal adenocarcinoma. Cancer Treat Rep 1984; 68:1055–1056.

78. Decker DA, Kish J, al-Sarraf M et al. Phase II clinical evaluation of AZQ in renal cell carcinoma. Am J Clin Oncol 1986; 9:126–128.

79. Fossa SD, Droz JP, Pavone-Macaluso MM, Debruyne FJ, Vermeylen K, Sylvester R. Vinblastine in metastatic renal cell carcinoma: EORTC phase II trial 30882. The EORTC Genitourinary Group. Eur J Cancer 1992; 28A(4–5):878–880.

80. Elson PJ, Kvols LK, Vogl SE, Glover DJ, Hahn RG, Trump DL, Carbone PP et al. Phase II trials of 5-day vinblastine infusion (NSC 49842), L-alanosine (NSC 153353), acivicin (NSC 163501), and aminothiadiazole (NSC 4728) in patients with recurrent or metastatic renal cell carcinoma. Invest New Drugs 1988; 6(2):97–103.

81. Crivellari D, Tumolo S, Frustaci S, Galligioni E, Figoli F, Lo Re G, Veronesi A, Monfardini S. Phase II study of five-day continuous infusion of vinblastine in patients with metastatic renal-cell carcinoma. Am J Clin Oncol 1987; 10(3):231–233.

82. Zeffren J, Yagoda A, Kelsen D et al. Phase I–II trial of a 5-day continuous infusion of vinblastine sulfate. Anticancer Res 1984; 4:411–414.

83. Kuebler JP, Hogan TF, Trump DL et al. Phase II study of continuous 5-day vinblastine infusion in renal adenocarcinoma. Cancer Treat Rep 1984; 68:925–926.

84. Tannock IF, Evans WK. Failure of 5-day vinblastine infusion in the treatment of patients with renal cell carcinoma. Cancer Treat Rep 1985; 69(2):227–228.

85. Wong PW, Yagoda A, Currie VE et al. Phase II study of vindesine sulfate in therapy for advanced renal cancer. Cancer Treat Rep 1977; 61:1727–1729.

86. Fossa SD, Denis L, Van Oosterom AT et al. Vindesine in advanced renal cancer: A study of the EORTC Genitourinary Tract Cancer Cooperative Group. Eur J Cancer Clin Oncol 1983; 19:473–475.

87. Valdisieso M, Bedikian AY, Bodey GP et al. Broad phase II study of vindesine. Cancer Treat Rep 1981; 65:877–879.

88. Valdisieso M, Richman S, Burgess AM et al. Initial clinical studies of vindesine. Cancer Treat Rep 1981; 65:873–875.

89. Canobbio L, Boccardo F, Guarneri D, Calabria C, Decensi A, Curotto A, Martorana G, Giuliani L. Phase II study of navelbine in advanced renal cell carcinoma [letter]. Eur J Cancer 1991; 27(6):804–805.

90. Oishi N, Berenberg J, Blumenstein BA, Johnson K, Rivkin SE, Bukowski RM, O'Bryan RM et al. Teniposide in metastatic renal and bladder cancer: a Southwest Oncology Group Study. Cancer Treat Rep 1987; 71(12):1307–1308.

91. Hire SA, Samson MK, Fraile RJ et al. Use of VM-26 as a single agent in the treatment of renal carcinoma. Cancer Clin Trials 1979; 2:293–295.

92. Pfiefle D, Renter N, Hahn R et al. Phase II trial of VM-26 in advanced measurable renal cell carcinoma. [Abstract] Proc Am Soc Clin Oncol 1984; 3:162 (abstract C-634).

93. Kish JA, Wolf M, Crawford ED, Leimert JT, Bueschen A, Neefe JR, Flanigan RC. Evaluation of low dose continuous infusion 5-fluorouracil in patients with advanced and recurrent renal cell carcinoma. A Southwest Oncology Group Study. Cancer 1994; 74(3):916–919.

94. Zaniboni A, Simoncini E, Marpicati P, Montini E, Ferrari V, Marini G. Phase II trial of 5-fluorouracil and high-dose folinic acid in advanced renal cell cancer. J Chemother 1989; 1(5):350–351.

95. Baiocchi C, Landonio G, Cacioppo C, Calgaro M, Cattaneo D, Ferrari M, Majno M. Continuous non chronomodulated infusion of floxuridine in

metastatic renal cell carcinoma (MRCC): report of 17 cases. Tumori 1996; 82(3):225–227.

96. Wilkinson MJ, Frye JW, Small EJ, Venook AP, Carroll PR, Ernest ML, Stagg RJ. A phase II study of constant-infusion floxuridine for the treatment of metastatic renal cell carcinoma. Cancer 1993; 71(11):3601–3604.

97. Von Roemeling R, Rabatin JT, Fraley EE, Hrushesky WJ. Progressive metastatic renal cell carcinoma controlled by continuous 5-fluoro-2-deoxyuridine infusion. J Urol 1988; 139(2):259–262.

98. Richards III F, Cooper MR, Jackson DV et al. Continuous 5-day (D) intravenous (IV) FUDR infusion for renal cell carcinoma (RCC): A phase I–II trial of the Piedmont Oncology Association. [Abstract] Proc Am Soc Clin Oncol 1991; 10:170.

99. Conroy T, Geoffrois L, Guillemin F, Luporsi E, Krakowski I, Spaeth D, Frasie V, Volff D. Simplified chronomodulated continuous infusion of floxuridine in patients with metastatic renal cell carcinoma. Cancer 1993; 72(7):2190–2197.

100. Dexeus FH, Logothetis CJ, Sella A, Amato R, Kilbourn R, Ogden S, Striegel A et al. Circadian infusion of floxuridine in patients with metastatic renal cell carcinoma. J Urol 1991; 146(3):709–713.

101. Damascelli B, Marchiano A, Spreafico C, Lutman R, Salvetti M, Bonalumi MG, Mauri M et al. Circadian continuous chemotherapy of renal cell carcinoma with an implantable, programmable infusion pump. Cancer 1990; 66(2):237–241.

102. Hrushesky WJ, Von Roemeling R, Lanning RM, Rabatin JT. Circadian-shaped infusions of floxuridine for progressive metastatic renal cell carcinoma. J Clin Oncol 1990; 8(9):1504–1513.

103. Huben RP. Advances in chemotherapy for renal cell carcinoma. Semin Urol 1992; 10:16–22.

104. Dimopoulous MA, Dexeus FH, Jones E et al. Evidence for additive anti-tumor activity and toxicity for the combination of FUDR and interferon alpha 2b (IFNa:Intron) in patients with metastatic renal cell carcinoma (RCC). [Abstract] Proc Am Assoc Cancer Res 1991; 32:186.

105. Budd GT, Murphy S, Klein E et al. Time-modified infusion of floxuridine in metastatic renal cell carcinoma (MRCC). [Abstract] Proc Am Assoc Cancer Res 1992; 33:220.

106. Marsh RD, Agaliotis D. Treatment of metastatic renal cell carcinoma with 5FUdr circadian shaped infusion. [Abstract] Proc Am Soc Clin Oncol 1992; 11:207.

107. Merrouche Y, Negrier S, Lanier F et al. Phase II study of continuous circadian infusion FUDR in metastatic renal cell cancer (RCC). [Abstract] Eur J Cancer Clin Oncol 1991; 27:(suppl 5)S102.

108. Poorter RL, Bakker PJM, Kurth KH. Circadian modulated continuous infusion of FUDR in patients with disseminated renal cell cancer (RCC). [Abstract] Eur J Cancer 1993; 29:(suppl 6)116.

109. Weissbach L, de Mulder P, Osieka R et al. Phase II trial of gemcitabine in renal cancer. [Abstract] Proc Am Soc Clin Oncol 1992; 11:219.

110. de Mulder PH, Weissbach L, Jakse G, Osieka R, Blatter J. Gemcitabine: a phase II study in patients with advanced renal cancer. Cancer Chemother Pharmacol 1996; 37(5):491–495.

111. Mertens WC, Eisenhauer EA, Moore M, Venner P, Stewart D, Muldal A, Wong D. Gemcitabine in advanced renal cell carcinoma. A phase II study of the National Cancer Institute of Canada Clinical Trials Group. Ann Oncol 1993; 4(4):331–332.

112. Witte RS, Elson P, Bryan GT, Trump DL. Trimetrexate in advanced renal cell carcinoma. An ECOG phase II trial. Invest New Drugs 1992; 10(1):51–54.

113. Sternberg CN, Yagoda A, Scher H, Bosl G, Dershaw D, Rosado K, Houston C et al. Phase II trial of trimetrexate in patients with advanced renal cell carcinoma. Clinical Community Oncology Program. Eur J Cancer Clin Oncol 1989; 25(4):753–754.

114. Shevrin DH, Lad TE, Kilton LJ, Cobleigh MA, Blough RR, Weidner LL, Vogelzang NJ. Phase II trial of fludarabine phosphate in advanced renal cell carcinoma: an Illinois Cancer Council Study. Invest New Drugs 1989; 7(2–3):251–253.

115. Balducci L, Blumenstein B, Von Hoff DD, Davis M, Hynes HE, Bukowski RM, Crawford ED. Evaluation of fludarabine phosphate in renal cell carcinoma: a Southwest Oncology Group Study. *Cancer Treat Rep* 1987; 71(5):543–544.

116. Law TM, Mencel P, Motzer RJ. Phase II trial of liposomal encapsulated doxorubicin in patients with advanced renal cell carcinoma. *Invest New Drugs* 1994; 12(4):323–325.

117. Fossa SD, Wik B, Bae E, Lien HH. Phase II study of 4'-epi-doxorubicin in metastatic renal cancer. *Cancer Treat Rep* 1982; 66(5):1219–1221.

118. Benedetto P, Ahmed T, Needles B, Watson RC, Yagoda A. Phase II trial of 4'epi-adriamycin for advanced hypernephroma. *Am J Clin Oncol* 1983; 6(5):553–554.

119. Scher HI, Yagoda A, Ahmed T, Budman D, Sordillo P, Watson RC. Phase-II trial of 4-demethoxydaunorubicin (DMDR) for advanced hypernephroma. *Cancer Chemother Pharmacol* 1985; 14(1):79–80.

120. Gams RA, Nelson O, Birch R. Phase II evaluation of mitoxantrone in advanced renal cell carcinoma: a Southeastern Cancer Study Group Trial. *Cancer Treat Rep* 1986; 70(7):921–922.

121. Taylor SA, Von Hoff DD, Baker LH et al. Phase II clinical trial of mitozantrone in patients with advanced renal cell carcinoma: a Southwest Oncology Group study. *Cancer Treat Rep* 1984; 68:919–920.

122. Van Oosterom AT, Fossa SD, Pizzocaro G, Bergerat JP, Bono AV, De Pauw M, Sylvester R. Mitoxantrone in advanced renal cancer: a phase II study in previously untreated patients from the EORTC Genito-Urinary Tract Cancer Cooperative Group. *Eur J Cancer Clin Oncol* 1984; 20(10):1239–1241.

123. DeJager R, Cappelaere P, Armand JP et al. An EORTC phase II study of mitoxantrone in solid tumors and lymphomas. *Eur J Cancer Clin Oncol* 1984; 28:1369–1375.

124. Schneider RJ, Woodcock TM, Yagoda A. Phase II trial of 4'-(9-acridinylamino)methanesulfon-m-anisidide (AMSA) in patients with metastatic hypernephroma. *Cancer Treat Rep* 1980; 64(1):183–185.

125. Van Echo DA, Markus S, Aisner J, Wiernik PH. Phase II trial of 4'-(9-acridinylamino)methanesulfon-m-anisidide (AMSA) in patients with metastatic renal cell carcinoma. *Cancer Treat Rep* 1980; 64(8–9):1009–1010.

126. Amrein PC, Coleman M, Richards F et al. Phase II study of amsacrine in metastatic renal cell carcinoma. *Cancer Treat Rep* 1983; 67:1043–1044.

127. Earhart RH, Elson PJ, Rosenthal SN et al. PALA and AMSA for renal cell carcinoma. *Am J Clin Oncol* 1983; 6:555–560.

128. Scher HJ, Schwartz S, Yagoda A et al. Phase II trial of bisantrene for advanced hypernephroma. *Cancer Treat Rep* 1982; 66:1653–1655.

129. Myers JW, Von Hoff DD, Coltman CA et al. Phase II evaluation of bisantrene in patients with renal cell carcinoma. *Cancer Treat Rep* 1982; 66:1869–1871.

130. Evans WK, Shepherd FA, Blackstein ME et al. Phase II evaluation of bisantrene in patients with advanced renal cell carcinoma. *Cancer Treat Rep* 1985; 69:727–728.

131. Spicer D, Daniels J, Skinner D et al. Phase II study of bisantrene administered weekly in patients with advanced renal cell carcinoma. [Abstract] *Proc Am Soc Clin Oncol* 1985; 4:101.

132. Elson PJ, Earhart RH, Kvols LK, Spiegel R, Keller AM, Kies MS, Davis TE et al. Phase II studies of PCNU and bisantrene in advanced renal cell carcinoma. *Cancer Treat Rep* 1987; 71(3):331–332.

133. Tait N, Abrams J, Egorin MJ et al. Phase II carboplatin (CBDCA) for metastatic renal cell cancer with a standard (SD) and a calculated (CD) dose according to renal function. [Abstract] *Proc Am Soc Clin Oncol* 1988; 7:125.

134. Trump DL, Elson P. Evaluation of carboplatin (NSC 241240) in patients with recurrent or metastatic renal cell carcinoma. *Invest New Drugs* 1990; 8(2):201–203.

135. Sternberg C, Yagoda A, Ahmed T et al. Phase II trial of elliptinium in advanced renal cell carcinoma and carcinoma of the breast. *Anticancer Res* 1985; 5:415–418.

136. Caille P, Mondesir JM, Droz JP, Kerbrat P, Goodman A, Ducret JP, Theodore C et al. Phase II trial of elliptinium in advanced renal cell carcinoma. *Cancer Treat Rep* 1985; 69(7–8):901–902.

137. Droz JP, Theodore C, Ghosn M, Lupera H, Piot G, De Forges A, Klink M et al. Twelve-year experience with chemotherapy in adult metastatic renal cell carcinoma at the Institut Gustave-Roussy. *Semin Surg Oncol* 1988; 4(2):97–99.

138. Child JA, Bono AV, Fossa SD et al. An EORTC phase II study of methylglyoxal bis-guanylhydrazone in advanced renal cell cancer. *Eur J Cancer Clin Oncol* 1982; 18:85–87.

139. Todd RF, Garnick MB, Canellos GP et al. Phase I–II trial of methyl-GAG in the treatment of patients with metastatic renal adenocarcinoma. *Cancer Treat Rep* 1981; 65:17–20.

140. Fuks AZ, Van Echo DA, Aisner J. Phase II trial of methyl-G (methyl-glyoxal bis-guanylhydrazone) in patients with metastatic renal cell carcinoma. *Cancer Clin Trials* 1981; 4:411–414.

141. Knight WA, Drehlichman A, Fabian C et al. Mitoguazone in advanced renal carcinoma: A phase II trial of the Southwest Oncology Group. *Cancer Treat Rep* 1983; 67:1139–1140.

142. Zeffren J, Yagoda A, Watson RC et al. Phase II trial of methylglyoxal bisguanylhydrazone in advanced renal cancer. *Cancer Treat Rep* 1981; (65):525–527.

143. Kerr DJ, Rustin GJ, Kaye SB, Selby P, Bleehen NM, Harper P, Bramptom MH. Phase II trials of rhizoxin in advanced ovarian, colorectal and renal cancer. *Br J Cancer* 1995; 72:1267–1269.

144. Motzer RJ, Nanus DM, O'Moore P, Scher HI, Bajorin DF, Reuter V, Tong WP et al. Phase II trial of suramin in patients with advanced renal cell carcinoma: treatment results, pharmacokinetics, and tumor growth factor expression. *Cancer Res* 1992; 52(20):5775–5779.

145. La Rocca RV, Stein CA, Danesi R, Cooper MR, Uhrich M, Myers CE. A pilot study of suramin in the treatment of metastatic renal cell carcinoma. *Cancer* 1991; 67(6):1509–1513.

146. Walpole ET, Dutcher JP, Sparano J, Gucalp R, Einzig A, Paietta E, Ciobanu N et al. Survival after phase II treatment of advanced renal cell carcinoma with taxol or high-dose interleukin-2. *J Immunother* 1993; 13(4):275–281.

147. Einzig AI, Gorowski E, Sasloff J, Wiernik PH. Phase II trial of taxol in patients with metastatic renal cell carcinoma. *Cancer Invest* 1991; 9(2):133–136.

148. Bruntsch U, Heinrich B, Kaye SB, de Mulder PH, van Oosterom A, Paridaens R, Vermorken JB et al. Docetaxel (Taxotere) in advanced renal cell cancer. A phase II trial of the EORTC Early Clinical Trials Group. *Eur J Cancer* 1994; 30A(8):1064–1067.

149. Law TM, Ilson DH, Motzer RJ. Phase II trial of topotecan in patients with advanced renal cell carcinoma. *Invest New Drugs* 1994; 12(2):143–145.

150. Lupera H, Theodore C, Ghosn M, Court BH, Wibault P, Droz JP. Phase II trial of combination chemotherapy with dacarbazine, cyclophosphamide, cisplatin, doxorubicin, and vindesine (DECAV) in advanced renal cell cancer. *Urology* 1989; 34(5):281–283.

151. Guimaraes JL, Ghosn M, Ostronoff M, Azab M, Theodore C, Droz JP. Phase II trial of methyl-gag and melphalan in metastatic adult renal cell carcinoma. *Cancer Invest* 1990; 8(6):623–624.

152. Small EJ, Frye JW, Wilkinson MJ, Carroll PR, Ernest ML, Stagg RJ. A phase I/II study of alternating constant rate infusion floxuridine with constant rate infusion vinblastine for the treatment of metastatic renal cell carcinoma. *Cancer* 1994; 73(11):2803–2807.

153. Jekunen A, Pyrhonen S. A combination of vinblastine and doxorubicin with interferon alpha. *Am J Clin Oncol* 1996; 19(4):384–385.

154. Murphy BR, Rynard SM, Pennington KL, Grosh W, Loehrer PJ. A phase II trial of vinblastine plus dipyridamole in advanced renal cell carcinoma. A Hoosier Oncology Group Study. *Am J Clin Oncol* 1994; 17(1):10–13.

155. Schwartsmann G, Medina de Cunha F, Silveira LA, Salgado G, Thereza MS, Vinholes J, Preger P, Segal F. Phase II trial of vinblastine plus nifedipine (VN) in patients with advanced renal cell carcinoma (RCC). Brazilian Oncology Trials Group [letter]. *Ann Oncol* 1991; 2(6):443.

156. Agarwala SS, Bahnson RR, Wilson JW, Szumowski J, Ernstoff MS. Evaluation of the combination of vinblastine and quinidine in patients with metastatic renal cell carcinoma. A phase I study. *Am J Clin Oncol* 1995; 18(3):211–215.

157. Overmayer B, Fox K, Tomaszewski J et al. A phase II trial of R-verapamil and infusional vinblastine (Velban) in advanced renal cell carcinoma. *Proc Am Soc Clin Oncol* 1993; **12**:251(abstract).

158. Motzer RJ, Lyn P, Fischer P, Lianes P, Ngo RL, Cordon-Cardo C, O'Brien JP. Phase I/II trial of dexverapamil plus vinblastine for patients with advanced renal cell carcinoma. *J Clin Oncol* 1995; **13**(8):1958–1965.

159. Mickisch GH, Noordzij MA, vd Gaast A, Gebreamlack P, Kohrmann KU, Mogler-Drautz E, Kupper H, Schroder FH. Dexverapamil to modulate vinblastine resistance in metastatic renal cell carcinoma. *J Cancer Res Clin Oncol* 1995; **121**(suppl 3):R11–R16.

160. Rodenburg CJ, Nooter K, Herweijer H et al. Phase II study of combining vinblastine and cyclosporin-A to cicumvent multidrug resistance in renal cell cancer. *Ann Oncol* 1991; **2**:305–306.

161. Warner E, Tobe SW, Andrulis IL, Pei Y, Trachtenberg J, Skorecki KL. Phase I–II study of vinblastine and oral cyclosporin A in metastatic renal cell carcinoma. *Am J Clin Oncol* 1995; **18**(3):251–256.

162. Berlin J, King AC, Tutsch K, Findlay JW, Kohler P, Collier M, Clendeninn NJ, Wilding G. A phase II study of vinblastine in combination with acrivastine in patients with advanced renal cell carcinoma. *Invest New Drugs* 1994; **12**(2):137–141.

163. Kakehi Y, Yoshida O, Segawa T, Kanematsu A, Hiura M, Shichiri Y, Arai Y. [Intraarterial chemotherapy for metastatic renal cell carcinomas: combination with MDR-overcoming agents]. [Japanese]. *Hinyokika Kiyo – Acta Urol Jpn* 1994; **40**(10):925–929.

164. Presant CA, Kennedy P, Wiseman C, Gala K, Smith JD, Bouzaglou A, Farbstein M et al. Pilot phase II trial of amphotericin B and CCNU in renal and colorectal carcinomas. *Eur J Cancer Clin Oncol* 1986; **22**(3): 329–330.

165. Gigante M, Sorio R, Colussi AM, Sandrin A, De Appollonia L, Galligioni E, Freschi A et al. Effect of cyclosporine on teniposide pharmacokinetics and pharmacodynamics in patients with renal cell cancer. *Anticancer Drugs* 1995; **6**(3):479–482.

166. Paolorossi F, Villa S, Barni S, Tancini G, Andres M, Lissoni P. Second-line therapy with interferon-alpha plus vinblastine in metastatic renal cell cancer patients progressed under interleukin-2 subcutaneous immunotherapy. *Tumori* 1995; **81**(1):45–47.

167. Kriegmair M, Oberneder R, Hofstetter A. Interferon alfa and vinblastine versus medroxyprogesterone acetate in the treatment of metastatic renal cell carcinoma. *Urology* 1995; **45**(5):758–762.

168. Pizzocaro G, Piva L, Faustini M, Mangiarotti B, Nicolai N, Salvioni R, Milani A, Zanoni F. [Interferon and vinblastine in presumably operable metastases of renal carcinoma]. [Italian]. *Arch Ital Urol Androl* 1993; **65**(2):177–180.

169. Massidda B, Migliari R, Padovani A, Scarpa RM, Pellegrini P, Cortesi E, Usai E, Pellegrini A. Metastatic renal cell cancer treated with recombinant alpha 2a interferon and vinblastine. *J Chemother* 1991; **3**(6):387–389.

170. Merimsky O, Shnider BI, Chaitchik S. Does vinblastine add to the potency of alpha interferon in the treatment of renal cell carcinoma? *Mol Biother* 1991; **3**(1):34–37.

171. Schuster D, Schneider G, Ade N, Heim ME. [Combination of recombinant interferon alpha-2A and vinblastine in advanced renal cell cancer.]. *Onkologie* 1990; **13**(5):359–362.

172. Kellokumpu-Lehtinen P, Nordman E. Recombinant interferon-alpha 2a and vinblastine in advanced renal cell cancer: a clinical phase I–II study. *J Biol Resp Modif* 1990; **9**(4):439–444.

173. Palmeri S, Gebbia V, Russo A, Gebbia N, Rausa L. Vinblastine and interferon-alpha-2a regimen in the treatment of metastatic renal cell carcinoma. *Tumori* 1990; **76**(1):64–65.

174. Trump DL, Ravdin PM, Borden EC, Magers CF, Whisnant JK. Interferon-alpha-n1 and continuous infusion vinblastine for treatment of advanced renal cell carcinoma. *J Biol Resp Mod* 1990; **9**(1):108–111.

175. Sertoli MR, Brunetti I, Ardizzoni A, Falcone A, Guarneri D, Boccardo F, Martorana G et al. Recombinant alpha-2a interferon plus vinblastine in the treatment of metastatic renal cell carcinoma. *Am J Clin Oncol* 1989; **12**(1):43–45.

176. Schornagel JH, Verweij J, ten Bokkel Huinink WW, Klijn JG, de Mulder PH, Debruyne FM, van Deijk WA et al. Phase II study of recombinant interferon alpha-2a and vinblastine in advanced renal cell carcinoma. *J Urol* 1989; **142**(2:Pt 1):253–256.

177. Bergerat JP, Herbrecht R, Dufour P, Jacqmin D, Bollack C, Prevot G, Bailly G et al. Combination of recombinant interferon alpha-2a and vinblastine in advanced renal cell cancer. *Cancer* 1988; **62**(11):2320–2324.

178. Cetto GL, Franceschi T, Turrina G, Chiarion-Sileni V, Capelli MC, Bellini A, Paccagnella A et al. Recombinant alpha-interferon and vinblastine in metastatic renal cell carcinoma: efficacy of low doses. [Review]. *Semin Surg Oncol* 1988; **4**(3):184–190.

179. Fossa SD. Is interferon with or without vinblastine the 'treatment of choice' in metastatic renal cell carcinoma? The Norwegian Radium Hospital's experience 1983–1986. *Semin Surg Oncol* 1988; **4**(3):178–183.

180. Kellokumpu-Lehtinen P, Nordman E. Combined interferon and vinblastine treatment of advanced melanoma and renal cell cancer. *Cancer Detect Prevent* 1988; **12**(1–6):523–529.

181. Jacqmin D, Bergerat JP, Dufour P, Bollack C, Prevot G, Jurascheck F, Bailly G et al. [Medical treatment of metastatic cancer of the kidney with a combination of vinblastine and recombinant interferon alpha IIa. Result of a phase I–II trial]. [French]. *J Urol* (Paris) 1987; **93**(8):463–466.

182. Fossa SD, De Garis ST, Heier MS, Flokkmann A, Lien HH, Salveson A, Moe B. Recombinant interferon alfa-2a with or without vinblastine in metastatic renal cell carcinoma. *Cancer* 1986; **57**(suppl 8):1700–1704.

183. Figlin RA, deKernion JB, Maldazys J, Sarna G. Treatment of renal cell carcinoma with alpha (human leukocyte) interferon and vinblastine in combination: a phase I–II trial. *Cancer Treat Rep* 1985; **69**(3):263–267.

184. Noguchi S, Shuin T, Kubota Y, Masuda M, Yao M, Hosaka M. [Combination therapy with interferon-alpha and continuous infusion of 5-fluorouracil for advanced renal cell carcinoma]. [Japanese]. *Hinyokika Kiyo – Acta Urol Jpn* 1995; **41**(7):517–520.

185. Lopez Hanninen E, Poliwoda H, Atzpodien J. Interferon-alpha/5-fluorouracil: a novel outpatient chemo/immunotherapy for progressive metastatic renal cell carcinoma. *Cancer Biother* 1995; **10**(1):21–24.

186. Haarstad H, Jacobsen AB, Schjolseth SA, Risberg T, Fossa SD. Interferon-alpha, 5-FU and prednisone in metastatic renal cell carcinoma: a phase II study. *Ann Oncol* 1994; **5**(3):245–248.

187. Murphy BR, Rynard SM, Einhorn LH, Loehrer PJ. A phase II trial of interferon alpha-2A plus fluorouracil in advanced renal cell carcinoma. A Hoosier Oncology Group study. *Invest New Drugs* 1992; **10**(3):225–230.

188. Falcone A, Cianci C, Ricci S, Brunetti I, Bertuccelli M, Conte PF. Alpha-2B-interferon plus floxuridine in metastatic renal cell carcinoma. A phase I–II study. *Cancer* 1993; **72**(2):564–568.

189. Falcone A, Cianci C, Pfanner E, Lencioni M, Allegrini G, Antonuzzo A, Brunetti I, Ricci S, Conte PF. Treatment of metastatic renal cell carcinoma (MRCC) with constant rate floxuridine (FUDR) infusion plus recombinant alpha2B-interferon (IFN) (Meeting abstract). *Proc Am Soc Clin Oncol* 1996; **15**:A626.

190. Panetta A, Martoni A, Guaraldi M, Tamberi S, Casadio M, Lelli G, Pannuti F. Combined chemo-immuno-hormonotherapy of advanced renal cell carcinoma. *J Chemother* 1994; **6**(5):349–353.

191. Sella A, Logothetis CJ, Fitz K, Dexeus FH, Amato R, Kilbourn R, Wallace S. Phase II study of interferon-alpha and chemotherapy (5-fluorouracil and mitomycin-C) in metastatic renal cell cancer. *J Urol* 1992; **147**(3):573–577.

192. Wadler S, Einzig AI, Dutcher JP, Ciobanu N, Landau L, Wiernik PH. Phase II trial of recombinant alpha-2b-interferon and low-dose cyclophosphamide in advanced melanoma and renal cell carcinoma. *Am J Clin Oncol* 1988; **11**(1):55–59.

193. Konig HJ, Gutmann W, Weissmuller J. Ifosfamide, vindesine and recombinant alpha-interferon combination chemotherapy for metastatic renal cell carcinoma. *J Cancer Res Clin Oncol* 1991; **117**:(suppl 4):S221–S223.

194. Indrova M, Bubenik J, Jakoubkova J, Simova J, Jandlova T, Helmichova E, Benesova K et al. Subcutaneous interleukin-2 in combination with vinblastine for metastatic renal cancer: cytolytic activity of peripheral blood lymphocytes. *Neoplasma* 1994; **41**(4):197–200.

195. Kuebler JP, Whitehead RP, Ward DL, Hemstreet GP III, Bradley EC. Treatment of metastatic renal cell carcinoma with recombinant interleukin-

2 in combination with vinblastine or lymphokine-activated killer cells. [Review]. *J Urol* 1993; **150**(3):814–820.

96. Sella A, Kilbourn RG, Gray I, Finn L, Zukiwski AA, Ellerhorst J, Amato RJ, Logothetis CJ. Phase I study of interleukin-2 combined with interferon-alpha and 5-fluorouracil in patients with metastatic renal cell cancer. *Cancer Biother* 1994; **9**(2):103–111.

97. Stadler WM, Talabay K, Vogelzang NJ. Interleukin-2 (IL2), interferon-alpha (IFNA), and cis-retinoic acid (CRA): an effective outpatient regimen for metastatic renal cell carcinoma (RCC) (Meeting abstract). *Proc Am Soc Clin Oncol* 1996; **15**:A602.

198. Wersall JP, Masucci G, Hjelm AL, Ragnhammar P, Fagerberg J, Frodin JE, Merk K *et al*. Low dose cyclophosphamide, alpha-interferon and continuous infusions of interleukin-2 in advanced renal cell carcinoma. *Med Oncol Tumor Pharmacother* 1993; **10**(3):103–111.

25 Transitional cell carcinoma of the upper urinary tract: Incidence, etiology, epidemiology and genetics

S E Robbins and M Droller

Incidence and epidemiology

The vast majority of transitional cell cancers arise in the bladder, and comprise a fairly common malignancy, constituting the fourth most common in males in the USA and the ninth most common in females. In contrast, transitional cell cancers of the renal pelvis and ureter are comparatively rare, although their histologic appearance and clinical behavior have much in common with those of the bladder[1]. An estimated 6–7% of all primary malignant tumors of the kidney are transitional cell carcinoma (TCC) of either the renal pelvis or ureter[1]. Renal pelvic cancers account for the majority, with their incidence being 3–4 times that of ureteral tumors[3].

The incidence of renal urothelial cancer reaches a peak incidence in the sixth to seventh decade and occurs three times more commonly in male than females[4]. The age-adjusted incidence is 0.6/100 000 people. Racial distribution is predominantly white. The white:black ratio is 1 to 0.09[5]. The occurrence of TCC of the upper tracts and the bladder in patients less than 30 years of age has been reported to be infrequent, and even includes isolated cases in infants[6]. Reports of familial TCC involving three sib-

lings have also been reported[6]. TCC appears in each kidney with equal frequency but occurs bilaterally in only 2–4% of cases. Most ureteral tumors involve the lower third of the ureter. The literature reports a range of 60–74% occurring in the lower third, with no predilection for either side[8].

Statistics for upper tract transitional cell cancer are different for inhabitants of the Balkan countries. These individuals develop a nephropathy that may ultimately be associated with cancer of the renal pelvis. The cause of this nephropathy is obscure, although it has been postulated that it may be on account of increased concentration of radon and minerals in the drinking water[9]. Tumors in these patients are commonly multiple and tend not to be aggressive[10].

Etiology

Although the cause of urothelial cancer in the upper tract is unknown, it is likely to be similar to that of bladder cancer. Renal urothelial cancer occurs in association with primary bladder cancer in only 2–4% of patients. On the other hand, patients with initial renal urothelial cancer develop similar tumors within the bladder in 50–75% of cases[10]. These data imply that urothelial cancer is a field disease that may simultaneously or subsequently develop anywhere in the urinary tract. The reason that upper tract tumors occur less frequently when the tumor is initially seen in the bladder is not entirely understood[10]. Differences in urinary transit and storage time allowing for cell implantation and increased contact with carcinogens have been implicated.

The pathogenesis of malignant disease probably involves both genetic and environmental factors. It appears that a number of agents may be carcinogenic in individuals whose susceptibility may be enhanced by genetic mechanisms. These include cigarette smoking, analgesics, coffee, cyclophosphamide, occupational exposure and contact with certain contrast agents.

Cigarette smoking has been considered as the most important risk factor for TCC. Two known bladder carcinogens, 2-aminonaphthalene (2-AN) and 4-aminobiphenyl (4-ABP), and two suspected carcinogens, o-toluidine and aniline, are present in tobacco[13]. Population based cancer-control studies of renal pelvic and ureteral cancers found cigarette smoking to be associated with an overall 3.1 fold increase in risk, with long-term (> 45 years) smokers having a 7.2 times risk[14]. Attributable risk estimates indicate that approximately seven out of 10 cancers in the renal pelvis and ureter in men and four out of 10 in females may be caused by smoking. The risk appears higher for ureteral tumors than renal pelvic tumors and higher for renal pelvic than for bladder tumors[14].

An effect of cessation of smoking on cancer of the renal pelvis and ureter has also been shown. The decline in relative risk of 60–70% was consistent in both male and females after only 10 years of cessation. However, former smokers still have two times the risk for the development of these cancers than a person who has never smoked[14]. When the relative risk analysis is analyzed according to tobacco type, the relative risk associated with blonde (heat-cured) tobacco was 50% of those associated with black (air-cured) tobacco. It is postulated that nitrosamines are more concentrated in air-cured, black tobacco[17]. Neither the age of onset of smoking nor the type of cigarette smoked was found to be an important risk factor for the prediction of disease[18]. Conflicting data exists on the risks conferred by the depth of inhalation[19]. The use of filtered cigarettes, however, is associated with a lower risk of bladder cancer[20].

Occupational exposure has also been associated with TCC. Most occupational or chemical substances and their metabolites are excreted through the urinary tract and have direct contact with the bladder mucosa. Occupations including work with dyestuff products, rubber manufacture, plastic industry, textile and leather, metal, mining, pesticides, hair dressing and cooking[21] have each been associated with the development of these cancers. Although the carcinogens associated with occupational exposure remain unclear, 2-AN, 4-ABP and benzidine (associated with occupational exposure to dyestuff, textile and rubber) are considered to be human bladder carcinogens. o-Toluidine (used in rubber manufacturing), 4,4′ methylenebis (2-chloroaniline) (used in polyurethane manufacturing) and nitroaromatics (products of diesel fuel) may be associated with the risk of bladder cancer[21]. In 1934 Hueper showed that pre-neoplastic and neoplastic carcinoma of the bladder could be obtained (13/16 dogs) with subcutaneous and oral feeding of beta-naphthylamine. Tumors found were multiple and located in the dependent portion of the bladder, suggesting that prolonged contact of the mucosa with beta-naphthylamine is a necessary step in tumor production[23].

Occupational bladder cancer has been associated with slow acetylation by N-acetyltransferase (NAT). NAT activity found in mammalian cytosol acetylates arylamines and their oxidized metabolites and has been implicated in the metabolic detoxification of these substances to the ultimate carcinogen[24]. Two isozymes have been identified and each allele is associated with either fast or slow acetylation. There is a significant difference in the frequency of the slow acetylator phenotype between occupationally exposed bladder cancer patients and non-malignant controls. Homozygous slow acetylators accounted for 71.0% of occupationally exposed bladder cancer patients, as opposed to 65.4% in those who developed bladder cancer without occupational exposure, while only 44.1% in the non-malignant control group are homozygous slow acetylators. The proportion of slow acetylators is much higher amongst those bladder cancer patients with direct exposure to cigarette smoke than in the non-malignant control population (71% vs. 39%). The slow acetylator phenotype may therefore be a contributory risk factor in bladder carcinogenesis which acts through influencing individual response to environmental carcinogens[25], while a protective effect may be afforded by fast acetylation.

The metabolism of the essential amino acid L-tryptophan has been found to give rise to a group of substituted ortho-aminophenols, many of which have been found to be carcinogenic. Bryan et al. showed that surgically implanted pellets containing metabolites of tryptophan induced a statistically greater number of carcinomas than did controls in the mouse bladder[26]. The concentration of the metabolites has been shown to be greater in certain patients with bladder cancer than age matched controls. The EORTC GU group in a randomized trial failed to show an effect on the rate of bladder cancer recurrence when patients were given pyridoxine (vitamin B6), known to reduce the urinary levels of tryptophan metabolites[27].

Individuals who have used drugs containing phenacetin or acetaminophen on a regular basis for a period of greater than 3 years have experienced a fourfold increased risk for the development of TCC of the urinary system[28]. At least two explanations have been proposed for the role of analgesic consumption in causing carcinoma of the renal pelvis. The more popular belief is that phenacetin yields carcinogenic metabolic derivatives. This view is supported by several observations. In virtually all reported cases of analgesic-associated renal pelvic cancer the analgesic consumed has contained phenacetin as one of its ingredients. In addition hydroxylated derivatives of phenacetin resemble in chemical structure the carcinogens implicated in industrial and smoking associated carcinoma of the urinary tract. Furthermore N-hydroxyphenacetin has been shown to induce liver tumors and phenacetin has been shown to induce urothelial cancers when fed to rats[29]. In the latter of these studies, the total dosage of carcinogen was not accounted for. Only the duration of exposure appeared to be important. A latency period of up to 25 years has been suggested[30]. Consumption of analgesics was not found to increase the risk for the development of cancer of the ureter, but has been strongly associated with the development of cancer of the renal pelvis, with phenacetin-containing analgesics conferring a six times increase in relative risk. However, a synergistic effect of tobacco and analgesics has been indicated by an increased risk of 14.3% in people exposed to both[31].

An alternative view is that renal papillary necrosis, which is caused by excessive analgesic consumption, predisposes the kidney to the development of transitional-cell carcinoma[32]. Renal papillary necrosis has been found in a large number of patients with analgesic-associated renal pelvic tumors. It has been proposed that papillary necrosis may be an intrinsic step in the development of these tumors[33]. The reason for subsequent development of transitional cell carcinoma in individual kidneys heavily exposed to analgesics or with analgesic-induced renal papillary necrosis is not yet evident, but genetically determined variability of detoxifying enzyme systems, such as mixed function oxidases or N-acetyltransferase may be operative[34]. An alternative explanation, because of the apparently synergistic effect of tobacco and analgesics in causing renal pelvic cancer, is a smoking induced alteration in the metabolism of phenacetin[35].

In a population-based case-control study by Cole in 1971, relative risks of 1.3 in men and 2.5 in women for the development of TCC were reported for drinkers of one or more cups of coffee per day compared with those who drank less[36]. Subsequent studies have shown that people who drink in excess of seven cups per day had twice the relative risk for the development of upper tract tumors[37]. However based on the negative results of some studies and the small and inconsistent associations found in others, any relation is likely to be weak. Moreover, the positive associations reported may have been in part the result of incomplete control for cigarette smoking.

Cyclophosphamide, an alkylating chemotherapeutic agent, has been associated with the development of TCC of the upper tracts. As of 1987, only five cases had been reported in the literature. Acrolein, a metabolite of cyclophosphamide, may be the active agent[38] by alkylating nucleophilic nitrogen sites of DNA and leading to depurination and mistakes in base insertion during replication[39].

Use of thorium dioxide (Thorotrast) as a contrast agent for retrograde pyelography in the 1930s was also associated with the development of renal urothelial cancer. The agent is thought to induce tumors caused by X-ray emission[40].

Future research should clarify whether exposure to carcinogens is more concentrated in the renal pelvis and ureter than in the bladder, or whether the epithelium of the renal pelvis and ureter may be especially susceptible to the effects of carcinogens, either by the existence of a different enzymatic array or by a difference in different DNA repair mechanisms.

Genetics

There is compelling evidence that cancer arises via a multistep process. It is known that most carcinogens induce carcinogenic changes as the result of a direct interaction with DNA[41]. It has become apparent that loss of tumor suppressor gene function is widespread and implicated in the development of most malignancies. Carcinogenic agents appear to induce molecular changes or abnormalities in gene regulation that result in uncontrolled cell growth and proliferation of transformed stem cells[42]. Direct evidence for the participation of oncogenes and tumor suppressor genes in tumor initiation and promotion has been suggested[43].

Because of the low incidence of TCC of the upper tracts, there have been no detailed genetic analyses of these tumors. We must therefore draw conclusions based on similarities to that of TCC of the bladder.

Certain carcinogens in tobacco cause DNA damage and may produce specific mutations. p53, which acts as a tumor suppressor, is a common target for carcinogenic agents. Mutations at this point are reported to be the most frequent mutational abnormality in human cancer[44]. The function of p53 in controlling DNA repair may be subverted by mutation in the p53 gene, reducing the effectiveness of DNA surveillance and repair, leading to an increased risk of gene mutations and chromosomal rearrangements[45]. p53 gene mutations appear to be frequently associated with invasive high-grade bladder cancers and rarely with superficial and low-grade bladder cancers. This suggests that p53 gene mutation may be either a rather late event in tumor development or more likely may be involved in the development of those forms of bladder cancer that are likely to be progressive. Alternatively, the p53 gene mutation may also be responsible for the conversion of superficial into invasive cancer[46].

Soini *et al.* retrospectively looked at the presence of p53 in TCC of the bladder. They found 9% of grade 1, 35% of grade 2 and 89% of grade 3 specimens were positive for p53. They also showed that significantly more T2–T4 bladder cancers were p53 positive when compared with T1[47]. In looking at p53 over-expression and its association with progression in pT1 bladder tumors, Thomas *et al.* found that significantly more patients with high levels of p53 over-expression (>10% nuclear staining) progressed compared with tumors with less than 10% nuclear staining[48]. A correlation was found to grade, stage and presence of p53, which suggests that p53 mutation may be associated with the evolution of aggressive growth characteristics in transitional cell cancers or, alternatively, that p53 positive tumors are of a more aggressive type from the start[49]. O'Malley *et al.* analyzed p53 expression in bladder urothelium cultured from smokers and found an elevated expression of p53 from urothelium from smokers. They theorize that p53 may be an early event in bladder carcinogenesis induced by cigarette smoking[50].

Terrel *et al.* analyzed histopathologic features of renal pelvic TCC and found that 46% of cases demonstrated p53 over-expression. However the disease-specific 5 year survival rate for patients with p53 over-expression was 66% compared with 71% for those without p53 over-expression. The p53 over-expression also failed statistically to predict tumor recurrence and recurrence-free survival. Therefore, controversy remains in regard to the role of p53 in the assessment of patient outcome in transitional cell carcinoma[51].

The involvement of the Rb gene product in bladder progression and metastasis has been suggested by studies that have shown loss of heterozygosity of the Rb locus and alterations of this gene product in high grade tumors[52].

Cytogenic analysis of human bladder tumors has established that chromosome 9 abnormalities are frequent occurrences. Of these tumors 62% have been shown to have LOH of part of chromosome 9. Losses of heterozygosity of chromosomal arms in other than chromosome 9 (3p, 6q, 11p, 13q, 17p, 18q) have been commonly observed in high-grade, high-stage tumors. This evidence suggests that initial activation of chromosome 9 is an early event in bladder carcinogenesis and may be followed by multiple sequential inactivation of other tumor suppressor genes, which then lead to an invasive phenotype[52]. Defects in chromosome 9 may be the only abnormality found in low-grade, mucosally confined tumors. Since these appear for the most part not to progress, defects in this chromosome may lead exclusively to a proliferative diathesis in which tumor cells lack the ability to infiltrate the lamina propria and to metastasize.

An increasing understanding of the molecular nature of the neoplastic process and the biological potential that specific genetic changes may create will ultimately allow clinicians to become more precise in their ability to predict the biological potential of a particular cancer and apply various types of treatment in a more precise fashion[52].

References

1. Melamed MR, Reuter VE. Pathology and staging of urothelial tumors of the kidney and ureter. *Urol Clinics N Am*, 1993;**20**:2.
3. 1987 Annual Annual Cancer Statistics Review: Including Cancer Trends 1950–1985. National Institute of Health, National Cancer Institute, January 1988.
4. Gillenwater JY. *Adult and pediatric urology* (2nd ed.) Mosby Year Book, 1992.
5. Say CS, Hori JM. Transitional cell carcinoma of the renal pelvis: experience from 1940–1972 and literature review. *J Urol* 1974;**112**:438–442.
6. Hudson HC, Kramer SA *et al.* Transitional cell carcinoma of the renal pelvis: rare occurrence in young male. *Urology* 1981;**18**:284–286.
8. Ochsner MG, Brannan W *et al.* Transitional cell carcinoma of the renal pelvis and ureter: retrospective review of 40 patients. *Urology* 1974;**4**:392–396.
9. Petkovic SD. Epidemiology and treatment of renal pelvic and ureteral tumors. *J Urol* 1975;**114**:858–865.
10. Gillenwater JY. *Adult and pediatric urology* (2nd edn). Mosby Year Book, 1992.
13. Zhang ZF, Sarkis AS *et al.* Tobacco smoking, occupation and p53 nuclear overexpression in early bladder cancer. *Cancer Epidem Biomarkers and Prevention* 1994;**3**:19–24.
14. McLaughlin JK, Silverman DT *et al.* Cigarette smoking and cancers of the renal pelvis and ureter. *Cancer Res* 1992;**52**:254–257.
17. Vineis P, Esteve J, Terracini B. Bladder cancer and smoking in males: types of cigarettes, age at start, effect of stopping and interaction with occupation. *Int J Cancer* 1984;**34**:165–170.
18. Sorahan T, Lancashire RJ, Sole G. Urothelial cancer and cigarette smoking: Findings from a regional case-controlled study. *Br J Urol* 1994;**74**:753–756.
19. Buzzeo BD, Messing EM. Urothelial cancers of the upper tract. *Adv Urol* 1996;**9**.
20. Vineis P, Esteve J, Terracini B. Bladder cancer and smoking in males: Types of cigarettes, age at start, effect of stopping and interaction with occupation. *Int J Cancer* 1984;**34**:165–170.
21. Zhang ZF, Sarkis AS *et al.* Tobacco smoking, occupation and p53 nuclear overexpression in early bladder cancer. *Cancer Epid Biomarkers and Prevention* 1994;**3**:19–24.
23. Heuper WC, Wiley FH, Wolfe HD. Experimental production of bladder tumors in dogs by administration of beta-napthylamine. *J Indust Hygiene Toxicol* 1937;**20**(1):46–83.
24. Risch A, Wallace DM, Bathers S. Slow N-acetylation genotype is a susceptibility factor in occupational and smoking related bladder cancer. *Hum Mol Gen* 1995;**4**(2):231–236.
26. Bryan GT, Brown RR, Price JM. Mouse bladder carcinogenicity of certain tryptophan metabolites and other aromatic nitrogen compounds suspended in cholesterol. *Cancer Res* 1964;**24**:596–602.
27. Newling DW, Robinson MR *et al.* Tryptophan metabolites, Pyridoxine and their influence on the recurrence rate of superficial bladder cancer. *Eur Urol* 1995;**27**:110–116.
28. McLaughlin JK, Blot WJ *et al.* Etiology of cancer of the renal pelvis. *JNCI* 1983;**71**(2):287–291.

29. McCredie M, Ford JM, *et al.* Analgesics and cancer of the renal pelvis in New South Wales. *Cancer* 1982;**49**:2617–2625.

30. Steffens J, Nagel R. Tumors of the renal pelvis and ureter. *Br J Urology* 1988;**61**:277–283.

31. McCredie M, Stewart JH, Ford JM. Analgesics and tobacco as risk factors for cancer of the ureter and renal pelvis. *J Urol* 1983;**130**:28–30.

32. McCredie M, Ford JM *et al.* Analgesics and cancer of the renal pelvis in New South Wales. *Cancer* 1982;**49**:2617–2625.

33. McCredie M, Stewart JH, Carter J. Phenacetin and papillary necrosis: Independent risk factors for renal pelvic cancer. *Kidney Int* 1986;**30**:81–84.

34. McCredie M, Ford JM *et al.* Analgesics and cancer of the renal pelvis in New South Wales. *Cancer* 1982;**49**:2617–2625.

35. Kuntzman R, Pantuk EJ, Kaplan SA. Phenacetin metabolism: effect of hydrocarbons and cigarette metabolism. *Clin Pharmacol Ther* 1977;**22**:757–764.

36. Cole P. Coffee-drinking and cancer of the lower urinary tract. *Lancet* 1971;**i**:1335–1337.

37. Ross RK, Paganini-Hill A, Landolf J *et al.* Analgesics, cigarette smoking, and other risk factors for cancer of the renal pelvis and ureter. *Cancer Res* 1989;**49**:1045–1048.

38. Cohen SM, Garland EM *et al.* Acrolein initiates rat urinary bladder carcinogenesis. *Cancer Res* 1992;**52**:3577–3581.

39. Brenner DW, Schellhammer PF. Upper tract urothelial malignancy after cyclophosphamide therapy: a case report and literature review. *J Urol* 1986;**137**:1226–1227.

40. Gillenwater JY. *Adult and pediatric urology* (2nd edn). Mosby Year Book, 1992.

41. Zhang ZF, Sarkis AS *et al.* Tobacco smoking, occupation and p53 nuclear overexpression in early bladder cancer. *Cancer Epid Biomarkers and Prevention* 1994;**3**:19–24.

42. Jones PA, Droller MJ. Pathways of development and progression in bladder cancer: New correlations between clinical observations and molecular mechanisms. *Sem Urol* 1993;**11**(4):177–192.

43. Schamauz R, Cole P. Epidemiology of cancer of the renal pelvis and ureter. *JNCI* 1974;**52**(5):1431–1434.

44. Zhang ZF, Sarkis AS *et al.* Tobacco smoking, occupation and p53 nuclear overexpression in early bladder cancer. Cancer Epid, Biomarkers and Prevention 1994;**3**:19–24.

45. Mellon K, Wilkinson S *et al.* Abnormalities in p53 and DNA content in transitional cell carcinoma of the bladder. *Br J Urol* 1994;**73**:522–525.

46. Fujimoto K, Yamada Y *et al.* Frequent association of p53 gene mutation in invasive bladder cancer. *Cancer Res* 1992;**52**:1393–1398.

47. Soini Y, Turpeenniemi-Hujanen T *et al.* P53 immunohistochemistry in transitional cell carcinoma and dysplasia of the urinary bladder correlates with disease progression. *Br J Cancer* 1993; **68**:1029–1035.

48. Thomas DJ, Robinson MC *et al.* P53 expression, ploidy and progression in pT1 transitional cell carcinoma of the bladder. *Br J Urol* 1994;**73**: 533–537.

49. Soini Y, Turpeenniemi-Hujanen T *et al.* P53 immunohistochemistry in transitional cell carcinoma and dysplasia of the urinary bladder correlates with disease progression. *Br J Cancer* 1993;**68**: 1029–1035.

50. O'Malley JK, Lynch TH, *et al.* P53 protein expression and increased SSCP mobility shifts in the p53 gene in bladder urothelium cultured from smokers. *J Urol* (abstract 1763);**157**:4.

51. Terrell RB, Cheville JC *et al.* Histopathological features of p53 nuclear protein staining as predictors of survival and tumor recurrence in patients with trasitional cell carcinoma of the renal pelvis. *J Urol* 1995;**154**:1342–1347.

52. Jones PA, Droller MJ. Pathways of development and progression in bladder cancer: New correlations between clinical observations and molecular mechanisms. *Sem Urol* 1993;**11**(4):177–192.

26 Transitional cell carcinoma of the upper urinary tract: Presentation, diagnosis and staging

S J Savage and M J Droller

Presentation

The most common clinical presentation of upper tract urothelial carcinoma is gross hematuria, which occurs in 70–90% of patients, although it may also present with microscopic hematuria. This may occur with or without flank pain[1–4]. The flank pain may be sharp or dull, depending on the amount of obstruction and the acuteness of its development. Obstruction may be caused either by the cancer itself or by clot formation. Acute colicky flank pain is usually caused by the passage of blood clots, and may have radiation of the pain similar to that which occurs during the passage of a calculus. Alternatively, dull flank pain is usually caused by gradual obstruction from tumor growth. Total hematuria implicates the upper tract as the source of bleeding, whereas mid-stream hematuria may be more likely to implicate the bladder. Those patients who present with only microscopic hematuria require further study in order to identify upper tract urothelial tumors as the source of their bleeding.

At times, a patient may present with hematuria associated with trauma. Although trauma may indeed be the cause of hematuria, it is important to remember that trauma may cause bleeding from a pre-existing lesion. Thus, it is important to evaluate patients after any episodes of hematuria.

A flank mass may be detected in 10–20% of patients[2]. Constitutional symptoms, including weight loss, anorexia, fever and adenopathy, may be the initial presentation in 7–10% of patients. These symptoms represent advanced, usually metastatic, disease[3].

Diagnosis

The diagnosis of upper tract urothelial carcinoma generally relies on intravenous pyelography (IVP). The most common finding is a radiolucent filling defect which may be seen in 50–75% of cases (Figure 26.1). Non-visualization (10%) or hydronephrosis may also be seen, depending upon the location of the tumor and the degree of invasion and consequent obstruction. It may be difficult to differentiate a urothelial tumor from non-opaque calculi, blood clots, sloughed renal papillae, fungi or tuberculosis. Therefore, other radiologic diagnostic modalities may be necessary to establish the diagnosis. These include sonography, computerized tomography, magnetic resonance imaging and retrograde pyelography[5].

Cystoscopy may aid in visualizing the ureteral orifice from which the efflux of bloody urine may be seen. Retrograde pyelography is specifically useful in cases of non-visualization, incomplete filling of the ureter, and in the presence of multiple tumors[3].

Other imaging modalities have been used in the diagnosis of upper tract urothelial cancer, but have not proven to be as sensitive. A urothelial tumor in the renal collecting system may be suggested by ultrasonography if there

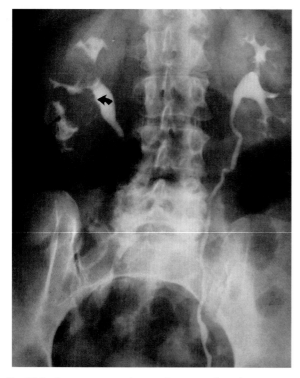

Fig. 26.1   Intravenous pyelogram demonstrating a large radiolucent filling defect in the right renal pelvis.

is dilatation of the collecting system. These lesions may be differentiated from calculi, due to the absence of acoustic shadowing from an echogenic focus (Figure 26.2). However, without distension, even large tumors (4–5 cm) infiltrating the renal pelvis may not be visualized[6].

Renal angiography has been used to distinguish renal cell carcinoma from transitional cell carcinoma, but is now rarely used to identify even hypernephromas. However, in cases when it presents with predominantly parenchymal involvement, it may be distinguished from renal cell carcinoma by the angiographic finding of encasement of the parenchymal vessels by tumor[7].

Computerized tomography (CT) is now widely used in diagnosing and staging upper tract urothelial tumors. CT has been shown to be less sensitive (68–86%) than urography in detecting upper tract urothelial tumors[8,9]. However, once a lesion is suggested on IVP, it is possible to change the contrast of the image, or make thin-section images in order to identify a greater percentage of lesions. CT scan with, and without, intravenous contrast may be most helpful in differentiating a ureteral tumor from a ureteral calculus[10]. This may be done by examining the radiodensity of the mass, which in the case of transitional cell carcinoma has attenuation values similar to that of soft tissue with an average density of 46 Hounsfield units[11,12]. Furthermore, these tumors do not frequently

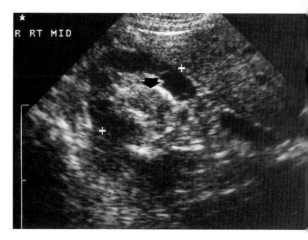

Fig. 26.2   Echogenic focus in the right renal pelvis without any evidence of acoustic shadowing.

disrupt the renal contour, or enhance with intravenous contrast (Figure 26.3). However, if the carcinoma is further advanced, it may be difficult to distinguish an invasive urothelial tumor from a parenchymal neoplasm[13].

In the evaluation of urothelial carcinoma it has become standard practice to examine urine for exfoliated cancer cells. Routine voided urine cytopathology has shown false-negatives in 80% of low-grade, low-stage tumors, while a rate as high as 40% false-negatives has been found even in high-grade lesions[3]. Selective cytology, which may be used when disease localization has not been established, has been found to provide a total sensitivity of 61%, with that for higher grade lesions approaching 75%[14]. However,

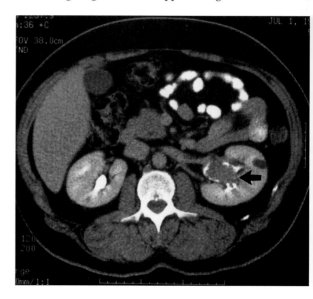

Fig. 26.3   CT scan demonstrating a mass in the right renal pelvis that does not enhance with contrast. Contrast can be seen in the surrounding areas of the collecting system.

even selective cytology via barbotage can give false-positive rates of 10% when only urolithiasis or inflammation are present, due to the similar appearance of sloughed cells from an inflammatory focus to that of cells from low-grade carcinoma.

In the past, retrograde cystoscopic brushing has been shown to provide a definitive diagnosis more often than voided or selective cytology[15]. In contrast to selective cytology, ureteroscopy will easily distinguish a calculus from a low-grade urothelial tumor. If direct vision is inconclusive, tissue sampling via ureteroscopy may be used. By performing cytopathologic examination on tissue sampled with cold-cup biopsy forceps, or a wire basket, diagnosis of urothelial tumors has been made possible with a reportedly marked increase in sensitivity[16,17].

Since Huffman et al.[18] reported on the endoscopic diagnosis of upper tract urothelial tumors, the technique has been used increasingly in establishing the diagnosis. Ureteroscopy offers the same opportunities that cystoscopy has offered for bladder tumors in allowing both direct visualization of the lesion in the upper tract and biopsy of the lesion. Sensitivity has been reported to be as high as 90%[19]. Furthermore, recent evidence suggests that p53 staining of endoscopically obtained specimens may increase sensitivity of diagnosis to 97%[20].

Percutaneous antegrade pyeloscopy should be avoided due to the theoretical possibility of tumor spillage and seeding.[21] Various reports, however, have described no evidence of tumor seeding with percutaneous approaches[20,3,22].

Staging

Staging systems for upper tract urothelial tumors are analogous to those used for bladder cancers. The most notable exception to this is that superficial and deep muscle invasion cannot be distinguished in the renal pelvis (Table 26.1).

Primary tumor stage has been found to be an excellent predictor of patient course and survival[23]. Stage has also been found to correlate closely with tumor grade[24].

$$pT_{a/T_1} \quad 51.8\% \text{ of pts} \rightarrow 91.1 \text{ months mean survival}$$
$$pT_{2/T_3} \quad 48.2\% \text{ of pts} \rightarrow 12.9 \text{ months mean survival}[23]$$

In examining the staging criteria for upper tract urothelial tumors, Guinan et al.[25] noted the anatomic difference between renal pelvic and ureteral tumors. T_3 tumors include those tumors invading the renal parenchyma and periureteral tissues. However, survival for T_3 of the ureter was 24% at 5 years[26–28], compared with 54% for T_3 renal pelvic carcinoma. Thus, it would be wise to consider T_3 renal pelvic and ureteral tumors separately.[25]

Fujimoto et al.[29] performed further examination of T_3 renal pelvic tumors. They identified decreased survival for patients in whom the tumor penetrated the basement membrane of the collecting system, versus those which

Table 26.1   TNM 1997 Classification – transitional cell carcinoma – renal pelvis and ureter

Jewett	Cummings	T – Primary tumor	Depth of invasion
		Tx	Primary tumor cannot be assessed
		T0	No evidence of primary tumor
0	I	Ta	Non-invasive papillary carcinoma
		Tis	Carcinoma in situ
A	II	T1	Tumor invades subepithelial connective tissue
B		T2	Tumor invades muscularis
		T3	
C	III	Renal pelvis	Tumor invades beyond muscularis into peripelvic fat or renal parenchyma
		Ureter	Tumor invades beyond muscularis into periureteric fat
D	IV	T4	Tumor invades adjacent organs or through the kidney into the perinephric fat
		N – Regional lymph nodes	
		Nx	Regional lymph nodes cannot be assessed
		N0	No regional lymph node metastasis
		N1	Metastasis in a single lymph node 2 cm or less
		N2	Metastasis in a single lymph node 2–5 cm, or multiple lymph nodes 5 cm or less in diameter
		N3	Metastasis in a lymph node more than 5 cm
		M – Distant metastasis	
		M0	No distant metastasis
		M1	Distant metastasis

simply infiltrated the collecting ducts. The significance of this, however, remains to be proven as infiltration, and thus poor survival, correlated with higher grade of the tumor.

Surgical staging provides a means to determine accurate prognoses for patients through survival after nephroureterectomy. It also allows the comparison between results of newer treatments for upper tract urothelial tumors. In order to predict patient survival as well as to help predict which patients may be most amenable to local excision, pre-operative staging is carried out routinely. These examinations include chest radiographs, CT scan, bone scan (in symptomatic patients) and, more frequently now, ureteroscopy. CT scan is the best imaging modality for pre-operative staging of upper tract urothelial tumors, but still has limited value in defining the extent of disease[17]. CT scan is not able to differentiate T_a from T_1 and T_2 lesions. CT sensitivity for parenchymal invasion is 75%, with a specificity of 43%. Its sensitivity for fat invasion is 67%, with a specificity of 44%[16]. Therefore, although it is the most useful imaging modality for pre-operative staging, CT is still not precise enough to use for management decisions.

Ureteropyeloscopy with biopsy may play an increasing role in the pre-operative evaluation and staging of patients with upper tract urothelial carcinoma. Actual staging of upper tract urothelial neoplasms may be difficult to perform, due to the inability to perform a deep biopsy without perforation. Presently, endoluminal ultrasound is being investigated as an adjunct for staging neoplasms, and has demonstrated submucosal invasion in some cases[30].

Endoscopic treatment of upper tract urothelial tumors necessitates close surveillance to diagnose recurrent tumors. In a compilation of various series of patients, there has been a local recurrence rate of 40% for renal pelvic tumors and 25% for ureteral tumors. Furthermore, asynchronous bladder tumors have been found in 39% of patients treated ureteroscopically[31].

Similarly, continued surveillance has been advocated in patients treated previously for carcinoma in situ of the bladder. After previous topical bladder therapy, a 15 month median time to relapse for distal ureteral carcinoma in situ was noted. This occurred in 29–35% of patients[32].

Carcinoma in situ of the renal pelvis and ureter is a diagnosis of exclusion. Patients with positive selective cytology and negative radiographic evaluation have been identified as having carcinoma in situ[33]. There is, however, some disagreement as to whether the upper urinary tract can be isolated from bladder contamination without resorting to a percutaneous approach when obtaining specimens for cytology[34].

Tumor grade correlates with tumor stage[5,24,28,40,43]. Therefore, in cases where a patient has a high-grade tumor

on biopsy, irrespective of CT scan results, greater caution may be taken in choosing local endoscopic excision rather than en bloc open surgical excision.

Further advances in immunohistochemical and molecular technology have made it possible to predict biologically aggressive urothelial tumors. DNA flow cytometry has shown correlations of ploidy with tumor grade and stage. In addition, the occasional patients with low-grade, low-stage tumors who also had DNA aneuploidy patterns have demonstrated significantly poorer survival than those with diploid patterns[35,36]. Thus, it may be wise to use DNA ploidy in planning conservative versus radical surgery.

Additional investigation has shown that p53 nuclear protein over-expression in bladder cancer may correlate with poorer survival[37–39]. However, when p53 expression was investigated in renal pelvic transitional cell carcinoma, it was not statistically associated with previously identified prognostic factors such as tumor grade and stage.

Conclusions

Upper tract urothelial carcinomas comprise only 5% of all urothelial malignancies, but represent an opportunity for the greatest amount of progress in diagnosis and treatment. Advances in molecular detection assays and endoscopic instruments promise to allow upper tract tumors and bladder tumors to be treated similarly. This may include diagnosis, initial treatment, intraluminal chemotherapy and surveillance of these tumors.

References

1. Cummings KB, Correa RJ, Gibbons RP, Stoll HM, Wheelis RF, Mason JT. Renal pelvic tumors. J Urol 1975;**126**:146.
2. Geerdsen J. Tumours of the renal pelvis and ureter. Symptomatology, diagnosis, treatment and prognosis. Scand J Urol Nephrol 1979;**12**:287.
3. McCarron JP, Mullis C, Vaughn ED. Tumors of the renal pelvis and ureter: Current concepts and management. Semin Urol 1983;**1**:75.
4. Booth CM, Cameron KM, Pugh RCB. Urothelial carcinoma of the kidney and ureter. Br J Urol 1980;**52**:430.
5. Batata M, Grabstald H. Upper urinary tract urothelial tumors. Urol Clin North Am 1976;**3**:79.
6. Yeh CS. In: Droller MJ (Ed.) Surgical management of urologic disease – an anatomic approach. Mosby-Yearbook 1992, St Louis, MO.
7. Mitty HA, Baron MG, Feller M. Infiltrating carcinoma of the renal pelvis: angiographic features. Radiology 1969;**92**:994.
8. McCoy J, Honda H, Resnicek M, Williams RD. Computerized tomography for detection and staging of localized and pathologically defined upper tract urothelial tumors. J Urol 1991;**146**:1500.
9. Planz B, George R, Adam G, Jakse G, Planz K. Computed tomography for detection and staging of transitional cell carcinoma of the upper tract. Eur Urol 1995;**27**:146.
10. Mendelson DS. In: Droller MJ (Ed.) Surgical management of urologic disease – an anatomic approach. Mosby-Yearbook 1992, St Louis, MO.
11. Lantz EJ, Hattery RR. Diagnostic imaging of urothelial cancer. Urol Clin North Am 1984;**11**:567.
12. Baghadassarian Gatewood OM, Goldman SM, Marshall FF et al. Computerized tomography in the diagnosis of transitional cell carcinoma of the kidney. J Urol 1982;**127**:876.

13. Bree RL, Schultz SR, Hayes R. Large infiltrating renal transitional cell carcinomas: CT and ultrasound features. *J Comput Assist Tomogr* 1990;**14**:381.

14. Zincke H, Aguilo JJ, Farrow GM, Utz DC, Khan AU. Significance of urinary cytology in the early detection of transitional cell cancer of the upper tract. *J Urol* 1976;**116**:781.

15. Gill WB, Lu CT, Thomsen S. Retrograde brushing: a new technique for obtaining histologic and cytologic material from ureteral renal pelvic and renal caliceal lesions. *J Urol* 1973;**109**:573.

16. Low RK, Moran ME, Anderson KR. Ureteroscopic cytologic diagnosis of upper tract lesions. *J Endourol* 1993;**7**:311.

17. Abdel-Razzak OM, Ehya H, Cubler-Goodman A, Bagley DH. Ureteroscopic biopsy in the upper urinary tract. *Urology* 1994;**44**:451.

18. Huffman JL, Morse MJ, Bagley DH *et al.* Endoscopic diagnosis and treatment of upper tract urothelial tumors. A preliminary report. *Cancer* 1985;**55**:1422.

19. Blute ML, Segura JW, Patterson DE. Ureteroscopy. *J Urol* 1985;**134**:1077.

20. Keeley FX, Bibbo M, McCue PA, Bagley DH. Use of p53 in the diagnosis of upper-tract transitional cell carcinoma. *Urology* 1997;**49**(2):181.

21. Tomera KM, Leary FJ, Zincke H. Pyeloscopy in urothelial tumors. *J Urol* 1982;**127**:1088.

22. Olesen S, Nielsen JB. Endoscopic diagnosis and treatment of urothelial tumors of the upper urinary tract. *Scand J Urol Nephrol* (-Suppl) 1995;**172**:11.

23. Huben RP, Mounzer AM, Murphy G. Tumor grade and stage as prognostic variables in upper tract urothelial tumors. *Cancer* 1988;**62**:2016.

24. Grabstald H, Whitmore WF, Melamed MR. Renal pelvic tumors. *JAMA* 1971;**218**:845.

25. Guinan P, Volgelzang NJ, Randazzo R *et al.* Renal pelvic transitional cell carcinoma: the role of the kidney in tumor-node-metastasis staging. *Cancer* 1992;**69**:1773.

26. Bloom NA, Vidone RA, Lytton B. Primary carcinoma of the ureter: a report of 102 new cases. *J Urol* 1970;**103**:590.

27. Heney NM, Nocks BN, Daly JJ *et al.* Prognostic factors in carcinoma of the ureter. *J Urol* 1981;**125**:632.

28. Batata MA, Whitmore WF, Hilaris BJ. Primary carcinoma of the ureter: a prognostic study. *Cancer* 1975;**35**:1626.

29. Fujimoto H, Tobisu K, Sakamoto M *et al.* Intraductal tumor involvement and renal parenchymal invasion of transitional cell carcinoma of the renal pelvis. *J Urol* 1995;**153**:57.

30. Bagley DH, Liu JB, Goldberg BB. The use of endoluminal ultrasound of the ureter. *Semin Urol* 1992;**10**:194.

31. Bagley DH. Treatment of upper urinary tract neoplasms. In: Smith AD (Ed.) *Smith's Textbook of Endourology*. Quality Medical Publications St Louis MO, 1996.

32. Herr HW, Whitmore WF Jr. Ureteral carcinoma in situ after successful intravesical therapy for superficial bladder tumors: incidence, possible pathogenesis and management. *J Urol* 1987;**138**:202.

33. Sarosdy MF, Pisters LL, Carroll PR *et al.* Bropiramine immunotherapy of upper urinary tract carcinoma in situ. *Urology* 1996;**48**(1):29.

34. Soloway MS. Intrarenal bacillus Calmette-Guerin therapy for upper urinary tract carcinoma in situ – Editorial comment. *J Urol* 1993; **149**:457.

35. Blute ML, Tsushima K, Farrow, GM, Therneau TM, Lieber MM. Transitional cell carcinoma of the renal pelvis: nuclear deoxyribonucleic acid ploidy studied by flow cytometry. *J Urol* 1988;**140**:944.

36. Al-Abadi H, Nagel R. Transitional cell carcinoma of the renal pelvis and ureter: prognostic relevance of nuclear deoxyribonucleic acid ploidy studied by slide cytometry: an 8-year survival time study. *J Urol* 1992; **148**:31.

37. Lipponen PK. Over-expression of p53 nuclear oncoprotein in transitional-cell bladder cancer and its prognostic value. *Int J Cancer* 1993;**53**:365.

38. Ye DW, Zheng JF, Qian SX, Ma YJ. Expression of p53 product in Chinese human bladder carcinoma. *Urol Res* 1993;**21**:223.

39. Furihata M, Inoue K, Ohtsuki Y, Hashimoto H, Teraio N, Fujita Y. High-risk human papillomavirus infections and overexpression of p53 protein as prognostic indicators in transitional cell carcinoma of the urinary bladder. *Cancer Res* 1993;**53**:4823.

40. Terrell RB, Cheville JC, See WA, Cohen MB. Histopathological features and p53 nuclear protein staining as predictors of survival and tumor recurrence in patients with transitional cell carcinoma of the renal pelvis. *J Urol* 1995;**154**:1342.

27 Transitional cell carcinoma of the upper urinary tract: Pathology

D Ansell

Pathology

The great majority of tumors of the renal pelvis and ureter are urothelial in origin. Other tumors are extremely rare, although there are a number of benign conditions which may be confused with urothelial malignancies and which should always be considered in a differential diagnosis.

The renal pelvis and ureter are lined by urothelium of similar appearance and histology to that found in the bladder and urethra. It therefore follows that tumors arising within this epithelium are likely to be very similar in their pathology and biology to those arising in the other two organs. Phenacetin abuse and Balkan nephropathy are particularly associated with urothelial tumors at this site but in other respects their etiology and natural history are similar to that of bladder cancer except some authors claim that the increased incidence of such tumors in males is not found at this site[1].

The mucosa of the upper urinary system is normally somewhat folded and this may lead to problems in the cytological interpretation of urine specimens or nephrostomy washouts obtained from this locality since the papillary structures detached from such an epithelium may be misinterpreted as well differentiated transitional cell carcinoma in cytologic assessment[2]. The nuclei of the urothelial cells in this region are also larger and more irregular than those seen more distally and this can lead to problems in the diagnosis of in situ carcinoma at resection margins, especially in frozen sections.

Benign tumors

Confusion and disagreement continues concerning whether or not a benign form of transitional cell tumor exists and if it does what proportion of non-invasive transitional cell tumors should be so called. Put in another way do true papillomas occur? However, as all well differentiated non-invasive transitional cell carcinomas of ureter and pelvis are cured by resection this can be considered to be of only academic interest in this portion of the urinary tract.

Inverted papilloma

This entity is controversial. Inverted papilloma was originally described as a solid pedunculated smooth surfaced spherical lesion occurring at the bladder trigone with a distinctive histologic appearance and which did not recur. They are composed of trabeculae of benign looking urothelium with a covering of continuous similar attenuated epithelium, the inner layer of cells is often columnar or cuboidal in appearance. The term is now often employed for tumors of a very similar histologic appearance which recur sometime after initial presentation. A number, if not all, of these recurrent lesions are most probably well differentiated transitional cell carcinomas with an inverted growth pattern. Certainly in my experience, despite what is written in publications and text books, differentiation between these two entities can be very difficult. However, reports continue to be published of recurrent inverted papillomas – the author has considerable difficulty in considering this to be a valid entity and is not convinced that this is a helpful diagnosis in this locality.

Transitional cell carcinoma

These tumors occur in various degrees of differentiation and are graded in an identical manner to that employed in the bladder. Similarly, the tumors will be diagnosed at varying stages of invasion and this will be reflected in the tumor stage. Like urothelial tumors elsewhere in the urinary tract they may be multiple at presentation or may occur before or after tumor is diagnosed in the bladder. This multicentricity necessitates removal of the whole of the ureter when urothelial cancer of the renal pelvis is removed surgically since if this is not done tumor may subsequently occur in the remaining ureter so-called 'stump carcinoma'.

Papillary carcinoma

Papillary transitional cell tumors most uncommonly occur as non-invasive lesions of ureter or pelvis and by growing into the lumen cause obstruction of pelvis to produce a variable degree of hydroureter or hydronephrosis (Figure 27.1). If longstanding such lesions will become complicated by infection and produce a pyonephrosis or pyelonephritis. These papillary non-invasive tumors are often multiple and are said to occur most commonly in the distal one-third of the ureter or in the extra-renal portion of the renal pelvis[2].

They have an identical histologic appearance to those tumors which arise in the bladder. Urothelial cells of a variable degree of differentiation line the surface of thin fibrovascular cores. The atypia of the urothelium and lack of significant connective tissue in the core differentiates tumor from papilliferous reactive conditions (see below). The histologic diagnosis of early invasion in these tumors can be extremely difficult and often controversial as the mere bulk of tumor in a restricted lumen may push groups of cells into the muscle wall simulating invasion and hence malignancy, but such groups of cells will have a rounded, well demarcated outline and not the irregular profile of true invasion. It is important correctly to interpret these findings as non-invasive tumors, unlike deeply invasive tumors, have an excellent prognosis; in Grabstadt's series[3], there were no tumor deaths unless tumor extended into peripelvic tissues[4].

Invasive carcinoma

The majority of these are poorly differentiated urothelial tumors. Some will be associated with a recognizable pap-

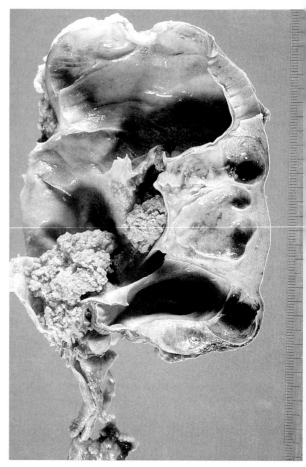

Fig. 27.1 Multiple papillary non-invasive transitional cell carcinomas of ureter and renal pelvis causing hydronephrosis.

illary element but in a significant number this will not be obvious and this may make precise diagnosis difficult in cases involving kidney only. As well as spreading into peripelvic or periureteric fat, tumors of the renal pelvis may infiltrate the renal parenchyma often spreading up tubules, a process that Dr Roger Pugh described as malignant ascending pyelonephritis. The majority of invasive urothelial tumors in the renal pelvis will be recognizable as of urothelial origin due to their location at the hilum, but larger tumors extensively invading the renal substance may be confused with renal tubular carcinomas especially of the sarcomatoid variety. This confusion often follows an imaging report of a lesion replacing a significant quantity of the renal substance in the manner of renal cell carcinoma. Extensive sampling, especially of adjacent pelvic urothelium, is necessary to reach a correct diagnosis in such cases and careful macroscopic scrutiny of the nature of the lining of the renal pelvis will often reveal areas with a papilliferous appearance (Figure 27.2) and microscopic examination of adjacent urothelium will often reveal flat in situ carcinoma. Occasional tumors which appear to be restricted to the renal medulla and which have a significant papillary component will turn out to be collecting duct carcinomas of the kidney[5].

Squamous cell carcinoma

A small percentage of renal pelvic carcinomas are true squamous cell carcinomas often with extensive keratin formation. Benign squamous metaplasia can frequently be seen in adjacent urothelium. In up to 50% of these cancers there are associated calculi and it is tempting to postulate that 'chronic irritation' by the calculus has produced squamous metaplasia, leading to leukoplakia and finally invasive squamous cell carcinoma (in a similar fashion to the progression of leukoplakia to squamous

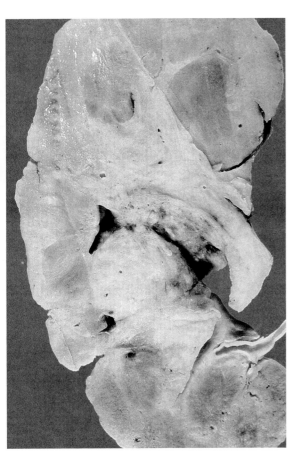

Fig. 27.2 Invasive transitional cell carcinoma of renal pelvis – there is much irregularity of adjacent urothelium indicating associated non-invasive tumor.

cell carcinoma of the bladder). However, a significant number of squamous cell cancers are not associated with calculi and Melamed[1] states that squamous metaplasia may actually be the cause of some calculi rather than the reverse.

Other primary tumors

True adenocarcinoma of the renal pelvis (as distinct from collecting duct carcinomas or renal cell carcinoma extending into the renal pelvis) is distinctly uncommon. They have to be distinguished from adenomatous metaplasia (see below) and are recognized by the carcinomatous nature of their nuclei and the fact that the majority of the tumor is within the lumen. Metastatic carcinoma will be situated predominantly in the wall and surrounding tissues of the ureter or pelvis. As in the bladder, glandular and, indeed, squamous areas may be seen in otherwise typical transitional cell carcinomas; these should be considered as transitional cell carcinomas with foci of glandular differentiation and not adenocarcinomas.

Similarly tumors with a prominent spindle, sarcomatoid or small cell component have been described in this location as they have in the bladder. Another particularly aggressive tumor termed renal medullary carcinoma known to be associated with sickle cell trait has been described recently[6].

Benign conditions simulating transitional cell carcinoma

Fibroepithelial polyp
These arborizing outgrowths of connective tissue with a covering of benign urothelium are most commonly found in the ureter in children. They have a very characteristic macroscopic appearance (Figure 27.3) but may be confused with papillary transitional cell carcinoma on radiologic appearances if occurring in adults. Histologically the abundant fibrovascular stromal core and low benign urothelial covering should not present any diagnostic difficulty.

Urothelial metaplasia
Various forms of metaplasia of urothelium, more commonly recognized in the bladder, may occur in the ureter and renal pelvis and produce papilliferous or polypoid lesions macroscopically resembling transitional cell neoplasms. Ureteritis cystica (Figure 27.4) may thus resemble multiple non-invasive tumors of the ureter as may adenomatous metaplasia (nephrogenic adenoma). Bullous and papillary cystitis (often called catheter tumor since

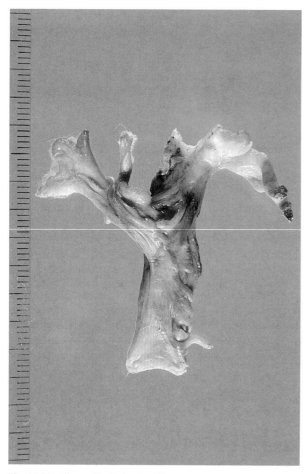

Fig. 27.3   Fibroepithelial polyp of ureter.

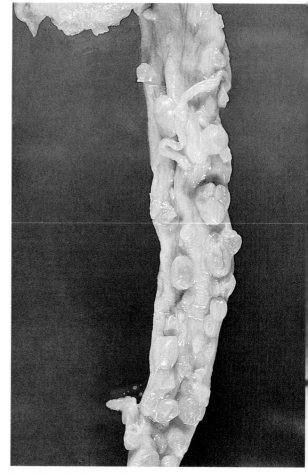

Fig. 27.4   Florid ureteritis cystica.

they are usually due to irritation from the tip of an indwelling urinary catheter) obviously do not really have a homologue in the ureter or renal pelvis.

Miscellaneous conditions

A number of uncommon conditions occasionally cause unilateral or bilateral ureteric obstruction and may mimic carcinoma[7]. Idiopathic retroperitoneal fibrosis can be a cause of bilateral ureteric obstruction and has to be differentiated from diffuse retroperitoneal tumors such as metastatic carcinoma, retroperitoneal sarcomas and not uncommonly malignant lymphoma. The advent of guided needle biopsy has enabled these conditions to be diagnosed in this site without recourse to open surgery in many cases.

Other causes are usually unilateral and here differentiation from tumor may be more of a problem. Both submucosal hematomas or isolated fibrotic strictures may be the result of a previously impacted calculus and the latter

may also be the late result of tuberculosis of the upper urinary tract.

Endometriosis and schistosomiasis although more commonly located in the bladder are occasionally situated in the ureter producing a localized stricture and, similarly, I have seen amyloid and malakoplakia of the ureter giving a macroscopic appearance of tumor.

References

1. Melamed MR, Reuter VE. Pathology and staging of urothelial tumors of the kidney and ureter. *Urol Clin North Am* 1993;**20**:333–347.
2. Murphy WM, Beckwith JB, Farrow GM. *Atlas of tumour pathology, 3rd series.* Fascicle 11. Tumours of the kidney, bladder and related structures. Armed Forces Institute of Pathology, Washington DC 1994, pp. 313–318.
3. Grabstadt H, Whitmore WF Jr, Melamed MR. Renal pelvic tumours. *JAMA* 1971;**218**:845–854.
4. Huben RP, Mounzer AM, Murphy GP. Tumour grade and stage as prognostic variables in upper tract urothelial tumours. *Cancer* 1988;**62**:2016–2020.

5. Fleming S, Lewi H. Collecting duct carcinoma of the kidney. *Histopathology* 1986;**10**:1131–1141.
6. Davis CJ Jr, Mostofi FK, Sesterhenn IA. Renal medullary carcinoma. The seventh sickle cell nephropathy. *Am J Surg Pathol* 1995;**19**(1):1–11.
7. Ordonez NG. Tumours of renal pelvis and ureter In: *Ackerman's Surgical Pathology*. Rosai J. St Louis, Missouri, Mosby, 1996; 1159–1163.

28 Transitional cell carcinoma of the upper urinary tract: Surgical treatment

Algorithm

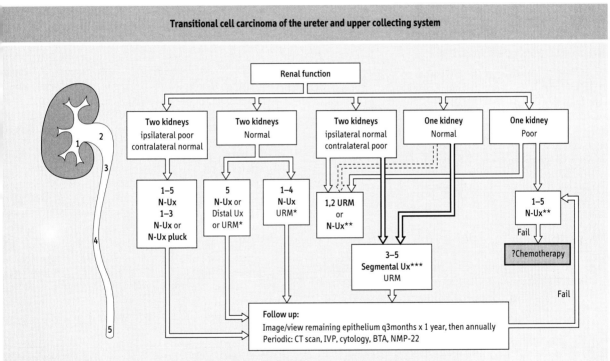

Transitional cell carcinoma of the ureter and upper collecting system

N-Ux, nephroureterectomy with 1cm cuff of bladder wall; Ux, ureterectomy; URM, ureteroscopic or percutaneous management.
1, major or minor calyces; 2, renal pelvis; 3, upper 1/3 ureter; 4, middle 1/3 ureter; 5, lower 1/3 ureter.
*Consider for isolated, low grade, easily accessible, papillary tumors. **dialysis.
***Possible primary re-anastomosis[3,4], bladder flap[4,5] consider ileal/appendiceal ureteral substitution[2–5], autotransplant with uretero (pyelo)-neocystostomy[2–4], Cutaneous diversion (ureterostomy, bowel conduit)[2–4].

28.1 Nephro-ureterectomy and partial ureterectomy

C R J Woodhouse

Introduction

The traditional treatment for renal pelvic and ureteric carcinoma was nephro-ureterectomy. Over the last 30 years, almost by accident, there has been a realization that such radical surgery is not always necessary. Improvements in pre-operative grading and staging now allow a more logical choice of operation.

Upper tract transitional cell carcinoma (TCC) behaves, grade for grade and stage for stage, in the same way as the disease in the bladder. The bladder should not be removed for a solitary well differentiated, non-invasive TCC and nor should the kidney.

Nephro-ureterectomy is indicated for invasive disease, poorly differentiated but superficial disease and for large or multifocal superficial disease.

Nephro-ureterectomy

Rationale

Upper tract TCC is a rare disease with a wide spectrum of behavior. It is hardly surprising that there are no controlled trial data to help management decisions. It has become accepted that the operation should include removal of the perinephric fat, the whole of the ureter and a cuff of bladder. Some also remove the adjacent retroperitoneal lymph nodes. How much of this is necessary remains unproven.

The ureter

Ureterectomy is the easiest part to justify. In surgery for TCC, parts of the urinary should only be left behind if they fulfil three criteria:

1. They are free of tumor (including in situ disease)
2. They retain some useful function
3. They can easily be followed up.

The ureter of a resected kidney fulfils none of these criteria and should always be removed. The ureteric recurrence rate is shown in Table 28.1.1[1-6]. Although the rates are not particularly high, it should be remembered that, at presentation, the recurrence is likely to be advanced and will probably prove fatal. Even when a radical nephrectomy has been performed for a presumed adenocarcinoma which ultimately turns out to be a TCC, a second operation should be carried out to remove the ureteric stump.

Table 28.1.1   Incidence of stump recurrence after subtotal ureterectomy for renal transitional cell carcinoma (cases/number at risk)

	Low grade/stage Unspecified	High grade/stage
Grabstald[1]	1/42	
Batata*[2]	4	3/11
Murphy[3]	1/15	
Booth[4]		7/65
Zincke and Neves[5]		6/20
Steffens and Nagel[6]		9/45

*11 cases in total at risk, distribution of grades not stated.

Similarly, in the rare circumstance where bladder TCC occurs in a patient who has had a nephrectomy in the past, any remaining ureteric stump is at risk of developing TCC[7]. It would be prudent at least to monitor such a blind ureter, if not to remove it.

The justification for removing a cuff of bladder is that it appears to reduce the incidence of subsequent bladder carcinoma. In a well documented and prospective series, the incidence of TCC was five of 17 cases with excision compared with 12 of 20 with no excision. Of the 17 cases that did suffer bladder recurrence, 12 were in the region of the resected ureteric orifice[8].

If a patient is known to have bladder carcinoma, it should be cleared endoscopically before nephrectomy to minimize tumor spillage.

Perinephric fat

In the current literature of renal pelvic carcinoma it is taken for granted that the perinephric fat and Gerotas fascia should be removed. As these renal coverings have no use, it is perfectly reasonable to do so even though the survival after this operation is often said to be poor. It must be accepted, however, that the justification is theoretical as no series compares the results of this operation with those of a simpler nephro-ureterectomy. The theoretical justification is much the same as that for adenocarcinoma of the kidney. About 38% of cases of renal pelvic TCC have invasion of the perinephric fat (or worse)[5,9]. The renal cortex is drained by a network of lymphatics that are widely anastomosed to those of the perinephric fat. While this would have less impact on the spread of a TCC than of an adenocarcinoma, the lymphatic flow is towards the periphery if there is any degree of urinary obstruction[10]. As any invasive TCC is likely to cause some obstruction, peripheral lymphatic flow should always be assumed.

The adrenal

The traditional operation of radical nephrectomy included resection of the ipsilateral adrenal. Even for adenocarcinoma, this is no longer considered essential. In renal TCC, the adrenal can be preserved unless the cancer field would be broken by so doing.

The regional lymph nodes

There are few things more controversial than regional lymphadenectomy for cancer. The conservatives will argue that removal of involved nodes does not cure patients and there is no need to remove uninvolved nodes. The radicals will argue that failure to remove the nodes misses the opportunity to cure those with small volume nodal disease and denies the clinician important prognostic information.

There can be no doubt that lymphadenectomy provides useful prognostic information. Those with positive nodes die more quickly than those with negative nodes.

The lymphatic drainage of the renal pelvis is to the hilar nodes. However, the renal cortical lymphatics anastomose with those of the retroperitoneum (see above). It is therefore possible for a TCC that deeply invades the parenchyma to have positive pelvic nodes while the hilar nodes are negative.

In adenocarcinoma of the kidney, the only controlled trial of radical nephrectomy with or without lymphadenectomy, has produced only preliminary results. No difference in survival was shown between the two groups[11]. This, of course, is a different disease.

In transitional cell carcinoma of the bladder, there are no relevant controlled trials. In an extensive review of the literature, Altwein concluded that there was no sound evidence that pelvic node dissection prolonged survival; occasional patients with small volume nodal disease might be cured[12]. This is the same disease as TCC of the kidney and the natural history seems to be the same in the two organs.

It is not justified to perform a radical node dissection for TCC of the kidney. Some local nodes may be sampled for prognostic information.

The operation

The intention of the operation is to remove the kidney, ureter and a cuff of bladder. The bladder should be free of TCC at the time of the operation. The patient should be free of metastases and have a locally resectable tumor.

The incision

There are almost as many approaches to this operation as there are authors in the field. The possibilities are given in Table 28.1.2. The choice of technique is influenced largely by personal prejudice. The whole specimen should be removed en bloc without dividing the ureter and so breaking the cancer field. The safest operations are performed with dissection under direct vision. Approaches

Table 28.1.2   Additional approaches to nephro-ureterectomy

Upper abdominal incision for the kidney. Catheterization of the ureter and intussusception through the bladder. Endoscopic resection of the uretero-vesical junction[13].
Flank incision for the kidney, separate Pfannensteil or gridiron for the ureter[14].
Preliminary endoscopic resection of the ureteric orifice. Upper abdominal incision for the kidney with 'rip and pluck' of the ureter[15].
Laparoscopic nephro-ureterectomy[16,17].

that involve 'ripping' and 'plucking' seem to transgress all good surgical principles.

Laparoscpic nephro-ureterectomy is a triumph of ingenuity and patience. For the present, it should only be conducted in specialist units. Its future will be controlled by its success or failure in curing patients.

The present author prefers a chevron incision that gives good access to the kidney, ureter and bladder and allows dissection under direct vision (Figure 28.1.1).

Renal dissection

The initial dissection is the same as that for radical nephrectomy for adenocarcinoma. The intestine overlying the kidney (ascending colon and duodenum on the right or descending colon on the left) are Kockerized to expose Gerotas fascia. On the left care should be taken not to damage the colonic blood supply which is tenuous at this point.

The fatty and nodal tissue over the great vessels is dissected to expose the renal vein. The nodal tissue is drawn laterally so that it can, eventually, be removed en bloc with the kidney.

A soft sling is put around the vein to control and protect it. Then the search for the renal artery begins. It can be frustrating, especially in a fat patient. The artery usually lies behind and slightly above the vein. Gentle dissection must be continued until the artery is found. Once defined, the artery can be ligated in continuity.

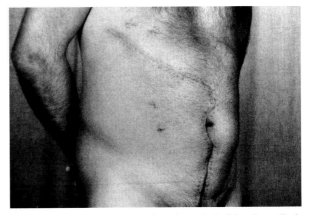

Fig. 28.1.1   Clinical photograph to show the incision for radical nephro-ureterectomy.

Once arterial control has been achieved, the vein is fully exposed, ligated and divided. This will further expose the artery which itself can be ligated and divided.

The dissection of Gerotas fascia can then continue with relatively little bleeding. The vessels to the adrenal are generally clipped with 'ligaclips' and divided. On the left, the greatest care must be taken to avoid damaging the spleen. Laterally, the fascia is incised and a finger can be passed behind the perinephric fat to lift the kidney off the psoas and posterior abdominal muscles.

As the lateral and medial dissections approach each other, the ureter and peri-ureteric connective tissue are seen. The ureter is mobilized by blunt dissection to the pelvis. The main blood supply comes from a branch of the internal iliac artery. This vessel can be clipped. Sharp dissection and division of the superior vesicle pedicle are usually needed to expose the uretero-vesical junction.

In thin patients it may be possible to define the uretero-vesical junction clearly enough to do a clean resection with a cuff of bladder. In most patients, however, it is safer to open the front of the bladder between stay sutures. The ureteric orifice can be circumcised under direct vision and the junction removed en bloc with the ureter. The local defect and the cystotomy are closed with absorbable sutures.

The abdominal wound is then closed in layers with non-absorbable sutures, with or without a drain.

Ureterectomy

Ureterectomy alone is very seldom required for upper tract TCC. Very small, low-grade tumors can be treated endoscopically[18]. Large, multiple and aggressive tumors usually require nephro-ureterectomy, or may be inoperable.

Up to 50% of patients will have other, synchronous, TCC which may dictate the overall management. In one series, nearly half the patients required a nephro-ureterectomy, regardless of the stage of the ureteric component of the disease. Most of the remainder were treated by local resection and end to end anastomosis or reimplantation. None of the conservatively treated patients died of cancer[19].

Conservative surgery was first suggested in a serious way in 1981 when the natural history was defined and the success of local resection in selected cases reported[20]. If the ureter is to be removed, the problem lies in reconstructing or replacing it. There are few hard and fast rules in a condition that is so rare and so diverse. The surgeon should be familiar with the basic principles and thereafter use wide imagination.

Patient and operation selection

Localized, single lesions

In patients with low-grade, non-invasive tumors, the involved segment can be locally resected.

For lesions in the upper third, the resection must be sufficiently localized that a tension-free, end to end anastomosis can be performed. Ideally the lower end should be anastomosed to the renal pelvis. If necessary, a flap of renal pelvis can be formed into a tube to bridge the gap (in the same manner as a Boari flap from the bladder).

It is surprising how much mobilization is required to achieve a tension-free anastomosis. It is important to mobilize the kidney from its upper attachments to liver or spleen, as well as to dissect the lower ureter.

For tumors in the middle third an end to end anastomosis may occasionally be possible. It is usually better to excise the whole lower ureter and do a transuretero-ureterostomy.

For the lower third of the ureter, a direct reimplant into the bladder, with or without a Boari flap, should always be possible.

Follow up

There is a strong association between upper tract and lower tract TCC (Table 28.1.3). The bladder cancer may be diagnosed concurrently or subsequently.

Bilateral upper tract TCC is rare. A few patients present with bilateral upper tract tumors, especially those with Balkan nephropathy or who have abused phenacetin. Once these patients have been excluded, however, subsequent contra-lateral renal or ureteric TCC is rare (Table 28.1.4).

Table 28.1.3   Relationship of upper tract to bladder transitional cell carcinoma

| Author | n | | Bladder carcinoma | | |
		Previous	Concurrent	Subsequent*	Notes
Grabstald[1]	70		37		
Murphy[3]	49		2	11	a
Murphy[25]	175		18	45	b
Booth[4]	203	45	39	27	
Cukier[26]	130		34	5	
Nocks[27]	68	7	9	14	c
Zincke[5]	62			30	
Anderstrom[19]	49	5	14	15	d

*Variable length of follow up.
Notes: a.   Grade 1 only b.   Grades 2–4 c.   Renal tumors only
d.   Ureteric tumors only

Table 28.1.4 Incidence of bilaterality of transitional cell carcinoma of the upper urinary tract

Author	n	Synchronous	Asynchronous	Notes
Grabstald[1]	70	3	2	
Batata[2]	41	0	1	d
Mazeman[28]	1118	23		
Murphy[3]	49	1	1	a
Murphy[25]	175	0	3	b
Booth[4]	203	2		
Nocks[27]	68	0	1	c
Zincke[5]	62	2	0	
Alderstrom[19]	49	1	5	d

Notes as for Table 28.1.3.

Follow up, therefore, is based on the search for recurrent TCC in the bladder and for metastatic disease.

The bladder surveillance is straightforward. If the patient has already had a bladder tumor, the frequency of cystoscopies is controlled by its grade and stage. The first cystoscopy is carried out at 3 months. If the bladder is clear, the next one is preferred at 9 months and annually thereafter. If the bladder has a recurrence, cystoscopies are carried out 3 monthly until a pattern is established and a decision is made about intra-vesical chemotherapy[21].

If there has never been a bladder cancer, it is more difficult to judge the frequency of cystoscopy. It is probably safest to cystoscope 3 monthly for the first year, 6 monthly in the second and annually thereafter. If a bladder carcinoma appears, it will, obviously, be treated according to its own grade and stage.

There is no point in looking for symptomless metastatic disease if no treatment will be offered for it. The development of successful cytotoxic chemotherapy for TCC has encouraged more active surveillance. If such treatment would be given, the search must include a chest X-ray, and imaging of the loco-regional nodes (see Chapter 3.2.4.3).

Surgery for bilateral disease or solitary kidneys

In bilateral synchronous disease it is usually possible to treat at least one side conservatively, even if the other requires a nephro-ureterectomy.

In patients with a solitary kidney, more drastic measures will be considered (though, perhaps, seldom used). It is possible to transplant the kidney, after clearance of the tumor on the bench, to the true pelvis and anastomose the renal pelvis directly to the bladder. The vessels are anastomosed to the internal iliacs. Such surgery has a 30% complication rate and may lead to loss of the kidney[22].

A safer procedure is to form an ileal conduit which is anastomosed directly to the renal pelvis. It is then poss-ible to endoscope the renal pelvis through the stoma and cauterize superficial recurrences. Alternatively, the ureter may be removed and replaced with tailored ileum. The technique of ileal replacement is important. If a poorly measured and untailored segment of ileum is used it tends to elongate and dilate with time. This leads to mucus retention and infection. Careful measurement, tailoring and the addition of an antireflux nipple have been shown to give superior results in a controlled trial[23]. Very occasionally the appendix can be used to replace some of the right ureter.

For superficial disease, the options discussed in the next section are appropriate section.

Occasionally, the surgeon may find himself considering the possibility of removing all of the remaining renal tissue and putting the patient on dialysis. Traditionally, this has a poor reputation. Recent reports have shown acceptable results of dialysis and even of transplantation up to 5 years post-surgery. Transplantation after 2 years tumor free has been suggested[24].

Prognosis

In such a rare condition with such wide variation in natural history, it is difficult to give any confident idea of prognosis. Patients who are candidates for nephro-ureterectomy are likely to have aggressive disease. Conversely, those having a ureterectomy are likely to have disease of low grade and stage.

Those with tumors invading no deeper than the lamina propria (T1), regardless of grade, are likely to be cured. Those with muscle or parenchymal invasion (T2 or 3) have about a 50% 5 year survival except poorly differentiated tumors, when it falls to about 10%. Virtually all patients with extension beyond the kidney will be dead in 2 years, regardless of grade[25].

References

1. Grabstald H, Whitmore WF, Melamed MR. Renal pelvic tumors. *JAMA* 1971;**218**:845–854.
2. Batata MA, Whitmore WF, Hilaris BS, Tokita N, Grabstald H. Primary carcinoma of the ureter: a prognostic study. *Cancer* 1975;**35**:1626–1632.
3. Murphy DM, Zincke H, Furlow WL. Primary grade I transitional cell carcinoma of the renal pelvis and ureter. *J Urol* 1980;**123**:629–631.
4. Booth CM, Cameron KM, Pugh RCB. Urothelial carcinoma of the kidney and ureter. *Br J Urol* 1980;**52**:430–435.
5. Zincke H, Neves RJ. Feasibility of conservative surgery for transitional cell carcinoma of the upper urinary tract. *Urol Clin N Am* 1984;**11**:717–724.
6. Steffens J, Nagel R. Tumors of the renal pelvis and ureter. *Br J Urol* 1988;**61**:277–283.
7. Cher ML, Milchgrub S, Sagalowsky AI. Transitional cell carcinoma of the ureteral stump 23 years after radical nephrectomy for adenocarcinoma. *J Urol* 1993;**149**:106–108.

8. Williams CB, Mitchell JP. Carcinoma of the renal pelvis: a review of 43 cases. *Br J Urol* 1973;**45**:370–376.

9. McDonald MW. Urothelial tumors of the upper urinary tract. In: de Kernion JB, Paulson DF (eds) *Genitourinary cancer management*. Lea & Febiger, Philadelphia, 1987, pp. 1–32.

10. Yoffey JM, Coutice FC. Lymph flow from the regional lymphatics. In *Lymphatics, lymph and the lymphomyeloid complex*. Academic Press, London, 1970, pp. 236–250.

11. Blom JHM, Schroder FH, Sylvester R, Hammond B. The EORTC Genitourinary Group: the therapeutic value of lymphadenectomy in conjunction with radical nephrectomy in non-metastatic renal cancer – results of an EORTC phase III study. *J Urol* 1992;**147**:422A.

12. Altwein JE. Radical cystectomy and pelvic node dissection in lymph node positive bladder cancer. In: Donohue JP (Ed.) *Lymph node surgery in urology*. Issis Medical Media, Oxford, 1995, pp. 51–62.

13. McDonald HP, Upchurch WE, Studerant CE. Nephroureterectomy: a new technique. *J Urol* 1952;**67**:804–809.

14. Blandy JP. Nephrectomy. In: *Operative urology*. Blackwell Scientific, Oxford, 1978, pp. 10–37.

15. Abercrombie GF, Eardley I, Payne SR, Walmesley BH, Vinnicombe J. Modified nephroureterectomy. Long term follow up with particular reference to subsequent bladder tumours. *Br J Urol* 1988;**61**:198–200.

16. Clayman RV, Kavoussi LR, Figenshau RS, Chandhoke PS, Albala DM. Laparoscopic nephroureterectomy: initial clinical report. *J Laparoendosc Surg* 1991;**1**:343–346.

17. Wilson BG, Deans GT, Kelly J, McCrory D. Laparoscopic nephrectomy: initial experience and cost implications. *Br J Urol* 1995;**75**:276–280.

18. Gerber GS, Lyon ES. Endourological management of upper tract urothelial tumors. *J Urol* 1993;**150**:2–7.

19. Anderstrom C, Johansson SL, Petersson S, Wahlqvist L. Carcinoma of the ureter: a clinicopathologic study of 49 cases. *J Urol* 1989;**142**:280–283.

20. Mills C, Vaughan ED. Carcinoma of the ureter: natural history, management and 5 year survival. *J Urol* 1983;**129**:275–277.

21. Morris SB, Shearer RJ, Gordon EM, Woodhouse CRJ. Superficial bladder cancer: timing of check cystoscopies in the first year. *Br J Urol* 1993;**72**:446–448.

22. Petterson S, Aamot P, Brynger H. *et al.* Extra corporeal renal surgery, autotransplantation and calicovesicostomy for renal pelvic and ureteric tumors. *Scand J Urol Nephrol* 1981;**60**:33–35.

23. Shokeir AA, Gaballah MA, Asamallah AA, Ghoneim MA. Optimization of replacement of the ureter by ileum. *J Urol* 1991;**146**:306–310.

24. Persad RA, Gillatt DA, Harrison P, Abrams PH. Dialysis in patients with upper urinary tract transitional cell carcinoma. *Br J Urol* 1992;**69**:577–579.

25. Murphy DM, Zincke H, Furlow WL. Management of high grade transitional cell carcinoma of the upper urinary tract. *J Urol* 1981;**125**:25–29.

26. Cukier J, Abourachid H, Pascal B, Suer JP, Merimsky E. Tumeurs de la voie excretrice haute. *J Urol* (Paris) 1981;**87**:57–66.

27. Nocks BN, Heney NM, Daly JJ *et al.* Transitional cell carcinoma of the renal pelvis. *Urology* 1982, pp. 472–477.

28. Mazaman E. Tumours of the upper urinary tract calyses, renal pelvis and ureter. *Eur Urol* 1976;**2**:120–128.

28.2 Percutaneous, ureteroscopic resection and novel approaches

E R Goldfischer and G S Gerber

Introduction

Transitional cell carcinoma (TCC) of the renal pelvis and ureter is relatively uncommon, accounting for less than 5% of all cases of TCC and only 6–8% of all upper urinary tract tumors[1,2]. While the standard treatment of upper urinary tract TCC is nephro-ureterectomy with the removal of a cuff of bladder surrounding the ipsilateral ureteral orifice[3,4], nephron-sparing surgery may be appropriate in certain situations. These include patients with tumor in a solitary kidney, bilateral synchronous tumors and renal insufficiency[5]. In addition, the development of innovative endoscopic technology, including smaller and flexible instrumentation, allows for an endoscopic approach to upper tract TCC either via a percutaneous or transurethral route[6]. Initially, endoscopic management was reserved for patients who would be unable to tolerate major surgery, but improved instrumentation that allows for more accurate and complete tumor ablation has led to more aggressive use of endoscopic techniques. While the risk of local recurrence and disease progression is higher than with open surgical resection, endoscopic treatment of upper tract TCC coupled with a rigid surveillance protocol has an important role in the management of this disease in selected patients[7,8,9].

Conservative open surgical treatment

Conservative approaches to the management of upper tract TCC have been reported since the 1940s[10–17]. In one of the earliest reports, Brown and Roumani treated a 75-year-old man with local excision of a medium-grade malignancy of the renal pelvis[10]. There was no evidence of tumor recurrence at 3 years follow up. Gibson reported results in two patients with low-grade TCC managed by wide local excision and reconstruction of the renal pelvis[11]. Both men died of unrelated causes 8–10 years later without recurrence. Petkovic managed 26 patients using the conservative techniques of pyelotomy, nephrotomy with wide caliceal splitting and/or partial nephrectomy[12]. Although no tumor recurrence was noted in any patient, only 5/26 (19%) patients were followed for more than 5 years making it difficult to assess the true efficacy of this conservative approach. Mufti *et al.* reported results of conservative surgical management in 58 patients with TCC of the renal pelvis and ureter[13]. Survival rates at 5 years were 100%, 62% and 0% for patients with grades 1, 2 and 3 tumors, respectively. In addition, only 1/34 (3%) patients with a solitary tumor had an ipsilateral recurrence as compared with 50% (12/24) of those with multifocal tumors. Previous, synchronous or subsequent TCC of the bladder was noted in 35% of patients in this series. Finally, Wallace *et al.* reported a 5 year survival rate of 83% in 14 patients with upper tract TCC managed conservatively[14].

Conservative surgical management of patients with TCC of the ureter has been attempted more frequently than in those with renal pelvic lesions since ureteral tumors, particularly those arising in the distal third of the ureter, tend to be smaller and are less often invasive than those in the renal pelvis. In many cases, segmental ureterectomy with ureteral reimplantation has been recommended as the treatment of choice for those with distal ureteral tumors[18–20]. Mills and Vaughan reviewed the records of 53 patients with primary ureteral carcinoma and found that the prognosis for patients with low-stage tumors was not enhanced by nephro-ureterectomy and hence recommended more conservative excision[21]. Similar results were reported by Zungri et al. in 73 patients with ureteral tumors[22]. Babaian and Johnson reported results in 44 patients with TCC of the ureter treated at a single institution[23]. Among patients with low-grade, superficial disease of the distal ureter managed by ureterectomy and reimplantation, all were alive without active disease at last follow up. Other investigators have also confirmed good results for patients treated in this fashion and it appears unlikely for tumor to recur proximal to the level of ureteral resection[24–26]. However, since TCC of the bladder may develop in up to 80% of patients with upper tract tumors followed for up to 10 years, long-term endoscopic surveillance is warranted[27–29].

Although conservative surgical management may be appropriate for patients with distal ureteral tumors, the role of this approach in those with upper and mid-ureteral malignancies is less clear. Mazeman managed 50 patients with proximal ureteral tumors by segmental ureterectomy and reported a 50% recurrence rate (including those in the bladder) after 3 years[24]. Similarly, Strong and Pearse noted a 30% recurrence rate in the ureter distal to the primary tumor after segmental resection in 47 patients with upper ureteral lesions[30]. Due to the significant incidence of recurrent tumor in the distal ureter, nephro-ureterectomy is most often recommended in those patients with malignancies arising proximal to the lower third of the ureter[23].

Percutaneous treatment of renal pelvic tumors

Although conservative treatment of patients with upper urinary tract TCC had been utilized for many years, the development and refinement of ureteroscopy and percutaneous techniques has given new impetus to this subject. While the first percutaneous nephrostomy tube was inserted in 1955, it was not until many years later that endoscopic advancements allowed for anything more than the establishment of drainage and rudimentary evaluation of the renal pelvis[31]. The results of percutaneous management of patients with urothelial tumors of the kidney have been reported by a number of investigators (Table 28.2.1)[32–39]. In the largest series to date, Jarrett et al. treated 34 patients (36 involved renal units) by percutaneous resection over a 9 year period[32]. Immediate nephro-

Table 28.2.1   Results of percutaneous treatment of renal pelvic tumors

Reference	No. Patients	Local recurrence rate No./total (%)	Follow up (months) Range/mean
Jarrett[32]	30	10/30 (33)	9–111/ 56
Patel[33]	26	6/26 (23)	1–100/ N/A
Plancke[34]	10	2/10 (25)	3–77/ 28
Tasca[36]	4	0/4 (0)	11–24/ N/A
Nurse[38]	16	7/16 (44)	5–54/ N/A
Webb[39]	7	4/7 (57)	12–33/ 21
Sharma[45]	1	0/1 (0)	3
Woodhouse[47]	4	1/4 (25)	7–36/ N/A

N/A = not available.

ureterectomy was performed in six cases due to the presence of aggressive disease and adjunctive therapy with Bacillus Calmette-Guérin (BCG) was given in 19 cases. With a mean follow up of 56.4 months, the recurrence rate was 18%, 33% and 50% for patients with grades 1, 2 and 3 tumors, respectively. All four patients with cancer related mortality had poorly differentiated tumors and a higher incidence of understaging and vascular complications were also seen in those with grade 3 disease. There was no significant improvement in survival in patients treated with BCG.

In another recent series of patients with TCC of the renal pelvis treated by percutaneous resection, Patel et al. used adjuvant radiation therapy in an attempt to improve local tumor control[33]. This was administered using either iridium wires or a high-dose iridium delivery system via the nephrostomy tube in 24/26 (92%) patients. With a mean follow up of 44.7 months, local recurrence was noted in six patients, while TCC of the bladder occurred in 11 patients. Although the 3 year local recurrence-free survival rate was 86%, only one patient in this series had grade 3 disease making it difficult directly to compare these results with those reported by other investigators. Therefore, the importance of post-operative irradiation in improving long-term outcome in patients with renal pelvic tumors treated by percutaneous resection remains unclear.

Overall, tumor grade appears to be the most important prognostic factor in patients with upper urinary tract urothelial tumors and correlates well with depth of invasion. In several large series of patients with upper tract tumors, more than 95% of those with grade 1 malignancy had disease confined to the mucosa[19,40]. Conversely, patients with high-grade TCC have an increased risk of tumor recurrence and development of metastatic disease. Therefore, conservative, percutaneous management of those with medium- to high-grade tumors should not be routinely considered in the presence of a normal contralateral kidney. An additional prognostic factor that may have a role in determining treatment of patients with TCC of the upper urinary tract is deoxyribonucleic acid (DNA) ploidy[41]. Although patients with aneuploid tumors had a median disease-free suvival of only 19 months compared with 59 months for those with diploid tumors in one series, this difference was not significant when a multivariate analysis was performed[42]. In addition, it is often difficult properly to perform flow cytometry on the small tissue specimens that can be obtained by endoscopic biopsy. Despite these limitations, it has been suggested that DNA ploidy may be useful in planning therapy in selected patients with urothelial tumors of the upper urinary trac[42].

Technique of percutaneous resection of renal pelvic tumors

As is true for most surgical procedures, a variety of techniques can be used successfully to resect renal pelvic tumors via a percutaneous approach. Initial access to the collecting system is critical to achieving a good result and must be tailored to the individual patient. In general, an upper or middle caliceal puncture is preferred since this allows for direct access to the ureteropelvic junction. In selected cases, however, alternative approaches may be needed based on intrarenal anatomy and tumor location. Once access is established, tract dilatation using a balloon catheter or progressive passage of rigid fascial dilators is performed based on surgeon preference and a working sheath is placed. Initially, a flexible or rigid nephroscope is inserted, the tumor and entire collecting system are visualized and cold-cup biopsies are taken adequately to stage and grade the tumor. No further treatment other than fulguration of the tumor base may be necessary in patients with small tumors, while careful resection of larger tumors using a loop electrode is often needed in those with greater tumor burdens. Resection in the renal pelvis can be difficult due to the limited space and thin pelviocalyceal lining and should be done with extreme caution to avoid significant parenchymal and vascular injury. A standard nephrostomy tube is placed at the completion of the procedure.

Some investigators have recommended the use of the Nd:YAG laser on an immediate or delayed basis to improve local tumor control[43]. Since the laser energy will penetrate up to several millimeters, treatment of the tumor base can be helpful in selected patients with superficially invasive disease. Such treatment has been advocated 7–10 days following the initial percutaneous resection at which time additional biopsies and washings for cytologic analysis can also be obtained[43]. This second-look procedure may be performed on an outpatient basis with limited intravenous sedation in selected patients. Finally, the nephrostomy tube may be removed when

there is no radiographic evidence of extravasation. Routine radiologic and endoscopic surveillance of the entire urothelium is performed at regular intervals postoperatively.

Complications of percutaneous treatment of renal pelvic tumors

Along with the risks of bleeding, infection and injury to surrounding organs that may generally occur with percutaneous renal surgery, other unique side effects may be seen in patients undergoing resection of renal pelvic tumors. The most important of these is seeding of the nephrostomy tract. In a group of 18 patients with indeterminate upper tract filling defects subsequently demonstrated to be transitional cell carcinoma, intraoperative pyeloscopy was performed followed by immediate nephro-ureterectomy[44]. In two patients, tumor recurred locally in the renal fossa within 6–36 months. Since both patients had low-grade, non-invasive lesions, it is likely that pyeloscopy led to seeding of the tumor. Sharma et al. also reported a case of nephrostomy tract infiltration in a 56-year-old male with a moderately differentiated renal pelvic tumor[45]. This patient underwent percutaneous resection followed 3 months later by nephro-ureterectomy due to rapid tumor recurrence. Histologic examination showed poorly differentiated TCC with transmural penetration of the tumor into the renal parenchyma and infiltration of the perirenal fat at the percutaneous nephrostomy tract site.

Despite concerns regarding tract seeding, other investigators have not found this to be a significant risk. In 33 patients in whom the collecting system was opened, McCarron et al. noted no local tumor recurrences[1]. Jarrett et al. reported no tract seeding in 36 renal units treated percutaneously, although autopsies were not performed on patients who died of metastatic disease and one patient with high-grade TCC found incidently during percutaneous stone extraction had a local tumor recurrence in the renal fossa 4 years later[32]. The risk of tumor tract seeding may be reduced by several measures. These include the use of sterile water as the irrigating fluid because of its osmotic-mediated cytolytic effect[44], post-operative local irradiation[33] and the use of a working sheath which prevents direct contact between malignant cells and flank tissues. In addition, the instillation of agents such as mitomycin C, thiotepa and BCG through the nephrostomy tube may help reduce the likelihood of tumor cell implantation, which has been demonstrated in mice to occur preferentially on cauterized mucosal surfaces[46]. While the overall risk of tumor tract seeding appears to be small, frequent radiographic follow up is important to rule out local recurrence.

Another concern in patients with renal pelvic tumors managed percutaneously is pyelovenous backflow during the procedure with introduction of tumor cells into the systemic circulation. The risk of this is unclear, but significant backflow can generally be avoided by keeping the irrigation bag less than 40 cm above the patient and by using an instrument that fits loosely through the working sheath to allow for a pop-off mechanism which helps prevent the development of elevated renal pelvic pressures[47]. The risk of significant bleeding also appears to be greater in patients undergoing tumor resection as compared with other percutaneous renal procedures. Transfusion was necessary in 53% (18/34) of patients treated by Jarrett et al.[32] In addition, four patients required embolization and nephrectomy was necessary in two patients due to persistent bleeding. Finally, the risk of explosion during endoscopic tumor fulguration leading to perforation of the collecting system with spillage of malignant cells can be reduced by minimizing the introduction of air into the irrigation system[48].

Ureteroscopic management of upper urinary tract tumors

Transurethral treatment of urothelial tumors of the renal pelvis and ureter is advantageous because violation of the collecting system is avoided thus obviating the risk of nephrostomy tract seeding (Table 28.2.2)[49-55]. However, ureteroscopic approaches necessitate the use of smaller instruments and access to portions of the renal pelvis and calyces are more difficult than via a percutaneous route in many cases. Despite these limitations, several investiga-

Table 28.2.2 Results of ureteroscopic treatment of renal pelvic and ureteral tumors

Reference	No. Patients	Local recurrence rate No./total (%)	Follow up (months) Range/mean
Renal pelvic tumors			
Andrews[48]	1	1/1 (100)	5
Blute[49]	5	1/5 (20)	12–48/ N/A
Huffman[50]	1	1/1 (100)	7
Inglis[51]	1	0/1 (0)	30
Grossman[52]	1	0/1 (0)	15
Ureteral tumors			
Blute[49]	13	2/13 (15)	6–50/ N/A
Huffman[50]	7	2/7 (28)	2–67/ N/A
Grossman[52]	7	4/7 (57)	4–36/ N/A
Schilling[53]	13	0/13 (0)	3–31/ 23
Carson[54]	8	0/8 (0)	6–40/ N/A
Gillon[55]	1	N/A	N/A

N/A = not available.

tors have reported succesful results in selected patients with upper tract TCC. Blute et al. treated 22 patients with renal pelvic tumors using a ureteroscopic approach.[49] The procedure was unsuccessful in three patients due to an inability to pass the rigid endoscope into the renal pelvis and an additional 12 patients underwent immediate nephro-ureterectomy. The remaining 10 patients were managed conservatively using open surgical, ureteroscopic or percutaneous resection and/or fulguration in two, five and three patients, respectively. The tumors managed percutaneously were larger (1.5–4.0 cm vs. 5–8 mm) and less well differentiated (grades 2–3 vs. grades 1–2) than those treated by ureteroscopy, suggesting that the latter approach may be most appropriate in those with smaller, low-grade lesions. With a median follow up of 20 months, local tumor recurrence was noted in only 1/8 patients managed solely by endoscopic means.

Although the role of ureteroscopy in the management of upper tract TCC remains unclear, diagnostic evaluation of the renal pelvis and ureter using small flexible and rigid instruments in patients with hematuria and radiographic filling defects of unclear etiology has become a standard approach[56,57]. Bagley et al. were able to visualize the entire renal collecting system with a flexible ureteroscope in 79% (23/29) of patients with indeterminate radiographic lesions[56]. The instrument could be advanced into the kidney and a diagnosis established in the majority of cases. In a later study, Bagley and his co-workers used flexible ureteroscopy to evaluate 62 patients with upper urinary tract filling defects[57]. A diagnosis of TCC was established in 25 patients and nine were treated endoscopically followed by BCG instillation. Long-term results were not available. In general, flexible ureteropyeloscopy allows for inspection of areas of the collecting system that are inaccessible to rigid instruments, particularly the lower pole calyces. Although therapeutic intervention has been limited to date, the development of small laser fibers and improved instrumentation are likely to increase the ability to manage small renal pelvic tumors via a transurethral approach.

Ureteroscopic management of ureteral tumors is generally easier than in patients with renal pelvic malignancy for several reasons. These include the generally smaller size and lower stage of ureteral lesions as well as easier access using larger, rigid instruments. In addition, the distal ureter is relatively immobile, with a thicker and better supported wall making biopsy and resection technically less difficult. Endoscopic management of ureteral lesions can be performed using cold-cup biopsy forceps and fulguration, specialized ureteroresectoscopes[55] or laser fulguration[49,53,54]. The use of laser photocoagulation of the tumor generally follows biopsy to establish the histologic grade and local tumor stage and offers the advantage of increased tissue penetration by the laser energy which may decrease the likelihood of local tumor recurrence. The neodymium:YAG laser has been used most commonly in patients with urothelial tumors of the upper urinary tract since the energy can be readily transmitted via a fiber in a fluid medium. The risk of ureteral perforation and injury using the Nd:YAG laser can be minimized by the use of reduced power settings of 25 watts, limiting treatment at a single site to less than 3 s and tangential application of laser energy[54]. Early reports using the Nd:YAG laser in small groups of patients with ureteral tumors have suggested a low incidence of local tumor recurrence and minimal morbidity (Table 28.2.2)[49,53,54]. However, the relative benefit of laser treatment versus standard electrocoagulation has not been tested and further study is necessary to determine the most efficacious and cost-effective approach in patients with ureteral tumors.

Laparoscopic resection

The use of laparoscopy to perform nephro-ureterectomy in patients with TCC of the upper urinary tract has been reported by several investigators[58–60]. In one of the largest series to date, McDougall et al. treated 10 patients with urothelial tumors using a transperitoneal approach.[58] Immediately prior to laparoscopy, transurethral unroofing of the distal ureter was performed to allow for complete removal of all urothelial tissue on the affected side. The mean operative time was 8.3 hours with minimal bleeding in most cases. However, one patient required open surgical exploration 7 hours after the laparoscopic procedure to control hemorrhage from the inferior edge of the adrenal gland. The length of hospital stay, interval until resumption of normal activity levels and post-operative analgesic use were significantly lower in the laparoscopy group than in a contemporary, consecutive group of patients treated by open nephro-ureterectomy at the same institution. Overall, the use of laparoscopy appears to lead to shortened recovery periods and convalescence periods compared with open surgery, although the prolonged operative times among a very experienced group of laparoscopic surgeons indicates the technical difficulty of performing laparoscopic nephro-ureterectomy. While improved technology and training may eventually allow this procedure to be performed on a wider basis, it appears that laparoscopic treatment of patients with upper urinary urothelial tumors is likely to be confined to specialty centers for the foreseeable future.

Conclusions

Although the outcome of conservative endoscopic management of the majority of patients with low-grade, upper urinary tract TCC is good, nephro-ureterectomy should be

performed in most cases for several reasons. These include the normal life expectancy of patients with a solitary kidney, the requirement for rigorous post-operative surveillance following endoscopic treatment and the low risk of metachronous tumor occurrence[19]. Surveillance protocols analogous to those used in patients following resection of bladder tumors should be used which would require ureteroscopy and/or pyeloscopy 2–4 times per year for several years. The need for frequent upper tract endoscopy, performed most commonly with regional or general anesthesia, may significantly outweigh the benefit of a renal parenchyma sparing approach in many cases. This may be particularly true for patients with renal pelvic tumors, which tend to be larger and are more often invasive and less well differentiated than ureteral lesions.

Overall, nephro-ureterectomy remains the procedure of choice for most patients with TCC of the upper urinary tract. An endoscopic approach should be considered in those patients with renal insufficiency, bilateral tumors, severe medical disease that precludes major surgery and a solitary kidney. While it has been suggested that conservative management of patients with low-grade, non-invasive tumors and a normal contralateral renal unit is appropriate in selected cases[11], the majority of such patients are best treated by nephro-ureterectomy which leads to a low risk of local recurrence and avoids the need for rigorous post-operative upper tract surveillance.

References

1. McCarron JP, Mills C, Vaughn D. Tumors of the renal pelvis and ureter: current concepts and management. *Sem Urol* 1983;1:75–81.
2. Krogh J, Kvist E, Rye B. Transitional cell carcinoma of the upper urinary tract: prognostic variables and post-operative recurrences. *Br J Urol* 1991;67:32–36.
3. Cummings KB. Nephroureterectomy: rationale in the management of transitional cell carcinoma of the upper urinary tract. *Urol Clin NA* 1980;7:569–578.
4. Catalona WJ. Urothelial tumors of the urinary tract. In: PC Walsh, AB Retik, TA Stamey and ED Vaughan, Jr (eds) *Campbell's urology* (6th edn). WB Saunders Co., Philadelphia, 2, chap. 28, pp. 1144–1145, 1992.
5. Gittes RF. Management of transitional cell carcinoma of the upper tract: case for conservative local excision. *Urol Clin NA* 1980;7:559–568.
6. Segura JW. Endourology. *J Urol* 1984;132:1079–1084.
7. Seaman EK, Slawin KM, Benson MC. Treatment options for upper tract transitional cell carcinoma. *Urol Clin NA* 1993;20:349–351.
8. Gerber GS, Lyon ES. Endourological management of upper tract urothelial tumors. *J Urol* 1993;150:2–7.
9. Blute M. Treatment of upper urinary tract transitional carcinoma. In: Smith AD (Ed.) *Smith's Textbook of Endourology*. Quality Medical Publishing, Inc. St Louis, 1, chap. 25, pp. 352–365, 1996.
10. Brown HE, Roumani GK. Conservative surgical management of transitional cell carcinoma of the upper urinary tract. *J Urol* 1974;112:184–191.
11. Gibson TE. Local excision in transitional cell tumors of the upper urinary tract. *J Urol* 1967;97:619–622.
12. Petkovic SD. Conservation of the kidney in operations for tumors of the renal pelvis and calyces. A report of 26 cases. *Br J Urol* 1972;44:1–8.

13. Mufti GR, Gove JRW, Badenoch DF et al. Transitional cell carcinoma of the renal pelvis and ureter. Br J Urol 1989;**63**:135–140.

14. Wallace DMA, Wallace DM, Whitfield HM, Hendry HN, Wickham JEA. The late results of conservative surgery for upper tract urothelial carcinomas. Br J Urol 1981;**53**:537–541.

15. Vest SA. Conservation surgery in certain benign tumors of the ureter. J Urol 1945;**53**:97–129.

16. Colston JAC, Arcadi JA. Bilateral renal papillomas: transpelvic electroresection within preservation of kidney contralateral nephrectomy: four year survival. J Urol 1955;**73**:460–467.

17. Carroll G. Bilateral transitional cell carcinoma of the renal pelvis. J Urol 1965;**93**:132–135.

18. Huffman JL, Bagley DH, Lyon ES, Morse MJ, Herr HW, Whitmore WF. Endoscopic diagnosis and treatment of upper-tract urothelial tumors. Cancer 1985;**55**:1422–1428.

19. Murphy DM, Zincke H, Furlow WL. Primary grade 1 transitional cell carcinoma of the renal pelvis and ureter. J Urol 1980;**123**:629–631.

20. Kretowski RC, Derrick FC Jr. Primary ureteral tumors: reconsideration and management. Urology 1973;**1**:36–39.

21. Mills C, Vaughan ED. Carcinoma of the ureter: natural history, management and 5-year survival. J Urol 1983;**129**:275–277.

22. Zungri W, Chechile G, Algaba F, Diaz I, Vila F, Castro C. Treatment of transitional cell carcinoma of the ureter: is the controversy justified? Eur Urol 1990;**17**:276–280.

23. Babaian RJ, Johnson DE. Primary carcinoma of the ureter. J Urol 1980;**123**:357–361.

24. Mazeman E. Tumours of the upper urinary tract calyces, renal pelvis and ureter. Eur Urol 1976;**2**:120–128.

25. Bloom MA, Vidone RA, Lytton B. Primary carcinoma of the ureter: a report of 102 new cases. J Urol 1970;**39**:590–598.

26. Johnson DE, Babaian RJ. Conservative surgical management for noninvasive distal ureteral carcinoma. Urology 1979;**13**:365–367.

27. Grabstald H, Whitmore WF Jr. Melamed MR. Renal pelvic tumors. JAMA 1971;**8**:845–853.

28. Williams CB, Mitchell JP. Carcinoma of the ureter: a review of 54 cases. Br J Urol 1973;**45**:377–387.

29. Murphy DM, Zincke H, Furlow WL. Management of high grade transitional cell cancer of the upper urinary tract. J Urol 1981;**125**:25–29.

30. Strong DW, Pearse HD. Recurrent urothelial tumors following surgery for transitional cell carcinoma of the upper urinary tract. Cancer 1976;**38**:2178–2186.

31. Goodwin WE, Casey WC, Woolf W. Percutaneous trochar (needle) nephrostomy in hydronephrosis. JAMA 1955;**157**:891.

32. Jarrett TW, Sweetser PM, Weiss GH, Smith AD. Percutaneous management of transitional cell carcinoma of the renal collecting system: 9-year experience. J Urol 1995;**154**:1629–1635.

33. Patel A, Soonawalla P, Shepherd SF, Dearnaley DP, Kellett MJ, Woodhouse CRJ. Long-term outcome after percutaneous treatment of transitional cell carcinoma of the renal pelvis. J Urol 1996;**155**:868–874.

34. Plancke HRF, Strijbos WEM, Delaere KPJ. Percutaneous endoscopic treatment of urothelial tumors of the renal pelvis. Br J Urol 1995;**75**:736–739.

35. Guz B, Streem SB, Novick AC, Montie JE, Zelch MG, Geisinger MA, Risuis B. Role of percutaneous nephrostomy in patients with upper urinary tract transitional cell carcinoma. Urology 1991;**37**:331–336.

36. Tasca A, Zattoni F. The case for a percutaneous approach to transitional cell carcinoma of the renal pelvis. J Urol 1990;**143**:902–905.

37. Streem SB, Pontes EJ. Percutaneous management of upper tract transitional cell carcinoma. J Urol 1986;**135**:773–775.

38. Nurse DE, Woodhouse CRJ, Kellett MJ, Dearnley DP. Percutaneous removal of upper tract tumors. World J Urol 1989;**7**:131–134.

39. Webb DR, Crosthwaire A, Angus D, Brown R, Kennedy D, Nunn I. The percutaneous treatment of upper urinary tract urothelial tumours. World J Urol 1989;**7**:135–137.

40. Heney NM, Nocks BN, Daly JJ, Blitzer PJ, Parkhurst EC. Prognostic factors in carcinoma of the ureter. J Urol 1981;**125**:632–636.

41. Corrado F, Ferri C, Mannini D, Corrado G, Bertoni F, Bacchini P, Lelli G et al. Transitional cell carcinoma of the upper urinary tract: evaluation of prognostic factors by histopathology and flow cytometric analysis. J Urol 1991;**145**:1159–1163.

42. Badalament RA, O' Toole RV, Kenworthy P, Young DC, Keyhani-Rofagha S, Simon J, Perez JF, Drago JR. Prognostic factors in patients with primary transitional cell carcinoma of the upper urinary tract. J Urol 1990;**144**:859–863.

43. Smith AD, Orihuela E, Crowley AR. Percutaneous management of renal pelvic tumors: a treatment option in selected cases. J Urol 1987;**137**:852–856.

44. Tomera KM, Leary FJ, Zincke H. Pyeloscopy in urothelial tumors. J Urol 1982;**127**:1088–1089.

45. Sharma NK, Nicol A, Powell CS. Track infiltration following percutaneous resection of renal pelvic transitional cell carcinoma. Br J Urol 1994;**73**:597–598.

46. Soloway MS, Masters S. Urothelial susceptibility to tumor cell implantation. Cancer 1980;**46**:1158–1163.

47. Woodhouse CRJ, Kellett MJ, Bloom HJG. Percutaneous renal surgery and local radiotherapy in the management of renal pelvic transitional cell carcinoma. Br J Urol 1986;**58**:245–249.

48. Andrews PE, Segura JW. Renal pelvic explosion during conservative management of upper tract urothelial cancer. J Urol 1991;**146**:407–408.

49. Blute ML, Segura JW, Patterson DE, Benson RC, Zincke H. Impact of endourology on diagnosis and management of upper urinary tract urothelial cancer. J Urol 1989;**141**:1298–1301.

50. Huffman JL, Bagley DH, Lyon ES, Morse MJ, Herr HW, Whitmore WF Jr. Endoscopic diagnosis and treatment of upper-tract urothelial tumors. A preliminary report. Cancer 1985;**55**:1422–1428.

51. Inglis JA, Tolley DA. Conservative management of transitional cell carcinoma of the renal pelvis. J Endourol 1988;**2**:27–30.

52. Grossman HB, Schwartz SL, Konnack JW. Ureteroscopic treatment of urothelial carcinoma of the ureter and renal pelvis. J Urol 1992;**148**:275–277.

53. Schilling A, Bowering R, Keiditsch E. Use of the neodymium:YAG laser in the treatment of ureteral tumors and urethral condylomata acuminata. Eur Urol 1986;**12**:30–33.

54. Carson C. Endoscopic treatment of upper and lower urinary tract lesions using lasers. Sem Urol 1991;**9**:185–191.

55. Gillon G, Nissekorn I, Slutzker D, Servadio C. Points of technique: the use of rigid paediatric resectoscope in the management of distal ureteral tumours. Br J Urol 1987;**59**:365–366.

56. Bagley DH, Huffman JL, Lyon ES. Flexible ureteropyeloscopy: diagnosis and treatment in the upper urinary tract. J Urol 1987;**138**:280–285.

57. Bagley DH, Rivas D. Upper urinary tract filling defects: flexible ureteroscopic diagnosis. J Urol 1990;**143**:1196–1200.

58. McDougall EM, Clayman RV, Elashry O. Laparoscopic nephro-ureterectomy for upper tract transitional cell cancer: the Washington University experience. J Urol 1995;**154**:975–980.

59. Kerbl K, Clayman RV, McDougall EM, Urban DA, Gill I, Kavoussi LR. Laparoscopic nephroureterectomy: evaluation of first clinical series. Eur Urol 1993;**23**:431–434.

60. Rassweiler J, Potempa DM, Henkel TO, Gunther M, Tschada R, Alken P. The technical aspects of transperitoneal laparoscopic nephrectomy (TLN), adrenalectomy (TLA) and nephroureterectomy. J Endourol 1992;**6**:S58.

29 Chemotherapy and immunotherapy for upper urinary tract transitional cell carcinoma

F S Freiha and M F Sarosdy

Introduction

Although transitional cell carcinoma is most often superficial and limited to the bladder, some patients have evidence of a 'field defect', with cancer found in the renal pelvis and ureter or in the prostatic or bulbar urethra[1–3]. Upper tract disease may include singly or a combination superficial papillary tumors, muscle-invasive disease, or carcinoma in situ (CIS). Upper tract involvement may precede the diagnosis of cancer in the bladder, or it may occur subsequent to the diagnosis and treatment of bladder cancer. Widespread disease is often associated with carcinoma in situ (CIS) of the bladder, as well as with grade III tumors and premalignant mucosal abnormalities such as dysplasia[2,4].

The exact incidence of upper tract tumors is difficult to ascertain, but there is a clear correlation between upper tract disease and superficial bladder cancer. Approximately 40% of patients who have upper tract cancer as the primary site of tumors will later develop secondary superficial bladder tumors[5]. Conversely, of those who present with bladder cancer as the primary site, 2–3% will later develop upper tract tumors[5,6]. Interestingly, Miller *et al.* reported that upper tract transitional cell carcinoma occurs much more frequently in those patients who appear to have been successfully treated with BCG for their bladder cancer, with upper tract disease seen in up to 13.4% of patients[7]. This higher incidence was attributed to the fact that most of their patients had known risk factors for developing upper tract lesions, including grade 3–4 lesions, carcinoma in situ (CIS), multiple tumors, T1 lesions and

prior failure of intravesical therapy. We have not noted such a high rate in our patients, despite substantially high success and substantially long duration of follow up after BCG therapy[8]. It should be noted that the incidence of concomitant ureteral CIS ranges up to 35% in patients undergoing cystectomy for CIS of the bladder[4].

An additional risk factor for upper tract tumors may be vesico-ureteral reflux in patients with superficial bladder cancer. Amar and Das reported 47 patients with a history of reflux and bladder cancer, 6.4% of whom developed upper tract tumors compared with only 0.44% of 222 patients without reflux[9].

Treatment

Tumors of the upper tract can be particularly difficult to treat, even after successful eradication of transitional cell carcinoma in the bladder by cystectomy or transurethral resection plus bacillus Calmette-Guérin (BCG) immunotherapy. This is true whether patients have papillary lesions or diffuse CIS. Previously, nephro-ureterectomy with inclusion of a cuff of bladder mucosa was considered standard care, particularly in patients with two normal kidneys. However, patients are occasionally encountered with disease in a solitary renal unit, with bilateral renal parenchymal disease, or with renal insufficiency in whom nephron-sparing procedures are needed. Furthermore, transitional cell carcinoma tends to be multifocal and contralateral renal involvement is rare[10]. It has also been noted that with less radical treatment, ipsilateral recurrence is high. Mostly anecdotal reports of partial ureterectomy and other renal-sparing approaches have shown that local recurrences of transitional cell carcinoma are seen in 16 to 29%[11,12].

Small, discrete, upper tract tumors may be managed through endoscopic means using either electrocautery or laser fulguration. Such conservative management is not unreasonable for small, low-grade, clearly papillary lesions, or in patients with solitary kidneys or renal insufficiency. Despite improving technology and increasing experience with endoscopic management, complete resection may not be possible. Topical treatment for residual papillary disease as well as CIS has been employed in growing numbers of patients, using both chemotherapy and BCG and a variety of routes of delivery.

Topical chemotherapy

Thiotepa

In 1980, Gittes first reported instillation of Thiotepa into the renal pelvis of patients with positive cytology, no evidence of bladder lesions, and negative upper tract radiologic studies (presumed CIS) via gravity drip into a ureteral catheter[13]. He reported conversion of positive to negative cytology and no toxicity. Concern about possible increased toxicity due to renal absorption of Thiotepa led Mukamel et al. to review their bladder cancer patients with reflux treated with intravesical Thiotepa and they reported no toxicity[14]. Powder et al. reported Thiotepa instillation into the renal pelvis of a patient with a solitary kidney via an Ommaya reservoir[15]. The patient received 4 monthly courses through the reservoir prior to removing it due to localized irritation. He subsequently received 6 monthly retrograde instillations. The patient remained free of recurrence for 6 years, and no side effects were reported. De Kock and Breytenback described a patient with a solitary kidney who developed a renal pelvic tumor[16]. Six weeks after resection of the lesion with primary ureteropyelostomy, the patient received 6 weekly and then 12 monthly retrograde Thiotepa instillations. He remained free of upper tract disease, though he developed a bladder recurrence 5 years later.

Thiotepa appears to be safe when used in the upper urinary tract. There have been no controlled studies assessing its efficacy.

Mitomycin C

Mitomycin C is active when given intravesically against residual disease and CIS, and has been reported to be effective in some upper tract tumors. Smith et al. reported two patients with recurrent bladder cancer and reflux who developed distal ureteral recurrences[17]. Both received 5 or 6 weekly intravesical instillations of mitomycin C then monthly treatments for 18 months. At 2 years, both patients were free of disease and no side effects were reported. Recently, Eastham and Huffman resected four ureteral and three renal pelvic tumors in patients with solitary kidneys or who were poor surgical candidates[18]. All were given topical mitomycin C. There were no reported complications. At 12 months, five were free of recurrence, one patient had a recurrence treated endoscopically, and one patient developed disease progression treated with radical cystectomy and distal ureterectomy.

Topical immunotherapy

Bacillus Calmette-Guérin (BCG)

By far, the most reported agent used in topical therapy of upper tract transitional cell carcinoma is BCG. This is in part due to the efficacy of intravesical BCG for the prophylaxis of bladder tumors and therapy of CIS. It has been well documented that the immunologic effects of BCG require direct contact of BCG with the tumor, and that the bacillus must bind to fibronectin receptors[19]. Several methods of instilling BCG have been used, including percutaneous[20–24], retrograde injection into a non-refluxing ureter[21,25], and intravesically[26,27] or into an ileal conduit[21] for refluxing ureters (Table 29.1.1).

The first report of topical BCG therapy was by Herr in 1985[26]. He reported a patient with a solitary pelvic kidney who underwent pelvectomy, ureterectomy, and autotransplantation with a pyelovesicostomy for a ureteropelvic junction pT2GIII papillary tumors and multifocal CIS. The patient then received 6 weekly courses of intravesical BCG and was free of recurrence with negative cytology at 13 months. Due to the concern of systemic absorption of BCG from upper tract instillation, Mukamel et al. tested the effect of the bacillus on the upper urinary tract in pigs[28]. They found no difference in the renal function, histologic examination, or stricture formation in renal units treated percutaneously with BCG as compared with those treated with only normal saline. No systemic side effects developed.

In another report, Mukamel et al. described 13 patients with reflux who were treated with intravesical BCG[29]. None had systemic complications and two had a decrease in renal function by radionucleotide studies which was attributed to the reflux itself and not the BCG. Several toxicities have been reported however, including severe sep-

Table 29.1.1 Methods of instillation of topical therapy

- Percutaneous
- Retrograde (no reflux)
- Intravesical (reflux)
- Ileal conduit (reflux)

ticemia[20], high fever requiring triple[25,27] or single[21] anti-tuberculin agent therapy, asymptomatic renal granuloma formation[22], and renal insufficiency[28].

The efficacy of topical BCG for upper urinary tract tumors is variable and not 100%. Shoenberg et al. reported ten patients with solitary kidneys and upper tract transitional cell carcinoma[21]. After resection of the tumors, all but one had topical BCG percutaneously (4), into a conduit (2), or intravesically with ureteral stents or known reflux (3). Six patients had no recurrence while one had recurrence at 19 months, one developed metastases at 15 months, and one died of disease progression. Vasavada et al. had eight patients with solitary kidneys and prior history of transitional cell carcinoma who developed upper tract tumors[28]. After resection of the index lesion, all had a 6 week course of percutaneous BCG. One patient developed a local recurrence and two developed metastases which were thought to be due to prior history of invasive transitional cell carcinoma.

Upper tract CIS has also been treated with topical BCG. Studer et al. reported eight patients with upper tract positive cytology and no evidence of lower tract lesions[20]. All received a 6 week course of percutaneous BCG, and cytology was repeated. If the cytology was positive, another course was given. Six patients had negative upper tract cytology at 12–24 months after one (4) to three (1) courses, one patient had negative cytology but a papillary tumor was resected, and one patient was unevaluable due to stopping BCG for severe septicemia after one instillation. Similarly, Sharpe et al. reported 11 patients with positive upper tract cytology and no bladder lesions presumed to have upper tract CIS[25]. All received 6 weekly courses of BCG via retrograde instillation. Four had negative cytology at 15–59 months, three required a second course of BCG and had negative cytology at 8–70 months, and one had only one instillation due to development of fever. One patient with bilateral disease required a nephro-ureterectomy on one side and had negative cytology on the other at 30 months, and two patients had disease progression.

Given all these reports, it appears that the topical use of BCG for upper urinary tract transitional cell carcinoma and CIS may decrease recurrences but with moderate toxicity. However, additional study is needed to determine the true impact on disease control and patient survival.

Two case reports have also suggested that autotransplantation with pyelovesicostomy to allow easy reflux of intravesical BCG into the pelvis might be successful, despite the heroic nature of such an effort[26,27].

Oral immunotherapy

Bropirimine

Bropirimine, an orally administered immunomodulator, has been shown to eliminate bladder CIS in approximately 50% of treated patients[30]. Recently, it has also been reported to be effective in upper tract CIS in 48% of patients who received at least 3 months of therapy[31]. In a multicenter study, 24 patients with negative upper tract radiographs and positive unilateral (19) or bilateral (5) cytology were treated. Among the 21 evaluable for response, 10 (48%) demonstrated conversion of positive cytology to negative. Five did so at the first evaluation after 12 weeks of treatment, while the other five required an additional 12 weeks to respond. Since bropirimine has not yet been evaluated for papillary tumors, its value in treatment or prophylaxis of upper tract tumors other than CIS is unclear.

Conclusion

Given the rarity of upper urinary tract transitional cell carcinoma and CIS, the optimal treatment is difficult to delineate. Few urologists would dispute the role of nephro-uretectomy with a bladder cuff in good surgical candidates with two normal kidneys and normal renal function. In the patient who is in need of renal sparing procedures, the high local recurrence rate has prompted investigators to add topical chemotherapeutic and immunologic therapy for prophylaxis or treatment of disease that remains after partial endoscopic resection. These agents seem to be efficacious with defined but acceptable toxicities. However, further work is needed to determine the best treatment.

References

1. Farrow GM, Utz DC, Rife CC. Morphological and clinical observations of patients with early bladder cancer treated with total cystectomy. *Cancer Res* 1976;**36**:2495–2501.
2. Althausen AF, Prout GR, Daly JJ. Non-invasive papillary carcinoma of the bladder associated with carcinoma in situ. *J Urol* 1976;**116**:575–580.
3. Farrow GM, Utz DC, Rife CC, Greene LF. Clinical observations on sixty-nine cases of in situ carcinoma of the urinary bladder. *Cancer Res* 1977;**37**:2794–2798.
4. Herr WH, Whitmore Jr WF. Ureteral carcinoma in situ after successful intravesical therapy for superficial bladder dumors: Incidence, possible pathogenesis and management. *J Urol* 1987;**138**:292–294.
5. Oldbring J, Glifberg I, Mikulowski P, Hellsten S. Carcinoma of the renal pelvis and ureter following bladder carcinoma: frequency, risk factors and clinicopathological findings. *J Urol* 1989;**141**:1311–1313.
6. Schwartz CB, Bekirov H, Melman A. Urothelial tumors of upper tract following treatment of primary bladder transitional cell carcinoma. *Urology* 1992;**40**:509–511.
7. Miller EB, Eure GR, Schellhammer PF. Upper tract transitional cell carcinoma following treatment of superficial bladder cancer with BCG. *Urology* 1993;**42**:26–30.
8. Cookson MS, Sarosdy MF. Management of stage T1 superficial bladder cancer with intravesical Bacillus Calmette-Guérin therapy. *J Urol* 1992;**148**:797–801.
9. Amar AD, Das S. Upper urinary tract transitional cell carcinoma in patients with bladder carcinoma and associated vesicoureteral reflux. *J Urol* 1985;**133**:468–471.

10. Seaman EK, Slawin KM, Benson MC. Treatment options for upper tract transitional cell carcinoma. *Urol Clin N Amer* 1993;**20**:349–354.

11. Wallace DMA, Wallace DM, Whitfield HN, Hendry WG, Wickham JEA. The late results of conservative surgery for upper tract urothelial carcinomas. *Br J Urol* 1981;**53**:537–541.

12. Nocks BN, Heney NM, Daly JJ, Perrone TA, Griffin PP, Prout Jr. GR. Transitional cell carcinoma of renal pelvis. *Urology* 1982;**19**:472–477.

13. Gittes RF. Management of transitional cell carcinoma of the upper tract: Case for conservative local excision. *Urol Clin N Amer* 1980;**7**:559–568.

14. Mukamel E, Glanz I, Nissenkorn I, Cytron S, Servadio C. Unanticipated vesicoureteral reflux: A possible sequela of long-term thio-tepa instillations to the bladder. *J Urol* 1982;**127**:245–246.

15. Powder JR, Mosberg Jr WH, Pierpont RZ, Tatoyan KB, Young Jr JD. Bilateral primary carcinoma of the ureter: Topical intraureteral thiotepa. *J Urol* 1984;**132**:349–352.

16. De Kock MLS, Breytenbach IH. Local excision and topical thiotepa in the treatment of transitional cell carcinoma of the renal pelvis: A case report. *J Urol* 1986;**135**:566–567.

17. Smith AY, Vitale PJ, Lowe BA, Woodside JR. Treatment of superficial papillary transitional cell carcinoma of the ureter by vesicoureteral reflux of mitomycin C. *J Urol* 1987;**138**:1231–1233.

18. Eastham JA, Huffman JL. Technique of mitomycin C instillation in the treatment of upper urinary tract urothelial tumors. *J Urol* 1993;**150**:324–325.

19. Ratliff TL. Bacillus Calmette-Guérin (BCG): Mechanism of action in superficial bladder cancer. *Urology* 1991;**37**(suppl 5):8–11.

20. Studer UE, Casanova G, Kraft R, Zingg EJ. Percutaneous BCG perfusion of the upper urinary tract for carcinoma in situ. *Prog Clin Biol Res* 1990;**350**:81–86.

21. Schoenberg MP, van Arsdalen KN, Wein AJ. The management of transitional cell carcinoma in solitary renal units. *J Urol* 1991;**146**:700–703.

22. Bellman GC, Sweetser P, Smith AD. Complications of intracavitary Bacillus Calmette-Guerin after percutaneous resection of upper tract transitional cell carcinoma. *J Urol* 1994;**151**:13–15.

23. Vasavada SP, Streem SB, Novick AC. Definitive tumor resection and percutaneous Bacille Calmette-Guérin for management of renal pelvic transitional cell carcinoma in solitary kidneys. *Urology* 1995;**45**:381–386.

24. Smith AD, Orihuela E, Crowley AR. Percutaneous management of renal pelvic tumors: A treatment option in selected cases. *J Urol* 1987;**137**:852–856.

25. Sharpe JR, Duffy G, Chin JL. Intrarenal Bacillus Calmette-Guérin therapy for upper urinary tract carcinoma in situ. *J Urol* 1993;**149**:457–460.

26. Herr HW. Durable response of a carcinoma in situ of the renal pelvis to topical Bacillus Calmette-Guérin. *J Urol* 1985;**134**:531–532.

27. Ransey JC, Soloway MS. Instillation of Bacillus Calmette-Guérin into the renal pelvis of a solitary kidney for the treatment of transitional cell carcinoma. *J Urol* 1990;**143**:1220–1222.

28. Mukamel E, Vilkovsky E, Hadar H, Engelstein D, Nussbaum B, Servadio C. The effect of intravesical Bacillus Calmette-Guérin therapy on the upper urinary tract. *J Urol* 1991;**146**:980–981.

29. Mukamel E, Layfield LJ, Hawkins RA, Dekernion JB. The effect of Bacillus Calmette-Guérin on the urinary system of pigs. *J Urol* 1988;**139**:165–169.

30. Sarosdy MF, Lamm DL, Williams RD *et al*. Phase I trial of oral bropirimine in superficial bladder cancer. *J Urol* 1992;**147**:31–33.

31. Sarosdy MF, Pisters LL, Carroll PR *et al*. Bropirimine immunotherapy of upper urinary tract carcinoma in situ. *Urology* 1996;**48**:28–32.

30 Rare renal tumors

W P Tongco, T Hodges, A Szmit and J W Basler

This chapter aims to incorporate renal tumors not discussed specifically in other parts of the text. An exhaustive review of anecdotal case reports would offer minimal benefit to the clinician. With few exceptions these tumors will be diagnosed on pathologic evaluation after extirpation. This chapter will review the most prevalent rare renal tumors to focus on early diagnosis and alterations in management. Various surgical and minimally invasive techniques for management of tumors are discussed in other chapters.

Renal medullary carcinoma

Termed the 'seventh sickle cell nephropathy' by Davis *et al.* (1995)[1], this represents one of the most aggressive and devastating cancers ever described. To date, all but one patient[2] diagnosed with renal medullary carcinoma have been African-American with sickle cell trait or sickle cell disease. Onset of this aggressive disease is early with a median age of 25 years. Common presenting symptoms include hematuria, flank pain and weight loss. Cough and dyspnea may be seen with pulmonary metastasis.

The diagnosis has only been made on pathologic evaluation but may be suggested by characteristic appearance on CT scan[3]. A review of the literature notes only one report of positive urine cytology for renal medullary carcinoma as means for possible early diagnosis[4].

Radiographically, renal medullary carcinoma arises centrally within the kidney. A reniform shape is often maintained but the involved kidney is uniformly enlarged. Renal medullary carcinoma has heterogeneous enhancement and displays an infiltrative pattern often invading the renal sinus, collecting system and renal vessels. Caliectasis can be seen. Satellite lesions in the renal cortex and metastatic lesions are often identified[5,6]. In at least one case[7] concurrent transitional cell carcinoma was identified in the same kidney though the metastatic disease was clearly medullary carcinoma.

The tumor arises from the calyceal epithelium and progresses in an infiltrative manner[1]. Grossly the tumor is yellow-tan with a reticular growth pattern and areas of focal necrosis. Microscopically the tumor is notable for diffuse glandular growth with microvilli lining the luminal surfaces. Inflammatory infiltrates and rhabdoid/plasmacytoid cells are also present[8]. Tumor cells stain positive for peanut agglutinin and luminal surfaces stain positively with antibodies to epithelial membrane antigen[9].

Because of its rarity, the nature of this tumor and the fact that many patients with sickle cell trait present frequently with hematuria and flank pain secondary to benign papillary necrosis, the diagnosis is almost always delayed. Renal medullary carcinoma is aggressive and to date universally fatal. The benefit of nephrectomy, if any, is not clear. The time from diagnosis, usually after nephrectomy, to death ranges from 1 to 15 months, and averages only 15 weeks. The longest known survivor (15 months from diagnosis) has been an adolescent treated aggressively with multimodal chemotherapy though he too succumbed to the disease[10]. Maintaining a high index of suspicion in evaluating sickle cell patients with hematuria and aggressive upper tract imaging may be the only way that we will ever identify a patient with curable disease.

Angiomyolipoma

Angiomyolipoma constitute only 1% of surgically confirmed renal tumors and are seen in two distinct clinical settings: sporadic (isolated) or in association with tuberous sclerosis[11,12]. The sporadic form accounts for approximately 80–90% of cases[13]. They are slow growing, benign lesions that often do not require surgery or even biopsy[11]. The sporadic form is typically seen in middle-aged patients (mean age 43 years) and is more common in women by at least a 4:1 ratio[14].

Although 60% of patients with angiomyolipomas are asymptomatic from the lesion, common presenting symptoms include: acute flank pain caused by spontaneous extrarenal hemorrhage. In 25% of cases, emergency laparotomy is needed because of either severe pain or life threatening bleeding. Currently, the most common presentation for patients with angiomyolipomas is incidental discovery during CT, and MRI performed for evaluation of suspected disease outside the genitourinary system.

Angiomyolipomas are composed of varying amounts of blood vessels, smooth muscle and fat. The typical angiomyolipoma most often has a prominent fat component, but all three tissue types must be seen for a diagnosis[15]. Malignant transformation, like calcification and necrosis are rare, but hemorrhage is frequent[11]. Angiomyolipoma is the cause for bleeding in 16–20% of patients with spontaneous perinephric hemorrhage[16].

Excretory urography demonstrates an expansile renal mass that cannot be distinguished from renal cell carcinoma. With sonography, an angiomyolipoma is more echogenic than the surrounding renal parenchyma but this may also be seen in 32% of small renal cell carcinomas[17]. CT is the examination of choice in patients in whom angiomyolipoma is suspected on the basis of sonographic appearances. On CT, angiomyolipomas appear as a well marginated, cortical, predominantly fat attenuated mass with heterogeneous soft tissue attenuation interspersed throughout the lesion[15]. Approximately 5% of angiomyolipomas do not show fat attenuation on CT scans and cannot be differentiated from renal cell carcinoma[18]. With MRI most angiomyolipomas can be clearly characterized because of the depiction of intramural fat[19].

Up to 80% of patients with tuberous sclerosis have angiomyolipomas, and these patients constitute up to 20% of all individuals with angiomyolipoma[11].

Small lesions discovered incidentally in asymptomatic patients do not usually prompt surgery for diagnosis or cure. Lesions larger than 4 cm in diameter are thought to have a significant risk of hemorrhage, potentially with hypotension or other associated morbidity, and are generally treated with elective resection. Asymptomatic patients with an angiomyolipoma approaching 4 cm in diameter are followed up annually with CT or US. Patients with lesions greater than 4 cm can be followed up at more frequent intervals, be treated with selective embolization, or undergo elective resection with renal-sparing surgery[20].

Oncocytoma

The incidence of oncocytoma is 3% to 7% of solid renal tumors, and can be found bilaterally in approximately 6%. Multiple oncocytomas within the kidneys are occasionally seen (termed: oncocytomatosis). The patient population demographics are similar to those for renal cell carcinoma with men being affected more often than women.

Oncocytomas are usually diagnosed incidentally since most are asymptomatic and, due to its relatively benign, non-invasive course, hematuria is rare.

Oncocytomas are composed of neoplastic cells with bright eosinophilic granules. The cell line of tumor origin is not known, but intercalated cells from the collecting system have been suggested. Grossly, oncocytomas are tan/brown, well encapsulated, with homogeneous tissues lacking necrosis or hemorrhage. A central, stellate scar is characteristically seen when the tumor is bivalved[21].

The diagnosis can be suggested pre-operatively if the central stellate scar can be imaged on CT, MRI or sonography. However, CT evaluation is often unable reliably to differentiate oncocytoma from adenocarcinoma. This is in part due to inhomogeneous uptake of contrast by oncocytoma[22]. MRI findings of a low intensity T1 homogeneous mass, increasing intensity on T2 images, stellate scar, capsule and lack of hemorrhage can be suggestive of oncocytoma[23]. Gross pathologic evaluation may be characteristic and diagnostic but histopathologic diagnosis can be challenging, since low-grade renal cell carcinoma may manifest oncocytic features.

Treatment of oncocytoma is usually resection since definitive pre-operative diagnosis is not often available to distinguish it from other malignant renal tumors. When the pre-operative index of suspicion is high, it is reasonable to perform nephron-sparing surgery in selected patients. Intra-operative frozen sections are advised to evaluate surgical margins and identify the rare oncocytoma with invasive properties. Observation may be appropriate in selected patients with the probable diagnosis of oncocytoma. In these cases needle biopsy may be helpful in confirming the diagnosis or at least suggesting a 'low-grade' tumor. Large oncocytomas have been followed for years without identifiable progression[21].

Juxtaglomerular cell tumor

Juxtaglomerular cell tumors (JGCT) are rare with a reported incidence in eight of 30 000 hypertensive patients. Patients present at an early age, mean of 22 years. The hallmark of the JGCT is the constellation of clinical characteristics related to secondary hyperaldosteronism; poorly controlled hypertension (mean diastolic BP of 134 mm Hg), hypokalemia (mean 2.8 mmol/l), and elevated renin[24]. Grossly, these tumors average ~24 mm in diameter, are well encapsulated, and are yellowish-gray in color without necrotic foci. Microscopically, solid sheets of round to polyhedral cells are seen in concentric patterns around capillaries, and separated by fibrous septa. Mast cells are scattered throughout the tumor. Mitotic figures are rarely encountered. Stains are positive for antibody to mouse renin[25].

Radiographic evaluation by CT scan reveals the JGCT to be isodense or hypodense on non-contrast imaging. Contrast CT will delineate the tumor as a well demarcated area of decreased contrast uptake. Similarly, angiography demonstrates JGCT as an area of hypo- or avascularity (Raynaud, 1985)[26].

Diagnosis is based on clinical stigmata of secondary hyperaldosteronism and renal mass. Other metabolically active tumors should be ruled out during the metabolic evaluation. Renal vein sampling lateralizes excess renin production in only 64%[24]. CT evaluation routinely delineates JGCT.

Pre-operatively, hypertension may be effectively controlled with ACE inhibitors such as captopril[27]. Treatment is by excision of the tumor. Nephron-sparing surgery appears to be appropriate management for JGCT. Haab *et al.* (1995)[24] reviewed eight patients treated with renal-sparing surgery. Due to tumor hypovascularity, the procedures were accomplished without renal pedicle clamping and none suffered excessive blood loss. In this series, tumor recurrence has not been noted at 98 month mean follow up. Hypertension and hypokalemia resolved in all patients within 1 week of removal of the JGCT.

Adenoma

The advances of abdominal imaging have produced a dilemma in the management of small (<3 cm) incidentally found renal tumors. The existence of benign small adenomatous renal tumors is in question. The existence of a small renal adenoma is now considered an early stage of renal carcinoma.

Diagnosis of renal adenoma is excluded if histopathologic evaluation demonstrates clear cells, mitotic activity, nuclear polymorphism or necrosis. Characteristic findings include basophilic or acidophilic cells with cellular and nuclear uniformity.

Current radiologic techniques are not always able to characterize small renal tumors. When neoplasm is suggested by radiography the tumor should be considered renal cell carcinoma and treated accordingly. Bosniak has followed renal tumors 3.5 cm or less with serial CT imaging[28]. Growth rates average 0.36 cm/yr, ranging from 0.0 to 1.1 cm/yr. At a mean follow up of 3.25 years there was no clinically evident metastatic disease. Twenty-six of 40 tumors were resected during the study. Close observation with routine radiographic examinations (annually) may be an acceptable alternative for patients incapable of tolerating surgery.

Leiomyoma

Approximately 5% of autopsy specimens exhibit renal leiomyomas, a rare, benign spindle cell tumor[29]. The average size of these tumors is less than 5 mm[30], whereas clinically apparent leiomyomas are much larger and less common. These lesions are more likely to be seen in middle-aged and older women (median age, 42 years)[29]. Leiomyomas have no metastatic potential, and are currently discovered as incidental findings in a large portion of cases but also occur with increased frequency in patients with tuberous sclerosis[11]. Tsujimura and co-workers[31] present just such a case in which a tuberous sclerosis patient with a renal leiomyoma which was detected incidentally during the investigation of a fever of unknown origin. Of those patients who present with clinical symptoms, more than 50% of the patients have a palpable mass or pain and 20% have haematuria[29].

Pathologically, leiomyoma of the kidney consists predominantly of smooth muscle cells without pleomorphism or nuclear atypia. Most are considered to be hamartomas[32]. A large number of these tumors contain fat which raises the possibility that they exist in a continuum with angiomyolipoma and lipoma[33]. Leiomyomas are well circumscribed, gray-white peripheral lesions[34] Among the clinically apparent lesions, 53% are subcapsular, 37% capsular, and 10% are attached to the renal pelvis[29]. Necrosis and hemorrhage are absent though those with a mean size of over 12 cm in diameter can contain hemorrhage (17%) and cystic degeneration (27%)[32].

Often diagnosis is an incidental finding on a radiographic study. Leiomyomas typically appear as well circumscribed, solid lesions. There may be a cleavage plane between the leiomyoma and the cortex and the lesion may be extremely exophytic or attached to the cortex by only a small stalk[29]. Irregular calcification may be seen in a minority of cases[35]. Pre-operative diagnosis of renal leiomyoma is difficult, but physicians should always consider this tumor in the differential diagnosis of peripheral renal tumors. Clinically symptomatic presentations are rare. An unusual presentation with exclusively gastrointestinal signs and symptoms (epigastric pain and melena) resulting from duodenal invasion has been reported[36].

Differentiation of leiomyoma from renal adenocarcinoma is not possible and the suspicion of a leiomyoma prompts surgical exploration for diagnosis[29]. Identification of a well circumscribed, peripheral renal mass, especially if it is small (less than 4 or 5 cm) and in a middle-aged woman, should allow one to suggest the diagnosis of a leiomyoma. This may allow the surgeon to prepare for a renal-sparing operation in selected cases. The prognosis after resection of these benign lesions is excellent[37].

Sarcoma

Primary renal sarcoma occurs in 1% of malignant renal tumors. Virtually all sarcomas have been identified as a primary renal tumor. Leiomyosarcoma is most common, seen in approximately 50% of renal sarcomas. Others include rhabdomyosarcoma, fibrosarcoma, osteosarcoma, chondrosarcoma, angiosarcoma and clear cell sarcoma. Leiomyosarcoma is most common in females in the third to fifth decades of life. Patients often present with symptoms of flank pain, abdominal mass and hematuria[38].

Pathologic findings are specific to each classification of sarcoma. Differentiating sarcoma from the sarcomatoid variant of renal cell carcinoma can be challenging. Sarcoma is suggested radiographically when the tumor arises from the renal capsule or sinus. Angiographically sarcomas are hypovascular or avacular[39]. Arterio-venous shunting, contrast pooling and tumor staining are seldom present.

Mainstay of treatment for all sarcomas is radical nephrectomy with en bloc excision of tumor. Recurrence is common and equally distributed between lung, renal fossa and multiple other sites. Of 21 patients with renal sarcoma, Vogelzang[38] noted only six that remained disease free. Sarcoma has remained relatively chemo-resistant. Doxorubicin based chemotherapy with radiotherapy has been shown to be effective in improving outcome. Ifosfamide and mesna have also shown promise in the treatment in soft tissue sarcomas[40].

Metastatic tumors

Nearly all tumors can metastasize to the kidney. Common primary malignancies include lymphoma, lymphoblastoma, gastrointestinal, lung, breast, and ovarian and (contralateral) renal cancer. Clinical symptoms related to the kidney are rare though flank pain and hematuria can be seen. Usually, manifestations of the primary tumor minimize the clinical significance of an isolated renal metastasis. Occasionally, the situation arises where it is necessary to determine if a renal mass is either a second primary malignancy or a solitary metastasis. Here, CT imaging has proven most beneficial. Metastases are usually isodense on non-contrast imaging with only slight enhancement after administration of IV contrast. In some cases, needle biopsy may be beneficial to aid in diagnosis.

Treatment is based on that for the primary tumor. Nephrectomy for metastases is usually for palliation when required at all. Renal embolization and/or radiotherapy may play a more important role in palliation of haematuria.

References

1. Davis CJ, Mostofi FK, Sesterhenn IA. Renal medullary carcinoma. The seventh sickle cell nephropathy. *Am J Pathol* 1995;**19**:1–11.

2. Kalyanpur A, Schwartz DS, Fields JM, Rayes-Mugica M, Keller MS, Gosche J, Renal medulla carcinoma in a white adolescent. *AJR Am J Roentgenol* 1997;**169**(4):1037–1038.

3. Pickhardt PJ. Renal medullary carcinoma: an aggressive neoplasm in patients with sickle cell trait. *Abdom Imaging* 1998;**23**(5):531–532.

4. Larson DM, Gilstad CW, Manson GW, Henry MR. Renal medullary carcinoma: report of a case with positive urinary cytology. *Diagnostic Cytopathol* 1998;**18**(4):276–279.

5. Avery RA, Harris JE, Davis CJ Jr, Borgaonkar DS, Byrd JC, Weiss RB. Renal medullary carcinoma: clinical and therapeutic aspects of a newly diagnosed tumor. *Cancer* 1996;**78**(1):128–132.

6. Davidson AJ, Choyke PL, Hartman DS, Davis CJ Jr. Renal medullary carcinoma associated with sickle cell trait: radiologic findings. *Radiology* 1995;**195**(1):83–85.

7. Figenshau RS, Basler JW, Ritter JH, Siegel CL, Simon JA, Dierks SM. Renal medullary carcinoma. *J Urol* 1998;**159**(3):711–713.

8. Adsay NV, deRoux SJ, Sakr W, Grignon D. Cancer as a marker of genetic medical disease: an unusual case of medullary carcinoma of the kidney. *Am J Surg Pathol* 1998;**22**(2):260–264.

9. Wesche WA, Wilimas J, Khare V, Parham DM. Renal medullary carcinoma: a potential sickle cell nephropathy of children and adolescents. *Pediat Pathol Lab Med* 1998;**18**(1):97–113.

10. Pirich LM, Chou P, Walterhouse DO. Prolonged survival of a patient with sickle cell trait and metastatic renal medullary carcinoma. *J Pediatr Hematol Oncol* 1999;**21**(1):67–69.

11. Wagner BJ, Wong-You-Cheong JJ, Davis CJ Jr. Adult renal hamartomas. *Radiographics* 1997;**17**(1):155–169.

12. Farrow GM, Harrison EG Jr, Utz DC, Jones DR. Renal angiomyolipoma: a clinicopathologic study of 32 cases. *Cancer* 1968;**22**:564–570.

13. Lemaitre L, Robert Y, Dubrulle F, Claudon M, Duhamel A, Danjou P, Mazeman E. Renal angiomyolipoma: growth followed up with CT and/or US. *Radiology* 1995;**197**:598–602.

14. Hajdu SI, Foote FW Jr. Angiomyolipoma of the kidney: report of 27 cases and review of the literature. *J Urol* 1989;**102**:396–401.

15. Sherman JL, Hartman DS, Friedman AC, Madewell JE, Davis CJ, Goldman SM. Angiomyolipoma: computed tomographic-pathologic correlation of 17 cases. *AJR* 1981;**137**:1221–1226.

16. Belville JS, Morgentaler A, Loughlin KR, Tumeh SS. Spontaneous perinephric and subcapsular renal hemorrhage: evaluation with CT, US, and angiography. *Radiology* 1989;**172**:733–738.

17. Forman HP, Middleton WD, Melson GL, McClennan BL. Hyperechoic renal cell carcinomas: increase in detection at US. *Radiology* 1993;**188**:431–434.

18. Wills JS. Management of small renal neoplasms and angiomyolipoma: a growing problem. *Radiology* 1995;**197**:583–586.

19. Uhlenbrock D, Fischer C, Beyer HK. Angiomyolipoma of the kidney. *Acta Radiol* 1988;**29**:523–524.

20. Oesterling JE, Fishman EK, Goldman SM, Marshall FF. The management of renal angiomyolipoma. *J Urol* 1986;**135**:1121–1124.

21. Lieber MM. Renal oncocytoma. *Urolog Clin N Am* 1993;**20**(2):355–359.

22. Davidson AJ, Hayes WS, Hartman DS, McCarthy WF, Davis CJ Jr. Renal oncocytoma and carcinoma: failure of differentiation with CT. *Radiology* 1993;**186**(3):693–696.

23. Shirkhoda A, Lewis E. Renal sarcoma and sarcomatoid renal cell carcinoma: CT and angiographic features. *Radiology* 1987;**162**(2):353–357.

24. Haab F, Duclos JM, Guyenne T, Plouin PF, Corvol P. Renin secreting tumors: diagnosis, conservative surgical approach and long-term results. *J Urol* 1995;**153**(6):1781–1784.

25. Hasegawa A. Juxtaglomerular cells tumor of the kidney: a case report with electron microscopic and flow cytometric investigation. *Ultrastructural Pathol* 1997;**21**(2):201–208.

26. Raynaud A, Chatellier G, Baruch D, Angel C, Menard J, Gausxe JC. Radiologic features of renin producing tumors. A report of two cases. *Ann Radiol* 1985;**28**:439.

27. Kashiwabara H, Inaba M, Itabashi A, Ishii J, Katayama S. A case of renin-producing juxtaglomerular cell tumor: effect of ACE inhibitor or angiotensin II receptor antagonist. *Blood Pressure* 1997;**6**(3):147–153.

28. Bosniak MA, Birnbaum BA, Krinsky GA, Waisman J. Small renal parynchymal neoplasms: further observations on growth. *Radiology* 1995;**197**(3):589–597.

29. Steiner M, Quinlan D, Goldman SM, Millmond S, Hallowell MJ, Stutzman RE, Korobkin M. Leiomyoma of the kidney: presentation of four new cases and the role of computerized tomography. *J Urol* 1990;**143**:994–998.

30. Farrow GM. Diseases of the kidney. In: Murphy WM (Ed.) *Urological pathology*. Saunders, Philadelphia, PA, 1989; pp. 409–482.

31. Tsujimura A, Miki T, Sugao H, Takaha M, Takeda M, Kurata A. Renal leiomyoma associated with tuberous sclerosis. *Urologia Internationalis* 1996;**57**(3):192–193.

32. Jenette CJ *Hetinstall's pathology of the kidney* (5th edn). Lippincott Raven Publishers, New York: 1998.

33. Millan JC. Tumors of the kidney. In: Hill GS (Ed.) *Uropathology*. Churchill Livingstone, New York, NY 1989, pp. 623–702.

34. Zagoria RJ, Dyer RB, Assimos DG, Scharling ES, Quinn SF. Spontaneous perinephric hemorrhage: imaging and management. *J Urol* 1991;**145**:468–471.

35. Fishbone G, Davidson AJ. Leiomyoma of the renal capsule. *Radiology* 1969;**92**:1006–1007.

36. Pontes JM, Leitao MC, Cabral JE, Portela F, Botelho J, Martins I, Freitas DS. Recurrence of a renal myogenic tumor presented as a duodenal ulcerated lesion. *Hepato-Gastroenterology* 1995;**42**(4):356–359.

37. Mohler JL, Casale AJ. Renal capsular leiomyoma. *J Urol* 1987;**138**:853–854.

38. Vogelzang NJ, Fremgen AM, Guinan PD, Chmiel JS, Sylvester JL, Sener SF. Primary renal sarcoma in adults. A natural history and management study by the American Cancer Society, Illinois Division. *Cancer* 1993;**71**(3):804–810.

39. Goldman SM, Hartman DS, Weiss SW. The varied radiographic manifestations of retroperitoneal malignant fibrous histiocytoma revealed through 27 cases. *J Urol* 1986;**135**(1):33–38.

40. Yalcin S, Barista I, Tekuzman G, Gullu I, Firat D. Dramatic response to Ifosfamide, mesna and doxorubicin chemotherapy regimen in an adult with clear cell carcinoma of the kidney. *J Urol* 1996;**155**(6):2024.

31 Adrenal tumors

C K Naughton and G L Andriole

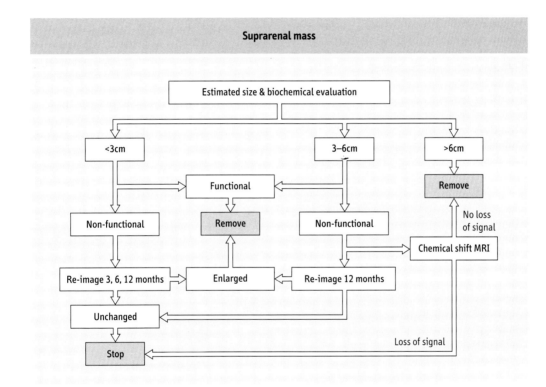

Fig. 31.1 A management and treatment algorithm for the incidental adrenal mass.

The adrenal gland

Our current understanding of the structure and function of the adrenal gland stems from the original recognition by Cuvier in 1805 that the gland consists of two parts, the mesoderm-derived cortex and the neural crest-derived medulla. The adult adrenal *cortex* is comprised of three zones: (1) an outer zona glomerulosa, responsible for exclusive synthesis of aldosterone, (2) a middle zona fasciculata, and (3) an inner zona reticularis. The inner two zones are involved in the synthesis of cortisol and androgens. The hypothalamic-pituitary-adrenal axis regulates hormone production. Hypothalamic corticotropin releasing factor (CRF) stimulates synthesis and secretion of adrenocorticotropic hormone (ACTH) from the anterior pituitary. ACTH binds to receptors in the adrenal cortex and cholesterol is cleaved in the cristae of the mitochondria to Δ5-pregnenolone. Pregnenolone exits the mitochondria and enters the smooth endoplasmic reticulum (SER) where it is shunted to three divergent pathways, for synthesis of glucocorticoid hormone (cortisol), mineralocorticoid hormone (aldosterone) or sex steroid hormone (dehydroepiandrosterone [DHEA]). The polyhedral cells of the adrenal *medulla* contribute approximately 10% of the total gland weight and contain core vesicles of epinephrine and norepinephrine.

These paired retroperitoneal organs may give rise to benign or malignant, functional or non-functional adrenal tumors. Currently most adrenal pathology is found unexpectedly. Therefore this chapter begins with evaluation of the incidental adrenal mass followed by a review of specific adrenal diseases.

The incidental adrenal mass

The widespread use of computed tomography (CT) has led to the discovery of non-functional adrenal 'incidentalomas' in 0.6% of abdominal CT scans[1]. The differential diagnosis of these benign appearing adrenal masses is shown in Table 31.1. The clinical challenge is to characterize a given lesion sufficiently enough to determine if therapy is necessary or if the lesion may be safely observed. The evaluation begins with a thorough history and physical examination followed by biochemical tests to determine the functional status of the lesion. Most biochemically inactive tumors less than 3 cm do not require therapy[2], while functioning tumors and those greater than 6 cm usually require intervention.

Initial biochemical screening should include serum electrolytes, urinary catecholamines, a 24 h urinary free cortisol and urinary 17-ketosteroids. Other provocative tests should be reserved for equivocal cases or when high clinical suspicion persists despite normal initial screening. Hypokalemia suggests an aldosterone-secreting tumor, that may be confirmed by measuring plasma renin and aldosterone excretion rates in response to salt loading. Determination of 24 h urinary vanillyl mandelic acid (VMA) and total metanephrines (TMN) during a hypertensive episode is the most sensitive screening method for pheochromocytoma. Patients with pheochromocytoma almost always excrete these metabolites at rates more than three times normal. However, both VMA and TMN may be increased by exogenous and/or endogenous catecholamines. Elevated urinary cortisol, along with loss of the normal diurnal plasma cortisol variation suggests Cushing's syndrome. Suppressed levels of ACTH suggest the presence of an adrenal neoplasm that is secreting cortisol; elevated levels of ACTH suggest pituitary dependent or ectopic ACTH sources. Adrenal carcinomas may have deficiencies in steroid producing enzymes[3], therefore, it is important to include the cortisol metabolites (urinary 17-ketosteroids) as part of the screening panel.

Dexamethasone stimulation tests[4] may detect subtle adrenal overactivity that may otherwise be overlooked. Such tests are shown on Table 31.2. The dexamethasone suppression test distinguishes pituitary from adrenal causes of hypercortisolism. The low dose overnight test is a quick and reliable screening test for Cushing's syndrome. If the morning plasma cortisol level is less than 5μg/dl, the syndrome is essentially excluded. In equivocal cases, the high-dose test should be performed. By increasing the dose of dexamethasone, ACTH can almost always be suppressed if Cushing's disease is present. This is reflected by a decrease of urinary 17-hydroxycorticosteroid (17OHCS) to 50% of baseline values. In contrast, among patients with other forms of Cushing's syndrome (such as adrenal tumors or etopic ACTH-secreting tumors), dexamethasone cannot suppress 17OHCS levels below 50%. The metyrapone stimulation test[4] differentiates ACTH-dependent (ACTH-producing tumors) from ACTH-independent (primary adrenocortical disease) etiologies. Normally this inhibitor causes a

Table 31.1 The differential diagnosis of an adrenal mass[21]

- Adenoma
- Adrenocortical carcinoma
- Aldosteronoma
- Cyst
- Ganglioneuroma
- Hemorrhage
- Metastatic tumors
- Myelolipoma
- Neuroblastoma
- Pheochromocytoma

Table 31.2   The dexamethasone suppression and metyrapone stimulation tests[4]

2a. Dexamethasone suppression tests

- **Low dose**
  - **Overnight test:** Dexamethasone 1 mg po at 11 pm; measure plasma cortisol and ACTH at 8 am the next day.

8 am cortisol	ACTH	Comments
<5 μg/dl	<20 pg/ml	Normal
5–10 μg/dl	–	Equivocal
>10 μg/dl	>20 pg/ml	Hypercortisolism

  - **Standard two-day test:** Dexamethasone 0.5 mg po Q6 h for 2 days; 24 h urine collections with measurements of urinary cortisol and 17OHCS, and plasma cortisol and ACTH.

Day	Urine cortisol	Urine 17OHCS	Plasma cortisol	Plasma ACTH	Comments
Day 0	20–90 μg/24 h	6–20 mg/24 h	8 am: 10–20 μg/dl 4 pm: 3–10 μg/dl	20–100 pg/ml	Baseline
Day 1					Baseline
Day 2	<20 μg/24 h	<2.5 mg/24 h	<5 μg/dl	<20 pg/ml	Normal
	>20 μg/24 h	>2.5 mg/24 h	>5 μg/dl	20–100 pg/ml	Cushing's disease
	>20 μg/24 h	>2.5 mg/24 h	>5 μg/dl	<20 pg/ml	Adrenal tumor
	>20 μg/24 h	>2.5 mg/24 h	>5 μg/dl	>100 pg/ml	Ectopic tumor

- **High dose**
  - **Standard two-day test:** Dexamethasone 2.0 mg po Q 6 h for 2 days; 24 h urine collections with measurements of urinary cortisol and 17OHCS, and plasma cortisol and ACTH.

Day	Urine cortisol	Urine 17OHCS	Plasma cortisol	Plasma ACTH	Comments
Day 0	20–90 μg/24 h	6–20 mg/24 h	8am: 10–20 μg/dl 4pm: 3–10 μg/dl	20–100 pg/ml	Baseline
Day 1					Baseline
Day 2	<10 μg/24 h	<2.5 mg/24 h	<5 μg/dl	<20 pg/ml	Normal
	<50% baseline	<50% baseline		<20 pg/ml	Cushing's disease
		6–20 mg/24 h			Adrenal tumor
		6–20 mg/24 h			Ectopic tumor

2b. Metyrapone stimulation tests

- **Overnight single-dose test:** Metyrapone 30 mg/kg po at 12 midnight; measure plasma 11-deoxycortisol, cortisol, and ACTH levels at 8 am the next day.
- **Standard three-day test:** Metyrapone 10 mg/kg po Q4 h x 6 doses; collect 24 h urine specimens for 17OHCS, plasma 11-deoxycortisol, cortisol and ACTH levels.

Plasma cortisol	11-deoxycortisol	ACTH	Urine 17OHCS	Comments
<10 μg/dl	7–22 μcg/dl	>75 pg.ml	2–3 × increase	Normal
	Large increase		2–4 × increase	Cushing's disease
			Decrease	Adrenal tumor
			Intermediate	Ectopic tumor

compensatory rise in ACTH secretion by the pituitary, causing the adrenal cortex to produce more cortisol precursors. Patients with Cushing's disease already have a 2–4 fold increase in urinary 17OHCS and a large increase in plasma 11-deoxycortisol. Patients with primary adrenocortical tumors show a fall in urinary 17OHCS because the chronic hypercortisolemia has suppressed hypothalamic CRH and pituitary ACTH synthesis. Patients with ectopic ACTH-secreting tumors show an intermediate response. Metyrapone in these patients causes a subnormal rise in urinary 17OHCS. Patients with chronic ectopic ACTH syndrome do not respond to metyrapone because the hypothalamic-pituitary axis is profoundly suppressed.

The evaluation and management of the incidentaloma is presented in Figure 31.1. In general, unilateral functioning tumors, regardless of size, should be surgically excised. Tumors equal to or greater than 6 cm should also be surgically removed because of the high likelihood of malignancy. Biochemical evaluation should be performed regardless of tumor size to determine if pre-operative therapy will be necessary, as in the case of pheochromocytoma. The treatment of non-functioning tumors between 3 and 6 cm remains controversial. Management options include observation with serial radiographs, surgical removal, or percutaneous biopsy. Observation is limited by the non-specific radiologic appearance of most incidental tumors. Surgical excision ensures certainty of histologic diagnosis but the potential for cure of an occasional primary cancer is estimated at 1 in 4000 for tumors greater than 1.5 cm[3]. Percutaneous needle biopsy does not ensure an accurate diagnosis. Therefore, non-functional incidentalomas between 3 and 6 cm need individualized management based on the patient's overall medical condition. If the patient is a poor surgical candidate or does not desire surgical intervention, repeat imaging of the mass in 12 months is appropriate. If the tumor grows on repeat studies, resection should be more strongly recommended. If the tumor is stable, no further studies are needed until clinical signs or symptoms prompt repeat biochemical testing or imaging. Although the MR appearance of adrenal cortical tumors is non-specific, most non-functioning adenomas have low signal intensity on both T_1 and T_2 weighted images, whereas some hyperfunctioning tumors have increased intensity on T_2 weighted images[5]. Most recently, chemical shift MR imaging[6] has been used to differentiate between adenoma and malignant masses. This technique utilizes the fact that most adenomas contain large amounts of lipid, corresponding to a loss of signal intensity on chemical shift MR images. In contrast, most malignant lesions do not contain lipid and therefore do not demonstrate signal intensity loss. If there is loss of signal intensity on chemical shift MR images of an adrenal mass, the diagnosis of adenoma can be made with 81% sensitivity and 100% specificity[6]. Surgical resection may be elected if there is no loss of signal intensity because of the possibility of malignancy.

Tumors of the adrenal cortex

Adrenocortical adenomas

Adrenocortical tumors are highly prevalent with 1.4% to 8.7% of cases from autopsy series demonstrating benign adenomas[3]. Benign tumors are usually less than 5 cm, weigh less than 200 g, and histologically resemble normal adrenal cells with nests and cords of cohesive vacuolated cells with abundant cytoplasm. Adenomas can be non-functional or functional and associated with various syndromes, such as hypercortisolism, hyperaldosteronism, and less commonly virilization. A recent report suggests that up to 50% of patients with incidentalomas have some evidence of subtle steroid overproduction if the more provocative tests are performed despite asymptomatology[7]. If left untreated, this overproduction can suppress the

hypothalamic-pituitary-adrenal (HPA) axis and impair the patient's ability to respond to stress.

CT images of benign tumors usually disclose a homogeneous lesion with smooth contour and well delineated margins, clearly distinct from surrounding structures[2], however, there are no CT findings to distinguish functioning versus non-functioning tumors[1]. Although size is a powerful predictor of malignancy as previously described, case reports of very large benign tumors and of small tumors with metastasis have been reported[8]. The majority of patients with these tumors are cured by surgical resection.

Adrenocortical carcinomas

Occult non-functioning adrenocortical carcinomas are rare with an annual incidence of 0.5–2.0 per million population[9]. They have a bimodal incidence: children less than 5 years of age and among adults during the third to fourth decades. Adrenocortical carcinoma is the most common cause of hypercortisolism in children. Women are affected twice as often as men. Sixty percent of carcinomas are functional with a greater proportion of biochemically active tumors in women. Adrenal carcinomas may occur as part of the hereditary cancer family complex **SBLA** (**S**arcoma, **B**reast and **B**rain tumors, **L**eukemia, **L**aryngeal carcinoma, and **L**ung cancer, **A**drenocortical carcinoma) where patients develop malignancies from all three germ cell-layers involving various sites[10]. Adrenal carcinomas account for about 3% of cancers in this syndrome and usually occur during childhood[11]. Despite extensive genetic studies in attempting to localize gene mutations in non-familial and familial adrenal carcinomas, there does not appear to be a consistent chromosomal defect.

Signs and symptoms of adrenal carcinoma are variable. Functioning tumors may present as a clinical syndrome based on overproduction of the particular adrenocortical hormone, whereas non-functioning carcinomas may be clinically silent or present with abdominal pain, increased abdominal girth, weight loss, weakness, anorexia, nausea, and headache. Adrenocortical carcinomas usually have heterogeneous internal architecture on CT scans and may invade surrounding structures[2]. Among standard histologic criteria differentiating adenoma from carcinoma, mitotic rate appears to be the best indicator of prognosis for adrenal carcinoma[8]. Immunohistochemical analysis with keratin and vimentin may be useful in separating adrenal tumors from other tumors, but have limited or no value in differentiating benign from malignant adrenal tumors. Similarly, studies of DNA content or ploidy to differentiate benign from malignant tumors remain unreliable.

The primary treatment of adrenocortical carcinoma is en bloc wide resection of the primary tumor, and in selected cases, resection of isolated metastases. In general, stage I and II tumors (i.e. those confined to the gland) are managed by surgical excision alone and stage III and IV are often debulked by surgery and subsequently treated with systemic chemotherapy. Inoperable cases require palliative chemotherapy or radiation therapy.

Stage I and II tumors are treated with en bloc excision of adjacent organs, often including the ipsilateral kidney, or portions of the pancreas and liver. Wide surgical exposure is necessary and is most often achieved via a chevron or thoracoabdominal incision. These lesions may be vascular, very large, and may invade adjacent soft tissue and organs. On the left, the descending colon is usually reflected inferiorly, with division of the splenocolic ligament and reflection of spleen and pancreas medially. The right adrenal gland is exposed by mobilization of the hepatic flexure of the colon and duodenum medially. Control of the vessels should be achieved prior to manipulation of the tumor. In patients with marked central obesity and a small tumor, the adrenal gland may be approached through the flank. Local recurrences may be treated by surgical excision if there is no evidence of metastases. Aggressive resection of recurrent disease in combination with chemotherapy was associated with longer survival compared with chemotherapy alone[12] (27 vs. 11 months).

Chemotherapeutic agents, including metyrapone, aminoglutethimide, ketoconazole and mitotane, may be used to control functional syndromes or to treat metastatic disease. Metyrapone has been used in cancer patients to control excess cortisol production, but may lead to hypokalemic alkalosis and hypertension. One to 3 g may be given daily in combination with other drugs that inhibit mineralocorticoid production, such as aminoglutethimide, but this approach has met with limited success in controlling symptoms of hypercortisolism.

Aminoglutethimide interferes with cortisol biosynthesis but also alters extra-adrenal metabolism of cortisol, decreasing urinary 17-hydroxycorticosteroid excretion disproportionately[13]. Thus plasma cortisol levels rather than urinary 17-hydroxycorticosteroid excretion should be used to gauge therapy. Replacement cortisone and mineralocorticoid is advisable since adrenal insufficiency may develop.

Mitotane (o,p'-DDD) [1,1-dichloro-2,2-bis(p-chlorophenylethanol)], a derivative of the insecticide DDD, inhibits cholesterol side chain cleaving enzyme and 11β-hydroxylase[14]. The original report of clinical effectiveness of mitotane in metastatic adrenal cancer patients was presented in a group of only 18 patients with objective remissions noted in 39% with average doses from 8 to 10 g/day for 6 to 8 weeks[15]. In a larger study of 138 patients, sponsored by the National Cancer Institute, control of steroid production was noted in 70% to 90% of patients and tumor regression in 34% to 61%, however these studies were not controlled, and duration of therapy and dosages were not standardized[16]. Luton et al.[17] showed control of endocrine hypersecretion in 75% of patients. Objective tumor regression was seen in eight of 37 patients treated with mitotane, five of whom showed ≥50%, but no improvement in overall survival. Review of 64 reports of mitotane use in adrenal cancer patients noted partial or complete responses in 194 of 551 patients (35%)[18]. There does not appear to be any benefit to mitotane in the adjuvant setting after surgical resection[17,19]. The toxicity of mitotane is substantial[20]. The most common side effects include nausea, vomiting, anorexia and diarrhea in over 70% of patients. Neurologic toxicity, in the form of depression, dizziness, confusion and headaches, is seen in over 40% of patients. Less common toxicities include skin rashes, hemorrhagic cystitis and proteinuria. Concomitant therapy with hydrocortisone and mineralocorticoids is recommended, especially if prolonged treatment is planned.

Chemotherapeutic agents commonly studied in the treatment of adrenal carcinoma include cisplatin alone or in combination with other agents. Response rates range between 10% and 30%[21]. Palliative radiation therapy on the order of 15 to 51 Gy given to 11 patients resulted in symptomatic relief[22] which has led to speculation of administering 30 to 45 Gy for palliation of symptoms and higher doses of 50–60 Gy to the post-operative tumor bed to provide long-term local control over residual microscopic disease at the primary site to prolong survival[23].

Tumors of the adrenal medulla
Pheochromocytoma

Pheochromocytomas may arise from the adrenal medulla or extra-adrenal sites. The autopsy incidence of this tumor is 0.3%[24]. These tumors may be benign or malignant and are associated with multiple endocrine neoplasia II (MEN II). MEN IIa is a hereditary, autosomal dominant predisposition to medullary thyroid carcinoma (MTC), pheochromocytoma and parathyroid hyperplasia. While nearly all patients develop MTC, only 50% develop pheochromocytoma or parathyroid hyperplasia. Usually pheochromocytomas in this syndrome are bilateral and multiple. MEN IIb is associated with MTC and pheochromocytoma, and multiple mucosal neuromas and ganglioneuromatosis. Because of this association, patients with MTC should be screened for pheochromocytoma. Five to ten per cent of patients with pheochromocytoma have neurofibromatosis (von Recklinghausen's disease) but <1% of all patients with neurofibromatosis have pheochromocytoma. Other neuroectodermal dysplasia syndromes associated with pheochromocytoma include tuberous sclerosis, Sturge-Weber syndrome and von

Hippel-Lindau disease. Pheochromocytoma may occur rarely in pregnancy and may present with eclampsia, paroxysmal hypertension, shock, or unexplained hyperpyrexia after delivery or death. The period of greatest risk is from the onset of labor to 48 h post-partum. If pheochromocytoma is diagnosed during the first or second trimester, surgical resection should be performed. If discovered during the third trimester, medical management is appropriate until planned delivery. Ten per cent of pheochromocytomas present in children less than 20 years of age. Boys before puberty are most commonly affected and have a higher likelihood of extra-adrenal lesions.

The clinical presentation includes hypertensive crisis, myocardial infarction, or cerebral vascular accident, but can also be more subtle, mimicking diabetes or hyperthyroidism. Hypertension is the most consistent sign but only half of patients have sustained hypertension. Most patients recognize paroxysmal precipitating factors, such as physical exercise, intercourse, micturition, high tyramine food ingestion, and drugs, such as histamine, nicotine and propranolol. Non-functioning tumors are uncommon and asymptomatic functioning tumors are rare.

Of sporadic pheochromocytomas 10–20% are malignant. Females are three times as likely to be affected than males. Sustained hypertension is the rule. There are no biochemical, gross or microscopic differences between benign and malignant tumors. The diagnosis of malignancy is established by presence of invasion of adjacent structures, nodal or distant metastases, usually to bone and liver. While earlier studies suggested extra-adrenal pheochromocytomas to be two to three times more likely than adrenal tumors to be malignant[25], more recent reports show that 10–15% of extra-adrenal tumors are malignant, similar to the rate among adrenal tumors[26].

Approximately 10–15% of pheochromocytomas are extra-adrenal and occur whereever chromaffin tissue is located. They may be found near sympathetic ganglion in the posterior mediastinum, in the paraganglia, bladder and the organ of Zuckerkandl, a vestigial structure located in the region of the inferior mesenteric artery, anterior aorta and aortic bifurcation. Pheochromocytomas of the bladder arise most frequently from the dome. Common signs and symptoms include hematuria and paroxysmal hypertensive episodes during micturition. Diagnosis is made by cystoscopy, which may itself elicit paroxysmal hypertension.

The *sine qua non* for establishing the diagnosis of pheochromocytoma is increased excretion rates of urinary epinephrine, norepinephrine and their metabolites, metanephrine, normetanephrine and vanillylmandelic acid. This elevation is observed in over 90% of patients with pheochromocytoma. False-positive elevations may be due to ingestion of coffee, tea, raw fruits and α-methyldopa. Stimulation and suppression tests aid in equivocal cases.

Glucagon 1.0–2.0 mg IV is administered to stimulate catecholamine release. This test is positive if the plasma catecholamine concentration increases at least threefold, or levels exceed 2000 pg/ml within 2–3 minutes of administration. If there is an increase in catecholamine levels but blood pressure remains normal, the clonidine suppression test may be employed. Theoretically, the autonomous release of catecholamines by pheochromocytoma would not be suppressed by clonidine. Normally, plasma norepinephrine and epinephrine are decreased to <500 ng/ml 2–3 hours after 0.3 mg clonidine is administered orally.

MR is considered non-specific for adrenal tumors except for pheochromocytomas (Figure 31.2) and offers advantages of avoiding ionizing radiation and intravenous contrast materials, preferable for pregnant patients. Typically pheochromocytomas display low signal intensity on T_1 weighted images and bright signal intensity on T_2 weighted images. The renal scanning agent ^{131}I-metaiodobenzylguanidine (^{131}I-MIBG) has been used to visualize pheochromocytomas pre-operatively and therapeutically for unresectable metastases[27]. More invasive techniques to localize pheochromocytomas include arteriography and adrenal venography. Great caution must be exercised if these studies are used since contrast medium can stimulate release of catecholamines and induce a hypertensive crisis. Adrenergic blockade with phenoxybenzamine (Dibenzyline) is recommended before these studies. These more invasive procedures may be employed when other non-invasive localizing procedures have failed or when exploration of a clinically functional tumor has been unsuccessful.

The primary treatment for pheochromocytoma is surgical resection. Pre-operatively, alpha blockade using phenoxybenzamine 10 mg orally twice daily with increasing increments of 10–20 mg/day to a total of 1 mg/kg is required to control blood pressure. Phentolamine 50 mg orally every 4 hours may also be used. The major side effects of α-blockade include postural hypotension, reflex tachycardia, nasal congestion and inability to ejaculate. Usually α-blockade in maintained 1 to 3 weeks pre-operatively. β-blockers, such as propranolol, should be considered if heart rate exceeds 140 beats/min, or if the patient has a history of arrhythmias. β-blockade should not be started until α-blockade is achieved, because uncurtailed β-effects inhibit epinephrine-induced vasodilatation, cause increased hypertension, create more heart strain, and predispose the patient to bradyarrhthymias and heart block. One scenario where pre-operative blood pressure treatment may be disadvantageous is if the tumor has not yet been localized pre-operatively despite imaging studies. In this case, the elevation in blood pressure response intraoperatively with the manipulation of tumor could provide a means for localization. If preoperative α-blockade is not administered, blood volume must be carefully monitored

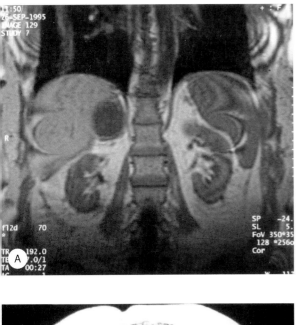

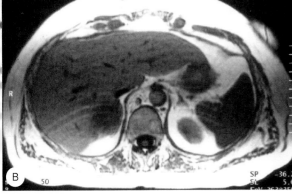

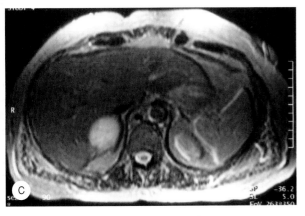

intra-operatively and 48 hours post-operatively since resection of pheochromocytoma essentially decreases circulating norepinephrine thereby resulting in vasodilatation and relative hypovolemia causing tachycardia.

Intensive intraoperative monitoring must be utilized during resection of a pheochromocytoma. Monitoring should include arterial line and central venous pressure recording, Foley catheter to measure urine output, and continuous electrocardiogram tracings. Induction with sodium thiopental in divided doses is usually recommended followed by nitrous oxide, oxygen and enflurane by mask. After deep anesthesia is achieved, pancuronium is administered. The trachea is sprayed with 4% lidocaine and the patient is intubated. General endotracheal anesthesia is maintained with enflurane, nitrous oxide and oxygen. The patient should be placed in slightly reversed Trendelenburg position so the lower extremities are used as volume capacitors during the procedure, with return to horizontal position after the tumor is excised, to aid in restoration of blood volume. Hypertensive episodes during removal of the tumor should be controlled with sodium nitroprusside. Cardiac arrhythmias caused by sudden increased catecholamine secretion with tumor manipulation are controlled with intravenous lidocaine and propranolol. Since profound hypotension due to vasodilatation is possible post-operatively, these patients should be observed in an intensive unit setting for 24 hours after surgery. Twenty-four hour urine for VMA and TMN may be performed one week or more after surgery. Persistent hypertension or sustained elevation in urinary catecholamines 2–3 weeks after surgery suggests residual pheochromocytoma.

Fig. 31.2 Magnetic resonance imaging of pheochromocytoma showing coronal (a) and axial (b) T_1 weighted images of a 4–5 cm adrenal mass displaying low signal intensity. Axial T_2 weighted image shows bright enhancement of the mass (c).

References

1. Glazer HS, Weyman PJ, Sagel SS, Levitt RG, McClennan BL. Nonfunctioning adrenal masses: incidental discovery on computed tomography. *AJR* 1982;**139**:81–85.
2. Mitnick JS, Bosniak MA, Megibow AJ, Naidich DP. Non-functioning adrenal adenomas discovered incidentally on computed tomography. *Radiology* 1983;**148**:495–499.
3. Copeland PM. The incidentally discovered adrenal mass. *Ann Int Med* 1983;**98**:940–945.
4. Orth DN, Kovacs WJ, Debold CR. The adrenal cortex. In Wilson JD and Foster DW (eds) *Williams textbook of endocrinology* (8th edn). WB Saunders Co, Philadelphia 1992. 575–592.
5. Remer BM, Weinfeld RM, Glazer GM, Quint LE, Francis IR, Gross MD, Bookstein FL. Hyperfunctioning and nonhyperfunctioning benign adrenal cortical lesions: characterization and comparison with MR imaging. *Radiology* 1989;**171**:681–685.
6. Korobkin M, Lombardi TH, Aisen AM. Characterization of adrenal masses with chemical shift and gadolinium-enhanced MR imaging. *Radiology* 1995;**197**:411–418.
7. Rosen HN, Swartz SL. Subtle glucocorticoid excess in patients with adrenal incidentaloma. *Am J Med* 1992;**92**:213–216.
8. Medeiros LJ, Weiss LM. New developments in the pathologic diagnosis of adrenal cortical neoplasms. *Am J Clin Pathol* 1992;**97**:73–83.

9. Cutler SJ, Young JL. Third national cancer survey: incidence data. Biometry Branch, Division of Cancer Cause and Prevention, National Cancer Institute 1975.

10. Lynch HT, Mulcahy GM, Harris RE, Guirgis HA, Lynch JF. Genetic and pathologic findings in a kindred with hereditary sarcoma, breast cancer, brain tumors, leukemia, lung, laryngeal, and adrenal cortical carcinoma. *Cancer* 1978;**41**:2055–2064.

11. Li FP, Fraumeni JF, Mulvihill JJ, Blattner WA, Dreyfus MG, Rucker MA, Miller RW. A cancer family syndrome in twenty-four kindreds. *Cancer Res* 1988;**48**:5358–5362.

12. Jensen IC, Pass HI, Sindelar WF, Norton JA. Recurrent or metatstatic disease in select patients with adrenocortical carcinoma. *Arch Surg* 1991;**126**:457–461.

13. Schteingart DE, Cash R, Conn JW. Amino-glutethimide and metastatic adrenal cancer. *JAMA* 1966;**198**:1007–1010.

14. Hoffman DL, Mattox VR. Treatment of adrenocortical carcinoma with o,p'-DDD. *Med Clin N Am* 1972;**56**:999–1012.

15. Bergenstal DM, Hertz R, Lipsett MB, Moy RH. Chemotherapy of adrenocortical cancer with o,p'-DDD. *Ann Intern Med* 1960;**53**:672–682.

16. Lubitz JA, Freeman L, Okun R. Mitotane use in inoperable adrenal cortical carcinoma. *JAMA* 1973;**223**:1109–1112.

17. Luton J, Cerdas S, Billaud L, Thomas G, Guilhaume B, Bertagna Z, Laudat M *et al.* Clinical features of adrenocortical carcinoma, prognostic factors, and the effect of mitotane therapy. *NEJM* 1990;**332**:1195–1201.

18. Wooten MD, King DK. Adrenal cortical carcinoma, epidemiology and treatment with mitotane and review of the literature. *Cancer* 1993;**72**:3145–3155.

19. Bodie B, Novick AC, Pontes JE, Straffon RA, Montie JE, Babiak T, Sheeler L, Schumacher P. The Cleveland Clinic experience with adrenal cortical carcinoma. *J Urol* 1989;**141**:257–260.

20. Gutierrez ML, Crooke ST. Mitotane (o,p'-DDD). *Cancer Treat Rev* 1980;**7**:49–55.

21. Bukowski RM, Klein EA. Adrenal and kidney cancers. In: Vogelzang NJ, Scardino PT, Shipley WU, Coffey DS (eds). *Comprehensive textbook of genitourinary oncology.* Williams & Wilkins, Baltimore, 1996. 125–153.

22. Percarpio B, Knowlton AH. Radiation therapy of adrenal cortical carcinoma. *Acta Rad Therapy Phys Bio* 1976;**15**:288–292.

23. Markoe AM, Serber W, Micaily B, Brady LW. Radiation therapy for adjunctive treatment of adrenal cortical carcinoma. *Am J Clin Oncol* 1991;**14**:170–174.

24. Sheps SG, Jiang N, Klee GG, van Heerden JA. Recent developments in the diagnosis and treatment of pheochromocytoma. *Mayo Clin Proc* 1990;**65**:88–95.

25. Remine WH, Chong GC, van Heerden JA, Sheps SG, Harrison EG. Current management of pheochromocytoma. *Ann Surg* 1974;**179**:740–748.

26. Pommier RF, Vetto JT, Billingsly K, Woltering EA, Brennan MF. Comparison of adrenal and extraadrenal pheochromocytomas. *Surgery* 1993;**114**:1160–1166.

27. Thompson NW, Allo MD, Shapiro B, Sisson JC, Beierwaltes W. Extra-adreanl and metastatic pheochromocytoma: the role of ^{131}I meta-iodobenzylguanidine (^{131}I MIBG) in localization and management. *World J Surg* 1984;**8**:605–611.

32 Retroperitoneal malignancies and processes

S B Bhayani, K Rockers, C K Naughton and J W Basler

Retroperitoneal tumour algorithm

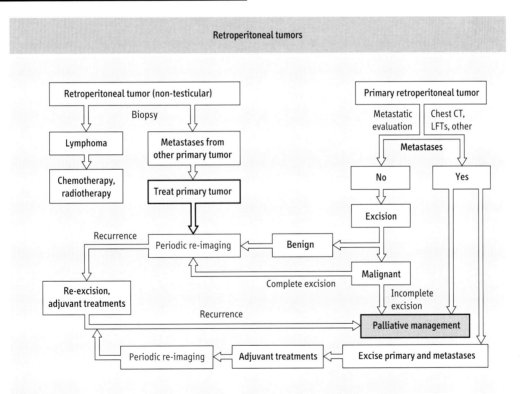

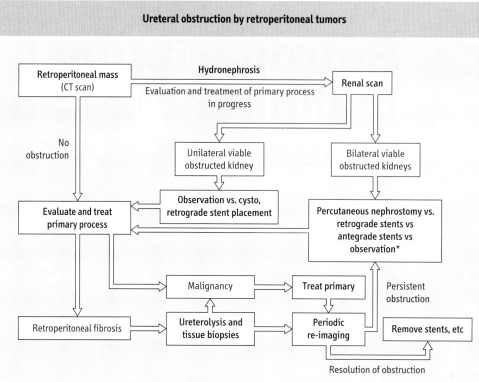

Ureteral obstruction by retroperitoneal tumors

*Consider counseling regarding this option if patient has poor prognosis for recovery.

The retroperitoneum has been anatomically defined as a potential space extending between the diaphragm and the pelvis. The posterior parietal peritoneum forms the anterior boundary, and the vertebral bodies, sacrum, psoas, quadratus lumborum, transversus abdominis and iliacus muscles form the posterior boundary. The retroperitoneum includes parts of the digestive, nervous, genitourinary, circulatory and skeletal systems. Major structures in the retroperitoneum include the kidneys, adrenal glands, ureters, bladder, aorta, inferior vena cava, pancreas, portions of duodenum and colon, lymph nodes, and various nerves and blood vessels[1].

Primary retroperitoneal tumors and tumors metastatic to the retroperitoneum present unique challenges. Primary tumors are often large, aggressive, and involve major retroperitoneal and intraperitoneal structures. Metastatic tumors tend to cause progressive ureteral obstruction. Urologists are commonly involved in the treatment of these malignancies; as such, a thorough understanding of these disease processes is essential. This chapter discusses primary retroperitoneal tumors and metastases to the retroperitoneum, with exclusion of primary tumors of the bowel, pancreas, and upper urinary tract.

Primary retroperitoneal tumors

Primary retroperitoneal tumors account for less than 1% of all malignancies[2]. The tumors exhibit various histopathologies, reflecting the diverse embryology and anatomy of the retroperitoneum. The tumors have been classified by their tissue type and origin (Table 32.1)[2,3]. Approximately 80% of retroperitoneal tumors are malignant[2]. In one recent series of 182 patients, sarcomas comprised 43% of primary retroperitoneal tumors, followed by lymphomas (23%), benign tumors (11%), undifferentiat-

ed malignant tumors (11%), carcinomas (8%) and germ cell tumors (4%)[4].

Primary retroperitoneal tumors generally present after reaching a sufficient size to compress or invade adjacent organs. The median time from onset of symptoms to treatment is 5 months and less than 20% of patients present within 2 months of symptoms[4,5]. Presenting features may be non-specific; however over 75% of patients have a palpable mass[6,7]. Common symptoms include abdominal pain, back pain, nausea, vomiting, and weight loss (Table 32.2)[4].

The diagnosis of retroperitoneal tumors has changed dramatically in the last two decades. Prior to the advent of computerized tomographic scanning (CT) and magnetic resonance imaging (MRI), radiologic diagnosis relied on the displacement of normal structures. Upper gastrointestinal series and barium enema studies are abnormal in 40–86% of cases, but they exhibit low sensitivity[4,5,7]. Intravenous pyelography shows ureteric obstruction or displacement in over 70% of cases[7]. Angiography suggests a large mass involving or compressing the aorta or inferior vena cava. Although some retroperitoneal tumors are poorly vascularized, aortography may show displacement or involvement of major arteries. Venography may reveal vena caval involvement[5,7].

Retroperitoneal tumors are most commonly diagnosed by CT and MRI. CT with intravenous and oral contrast can demonstrate the extent of tumor, including evidence of vascular and gastrointestinal invasion. MRI has the advantages of multiplanar imaging, and differentiation of tumor from fat (T1 weighted) and from muscle (T2 weighted). For the diagnosis of retroperitoneal sarcomas, MRI provides better prediction of resectability (96% vs. 75%) and superior sensitivity (95% vs. 73%) than CT[8].

If the diagnosis of the retroperitoneal tumor is not established with CT or MRI, percutaneous biopsy may be performed, with the known risk of tract seeding. Alternatively, open biopsy allows easy tumor accessibility and visualization, but care should be taken to avoid

Table 32.1 Primary tumors of the retroperitoneum, classified by tissue of origin[2,3]

Tissue of origin	Benign tumor	Malignant tumor
Fibrous	Fibroma	Fibrosarcoma
Adipose	Lipoma	Liposarcoma
Mucoid	Myxoma	Myxosarcoma
Muscle	Rhabdomyoma	Leiomyosarcoma, rhabdomyosarcoma
Vascular	Hemangioma, Hemangiopericytoma	Malignant hemangiopericytoma, angiosarcoma
Mesenchymal	Mesenchymoma	
Lymphatic	Lymphangioma	Lymphoma, lymphosarcoma, lymphangiosarcoma
Nervous	Schwannoma, chordoma	Malignant schwannoma, neuroblastoma
Chromaffin tissue	Extra-adrenal pheochromocytoma	Malignant pheochromocytoma

Table 32.2 Common presenting features of primary retroperitoneal tumors[4]

Presenting features	Patients (%)
Abdominal or flank mass	81
Abdominal pain	69
Weight loss	55
Loss of appetite	44
Increase in abdominal girth	35
Back pain	30
Nausea, vomiting	27
Constipation	19
Leg pain	15

intraoperative tumor spillage[9]. Laparoscopic biopsy may be possible in selected cases, but has not been widely reported.

Retroperitoneal sarcomas

Retroperitoneal sarcomas account for nearly half of primary retroperitoneal tumors. There is a slight male predominance[10,11]. Sarcomas affect all ages with 63% of patients less than 50 years of age[10]. Retroperitoneal sarcomas exhibit a variety of subtypes (Table 32.3); liposarcoma is the most common histologic subtype, followed by leiomyosarcoma and fibrosarcoma[2,10]. Overall survival reflects the aggressive nature of these tumors, with only 34% of patients surviving 5 years, and 18% of patients surviving 10 years[9].

The etiology of soft tissue sarcomas is largely unknown. Associations with dioxin, prior irradiation and herbicide exposure have been suggested[12–14]. In nearly all cases, no etiologic agent can be identified.

The American Joint Commission on Cancer stages soft tissue sarcomas by tumor grade, size, lymph node involvement and metastatic spread (Table 32.4)[15]. Clinical staging should include CT or MRI of the abdomen and pelvis, chest radiograph and bone scan. Angiography, intravenous pyelography and gastrointestinal studies should be considered if clinically relevant.

Complete surgical excision with negative margins affords the best prognosis for localized sarcoma[10,16]. Preoperatively all patients receive a mechanical and antimicrobial bowel preparation and ureteral stents should be placed in selected cases. A midline, chevron, or thoracoabdominal approach is indicated depending on tumor location. Pre-operative surgical planning is essential successfully to excise retroperitoneal sarcomas. The surgeon must be prepared to excise portions of any intraabdominal and retroperitoneal organ en bloc to achieve complete resection. In over 50% of cases major organs are sacrificed, most commonly the kidney, colon, spleen, or pancreas[6,17]. Major vascular resection is involved in over 10% of patients. Adequate resection may involve a team of surgical specialists including a urologic,

Table 32.3   Histologic subtypes of soft tissue sarcomas

Angiosarcoma
Fibrosarcoma
Hemangiopericytoma
Leiomyosarcoma
Liposarcoma
Malignant fibrous histiocytoma
Neurofibrosarcoma
Rhabdomyosarcoma
Undifferentiated sarcoma

Table 32.4   TNM staging of retroperitoneal soft tissue sarcomas[15]

G: Histopathologic grade
G1   Well differentiated
G2   Moderately differentiated
G3   Poorly differentiated

T: Tumor size
T1   Tumor 5 cm or less in greatest dimension
T2   Tumor more than 5 cm in greatest dimension

N: Regional lymph node involvement
N0   No regional lymph node metastasis
N1   Regional lymph node metastasis

M: Distant metastasis
M0   No distant metastasis
M1   Distant metastasis

Stages
I   G1–2, T1, N0, M0
IIA   G1–2, T2, N0, M0
IIB   G3, T1, N0, M0
III   G3, T2, N0, M0
IV   N1 or M1

vascular, general and occasionally a thoracic surgeon. Combined data from many series demonstrate that complete excision may be achieved in 53% of patients[9].

Complete resection is the most important predictor of improved survival[4,10,16,17]. After complete resection, the 5 year survival rate has been reported from 38% to 70%, with an average of nearly 50%[9,11,17,18]. Partial resection is strictly palliative, as it offers no survival advantage over biopsy alone[4,17].

After completeness of resection, tumor grade is the only other important predictor of outcome. One cumulative assessment of 129 patients showed a 5 year survival of 74% of patients with G1 tumors, compared with 24% of patients with G2 and G3 tumors[9]. In another series of 83 patients, the 12 year survival of low- and high-grade tumors were 81% and 43% respectively[16].

Retroperitoneal sarcomas tend to recur after complete resection. Local recurrences account for 75% of all recurrences[17,19]. A cumulative series of 204 patients demonstrated local recurrences of 40%, 72% and 91% at 2, 5 and 10 years following complete resection. Even after a 5 year disease-free interval, 40% of patients will recur in the subsequent 5 years[10]. High-grade tumors recur earlier (median of 15 months) than low-grade tumors (median of 44 months)[17]. After resection, patients require close surveillance for symptoms and signs of recurrence. Patients should be followed every 6 months with abdominal imaging (CT or MRI).

After a local recurrence has been identified, restaging is essential. If the metastatic evaluation is negative, re-excision of the recurrence is the treatment of choice. A complete resection rate of 44% has been reported for recurrent retroperitoneal sarcomas. Patients who underwent complete resection of local recurrences had a median survival of 48 months, compared with 15 months for unresectable recurrences[17].

Adjuvant chemotherapy for retroperitoneal tumors has not shown a survival benefit[9,11]. Although regiments with doxorubicin have been effective in extremity soft tissue sarcomas, the role of chemotherapy in primary retroperitoneal sarcomas has not been established[20].

The role of adjuvant external beam radiotherapy is controversial. While some reports suggest improved local control, other studies show no benefit[9,10,17,21,22]. Most studies have used doses of over 4000 rads to treat the retroperitoneum. At these doses, significant toxicity to the retroperitoneum and abdomen is recognized. Radiation enteritis occurs in up to 50% of patients. Other complications include radiation nephritis, ureteral stenosis, intraabdominal fistula and abscess formation[22]. Intraoperative radiotherapy (IORT) has also been used to treat retroperitoneal sarcomas. A prospective randomized trial by the National Cancer Institute compared IORT (2000 rads) with low-dose external beam therapy (3000–3500 rads) to high-dose external beam therapy (5000–5500 rads)[22]. No statistical significant difference in survival rates was found between the two groups, but the IORT group had significantly better local control and fewer gastrointestinal side effects. Unfortunately the IORT group did have an increased incidence of peripheral neuropathy; 33% of the patients had permanent weakness resulting in disability. Although retroperitoneal sarcomas may be radiosensitive, adjuvant radiotherapy has not yet been translated into a consistent survival advantage compared with surgery alone.

Retroperitoneal sarcomas most often metastasize to the lung and liver. Chemotherapeutic treatment of metastatic sarcoma with doxorubicin alone is as effective and has fewer side effects than combination chemotherapy with doxorubicin[23]. Overall, a 24% response rate was seen. Pulmonary metastatectomy has also been reported and pre-operative chemotherapy is recommended in these cases[24].

Retroperitoneal lymphoma

Retroperitoneal lymphoma accounts for nearly 25% of retroperitoneal tumors. Patients often present with constitutional symptoms and lymphadenopathy. Abdominal imaging may reveal a retroperitoneal mass and multiple enlarged lymph nodes. Although lymphoma is primarily a non-surgical disease, a tissue diagnosis may be required by open biopsy[25]. Hodgkin's lymphoma is generally treated with radiation therapy for limited stage disease, and chemotherapy for advanced stage disease. Some patients benefit from both treatment modalities. Non-Hodgkin's lymphomas are treated primarily by chemotherapy, with radiation used adjunctively in selected cases.

Treatment decisions for retroperitoneal tumors are based primarily on stage (see Algorithm).

Metastatic disease to the retroperitoneum and urological consequences

Metastatic disease in the retroperitoneum involving the genitourinary tract is rare. Most of the data on the subject have been compiled from post-mortem studies, the largest being MacLean and Fowler's review of 10 223 cases[26]. They found ureteral involvement by metastatic tumor in the retroperitoneum in only 0.38% of cases. In Abrams review of 1000 autopsies from patients with known carcinoma, he found ureteral involvement in 4.3% of cases[27]. Primary neoplasms from a variety of tissues may metastasize to the retroperitoneum, potentially causing serious urologic complications (Table 32.5).

Types of tumors

A variety of neoplasms have been reported to metastasize to the retroperitoneum. Secondary tumors in the retroperitoneum may involve the genitourinary system as follows: 1) metastatic malignancy in the periureteral lymph nodes and soft tissues, 2) metastatic malignancy in the ureteral wall, and 3) direct extension of pelvic malignancy to the retroperitoneum[28,29]. The pelvic organs are common sites

Table 32.5 Primary sites with potential extension or metastases to the retroperitoneum[28–30]

Genitourinary organs
Bladder
Cervix
Endometrium
Ovary
Prostate
Testis
Urethra
Uterus
Other organs
Breast
Colon
Gallbladder
Lung
Lymphoma
Melanoma
Pancreas
Rectum
Stomach

of primary neoplasms that involve the retroperitoneal structures, either by metastasis or by direct extension. Among the most common pelvic primary neoplasms are cancers of the cervix, prostate, bladder and ovary[29,30]. Excluding the pelvic organs, metastases from lymphomas and cancers of the breast, stomach, colon and lung are most common[28–31]. Primary tumors from many other sites have been reported including the pancreas, testicles, uterus, esophagus and gall bladder[28,29,31]. As would be expected, the histologic types of the metastatic lesions are those of the primary tumors, most commonly adenocarcinoma (60%) and squamous (16%) cell carcinoma[29].

Urologic manifestation of secondary retroperitoneal malignancy

The primary urologic manifestation of tumors in the retroperitoneum is ureteral obstruction. Metastatic tumor may involve any portion of the ureteral wall, and may cause mechanical luminal obstruction[29]. Hydronephrosis is common, occurring in over 70% of cases[28,29,31]. Ureteral obstruction may occur despite patent ureters, suggesting a functional impairment of the ureter by metastatic malignancies as well[33].

Ureteral involvement may be unilateral or bilateral, and occurs most frequently in the distal ureter[30]. When excluding tumors involving the ureters by direct extension, however, metastatic disease occurs with equal frequency in the upper, middle and lower portions of the ureters[29,32]. Over 90% of patients will have co-existent metastases to other organs and tissues at presentation of ureteral metastases[28,29].

Clinical presentation

Most patients with ureteral obstruction from retroperitoneal metastases present relatively soon after diagnosis of the primary tumor. In one series, 87% of patients required urinary diversion within 5 years of the diagnosis of the primary neoplasm. Sixty per cent required diversion in the first 2 years after diagnosis[34]. The clinical presentation of patients with genitourinary involvement by secondary malignancy may include symptomatology from the primary disease process, as well as urinary symptoms caused by ureteral obstruction. The most common genitourinary symptoms are flank or lumbar pain, occurring in up to 50% of patients[29,30]. This pain may be due to both ureteral colic and co-existing urinary tract infections that develop proximal to the obstruction, resulting in urosepsis[35]. Patients may also present with oliguria, anuria or symptoms of uremia, especially when both ureters or the lower urinary tract are involved[29,32]. When tumors involving the ureteral wall cause ulceration of the mucosa,

patients may present with gross hematuria[29,30]. Other reported symptoms include frequency, dysuria and incontinence[30–32] It is important to recognize, however, that a large proportion of patients with ureteral metastases are asymptomatic[28,30,31].

Although many patients with genitourinary involvement lack symptoms or suggestive physical findings, most patients will have laboratory abnormalities. Creatinine and blood urea nitrogen levels are frequently elevated, as are urinary protein levels on urinalysis[29–31]. Mucosal ulceration of the ureters leads to hematuria, which may be either gross or microscopic. Casts are often present in the urine, usually due to metastatic involvement of the kidney[31]. Urinalysis may reveal pyuria, and urine cultures are frequently positive, with *Escherichia coli* being the most common pathogen[30,31].

Diagnostic imaging

Ureteral obstruction due to metastatic disease may demonstrate a wide range of radiographic appearances depending on the level of obstruction, and the mechanism by which the tumor is causing obstruction. Several different diagnostic imaging methods are available to detect metastatic disease causing ureteral obstruction. Intravenous pyelography is a commonly utilized modality, and usually demonstrates some degree of hydronephrosis[32]. Antegrade or retrograde pyelography may be used to evaluate the ureteral obstruction. Imaging by CT scan allows visualization of the surrounding periureteral soft tissues, and provides localization of masses for needle biopsy. Metastatic disease in the retroperitoneum may appear as a well defined solitary mass, as an indistinct mass infiltrating retroperitoneal soft tissues, or it may resemble para-aortic lymphadenopathy. Using CT, over 90% of patients with ureteral obstruction secondary to metastatic disease will have identifiable masses at the point of obstruction that are amenable to percutaneous biopsy[35].

Other useful imaging modalities include lymphangiography and ultrasonography. Lymphangiography offers improved detection of metastatic disease in retroperitoneal lymph nodes over CT, especially in normal-sized nodes[36]. In a series of 96 patients with ovarian carcinoma in whom lymphangiography and lymph node biopsy were performed, lymphangiography demonstrated a sensitivity of 80.5% and a specificity of 100% in detecting retroperitoneal lymph node metastases[37]. Ultrasonography has also proven useful with a reported sensitivity of 76% for the detection of macroscopic retroperitoneal lymph node metastases. When used together, CT and ultrasound have a combined sensitivity of 90% for the detection of macroscopic lymph node metastases[38].

Treatment and prognosis

Surgical management

Transperitoneal midline incision with en bloc excision of tumor is the preferred approach in most cases. This approach allows inspection and removal of adjacent organs, such as the kidney, colon and spleen, if necessary. For this reason pre-operative bowel preparation is recommended. Although the entire tumor may not be resectable, aggressive debulking may relieve symptoms and improve response to adjuvant therapy. The margins of resection should be identified with surgical clips to guide the administration of post-operative radiation therapy. Long-term follow-up should be maintained because of high recurrence rates.

Secondary retroperitoneal tumor involvement occurs in two ways: 1) direct extension of an adjacent malignancy, or 2) metastases to retroperitoneal lymph nodes from breast, stomach, lung, pancreas, colon primaries and lymphoma. Tumors that directly extend into the retroperitoneum, such as those arising from the cervix, endometrium, bladder, prostate, sigmoid and rectum, usually compress the lower one-third of ureter. Metastases to retroperitoneal periureteral lymphatics tend to encase the ureter causing obstruction, displacement and angulation. Symptoms of retroperitoneal involvement may be masked by the primary tumor, but flank pain, sepsis and fever may be present. If both ureters are obstructed, the patient may develop oliguria/anuria, and azotemia. Progressive fibrosis may lead to obstruction of the vena cava or iliac veins causing thrombophlebitis. CT or MR imaging may aid in delineation of hydronephrosis.

The mainstay of treatment for ureteral obstruction secondary to metastatic malignancy in the retroperitoneum is palliative diversion. The decision to divert must be made with consideration of other factors including the patient's current clinical condition, age, previous history, the tumor grade and stage, and the prognosis[39,40].

Temporary and permanent diversion techniques are available. A ureteral stent is adequate for simple, temporary diversion. A nephrostomy tube may be placed if stenting is not feasible. Both stents and nephrostomy tubes will require periodic changes. If reversal of diversion is unlikely and the patient is a surgical candidate, permanent diversion with an ileal conduit or ureterostomy may be considered[40]. Intubated ureterotomy and transureteroureterostomy have also been performed, but with increased complications including urinary extravasation and sepsis[40].

Not surprisingly, the prognosis for patients with metastatic disease causing ureteral obstruction is poor. Of patients 40–55% who require urinary diversion will never leave the hospital, and most die within the first 6 months following the diagnosis of ureteral obstruction[32,34,39]. Still, some patients may survive for 2 years or more. Specifically, patients with metastatic prostate cancer tend to live longer following urinary diversion than patients with other primary tumor sources[34,39].

Retroperitoneal fibrosis

Retroperitoneal fibrosis is an inflammatory, fibrotic process that frequently produces ureteral obstruction. It is a rare condition with an estimated prevalence of one case per 200 000 people[41]. Grossly, retroperitoneal fibrosis appears as a dense grayish white plaque of fibrous tissue that is centered over the anterior surfaces of the fourth and fifth lumbar vertebrae, and extends to the aorta, vena cava and common iliac vessels[41,42]. The histologic appearance shows active chronic inflammation with lymphocytes, macrophages and plasma cells among a matrix of fibroblasts and collagen bundles. Later in the process, the tissue shows more scarring with fewer cells and tissue calcifications[43].

Two-thirds of the cases of retroperitoneal fibrosis are idiopathic[44]. Other causes include retroperitoneal injury, infections, pharmaceuticals and fibrosis associated with aortic aneurysms (Table 32.6)[45,46]. Retroperitoneal malignancy is an important cause, and accounts for approximately 8% of cases[44]. Malignancies most often associated with fibrosis include those that induce a strong desmoplastic response in the retroperitoneum. These include lymphomas, sarcomas, carcinoid tumors, and carcinomas of the breast, lung, stomach, colon, kidney, bladder, prostate and cervix[43].

Retroperitoneal fibrosis most commonly presents in the fifth or sixth decades of life, and shows a male to female ratio of 2–3 : 1[44,45]. The presenting signs and symptoms are often poorly localized and non-specific. The most common symptom is pain, either in the back, flank, or abdomen[44]. Patients may also present with general malaise, weight loss, vomiting, polydipsia and oliguria[42]. Physical examination may reveal an abdominal mass, hypertension, fever or peripheral edema. Laboratory abnormalities frequently include elevated blood urea nitrogen, creatinine, and erythrocyte sedimentation rate. Pyuria and positive urine cultures are often present[42,44,45].

Intravenous pyelography of patients with retroperitoneal fibrosis will show either unilateral or bilateral hydronephrosis in over 85% of cases[44]. Medial deviation of the ureters may be present. Another finding is smooth, extrinsic narrowing of the ureters near the lower lumbar vertebrae or upper sacrum[41]. CT or MRI may show a sheet of soft tissue surrounding the aorta, vena cava and ureters. It is important to realize, however, that CT cannot reliably distinguish benign fibrosis from fibrosis secondary to malignancy[48]. Additionally, if CT is used to guide needle

403

Table 32.6   Postulated causes of retroperitoneal fibrosis[41,42,44,47]

Malignancy
  Carcinoid tumors
  Periureteral metastatic disease
  Primary retroperitoneal tumor

Retroperitoneal injury
  Appendicitis
  Fat necrosis
  Hemorrhage
  Radiation
  Ragional enteritis
  Ruptured diverticulitis
  Surgery
  Trauma
  Urinary extravasation

Infectious agents
  Actinomycosis
  Brucellosis
  Genitourinary tract infection
  Histoplasmosis
  Tuberculosis

Pharmaceuticals
  Bromocriptine
  Lysergic acid
  Methysergide

Miscellaneous inflammation
  Aortitis
  Gerota's fasciitis
  Mesenteric panniculitis
  Pancreatic pseudocyst
  Sclerosing fibrosis
  Vasculitis
  Weber-Christian panniculitis

Idiopathic

Autoimmune

biopsy, it is important to note that false-negatives are commonly due to the wide dispersion of metastatic cells within the fibrous plaque[41]. Other imaging studies that may be useful in diagnosis include ultrasonography, lymphangiography, inferior vena cavography, and antegrade or retrograde pyelography[41,48].

Resolution of ureteral obstruction due to retroperitoneal fibrosis has been shown with steroid management[47], however surgical exploration with ureterolysis is required in most cases. A transabdominal approach through a midline incision is recommended since the process is usually bilateral. To expose the entire retroperitoneal area and both ureters simultaneously, the posterior peritoneum is incised between the duodenum and the inferior mesenteric vein. The fibrous tissue is sampled for frozen section. Ureterolysis begins with blunt dissection immediately adjacent to the ureteral adventitia. Bilateral dissection should be performed even in the case

of unilateral obstruction, because later involvement of the contralateral ureter is almost inevitable. After lysis, the ureters may be transplanted intraperitoneally, transposed laterally separated from the fibrosis by intervening retroperitoneal fat, or wrapped with omental fat. If the fibrotic process has invaded the ureter, resection of the affected segment with ureteroureterostomy may be necessary. Post-operative ureteral catheters are used. Satisfactory outcome is expected if pre-operative renal impairment is not severe, however close follow up is important to rule out progression or recurrence of disease. The ureteral catheters are usually removed in 4–6 weeks following a renal scan to ensure absence of obstruction. Following stent removal, a repeat renal scan or an ultrasound is obtained in 1–2 months to rule out hydronephrosis. Serum creatinine may be used to follow the patient in the long term.

The prognosis for patients with retroperitoneal fibrosis is variable. Occasionally, patients will have spontaneous resolution of ureteral obstruction[45]. Most patients, however, will require surgical or medical intervention. While the prognosis for patients with benign fibrosis may be favorable, the prognosis is poor for patients with malignant retroperitoneal fibrosis; few patients survive beyond 6 months[43]. Regular follow up with imaging studies such as IVP, CT scan, and renal scintigraphy is recommended[42].

References

1. Sittig KM, Rohr MS, Mcdonald JC. Abdominal wall, umbilicus, peritoneum, mesenteries, omentum, and retroperitoneum. In: Sabistion DC, Lyerly HK (eds) *Textbook of surgery* (15th edn). WB Saunders Co: Philadelphia, 1997, pp. 809–823.
2. Armstrong JR, Cohn I. Primary malignant retroperitoneal tumors. *Am J Surg* 1965;**110**:937–945.
3. Ackerman, LV. Atlas of tumor pathology. Section V. Fascicles 23 and 24: Tumors of the retroperitoneum, mesentery, and peritoneum. Washington DC, Armed Forces Institute of Pathology, 1954:12–13.
4. Pinson CW, ReMine SG, Fletcher WS *et al.* Long-term results with primary retroperitoneal tumors. *Arch Surg* 1989;**124**:1168–1173.
5. Bryant RL, Stevenson DR, Hunton DW *et al.* Primary malignant retroperitoneal tumors. *Am J Surg* 1982;**144**:646–649.
6. Serio G, Tenchini P, Nifosi, F *et al.* Surgical strategy in primary retroperitoneal tumors. *Br J Surg* 1989;**76**:385–389.
7. Wagenknecht LV, Schumpelick V, Winkler R. Urological aspects of primary retroperitoneal tumors. *Eur Urol* 1976;**2**:15–20.
8. Bland KI, McCoy DM, Kinard RE *et al.* Application of magnetic resonance imaging and computerized tomography as an adjunct to the surgical management of soft tissue sarcomas. *Ann Surg* 1987;**205**:473–481.
9. Storm FK, Mahvi DM. Diagnosis and management of retroperitoneal soft tissue sarcoma. *Ann Surg* 1991;**214**:2–10.
10. Heslin MJ, Lewis JJ, Nadler E *et al.* Prognostic factors associated with long term survival for retroperitoneal sarcoma: implications for management. *J Clin Onc* 1997;**15**:2832–2839.
11. Glenn J, Sindelar WF, Kinsella T *et al.* Results of multimodality therapy of resectable soft tissue sarcomas of the retroperitoneum. *Surgery* 1985;**97**:316–325.

12. Wingren G, Fredrikson M, Brage HN *et al.* Soft tissue sarcoma and occupational exposures. *Cancer* 1990;**66**:806.

13. Bailar JC. How dangerous is dioxin. *N Engl J Med* 1991;**324**:260–262.

14. Laskin WB, Silverman TA, Enzinger FM. Post radiation soft tissue sarcomas: an analysis of 53 cases. *Cancer* 1988;**62**:2330–2340.

15. Fleming ID, Cooper JS, Henson DE *et al. AJCC Cancer Staging Manual* (5th edn). Lippincott-Raven, Philadelphia, 1997, pp. 149–156.

16. Singer S, Corson JM, Demetri GD *et al.* Prognostic factors predictive of survival for truncal and retroperitoneal soft-tissue sarcoma. *Ann Surg* 1995;**221**:185–195.

17. Jaques DP, Coit DG, Hajdu SI *et al.* Management of primary and recurrent soft tissue sarcoma of the retroperitoneum. *Ann Surg* 1990;**212**:51–59.

18. Zornig C, Weh HJ, Krall A *et al.* Retroperitoneal sarcomas in a series of 51 adults. *Eur J Surg Onc* 1992;**18**:475–480.

19. Potter DA, Glenn J, Kinsella T *et al.* Patterns of recurrence in patients with high grade soft tissue sarcomas. *J Clin Onc* 1985;**3**:353–366.

20. Rosenberg SA, Tepper J, Glatstein E *et al.* Prospective randomized evaluation of adjuvant chemotherapy in adults with soft tissue sarcomas of the extremeties. *Cancer* 1983;**52**:424–434.

21. Bevilacqua RG, Rogatko A, Hajdu SI *et al.* Prognostic factors in primary retroperitoneal soft tissue sarcomas. *Arch Surg* 1991;**126**:328–334.

22. Sindelar WF, Kinsella TJ, Chen PW *et al.* Intraoperative radiotherapy in retroperitoneal sarcomas. *Arch Surg* 1993;**128**:402–410.

23. Santoro A, Tursz T, Mouridsen H *et al.* Doxorubicin versus CYVADIC versus doxorubicin plus ifosfamide in first line treatment of advanced soft tissue sarcomas: a randomized study of the European Organization for Research and Treatment of Cancer Soft Tissue and Bone Sarcoma group. *J Clin Onc* 1995;**13**:1537–1545.

24. Sondak K, Economou JS, Eilber FR. Soft tissue sarcomas of the extremity and retroperitoneum: advances in management. *Adv Surg* 1991;**24**:333–359.

25. Eyre HJ, Farver ML. Hodgkin's disease and non-Hodgkin's lymphomas. In: Holleb AI, Fink DJ, Murphy GP (eds) American Cancer Society Textbook of Clinical Oncology, Atlanta, 1991:377–396.

26. MacLean JT, Fowler VB. Pathology of tumors of the renal pelvis and ureter. *J Urol* 1956;**75**:384–414.

27. Abrams HL, Spiro R, Goldstein N. Metastases in carcinoma – analysis of 1000 autopsied cases. *Cancer* 1950;**3**:74–84.

28. Cohen WM, Freed SZ, Hasson J. Metastatic cancer to the ureter: a review of the literature and case presentations. *J Urol* 1974;**112**:188–189.

29. Presman D, Ehrlich L. Metastatic tumors of the ureter. *J Urol* 1948;**59**:312–325.

30. Richie JP, Withers G, Ehrlich RM. Ureteral obstruction secondary to metastatic tumors. *Surg Gyn Obstet* 1979;**148**:355–357.

31. Klinger ME. Secondary tumors of the genito-urinary tract. *J Urol* 1951;**65**(1):144–153.

32. Grabstald H, Kaufman R. Hydronephrosis secondary to ureteral obstruction by metastatic breast cancer. *J Urol* 1969;**102**:569–576.

33. Kay RG. Metastatic malignant, functional, post-renal anuria. *Br J Urol* 1962;**34**:194–199.

34. Brin EN, Schiff M Jr, Weiss RM. Palliative urinary diversion for pelvic malignancy. *J Urol* 1975;**113**:619–622.

35. Megibow AJ, Mitnick JS, Bosniak MA. The contribution of computed tomography to the evaluation of the obstructed ureter. *Uro Rad* 1982;**4**:95–104.

36. Jing B, Wallace S, Zornoza J. Metastases to retroperitoneal and pelvic lymph nodes – computed tomography and lymphangiography. *Rad Clin N Amer* 1982;**20**(3):511–530.

37. Musumeci R, De Palo G, Kenda R *et al.* Retroperitoneal metastases from ovarian carcinoma: reassessment of 365 patients studied with lymphography. *Am J Rad* 1980;**134**:449–452.

38. Damgaard-Pedersen K, Von der Maase H. Ultrasound and ultrasound guided biopsy, CT and lymphography in the diagnosis of retroperitoneal metastases in testicular cancer. *Scan J Urol Nephr* 1991;**137**:139–144.

39. Chisholm GD, Shackman R. Malignant obstructive uraemia. *Br J Urol* 1968;**40**:720–726.

40. Sharer W, Grayhack JT, Graham J. Palliative urinary diversion for malignant ureteral obstruction. *J Urol* 1978;**120**:162–164.

41. Amis ES Jr. Retroperitoneal fibrosis. *Am J Rad* 1991;**157**:321–329.

42. Higgins PM, Aber GM. Idiopathic retroperitoneal fibrosis – an update. *Digestive Dis* 1990;**8**:206–222.

43. Kottra JJ, Dunnick NR. Retroperitoneal fibrosis. *Rad Clin N Amer* 1996;**34**(6):1259–1275.

44. Koep L, Zuidema GD. The clinical significance of retroperitoneal fibrosis. *Surg* 1977;**81**(3):250–257.

45. Lepor H, Walsh PC. Idiopathic retroperitoneal fibrosis. *J Urol* 1979;**122**:1–6.

46. Rault R, Kapoor W, Kam W. Perianeurysmal fibrosis and ureteric obstruction: case report and review of literature. *Clin Nephr* 1982;**18**(3):159–162.

47. Talner LB. Specific causes of obstruction. In Pollack HM (Ed.) *Clinical Urography – An Atlas and Textbook of Urological Imaging.* Philadelphia, W. B. Saunders Company, 1990, pp. 1665–1675.

48. Tiptoft RC, Costello AJ, Paris AMI, Blandy JP. The long-term follow up of Idiopathic retroperitoneal fibrosis. *Br J Urol* 1982;**54**:620–624.

Pathology of adrenal and retroperitoneal tumors

D J M DiMaio

Tumors of the adrenal cortex

One of the side effects of computerized tomography (CT) has been the incidental detection of masses in the adrenal gland. Adrenal gland lesions have been detected in 0.4% to 4.3% of patients who underwent CT scanning for reasons other than suspected adrenal disease[1]. In large autopsy studies of patients dying without pre-mortem suspicion of adrenal disease, masses have been found in 1.4% to 8.7% of the cases. The vast majority of masses in the adrenal gland are benign, a fact to keep in mind when discussing the adrenal gland[1].

Adenoma

The most commonly encountered mass in the adrenal cortex is the adenoma. Autopsy studies have found adenomas in 2% to 9% of the population[2]. Clinically detected adenomas have been discovered in patients ranging from 31 to 71 years old (mean 58)[3]. Adenomas may range in size from 1 to 9 cm with 90% 2 to 5 cm in maximum diameter[2]. Upon gross examination, adenomas have a yellow fleshy color due to the presence of lipid[4]. Microscopically, adenomas are either encapsulated or pseudoencapsulated with the cells typically arranged in small nests. The majority of the cells have clear or foamy cytoplasms due to the presence of abundant lipids (Figure 33.1). Mitotic figures are rare and tumor necrosis extremely uncommon[3]. Some cytologic atypia may be seen[4]. The histologic distinction between an adenoma and adenocarcinoma can be very difficult at times and will be discussed subsequently.

Clinically, adenomas can be divided into functional (they respond to feedback inhibition) and non-functional (they do not respond to feedback inhibition). Histologically, however, both types look the same. Functional adenomas can produce clinical syndromes such as Conn's syndrome, Cushing's syndrome, virilization or feminization. It sometimes can be difficult to distinguish a functional adenoma from cortical nodular hyperplasia, especially if one of the nodules in cortical nodular hyperplasia becomes much larger then the rest[4]. Both processes may look identical microscopically. Because of its excess corticosteroid secretion a functional adenoma will present with bilateral atrophy of the residual adrenal cortex while cortical nodule hyperplasia will present with bilaterally diffuse nodularity.

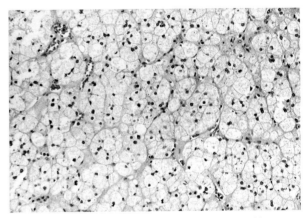

Fig. 33.1 Cortical adenomas are composed of cells with abundant clear foamy cytoplasm. The nuclei are small and lack significant atypia. Thin bands of fibrosis separate the cells into nests (hematoxlyin and eosin, 200 ×).

Adenocarcinoma

The most important differential diagnosis of an adenoma is cortical adenocarcinoma. Cortical carcinomas represents 5% of all adrenal neoplasms[2]. Differentiating a cortical carcinoma from an adenoma can be difficult. There are, however, certain clinical, gross and microscopic findings which in combination with each other help to distinguish the vast majority of carcinomas from adenomas.

Patients with carcinoma tend to be younger (median 41 years, range 5 months to 66 years) than those with adenomas[3]. Carcinomas occur slightly more often in the left adrenal gland (53%) and are rarely bilateral (2% to 4%)[5,6]. They tend to be larger than adenomas with 90% of adenomas between 2 and 5 cm and 80% of carcinomas greater than 6 cm[2]. The difference in size can be utilized predominately to differentiate between adenomas and carcinomas. One study, using a 5 cm cut-off for adenomas, provided a 93% sensitivity and a 64% specificity for distinguishing between an adenoma and a carcinoma[1].

Histologically, the cells in carcinoma tend to have eosinophilic cytoplasm and be arranged in either solid sheets or a trabecular pattern. In contrast cells in adenomas have abundant clear foamy cytoplasm and are arranged in small nests. Carcinomas also tend to have more mitotic figures (>4 per 10 high power field) than adenomas (<2 per 10 high power field)[3]. One study showed a correlation between mitotic rate and clinical outcome in patients with carcinoma. Patients whose tumors had a mitotic rate of greater than 20 per 10 high power fields were disease free for 14 months. In comparison, those patients with a mitotic rate of less than 20 per 10 high power field were disease free for 58 months[7]. The presence of tumor necrosis is common in carcinomas and extremely rare in adenomas[3,7]. Other features that may be seen in carcinomas to help distinguish them from adenomas include prominent nuclear atypia, vascular and capsular invasion[6,7].

Like adenomas, carcinomas may be functional or nonfunctional. They may secrete glucocorticoids, androgens, mineralocorticoids and estrogens. Functional tumors are more common in women (70%) than men (40%) and more often in patients under 30 years (84.7%)[5]. The func-

tional status has little effect on survival, however[6,7]. At time of diagnosis, up to 50% of patients may have metastatic disease. The most common metastatic sites include the liver, local lymph nodes, bone and lung[8]. Five and 10 year survival is 30% and 10%, respectively, with 50% of patients dead in less than 2 years[6].

Myelolipoma

Myelolipomas are rare benign tumors that may occur in either the adrenal cortex or the medulla. Their prevalence is 0.08% to 0.2%[9]. While most myelolipomas range in size from 2 to 9 cm they have been reported up to 34 cm in diameter[10]. They typically present in the fifth to sixth decade of life[11]. They are composed of mature adipose cells and scattered islands of hematopoietic cells (myeloid tissue). The ratio of adipose tissue to myeloid tissue varies. Although the origin of these tumors is unknown, the most widely accepted theory is that they are a result of metaplasia of the reticuloendothelial cells of the capillaries in response to a stimulus such as necrosis, infection or stress[11]. High ACTH levels may also play a role in their pathogenesis[12].

Neuroblastic tumors

There are three types of neuroblastic tumors: neuroblastomas, ganglioneuroblastomas and ganglioneuromas[13]. The main difference between these three tumors lies in the amount of immature (neuroblasts) and mature (ganglions) neural elements present. Neuroblastomas are almost exclusively composed of neuroblasts with only a minimal amount of ganglioneuromatous element (ganglion and Schwann cells): ganglioneuroblastomas of more than a 50% ganglioneuromatous element and ganglioneuromas exclusively of a ganglioneuromatous element with no neuroblasts present[14]. Both neuroblastomas and ganglioneuroblastomas have been further subdivided based upon the distribution of the mature and immature components (Table 33.1).

The median age of presentation of neuroblastomas is 2 years with 90% presenting at less than 5 years. They are the most common extracranial neoplasm of children re-

Table 33.1 Classification of Neuroblastomas and ganglioneuroblastomas

Neuroblastomas	
Undifferentiated NB[1]	Only neuroblasts present
Poorly differentiated NB	Neuroblasts with occasional diffusely scattered ganglion/Schwann cells
Differentiating NB	Neuroblasts with a well defined nodule of ganglions/Schwann cells
Ganglioneuroblastomas	
Nodular GNB[2]	>50% ganglioneuromatous element with rare discrete nodules of neuroblasts
Intermixed GNB	Predominantly ganglioneuromatous elements with mixture of neuroblasts
Borderline GNB	Almost exclusively ganglioneuromatous elements with rare neuroblasts

[1] NB Neuroblastoma. [2] GNB Ganglioneuroblastoma.

presenting 8% of pediatric malignancies[15]. Neuroblastomas are circumscribed tumors that may range in size from microscopic nodules in the adrenal gland to large tumors filling the abdominal cavity. They are gray-white with areas of necrosis, hemorrhage and small cyst formation[4]. Microscopically, neuroblastomas are composed of sheets of neuroblasts with very little cytoplasm and round hyperchromatic nuclei (Figure 33.2). As the tumor becomes more differentiated, the cellularity decreases and the amount of extracellular matrix increases. The matrix is composed of eosinophilic nerve fibers. Approximately 30% of neuroblastomas will have Homer-Wright rosettes[4]. These rosettes are neuroblasts arranged in a ring with the center of the ring filled with eosinophilic nerve fibers. Occasionally ganglion cells may be seen. Ganglion cells are much larger then neuroblasts and have abundant eosinophilic cytoplasm, a vesicular nucleus and a prominent nucleoli. As neural tumors mature they take on more of the histologic features of ganglion cells and less of those of neuroblasts. At the time of diagnosis, 66% of the patients will have metastatic disease[15]. The most common metastatic sites include bone, lymph nodes and liver[4]. Cytogenetic testing of the tumor for the number of copies of the oncogene N-myc can be helpful in predicting the behavior of the tumor. Patients with tumors that have greater than 10 copies of the oncogene have a worse prognosis[15].

Ganglioneuroblastomas usually present before 10 years of age. Their gross appearance can resemble a neuroblastoma. Histologically they differ from neuroblastomas by having more mature neural elements present and only a small number of neuroblasts. Clinically these are localized tumors with a more favorable prognosis than that of a neuroblastoma[14].

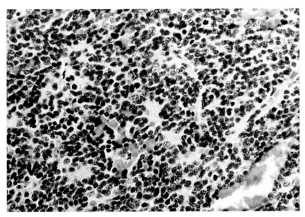

Fig. 33.2 Neuroblastomas are composed of cells with uniform hyperchromatic nuclei and minimal cytoplasm. The tumor is hypercellular. Some of the neuroblasts are arranged in rings (Homer-Wright rosettes) with central eosinophilic nerve fibers (hematoxlyin and eosin, 200×)

Ganglioneuromas are benign well circumscribed tumors typically found in children older than those with neuroblastomas. Ganglioneuromas are composed of ganglion cells and Schwann cells and contain no neuroblasts.

Pheochromocytoma

Pheochromocytomas are rare tumors of the adrenal medulla that typically present between 25 to 55 years of age[16]. While the majority of pheochromocytomas are sporadic in origin, approximately 10% are associated with syndromes such as multiple endocrine neoplasms Type 2a and 2b, neurofibromatosis, von Hippel-Lindau disease and cerebellar hemangioblastomas[16–18]. Those occurring in patients with a familial syndrome tend to occur at a younger age and are more often bilateral than those seen in non-familial (sporadic) cases[16]. Pheochromocytomas are well circumscribed tumors that vary from gray to red with areas of hemorrhage, cyst formation and calcifications seen in larger tumors.

One of the major problems in dealing with a pheochromocytoma is in determining whether it will behave in a benign or malignant fashion. Except for the presence of metastatic disease, there are no reliable gross or microscopic findings that can distinguish between a benign and a malignant pheochromocytoma. Malignant pheochromocytomas make up only 2% to 8% of all pheochromocytomas[19,20]. When located outside the adrenal gland, where they are typically referred to as paragangliomas, the incidence of malignancy increases to 30%[19].

In a study of 60 cases, benign pheochromocytomas had a mean weight of 156.5 g; malignant pheochromocytomas had a mean weight of 759 g (range 35 to 2700 g)[18]. One gross finding that has been associated with malignancy is a coarse nodularity of the primary tumor[21]. Histologically, pheochromocytomas (both benign and malignant) are typically composed of large cells with acidophilic to basophilic granular cytoplasm. The cells may be small and even spindled at times, though tumors with numerous small cells are more likely to be malignant than those with large cells[16]. The cells may be arranged in a variety of architectural patterns including alveolar (Zellballen), trabecular and diffuse sheets of cells. Although the alveolar pattern is the most common, a mixture of patterns may exist in any one tumor. Nuclear and cellular pleomorphism is common and should not be used as an indicator of malignancy. Intracytoplasmic and extracytoplasmic hyaline globules are commonly seen in benign tumors and less in malignant tumors[21]. The presence of large areas of tumor necrosis is more often seen in malignant tumors. Less helpful features used to differentiate benign from malignant pheochromocytomas include increased mitotic rate, capsular and vascular invasion. The 5 year survival for malignant pheochromocytomas is 25%[22].

Retroperitoneal tumors

Primary retroperitoneal tumors are extremely rare neoplasms that represent only 0.1% to 0.3% of all tumors[23–25]. Their rate of malignancy ranges from 70% to 90%[25–27]. Primary retroperitoneal tumors are defined as those tumors originating in the retroperitoneal space other than a tumor of the kidney, ureter, pancreas or adrenal gland. Malignant tumors of the retroperitoneum can arise from tissue of mesodermal (75%) or neuroectodermal origin (24%) or from embryonic remnants (1%)[28]. While primary lymphomas of the retroperitoneum do exist, most retroperitoneal lymphomas represent a systemic disease and as such will not be discussed in this chapter[29]. A list of both benign and malignant tumors seen in the retroperitoneum is provided in Table 33.2.

Retroperitoneal sarcomas

While interesting from an academic point of view, the histologic type of sarcoma, size of the tumor and the gender of the patient are generally not helpful in predicting a patient's outcome[30–32]. The variables that have been associated with death from disease are metastases, high-grade tumors and T3 tumors[30]. Tumor grade is one of the strongest predictors of long-term survival and is typically divided into three grades (1 through 3) corresponding to well, moderate or poorly differentiated. Histologic criteria used in the grading of sarcomas include the degree of cellularity, cellular pleomorphism, mitotic activity and extent of necrosis. The more cellularity, pleomorphism, mitotic activity or necrosis that exists, the higher the grade of the sarcoma[33]. Some sarcomas, such as angiosarcomas and synovial cell sarcoma, are automatically high-grade (Grade 3) neoplasms. Retroperitoneal sarcomas

Table 33.2   Retroperitored tumors

Benign retroperitoneal tumors
Lipoma
Schwannoma
Ganglioneuroma
Paraganglioma

Malignant retroperitoneal tumors
Liposarcoma
Leiomyosarcoma
Malignant fibrous histiocytoma
Malignant peripheral nerve sheath tumor
Neuroblastoma/ganglioneuroblastoma
Paraganglioma
Rhabdomyosarcoma
Angiosarcoma
Fibrosarcoma
Hemangiopericytoma
Germ cell tumors
Lymphoma
Synovial sarcoma
Mesothelioma

generally present between the fifth and sixth decades of life[33–34]. They tend to be locally aggressive neoplasms that spread along fascial planes and vessels for long distances. By compressing surrounding structures and causing local tissue reaction they give the false impression of being encapsulated. They typically metastasize via blood vessels to the lung (30–56%), liver (22–56%), bladder (18–19%) and bone (10%)[28].

The incidence of certain types of sarcomas has been changing over the past 20 years. With advances in immunohistochemistry and the recognition of new entities, such as malignant fibrous histiocytomas and malignant peripheral nerve sheath tumors, once commonly diagnosed tumors such as fibrosarcomas are rare. For these reasons, it is difficult to determine the true percentage of various retroperitoneal sarcomas. The most common malignant retroperitoneal neoplasms, however, are most likely liposarcomas, leiomyosarcomas and malignant fibrous histiocytomas[35].

Liposarcoma

In most studies, liposarcomas are the most common retroperitoneal sarcomas[28,29,34]. They are typically larger than other sarcomas at the time of diagnosis with an average diameter of 20 cm[36]. Their variable gross appearance is a reflection of their variable histologic subtypes. They may range from resembling a typical lipoma (well differentiated liposarcoma) to being gray-white and slimy (myxoid). There are five histologic subtypes of liposarcoma: well differentiated; myxoid; round cell; de-differentiated and pleomorphic liposarcoma. The one thing that all five subtypes have in common is the presence of lipoblasts. Lipoblasts are pleomorphic cells with hyperchromatic irregular nuclei and a vacuolated cytoplasm (Figure 33.3). The well differentiated

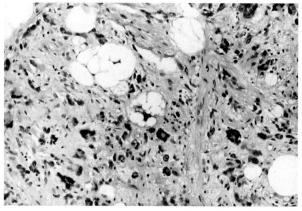

Fig. 33.3   This pleomorphic liposarcoma is composed of cells with prominent nuclear atypia. In the center of the picture is a lipoblast. The presence of lipid droplets in the cytoplasm is causing scalloping of the nucleus (hematoxlyin and eosin, 200 ×).

variant may resemble a lipoma with scattered lipoblasts or there may be prominent areas of inflammation or fibrosis. The myxoid type has an abundant myxoid background and a prominent plexiform network of capillaries. The round cell variant has numerous small rounded cells with vesicular nuclei and a high nuclear to cytoplasmic ratio. Histologically they may resemble lymphoma. The pleomorphic variant is composed of extremely atypical and bizarre cells. Finally, the de-differentiated variant is characterized by the presence of both a well differentiated and a poorly differentiated component in the same tumor or in the primary and the recurrent tumor. The well differentiated and the pleomorphic subtypes are the most common in the retroperitoneum. The round cell and the pleomorphic variants, however, are the most aggressive and are associated with a worse prognosis[35].

Leiomyosarcoma

Almost all tumors of smooth muscle origin in the retroperitoneum are malignant. They occur more often in females and have an average diameter of 11 cm[36]. Grossly they are white-gray with occasional areas of hemorrhage and necrosis. The typical cell is spindled shaped with a centrally placed 'cigar shaped' nucleus and prominent eosinophilic cytoplasm. As the tumor becomes less well differentiated, the nuclear to cytoplasmic ratio increases and the nucleus becomes more atypical and hyperchromatic. Multinucleated giant cells are common (Figure 33.4). Features of malignancy include significant mitotic activity, nuclear atypia, vascular invasion and necrosis.

Malignant fibrous histiocytoma

Malignant fibrous histiocytomas are relatively newly described entities and, as such, are not even listed in many of the older papers reviewing the types of retroperitoneal neoplasms. In more recent reviews, however, they are listed as one of the more common types of retroperitoneal tumors[35,36]. In the retroperitoneum, they predominantly occur in older men (mean age 64 years)[36]. There are four histologic subtypes of malignant fibrous histiocytomas: storiform-pleomorphic; myxoid; giant cell and inflammatory[37]. The storiform-pleomorphic type has atypical spindle cells arranged in a cartwheel or storiform pattern. In other areas, bizarre pleomorphic giant cells with abundant cytoplasm are present. In the myxoid variant, over 50% of the tumor appears myxoid while the remainder may resemble the storiform-pleomorphic variant. In the giant cell variant, dense bands of fibrosis surround islands of fibroblasts, histiocytes and osteoclast type giant cells. The inflammatory subtype is composed histiocytes containing abundant lipid. The histiocytes range from bland to highly atypical with enlarged pleomorphic nuclei. A prominent acute and chronic inflammatory infiltrate is also present. The inflammatory subtype is the most common in the retroperitoneum.

Miscellaneous retroperitoneal tumors

Numerous other types of tumors arise in the retroperitoneum and are listed in Table 33.2. Malignant peripheral nerve sheath tumor is the new name applied to tumors previously listed as neurofibrosarcoma or malignant schwannoma. All types of germ cell tumors can also occur as primary retroperitoneal tumors. Histologically they resemble those seen in the testicle[38–39]. Tumors described occurring as primary adrenal neoplasms such as neuroblastomas and paragangliomas (pheochromocytomas) also occur as primary retroperitoneal tumors. While retroperitoneal tumors are uncommon, the differential diagnosis for a retroperitoneal mass can be long and complicated.

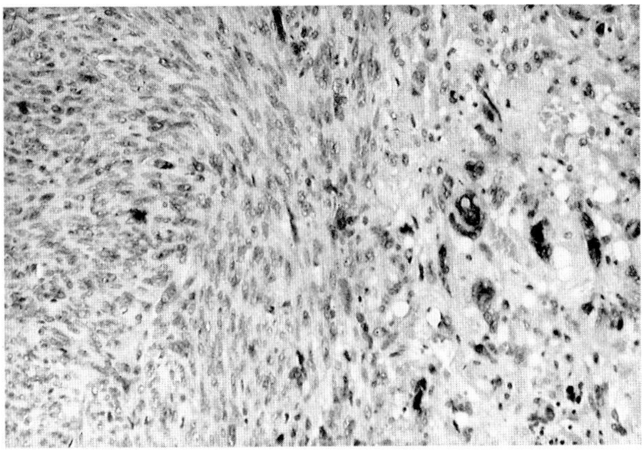

Fig. 33.4 This leiomyosarcoma has typical areas of spindle cells with cigar shaped nuclei adjacent to areas of prominent nuclear atypia (hematoxlyin and eosin, 200 ×).

References

1. Terzolo M, Ali A, Osella G, Mazza E. Prevalence of adrenal carcinoma among incidental discovered adrenal masses. *Arch Surg* 1997;**132**:914–919.
2. Roubidoux M, Dunnick NR. Adrenal cortical tumors. *Bull NY Acad Med* 1991;**67**:119–130.
3. Evans HL, Vassilopoulou-Sellin R. Adrenal cortical neoplasms: a study of 56 cases. *AMJ Clin Path* 1996;**105**:76–86.
4. Silverman ML, Lee AK. Anatomy and pathology of the adrenal gland. *Urol Clin North Am* 1989;**16**:417–432.
5. Wooten MD, King DK. Adrenal cortical carcinoma: epidemiology and treatment with mitotane and a review of the literature. *Cancer* 1993;**72**:3145–3155.
6. Samaan NA, Hickey RC. Adrenal cortical carcinoma. *Semin Oncol* 1987;**14**:292–296.
7. Medeiros LJ, Weiss LM. New development in the pathologic diagnosis of adrenal cortical neoplasms. *Am J Clin Path* 1992;**97**:73–83.
8. Zografos GC, Driscoll DL, Kapakousis CP, Huben RP. Adrenal adenocarcinoma: a review of 53 cases. *J Surg Oncol* 1994;**55**:160–164.
9. Dieckmann KP, Hamm B, Pickartz H. Adrenal myelolipoma: clinical, radiologic, and histologic features. *Urology.* 1987;**29**:1–8.

411

10. Bayram F, Atasoy KC, Yalcin B, Salih M, Hekimoglu K, Uysal AR, Evcik E. Adrenal myelipoma: case report with a review of the literature. *Aus Radiol* 1996;**40**:68–71.
11. Copher JC, Souza JW, Erickson DJ, Dalton ML, Rogers JJ. Myelolipoma of the adrenal gland: a case report. *South Med J* 1995;**88**:635–638.
12. Umpierrez MB, Fackler S, Umpierrez GE, Rubin J. Adrenal myelolipoma associated with endocrine dysfunction: review of the literature. *Am J Med Sci* 1997;**314**:338–341.
13. Joshi VV, Silverman JF. Pathology of neuroblastic tumors. *Semin Diagn Pathol* 1994;**11**:107–117.
14. Joshi VV, Cantor AB, Altshuler G *et al*. Conventional versus modified morphologic criteria for ganglioneuroblastoma: a review of cases from the pediatric oncology group. *Arch Pathol Lab Med* 1996;**120**:859–865.
15. Abramson SJ. Adrenal neoplasms in children. *Radiol Clin North Am* 1997;**35**:1415–1453.
16. Capella C, Riva C, Cornaggia M, Chiaravalli AM, Frigerio B. Histopathology, cytology and cytochemistry of pheochromocytomas and paragangliomas including chemodectomas. *Path Res Pract* 1988;**183**:176–187.
17. Lamovec J, Frkovic-Grazio S, Bracko M. Nonsporadic cases and unusual morphological features in pheochromocytoma and paraganglioma. *Arch Pathol Lab Med* 1998;**122**:63–68.
18. Medeiros LJ, Wolf BC, Balogh K, Federman M. Adrenal pheochromocytomas: a clinicopathological review of 60 cases. *Hum Pathol* 1985;**16**:580–589.
19. Melicow MM. One hundred cases of pheochromocytoma (107 tumors) at the Columbia-Presbyterian Medical Center 1926–1976: a clinicopathological analysis. *Cancer* 1977;**40**:1987–2004.
20. van Heerden JA, Sheps SG, Hamberger B *et al*. Pheochromocytoma: current status and changing trends. *Surgery* 1982;**91**:367–373.
21. Linnoila RI, Keiser HR, Steinberg SM, Lack EE. Histopathology of benign versus malignant sympathoadrenal paragangliomas: clinicopathologic study of 120 cases including unusual histologic features. *Hum Pathol* 1990;**21**:1168–1180.
22. Goldfarb DA. Surgical adrenal disorders. *Semin Nephrol* 1994;**14**:570–579.
23. Pack GT, Tabah GJ. Primary retroperitoneal tumors: a study of 120 cases. *Surg Gynecol Obstet* 1954;**99**:209–231.
24. Bek V. Primary retroperitoneal tumors. *Neoplasma* 1970;**17**:253–263.
25. Wagenknecht LV, Schumpelick V, Winkler R. Urologic aspects of primary retroperitoneal tumors. *Eur Urol* 1976;**2**:15–20.
26. Scanlan DB. Primary retroperitoneal tumors. *J Urol* 1959;**81**:740–745.
27. Braasch JW, Mon AB. Primary retroperitoneal tumor. *Surg Clin North Am* 1967;**47**:3.
28. Van Dam PA, Lowe DG, McKenzie-Gray B, Shepherd JH. Retroperitoneal soft tissue sarcomas: a review of the literature. *Obstet Gynecol Surv* 1990;**45**:670–682.
29. Felix E, Wood DK, Das Gupta TK. Tumors of the retroperitoneum. *Curr Probl Cancer* 1981;**6**:1–47.
30. Dalton RR, Donohue JH, Mucha P *et al*. Management of retroperitoneal sarcomas. *Surgery* 1989;**106**:725–733.
31. Jaques DP, Coit DG, Hajdu SI, Brennan MF. Management of primary and recurrent soft tissue sarcoma of the retroperitoneum. *Ann Surg* 1990;**212**:51–59.
32. Bevilacqua RG, Rogatko A, Hajdu SI, Brennan MF. Prognostic factors in preimary retroperitoneal soft tissue sarcomas. *Arch Surg* 1991;**126**:328–334.
33. McGrath PC. Retroperitoneal sarcomas. *Semin Surg Oncol* 1994;**10**:364–368.
34. Storm FK, Mahvi DM. Diagnosis and management of retroperitoneal soft tissue sarcoma. *Ann Surg* 1991;**214**:2–10.
35. Engelken JD, Ros PR. Retroperitoneal MR Imaging. *MRI Clin North Am* 1997;**5**:165–178.
36. Lane RH, Stephens DH, Reiman HM. Primary retroperitoneal neoplasms: CT findings in 90 cases with clinical and pathologic correlation. *AJR* 1989;**152**:83–89.
37. Enzinger FM. Malignant fibrous histiocytoma 20 years after Stout. *Am J Surg Pathol* 1986;**10**:43.
38. Hainsworth JD, Greco FA. Extragonadal germ cell tumors and unrecognized germ cell tumors. *Semin Oncol* 1992;**19**:119–127.
39. Choyke PL, Hayes WS, Sesterhenn IA. Primary extragonadal germ cell tumors of the retroperitoneum: differentiation of primary and secondary tumors. *Radiographics* 1993;**13**:1365–1375.

PART FOUR
Testicular cancer

Chapter 34
Incidence, etiology, epidemiology and genetics

Chapter 35
Pathology

Chapter 36
Presentation, diagnosis and staging

Chapter 37
Carcinoma in situ

Chapter 38
Non-seminomatous germ-cell tumors

38.1 Germ cell tumors: surveillance and adjuvant chemotherapy

38.2 Surgical treatment in retroperoperitoneal lymphadenectomy

38.3 Practical approaches to use of chemotherapy

Chapter 39
Seminomatious germ cell tumor

39.1 Treatment of seminomas

39.2 Radiotherapy

39.3 Background, rationale and results from use of chemotherapy in metastatic and localized seminoma

Chapter 40
Non-germ cell testicular tumors

34 Incidence, etiology, epidemiology and genetics

A Heidenreich and J W Moul

Incidence

Although testicular cancer accounts for only about 1% of all human neoplasms, it is the most common malignancy among white males in the age group of 15 to 45 years and accounts for approximately 23% of all cancers in this group[1]. Ninety per cent to 95% of testicular tumors are malignant germ cell tumors; the other 5% to 10% represent a heterogeneous group of malignant and benign tumors derived from the interstitium or representing metastases from different primaries[2]. It is estimated that 6000 new cases of testicular germ cell tumors have been diagnosed in 1993 and approximately 350 deaths related to testicular cancer have been reported in 1993[3]. The life time probability of developing testicular cancer is approximately 0.2% and 0.4% in whites and it is significantly lower in blacks[1].

Annual age standardized incidence rates of testicular germ cell tumors for American white males was 4.1 per 100 000 from 1979 to 1981 which was more than twice as much as the rate of 2.0 per 100 000 from 1937 to 1939[1,4]. The average age adjusted incidence rate among blacks, however, remained unchanged during the last 50 years with 0.9 per 100 000 from 1937 to 1939 and 0.8 per 100 000 from 1979 to 1981[1,4].

Despite the rising incidence rates the age-adjusted mortality rates decreased significantly during the last 20 years. Age-adjusted mortality rates for males 15 to 44 years of age was similar for the time periods 1950 to 1954 and 1970 and 1974 with a rate of 1.3 and 1.4 per 100 000 and year, respectively. However, mortality rates decreased significantly to 1.0 per 100 000 from 1975 to 1979[1,4]; decline of mortality rates reflects the introduction of cisplatin to chemotherapeutic regimens thereby achieving overall cure rates, even in advanced disease, of approximately 80%[7]. Mortality rates did not differ significantly among black and white patients[4].

Similar diverging trends in incidence and mortality of testicular cancer have been noted in the white population of central and northern Europe, especially in Denmark where age-adjusted incidence rose from 3.1 per 100 000 from 1943 to 1947 to 8.0 per 100 000 from 1978 to 1982[6]. Data collected by Schottenfeld *et al.*[4] demonstrate a wide variability of age-adjusted incidence rates of adult germ cell tumors among the world population. Average incidences are highest in Denmark, Norway and Germany; it is intermediate in the United States and Great Britain and incidence rates are lowest in Africa, Japan and China.

Testicular germ cell tumors in children are even more rare than adult germ cell tumors. The age-adjusted incidence rate is approximately 0.5 to 2.0 per 100 000 children and has remained stable during the last 50 years. Interestingly, pediatric germ cell tumors do not reveal racial differences in incidence rates as adult tumors do[8].

Age

A small peak in the incidence is noted for males under the age of 5 years, followed by a significant decline to 0.1 for children of age 5 to 14 years[1,4,5]. The peak incidence occurs between 15 and 44 years of age with men between 25 and 34 years demonstrating the apex of the peak. Age-adjusted incidence in this group is as high as 11.6 per 100 000. In men between 45 and 60 years of age incidence declines before a new peak develops in men over the age of 60 years[4,5].

Increase of annual incidence rates has been shown to vary between different age groups. No increase has occurred in children (0–14 years) and in adults older than 65 years; however, a fourfold increase has been observed in young adults between 15 and 24 years and a twofold increase was reported for men between 25 and 64 years of age since 1943.

Rise in incidence did not affect seminomas and non-seminomatous germ cell tumors to the same degree as could be demonstrated by Osterlind[6]: over a 40 year period seminomas accounted for about 52% whereas the percentage of NSGCT rose from 33% to 44%. Since the incidence of unspecified testicular tumors decreased during the same time period, the rise in incidence of NSGCT is probably an epidemiologic epiphenomenon and does represent a true increase in incidence.

Racial differences

Incidence rates for testicular cancer vary significantly between different ethnical groups even within the same geographic regions[1,4,5]. Highest incidence rate have been described for Scandinavia, Germany and Switzerland (4.1 per 100 000) whereas blacks, with the exception of New Zealand Maori, show the lowest incidence rates (0.8 per 100 000) independent of the geographic area they are living in; Chinese and Japanese men have slightly higher annual incidence rates (1.0 per 100 000) than black Americans, but still significantly lower rates than whites. No consistent significant differences exist with regard to histologic subgroups or laterality in blacks. However, in contrast to the low incidence of testicular germ cell tumors a higher incidence of interstitial testis tumors has been reported for blacks. Although annual incidence rates are four to five times higher in whites, age-adjusted incidence rates are similar in white and black Americans regarding childhood testicular cancer. Additionally, blacks demonstrate the same age-dependent incidence peaks as whites with the apex of the peak between ages 15 and 44. Regarding prognosis blacks and whites appear to have similar outlooks and mortality rates do not differ between both groups[9].

Involvement of genetic factors has been suggested as possible explanation for racial differences in incidence rates since migration did not alter the incidence rates in blacks.

Occupation

Several studies have indicated a positive correlation between socioeconomic status and the risk of testicular cancer[10–12]. The risk was highest in adults of high socioeconomic status or education, whereas the risk generally was lower in men with manual occupations. Although an occupational carcinogen has not been identified, the United Kingdom Testicular Cancer Group[13] reported that lack of exercise and sedentary lifestyle – typical features of the non-manual profession – may double the risk of testicular cancer. On the other hand, several studies have reported an increased risk for testicular cancer in farmers, foresters and fishermen with tumors developing at older ages suggesting an occupational risk factor[10,11].

It is unlikely that the current or most recent occupation is etiologically important since testicular tumors peak in young adulthood. With neoplasms developing at this age, one might consider carcinogens, dietary factors or behaviors in utero, early childhood or adolescence to be etiologically more important as has been demonstrated for high intake of dietary fat[14], milk in adolescence[15] and sedentary living[13,16]. In this context, several studies have indicated that elevated maternal estrogen levels during the first trimester of pregnancy may permanently alter the germ cells and cause urogenital abnormalities such as cryptorchidism, inguinal hernias and hypospadias[33].

Frequency, histology, laterality and bilaterality

Germ cell tumors account for about 90% to 95% of all testicular neoplasms with seminomas accounting for approximately 60% of all germ cell tumors whereas non-seminomatous germ cell tumors (NSGCT) account for the remainder[2]. Over a 50 year time period the incidence rate for seminomas increased in men 25 to 64 years old[1]; however, it remained constant in young adults 15 to 24 years of age. NSGCT demonstrate a different age pattern: peak incidence occurs in men 15 to 24 years old and then gradually decreases for each subsequent age category. During the last 50 years the incidence for NSGCT rose almost 130%.

Most germ cell tumors develop unilaterally with right sided tumors being slightly more common than left sided tumors (57% versus 42%)[16]. Approximately 3.5% of all testicular germ cell tumors develop bilaterally; the vast majority of bilateral germ cell tumors occurs metachronously with time intervals of up to 32 years. Similar rather than different histology predominates in bilateral testis tumors. In a recent series[17], bilateral seminomas (32%) and bilateral non-seminomas (34%) were the most common histologic findings; germ cell tumors of different histology were found in 40% of the cases. These findings are in contrast with the series of Bach et al.[18] who reported bilateral seminoma in 48% and germ cell tumors of different histology in only 15%. However, the recent series included only patients diagnosed after 1985 and resembles the incidence data with increasing numbers of NSGCT among testicular neoplasms. The prevalence of bilateral germ cell tumors is in accordance with the frequency of contralateral carcinoma in situ in patients with unilateral testis tumors which is reported at between 4.5% and 6.6%[19,20].

Etiology of adult germ cell tumors

Experimental and clinical evidence support the evidence that heredity, congenital and environmental factors are involved in the etiology of testicular germ cell tumors.

Cryptorchidism

Since the initial observation of an interrelationship between testicular maldescent and testicular cancer development by Pott in the 18th century, many studies have demonstrated an increased risk for malignant germ cell tumors in patients with cryptorchidism[16,21–25]. Various series described that 3% to 12% of all testis tumors arise in cryptorchid testes. A recent case-control study performed by the United Kingdom Testicular Cancer Study Group (UKTCSG)[13] reported the most significant risk for patients with bilateral cryprochidism (overall odds ratio 3.82 (95% confidence interval 2.24 to 6.52)) whereas unilateral testicular maldescent is associated with only a moderate risk (overall odds ratio 2.71 (95% confidence interval 1.55 to 4.72)). In former series the estimated risk of testicular tumorigenesis in men with a history of testicular maldescent was calculated to be 48 times that of men with normally descended testes. However, the cited case-control studies indicate that the risk to develop a testicular malignancy ranges from two to 11 times greater among patients with cryptorchidism than among the male population in general. The higher risk estimates of earlier studies might have been derived from recall biases since the data most often included patients with retractile testes or late descending testicles.

According to six large case-control studies[16,21–25] 10% to 25% of men with unilateral cryptorchidism develop a germ cell tumor in the contralateral normally descended testis. These data are slightly higher than the reported frequency of CIS in the cryptorchid testis and its normal counterpart which ranges from 2% to 8%[19,20]. However, one must note that the diagnosis of CIS in prepubertal testes is difficult so that a few cases might be missed on initial screening.

Despite the strong association between cryptorchidism and testicular cancer, the causative factors are still not fully understood. Several factors such as abnormal cell morphology, elevated intrascrotal temperature, endocrine dysfunction and gonadal dysgenesis may play a role. In this context, the UKTCSG[13] developed an interesting general hypothesis: testicular atrophy with reduced spermatogenesis as a direct result of cryptorchidism leads to increased exposure of the testis to gonadotropins due to testicular-hypophysis-hypothalamus feedback. Increased intratesticular concentrations of gonadotropins after puberty cause increased rates of germ cell mitosis which might influence tumor development.

Inguinal hernia

A relationship between inguinal hernia and testicular cancer has been described in several case-control studies; however, in most studies the risk for cancer development was elevated primarily in those men whose hernias occurred at a young age (< 15 years) or in men with associated ipsilateral cryptorchidism[16,25]. In studies examining men without testicular maldescent who reported having had a herniorrhapy no substantial excessive risk of testicular cancer has been described.

Vasectomy

The idea that vasectomy might be an important risk factor of testicular cancer has been discussed for many years although germ cell tumors commonly occur before the age vasectomy usually is performed. A comprehensive review of nine studies[13,26] examining the relationship between vasectomy and testis cancer demonstrates that only two studies observed an increased risk for tumor development[23,27]. However, the short interval of less than 2 months between surgery and manifestation of testis cancer questions the causal relationship.

Infertility

Much has been reported about the association of infertility and testicular cancer mainly based on the increased prevalence of CIS among subfertile and infertile men and the finding of defective spermatogenesis in both subfertile men and patients with germ cell tumors. If gonadal function with resultant subfertility plays a role in the etiology of testicular cancer, patients should have experienced problems in procreating prior to cancer diagnosis. Excluding patients with cryptorchidism, all of whom are likely to be subfertile, the association of infertility and testis cancer is only of borderline significance and most patients with testicular cancer do not have significantly decreased fertility potential[13,28].

Hormones

The peak incidence of testicular cancer in young adulthood suggests that gestational development and exogenous influences during infancy and early puberty might be involved in testicular cancer pathogenesis. Sex hormones have long been suspected to represent such exogenous factors and might be important in the development of CIS and in the transition from CIS to invasive cancer. Excessive bioavailable estrogens, insufficient androgens and high concentrations of gonadotropins have been shown to be associated with genital disorders such as cryptorchidism, testicular hypoplasia, infertility and testicular cancer. Although maternal exposure to diethylstilbestrol (DES) and other estrogen based treatment during pregnancy has been suggested to be important in testicular tumorigenesis[28], large epidemiologic studies have not demonstrated convincing results and failed to find a statistically significant relative risk ratio of prenatal DES exposure and testis cancer[30].

However, it has been demonstrated that elevated maternal estrogen levels during the first weeks of gestation, and therefore during the critical period for urogenital differentiation, might be an important mechanism. Excessive bioavailable estrogens due to low sex hormone binding globulin concentrations, higher amounts of free estradiol or increased concentrations of total estrogens may permanently alter germ cells which are later stimulated to mitotic division by gonadotropins.

Low androgen state has been associated with germ cell tumors and CIS; however, the incidence of primary germ cell tumors in disorders with low testosterone levels such as Klinefelter's syndrome is low whereas the incidence of extragonadal germ cell tumors is very high[32]. This association might result from inhibition of germ cell migration during urogenital differentiation due to low androgen state during gestation. Therefore, the role of androgens in germ cell tumor development remains questionable.

Gonadotropins have been implicated in the development of testis cancer since the peak secretion occurs during early infancy and at puberty thereby resembling the peak incidence of testicular germ cell tumors. In addition, germ cell tumors have not been described in patients with hypogonadotropic hypogonadism, e.g. Kallmann's syndrome, despite a high frequency of cryptorchidism[33].

Trauma

Trauma or injuries to the scrotum, horseback riding as well as tight underwear have long been suggested as contributing factors in testicular tumorigenesis[34]. However, large case-control studies have failed to identify a significantly relative risk for these factors and testicular cancer. Investigators conclude that any type of trauma to the enlarged testicle prompts subjects to seek medical care thereby increasing the frequency of diagnosis of testicular cancer in testicular trauma patients[35]. Large case-control studies have also not been able to identify elevated scrotal temperature as a significant risk factor for germ cell tumor development.

Infectious diseases

Since the epidemiology of testicular cancer resembles epidemiologic data of cancers of viral origin such as young adult-type Hodgkin's disease, it has been speculated that

viruses such as cytomegalo-virus (CMV) or Epstein-Barr virus (EBV) might be involved in testicular tumorigenesis[36]. However, results are based on elevated serum titers only and not on diagnosis of intratesticular or intratumoral virus DNA.

With respect to mumps orchitis, inconsistent findings have been reported in the literature with some studies demonstrating a positive correlation and others showing no correlation. Interestingly, case-control studies performed by the same authors[37,38] in different patient populations came to completely contradictory results which underline the problem of recall bias in epidemiologic studies if subjects are only asked if mumps involved the testis and a physical examination (atrophy) is not performed.

Prenatal and perinatal risk factors

Since testicular cancer demonstrates a peak in young adults it has been thought that exogenous factors during gestational development might be involved in tumorigenesis. Several case-control studies described a three to 13-fold elevated relative risk for testicular cancer associated with a birth weight of less than 6 lbs.[31,39] or premature delivery[40]. A slightly increased risk was associated with unusual bleeding or spotting, treated or untreated nausea, and consumption of cigarettes and alcohol during pregnancy.

Genetics

Cytogenetic studies

The presence of isochromosome 12p [i(12p)] represents a characteristic chromosomal anomaly in testicular germ cell tumors of all histologic subtypes and all locations and was first described by Atkin and Baker[41]. They found that most testicular tumors contained extra copies of the short arm of chromosome 12 and they suggested that genetic alterations might be responsible for the development of testicular neoplasms. Since that time numerous studies have confirmed these results[42,43] and the number of extra copies of chromosome 12 short-arm in tumor cells could even be correlated with the prognostic outcome of these tumors[44].

Comparing the incidence of i(12p) in seminomas and nonseminomatous testicular germ cell tumors it was shown that nonseminomas demonstrate a significantly higher copy number (75%) than seminomas (7%) when tumor biopsy specimens were studied by flourescence in situ hybridization. However, the clinical importance of this finding still remains to be determined.

Despite the numerous cytogenetic studies little is known about the role of i(12p) in tumor development. Questions have been raised whether an amplification of oncogenes located on 12p (e.g. K-ras, cyclin D2) or concomitant loss of tumor suppressor genes on 12q might contribute to testicular tumorigenesis. Nevertheless, i(12p) seems to be important in the pathogenesis of male testicular germ cell tumors.

Structural changes common to all types of testicular germ cell tumors in addition to the i(12p) iso-chromosome affect the 12p, 17q, 1p, 1q, 9p, 22q, 6q, and 7p regions. However, none of these chromosomal anomalies occurs as frequently as the i(12p).

Oncogenes

Several proto-oncogenes such as K-ras, hst-1, int-2, c-kit and its ligand stem cell factor have been studied for their putative involvement in testicular germ cell tumorigenesis.

With regard to K-ras and N-ras only a low frequency of mutations have been detected in adult testicular cancer[42,45]. Therefore, mutations of the ras genes are not believed to play a major role in testis carcinogenesis and do not appear to be a useful clinical or prognostic marker.

The proto-oncogenes hst-1 and c-kit have been shown to be expressed in some but not all testicular tumors[46]. Whereas only 4% of all seminomas and none of the benign testicular tissue specimens tested did express hst-1, approximately 80% of all non-seminomas expressed hst-1. In contrast, the proto-oncogene c-kit, which encodes for a cell surface protein that is a tyrosine kinase growth factor receptor, has been shown to be expressed predominantly in seminomatous germ cell tumors (78%) and only in about 7% of the non-seminomatous tumors. In addition, it has been shown that c-kit is only expressed in testicular parenchyma with intact spermatogenesis but expression was decreased or absent with altered spermatogenesis. Based on these findings it was suggested that c-kit expression might be decreased or even lost during differentiation from normal testicular tissue to seminomas and non-seminomas. The interaction of stem cell factor (SCF) – the natural ligand of c-kit – with c-kit is said to be critical in the development of hematological, gonadal and pigment stem cells. However, a heterogeneous expression of SCF was noted in germ cell tumors with absent SCF expression at the RNA level in all germ cell tumors investigated. SCF protein was expressed in tumor cells of seven of the 18 GCTs investigated[47].

The human mouse double minute 2 (mdm 2) gene might be another proto-oncogene with tumorigenic activity in human germ cell tumors. Mdm-2 gene encodes for a cellular protein that forms a complex with the mutant and wild type p53 protein and modulates its activity. Overexpression of the mdm-2 gene in cells increases their tumorigeneic potential and overcomes the growth inhibitory activity of p53. The expression of mdm-2 might be of particular interest in testis cancer since overexpression of the wild type p53 has been implicated in the pathogenesis of germ cell tumors. However, none of the studies performed so far showed evidence of mdm-2 gene amplifications and it was concluded that the mdm-2 gene is rarely mutated in germ cell tumors. Other factors must be responsible for the induction of malignancy[48].

The bcl-2 gene encodes for an inner mitochondrial membrane protein which was first discovered in human B cell lymphoma[59]. Studies in hematopoietic cells have demonstrated that bcl-2 protein can inhibit apoptosis induced by chemotherapeutic agents such as cisplatin, the most effective drug in testicular cancer[7]. In addition, it has been shown that overproduction of bcl-2 can overcome the growth inhibitory effect of p53[50]. Given this functional relationship of bcl-2 and p53 the immunohistochemical expression of bcl-2 and p53 in germ cell tumors was studied recently[51]. Whereas an increased protein expression for p53 was detected, no bcl-2 protein was expressed in seminomas or non-seminomas. This relationship – high p53 expression, low bcl-2 expression – might explain the high chemosensitivity of germ cell tumors, but it also demonstrates that bcl-2 does not appear to be involved in testicular tumorigenesis.

Another example of significant differential expression of proto-oncogenes in adult testicular germ cell tumors has been described for the PTHLH gene[52], which is mapped to the short arm of chromosome 12. The PTHLH gene was expressed in all testis tumors containing seminomatous and choriocarcinomatous elements whereas it was not detected in embryonal carcinomas or teratomas. However, the exact role of PTHLH gene in testicular carcinogenesis remains to be established.

Tumor suppressor genes (TSG)

With regard to TSG only a few detailed studies have been performed in testicular germ cell tumors. With respect to the retinoblastoma (RB) gene no gross alterations of the gene structure or the copy number could be detected[53]. On the other hand, significantly decreased expression of RB mRNA has been found in all germ cell tumors studied so far; the RB protein product was absent in undifferentiated tumors such as seminomas, embryonal carcinomas and choriocarcinomas but it was present in differentiated mature teratoma cells of all teratocarcinomas and mixed tumors. Although it was suggested that the RB protein was regulated by phosphorylation and an additional regulatory mechanism of the RB gene might occur at the transcript level, subtle microdeletions or mutations at the DNA levels could not be excluded and more study is needed.

Alterations of the p53 TSG in testicular germ cell tumors have been studied by several groups since point mutations, allelic loss, rearrangements and deletions have been described for a variety of human cancers[42,43]. On the protein level all studies have described an increased p53 expression which has been thought to represent mutant p53[54]. The half-life of the p53 wild type protein product is very short and virtually not detectable by immunohistochemistry. However, mutations of the p53 gene results in a stabilization of the protein with prolonged half-life. Despite increased p53 protein expression in adult testicular germ cell tumors, mutations of the coding regions of p53 are extremely rare and it has been suggested that post-translational alterations rather than intragenic mutations might stabilize the p53 protein for immunohistochemical detection[55].

The TSG p16 encodes for a cell cycle regulatory protein that binds to cyclin dependent kinase 4 and inhibits the catalytic activity of the CDK4/cyclin D complexes which control the transit from G1-phase to S-phase of the cell cycle. Inactivation of p16 might result in unregulated activity of CDK4/cyclin D complexes leading to loss of growth control as has been demonstrated in a variety of human neoplasms. So far only one study has examined adult testicular germ cell tumors for genetic alterations of p15 and p16[56]. Whereas no gross deletions or rearrangements for p15 and p16 could be detected by Southern Blot analysis, an unusual high frequency (33%) of mutations of the p16 protein coding region was observed in tumor samples but not in matching normal controls. These results suggested that p16 alterations might be involved in testicular carcinogenesis.

Conclusion

The incidence of testicular germ cell tumors has been rising for the last four decades making them the most common malignancy in young adults 15 to 35 years of age. Due to improved chemotherapeutic regimes, overall cure rates of approximately 80% have been achieved and mortality rates declined significantly during the last 20 years. Cryptorchidism is the best etiologically established risk factor for the development of testicular cancer. The peak incidence of testicular cancer after puberty suggests that events occuring during infancy or early childhood including endocrinological factors may play a role in the pathogenesis of germ cell tumors; however, their exact contribution to tumorigenesis remains to be established. Since the incidence of testis cancer has risen predominantly in the white population, environmental factors might influence tumor development in genetically susceptible individuals.

With regard to genetic alterations, activation of cellular oncogenes and loss of function of tumor suppressor genes appear to be key events in the pathogenesis of human testicular germ cell tumors. Altered forms of these genes or their protein products may have the potential to provide not only new information on the carcinogenesis of testis cancer but they may also provide a new generation of cancer markers. However, further studies have to be performed to apply oncogenes and tumor suppressor genes as predictors of prognostic information or to use genetic alterations, overabundance or absence of one of these genes, as a basis for therapeutic intervention.

References

1. Brown LM, Pottern LM, Hoover RN, Devesa SS, Aselton P, Flannery JT. Testicular cancer in the United States: trends in incidence and mortality. *Int J Epidemiol* 1986;**15**:164–170.
2. Mostofi FK, Sobin LH. *Histological typing of testis tumors.* Geneva, Switzerland: World Health Organization, 1977.
3. Boring CC, Squires TS, Tong T. *CA Cancer J Clin* 1993;**43**:7–6.
4. Schottenfeld D, Warshauer ME, Sherlock S, Zauber AG, Leder M, Payne R. The epidemiology of testicular cancer in young adults. *Am J Epidemiol* 1980;**112**:232–246.
5. Buetow SA. Epidemiology of testicular cancer. *Epidem Rev* 1995;**17**:433–449.
6. Øterlind A. Diverging trends in incidence and mortality of testicular cancer in Denmark, 1943–1982. *Br J Cancer* 1986;**53**:501–505.
7. Einhorn LH. Treatment of testicular cancer: a new and improved model. *J Clin Oncol* 1990, pp. 1777–1781.
8. Kay R. Prepubertal testicular tumor registry. *J Urol* 1993;**150**:671–674.
9. Moul JW, Schanne FJ, Thompson IM, Frazier HA, Teretsman SA, Wettlaufer JN, Rozanski TA, Stack RS, Kreder KJ, Hoffman KJ. Testicular cancer in blacks. *Cancer* 1994;**73**:388–93.
10. Pearce N, Sheppard RA, Howard JK, Fraser J, Lilley BM. Time trends and occupational differences in cancer of the testis in New Zealand. *Cancer* 1987;**59**:1677–1682.
11. Swerdlow AJ, Skeet RG. Occupational associations of testicular cancer in south east England. *Br J Ind Med* 1988;**45**:225–230.
12. Harding M, Hole D, Gillis C. The epidemiology of non-seminomatous germ cell tumours in the west of Scotland 1975–89. *Br J Cancer* 1995;**72**:1559–1562.
13. United Kingdom Testicular Cancer Study Group. Aetiology of testicular cancer; association with congenital abnormalities, age at puberty, infertility and exercise. *BMJ* 1994;**308**:1393–1399.
14. Armstrong B, Doll R. Environmental factors and cancer incidence and mortality in different countries with special reference to dieatry practices. *Int J Cancer* 1975;**15**:617–631.
15. Davies TW, Ruha W, Palmer CR. Diet and testicular cancer. *J Epidemiol Community Health* 1993;**47**:399 (Abstract).
16. Pottern LM, Morris Brown L, Hoover RN, Javadpour J, O'Connel KJ, Stutzman RE, Blattner WA. Testicular cancer risk among young men: role of cryptorchidism and inguinal hernia. *JNCI* 1985;**74**:377–81.
17. Heidenreich A, Neubauer S, Engelmann UH. Bilateral testicular germ cell tumors: prevalence, histology and implication for therapy. *J Urol* submitted.
18. Bach DW, Weißbach L, Hartlapp JH. Bilateral testicular tumor. *J Urol* 1983;**129**:989–991.
19. Giwercman A, Skakkebaek NE. Carcinoma in situ testis: biology, screening, and management. *Eur Urol* 1993;**23**:19–21.
20. Heidenreich A, Beckert R, Vietsch Hv, Engelmann UH. Screening, diagnosis and therapy of testicular intraepithelial neoplasia. *Akt Urol* 1995;**26**:175–180.
21. Pike MC, Chilvers C, Peckham MJ. Effect of age at orchidopexy in risk of testicular cancer. *Lancet* 1986;**i**:1246–1248.
22. Strader CH, Weiss NS, Daling JR, Karagas MR, McKnight B. Cryptorchidism, orchiopexy, and the risk of testicular cancer. *Am J Epidemiol* 1988;**127**:1013–1018.
23. Thornhill JA, Conroy RM, Kelly DG, Walsh A, Fennelly JJ, Fitzpatrick JM. An evaluation of predisposing factors for testis cancer in Ireland. *Eur Urol* 1988;**14**:429–433.

24. Benson RC, Beard CM, Kelalis PP, Kurtland LT. Malignant potential of the cryptorchid testis. *Mayo Clin Proc* 1991;**66**:372–378.

25. Prener A, Engholm G, Jensen OM. Genital anomalies and risk for testicular cancer in Danish men. *Epidemiology* 1996;**7**:14–19.

26. Lynge E, Knudsen NB. Vasectomy and testicular cancer: epidemiological evidence of association. *Eur J Cancer* 1993;**29**A:1064–1066.

27. Strader CH, Weiss NS, Daling JR. Vasectomy and the incidence of testicular cancer. *Am J Epidemiol* 1988;**128**:56–63.

28. Johnson DE, Fueger JJ, Alfaro PJ, Spitz MR, Newell GR. Subfertility: an etiologic factor in development of testicular cancer? *Urology* 1987;**30**:199–200.

29. Conley GR, Sant GR, Ucci AA, Mitcheson HD. Seminoma and epididymal cyst in a young man with known diethylstilboestrol exposure. *JAMA* 1983;**249**:1325–1326.

30. Moss AR, Osmond D, Bachetti P, Yorti FM, Gurgin V. Hormonal risk factors in testicular cancer. *Am J Epidemiol* 1986;**124**:39–52.

31. Depue RH, Pike MC, Henderson BE. Estrogen exposure during gestation and risk for testicular cancer. *JNCI* 1983;**71**:1151–1155.

32. Heidenreich A, Wilbert DM, Schäfer R, Vietsch H. Mature teratoma of the testis associated with Klinefelter's syndrome. *Akt Urol* 1993;**7**:293–296.

33. Rajpert-de Meyts E, Skakkebaek NE. The possible role of sex hormones in the development of testicular cancer. *Eur Urol* 1993;**23**:54–61.

34. Coldman AJ, Elwood JM, Gallagher RP. Sports activities and risk of testicular cancer. *Br J Cancer* 1982;**46**:749–756.

35. Moul JW. Early and accurate diagnosis of testicular cancer. *Probl Urol* 1994;**8**:58–66.

36. Algood CB, Newell GR, Johnson DE. Viral etiology of testicular tumors. *Urology* 1988;**139**:308–310.

37. Brown LM, Pottern LM, Hoover RN. Testicular cancer in young men: the search for causes of the epidemic increase in the United States. *J Epidemiol Comm Health* 1987;**41**:349–354.

38. Brown LM, Pottern LM, Hoover RN. Prenatal and perinatal risk factors for testicular cancer. *Cancer Res* 1986;**46**:4812–4816.

39. Henderson BE, Benton B, Jing J, Yu M, Pike MC. is factors for cancer of the testis in young men. *Int J Cancer* 1979;**23**:598–602.

40. Atkin NB, Baker MC. Specific chromosome change, i(12p) in testicular tumors? *Lancet* 1082;**2**:1349–1351.

41. Sandberg AA, Meloni AM, Suijkerbuijk. Reviews of chromosome studies in urological tumors. III. Cytogenetics and genes in testicular tumors. *J Urol* **155**:1531–1556.

42. Moul JW, Heidenreich A. Future directions in testicular cancer. In: Ernsthoff MC, Heaney JA, Peschel RE (eds) *Urologic cancer*, Chapter 44, Section 4, Norton Medical Books, in press.

43. Bosl GJ, Dmitrovsky E, Reuter VE, Samaniego F, Rodriguez E, Geller NJ, Chaganti RS. Isochromosome of chromosome 12: clinically useful marker for male germ cell tumors. *J Natl Cancer Inst* 1989;**81**:1874–1879.

44. Moul JW, Theune SM, Chang EH. Detection of ras mutations in archival testicular germ cell tumors by polymerase chain reaction and oligonucleotide hybridization. *Genes, Chrom Cancer* 1992;**5**:109–113.

45. Strohmeyer T, Peter S, Hartmann M, Munemitsu S, Ackermann R, Ullrich A, Slamon DJ. Expression of the hst-1 and c-kit protooncogenes in human testicular germ cell tumors. *Cancer Res* 1991;**51**:1811–1815.

46. Strohmeyer T, Reese D, Press M, Ackermann R, Hartmann M, Slamon DJ. Expression of the c-kit proto-oncogene and its ligand stem cell factor in normal and malignant human testicular tissue. *J Urol* 1995;**153**:511–519.

47. Strohmeyer T, Fleischaker M, Imal Y, Slamon DJ, Koeffler P. Status of the p53 tumor suppressor gene and the mdm-2 gene in human testicular tumors. *J Urol* 1993;**149**:311A.

48. Tsujimoto Y, Cossman J, Jaffe E, Croce C. Involvement of the bcl-2 gene in human follicular lymphoma. *Science* 1985;**228**:1440–1443.

49. Eliopoulos AG, Kerr DJ, Herod J, Hodgkins L, Krajewski S, Reed JC, Young LS. The control of apoptosis and drug resistance in ovarian cancer: influence of p53 and bcl-2. *J Clin Oncol* 1995;1217–1228.

50. Heidenreich A, Schenkman WS, Sesterhenn IA, Mostofi KF, Moul JW, Srivastava S, Engelmann UH. Immunohistochemical and mutational analysis of the p53 tumor suppressor gene and the bcl-2 oncogene in primary testicular germ cell tumours. *APMIS.* 1998;**106**:90–9

51. Shimogaki H, Kitazawa S, Maeda S, Kamidono S. Variable expression of hst-1, int-1 and parathyroide hormone-related protein in different histological types of human testicular germ cell tumors. *Cancer J* 1993;**6**:81–85.

52. Strohmeyer T, Reissmann P, Cordon-Cardo C, Hartmann M, Ackermann R, Slamon DJ. Correlation between retinoblastoma gene expression and differentiation in human testicular tumors. *Proc Natl Acad Sci USA* 1991;**88**:6662–6666.

53. Lewis DJ, Sesterhenn IA, McCarthy WF, Moul JW. Immunohistochemical expression of p53 tumor suppressor gene protein in adult germ cell testis tumors: clinical correlation in stage I disease. *J Urol* 1994;**152**:418–423.

54. Schenkman NS, Sesterhenn IA, Washington L, Tong YA, Weghorst CM, Buzard GS, Srivastava S, Moul S. Increased p53 protein does not correlate to p53 gene mutations in microdissected human testicular germ cell tumors. *J Urol* 1995;**154**:617–621.

55. Heidenreich A, Gadipatti J, Moul JW, Srivastava S. Mutations of the tumor suppressor genes p15 and p16 are rare in human testicular germ cell tumors. *Proc Am Ass Cancer Res* 1996;**37**:586.

35 Pathology

P Harnden and M C Parkinson

Classification

The classification of germ cell tumors has been a matter of debate for more than 20 years, which probably indicates that no one classification is ideal. However, differences between the two main classifications, from Britain and the WHO, are more apparent than real and correlations can easily be drawn between the two (Table 35.1).

The separation of seminomas from teratomas is common to both. It is in the subdivision of teratomas that there

Table 35.1 Correlations between the British and the WHO classifications

British classification	WHO classification
Intratubular germ cell neoplasia[1]	Intratubular uncommitted malignant germ cell
Seminoma Classical	Same
	Seminoma with high mitotic index
Spermatocytic[2]	Same
Malignant teratoma differentiated	Teratoma Mature
	Immature
Malignant teratoma intermediate[3]	Embryonal carcinoma + teratoma
Malignant teratoma undifferentiated[4]	Embryonal carcinoma
Malignant teratoma trophoblastic[5]	Choriocarcinoma
Combined tumor: seminoma + teratoma	
Yolk sac tumour	Same

Notes:
1   This is the term most commonly used for the precursor lesion of germ cell tumors, which had not been identified when the classification was devised. It refers to malignant transformation of the germinal epithelium lining the tubule, as distinct from 'intratubular spread of germ cell neoplasia'.
2   Whilst a subdivision of seminoma, it must be recognized that spermatocytic seminomas are unique morphologically and clinically.
3   This refers to tumors which have a mixture of differentiated and undifferentiated elements.
4   This may include areas with yolk sac differentiation.
5   This may contain either differentiated or undifferentiated teratoma but is identified by the presence of syncytiotrophoblast and cytotrophoblast in the characteristic biphasic arrangement.

appear to be major differences. In Britain, the aim was for a clinically relevant classification. It recognized that a variety of morphological patterns often occurred in combination as well as separately and could usefully be grouped together for treatment and prognostic purposes[1]. However, it must be remembered that the treatment current to the era was orchidectomy and radiotherapy. In contrast, the WHO classification[2] relates to descriptive morphology in which each tumor component is identified separately. This gives maximum information in trial pathology where the aim is to seek correlations between the presence of different components, disease course and response to new forms of therapy. Unfortunately, despite being presented as an international collaborative effort, the WHO classification failed to bridge transatlantic differences. We hope that these differences will be resolved in the forthcoming revision.

It is important to be clear about why we attempt to classify tumors in general and germ cell tumors in particular. From a pathologist's point of view, it is important to recognize the spectrum of morphologic appearances associated with germ cell tumors, so that a neoplasm can be correctly identified to be of germ cell origin. The second purpose is to place the patient into a prognostic group based on morphologic or other factors so that the most appropriate therapy can be given. In a broader context, classifications are useful for epidemiologic purposes and for the communication and comparison of results. It is difficult to devise a single classification which fulfils all those objectives, since 'prognostic' classifications tend to include broader categories than descriptive classifications, and it is perhaps appropriate that both types co-exist.

The advent of modern chemotherapy has transformed prognosis in germ cell tumors since the British classification was devised. The main subdivision between seminomas and teratomas appears still to be valid (most international publications divide cases into seminomas and 'non-seminomatous germ cell tumors') but within teratomas, undifferentiated teratoma or teratoma tro-phoblastic no longer carry the dire prognosis of

423

'pre-cisplatin' days. Current problems in the treatment of germ cell tumors are threefold: the identification of tumors in a good prognostic category in order to reduce treatment intensity thereby minimizing the short- and long-term side effects associated with chemo- or radiotherapy; the identification of tumors that will not respond to conventional treatment in order to offer more intensive therapy before tumor burden becomes too great; and the prediction of residual teratoma differentiated or the malignant (carcinomatous, sarcomatous or lymphomatous/ leukemic) transformation of such elements post-chemotherapy.

In this chapter we will first describe the diagnostic features of germ cell tumors and their differential diagnosis before reviewing prognostic indicators.

Diagnosis

Intratubular germ cell neoplasia (ITGCN)

Clinical significance

The association between atypical cells in seminiferous tubules and subsequent development of a germ cell tumor was first described as early as 1965[3], although the acceptance that this lesion represents the precursor lesion to all germ cell tumors came later.

The diagnosis is made in two main situations: in orchidectomy specimens where ITGCN is identified in the tubules adjacent to the tumor, and in testicular biopsies performed in the context of infertility, testicular dysgenesis, an apparent retroperitoneal primary or germ cell tumor of the contralateral testis. The diagnosis of ITGCN on biopsy may lead to treatment as progression to invasive germ cell tumors (seminoma and teratoma) has been documented in 50% of patients within 5 years[4]. Treatment has included close surveillance, chemotherapy, radiotherapy and orchidectomy. Currently, radiotherapy is the favored option as some Leydig cell function is retained. ITGCN has been shown to persist following chemotherapy[5]

Pathology

The diagnosis rests on the identification of bizarre cells with large, irregular nuclei, coarse chromatin, prominent nucleoli and clear cytoplasm (Figure 35.1). These cells are close to the tubular basement membrane, and often form a ring of contiguous cells pushing the remaining Sertoli cells towards the center of the tubule. The distribution of ITGCN may be patchy, raising issues of biopsy sampling. Sampling of the area near the rete testis has been recommended in atrophic testes[6], but consideration must be given to preservation of function given that scarring of the rete and epididymis may affect sperm transport.

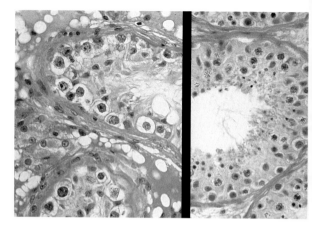

Fig. 35.1 Comparison between ITGCN (left) and normal spermatogenesis (right).

Seminoma

Macroscopy

The cut surface is pale, white and uniform, in contrast to teratomas (Figure 35.2), although variable degrees of nodularity can be seen because of the presence of fibrous septae, and foci of necrosis are quite common.

Microscopy

The nuclei have irregular outlines with coarse chromatin and one or more nucleoli. The cytoplasm is clear to eosinophilic depending on the glycogen content and fixation. Cell boundaries are well defined. The cells are arranged in sheets or cords separated by fibrous stroma containing a lymphocytic infiltrate predominantly of T cells (Figure 35.3). Up to 50% of tumors are associated

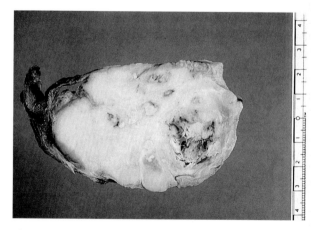

Fig. 35.2 Combined tumor showing differences between seminoma (left) and MTU (right).

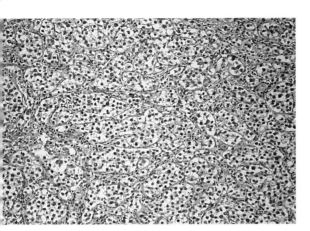

Fig. 35.3 Classical seminoma.

with a prominent granulomatous response. Scattered syncytiotrophoblastic cells, the source of human chorionic gonadotrophin (HCG) production, may be present.

Spermatocytic seminoma

Macroscopy
The cut surface is cream or even yellow rather than the white of classical seminomas and of edematous or gelatinous appearance. Cyst formation may be seen, particularly in larger tumors.

Microscopy
There is a diffuse, sheet-like pattern of growth with very little stroma, unlike the packeted appearance of the classical seminoma. Interstitial edema may lead to cyst formation. Variation in cell size is more marked and in fact the diagnosis of spermatocytic seminoma rests on the identification of three cell types. The most abundant cell type is medium in size with dispersed chromatin, and the second cell type consists of smaller cells with condensed nuclei. Both types of cell have scant but deeply eosinophilic cytoplasm which does not contain glycogen. Finally, there are cells containing giant nuclei or three or four large nuclei with finely granular or filamentous chromatin, morphologically distinct from the syncytiotrophoblastic cells of classical seminomas. Mitoses are frequent, and abnormal forms may be present. A lymphocytic or granulomatous reaction are typically not seen. Spermatocytic seminomas are not associated with ITGCN but intratubular spread is common. On the rare occasions where the diagnostic features described are not present, staining for PLAP may be helpful in the distinction from classical seminoma since spermatocytic seminomas do not express this marker.

Spermatocytic seminomas may occasionally be associated with a sarcoma, the clinical course being determined by the sarcomatous component as pure spermatocytic seminomas rarely if ever metastasize. In contrast to the classical type, the spermatocytic form is not associated with other germ cell tumors.

Malignant teratoma undifferentiated (MTU)

Macroscopy
Many tumors are large and may extend to the tunica albuginea or epididymis. The cut surface is soft and pale grey, often with extensive necrosis and hemorrhage (Figure 35.2).

Microscopy
The tumors may show a solid growth pattern with cohesive, pleomorphic cells containing clumped chromatin and lacking well-defined cell boundaries. Cytoplasm is amphophilic or eosinophilic rather than clear. Poorly formed glands, pseudopapillary structures and cleft-like spaces may also be present (Figure 35.4). Stroma, which can be abundant, may separate the islands of malignant germ cells. Necrosis and hemorrhage are typically seen.

Malignant teratoma differentiated (MTD) or pure teratoma

Macroscopy
The cut surface is generally cystic and mucoid. Hemorrhage and necrosis are typically absent.

Microscopy
The cysts are lined by a variety of epithelial cell types and the intervening stroma may contain any type of tissue including bone, cartilage and neural tissue. In some cases, these tissues may not be fully developed: neural tissue is the most commonly encountered immature tissue, and

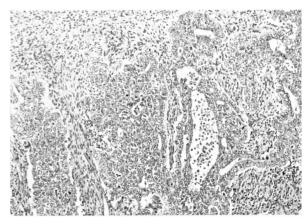

Fig. 35.4 Malignant teratoma undifferentiated.

425

pseudorosettes and rosettes as seen in neuroblastomas may be present. Tumors that contain such elements are classified as immature teratomas in the WHO classification, but are contained within the MTD category in the British, as the prognosis is the same.

In adults, these tumors are malignant despite their relatively bland histology. ITGCN is usually identified in adjacent tubules. In children, these tumors are biologically benign and treated by orchidectomy alone.

Malignant teratoma intermediate (MTI)

Macroscopy
Appearances vary but there is generally a mixture of cystic and solid areas with areas of hemorrhage and necrosis.

Microscopy
The diagnosis is made by the identification of both differentiated elements and undifferentiated teratoma, as described above. Yolk sac tumor (YST) and solitary syncytiotrophoblasts may also be present, so that AFP and HCG may be useful serum markers.

Malignant teratoma trophoblastic (MTT)

Macroscopy
The center of the tumor is generally hemorrhagic and necrotic and only a thin rim of tumor may remain at the periphery, so that extensive sampling may be required to identify the characteristic pattern.

Microscopy
The diagnosis can only be made if both syncytio- and cytotrophoblast are present and arranged in the characteristic biphasic pattern where the syncytiotrophoblasts are 'capping' the cytotrophoblast resulting in alternating layers of both types of cells. Cytotrophoblastic cells are round, with a single nucleus, scant cytoplasm and relatively high mitotic activity. Syncytiotrophoblastic cells have a variable, very irregular shape, multiple nuclei and abundant dense cytoplasm. Extensive vascular invasion is often present.

Yolk sac tumor (YST)

Macroscopy
The surface is greyish-white and soft with a mucoid appearance and areas of necrosis and hemorrhage. As yolk sac tumors are generally found in association with other germ cell components in the adult testis, the macroscopic appearance will vary with the nature of those components.

Microscopy
An increasing number of patterns have been described as representing yolk sac differentiation[7]. One of the most common patterns is the microcystic pattern where cysts lined by a single layer of flattened or cuboidal epithelium with often vacuolated cytoplasm are set in an edematous, poorly cellular myxoid stroma. In the reticular pattern, there are interconnecting cords of cells producing a rather delicate, 'lacy' appearance. The characteristic Schiller-Duval or glomeruloid bodies consist of a fibrovascular core covered by tumor cells projecting into a cystic space. Although diagnostic of yolk sac differentiation, they are relatively uncommon. The morphologic separation of YST and MTU is not always clear cut, probably because many undifferentiated tumors show early yolk sac differentiation. Moreover we suspect that the approach to distinguishing these two neoplastic elements varies between pathologists. Immunocytochemistry may help in so much as positivity for CD30 is said to identify MTU[8], whilst expression of alpha fetoprotein (AFP) is seen with yolk sac differentiation.

Differential diagnoses

Immunocytochemical markers which may be useful in the distinction between normal and malignant germ cells, seminoma and teratoma and germ cell from non-germ cell primary testicular tumors are summarized in Table 35.2. As with all immunocytochemistry, results must be validated in individual laboratories as differences in fixation, processing, methodology, choice of antibody will influence the results.

Germ cell tumors versus non-germ cell tumors
ITGCN can usually be identified in the tubules adjacent to germ cell tumors, with the exception of spermatocytic seminomas and teratomas differentiated in pre-pubertal males. Germ cell tumors stain positively for placental alkaline phosphatase (PLAP) and negatively for epithelial membrane antigen (EMA): occasional adenocarcinomas can be PLAP positive but are usually also EMA positive. Positivity for PLAP distinguishes germ cell tumors from lymphomas, which are generally positive for the common leukocyte antigen CD, and from Sertoli and Leydig cell tumors (see Table 35.2).

ITGCN versus degenerate germ cells
This usually arises when the specimen has been imperfectly fixed. Difficulties may also arise in the interpretation of the testes of elderly men on estrogens. Degenerate cells are often large and ballooned, but their nuclei are generally small and condensed rather than large and pleomorphic. In cases of doubt, distinction can be made by

Table 35.2 Immunocytochemistry in testicular neoplasms

	PLAP	Cytokeratins	Vimentin	CD30
Normal germ cells	**negative** in adults			negative
Intratubular germ cell neoplasia	positive	8,18		negative
Undifferentiated teratoma	positive	8, 18, **19**	mostly negative	**positive**
Seminoma	positive	8, 18, **4, 17**	some positive	positive
Malignant teratoma trophoblastic	positive	7		negative
Yolk sac tumor	positive	8, 18		negative
Leydig cell tumor	**negative**	negative	positive	negative
Sertoli cell tumor	**negative**	positive	positive	negative

Notes:

1   AFP may be positive in yolk sac tumors and may also be expressed in teratomas showing enteric differentiation. The beta subunit of HCG is positive in syncytiotrophoblastic cells. In practise, the authors have found these markers to be of little value over and above detailed morphologic examination.

2   The various elements of MTD express the markers normally associated with those tissues, such as cytokeratin 14 for squamous epithelium or cytokeratin 20 for glandular enteric mucosa.

immunocytochemistry since malignant germ cells, unlike normal germ cells, express PLAP.

ITGCN versus spermatogenic arrest at spermatogonia stage

A more practical problem encountered in biopsies from young men in the context of infertility is the distinction between malignant germ cells and maturation arrest at the spermatogonia stage. Such spermatogonia form a ring at the tubule periphery in the absence of more mature spermatogenic cells. The normal nuclear size of these cells (in contrast to ITGCN) may not be initially appreciated as normal spermatogenesis is not usually present for comparison. Immunostaining for PLAP is again extremely useful for identifying malignant germ cells.

ITGCN versus intratubular spread of neoplasia

Invasive germ cell tumors may spread through tubular lumens but, in contrast with ITGCN, fill and distend tubules and may show necrosis. This is only rarely seen in biopsies from patients whose tumors are impalpable.

Granulomatous seminoma versus granulomatous orchitis

The granulomatous reaction within some seminomas may be so marked as to obscure tumor cells. Extensive sampling is required before rendering the diagnosis of gran-

ulomatous orchitis. A reticulin preparation may help to identify residual tubular structures to assess the distribution of the inflammation: interstitial (corresponding to the tumor) in seminoma rather than centered on tubules as in granulomatous orchitis. Immunocytochemical staining for PLAP may also be useful in identifying seminoma cells within the inflammatory infiltrate and ITGCN which is generally present in seminomas. However, in cases with extensive tubular destruction, it may be necessary to take sections from the hilum to demonstrate Pagetoid spread of malignant germ cells within the rete testis.

Seminoma versus undifferentiated teratoma

Examination at low power is useful in identifying the clefts and papillae seen in undifferentiated teratoma versus the packeted appearance of seminomas, with islands of cell separated by fibrovascular stroma. A reticulin preparation may help in that respect. Seminoma cells also tend to have clearer cytoplasm and better defined cytoplasmic membranes whereas MTU cells tend to overlap and be more cohesive. Immunostains for cytokeratins may be helpful, but positivity for CD30 more reliably identifies MTU (Table 35.2).

Seminoma versus yolk sac tumor

The presence of edema within seminomas may lead to the development of cystic spaces. However, these spaces contain loose cells in seminomas and are generally empty in YSTs, and the cytology of the lining cells distinguishes seminoma (see above).

Seminoma versus malignant teratoma trophoblastic

The presence of syncytiotrophoblastic cells may raise the possibility of MTT but the presence of cytotrophoblast and the distinctive biphasic arrangement are lacking, as is significant hemorrhage.

Seminoma versus Sertoli cell tumor

One of the rare morphologic variants of seminoma consists of tubular or tubulopapillary structures lined by a single layer of cells separated by fibrovascular septae. Designated as tubular seminoma, it is however not clear whether these are true tubules or pseudotubules formed by loss of central cells in a small nest of seminoma cells. The confusion with a Sertoli cell tumor can be avoided by adequate sampling of the tumor since foci of classical seminoma are invariably present[9]. Furthermore, the cytology of Sertoli cells is generally bland, without the large nucleoli seen in seminoma cells, nuclei tend to be elongated and the cytoplasm contains lipid rather than glycogen.

427

Finally Sertoli cell tumors lack the lymphocytic infiltrate seen in seminomas, are not associated with ITGCN and do not express PLAP.

MTD versus epidermal cyst

Malignant teratoma differentiated may occasionally contain a restricted range of tissues. If the only element present, despite adequate sampling, is a cyst lined by squamous epithelium, it is important to consider the possibility of an epidermal cyst, a totally benign entity. The diagnosis of MTD can be made on the identification of skin appendages associated with the squamous epithelium and/or the presence of ITGCN in adjacent tubules.

True vascular involvement versus artefactual spread

The presence of vascular invasion has been identified as a risk factor for the development of metastatic disease (see below) but artefactual spread during specimen dissection and processing is a common problem because of the lack of cohesiveness of germ cell tumors. Meticulous handling of the specimen should reduce this risk, and the importance of sampling the cord before the testis is bisected is stressed. True vascular invasion has been defined as tumor plugs that were attached to the vessel wall and/or conformed to the shape of the vascular lumen and pseudovascular invasion as poorly cohesive cells not attached to the vessel wall or conforming to the vessel shape[10]. The difficulty is that these definitions are to some extent arbitrary and were not tested against clinical outcome in terms of the development of metastases. Furthermore, in our experience, 'pseudo-vessels' can be created by the retraction of islands of invasive tumor leaving a 'pseudo-lumen', so that endothelial markers are required to confirm the nature of the space. CD31 or CD34 are more universally expressed by endothelial cells whereas factor VIII related antigen is generally negative in lymphatics.

Prognostic indicators

Clinical stage I disease

Seminoma

The identification of a separate group of 'anaplastic' seminomas based predominantly on a higher mitotic index is controversial. The distribution of the proliferative compartment in seminomas has been shown to be dependent on tumor geometry and size[11]. In keeping with this, high mitotic activity has been found to be predictive of relapse in univariate analysis but was not an independent predictor in multivariate analysis because associated with tumor size[12]. This study confirmed the high risk associated with

tumors of more than 6 cm[13]. The 4 year relapse free survival on surveillance was 94% for tumors less than 3 cm, 82% for tumors between 3 and 5.9 cm, dropping to 64% for tumors of 6 cm or more[12].

The issue of vascular invasion is also controversial. Vascular invasion was more commonly seen in patients with pathologic stage II or greater disease[13] but this was not confirmed subsequently[12].

Teratoma

A retrospective Medical Research Council (MRC) study identified the presence of MTU or venous or lymphatic invasion and the absence of YST as risk factors for the development of metastatic disease[14]. The prospective study conducted by the MRC to test their initial findings confirmed their importance: patients with none of the risk features had a 100% 2 year relapse-free rate falling to 81% if one and 53% if any three or all four were present[15]. The successful results of treating the high-risk group with short-course chemotherapy is well established[16]. The presence of vascular invasion and the percentage volume of MTU have been demonstrated as significant risk factors in other retrospective studies[17] and have become widely accepted as the prognostic factors in stage I disease.

A specific issue is that of the development of metastases containing differentiated elements since these are not sensitive to chemotherapy. If this could be predicted, such high-risk patients could be directed towards RLND rather than post-orchidectomy chemotherapy. The only pathologic predictor identified so far is the presence of MTD in the orchidectomy specimen[18]. The factors that govern the malignant transformation of differentiated elements are largely unknown.

Studies have shown statistically significant differences in flow cytometric parameters and levels of proliferation as judged by immunocytochemical markers between pathological stage I tumors and tumors in patients with metastases[17,19]. However, the overlap in values was such that the discriminatory value of these parameters for individual patients is not proven.

Clinically advanced disease

Attention has focused on metastatic 'non-seminomatous' germ cell tumors rather than seminoma. In the study conducted through the European Organization for Research on Treatment of Cancer[20], prognostic groups were based on three variables after multivariate analysis of the data: trophoblastic elements in the primary tumor, serum concentration of AFP, and lung metastasis by size and number. Univariate analysis of the data collected through the MRC[21] showed that invasion of the lower spermatic cord, absence of ITGCN, fibrous tissue and/or MTU and the presence of trophoblastic elements conferred a poorer prognosis. Multivariate analysis confirmed that the absence of MTU and fibrous tissue in the primary tumor, but not presence of trophoblastic elements, were independent predictors of poorer survival. Nevertheless, the MRC chose to base their definition of a poor prognosis group entirely on clinical variables[22].

Chapter submitted in 1996.

References

1. *Pathology of the testis.* Oxford: Blackwell, 1976.

2. WHO. *Histological typing of testis tumours.* International histological classification of tumors. No. 16. Geneva: World Health Organization, 1977.

3. Bunge RG, Bradbury TJ. An early human seminoma. *JAMA* 1965;**193**:960–962.

4. Burke AP, Mostofi FK. Intratubular malignant germ cells in testicular biopsies: clinical course and identification by staining for placental alkaline phosphatase. *Mod Pathol* 1988;**1**:475–479.

5. Bottomley D, Fisher C, Hendry WF, Horwich A. Persistent carcinoma in situ of the testis after chemotherapy for advanced testicular germ cell tumors. *Br J Urol* 1990;**66**:420–424.

6. Nistal M, Codesal J, Paniagua R. Carcinoma in situ of the testis in infertile men. A histological, immunocytochemical, and cytophotometric study of DNA content. *J Pathol* 1989;**159**:205–210.

7. Ulbright TM, Roth LM, Brodhecker CA. Yolk sac differentiation in germ cell tumors. A morphologic study of 50 cases with emphasis on hepatic, enteric, and parietal yolk sac features. *Am J Surg Pathol* 1986;**10**:151–164.

8. Latza U, Foss HD, Durkop H et al. CD30 antigen in embryonal carcinoma and embryogenesis and release of the soluble molecule. *Am J Pathol* 1995;**146**:463–471.

9. Zavala-Pompa A, Ro JY, el-Naggar AK et al. Tubular seminoma. An immunohistochemical and DNA flow-cytometric study of four cases. *Am J Clin Pathol* 1994;**102**:397–401.

10. Nazeer T, Ro JY, Kee KH, Ayala AG. Spermatic cord contamination in testicular cancer. *Mod Pathol* 1996;**9**:762–766.

11. Rabes HM, Schmeller N, Hartmann A, Rattenhuber U, Carl P, Staehler G. Analysis of proliferative compartments in human tumors. II. Seminoma. *Cancer* 1985;**55**:1758–1769.

12. Jacobsen GK, von der Maase H, Specht L et al. Histopathological features in stage I seminoma treated with orchidectomy only. *J Urol Pathol* 1995;**3**:85–94.

13. Marks LB, Rutgers JL, Shipley WU et al. Testicular seminoma: clinical and pathological features that may predict para-aortic lymph node metastases. *J Urol* 1990;**143**:524–527.

14. Freedman LS, Parkinson MC, Jones WG et al. Histopathology in the prediction of relapse of patients with stage I testicular teratoma treated by orchidectomy alone. *Lancet* 1987;**ii**:294–298.

15. Read G, Stenning SP, Cullen MH et al. Medical Research Council prospective study of surveillance for stage I testicular teratoma. Medical Research Council Testicular Tumors Working Party. *J Clin Oncol* 1992;**10**: 1762–1768.

16. Cullen MH, Stenning SP, Parkinson MC et al. Short-course adjuvant chemotherapy in high-risk stage I nonseminomatous germ cell tumors of the testis: a Medical Research Council report. *J Clin Oncol* 1996;**14**:1106–1113.

17. Fernandez EB, Sesterhenn IA, McCarthy WF, Mostofi FK, Moul JW. Proliferating cell nuclear antigen expression to predict occult disease in clinical stage I nonseminomatous testicular germ cell tumors. *J Urol* 1994;**152**:1133–1138.

18. Foster RS, Baniel J, Leibovitch I et al. Teratoma in the orchiectomy specimen and volume of metastasis are predictors of retroperitoneal teratoma in low stage nonseminomatous testis cancer. *J Urol* 1996;**155**:1943–1945.

19. Albers P, Ulbright TM, Albers J et al. Tumor proliferative activity is predictive of pathological stage in clinical stage A nonseminomatous testicular germ cell tumors [see comments]. *J Urol* 1996;**155**:579–586.

20. Stoter G, Sylvester R, Sleijfer DT et al. Multivariate analysis of prognostic factors in patients with disseminated nonseminomatous testicular cancer: results from a European Organization for Research on Treatment of Cancer Multiinstitutional Phase III Study. *Cancer Res* 1987;**47**:2714–2718.

21. Mead GM, Stenning SP, Parkinson MC et al. The Second Medical Research Council study of prognostic factors in nonseminomatous germ cell tumors. Medical Research Council Testicular Tumour Working Party. *J Clin Oncol* 1992;**10**:85–94.

22. Mead GM, Stenning SP. Prognostic factors in metastatic non-seminomatous germ cell tumors: the Medical Research Council studies. *Eur Urol* 1993;**23**:196–200.

36 Presentation, diagnosis and staging

M I Johnson and F C Hamdy

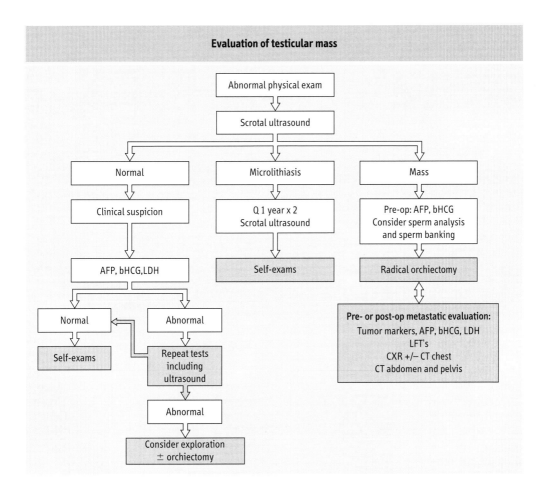

Evaluation of testicular mass

Abnormal physical exam → Scrotal ultrasound

- Normal → Clinical suspicion → AFP, bHCG, LDH
  - Normal → Self-exams
  - Abnormal → Repeat tests including ultrasound → Abnormal → Consider exploration ± orchiectomy
- Microlithiasis → Q 1 year x 2 Scrotal ultrasound → Self-exams
- Mass → Pre-op: AFP, bHCG Consider sperm analysis and sperm banking → Radical orchiectomy ↕ Pre- or post-op metastatic evaluation: Tumor markers, AFP, bHCG, LDH LFT's CXR +/− CT chest CT abdomen and pelvis

Presentation

Testicular cancer accounts for approximately 1% of all male neoplasms. The incidence peaks between 20 and 40 years of age and is around nine per 100 000 population, the incidence has increased rapidly over the past 20 years.

Groups at increased risk of developing testicular cancer include patients with testicular maldescent (four- to tenfold increase), previous contralateral testicular tumor (24-fold increase) and affected first degree relative (sixfold increase)[1].

Testicular tumors most commonly present as a painless swelling or mass in the testis. It may cause mild discomfort, but in around 10% of cases it presents as pain of acute onset. A firm, hard or fixed area within the tunica albuginea is considered suspicious until proved otherwise. There may be a secondary hydrocele which may be aspirated to allow palpation of the underlying testis.

Approximately 10% of patients will present with metastases, the primary tumor being occult or having regressed. The presenting features include palpable supraclavicular or abdominal nodes, abdominal or back pain from retroperitoneal nodes, respiratory symptoms from lung metastasis, bone pain from skeletal metastasis, central and peripheral nervous symptoms from metastatic involvement and weight loss.

Gynecomastia is present in 5% of patients with germ cell tumors and suggests a functioning tumor with either excess oestrogen production or androgen deficiency.

Delay in diagnosis is common and usually results from a delay in the patients seeking advice. How this affects overall survival is unclear but the tumor burden in teratoma may double every 5 days, so increasing public awareness is an important goal[2].

Diagnosis

Clinical examination allied to a high degree of suspicion remains the mainstay for the diagnosis of testicular tumors. Ultrasound scanning of the testes can help in patients who are difficult to assess clinically and may differentiate between tumor and inflammatory disease. Ultrasound can also identify clinically occult testicular masses in patients who present with metastases, differentiating this group from true extragonadal germ cell tumors. The contralateral testis should also be examined by ultrasound to exclude bilateral tumors, which occur in around 1% of cases[3].

As soon as a suspicious mass is found within the testis the diagnosis should be confirmed by inguinal orchidectomy; this provides a histologic diagnosis and establishes local control. Biopsy should never be performed through the scrotal skin as this risks local recurrence and dissemination to the inguinal lymph nodes. In view of the rapid growth rate of testicular tumors, orchidectomy should be performed urgently.

Patients may present with extensive life threatening metastatic disease, the diagnosis may then be made by assay of tumor markers and fine needle aspiration or biopsy of a metastasis. In these cases orchidectomy may not be part of the initial management.

The serum concentration of the tumor markers β human chorionic gonadotrophin (βhCG), alpha-fetoprotein (AFP) and lactic acid dehydrogenase (LDH) should be determined before orchidectomy to help with staging, prognosis and monitoring of treatment.

At orchidectomy the spermatic cord is soft clamped at the level of the deep inguinal ring before manipulating the involved testis. If the macroscopic appearance is uncertain the testis can be explored by opening it through the anti-mesenteric border after isolating it from the operative field. Frozen section can then be performed if necessary and if this proves benign the testis can be closed and replaced within the scrotum. Frozen sections of the testis can be difficult to interpret and is rarely required in practice.

Orchidectomy if indicated is then performed after doubly ligating the cord at the deep ring. Meticulous hemostasis is essential as a hematoma may delay subsequent chemotherapy or radiotherapy.

It is standard practice in several countries including the UK to perform a small open biopsy of the contralateral testis to exclude concomitant intratubular germ cell neoplasia, which is present in around 5% of men undergoing orchidectomy for tumor. Biopsy should always be performed if the testis is small or there is a history of testicular maldescent.

Ninety-five per cent of testicular tumors are of germ cell origin and divide broadly into seminomas and non-seminomatous germ cell tumors (NSGCT). The remaining cases being lymphoma (4%) and a variety of rare tumors (1%). Of the germ cell tumors 40% are pure seminoma, the remaining are NSGCT.

Staging

Histologic examination of the excised testis allows assessment of tumor type and the extent of local spread including presence of cord involvement and lymphovascular invasion. Following the histologic confirmation staging is performed, guided by the findings of clinical examination. Staging involves measurement of the serum level of tumor markers and imaging studies, principally computed tomography (CT).

Tumor markers for testicular cancer are in two main groups, the oncofetal proteins βhCG and AFP and cellular enzymes LDH and PLAP. Elevated AFP (>10 iu/l) or βhCG (>5 iu/l) occurs in 80% of metastatic and 57% of stage 1 NSGCTs of the testis. In seminomas the βhCG is elevated in less than 20% of all cases and indicates the presence of trophoblastic elements. An elevated AFP in the absence of hepatic involvement indicates non-seminomatous elements. The tumor markers βhCG and AFP should not replace a tissue diagnosis as they lack sensitivity and specificity, however elevation of both is rare except in germ cell tumors[4].

LDH is elevated in 27% of stage 1 and 55% of metastatic seminomas, but its lack of sensitivity and specificity make its value limited. Greatly raised LDH levels (> 2000 u/l) are reliable as markers and rising levels a good indicator of recurrence in seminoma.

Abdominal, pelvic and thoracic CT scanning should be included in the initial staging of all germ cell tumors. Retroperitoneal lymph node involvement is defined by size criteria, and CT is unable to detect microscopic tumor deposits. Lymphography is no longer routine but may have a role in the assessment of equivocal nodes in patients with normal tumor markers when follow up CT scan is not acceptable.

Chest radiography though not as sensitive as CT is a useful baseline at the time of initial staging, and can be repeated more frequently than CT during follow up. Ultrasound examination has little role in the detection of retroperitoneal disease but can help to clarify equivocal hepatic lesions identified by CT. Cranial imaging by CT or magnetic resonance imaging is not done routinely in asymptomatic patients. Asymptomatic cerebral metastases may be seen in patients with multiple metastases (greater than 20 lung metastases) or greatly raised βhCG (over 20 000 iu/l)[5].

In the USA and some European countries a staging retroperitoneal lymph node dissection is performed in patients with no evidence of lymph node metastases, though this is not standard practice in the UK. When this surgery is compared with careful surveillance the overall long-term survival appears similar.

There are a variety of clinical staging classifications, in the UK the Royal Marsden Hospital staging classification is almost universal (Table 36.1), within this classification identical criteria are used for all germ cell tumors.

As a result of the wide variety of measurable parameters affecting prognosis, no consensus had emerged on a unifying staging system. The International Germ Cell Cancer Collaborative Group (IGCCCG) was formed in 1991 and analysed a large number of patientsw with both seminoma and non-seminoma treated with chemotherapy including cisplatin[6]. The classification places patients into three prognostic groups based on a variety of factors measured prior to chemotherapy (Table 36.2).

Pathologic staging of germ cell tumors of the testis can be performed according to the TNM classification[7].

The regional lymph nodes are the abdominal para-aortic, pre-aortic, inter-aortocaval, pre-caval, paracaval, retrocaval and retroaortic nodes. Nodes along the spermatic vein should be considered regional. Laterality does not affect the N classification. The intrapelvic nodes and the inguinal nodes are considered regional after scrotal or inguinal surgery.

pTN Pathological Classification

pT – Primary tumor

pTX Primary tumor cannot be assessed (if no radical orchidectomy has been performed TX is used)

pT0 No evidence of primary tumor

pTis Intratubular germ cell neoplasia

pT1 Tumor limited to testis and epididymis without vascular/lymphatic invasion; tumor may invade tunica albuginea but not tunica vaginalis

pT2 Tumor limited to testis and epididymis with vascular/lymphatic invasion or tumor extending through tunica albuginea with involvement of tunica vaginalis

pT3 Tumor invades spermatic cord with or without vascular/lymphatic invasion

pT4 Tumor invades scrotum with or without vascular/lymphatic invasion

pT – Regional Lymph Nodes

pNX Regional lymph nodes cannot be assessed

Table 36.1 The Royal Marsden Hospital Staging Classification for testicular germ cell tumors

Stage		Definition
I		No evidence of metastases
IM		Rising serum markers with no other evidence of metastases
II		Abdominal lymphadenopathy
	A	<2 cm
	B	2–5 cm
	C	>5 cm
III		Supradiaphragmatic lymphadenopathy
	M	Mediastinal
	N	Supraclavicular/cervical/axillary
	O	No abdominnnal disease
	ABC	Nodes as defined in stage II
IV		Extralymphatic metastases
	Lung	
	L1	≤3 lung metastases
	L2	>3 lung metastases all <2cm
	L3	>3 metastases with 1 or more >2cm
	H+	Liver metastases
	Br+	Brain metastases
	Bo+	Bone metastases

Table 36.2   The International Germ Cell Consensus Classification

Good Prognosis

Non-seminoma	*Seminoma*
Testis/retroperitoneal primary	Any primary site
and	*and*
No non-pulmonary visceral metastases	No non pulmonary visceral metastases
and	*and*
Good markers – all of	Normal AFP, any hCG, any LDH
AFP <1000 ng/ml and	
βhCG <5000 iu/l (1000 ng/ml) and	
LDH <1.5 × upper limit of normal	
56% of non-seminomas	90% of seminomas
5 year PFS 89%	5 year PFS 82%
5 year survival 92%	5 year survival 86%

Intermediate Prognosis

Non-seminoma	*Seminoma*
Testis/retroperitoneal primary	Any primary site
and	*and*
No non-pulmonary visceral metastases	Non-pulmonary visceral metastases
and	*and*
Intermediate markers – any of:	Normal AFP, any hCG, any LDH
AFP > 1000 and < 10 000 iu/l or	
hCG >5000 and < 50 000 iu/i or	
LDH > 1.5 × N and < 10 × N	
28% of non-seminomas	10% of seminomas
5 year PFS 75%	5 year PFS 67%
5 year survival 80%	5 year survival 72%

Poor Prognosis

Non-seminoma	*Seminoma*
Mediastinal primary	
or	
Non-pulmonary visceral metastases	
or	
Poor markers – any of:	
AFP >10 000 ng/ml or	No patients classfied as poor prognosis
hCG > 50 000 iu/l (10 000 ng/ml) or	
LDH > 10 × upper limit of normal	
16% of non-seminomas	
5 year PFS 41%	
5 year survival 48%	

PFS – Progression free survival.

pN0   No regional lymph node metastasis

pN1   Metastasis with lymph node mass 2 cm or less in greatest dimension and 5 or fewer positive nodes none more than 2 cm in greatest dimension

pN2   Metastasis with a lymph node mass more than 2 cm but no more than 5 cm in greatest dimension; or more than 5 nodes positive, none more than 5 cm; or evidence of extranodal extension of tumor

pN3   Metastasis with a lymph node mass more than 5 cm in greatest dimension

Conclusions

Testicular cancer is uncommon, but vitally important as it is the most common malignancy in men aged between 20 and 34 years old. Increasing public awareness and knowledge of the tumor's high cure rate, will allow prompt diagnosis and earlier treatment, with possible improved response. Testicular self-examination should be encouraged. The possibility of a tumor presenting with pain should be borne in mind, and if there is any suspicion testicular ultrasound should be performed. When diagnosed a patient with a testicular tumor requires thorough accurate staging in order that optimal treatment can be given and allow comparison between treatment and response in different centers.

References

1.   Buetow SA. Epidemiology of testicular cancer. *Epidemiol Rev* 1995;**17**(2):433–449.
2.   Horwich A. *Testicular cancer. Investigation and management.* London, Chapman and Hall Medical, 1991.
3.   Berthelsen JG, Skakkebaek NE, Maase H, Sorenson BL, Mogensen P. Screening for carcinoma in situ of the contralateral testis in patients with germinal testicular cancer. *BMJ* 1982;**285**:1683–1686.
4.   Doherty AP, Bower M, Christmas TJ. The role of tumor markers in the diagnosis and treatment of testicular germ cell cancers. *Br J Urol* 1997;**79**:247–252.
5.   MacVicar D. Staging of testicular germ cell tumours (review). *Clin Radiol* 1993;**47**(3):149–158.
6.   (IGCCCG) IGCCG. International Germ Cell Consensus Classification. A Prognostic Factor-Based Staging for Metastatic Germ Cell Cancers. *J Clin Oncol* 1997;**15**(2):594–603.
7.   Hermanek P, Hutter RVP, Sobin LH, Wagner G, Wittekind C. *TNM atlas* (4th edn) Springer-Verlag, Berlin, 1997.

37 Carcinoma in situ

S Fosså and E H Wanderås

Definition

Intratubular germ cell neoplasia (ITGCN), or carcinoma in situ (CIS) of the testis, is a pre-invasive lesion of the seminiferous tubules with a high tendency to progress to invasive germ cell cancer.

Characteristics and origin

ITGCN is suggested to proceed all types of germ cell neoplasms except spermatocytic seminoma and is frequently observed in the tissue adjacent to malignant testicular tumors (Figure 37.1)[1]. If not treated, about 50% of adults with ITGCN will develop invasive germ cell cancer within 5 years[2,3]. Spontaneous regression of ITGCN has never been observed, and it is suggested that with time nearly all cases of ITGCN will become invasive. Development of germ cell neoplasms in testicles with a prior negative biopsy is rare[2,4], though ITGCN may not be as diffusely distributed within the testis as earlier believed[5].

ITGCN cells are most often triploid[6] or almost tetraploid[7] and are, based on ultrastructural studies, believed to develop by polyploidization from dysplastic pre-spermatogenic cells (gonocytes or pre-spermatogonia),

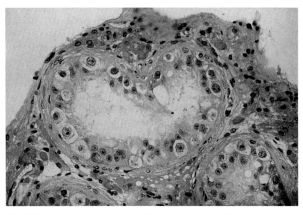

Fig. 37.1   Intratubular germ cell neoplasia (ITGCN) of the testis. Tubuli containing large atypical germ cells and smaller Sertoli cells.

primarily in fetal life[8]. This is also supported by immunohistochemical methods, as example by expression of placental like alkaline phosphatase (P1AP) in gonocytes, ITGCN cells and also in malignant germ cells[9,10].

Prevalence of ITGCN

In Denmark, harboring the highest incidence of testicular cancer in the world, the prevalence of ITGCN in the general population is estimated to be in the range of 0.5–1%[11].

Non-malignant conditions

In males with cryptorchidism and no previous germ cell cancer, the prevalence of ITGCN is about 2%[4], and in men with infertility 0.5–1%[3]. In a review of 102 cases with various intersex states including a Y-chromosome in the karyotype, the prevalence of ITGCN was 6%[12].

Previous germ cell malignancy

In patients with testicular cancer, ITGCN is found in the contralateral testis in 5–6%[2,13]. The risk is believed to be especially high in patients with maldescent, testicular atrophy, low sperm density ($<10 \times 10^6$/ml)[14] or familial testicular cancer.[15] As many as 35% of men with assumed primary extragonadal germ cell cancer are claimed to have ITGCN in one or both gonads[16].

A total of 35–45% of all patients with testicular cancer is believed to belong to one or more high risk groups[17]. According to data from the Norwegian Radium Hospital 12.5% (92/738) of patients with germ cell cancer have a history of maldescent and 14% (87/615) record infertility problems.

Screening

At the present time no strict recommendations exist for screening of males without germ cell cancer, displaying maldescent, infertility problems or genetic predisposition. In cryptorchid males the best time for biopsy would be between 18 and 20 years, as ITGCN cells are easier distinguished in adult testicles, and the risk of germ cell cancer is very low before this age. More data on the prevalence of ITGCN in infertile men and in first degree relatives of patients with germ cell cancer are necessary before it can be decided whether they should be screened. All adolescents with intersex bearing a Y-chromosome should be offered a screening biopsy.

In patients with unilateral testicular cancer many centers now routinely perform a biopsy of the contralateral testis either in all patients or only in risk groups (testicular atrophy, azo- or oligozoospermia, history of maldescent, genetic predisposition and age lower than 30 years). In addition a screening biopsy should be considered in men with assumed extragonadal germ cell cancer. However, the clinical significance of such early diagnosis of ITGCN is still under discussion.

Diagnostics

Patients with ITGCN of the testis are usually asymptomatic. The involved testis, however, is often small,[18] with soft consistency. Infertility might be a problem.

In local anesthesia a surgical biopsy (3×3×3× mm), preferably from the lateral part of the cranial pole of the testis, can be performed as an outpatient procedure. Stieve's or Bouin's fluid are recommended as fixative.

Other invasive diagnostic methods for demonstration of ITGCN are fine-needle aspiration[19] and TRU-CUT or Biopty-Gun biopsy. In a previous series[20] the latter method seems to be as sensitive as open biopsy.

Immunostaining of cell markers
Polyclonal antibodies against PIAP are rather sensitive and specific markers of ITGCN cells[9] and can be used on formaldehyde fixed material. Other markers of ITGCN are monoclonal antibodies against M2A and 43-9F[9].

DNA-flow cytometry
In contrast to the normal euploid spermatogonia ITGCN cells are highly aneuploid and may be detected by flow cytometry[7]. Nevertheless, aneuploid cells are not necessarily

malignant and are found in cryptorchid testes[21]. The low sensitivity of this method is a great disadvantage.

Seminal fluid analyses
ITGCN cells may or may not be present in the seminal fluid in patients with testicular ITGCN. In a study using seminal fluid[22], in situ hybridization has visualized numerical aberrations in chromosome 1, frequently present in DNA of germ cell cancer and ITGCN cells.

At the Norwegian Radium Hospital a biopsy of the contralateral testis was performed in patients with testicular cancer if one or more of the following risk factors were present: testicular volume <12 ml (normal 15–32 ml), history of cryptorchidism, or father or brother having had testicular cancer. ITGCN was found in 15 of 120 patients (12.5%) and microinvasive testicular cancer in one patient (Table 37.1). As also demonstrated elsewhere[14,18], the patients with ITGCN in contralateral testis were younger than those without, and FSH was often elevated. The cumulative risk of developing invasive germ cell cancer was 67% after 5 years (95% confidence interval 32–100%) (Figure 37.2).

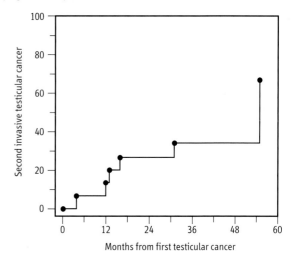

Fig. 37.2   Diagnosis of 2nd invasive testicular cancer in 15 patients with ITGCN in the contralateral testis.

Table 37.1   Characteristics of 15 patients with ITGCN in contralateral testis diagnosed in a high-risk group of patients with unilateral testicular cancer

Age at primary testicular cancer Mean (range), years	Maldescent No.	Testicular volume mean (range) ml	Infertility* No.	FSH† >12 iE/l No.	Sperm count‡ 0/≤5 / >5 x 10⁶/ml No.
26.0 (18.2–41.7)	7 / 15	8.7 (4.8–14.0)	5 / 7	9 / 13	8 / 4 / 1

*Not assessable in eight patients. †FSH after unilateral orchidectomy before further treatment excluding two patients with elevated HCG. ‡Not done in two patients.

Management

Dependent on the clinical situation, ITGCN should be managed by orchidectomy, irradiation or close follow up. The management is highly dependent on whether the condition is unilateral or bilateral.

Unilateral orchidectomy is recommended for unilateral ITGCN associated with infertility or maldescent[23]. If ITGCN is diagnosed in a pre-pubertal boy, it may be sufficient to institute close follow up and confirm the diagnosis in a repeat biopsy after puberty before performing an orchidectomy. Testicular irradiation should be considered for bilateral disease. In patients with a previous unilateral testicular cancer, testicular irradiation or orchidectomy represents alternative treatment modalities for ITGCN. When some sperm production is present in a patient with ITGCN who wishes to father children, the development of ITGCN may be followed by repeat biopsies for some time. Multiple semen cryopreservations are to be offered to such a patient.

The target irradiation dose necessary to eradicate ITGCN has not been finally clarified. Today many centers use a dose of 2 Gy × 10 delivered during 2 weeks. This dose safely removes ITGCN[24], but produces irreversible sterility with a 'Sertoli cell only' picture microscopically, and some impairment of Leydig cell function[24,25]. Androgen replacement therapy, on the other hand, is only occasionally indicated.

Cisplatin based chemotherapy is too toxic as treatment of a pre-invasive disease. Such treatment does not eradicate ITGCN permanently[26], but may delay the development of invasive testicular cancer. Patients who receive cisplatin based chemotherapy due to metastatic germ cell cancer should have close follow up of their contralateral testis if ITGCN has been demonstrated initially.

Conclusion

ITGCN is suggested to proceed all types of germ cell cancer probably except spermatocytic seminoma. ITGCN is found in 0.5–1% of the general population and in 5–6% of patients with unilateral testicular cancer, the prevalence being higher if one or more additional risk factors are present. The significance of screening risk groups is not fully clarified. When diagnosed, a patient with ITGCN should be offered treatment with orchidectomy, irradiation or close follow up.

References

1. Jacobsen GK, Henriksen OB, von der Maase H. Carcinoma in situ of testicular tissue adjacent to malignant germ-cell tumors: a study of 105 cases. *Cancer* 1981;**47**:2660–2662.

2. von der Maase H, Rörth M, Walbom Jörgensen S *et al.* Carcinoma in situ of contralateral testis in patients with testicular germ cell cancer: study of 27 cases in 500 patients. *Br Med J Clin Res Ed* 1986;**293**:1398–1401.

3. Bettocchi C, Coker CB, Deacon J, Parkinson C, Pryor JP. A review of testicular intratubular germ cell neoplasia in infertile men. *J Androl* 1994;**15**(suppl 1):14S–16S

4. Giwercman A, Bruun E, Frimodt Möller C, Skakkebaek NE. Prevalence of carcinoma in situ and other histopathological abnormalities in testes of men with a history of cryptorchidism. *J Urol* 1989;**142**:998–1001.

5. Loy V, Wigand I, Dieckmann KP. Incidence and distribution of carcinoma in situ in testes removed for germ cell tumor: possible inadequacy of random testicular biopsy in detecting the condition [see comments]. *Histopathology* 1990;**16**:198–200.

6. Giwercman A, Clausen OP, Skakkebaek NE. Carcinoma in situ of the testis: aneuploid cells in semen. *Br Med J Clin Res Ed* 1988;**296**:1762–1764.

7. Nistal M, Codesal J, Paniagua R. Carcinoma in situ of the testis in infertile men. A histological, immunocytochemical, and cytophotometric study of DNA content [see comments]. *J Pathol* 1989;**159**:205–210.

8. Gondos B. Ultrastructure of developing and malignant germ cells. *Eur Urol* 1993;**23**:68–74.

9. Giwercman A, Cantell L, Marks A. Placental-like alkaline phosphatase as a marker of carcinoma-in-situ of the testis. Comparison with monoclonal antibodies M2A and 43-9F. *APMIS* 1991;**99**:586–594.

10. Skakkebaek NE, Berthelsen JG, Giwercman A, Müller J. Carcinoma-in-situ of the testis: possible origin from gonocytes and precursor of all types of germ cell tumors except spermatocytoma. *Int J Androl* 1987;**10**:19–28.

11. Giwercman A, Müller J, Skakkebaek NE. Prevalence of carcinoma in situ and other histopathological abnormalities in testes from 399 men who died suddenly and unexpectedly. *J Urol* 1991;**145**:77–80.

12. Ramani P, Yeung CK, Habeebu SS. Testicular intratubular germ cell neoplasia in children and adolescents with intersex. *Am J Surg Pathol* 1993;**17**:1124–1133.

13. Loy V, Dieckmann KP. Prevalence of contralateral testicular intraepithelial neoplasia (carcinoma in situ) in patients with testicular germ cell tumor. Results of the German multicentre study. *Eur Urol* 1993;**23**:120–122.

14. Harland SJ, Cook PA, Fosså SD *et al.* Quantifying risk of contralateral testicular carcinoma in situ (CIS) in patients with testicular cancer – an MRC study. *Proc ASCO* 1996;**15**:239.

15. Heimdal K, Olsson H, Tretli S, Flodgren P, Børresen A, Fosså SD. Familial testicular cancer in Norway and Southern Sweden. *Br J Cancer* 1996;**73**:964–969.

16. Daugaard G, Rörth M, von der Maase H, Skakkebaek NE. Management of extragonadal germ-cell tumors and the significance of bilateral testicular biopsies. *Ann Oncol* 1992;**3**:283–289.

17. Giwercman, A. Carcinoma-in-situ of the testis: screening and management 1992; University of Copenhagen, Denmark; Thesis.

18. Dieckmann KP, Loy V. Management of contralateral testicular intraepithelial neoplasia in patients with testicular germ-cell tumor. *World J Urol* 1994;**12**:131–135.

19. Brackenbury ET, Hargreave TB, Howard GC, McIntyre MA. Seminal fluid analysis and fine-needle aspiration cytology in the diagnosis of carcinoma in situ of the testis. *Eur Urol* 1993;**23**:123–128.

20. Heikkila R, Heilo A, Stenwig AE, Fossa SD. Testicular ultrasonography and 18G biopty biopsy for clinically undetected cancer or carcinoma in situ in patients with germ cell tumors. *Br J Urol* 1993;**71**:214–216.

21. Muller J, Skakkebaek NE. Abnormal germ cells in maldescended testes: a study of cell density, nuclear size and deoxyribonucleic acid content in testicular biopsies from 50 boys. *J Urol* 1984;**131**:730–733.

22. Giwercman A, Hopman AH, Ramaekers FC, Skakkebaek NE. Carcinoma in situ of the testis. Detection of malignant germ cells in seminal fluid by means of in situ hybridization. *Am J Pathol* 1990;**136**:497–502.

23. von der Maase H, Giwercman A, Muller J, Skakkebaek NE. Management of carcinoma-in-situ of the testis. *Int J Androl* 1987;**10**:209–220.

24. Giwercman A, von der Maase H, Berthelsen JG, Rorth M, Bertelsen A, Skakkebaek NE. Localized irradiation of testes with

437

carcinoma in situ: effects on Leydig cell function and eradication of malignant germ cells in 20 patients. *J Clin Endocrinol Metab* 1991;**73**:596–603.

25.   Shalet SM, Tsatsoulis A, Whitehead E, Read G. Vulnerability of the human Leydig cell to radiation damage is dependent upon age. *J Endocrinol* 1989;**120**:161–165.

26.   Fossa SD, Aass N. Cisplatin-based chemotherapy does not eliminate the risk of a second testicular cancer. *Br J Urol* 1989;**63**:531–534.

38 Non-seminomatous germ-cell tumors

Algorithm

Testicular tumor algorithm

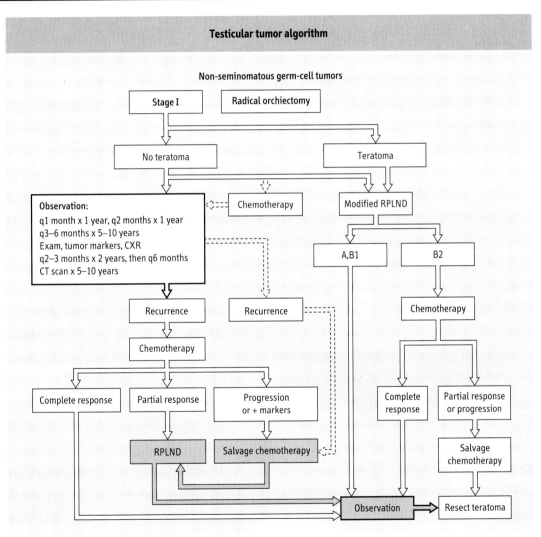

Non-seminomatous germ-cell tumors

Stage I

Radical orchiectomy

No teratoma

Teratoma

Observation:
q1 month x 1 year, q2 months x 1 year
q3–6 months x 5–10 years
Exam, tumor markers, CXR
q2–3 months x 2 years, then q6 months
CT scan x 5–10 years

Chemotherapy

Modified RPLND

A,B1

B2

Recurrence

Recurrence

Chemotherapy

Chemotherapy

Complete response

Partial response

Progression
or + markers

Complete
response

Partial response
or progression

RPLND

Salvage chemotherapy

Salvage
chemotherapy

Observation

Resect teratoma

439

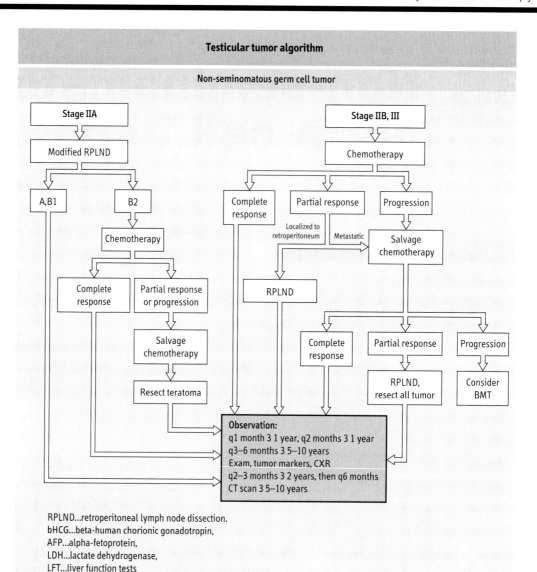

Testicular tumor algorithm

Non-seminomatous germ cell tumor

RPLND...retroperitoneal lymph node dissection.
bHCG...beta-human chorionic gonadotropin,
AFP...alpha-fetoprotein,
LDH...lactate dehydrogenase,
LFT...liver function tests

38.1   Germ cell tumors: Surveillance and adjuvant chemotherapy

M Cullen

Introduction

Approximately 50% of patients with non-seminomatous germ cell tumors of the testis (NSGCTT) present with stage I disease[1]. In the last 30 years there have been important changes in the management of these patients. Elective treatment of the retroperitoneal area with radio-therapy (in the UK and Denmark) or with surgery (in the USA and most of Europe) reduced the recurrence rate in this area but disseminated relapse remained a problem. The advent of cisplatin based combination chemotherapy in the early 1970s offered the real prospect of cure for all relapsing stage I cases. However, the myelosuppression of chemotherapy in patients who had received radical para-aortic and pelvic radiotherapy was a significant problem, as was ejaculatory impotence in cases having elective retroperitoneal lymph node dissection (RPLND). This, plus the widespread use of CT scanning and tumor marker (AFP, HCG) assays to monitor disease recurrence, encouraged Peckham to suggest a policy of close surveillance in stage I NSGCTT with chemotherapy at the first sign of relapse[2]. The vast majority of cases are cured with this approach, despite a relapse rate of around 30%[3]. Consequently, unlike most other tumors, where the principal aim is still to achieve higher cure rates, the questions surrounding the management of early stage testis cancer involve finding better ways of curing virtually every case.

Radiotherapy is no longer practised in this setting and developments in retroperitoneal surgery are presented in the next section. This chapter discusses developments in surveillance and adjuvant chemotherapy.

Surveillance in stage I NSGCTT

The initial report of surveillance[2] was soon followed by others from the United Kingdom[4] and data from these studies were subsequently incorporated into a retrospective, multicenter study coordinated by the United Kingdom Medical Research Council. At the same time (January 1984) a prospective study was initiated. These now form by far the largest group of cases of stage I NSGCTT, managed consistently on a surveillance policy, in the world.

Medical Research Council studies

Retrospective study

Between 1979 and 1983, 259 patients had entered this study, which was first reported by Freedman *et al.* in 1987[5]. All had histologically verified stage I teratoma, and had been treated with orchidectomy alone. The median follow up was 54 months, and 90% of cases had been followed for more than 2 years. Seventy patients (27%) relapsed, 53 within the first 12 months after orchidectomy. After 18 months the risk of relapse decreased to about 4% per year. The overall relapse-free rate at 4 years was 68% with three deaths.

Prospective study

The MRC prospective surveillance study opened in 1984. Three hundred and seventy-three eligible patients from 16 UK and one Norwegian centers entered the prospective study[5]. Follow up attendances after staging investigations were at monthly intervals for the first year, 2 monthly for the second and 3 monthly in the third. Assessment consisted of clinical examination, AFP and HCG assay, and chest X-ray at each visit. Marker investigations were performed more frequently if there was clinical need. CT scanning was performed at each center according to one of two schedules: at alternate visits for the first 2 years, or at 2, 6, 8 and 12 months. Treatment of relapse was dependent on stage. The median follow up time on those patients who were relapse-free was 37 months. Ninety-four per cent of cases had been followed up for more than 2 years.

One hundred patients (27%) relapsed of whom 78 (80%) were in the first 12 months following orchidectomy. The overall relapse free curve is shown in Figure 38.1.1. The curve was virtually identical to that for the retrospective study, and again the annual risk of relapse appeared to drop sharply after the first 12 months following orchidectomy, and continued to decline in the second and subsequent years. The 2 year actuarial relapse-free rate was 75%, dropping to only 72% 5 years after orchidectomy. The latest relapse to have occurred was 44 months after orchidectomy.

Following relapse, chemotherapy was given according to the usual practise of the referring center, and all but four were alive and disease free at the time of reporting. The 4 year survival rate for mortality from all causes was 98%, and for tumor mortality 99%.

Other studies of surveillance

Over 1000 patients have been reported from 12 studies in which a surveillance policy has been adopted following orchidectomy for stage I NSGCTT. Over half the patients

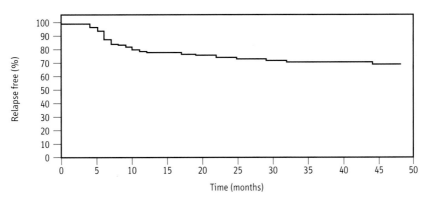

Fig. 38.1.1 Stage 1 non seminoma free survival on surveillance.

have been in MRC studies. The schedules of surveillance have not differed substantially from those employed in the MRC studies and the results have been remarkably similar. These have recently been reviewed[3]. With median follow up times of 30–40 months relapse rates have been 27% in both MRC studies and 28% in the other smaller series combined. Furthermore complete response rates in relapsing cases were 96% in both MRC studies and 95% in the rest.

Drawbacks of surveillance

On the face of it, surveillance would seem to be an almost perfect management policy in that the majority of cases escape treatment (other than orchidectomy) altogether, whilst the minority who relapse will be detected at an early stage and treated with curative chemotherapy. However, some patients find the process of surveillance to be stressful[6]. Frequent examinations, CT scans and tumor marker analyses remind patients of their cancer history and of their continuing risk of relapse. This has been called the 'Damocles syndrome'. There are other drawbacks to surveillance. The most important of these is that excellent patient compliance is essential. This may be a problem in a largely young population who may have less well developed feelings of responsibility for their own health than older patients, and whose occupations may be less stable geographically. A recent population based study in Scotland revealed a defaulting rate of over 25% amongst a group of stage I teratoma patients[7]. This may partly explain the rather high proportion of cases in which recurrent disease has been advanced at the time of detection[8]. In addition, some patients on surveillance may experience problems in relation to employment, housing, mortgages, life insurance or adoption which are greatly reduced if they have successfully completed adjuvant therapy and are thus more likely to remain in uninterrupted good health.

Adjuvant chemotherapy

Adjuvant chemotherapy is a clear alternative policy for stage I NSGCTT but the toxicity of chemotherapy is such that its applicability would be influenced by the proportion of patients who received treatment unnecessarily. Clearly adjuvant chemotherapy with significant toxicity would not be appropriate for a population of patients with a very small risk of recurrence. Arguably the most important information to emerge from the UK MRC studies of surveillance is the histologic prognostic scoring, allowing distinct categories of patients to be identified who have different risks of recurrence.

The retrospective study of surveillance highlighted four histologic factors within the primary tumor which carried independent prognostic significance[4]. These were: tumor invasion of testicular veins; tumor invasion of testicular lymphatics; presence of undifferentiated cells; and absence of yolk sac elements. The presence of any three or all four of these factors identifies a high-risk group of stage I NSGCTT patients with a chance of recurrence around 50% (Figure 38.1.2). The subsequent prospective study validated this prognostic index and allowed the identification of a group of patients to whom adjuvant chemotherapy might be offered[5]. Data from surgically treated stage II cases suggested that two courses of BEP (bleomycin, etopside, cis-platinum) would be sufficient adjuvant therapy[9]. Furthermore, the long-term toxicity of chemotherapy for NSGCTT seems to be related to total dose administered[10]. Hence just two courses were likely to be acceptable to a patient population where about half of those included would not develop metastatic disease.

MRC adjuvant chemotherapy study

Based on the above observations the UK MRC launched a study of adjuvant chemotherapy (BEP × 2) in October 1987[11]. Patients with newly diagnosed stage I (i.e. CT scan

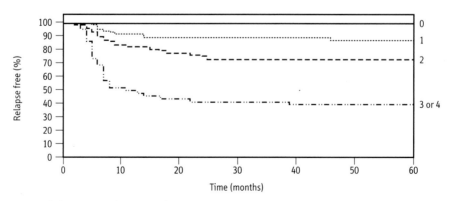

Fig. 38.1.2   MRC prognostic factor soure for relapse free nurvial for stage 1 non seminoma on surveillance.

Table 38.1.1   Surveillance protocol for orchiectomy-only treatment option based on MRC study protocol

Radical inguinal orchietctomy
(favorable pathology, evaluable markers)

First year (relapse rate ~ 21% of initial group):
Q 1 month examination, AFP, HCG (optional PALP, LDH), CXR
Q 2 month CT chest, abdomen & pelvis

Second year (relapse rate ~ 4% of initial group):
Q 2 month examination, AFP, HCG (optional PALP, LDH), CXR
Q 4 month CT chest, abdomen & pelvis

Third year:
Q 4 month examination, AFP, HCG (optional PALP, LDH), CXR
Q 6 month CT chest, abdomen & pelvis

Fourth year:
Q 6 month examination, AFP, HCG (optional PALP, LDH), CXR
Q 6 month CT chest, abdomen & pelvis

Fifth year (relapse rate ~ 2% of initial group during yrs 3–5):
Q 6 month examination, AFP, HCG (optional PALP, LDH), CXR
Q 6 month CT chest, abdomen & pelvis

Sixth year (and beyond):
Q 12 month examination, AFP, HCG (optional PALP, LDH), CXR
Further imaging as clinically indicated.

Relapses treated with standard chemotherapy.
Observation protocol not recommended for poor prognosis histologic findings or when markers cannot be assessed or were not elevated initially.

Table 38.1.2   NSGCTT treatment protocol

Radical inguinal orchiectomy
confirm pathology NSGCTT
assess risk factors for poor prognosis

1. Venous invasion
2. Lymphatic invasion.
3. Undifferentiated cells
4. Absence of yolk sac elements

Low risk	High risk
(0–2 risk factors)	(3–4 Risk Factors)
Surveillance protocol:	Adjuvant chemotherapy
Exam	(BEP × 2–4 cycles)
Tumor markers	**Then:** Exam,
CT (Chest/abd/pelvis)	Tumor markers
Schedule:	CT (Chest/abd/pelvis)
F/U per Table 1	**Schedule:**
	F/U per Table 1

of chest, abdomen and pelvis showing no metastases and normal AFP and HCG) NSGCTT were eligible if any three or all four of the high risk histopathologic features described above were present in the primary tumor. The study was set up as a non-randomized phase II study with strict early stopping rules in the event of an unacceptably high (>5%) recurrence rate.

Chemotherapy consisted of two courses of standard cisplatin, etoposide and bleomycin. In addition to standard short-term toxicity evaluation, longer-term toxicity problems were studied. These included fertility assessments, lung function studies and audiometry. One hundred and fourteen eligible patients were included with a median follow up time of 4 years.

Sperm analysis showed no consistent reduction in sperm density or percentage of motile forms, and lung function studies revealed no clinically significant respiratory dysfunction.

After a median follow up time of 4 years there were two relapses. Following central histopathologic review of diagnostic material (undertaken without knowledge of clinical outcome) one of these was re-classified as adenocarcinoma of the rete testis rather than a germ cell neoplasm. The other case relapsed 7 months after adjuvant chemotherapy, and eventually died with resistant NSGCTT 27 months after first recurrence.

Other studies of adjuvant chemotherapy

There have been other smaller studies of adjuvant chemotherapy in stage I NSGCTT. The most mature study[12] includes 29 cases which had been followed up for more than 2 years. They were selected on the basis of venous invasion (VI) alone, and the authors do not comment on the expected recurrence rate in patients with VI according to their histologic definition. Eligible patients received two courses of standard BEP. With a median follow up of 79 months there had been two recurrences. Long-term toxicity data were based on comparisons between 25 adjuvant chemotherapy cases and a control group managed by surveillance. No significant differences were noted between the two groups with respect to gonadal function, hearing and lung function. The study from Studer *et al.* has 43 patients selected on the basis of slightly different, unvalidated high-risk criteria[13], and it is not possible to estimate what the relapse rate without chemotherapy would have been. After a median follow up of 42 months there was just one recurrence consisting of mature teratoma treated surgically. Oliver *et al.* reported a pilot study with 22 cases, which were selected using MRC criteria, but those with only two high-risk factors (equivalent to a recurrence risk of less than 25%) were also eligible[14].

Management preferences

The results of these studies of adjuvant chemotherapy, particularly the MRC study, suggest that two quite different management options: namely, surveillance with four courses of BEP for those who relapse; and adjuvant chemotherapy with two courses of BEP for all, produce similar high levels of cure in stage I NSGCTT. In Birmingham we then embarked on a study to investigate which approach patients prefer[15]. Questionnaires were given to newly diagnosed teratoma patients, to patients with previous experience of the two options and to non-cancer controls, including specialist testicular tumor oncologists. Risks of recurrence ranging from 10% to 90% were explained and participants were asked to choose between immediate adjuvant chemotherapy, surveillance, or for the doctor to decide, at each risk level. Questionnaires were returned by 207 subjects (98% compliance) in nine groups with differing prior experience and present predicament.

The most striking finding was the very wide range of risk thresholds at which subjects' management preference changed, within apparently homogeneous groups. For instance, one (of 18) newly diagnosed patient opted for surveillance at all recurrence risk thresholds of 50% and below, whereas in four others the upper limit of range of risk for making this choice was as low as 10%. Similarly among 29 patients with prior experience of surveillance (without relapse), the upper threshold for choosing that management option was 50% risk of recurrence, whereas five of this group preferred adjuvant chemotherapy even at the lowest (10%) risk level. The range of choices was wider in those 38 patients who had prior experience of BEP chemotherapy, one of whom preferred surveillance even at the 90% chance of recurrence, but 10 selected adjuvant chemotherapy at the lowest (10%) risk. Interestingly, the most diverse group of all was the specialist testicular tumor oncologists. Two of the 17 opted for surveillance up to and including the highest (90%) risk of recurrence, but one preferred adjuvant chemotherapy at the 10% risk, and three at 20%. Cancer patients tended to want the doctor to decide more frequently than non-cancer controls.

The implication of these findings is that germane experience and knowledge have less influence on decision making than other factors. These factors are likely to be linked to differences in personality that may be common to all groups. Therapeutic research tends to be directed towards identifying a single best management strategy for each disease situation. Perhaps, instead, we should be prepared to accept that, as the range of treatment options widens, there may no longer be a best option for a particular patient population, but rather an optimum management plan for each individual. As treatment improves it will become more important to offer patients alternative strategies, with similar principal outcomes, and to help those who wish to choose for themselves to do so. At the same time we must recognize that some will wish to delegate these decisions to doctors who, in turn, will have as broad a range of personalities, and hence favor as wide a range of choices as their patients.

Conclusions

Elective radiotherapy no longer has a place in the management of stage I NSGCTT. The role of elective retroperitoneal lymph node dissection is being re-evaluated in the light of its failure to prevent relapse elsewhere and hence the requirement for ongoing surveillance, the associated morbidity, and the established place of surveillance alone, post-orchidectomy. As a management option surveillance itself has distinct drawbacks. Short course adjuvant chemotherapy overcomes many of these drawbacks and has recently been shown to be effective, free from significant long-term toxicity, and the preferred option by some patients.

References

1. Fossa SD, Horwich AH. The staging and treatment of testicular cancer: management of stage I disease. In: Smith PH (Ed.) *Combination therapy in urological malignancy*. Springer Verlag, London, 1989, pp. 173–189.
2. Peckham MJ, Barrett A, Husband JE, Hendry WF (1982) Orchidectomy alone in testicular stage I non-seminomatous germ-cell tumors. *Lancet* 1982;**ii**:678–680.
3. Cullen MH. Management of stage I non-seminoma: surveillance. In: Horwich A (Ed.) *Testicular cancer investigation and management* (2nd edn). Chapman and Hall Medical, London (1996).
4. Freedman LS, Parkinson MC, Jones WG, Oliver RTD, Peckham MJ, Read G, Newlands ES, Williams CJ (1987) Histopathology in the prediction of relapse of patients with stage I testicular teratoma treated by orchidectomy alone. *Lancet* 1987;**ii**:294–298.
5. Read G, Stenning SP, Cullen MH *et al.* Medical Research Council prospective study of surveillance for stage I testicular teratoma. *J Clin Oncol* 1992;**10**:1762–1768.
6. Moynihan C (1987) Testicular cancer: the psychosocial problems of patients and their relatives. *Cancer Surveys* 1987;**6**:477–510.
7. Howard GCW, Clarke K, Elia MH *et al.* A Scottish National Audit of current patterns of management for patients with testicular non-seminomatous germ cell tumors. *Br J Cancer* 1996;**72**:1303–1306.
8. Sogani PC, Whitmore WF Jr, Herr HW *et al.* Orchiectomy alone in the treatment of clinical stage I nonseminomatous germ cell tumor of the testis. *J Clin Oncol* 1984;**2**:267–270.
9. Williams SD, Stablein DM, Einhorn LH *et al.* Immediate adjuvant chemotherapy versus observation with treatment at relapse in pathological stage II testicular cancer. *N Engl J Med* 1987;**317**:1433–1438.
10. Stuart NSA, Woodroffe CM, Grundy R, Cullen MH. Long-term side-effects of chemotherapy for testicular cancer: the cost of cure. *Br J Cancer* 1990;**61**:479–484.
11. Cullen MH, Stenning SP, Parkinson MC, Fossa SD, Kaye SB, Horwich AH, Harland SJ, Williams MV, Jakes R. Short course adjuvant chemotherapy in high risk stage 1 non-seminomatous germ cell tumors of the testis (NSGCTT): an MRC study report. *J Clin Oncol* 1996;**14**:1106–1113.
12. Pont J, Albrecht W, Postner G, Sellner F, Angel K, Holtl W. Adjuvant chemotherapy for high risk clinical stage I nonseminomatous testicular germ cell cancer: long-term results of a prospective trial. *J Clin Oncol* 1996;**14**:441–448.
13. Studer UE, Fey MF, Calderoni A, Kraft R, Mazzucchelli L, Sonntag RW. Adjuvant chemotherapy after orchidectomy in high-risk patients with clinical stage I non-seminotous testicular cancer. *Eur Urol* 1993;**23**:444–449.
14. Oliver RTD, Raja MA, Ong J, Gallagher CJ. Pilot study to evaluate impact of a policy of adjuvant chemotherapy for high risk stage I malignant teratoma on overall relapse rate of stage 1 cancer patients. *J Urol* 1992;**148**:1453–1456.

15. Cullen MH, Billingham L, Cook J, Woodroffe C. Management preferences in stage I non-seminomatous germ cell tumors of the testis: an investigation among patients, controls and oncologists. *Br J Cancer* 1996;**74**:1487–91.

38.2   Surgical treatment

R S Foster and J P Donohue

Radical orchiectomy

Most solid testicular masses in young men will represent germ cell tumors. The remainder are Sertoli cell tumors, Leydig cell tumors or inflammatory masses. Two aspects of germ cell tumors of the testicle argue for radical orchiectomy as the preferred mode of initial treatment: the propensity of these tumors to implant and the ability to cure patients with metastatic disease surgically. That is, since tumor spillage at the time of surgical treatment can potentially contaminate another lymphatic drainage area and since these tumors can be cured by surgical removal of such a lymphatic drainage area, any maneuver to decrease spillage and potential contamination of a secondary lymphatic drainage area is preferred. Radical inguinal orchiectomy (as opposed to transscrotal orchiectomy) limits the amount of surgical manipulation in the area immediately adjacent to the tumor and therefore decreases the chance of tumor spillage.

Spillage of tumor at the time of orchiectomy may necessitate additional therapy such as chemotherapy which would otherwise have been unnecessary[1]. Additionally, though surgical removal of inguinal lymph nodes is certainly possible and necessary in some cases, inguinal lymphadenectomy is associated with moderate morbidity such as flap necrosis and lymphedema[2]. Therefore, since the morbidity of inguinal orchiectomy is no greater than transscrotal orchiectomy and since inguinal orchiectomy decreases the likelihood of tumor spillage, radical inguinal orchiectomy is the preferred mode of treatment of primary testicular germ cell tumors.

Rationale for retroperitoneal lymph node dissection (RPLND)

Low-stage disease

Nerve sparing RPLND in low-stage non-seminomatous testis cancer confers several potential benefits to the patient[3,4]. These benefits include the following. First by performing nerve sparing RPLND patients are effectively staged. In clinical stage I the 30% of patients who in fact are pathologic stage II are identified early in the course of

treatment. For clinical stage II the 23% of patients who in fact are pathologic stage I are also identified and spared further unnecessary therapy[4]. Second, for those low-stage patients found to have retroperitoneal disease, the removal of this disease surgically confers a likelihood of long-term cure of 50% to 70%, depending on the volume of retroperitoneal disease removed[3,4]. Therefore, effective therapy has been performed early in the course of management.

A third benefit of RPLND is to eliminate the retroperitoneum as a site of recurrence. Radiographic monitoring of the retroperitoneum is notoriously difficult. Furthermore, for the patient it is time consuming and expensive. By performing RPLND the retroperitoneum is eliminated as a site of recurrence. Hence, follow up after RPLND does not involve CT scanning of the abdomen. This confers benefit in terms of quality of life for the patient and minimization of cost. The fourth benefit of RPLND in low-stage disease is the ensuing reduction in the intensity of follow up. For pathologic stage I patients follow up includes chest X-ray and marker determinations every other month for 1 year and every 4 months for the second year[5]. At Indiana University we have not noted a late recurrence (beyond 2 years) in this group of patients. For pathologic stage II patients who elect to be followed and not receive adjuvant chemotherapy, follow up includes a chest X-ray and marker determinations monthly for 1 year and bi-monthly for the second year. Thereafter, these patients are followed yearly with a chest X-ray, physical examination and marker determination. Hence, although follow up is necessary after RPLND the intensity of follow up is much less, making patient compliance with a rigoros follow up schedule less of a necessity. This clearly has benefits for the patient.

A further benefit of RPLND is to minimize patient anxiety. Many studies have shown that patient anxiety is a problem in patients managed on a surveillance scheme[6,7]. The psychological burden to a patient in knowing that he may have metastatic disease but is simply being observed for this is sometimes great. By staging and treating the patient at the time of RPLND the patient is treated effectively and can be accurately appraised of the chance of recurrence and long-term cure.

Nerve-sparing RPLND preserves emission and ejaculation[8,9]. Nerve-sparing RPLND also reduces the chance of the patient ultimately requiring chemotherapy. Therefore, nerve-sparing RPLND minimizes any therapy related effects on fertility which is certainly a consideration in this group of young patients. Recent analysis showed that if emission and ejaculation can be preserved at the time of RPLND, RPLND (as opposed to surveillance) minimizes any therapy related effects on fertility[10].

Finally, RPLND in low-stage non-seminomatous testis cancer decreases the likelihood of late recurrence (recurrence beyond 2 years after initial successful therapy). This is not only important in terms of minimizing the intensity of follow up in these patients, it also has implications on long-term survival. It has been shown that the likelihood of long-term cure following treatment of late recurrence is only around 40%[11]. Therefore, minimization of the propensity for late recurrence is appealing, not only in terms of minimizing follow up but also has implications in terms of overall survival.

High-stage disease

Post-chemotherapy RPLND is generally performed in patients who experience a partial remission after initial systemic chemotherapy. Partial remission is defined as normalization of serum alpha fetoprotein and beta HCG in conjunction with radiographic persistence of retroperitoneal disease. After primary chemotherapy, resection of these retroperitoneal masses will yield teratoma pathologically in 45%, necrosis/fibrosis in approximately 45%, and persistent germ cell cancer in approximately 10%.

Post-chemotherapy RPLND performs a staging function. The finding of necrosis/fibrosis effectively confirms a good response to chemotherapy and confers an excellent long-term prognosis. The finding of teratoma or carcinoma indicates a less than complete clinical response.

Surgical removal of teratoma or carcinoma at the time of post-chemotherapy RPLND is therapeutic[12]. Teratoma is not chemo-sensitive; surgical removal is curative. The finding of carcinoma in the post-chemotherapy RPLND specimen provokes the administration post-operatively of two further courses of cisplatin based chemotherapy if the patient received primary chemotherapy alone prior to the RPLND. Alternatively, if the patient had received 'salvage' chemotherapy prior to the RPLND, no further post-operative chemotherapy is administered[13]. Therefore, surgical removal of carcinoma at the time of RPLND also offers therapeutic value.

A small group of post-chemotherapy RPLND patients undergo what is termed 'desperation' RPLND. This highly selected group of patients are those in whom multiple chemotherapeutic regimens have failed in eradicating carcinoma from the retroperitoneum. Patients who have disease localized to the retroperitoneum in one site and who have failed all previous chemotherapy are eligible to undergo desperation RPLND. Approximately 33% of these patients are long-term survivors[14]. Hence, even in some groups of patients highly refractory to chemotherapy surgical removal of retroperitoneal disease confers benefits.

Technique

Basic technique

The cornerstone of retroperitoneal lymph node dissection is based on the idea that the great vessels are mobilized completely and moved away from the tumor after which the tumor and lymphatic tissue is resected off the posterior body wall. This concept of the operation is known as the 'split and roll' and has been popularized by Donohue[15]. By considering this procedure as mobilization of the great vessels followed by removal of tumor and lymphatic tissue the procedure is standardized and is not an ad hoc removal of palpable tumor tissue at the time of the operation. This enables the technique to be reproduced and allows the procedure to be taught effectively.

Therefore, RPLND has become a three step procedure: 1) delineation of the appropriate template of resection; 2) mobilization of great vessels, renal arteries and veins, and relevant neural structures; 3) removal of lymphatic zones from the posterior body wall taking care to control lumbar arteries and veins as they penetrate the posterior body wall medial to the sympathetic chain.

The technique of full bilateral RPLND will be described. After a midline laparotomy the retroperitoneum is palpated. Based on the volume of retroperitoneal disease, the decision is made as to which template to employ. For a full bilateral RPLND an incision is then made in the posterior peritoneum from the epiploic foramen of Winslow distally around the cecum extending cephalad to the ligament of Treitz (Figure 38.2.1). The inferior mesenteric vein is divided between silk ties. The cecum and root of the small bowel along with the right colon is then reflected up off the retroperitoneum and placed in a bowel bag retracted onto the patient's chest. The borders of a full bilateral template include the crura of the diaphragm superiorly, the bifurcation of the common iliac arteries inferiorly, and the ureters laterally (Figure 38.2.2). The split maneuver is then begun by using either a right-angle clamp with cautery or Metzenbaum scissors to split the lymphatic tissue overlying the surface of the aorta at the 12:00 position (Figure 38.2.3). This tissue is then rolled medially and laterally which eventually exposes the lumbar arteries. These are mobilized and divided between silk ties. A similar maneuver is performed over the left renal vein and after the tissue is rolled inferiorly, the origin of the left gonadal vein is divided between silk ties. A lumbar vein exists in this location around 40% of the time and is also divided between ties. The left renal artery is identified and dissected from lymphatic and tumorous tissue.

Attention is then turned to the vena cava. The split maneuver is performed over the vena cava after which the tissue is rolled medially and laterally exposing lumbar veins (Figure 38.2.4). These are also divided between silk ties. The vena cava and left renal vein are retracted anteriorly which exposes the right renal artery which is dissected from lymphatic and tumorous tissue. The crus of the diaphragm may be seen posteriorly. In rolling tissue from the vena cava the origin of the right gonadal vein is identified and divided between silk ties. Inferiorly tissue is rolled from the common iliac arteries and veins. Any rel-

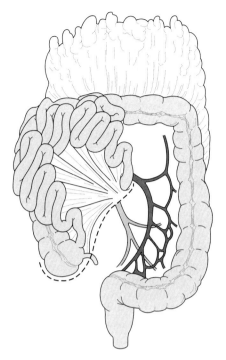

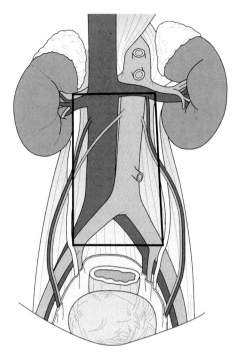

Fig. 38.2.1 Retroperitoneal incision for exposure of right side of retroperitoneun.

Fig. 38.2.2 Template used for full bilateral retroperitoneal lymph noe dissection.

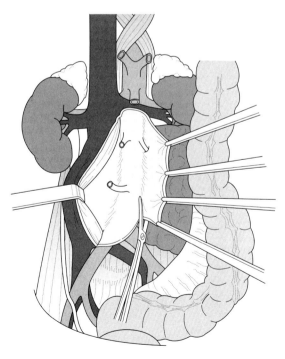

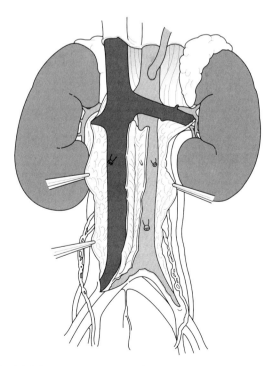

Fig. 38.2.3 The split maneuver at the 120' clock position on the aorta is used to expose the aorta and lead to vascular control.

Fig. 38.2.4 The split at the 120' clock position has been accoplished on the aorta and the vena cava.

447

evant lumbars are identified and divided between silk ties. The ureters are then mobilized laterally leaving the only remaining attachments of lymphatic and tumorous tissue posteriorly. The left periaortic, interaortocaval, right paracaval, and interiliac zones of lymphatic and tumor tissue are then harvested from the posterior body wall using cautery. Lumbar arteries and veins are identified as passing into the posterior body wall medial to the sympathetic chain. Clips, cautery, or suture ligatures are used to control these vessels as they pass into the posterior body wall.

Therefore, Full bilateral RPLND involves resection of four lymphatic zones: the left periaortic, interaortocaval, right paracaval and interiliac (Figure 38.2.5). Both more limited and more global zones of resection of lymphatic tissue are appropriate based on the clinical situation. These clinical situations are further discussed below.

Low-stage modifications

The site of metastasis in the retroperitoneum is dependent on two factors: the volume of metastasis and the side

of the testicular primary. This information was developed from mapping studies done in patients with low-stage disease who had historically undergone full bilateral RPLND.[16] These studies proved that full bilateral RPLND is not necessary for patients who have minimal metastasis to the retroperitoneum. Therefore, based on clinical staging and palpation of the retroperitoneum at the time of laparotomy, the so-called modified templates may be used if the volume of metastasis is judged to be relatively low (Figures 38.2.6 and 38.2.7). Advantages of a modified template dissection include decreased time required for the procedure, less post-operative ileus, and possible maintenance of emission and ejaculation even if nerve-sparing modifications are not used.

A further modification of technique in low-stage disease is the use of nerve-sparing techniques. Nerve sparing in conjunction with a modified template effectively preserves emission and ejaculation at the 99% level[8]. This allows patients to benefit from the staging and therapeutic aspect of RPLND without being subjected to the loss of emission and ejaculation.

Though variability exists in the course of retroperitoneal efferent sympathetic fibers, several operative maneuvers are

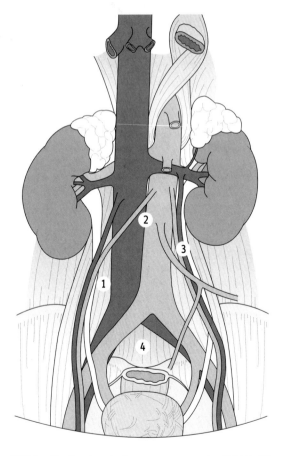

Fig. 38.2.5   The four lymphatic zones are reseced at RPLND: (1) right paracaval: (2) interaortocaval: (3) left periaortic: (4) interiliac.

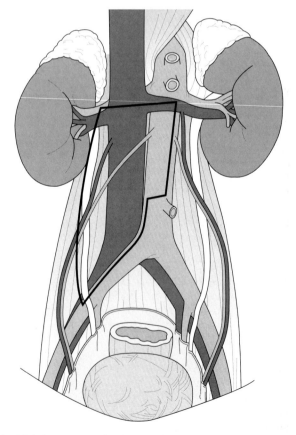

Fig. 38.2.6   Template for right modified nerve-sparing RPLND.

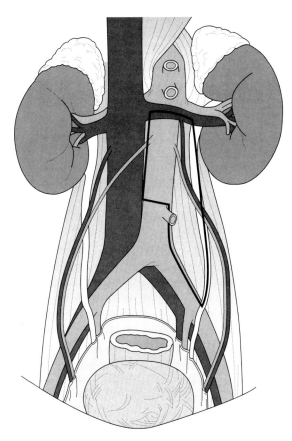

Fig. 38.2.7 Template for left modified nerve-sparing RPLND.

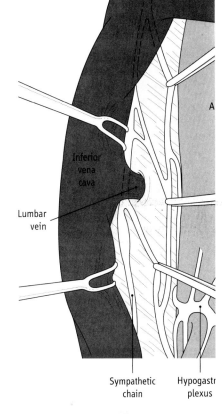

Fig. 38.2.8 Depiction of interaortocaval sympathetic fibers and their relationship to the vena cava.

available to allow accurate definition and dissection of these fibers prior to removal of relevant lymphatic tissue. The right-sided sympathetic efferent fibers course posterior to the vena cava from the sympathetic chain, passing into the interaortocaval zone from which they extend over the aortic bifurcation into the pelvis. These fibers may be identified and placed in vessel loops as they pass over the aortic bifurcation. Similarly, these fibers may be identified as they course immediately superior to lumbar veins near the right sympathetic chain. (Figure 38.2.8) Characteristically, three or four fibers from the sympathetic chain coalesce in the interaortocaval zone to create a larger trunk which passes into the pelvis.

For a low-stage dissection in a patient with a left testis tumor the left colon is mobilized medially in order to expose the left periaortic zone. Left-sided sympathetic efferent fibers are seen coursing over the left common iliac artery and may be dissected and placed in a vessel loop. These fibers are then followed superiorly where they penetrate the left periaortic lymphatic tissue and meet the sympathetic chain. These fibers are fully dissected and placed in vessel loops prior to mobilizing the aorta, dividing the lumbars and resecting the lymphatic tissue.

High-stage modifications

The template of dissection to be used in a post-chemotherapy RPLND is dependent upon the volume and site of metastatic disease. If only retroperitoneal disease exists, a standard full bilateral RPLND is performed. However, not uncommonly these post-chemotherapy patients will have retrocrural, pelvic or mediastinal disease. Hence, the standard full bilateral template may not be adequate in this group of patients. Retrocrural and mediastinal tumors may necessitate chevron or thoracoabdominal incisions. Approaching retrocrural disease may require full mobilization of the liver (Langenbach maneuver, Figure 38.2.9) or the spleen, stomach and tail of the pancreas (Figure 38.2.10). The operative incision and technique must be highly individualized based on the clinical situation and the volume and site of tumor. Nonetheless, the standard paradigm of split and roll and mobilization of vessels away from the tumor followed by

449

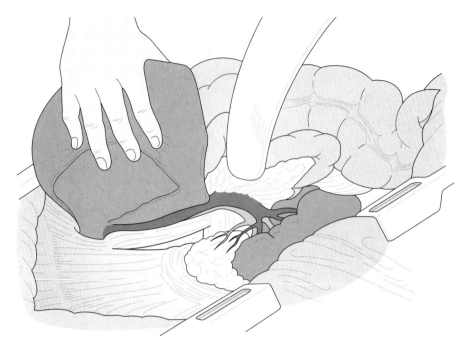

Fig. 38.2.9   Mobilization of the liver to expose the right retrocrural area is depicted.

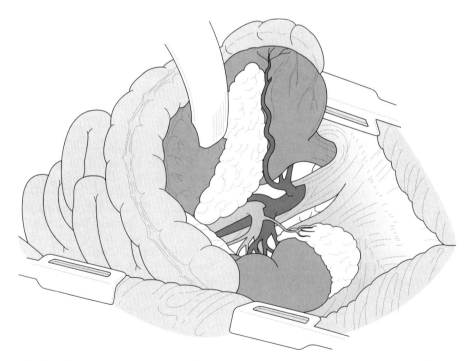

Fig. 38.2.10   Mobilization of the spleen, pancreas, and left colon is illustrated in order to expose the left retrocrural area.

removal of tumor remains the mainstay of technique, even in the retrocrural area and mediastinum.

Results

Results of RPLND in low-stage disease at Indiana University are presented in Tables 38.2.1 and 38.2.2. It is apparent that RPLND effectively stages the patient accurately but also provides therapy for those patients found to have retroperitoneal disease. Pathologic stage II patients who elect post-operative adjuvant chemotherapy have a very low chance of experiencing a subsequent recurrence. Indeed, follow up in this group of patients may be much less intense since recurrence is extremely unlikely[5].

Morbidity in low-stage disease

Primary RPLND for low-stage testicular cancer is accompanied by very low morbidity[17]. Published experience

Table 38.2.1   RPLND in clinical stage A

Extent of disease (Pathologic stage)	Patients No. (%)	Relapse No. (%)	Survival (%)	Deaths
Stage A	266 (70)	31 (12)	99.2	2*
Stage B No adjuvant	64 (17)	22 (34)	98.4	1†
Stage B Plus adjuvant	48 (13)	0 (0)	100	0
Total	378	53 (14)	99.2	3

Patients' age
N = 378. Mean 28.3. years. < 12 years = 5 (1.3%).

Time to follow up (months)
N = 374. Mean 74.4. Highest 153.0. Lowest 18.2. Range 134.8.

* Two deaths, 1 cancer, 1 operative complication.
† One cancer death.

Table 38.2.2   RPLND in clinical stage B

Disease extent	Patients No. (%)	Relapse No. (%)	Survival %	Deaths No.
Path. A	32 (23)	2 (6)	100	0
Path. B No Adj.	49 (35)	18 (37)	96	2
Path. B + 'Adj Rx'	59 (42)	0	98.3	1
All cases	140	20 (14)	98	3

3 deaths: 1 cancer, 1 postoperative, 1 chemotherapy-related.
For abbreviations see Table 38.2.1.

suggests the only long-term source of morbidity is an approximate 1% chance of experiencing a subsequent small bowel obstruction. On the other hand, fertility is not affected nor do most patients experience the potential morbidity of full-dose chemotherapy. In the short term, hospitalization averages 4 days and return to employment is usually attained in 4 weeks.

Morbidity in high-stage disease

The Indiana University experience with post-chemotherapy RPLND was recently presented[12]. Analysis of this experience revealed that the entire group of post-chemotherapy RPLND patients can be stratified into 'good-risk' and 'poor-risk' groups.

The good-risk group consists of patients who present for post-chemotherapy RPLND after only three or four courses of induction chemotherapy. These patients have experienced a partial remission which consists of normalization of serum alpha fetoprotein and beta HCG but with persistence of radiographic retroperitoneal disease. These patients have an overall survival of 95%.

The poor-risk group of post-chemotherapy RPLND patients consist of those patients who have one or more of the following characteristics: 1) redo RPLND; 2) desperation RPLND; 3) RPLND after primary and salvage chemotherapy; 4) incomplete RPLND (defined as lack of normalization of tumor markers after RPLND or immediate elevation of serum markers shortly after post-chemo RPLND). Patients in these categories have only a 70% chance of long-term survival.

Conclusions

Retroperitoneal lymph node dissection is a step wise procedure performed by a systematic approach. It is teachable and reproducible. As modifications have ensued in low-stage disease the procedure has retained its ability accurately to stage and treat testis cancer patients. Similarly, these modifications to technique over the years have resulted in a minimization of morbidity, especially in terms of fertility considerations (preservation of emission and ejaculation) and minimization of immediate post-operative morbidity (no nasogastric depression, short hospitalization time).

Although post-chemotherapy RPLND is more morbid than RPLND performed for low-stage disease, the staging and therapeutic benefits outweigh its morbidity. Still, post-chemotherapy RPLND can represent a very challenging procedure; the surgeon contemplating post-chemotherapy RPLND must be well versed in techniques of surgical exposure through various incisions, liver and splenic mobilization, and techniques of vascular control and repair.

References

1. Leibovitch I, Baniel J, Foster RS, Donohue JP. The clinical implications of procedural deviations during orchiectomy for nonseminomatous testis cancer. *J Urol* 1995;**154**:935–939.
2. Whitmore WF, Vagiwala MR. A technique of ileoinguinal lymph node dissection for carcinoma of the penis. *Surg Gynecol Obstet* 1984;**159**:573.
3. Donohue JP, Thornhill JA, Foster RS, Rowland RG, Bihrle R. Retroperitoneal lymphadenectomy in clinical stage A testis cancer (1965–1989): Modifications of technique and impact on ejaculation. *J Urol* 1993;**149**:237–243.
4. Donohue JP, Thornhill JA, Foster RS, Rowland RG, Bihrle R. Clinical stage B nonseminomatous germ cell testis cancer: The Indiana University experience (1965–1989) using routine primary retroperitoneal lymph node dissection. *Eur J Cancer* 1995;**31A**:1599–1604.
5. Sharir S, Foster RS, Jewett MA, Sturgeon J, Moore M, Donohue JP. Optimizing follow up for early stage nonseminomatous testicular cancer. Proceedings of the American Urological Association Annual Meeting. Orlando, FL: 1996: Abstract #67.
6. Cullen MH, Stenning SP, Parkinson MC, Fossa SD, Kaye SB, Horwich AH, Harland SJ *et al.* Short course adjuvant chemotherapy in high risk stage I nonseminomatous germ cell tumors of the testis: a Medical Research Council report. *J Clin Oncol* 1996;**14**:1106–1113.
7. Cullen M. Management of stage I nonseminoma: surveillance and chemotherapy. In: Horwich A (Ed.) *Testicular cancer: investigation and management* 1991:149.
8. Donohue JP, Foster RS, Rowland RG, Bihrle R, Jones JA, Geier GE. Nerve sparing retroperitoneal lymphadenectomy with preservation for ejaculation. *J Urol* 1990;**144**:287–292.
9. Jewett MA, Kong YP, Goldberg SD, Sturgeon JF, Thomas GM, Alison RE, Gospodarowicz MK. Retroperitoneal lymphadenectomy for testis tumor with nerve sparing for ejaculation. *J Urol* 1988;**139**:1220–1224.
10. Langenstroer P, Rosen MA. A decision analysis model for fertility preservation in stage A nonseminomatous germ cell tumors (NSGCT) of the testis. Proceedings of the American Urological Association Annual Meeting. Orlando, FL. 1996; Abstract #945.
11. Baniel J, Foster RS, Gonon R, Messemer JE, Donohue JP, Einhorn LH. Late relapse of testicular cancer. *J Clin Oncol* 1995;**13**:1170–1176.
12. Donohue JP, Foster RS, Leibovitch I, Bihrle R, Rowland RG, Wahle GR, Einhorn LH. Retroperitoneal lymph node dissection for post chemotherapy residual masses (PCRPLND) in patients with advanced testis cancer. Review of the Indiana University experience 1974–1994. Proceedings of the American Urological Association Annual Meeting. Orlando, FL. 1996; Abstract #66.
13. Fox E, Weathers T, Williams SD *et al.* Outcome analysis for patients with persistent germ cell carcinoma in post chemotherapy retroperitoneal lymph node dissections. *J Clin Oncol* 1993;**11**:1294–1299.
14. Murphy B, Breeden E, Donohue JP *et al.* Surgical salvage of chemorefractory germ cell tumors. *J Clin Oncol* 1993;**11**:324–329.
15. Donohue JP. Retroperitoneal lymphadenectomy: the anterior approach including bilateral suprarenal hilar dissection. *Urol Clin N Am* 1977;**4**:509–521.
16. Donohue JP, Zachary J, Maynard B. Distribution of nodal metastases in nonseminomatous testis cancer. *J Urol* 1982;**128**:315–320.
17. Baniel J, Foster RS, Rowland RG, Bihrle R, Donohue JP. Complications of primary retroperitoneal lymph node dissection. *J Urol* 1994;**152**:424–427

38.3 Practical approaches to the use of chemotherapy

R T D Oliver

Since the success from use of chemotherapy to treat chorio-carcinoma in women in the late 1950s, patients with metastatic non-seminomatous testicular germ cell cancers have been a test bed that has made a significant contribution to the development of chemotherapy for adult cancers. Today, compared with other cancers there is an almost embarrassing excess of choice for first, second and third line treatment and in excess of 85% of metastatic disease patients achieve durable primary long-term disease-free survival and in excess of 95% of all cases survive[1,2].

Much of the work on chemotherapy in testis cancer has been in patients with metastatic non-seminoma. However, with evidence that non-seminomas arise by clonal evolution from non-seminomas[3], the chapter will also review the observations that have been made from chemotherapy of seminoma.

Chemotherapy in the primary management of germ cell cancers

Before the advent of cisplatin early diagnosis and immediate orchidectomy were paramount. Today less attention is paid to this issue and there has been a tendency to treat these patients as less of an emergency. There is some evidence to support this attitude as today the overall results are so good[5] with more than 95% cured that it is difficult to see any gain from reduction in delay in terms of overall survival[1]. However when delay (Table 38.3.1) is correlated with stage which directly correlates with the amount of treatment needed, it is clear that there is still a direct relation between delay and extent of disease (Table 38.3.2). A further demonstration of the significance of delay comes from analysis of extent of delay in those needing salvage chemotherapy and those cured by primary chemotherapy. With average delay in those needing bone marrow transplant (6.2 months) being nearly double that of those cured by primary chemotherapy (3.4 months), it is clear that avoidance of delay in diagnosis is still of primary importance in management of this disease.

A further factor justifying attention to delay is the rare occurrence (1–2% of metastatic cases) of hurricane growth of these tumors after orchidectomy. Examples of this are a patient who developed acute respiratory failure within 2 weeks of orchidectomy, a patient who developed Budd–Chiari hepato-renal shut down from para-aortic lymph node metastasis invasion of vena cava, hepatic and renal veins within 2 weeks of initial histologic diagnosis; a patient who developed lower limb venous infarction from a low para-aortic lymph node mass invading the bifurcation of the vena cava but also spreading up the vena cava causing hepato-renal failure and died within 2 weeks of presentation without being able to have any chemotherapy.

The lesson from the analysis of effect of delay and extent of spread and the anecdotes on hurricane growth is that it

Table 38.3.1 Influences of changes in pre-orchidectomy delay on cure of testis germ cell cancer 1978–1984

Delay	1978–1983 Proportion in cohort (%)	(n=113) Currently nem (%)	1984–1988 Proportion in cohort (%)	(n=155) Currently nem (%)	1989–1994 Proportion in cohort (%)	(n=185) Currently nem (%)
<1 month	17	89 (n=19)	23	94 (n=36)	31	100 (n=57)
2–3 months	30	79 (n=34)	36	93 (n=56)	28	98 (n=52)
4–11 months	33	81 (n=37)	24	89 (n=37)	32	100 (n=59)
>12 months	20	57 (n=23)	17	89 (n=26)	9	94 (n=17)
All cases Median delay/ Currently nem Median tumor size			4 months/77% 4.8 cm	3 months/92% 4.5 cm	3 months/98% 4.0 cm	

Table 38.3.2 Delay and proportion true stage 1 testis cancer

Months delay	No of cases	Proportion stage 1 (%)	Relapse on surveillance (%)	Proportion true stage 1 (%)
<1	40	80	18	66
1–2	70	60	26	44
2–3	143	46	29	33
<3	200	45	38	28

is vital that all clinicians involved in diagnosis of this disease must be aware of these possibilities and prepared to organize for the patients to be treated as an emergency. In such a circumstance it may be necessary to make the diagnosis on the basis of the clinical situation and tumor markers which can be performed as an emergency using the urinary pregnancy test with or without a fine needle biopsy depending on the circumstance.

A further factor which has made it of considerable importance to consider medical management before orchidectomy is the issue of fertility. There is now evidence that 10% of patients presenting with a primary testis tumor have no sperm production from the contralateral testis and orchidectomy of patient with a small tumor in a testis with a normally functioning rim of germ cells can lead to induction of infertility in these patients and a 50% reduction of sperm count in half of the other patients, demonstrating the importance of not carrying out orchidectomy unnecessarily in patients who are going to have to proceed to chemotherapy. It is important in such cases that at least some thought is given to preserving sperm before any treatment, i.e. chemotherapy or orchidectomy, is undertaken.

Practical issues with use of chemotherapy for treating germ cell cancers

While there is little doubt that following the standard bleomycin-etoposide-cisplatin regimen is not particularly complex, it is the actual decision taking over the period of treatment that is crucial to the success of the treatment. This is the reason that it is of paramount importance that these patients are treated in major centers treating adequate numbers of patients to gain sufficient experience in the minutiae of treatment. All major centers have demonstrated improvement in results as a result of the experience of using the regimen[5,6]. This experience relates to management issues such as the need to ensure that the treatment is timed according to the 21 day schedule, to ensure that treatment related death is avoided by intensive treatment of neutropenic sepsis and in particularly at risk patients using antibiotic prophylaxis over the neutropenic phase, avoiding aminoglycoside use or having extremely careful dosage control if this is the only antibiotic that can be used as this agent is synergistic with cisplatin and in the past has led to patients having to be put onto hemodialysis. A recently identified risk has been the use of intravenous contrast in the week after cisplatin. Monitoring for cisplatin induced magnesium leak in sick patients and adjusting bleomycin dosage in the event of any cisplatin induced reduction of renal function to avoid bleomycin lung are often critical aspects of management. Finally once cured as well as monitoring for relapse on follow up, it is also important to assess testicular function and organize testosterone replacement for any patients with Leydig cell failure. This occurs in the majority of patients in the first 6 months after chemotherapy, and for some of these patients a short period of monthly intramuscular testosterone replacement helps. Only a small minority requires continuous replacement.

Selection of patients for chemotherapy

In the late 1970s, when cisplatin based curative treatment first became available, treatment was restricted to patients with blood borne metastatic M+ disease or those who had failed conventional local treatment with surgery or radiation for node-positive patients. These were initially mainly non-seminomas as whole lung radiation could cure a proportion of seminomas with lung metastases. As confidence grew in the durability of cures and it became apparent that previously irradiated patients had higher risks of neutropenic deaths, nodal disease N+ patients in centers using radiotherapy began receiving chemotherapy first. With increasing recognition of the value of post-chemotherapy surgery for establishing when it was safe to stop chemotherapy this began to be increasingly used in these centers and it is now the practice in our centre to use chemotherapy for all patients with metastatic non-seminoma with early surgery for localized disease if there is marker response but no obvious shrinkage by d 21[7]. If the markers fail to respond salvage chemotherapy is usually the treatment of choice, though in patients with α-fetoprotein positive disease there is a subgroup who become long-term cured following surgery alone despite persistent viable malignancy.

Choice of chemotherapy for non-seminoma

It was the demonstration that etoposide cisplatin produced 37% continuous disease-free survival after failure of PVB[7] that led to etoposide being substituted for vinblastine and proving significantly better as first line therapy in both good and poor risk patients[8]. Subsequently three salvage strategies of BEP failures have been explored in reasonable numbers[9]. Velbe, ifosfamide and cisplatin (VIP) was the first and although it salvaged 24% of BEP failures, it failed to improve survival over BEP when used in a randomized trial.

Two strategies of dose intensification have been explored in salvage setting. The first used 'horizontal' dose intensification with weekly bleomycin, oncovin and cisplatin (BOP). This uses doses similar to those standard regimens. When used as first line salvage it does not show cross-resistance with the other standard salvage regimen (VIP) and 47% achieve primary salvage and 60% are salvaged overall after 3rd line regimens.

However when BOP was combined with VIP as a first line regimen (BOP/VIP) it failed to demonstrate any superiority over BEP in poor risk patients.

Currently most research on salvage treatment internationally is being made on the effects of 'vertical' dose intensification using one to four high-dose treatments with chemotherapy and peripheral blood stem cell rescue[10]. Although this approach is currently being investigated in a randomized trial against VIP without high dose, to date there is no evidence that it is better than BEP which remains the universal standard today.

Several drugs both old and new (methotrexate, paclitaxel and gemcitabine) are working after failed high dose and hold promise that there will be even further progress in the future.

In addition to new chemotherapy regimens there is increasing recognition that surgery can salvage patients with localized chemotherapy resistant disease[11]. There are several reports of durable relapse-free survival after RPLND of patients with persistent tumor marker elevation after chemotherapy. However reports of accelerated tumor recurrence after surgery if done in totally unresponsive patients[12],

emphasizes the importance of case selection for such surgery. An example of this is shown in Fig. 38.1–38.4.

Trials in good and poor risk non-seminoma patients

Today using level of α-fetoprotein, β-human chorionic gonadotrophin and lactic dehydrogenase with extent of disease it is possible to define three prognostic groups for outcome after chemotherapy[5,6,13].

Three principal questions have been addressed in the good risk patients (Table 38.3.3), i.e. dropping bleomycin because of the risk of mortality from bleomycin lung, changing cisplatin to carboplatin because of oto- and nephrotoxicity and reducing treatment from four courses to three. Only the last of these has proven safe[14].

Despite several phase two studies suggesting that there are regimens better than BEP in poor risk patients (Table 38.3.4), for no regimen tested in poor risk patients to date

Table 38.3.3   Overview of trials in good-risk patients

	Number of trials	Number of cases	Progression free (%)
Platinum combination			
+Bleomycin	4	434	86
−Bleomycin	4	425	77
Combination plus			
Cisplatin	3	256	91
Carboplatin	3	240	79
Number of courses			
BEP × 4	1	96	92
BEP × 3	1	88	92

BEP bleomycin, etoposide and cisplatin:

Table 38.3.4   Comparison of BEPq21 and Phase II studies of accelerated cisplatin (nq<14) regimens versus high-dose regimens as first line therapy in 'poor risk' non-seminoma

	No. of cases	Progression free (%)	Toxic deaths (%)
BEP	81	77	4
BOP	58	83	NA
BOP/VIP	91	63	2
C-BOP/BEP	91	82	7
MD Anderson	22	82	Nil
HD VIP x 4	141	68	8
VIP + HD	30	50	NA
VIP v.	145	64	3
PEB	141	60	4
BOP-VIP v.	185	53	8
BEP	185	60	3

NA = not applicable.

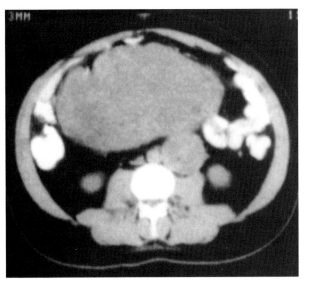

Fig. 38.3.1 Pre chemotherapy CT scan of abdominal mass.

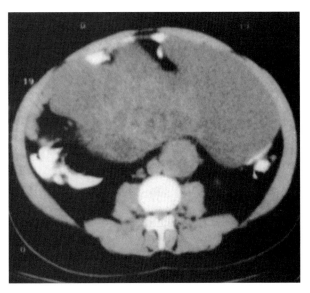

Fig. 38.3.2 Post-chemotherapy CT scan same patient.

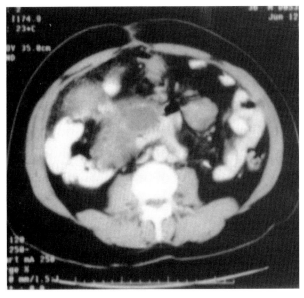

Fig. 38.3.3 4 weeks Port RPLND CTscan same patient.

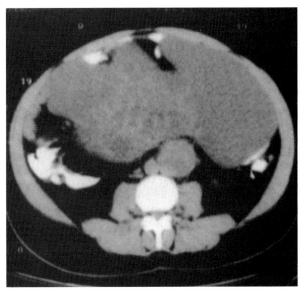

Fig. 38.3.4 8 weeks Post RPCND CT scan 1 week prior to death with absolute chemotherapy resistance.

has there been significant progression-free survival advantage and all have to a greater or lesser extent increased toxicity problems, including treatment related mortality[16].

Late events

Apart from the treatment-related mortalities discussed in the previous section, the most serious treatment related event seen in these patients has been etoposide-associated leukemia. Although this has been predominantly in patients who have accumulated a high dose over a long period of treatment, it has occurred in patients with low doses[17]. Interestingly the ultra high doses used with stem cell rescue do not seem to be associated with any increased risk over conventional doses. With radiation induced secondary cancers it is known that most of the risk is associated with low-dose prolonged treatment. So far follow up after etoposide is too short to exclude any risk in terms of late solid cancers. As has been seen after radiation the risk of solid tumors[18] does not develop until 10–20 years have passed. This issue is of some importance when one contemplates using etoposide in adjuvant setting (vide infra).

Gonadal toxicity is one other area where there is increasing information. It is now becoming clear that the majority (c. 80%) of patients treated with bleomycin, etoposide and cisplatin recover spermatogenesis, though in about one in three it is delayed beyond the conventionally stated time of 2 years and can return as late as 5 years[19]. Of interest about 20% of patients with absolute azoospermia prior to chemotherapy can recover normo-spermic counts while some with normal spermic counts never recover. It is thought that in the majority of the former hCG is suppressing spermatogenesis, though some effect of chemotherapy on pre-existing in situ carcinoma has not been excluded as yet. In fitting with the poorer cure of metastases by regimens using carboplatin, spermatogenesis recovery is generally 6–12 months quicker after carboplatin than cisplatin[19].

Role of chemotherapy in stage 1 and 2 non-seminoma

Stage 2 disease

In the USA two courses of chemotherapy are used as an adjunct to surgery in the management of early stage 2a/b tumors. In the UK chemotherapy has been primary management for small volume stage 2 cases with salvage surgery for patients left with residual disease after achieving marker remission with similar results to those achieved by surgery[3]. In the UK there has been a tendency to leave residual masses after chemotherapy rather than doing post-treatment surgical staging and this has been identified as one factor that may reduce cure[20]. It would seem that given the fact that more than 50% of tumor bulk can disappear after one course of chemotherapy[7] and the observation that ejaculatory nerve damage is more frequent when removing large masses while chemotherapy induced loss of spermatogenesis is also increased the longer treatment is continued[19] that one course of chemotherapy follow by d 21 scanning should be the standard strategy for stage 2 cases. Treatment should then be based on response, with those showing less than 50% response prepared for surgery early after 2–3 courses unless a delayed response is seen while the rest are allowed to complete three courses of chemotherapy. It is of course incumbent on any center that uses the medical approach to stage 2 disease not to treat on the basis of a small para-aortic mass on CT alone unless it is enlarging or there are rising tumor markers as it is known from surgical series that

10% of patients staged as stage 2 on CT scan have enlarged nodes due to reactive hyperplasia[20,21].

Chemotherapy for stage 1 disease

In the course of the last 40 years the relapse rate for stage 1 non-seminoma after radiotherapy fell from 55% to 15% due to the advent of improvements in staging from lymphangiogram, CT scan and tumor markers[22]. Until recently in the UK it was conventional to define stage 1 disease as any patient with less than 2 cm lesion visible on CT scan. With the increasing accuracy of spiral CT scans it is possible to define many smaller lesions. Though the chances of malignancy is known to increase with increasing size, use of a full lymph node dissection to prove this is increasingly accepted as 'overkill' as the risk of relapse remains 10% after surgery[23]. However laparoscopic retroperitoneal lymph node dissection from PET scanning and new approaches to immunohistochemistry of the primary tumor are improving the prediction of relapse. The critical issue is whether we have achieved enough precision in diagnosis of early metastatic risk to justify adjuvant chemotherapy (Table 38.3.5). As the risk of relapse after adjuvant therapy is very low, and salvage of such relapse is good this is increasingly used as the standard approach. Despite this standard treatment is still unresolved. Reduced hair loss after BOP regimens is one factor in increasing interest in this combination instead of BEP. The 100% relapse free results after RPLND plus single agent actinomycin D or mithramycin in historic studies suggest that there would be justification for single agent chemotherapy regimens in good risk situations.

Testis conservation with chemotherapy

Despite the overall cure of testes cancer being so high until recently it was thought that the risks of second cancers from carcinoma in situ precluded the use of chemo-

Table 38.3.5   Adjuvant studies for stage 1 non-seminoma

	No. of cases		Relapse free (%)	Survival (%)
RPLND	263	(unselected)	89	97
Radiotherapy	73	(unselected)	85	97
+ RPLND Neo adj Actinomycin	42	(unselected)	95	100
RPLND + mithramycin	21	(unselected)	100	100
Rad/Velbe/Bleo	16	(poor risk)	87	94
BEP × 2	216	(poor risk)	97	99
BEP × 1	44	(poor risk)	93	100
BOP q14	115	(poor risk)	98	99
BOP q10	33	(poor risk)	100	100

therapy for testes conservation. With evidence that 75% of patients with germ cell cancer are subfertile, evidence that atrophy is a major risk factor for testis cancer development[24] and a report that one in 10 patients with sperm in ejaculate pre-orchidectomy actually became azoospermic after orchidectomy[25] more attention is being paid to this issue[1,26,27].

In one small series 14 of 42 with metastases and three of 10 with stage 1 tumor were salvaged by chemotherapy though there has been two recurrences salvaged by orchidectomy. So far there has been one pregnancy and two others have recovered spermatogenesis.

Chemotherapy for seminoma

It is now more than 50 years since the classical paper by Friedman[28] which demonstrated that patients with metastatic seminoma had more lasting complete remissions with lower doses of radiation than malignant teratoma/non-seminoma, led to adjuvant radiation becoming the standard treatment for stage 1 seminoma. This occurred in the late 1950s/early 1960s with the cure increasing from 90–95% in most recently treated cohorts of patients[29]. Because relapse has occurred in patients as late as 9 years after orchidectomy alone and patients have presented with signs and symptoms of spinal cord compression as first manifestation of relapse, the need for use of adjuvant treatment has been accepted by most physicians involved in treatment of these patients. Because of the high success rates with radiation, this has remained the standard treatment for stage 1 seminoma[29].

As mentioned earlier when cisplatin chemotherapy first begun to be used in metastatic non-seminoma because of the exquisite radio-sensitivity of seminoma, chemotherapy was being used as an even more last resort treatment in seminoma than in non-seminoma. This was illustrated by the use of whole lung radiation for seminoma lung metastases as this cured over 50% of patients with lung metastases. As a consequence some of the early reports suggested that outcome of metastatic seminoma after cisplatin based chemotherapy in seminoma was worse than in non-seminoma. It has only been in the last few years that data has clearly emerged demonstrating that when using single agent platinum or BEP as first line and VIP or BOP as second treatment the results from cisplatin based chemotherapy treatment of seminoma are substantially better than that from treatment of non-seminoma and this is most pronounced when single agent cisplatin is used (Table 38.3.6). The importance of pure seminoma histology as an independent good risk factor for response to cisplatin based therapy has only recently been incontrovertibly confirmed[6,13].

Table 38.3.6 Differential chemosensitivity of seminoma and non-seminoma

	Seminoma (%)	Non-seminoma (%)
Cisplatin as first line	90	10
Carboplatin as first line	78	NA
BEP as first line	95	85
VIP as salvage	67	24
BOP as salvage	85	47

NA = not applicable.

Although the MRC trial TE12 set up to compare single agent versus combination therapy in seminoma it was terminated because of poor results when carboplatin was used in non-seminoma and a non-significant excess of relapses developed in the carboplatin arm. Subsequently analysis showed no significant difference in relapse rate[30]. Recent in vitro studies suggest that oxaliplatin, a new platinum analog is better than either cisplatin or carboplatin. Given increasing anxiety about etoposide related leukemia and questions about cancers after radiation there is clearly a case for further investigation of single agent platinum analogs in seminoma. This needs to be both in metastatic disease but also in stage 1 disease[31] where one course of carboplatin has been given to 134 patients and there has only been one relapse. Given this apparently lower relapse rate than radiation and its potential to be less toxic, this is being assessed in the latest MRC trial (TE20). Currently more than 1400 patients have been recruited but it will be some time before we get any indication as to the comparative impact on relapse-free survival and even longer in respect of late events.

Clinical significance of excessive chemo-sensitivity of seminoma over non-seminoma

With increasing evidence that non-seminoma can develop by clonal evolution from non-seminoma[3] and with evidence that a p53 related mechanism could be involved in the greater chemo-sensitivity of germ cell cancers, there is clearly more to be learnt from further study of the molecular basis of germ cell cancer chemo-sensitivity. As well as helping design molecular approaches to treatment of common solid cancers, it might also help to develop ideas to counteract the continuing anxiety over the declining sperm count that has become increasingly associated with the rising incidence of testis cancer.[24]

457

Conclusions

Bleomycin 30 mg d 2, 9, 19, etoposide 165 mg/m^2 d 1–3 or 100 mg/m^2 d 1–5, cisplatin 50 mg/m^2 d 1–2 or 20 mg/m^2 d 1–5 has been established as the standard regimen for all cases of metastatic non-seminoma with in excess of 85% durable relapse-free survival. There are at least three established salvage regimens, VIP, weekly BOP and high-dose chemotherapy that have salvaged patients who fail first line treatment. Despite increasingly strict criteria for definition of poor risk as well as evidence that patients are being diagnosed earlier with less advanced disease, no regimen has done better than BEP when used as first line therapy. With paclitaxel and gemcitabine showing activity there may be newer regimens in the near future.

So far apart from a possible excess of acute myeloid leukemias after high cumulative doses of etoposide there have been no serious late events. However more detailed and more prolonged follow up is required to exclude late solid cancer and vascular problems.

Chemotherapy with salvage surgery or surgery with adjuvant/salvage chemotherapy produce equivalent survival for patients with early stage 2 disease. The recent introduction of a policy of D21 CT assessment of response provides the most cost-effective approach to reduce exposure to chemotherapy in these patients.

Low toxicity chemotherapy regimens are also becoming established as adjuvants for high-risk stage 1 patients because of their low risks of relapse (less than 4%). Encouraged by these results and the increasing recognition of the need to conserve germinal epithelium in patients 75% of who will have subfertile levels of sperm count there is increasing interest in the use of chemotherapy for testis conservation.

Multivariate analysis and phase 2 studies in first line and salvage patients has demonstrated that pure seminoma is a predictor of a more favorable response to both single agent and combination chemotherapy. A further demonstration of this exquisite chemo-sensitivity of seminoma comes from data on use of one course of carboplatin as adjuvant in 134 patients, with a solitary relapse comparing favorably to the 4% relapse in the contemporarily treated series receiving radiation. Further confirmation from randomized comparison with radiation is now in progress.

References

1. Oliver R, Ong J, Blandy J, Altman D. Testis conservation studies in germ cell cancer justified by improved primary chemotherapy response and reduced delay 1978–1994. *Br J Urol* 1996;**78**:119–124.
2. Bosl GJ, Motzer RJ. Testicular germ cell cancer. *New Engl J Med* 1997;**337**:242.
3. Oliver RTD, Leahy M, Ong J. Combined seminoma/non-seminoma should be considered as intermediate grade germ cell cancer (GCC). *Eur J Cancer* 1995;**31A**:1392–1394.
5. Peckham MJ, Barrett A, Husband JE, Hendry WF. Orchidectomy alone in testicular stage I non-seminomatous germ-cell tumors. *Lancet* 1982;**ii**(8300):678–680.
6. Mead GM, Stenning SP, Cullen MH *et al.* The Second Medical Research Study of prognostic factors in nonseminomatous germ cell tumors. *J Clin Oncol* 1992;**10**(1):85–94.
7. Tsetis D, Sharma A, Easty M, Brown I, Oliver R, Chan O. Potential of limited d21 post chemotherapy in predicting need for post chemotherapy surgery in nonseminomatous testicular germ cell cancer. *Urologia Internationalis* 1996;**61**:22–26.
8. Williams SD, Birch R, Einhorn LH, Irwin L, Greco F, Loehrer PJ. Treatment of disseminated germ-cell tumors with Cisplatin, Bleomycin, and either Vinblastine or Etoposide. *New Engl J Med* 1987;**316**(23):1435–1440.
9. Oliver R. Future trials in Germ Cell Malignancy (GCM) of the testis. *Eur J Surg Oncol* 1997;**23**:117–122.
10. Beyer J, Kingreen D, Krause M. Long term survival of patients with recurrent or refractory germ cell tumors after high dose chemotherapy. *Cancer* 1997;**79**:1605–1610.
11. Ravi R, Ong J, Oliver RTD, Badenoch DF, Fowler CG, Hendry WF. Surgery as salvage therapy in chemotherapy resistant nonseminomatous germ cell tumors. *Br J Urol* 1998;**81**(6):884–888.
12. Lange P, Hekmat K, Bosl G, Kennedy B, Fraley E. Accelerated growth of testicular cancer after cytoreductive surgery. *Cancer* 1980;**45**(6):1498–1506.
13. Bajorin DF, Sarosdy MF, Pfister DG *et al.* Randomized trial of etoposide and cisplatin versus etoposide and carboplatin in patients with good-risk germ cell tumors: a multi-institutional study. *J Clin Oncol* 1993;**11**:598–606.
14. Bajorin DF, Mazumdar M, Meyers M *et al.* Metastatic germ cell tumors: modeling for response to chemotherapy. *J Clin Oncol* 1998;**16**(2):707–715.
15. Bokemeyer C, Harstrick A, Metzner B *et al.* Sequential high dose VIP-chemotherapy plus peripheral stem cell (PBSC) support for advanced germ cell cancer. *Ann Oncol* 1996;**7**(suppl 5):55(abstract 259).
17. Boshoff CB, Begent RHJ, Oliver RTD *et al.* Secondary tumors following etoposide containing therapy for germ cell cancer. *Ann Oncol* 1995;**6**(1):35–40.
18. Travis L, Rochelle E, Curtis H, Per H, Hollowaty E. Risk of second malignant neoplasms among long term survivors of testicular cancer. *J Nat Cancer Inst* 1997;**89**:1429–1439.
19. Lampe H, Horwich A, Norman A, Nicholls J, Dearnaley DP. Fertility after chemotherapy for testicular germ cell cancers. *J Clin Oncol* 1997;**15**(1):239–245.
20. Stenning S, Parkinson MC, Fisher C *et al.* Postchemotherapy residual masses in germ cell tumor patients. *Cancer* 1998;**83**:1409–1419.
21. Pizzocaro G, Nicolai N, Salvoni R. Comparison between clinical and pathological staging in low stage non seminomatous germ cell testicular tumors. *J Urol* 1992;**148**:76.
22. Oliver RTD, Hope-Stone HF, Blandy JP. Justification of the use of surveillance in the management of stage 1 germ cell tumors of the testis. *Br J Urol* 1983;**55**:760–763.
23. Donohue JP, Thornhill JA, Foster RS, Rowland RG, Bihrle R. Primary retroperitoneal lymph node dissection in a clinical stage A non-seminomatous germ cell testis cancer. Review of the Indiana University experience 1965–1989. *Br J Urol* 1993;**71**:326–335.
24. Oliver R. Epidemiology of testis cancer. *Comprehensive Textbook of Genito-Urinary Oncology* 1999.
25. Petersen PM, Skakkebaek NE, Giwercman A. Gonadal function in men with testicular cancer: biological and clinical aspects. *Apmis* 1998;**106**(1):24–34; discussion 34–36.
26. Nargund V, Oliver R, Ong J, Sohaib S, Reznek R, Badenoch D. Chemotherapy ± partial orchidectomy for testis conservation in patients with germ cell cancer (GCC): is it safe, is it justified? *J Urol* 1999.
27. Heidenreich A, Holtl W, Albrecht W, Pont J, Engelmann UH. Testis-preserving surgery in bilateral testicular germ cell tumors. *Br J Urol* 1997;**79**(2):253–257.
28. Friedman M. Supervoltage roentgen therapy at Walter Reed General Hospital. *Surg Clin N Am* 1944;**24**(6):1424–1432.

29. Zagars G. Stage I testicular seminoma following orchidectomy – to treat or not to treat. *Eur J Cancer* 1993;**29A**:1923–1924.

30. Horwich A, Sleijfer D, Fossa S *et al.* A trial of carboplatin-based combination chemotherapy in good prognosis metastatic testicular non seminoma, 1994.

31. Oliver R, Edmonds P, Ong J, Ostrowski M, Jackson A. Pilot studies of 2 and 1 course Carboplatin as adjuvant for Stage I seminoma: should it be tested in a randomized trial against radiotherapy? *Int J Rad Oncol Biol, Phys* 1994;**29**(1):3–8.

39 Seminomatous germ cell tumor

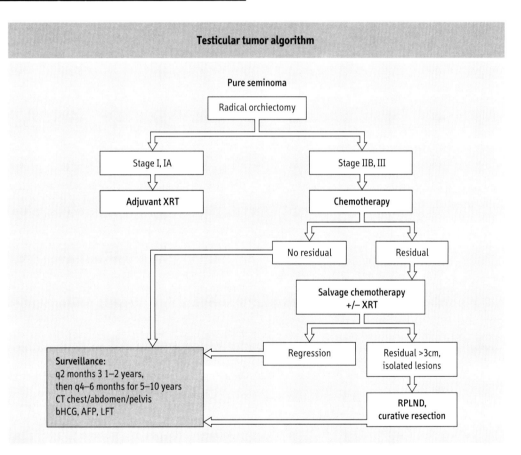

Testicular tumor algorithm

Pure seminoma

Radical orchiectomy

Stage I, IA → Adjuvant XRT

Stage IIB, III → Chemotherapy → No residual / Residual

Salvage chemotherapy +/− XRT → Regression / Residual >3cm, isolated lesions → RPLND, curative resection

Surveillance:
q2 months 3 1–2 years,
then q4–6 months for 5–10 years
CT chest/abdomen/pelvis
bHCG, AFP, LFT

39.1   Treatment of seminomas

R S Foster and J P Donohue

Introduction

Surgical therapy is not a major component of the treatment of seminomas. There are two basic reasons for this. The first reason is the exquisite sensitivity of seminomas to radiation therapy. This sensitivity of seminomas to external beam radiation is fairly uniform and consistent. Hence, the treatment of lower volume regional metastasis is characteristically radiation therapy. The second reason surgical therapy is not a large component of the treatment of seminomas is the similar exquisite sensitivity of seminoma to cisplatin based chemotherapy. Because chemo-resistant elements such as teratoma are not a component of pure seminoma, and since seminoma is very sensitive to cisplatin based chemotherapy, the likelihood of finding persistent radiographic tumor after chemotherapeutic treatment of seminoma is quite low. However, when this situation occurs (persistent radiographic disease after full-dose chemotherapeutic treatment of seminoma), there is controversy in management as will be discussed below.

Radical inguinal orchiectomy

The reasons for performing radical inguinal orchiectomy in seminoma are the same as for non-seminoma. Briefly, an inguinal incision decreases the possibility of tumor spillage at the time of orchiectomy since the incision is well away from the tumor itself. If tumor spillage were to occur after a scrotal incision, another lymphatic area (inguinal lymph nodes) would possibly be contaminated by such a maneuver. Since the treatment of low volume seminoma involves radiotherapy to the site of lymphatic metastasis, radiotherapy would have to be given not only to the retroperitoneal nodes but also the inguinal nodes. Therefore, it is safest and appropriate to perform radical inguinal orchiectomy for a presumed seminoma as opposed to scrotal orchiectomy.

After chemotherapy

The appropriate therapy of higher volume metastatic seminoma is cisplatin based chemotherapy. Typically such therapy is effective in itself with most patients experiencing complete resolution of radiographic disease. However, some patients are found to have residual radiographic disease after full-dose chemotherapeutic treatment of metastatic seminoma. Typically these are patients who present with very high volume disease at the time of discovery. Significant controversy exists as to whether or not these residual masses should be excised.

Most centers generally observe residual radiographic masses after full-dose chemotherapeutic treatment of seminoma. There is a reasonable rationale for this. First, there is an extensive desmoplastic reaction in the area of metastatic seminoma and surgical removal is generally much more difficult compared with non-seminoma. Therefore, adequately and completely excising these residual masses is problematic compared with non-seminoma. Secondly, most centers have observed a very low probability of progression if such patients are observed. For instance, 21 patients who had an evaluable residual radiographic mass after chemotherapy at Indiana University were evaluated for evidence of progression[1]. Patients were stratified into two separate groups; greater than 3 cm maximal transverse diameter and less than 3 cm maximal transverse diameter. Of nine patients with residual mass greater than 3 cm one relapse occurred. This patient is a long-term survival after treatment with salvage chemotherapy. Of 12 patients with residual masses less than 3 cm in greatest transverse diameter, there have been two relapses. One patient was treated with salvage chemotherapy and is a long-term survivor; the other patient was similarly treated with salvage chemotherapy but eventually relapsed and died of disease. Of the entire group of 21 patients, three patients were subjected to postchemotherapy surgery. Necrosis and fibrosis was found in all three patients.

In contrast, Motzer and associates reported on 23 patients with significant residual radiographic abnormalities after treatment for metastatic seminoma with cisplatin based chemotherapy[2]. Fourteen of these patients had masses 3 cm or greater in size. Of the 23 patients, 19 underwent surgical exploration and five were found to have significant findings other than fibrosis. Four of these patients had viable seminoma and one had teratoma. Therefore, the Memorial Sloan-Kettering recommendation has been to biopsy residual radiographic abnormalities if the residual disease measured 3 cm or greater.

This issue of whether or not surgically to explore patients with residual radiographic disease of 3 cm or greater remains unresolved. However, since these patients represent such a small number of the overall patients presenting with seminoma, fortunately this question does not arise commonly. The treatment of such patients should be based upon the entire clinical situation, adequacy of the chemotherapy, and the potential morbidity of an operation in an individual patient.

References

1. Schultz S, Einhorn L, Conces D, Williams S, Loehrer P. Management of post chemotherapy residual mass in patients with advanced seminoma: Indiana University experience. *J Clin Oncol* 1989;7:1497–1503.

2. Motzer R, Bosi G, Heelan R *et al.* Residual mass: an indication for further therapy in patients with advanced seminoma following systemic chemotherapy. *J Clin Oncol* 1987;**5**:1065–1070.

39.2 Radiotherapy

W G Jones

Introduction

Radiotherapy has played a part in the management of seminoma testis as a post-orchidectomy treatment for nearly 70 years[1]. The management of, and treatment results for, germ cell tumors have improved considerably in the last two decades[2] due to: improved specificity in the histologic diagnosis; improved radiologic imaging (especially CT scanning); use of serum tumor markers (α-fetoprotein, human chorionic gonadotrophin and lactic dehydrogenase); and, most importantly, the development of effective chemotherapy, and additionally improvements in medical care, e.g. $5HT_3$ antagonist anti-emetics and colony stimulating factors. Delightfully, seminoma testis appears to be as responsive to chemotherapy as it is to radiotherapy and even patients with grossly metastatic tumors can now be cured[3–5], the overall cure rate for this disease being in excess of 95%[2,6–11]. In recent years the main thrust of research into the management of seminoma has been to try to improve the acceptability, convenience and cost-effectiveness of therapy, and the reduction of toxicity, while maintaining such excellent outcome statistics[2].

Immediate management

The modes of presentation, investigation, surgical management, histologic confirmation and staging have been discussed in earlier chapters, but a few important points must be reiterated here.

Serum tumor markers

Blood for serum tumor markers should be taken before the orchidectomy and the estimations repeated after. Patients with raised α-fetoprotein levels must have their histology reviewed and be treated as for teratoma. Seminomas do not produce this marker.

Fertility

The wishes of the patient regarding the preservation of fertility should be determined and semen cryopreservation offered if the patient wishes to maximize his chances of siring (further) children. Since seminoma occurs mainly in an older age group (approximately 10 years) than patients with teratoma testis, it is found that many couples may have already decided they do not want further children, so the take-up rate for sperm storage is often lower than in the teratoma group.

Surgery

An inguinal incision should be used for the orchidectomy since this reduces the likelihood of scrotal contamination with tumor and also allows the high ligation of the spermatic cord. Scrotal orchidectomy or indeed prior inguinal scrotal surgery related to maldescent of the testes can potentially open alternative lymphatic drainage pathways and may require a modification to the radiotherapeutic technique applied when post-orchidectomy treatment is delivered[12,13].

Post-surgery treatment

Referral to a specialist (regional) cancer center for further investigation and treatment is mandatory, in view of the rarity of this disease, so that expertise can be developed and maintained.

Staging

Refinements in radiologic techniques now allows very accurate anatomical staging of testicular tumors. The Royal Marsden Hospital staging system is still commonly in use for seminoma cases in the United Kingdom and Europe (Table 39.2.1)[11]. It is important to know that there are small but subtle differences in staging systems used around the world, although the majority of systems commonly define stage 1 as tumor confined to the testis without any clinical or radiologic evidence of spread and with normalized post-orchidectomy tumor markers.

Table 39.2.1 Royal Marsden Hospital staging classification for testicular tumors (modified)

Stage		
1		No clinical or radiological evidence of metastases.
1m		No clinical or radiological evidence of metastases, but serum tumor marker(s) raised.
2		Metastases confined to abdominal nodes:
	2A	Maximum diameter of nodes <2 cm
	2B	Maximum diameter of nodes 2–5 cm
	2C	Maximum diameter of nodes 5–10 cm
	2D	Maximum diameter of nodes >10 cm
3		Involvement of supra diaphragmatic nodes. No extralymphatic metastases.
4		Extralymphatic metastases. Suffixes denote site.
	L	= lung
	H	= liver
	B	= bone
	BM	= bone marrow
	C	= brain/CNS
	S	= skin

Therapeutic options

Since seminoma is exquisitely radio-sensitive and rarely spreads beyond the retroperitoneal lymph nodes[14], adjuvant radiotherapy to the para-aortic and pelvic nodes has been standard practice for many decades[7,9,10,14–16]. There is a decrease in the curability with increasing bulk of metastatic disease[14,16,17]. With the advent of effective chemotherapy of the same or similar nature to that used for teratoma, patients with bulky or extra-nodal metastases are managed by this modality. There is some controversy as to the level of cut-off with increasing stage as to when patients should be treated with chemotherapy. Certainly patients with stage 2C or greater stage disease are best managed in this way[16,17], but since the cure rates for radiotherapy for stage 2B disease are worse than 90%, some believe that chemotherapy should be given for patients with metastases >3 to 3.5 cm in transverse diameter. There is the argument that chemotherapy should be used for all stages of this disease and especially as adjuvant therapy for stage I disease (Chapter 39.3)[5].

Since the great majority of patients with stage 1 disease have been cured by their orchidectomy and have no metastases, surveillance is being investigated as an option for the management of these patients[18–22]. Surveillance, as for testicular teratoma, is a very intensive way of following these patients who must comply with the investigation schedule. There are concerns that unlike surveillance for teratoma, because the disease is more slowly growing, relapses for seminoma patients could be very late and more difficult to detect since tumor markers are rarely raised and are of little use in follow up[18]. For the moment, surveillance techniques belong solely in the research sphere of large cancer centers[20,22].

Radiotherapy

Stage 1
Approximately 80% of all seminoma patients fall into this category[2,6,7,18–20]. Evidence from surgical staging series and surveillance series suggests that the incidence of undetected retroperitoneal metastases in stage 1 subjects is less than 20%[10,20,21,23]. However, because of the historically excellent results of post-orchidectomy para-aortic and pelvic node irradiation and the very low morbidity of this treatment, adjuvant radiotherapy remains the treatment of choice, despite 80% of patients being treated unnecessarily, with an expected survival >98%.[6–9,11,14,16,19,24,25].

Radiotherapy dose
Seminoma is exquisitely radio-sensitive and total doses ranging from between 25 to 40 Gy in 13 to 20 daily fractions have been employed in treatment[2,6,8,9]. Relapse within the irradiated area is a rare event. There has been an increasing trend to use doses towards the lower end of the spectrum quoted above and, in 1989 at the International Testicular Cancer Consensus Conference in Hull, UK, a recommendation was made that a total dose of 25 Gy in 15 to 20 fractions was suitable for the management of stage 1 seminoma[2]. The MRC is currently conducting a study (TE18) comparing 20 Gy mid plane dose (MPD) in 10 fractions versus (what is regarded in the UK as the standard treatment of) 30 Gy MPD in 15 fractions, with the aims of reducing toxicity, improving acceptability and cost-effectiveness of treatment. This strategy was adopted following the publication of results of series of patients treated with reduced dose from Manchester[26] and from France[27].

Stage 2 disease
As stated above, the results of treatment worsen with progressive increase in stage and chemotherapy is now the treatment of choice for patients with bulky stage 2B disease or greater[2,11,14]. However patients with low volume metastases in the retroperitoneal lymph nodes, as seen on CT scanning, are eminently curable using the same techniques as described above, but perhaps with a very modest increase in total dose (35 Gy in 15–20 fractions).

Supra-diaphragmatic irradiation
Historically prophylactic mediastinal and supraclavicular irradiation was sometimes given particularly for patients with bulky stage 2 disease for fear of supra-diaphragmatic spread. There is now clear evidence that this practice should be abandoned particularly since there is now effective chemotherapy available for the management of patients with this condition[9,11,17]. Prophylactic mediastinal irradiation carried with it a very high incidence of cardiac toxicity[9]. By the irradiation of an increased volume of bone marrow there was a danger of increased toxicity for any salvage chemotherapy if this was required later.

Response to treatment of bulky seminomas
Occasionally, following radiotherapy, but more particularly following chemotherapy for bulky seminomatous metastases in the retroperitoneum and elsewhere the disease is slow to regress radiologically with some masses taking up to 2 years or more to disappear completely. Some authors have suggested that patients should receive radiation following chemotherapy treatment in order to bring about rapid resolution of the masses[11,28]. However, there is now some controversy over this approach particularly

since the potential long-term hazards increase when both radiotherapy and chemotherapy are used sequentially.

Other indications for radiotherapy

There appears to be a subgroup of patients with seminoma who develop rather atypical patterns of disease which can be indolent to chemotherapy treatment. The exquisite sensitivity of seminoma to radiation allows some of these patients to be salvaged with local radiotherapy, for example, to the brain, bone, etc.

Radiation toxicity

Acute toxicity

Although the acute side effects of radiation for patients undergoing either para-aortic strip or dog-leg radiotherapy are extremely low[10,29], surprisingly these have not been accurately documented in a prospective way. The MRC study TE18 is hoping to document the side effects of the treatment by asking the patients to fill in a daily diary card and also to complete quality of life questionnaires. The acute side effects of treatment are as follows:

1 Fatigue   This is a very variable side effect with some patients complaining that they feel fatigued for many months after treatment and others not apparently noticing any difference in their well-being. Psychological factors may be playing a part in the former group of patients.
2 Gastrointestinal Patients complain of variable amounts of anorexia, nausea and vomiting[30] and many radiotherapists now prescribe antiemetics prophylactically. Occasionally the use of a $5HT_3$ antagonist is required for patients with acute vomiting who are not responsive to more usual (and less expensive) antiemetic preparations.
3 Hematologic   Patients are usually monitored with weekly blood counts during treatment and rarely a depression of the white cell count or platelet count is seen.[16,31] However, with more abbreviated radiotherapy fields being employed now, this phenomena is likely to be seen far less often unless the patient has a predisposing medical condition.

Long-term toxicity

With modern radiotherapy facilities and the application of improved radiation techniques the risk of irradiation-induced nephro-, cardiac-, and neuro-toxicity are extremely small[16,31]. There is a suggestion that there may be a reduction of sexual function in some patients following treatment[15,32]. However there are concerns regarding gastrointestinal toxicity, gonadal toxicity and

carcinogenesis. The suggestion that (possibly carcinogenic) chemotherapy should replace radiotherapy, especially for stage 1[5], must be tempered by the fact that there is long-term follow up data for radiotherapy patients but not for chemotherapy patients yet, especially for treatment related carcinogenesis, a process which may take 20 to 30+ years.

Gastrointestinal toxicity

Following infra-diaphragmatic radiotherapy there is slight increase in long-term gastrointestinal effects such as dyspepsia, acid reflux, etc. with patients having pre-treatment problems being at higher risk than those without. Peptic ulceration was observed in 4% to 9% of irradiated patients[7,15,31,33]. Since there has been a great improvement in the medical management of peptic ulceration in recent times, this toxicity problem will probably assume a lesser importance.

Gonadal toxicity

As stated above, with modern radiation techniques the gonadal dose following abdominal irradiation is usually less than 0.5 Gy[7]. This results in reduction in spermatogenesis for about 1 to 2 years with a gradual subsequent increase in sperm count[30]. However sperm storage should be offered to those wishing to maximize their chances of fathering (further) children. Leydig cell function (and thus hormone production) is not affected by such small doses of radiation.

Second cancer induction

It has now become evident that the relative risks of developing second malignancies following irradiation for seminoma of the testis may be slightly elevated[9,10,34–41]. The reported types of second malignancies are: leukemia, lung cancer, gastric and colon cancers, bladder cancer, melanoma and soft tissue sarcoma[40]. Some studies (mainly institution-based) have shown no evidence of increased risk[34,35,39], whereas others have[36,37,40]. It is currently impossible accurately to determine what proportion of any increased risk of second cancer incidence is due to radiation therapy. An MRC retrospective study (TER1) has recently been activated and may provide better data in due course.

Extra-gonadal seminomas

Extra-gonadal germ cell tumors can arise in the retroperitoneum, mediastinum, base of brain and sacrococcygeal areas. Surgery, chemotherapy and radiation treatment, either alone or in combination, are used in the treatment of these rather rare extra-testicular tumors.

Conclusions

Radiotherapy has an important part to play in the adjuvant therapy of seminoma of the testis following orchidectomy. However, its role is less than it was a number of years ago because of the advent of chemotherapy which is now used routinely for patients with bulky nodal or extra-nodal metastatic disease. Chemotherapy is also being considered in the adjuvant treatment of stage 1 disease. The favorable results achieved with radiotherapy for seminoma with very high local control and survival rates with minimal morbidity make it difficult for alternative therapies to be considered. The current thrust of research is to investigate reducing the amount of therapy required to maintain these results both in terms of the volume of tissue to be treated and by reducing the overall radiation dose.

References

1. Desjardins AU, Squire FH, Morton SA. Radiotherapy for tumors of the testis. *Am J Roentgenol* 1929;**22**:137–146.
2. Thomas G, Jones W, van Oosterom A, Kawai T. Consensus statement on the investigation and management of testicular seminoma 1989. In: Newling DWW, Jones WG (eds) *EORTC genitourinary group monograph 7: prostate cancer and testicular cancer* (Progress in Clinical and Biological Research, Vol. 357). Wiley-Liss, New York, 1990, pp. 285–294.
3. Logothetis CJ, Samuels ML, Ogden SL *et al.* Cyclophosphamide and sequential cis-platin for advanced seminoma: long term follow-up in 52 patients. *J Urol* 1987;**138**:789–794.
4. Horwich A, Dearnaley DP, Duchesne GM *et al.* Simple nontoxic treatment of advanced metastatic seminoma with carboplatin. *J Clin Oncol* 1989; **7**:1150–1156.
5. Oliver RTD, Edmonds PM, Ong JYH *et al.* Pilot studies of 2 and 1 course carboplatin as adjuvant for stage 1 seminoma: should it be tested in a randomised trial against radiotherapy? *Int J Radiat Oncol Biol Phys* 1994;**29**:3–8.
6. Thomas GM. Controversies in the management of testicular seminoma. *Cancer* 1985;**55**:2296–2302.
7. Hamilton C, Horwich A, Easton D, Peckham MJ. Radiotherapy for stage 1 seminoma testis: results of treatment and complications. *Radiother Oncol* 1986;**6**:115–120.
8. Doornbos JF, Hussey DH, Johnson DE. Radiotherapy for pure seminoma of the testis. *Radiology* 1975;**116**:401–404.
9. Hanks GE, Peters T, Owen J. Seminoma of the testis: long term beneficial and deleterious results of radiation. *Int J Radiat Oncol Biol Phys* 1992;**24**:913–919.
10. Vallis KA, Howard GCW, Duncan W, Cornbleet MA, Kerr GR. Radiotherapy for stages I and II testicular seminoma: results and morbidity in 238 patients. *Br J Radiol* 1995;**68**:400–405.
11. Ball D, Barrett A, Peckham MJ. The management of metastatic seminoma testis. *Cancer* 1982;**50**:2289–2294.
12. Busch FM, Sayegh ES. Some uses of lymphangiography in the management of testicular tumors. *J Urol* 1965;**93**:490–495.
13. Ray B, Steven I, Hajdu SI, Whitmore WF. Distribution of retroperitoneal lymph node metastases in testicular germinal tumors. *Cancer* 1974;**33**:340–348.
14. Read G, Robertson AG, Blair V. Radiotherapy in seminoma of the testis. *Clin Radiol* 1983;**34**:469–473.
15. Fosså SD, Aass N, Kaalhus O. Long term morbidity after infradiaphragmatic radiotherapy in young men with testicular cancer. *Cancer* 1989;**64**:404–408.
16. Duncan W, Munro AJ. The management of testicular seminoma: Edinburgh 1970–1981. *Br J Cancer* 1987;**55**:443–448.
17. Gregory C, Peckham MJ. Results of radiotherapy for stage II testicular seminoma. *Radiother Oncol* 1986;**6**:285–292.
18. Duchesne GM, Horwich A, Dearnaley DP *et al.* Orchidectomy alone for stage 1 seminoma of the testis. *Cancer* 1990;**65**:1115–1118.
19. Thomas GM, Sturgeon JF, Alison R *et al.* A study of post-orchidectomy surveillance in stage 1 testicular seminoma. *J Urol* 1989;**142**:243–247.
20. Warde PR, Gospodarowicz MK, Goodman PJ *et al.* Results of surveillance in stage 1 testicular seminoma. *Int J Radiat Oncol Biol Phys* 1993;**27**:11–15.
21. von der Maase H, Specht L, Jacobsen GK *et al.* Surveillance following orchidectomy for stage 1 seminoma testis. *Eur J Cancer* 1993;**29A**:1931–1934.
22. Ramakrishnan S, Champion AE, Dorreen MS, Fox M. Stage I seminoma testis: is post-orchidectomy surveillance a safe alternative to routine postoperative radiotherapy? *Clin Oncol* 1992;**4**:284–286.
23. Donohue JP. Metastatic pathways of non-seminomatous germ cell tumors. *Sem Urol* 1984;**11**:217–219.
24. Shultz HP, von der Maase A, Rørth M *et al.* Testicular seminoma in Denmark 1976–1980. *Acta Radiol Oncol* 1984;**23**:263–270.
25. Zagars GK, Babaian RJ. Stage 1 testicular seminoma: rationale for post-orchidectomy radiation therapy. *Int J Radiat Oncol Biol Phys* 1987;**13**:155–162.
26. Read G, Johnston RJ. Short duration radiotherapy in stage 1 seminoma of the testis: preliminary results. *Clin Oncol* 1993;**5**:364–366.
27. Giacchetti S, Raoul Y, Wibault P, Droz J-P, Court B, Eschwege F. Treatment of stage 1 testis seminoma by radiotherapy: long-term results – a 30-year experience. *Int J Radiat Oncol Biol Phys* 1993;**27**:3–9.
28. Ravinthiran T, Jones WG. Chemotherapy for advanced and recurrent metastatic seminoma. In: Jones WG, Milford Ward A, Anderson CK (eds) *Germ cell tumours* II. Pergamon Oxford, 1986; p. 239.
29. Aass N, Fosså SD, Høst H. Acute and subacute side effects due to infra-diaphragmatic radiotherapy for testicular cancer: a prospective study. *Int J Radiat Oncol Biol Phys* 1992;**22**:1057–1064.
30. Fosså SD, Horwich A, Russell JM, Roberts JP, Jakes R, Stenning S. Optimal field size in adjuvant radiotherapy (XRT) of stage 1 seminoma – a randomised trial. *Proc ASCO* 1996;**15**:239(abstract 595).
31. Coia LR, Hanks GE. Complications from large field intermediate dose infradiaphragmatic radiation: an analysis of the patterns of care outcome studies for Hodgkin's disease and seminoma. *Int J Radiat Oncol Biol Phys* 1988;**15**:29–35.
32. Tinkler SD, Howard GCW, Kerr GR. Sexual morbidity following radiotherapy for germ cell tumors of the testis. *Radiother Oncol* 1992;**25**:207–212.
33. Hamilton C, Horwich A, Bliss JM, Peckham MJ. Gastrointestinal morbidity of adjuvant radiotherapy in stage 1 malignant seminoma of the testis. *Radiother Oncol* 1987;**10**:85–90.
34. Fosså SD, Langmark F, Aass N, Andersen A, Lothe R, Børresen AL. Second non-germ cell malignancies after radiotherapy for testicular cancer with or without chemotherapy. *Br J Cancer* 1990;**61**:639–643.
35. Horwich A, Bell J. Late mortality after radiotherapy for stage 1 seminoma of the testis. *Eur J Cancer* 1991;**6**:639.
36. van Leeuwen FE, Stiggelbout AM, van Belt-Dusebout AW *et al.* Second cancer risk following testicular cancer: a follow-up study of 1909 patients. *J Clin Oncol* 1993;**11**:415–424.
37. Møller H, Mellemgaard A, Jacobsen GK, Pedersen D, Storm HH. Incidence of second primary cancer following testicular cancer. *Eur J Cancer* 1993;**5**:672–676.
38. Hay JH, Duncan W, Kerr GR. Subsequent malignancies in patients irradiated for testicular tumors. *Br J Radiol* 1984;**57**:597–602.
39. Chao CK, Lai PP, Michalski JM, Perez CA. Secondary malignancy among seminoma patients treated with adjuvant radiation therapy. *Int J Radiat Oncol Biol Phys* 1995;**33**:831–835.
40. Jacobsen GK, Mellemond A, Engelholm SA, Moller H. Increased incidence of sarcoma in patients treated for testicular seminoma. *Eur J Cancer* 1993;**29A**:664–668.
41. Kaldor JM, Day NE, Band P *et al.* Second malignancies following testicular cancer, ovarian cancer and Hodgkin's disease: an international collaborative study among cancer registries. *Int J Cancer* 1987;**39**:571–585.

39.3 Background, rationale and results from use of chemotherapy in metastatic and localized seminoma

R T D Oliver

It is now more than 50 years since the classical paper by Friedman (1944)[1], demonstrating that patients with metastatic seminoma had more lasting complete remissions with lower doses of radiation than malignant teratoma/non-seminoma, led to adjuvant radiation becoming the standard treatment for stage 1 seminoma. This occurred in the late 1950s/early 1960s with the cure increasing from 90–95% in most recently treated cohorts of patients[2]. Because relapse has occurred in patients as late as 9 years after orchidectomy alone[3], and patients have presented with signs and symptoms of spinal cord compression as first manifestation of relapse, the need for use of adjuvant treatment has been accepted by most physicians involved in treatment of these patients. Because of the high success rates with radiation, this has remained the standard.

Given this success, there has been considerable resistance and incredulity that there might be a need to change a winning formula.

It is the aim of this chapter to:

1. Review the problems associated with late events after radiation that provide in part a justification for considering alternates
2. Review what we understand about biology of seminoma and its development and why this suggests that chemotherapy may be better than radiation.
3. Review data on use of chemotherapy versus radiation for metastatic disease and why it justifies study of single agent carboplatin as adjuvant instead of radiation.
4. The results of two versus one course adjuvant carboplatin
5. Where next and in particular could we do without orchidectomy.

Problems associated with late events after radiation that provide in part a justification for considering alternatives

The most recent publication from a British center[4] did not observe a major increase in risk of second cancer from use of radiation as adjuvant in stage 1 seminoma, although with less than 50% followed for more than 10 years in that study and data showing that there was a non-significant excess of deaths in those followed for more than 10 years,

the observations from Van Leeuwen[5] carry greater weight. They show in a study of non-seminoma and seminoma that an excess of second non-germ cell cancer only begins to be seen after 10 years and by 20 years has occurred in 20% of those followed. A similar observation emerged from the study by Duncan et al.[6]. Admittedly, in the Van Leeuwen study, the patients receiving the lower dose of radiation used to treat seminoma had less incidence but a 3.2-fold increased risk is still not negligible (Table 39.3.1). Given the steep dose response indicated by the 7-fold increased risk for those receiving the higher dose used for malignant teratoma, it is possible that the current trials using smaller fields and lower doses may well further reduce the risks.

Our own studies in this area with 58% dead at 30 years compared with 28% expected on the basis of UK statistics have confirmed the importance of long follow up but also emphasizes that it is not only late cancer deaths that occur more frequently in patients treated by radiation (Table 39.3.2). Because of the large impact of social factors on life expectancy only by having matched control population from the same area will it be possible unequivocally to confirm this difference. Despite this it is not clear whether these excess cancers are radiation related or simply a reflection of the degree of biological unfitness of patients with seminoma. Only by collecting similar late follow up data on the more than 600 cases in the literature of stage 1 seminoma treated by orchidectomy and surveillance will it be possible to address this issue though to prove it conclusively would need a randomized control trial.

New ideas on the biology of seminoma and its development and why this suggests that chemotherapy may be better than radiation

That all germ cell cancer with the notable exception of spermatocytic seminoma and mature teratoma in children arises from malignant transformation of spermatogonia via a carcinoma in situ (CIS) stage is now increasingly accepted through the work of Skakkebaek's group[7]. They

Table 39.3.1 Dose and development of stomach cancer on 10–15 year follow up of 5 year survivors after radiation for germ cell cancer[5]

	Number treated	Observed/expected in 5 year survivors	Relative risk
Seminoma (<30 cGY)	874	4/1.3	3.2
Non-seminoma (40–50 cGY)	992	5/0.2	26.3

Table 39.3.2   Royal London Hospital cumulative risk of death in stage 1 seminoma after radiation and surveillance (Oliver and Ong, unpublished)

	10 year (%)	20 year (%)	30 year (%)
Radiation series (n=137)			
Germ cell cancer death	4	4	4
2nd non-germ cell cancer death	2	13	33
Non-cancer death	4	7	21
All deaths	10	24	58
Surveillance series (n=74) 1983–85			
Germ cell cancer deaths	3	NA	NA
2nd non-germ cell cancer deaths	1	NA	NA
Non-cancer deaths	1	NA	NA
All deaths	5	NA	NA
Expected deaths (all causes 36-year-old male born in UK in 1979)	2	9	28

NA = not applicable.

demonstrated that CIS can be detected in all groups with a high risk of germ cell cancer such as cryptorchids, infertile males and inter sex cases as well as the contralateral testis of patients who have had a previous germ cell cancer. The most convincing evidence for the link between CIS and active cancer is the fact that CIS is demonstrated in residual normal tubules in more than 90% of testes removed with a proven germ cell cancer.

The observation that the DNA content of CIS cells is near tetraploid and that there is a loss of chromosome material in progression from seminoma (Table 39.3.3) to non-seminoma is the most clear evidence to support the concept that clonal evolution in association with loss of suppressor genes could be a factor in linking all the germ cell cancers as a single group of diseases[8]. The clinical behavior showing combined seminoma and non-seminoma as being intermediate between seminoma and pure non-seminoma (Table 39.3.4) would fit with this concept of clonal evolution and support the idea that seminoma is a grade 1 or well differentiated germ cell cancer (G1 GCC) with respect to its cell of origin. Pure non-seminoma without cells resembling the differentiated stem cell would be considered as undifferentiated or grade 3 germ cell cancer (G3 GCC), while combined seminoma/non-seminoma would be considered as grade 2 (G2 GCC) or intermediate germ cell cancer[8].

Although these observations help to explain the relationship between seminoma and the embryonal carcinoma elements, the occurrence of extra-embryonic tissue such as trophoblast, yolk sac or fetal cartilage, glandular or neural elements is not so easily explained. The frequency with which immunocytochemistry identifies these elements in other solid tumors[9], and classifies them as metaplastic components provides a nomenclature that could be combined with grading in germ cell cancer classification. That GCC with these somatic ele-

Table 39.3.3   DNA index and development of germ cell tumors sub-type

	CIS component	Tumor component
Primary CIS	2.01	NA
Seminoma	1.59	1.64
Combined Tumors	1.62	1.61
Non-seminoma	1.53	1.43

Table 39.3.4   Combined tumors as an intermediate prognosis subgroup of testicular germ cell tumors

	Seminoma n=248	Combined seminoma non-seminoma n=116	Non-seminoma n=241
Median age stage 1	36 years	31 years	29 years
Median age metastatic patients	42 years	37 years	29 years
Proportion presenting in stage 1	79%	51%	41%
Relapse stage 1 after adjuvant chemotherapy	1%	6%	0%
Relapse stage 1 after surveillance only	23%	31%	38%
Primary cure of all metastatic patients	91%	93%	86%
Proportion of metastatic cases with high markers	0%	16%	21%
Cure rate low markers	91%	94%	92%
Cure rate high markers	–	89%	65%

ments have a higher level of loss of heterzygosity than other GCC[10], provides a justification for considering the clonal grading evolution and fetal/somatic tissue differentiation as two separate dimensions of the pathologic classification relevant to the prognosis of germ cell cancer metastasis.

There is increasing evidence for common factors linking declining sperm count and rising incidence of testicular cancer. The occurrence of subfertile levels of sperm count in 60–70% of patients with testis cancer compared with 20–25% of the normal population and the observation of the association with elevated FSH levels in 40% of patients with testis cancer and an enhanced risk of such patients developing second germ cell cancers, is the most convincing data explaining this association. Loss of feedback suppression of gonadotrophin leading to reduced time for DNA repair in the spermatogonia has been proposed as the final common pathway linking declining sperm count and rising testis cancer[11].

Recent epidemiology studies from the UK Testicular Cancer Study Group have provided some evidence to support the view that genetic, viral, chemical and trauma factors can, possibly by inducing testicular atrophy, influence germ cell cancer development and that an endocrine mechanism via the hypothalamic gonadal axis may be the final common pathway[12–14]. That the hypothalamic gonadal axis is known to be affected by exercise could explain the increased risk of a sedentary lifestyle reported by Forman et al. and this could also be one factor contributing to the marked sperm count difference recently reported between sperm donors from New York and California[15,16].

Recently, there have been new observations from the laboratory that help to explain the exquisite sensitivity of normal and malignant germ cells to chemical insults whether environmental or therapeutic.

Expression of p53 and Bcl 2 are known to be two critical factors in regulating cell proliferation and suppressing apoptosis. Under normal conditions, very little or no p53 is detectable in normal cells, though because its function is primarily to act as the guardian of the genome, this changes rapidly when cells are exposed to DNA damage or mutation[17]. Under such circumstances p53 is rapidly induced and causes mitotic arrest until the DNA damage is repaired or if it is too great to repair, switches on programmed cell death (apoptosis) via p21 ras pathway which is blocked in some malignancies by inappropriate expression of Bcl-2. Heat shock protein (HSP70) is a critical factor required at this stage for stabilization and hence functional activity of p53. The demonstration that heat induces apoptosis of germ cells via a p53 mechanism[18] could go a long way to explain the association between testis cancer and a sedentary lifestyle.

Mutation of p53 gene has been known to be a frequent event in common adult cancers and in most cases this correlates with poor prognosis and poor response to chemotherapy and radiotherapy[19]. In most of these cases mutation leads to overexpression of non-functional p53 protein which, because it is not eliminated by normal breakdown processes, can be detected using immuno-histochemistry.

Recently it has become clear that not all p53 detectable by immuno-histochemistry in tumor cells is mutated. This phenomenon has been most noticeable in germ cell cancers of the testis, i.e. both seminomas and non-seminomas. Sequencing of p53 gene in these tumors and studies of apoptosis have proven that the gene is fully functional and active[20]. Schwartz et al.[21] by demonstrating that p53 is switched on during normal spermatogenesis have demonstrated a possible reason why non-mutated p53 expression is universal in spermatogenesis. These authors demonstrated that p53 is only detectable during the brief period that the tetraploid pachytene primary spermatocyte is in existence and this is presumably responsible for a final check of the genome prior to meiosis. The observation that this tetraploid cell may be the primary stem cell

for all germ cell cancers (Table 39.3.3) provides an explanation for why unmutated p53 is so overexpressed in all germ cell cancers. Some authors studying other tumor types which have non-mutated p53 constitutively expressed have noted that they retain sensitivity to chemotherapy and radiotherapy. p53 functionally expressed in a tetraploid dose and requiring little triggering to undergo apoptosis could go a long way to explaining why germ cell cancers are so exquisitely sensitive to radiation and chemotherapy. Our own studies (Nouri and Oliver, in preparation) demonstrate that there is a clonal trend for reduction of p53 and increasing Bcl-2 expression between primary seminoma and pure non-seminoma.

Review data on use of single agent or combination chemotherapy versus radiation for metastatic disease

Prognostication of metastatic seminoma on the basis of response to combination therapy

Because of the relative rarity of patients with metastatic seminoma there have been very few studies reporting more than 50 patients. The occasion of the setting up of the International Germ Cell Cancer Collaborative Group enabled information on more than 10 times that number of cases to be studied (Table 39.3.5). Although the impact of age, era when treated, the presence of lung or visceral non-lung metastases such as liver, bone and brain as well as a history of previous radiation had a similar poor prognostic effect to that demonstrated in studies of non-seminoma, tumor markers particularly LDH and hCG were less impressive risk factors than in non-seminoma as was the presence of a mediastinal or retroperitoneal primary[22].

In a subset of this data, i.e. that from the UK MRC collaborating centers[23], more information was available on chemotherapy regimen (Table 39.3.6). The apparently better survival of patients treated with bleomycin, etoposide, cisplatin (BEP) could be a factor in the continued improvement in the 1990 onward treated patients in the IGCCG as though 96% cure of patients with metastatic seminoma with this regimen was reported in 1985[24] it did not become widely used immediately. This was because of studies into the use of regimens without bleomycin.

The high cure rate with BEP leaves very little margin for prognostication. It might seem scientifically unsound to consider the 4% worse (92%) survival in the reports of seminoma patients treated with etoposide and cisplatin[25] as clinically significantly worse even if it isn't statistically so. The dropping of bleomycin is a difficult issue to resolve. In non-seminoma it is increasingly accepted that it is

Table 39.3.5   International Germ Cell Cancer Collaborative Group Prognostic Factors for Metastatic Seminoma (Mead & Stenning, in preparation)

		No. of cases	5 Year progression free (%)
Age			
	<30	146	86
	30–50	415	81
	>50	99	73
Primary site			
	Testis	559	80
	Mediastinal	41	80
	Retroperitoneum	45	88
	Other	15	88
Lung mets			
	No	543	81
	Yes	78	67
Visceral met (non-lung)			
	No	508	81
	Yes	64	67
HCG m/l			
	<5000	526	79
	5000–50 000	9	67
	>50 000	6	50
Years treated			
	<1985	221	80
	1985–89	355	85
	>1989	84	91
Radiation before chemotherapy			
	Nil	342	83
	Yes	103	74
LDH			
	<1.5 × n	226	87
	1.5–10	213	77
	>10	24	83

Table 39.3.6   MRC Testicular Tumor Working Party Prognostic Factors for Metastatic Seminoma (Fossa et al. Eur J Cancer submitted)

		No. of cases	3 Year progression free (%)
Stage 2/3 (no radiation)			
	BEP	39	95
	Other	85	86
Lung ± nodes (no radiation)			
	BEP	3	100
	Other	17	71
Liver/bone/brain ± node ± lung (no radiation)			
	BEP	3	33
	Other	8	75

unsafe to omit bleomycin. Despite early warnings of high relapse rates in good risk patients from phase 2 studies[26,27] and preliminary reports that use of prolonged infusion

bleomycin instead of the rapid IV bolus of the Einhorn regimen was a better way of reducing bleomycin lung deaths[27,28], it has taken four trials involving 859 patients all of which had worse survival in the arm without bleomycin with an overall 9% worse survival without bleomycin before a consensus has been reached that it is perhaps not safe to eliminate bleomycin from combination therapy even in good risk patients. Although only two of these trials had a statistically significant difference, one of the others compared EP to VAB-6 as a control arm. As this later regimen has, unlike BEP[29], not been proven to be any better than BVP, equivalence in this trial could be misleading.

In view of this albeit minor difference, given the added safety from use of bleomycin by infusion, it would seem prudent to continue using bleomycin for patients with both metastatic seminoma and non-seminoma, but making sure treatment is by infusion rather than bolus, that the total dose is kept below 270 mg and that the use of bleomycin is drastically reduced if there is any fall off in renal function while on treatment[30].

Despite the excellent result with BEP, there is a need to resolve the issue as to whether histology should play any role in discrimination of treatment or, as is currently the case for non-seminoma, whether prognostication should be totally based on tumor marker levels and volume/site of metastases. The strongest advocates of this have been the Memorial Group[25]. Given that there are differences between seminoma and non-seminoma as demonstrated for some of the prognostic factors presented in Table 38.4.5, as most of the Memorial prognostication has been based on their VAB-6 trials in seminoma and non-seminoma and as this combination has not been proven to be significantly better than BVP in contrast to the situation with BEP[29] there is a need for more data on this issue comparing seminoma, combined and pure non-seminoma patients who have been treated with BEP without any previous chemotherapy or radiation before the issue can be resolved. The opportunity to do this is presented by the current MRC/EORTC good risk protocol which compares a 3 versus 5 day regimen of BEP chemotherapy and three versus four courses of treatment in seminoma and non-seminoma.

Prognostic factors and single agent platinum for lymph node metastatic stage 2 and 3 seminoma

One of the most important issues of prognostication for metastatic seminoma patients which needs to be resolved relates to whether it is possible to identify a subgroup in whom single agent platinum therapy is justified[31]. Cisplatin, vinblastine and bleomycin (PVB) combination chemotherapy became standard for metastatic seminoma after only two patients (one a long-term survivor) had been treated with single agent cisplatin in the initial phase 2 study which consisted primarily of patients with metastatic non-seminoma[32]. In 1980 Samuels reported on five patients treated with weekly cisplatin 100 mg/m[2] and then changed to cisplatin plus cyclophosphamide[33,34]. Our own unit explored conventional cisplatin dosage of 100 mg/m[2] every 3 weeks and then changed to carboplatin when that drug became available[35,36]. Table 38.4.7 summarizes the admittedly far too small series treated by either cisplatin alone or carboplatin alone. After cisplatin 100% of stage 2C/3 patients (n=12) achieved durable progression-free survival, while after carboplatin it has only been 73% (n=85). There were two factors which possibly explain the poor performance of carboplatin. First, in two of the studies[37,38] most of the patients received their treatment every 4 weeks. Only 70% of these patients achieved durable primary progression free survival compared with 83% in the smaller series treated with a similar dose every 21 days. Substantially higher doses of carboplatin have now been safely used in ovarian cancer patients. As Horwich et al.[37] salvaged 12/14 of carboplatin failures using weekly bleomycin, oncovin and cisplatin, Schmoll et al.[38] salvaged 10/12 carboplatin failures using PEI and our group salvaged 2/3 carboplatin failures using BEP[31], giving an overall survival of single agent treated patients of 95%, it would seem justified further to explore single agent carboplatin as an alternative to BEP given that this approach reduces the cost of treatment by at least two-thirds, to say nothing of the reduced toxicity. The debate revolves around whether the level of quality of life gain for the 75–90% who avoid the extra toxicity of immediate combination treatment exceeds the extra toxicity for the 10–25% extra who have to have more intensive treatment of relapse.

The MRC trial TE12 which compared carboplatin versus etoposide cisplatin was set up to investigate this issue. It was terminated in November 1993 when there was a non-significant excess of relapses in the carboplatin arm. This was because the protocol review committee, worried by the results from a large trial in non-seminoma where there had been a significantly worse progression-free sur-

vival in the carboplatin combination arm compared with those receiving cisplatin combination[39], felt it inappropriate to allow the trial to proceed until more information was available. Although a further interim analysis has still not shown a significant difference in relapse rate[40] the trial data is currently in the process of maturing and will be analysed in a year's time when all patients will have been followed for 4 years. In the mean time given the phase 2 data presented in Table 39.3.7, further exploration of single agent studies in stage 2/3, i.e. N+, M0 seminoma is undoubtedly justified. As there is such poor survival of M+ seminoma cases, whether lung or other visceral sites (see Tables 39.3.5 and 39.3.6) it would be prudent to treat these cases like good risk non-seminoma to establish if there is any difference in responsiveness between pure seminoma, combined tumors and pure non-seminoma, by including them in the next European good risk trial comparing three versus four courses of BEP and 2 versus 5 days of cisplatin treatment.

Is there still a place for radiation in patients with small volume metastatic seminoma?

The very high cure rate of stage 2CD/3 seminoma discussed in the previous section even with single agent platinum drugs makes it very difficult to justify further studies of radiation as first line therapy in these patients. The most recent publication (Table 39.3.8) suggests that primary cure with radiation in such patients is 20% worse. As cure by chemotherapy of relapse patients after radiotherapy is more difficult than untreated cases (Table 39.3.6), and there is no evidence of any gain from adding radiation to sites of bulky diseases (Table 39.3.9) in a retrospective

Table 39.3.8 Ontario Cancer Institute Radiotherapy for Stage II Seminoma (Gospodarowicz et al. 1994)

	No. of cases	Nem > 2 year
Lymphangiogram positive stage IIa (<2 cm)	13	100%
CT scan stage II a + b (≤ 5 cm)	43	86%
CT scan stage II c + d (> 5 cm)	16	44%

Table 39.3.7 Single agent platinum studies for metastatic semonoma

		Progression free		Overall primary cure	Current NEM
		Stage 2 and 3	Stage 4		
Oliver et al. 1984	cisplatin q21	12/12	1/4	} 82%	88%
Oliver et al. 1990	carboplatin q21	15/18	nil		
Schmoll et al. 1993[38]	carboplatin q28	27/36	3/6	71%	95%
Horwich et al. 1992[37]	carboplatin q28	20/31	7/10	68%	94%

Table 39.3.9 Impact of radiation on metastatic seminoma response to chemotherapy[46]

	No. of cases	3 Year progression-free survival
No. radiation	155	85%
Radiation to bulk sites post chemotherapy	87	87%
Relapse after radiation	49	65%

review of more than 300 patients, there can be little justification for use of radiation today even in patients with small volume metastases. In the past, many of the reports on the use of radiotherapy in seminoma patients with small volume seminoma metastases less than 2 cm showed very little difference from the relapse rate of stage 1 seminoma. As the data in Table 39.3.8 suggests one factor in this might have been the use of lymphography which detected more false positives than CT.

The results of 2 versus 1 course adjuvant carboplatin

It is now clear that single agent cisplatin (and now more recently carboplatin when used in a dose of greater than AUC 6.5 corrected for surface area), while possibly not quite as good as combination BEP, produces such a high complete response rate that is at least as good as compared with those achieved using radiation (Table 39.3.8). Having first appreciated this 12 years ago, I decided that future adjuvant studies in stage I seminoma should use fewer courses of the more effective agent than continued modified usage of the less effective agent, i.e. radiotherapy.

These stage I seminoma adjuvant studies began using cisplatin, but after the first four patients we switched to carboplatin. Initially from 1984 to 1988 patients received two courses but subsequent patients have received one course[40]. With 119 patients treated and median follow up now greater than 4 years there have been two relapses both in cohort of 54 patients receiving two courses. With other centers now reporting similar results, it is clear that there is a need to extend these results. The recent launch of the MRC Te20 is an attempt to examine this by randomizing between radiation and a single course of carboplatin. Given the problem of late relapse of seminoma patients on surveillance and our experience of one patient presenting with paraplegia at 8 years on surveillance, it was felt that surveillance should not be an arm of this study. Prolonged follow up from 15–20 years will be necessary to assess late events.

Might it be possible to do without orchidectomy as primary diagnostic procedure?

The absence so far of second germ cell cancers in the contralateral testis in the patients treated with adjuvant carboplatin[40], taken with the ease of salvage of carboplatin failures with second line regimens,[41] provides courage to consider extending the use of chemotherapy to preserve the testis instead of the routine use of orchidectomy as at present, particularly in patients with a tumor in a solitary testis.

It is now increasingly accepted that cisplatin chemotherapy treated testicular germ cell cancer patients have a reduced risk of contralateral testis cancer compared with radiation or surgically treated patients[42]. In addition there is some new information[43] suggesting that etoposide containing combinations may be more efficient than bleomycin vinblastine cisplatin in crossing the presumptive 'blood testis barrier'. The encouraging preliminary results[44] from use of this combination as neo-adjuvant treatment before orchidectomy (Table 39.3.10) could eliminate the need for routine orchidectomy in the majority of patients who have chemotherapy for advanced metastases. With recognition that more than 70% of patients have suboptimal sperm production from their remaining so called 'normal' testis,[11] there is a need for greater awareness amongst urologists that it is safe to increase the proportion of patients with metastases diagnosed through needle biopsy of metastatic sites in order to try to conserve residual germinal epithelium. Extension of such testis conservation studies to patients without metastases is clearly justified for patients with tumors in solitary testis, given the observation that such patients can recover fertility[45]. Our recent experience suggests that for such patients with seminoma it might even be possible to use single agent carboplatin only.

Conclusions

Despite primary cure of more than 90% of all patients presenting with seminoma using a policy of primary radiotherapy for all cases, late events at 15–30 years have justified exploration of alternative approaches.Cytogenetics studies in seminoma (3.6n DNA contact) and non-seminoma (2.8N DNA contact) suggest that clonal evolution occurs from a near tetraploid carcinoma in situ stage. As data from studies of normal spermatogonia demonstrate that p53 is switched on in the tetraploid cell that precedes meoisis there is increasing interest in investigating how much the over-expression of non-mutated p53 demonstrable in most germ cell cancers contributes to their differentiated chemosensitivity. These observations have provided strong retrospective justification for continued study of the role of single agent platinum in treatment of

Table 39.3.10 Clinical/pathologic response of primary and metastases to systemic chemotherapy

	Chemotherapy regimen	No. of cases	Primary CR	Metastases CR
Greist et al. 1994	PVB	20	85%	90%
Chong et al. 1986	PVB	16	75%	81%
Oliver et al. 1995	BEP	15	87%	87%
	Other cisplatin	16	67%	75%
TOTAL		67	81%	84%

both lymph node, metastatic and stage I seminoma. However, limited evidence that patients with blood-borne seminoma metastases have a prognosis equivalent to that of non-seminoma, justifies treatment of such patients in non-seminoma trials to establish whether histology does provide prognostic information. With more than 250 patients in phase 2 studies of adjuvant carboplatin worldwide and only four relapses observed to date, the planned trial comparing this approach with radiotherapy is clearly justified and needs to be continued for 15–20 years to investigate late events. Preliminary observations on the effects of such treatment in primary tumors is providing the first evidence that questions the need for use of orchidectomy for diagnostic purposes, particularly in patients with tumors in a solitary testis.

References

1. Friedman M. Supervoltage roentgen therapy at Walter Reed General Hospital. *Surg Clin N Am* 1944;**24**(6):1424–1432.

2. Zagars G. Stage I testicular seminoma following orchidectomy – to treat or not to treat. *Eur J Cancer* 1993;**29A**:1923–1924.

3. Warde P, Gospodarowicz MK, Panzarella T *et al.* Stage I testicular seminoma: results of adjuvant irradiation and surveillance. *J Clin Oncol* 1995;**13**(9):2255–2262.

4. Horwich A, Bell J. Mortality and cancer incidence following radiotherapy for seminoma of the testis. *Radiother Oncol* 1994;**30**(3):193–198.

5. van Leeuwen FE, Stiggelbout AM, Vandenbeltdusebout AW *et al.* Second tumors after radiation treatment of testicular germ-cell tumors. *J Clin Oncol* 1993;**11**:2286–2287.

6. Hay JH, Duncan W, Kerr GR. Subsequent malignancies in patients irradiated for testicular tumors. *Br J Radiol* 1984;**57**:597–602.

7. Giwercman A, von der Maase H, Skakkebaek NE. Epidemiological and clinical aspects of carcinoma in situ of the testis. *Eur Urol* 1993;**23**:104–114.

8. Oliver RTD, Leahy M, Ong J. Combined seminoma/non-seminoma should be considered as intermediate grade germ cell cancer (GCC). *Eur J Cancer* 1995;**31A**:1392–1394.

9. Oliver RTD, Nouri AME, Crosby D *et al.* Biological significance of Beta hCG, HLA and other membrane antigen expression on bladder tumors and their relationship to tumor infiltrating lymphocytes (TIL). *J Immunogenetics* 1989;**16**:381–390.

10. Murty V, Bosi G, Houldsworth J *et al.* Allelic loss and somatic differentiation in human male germ cell tumors. *Oncogene* 1994;**9**:2245–2251.

11. Oliver RTD. Atrophy, hormones, genes and viruses in aetiology of germ cell tumors. *Cancer Surveys* 1990;**9**(2):263–268.

12. Forman D, Chilvers C, Oliver R, Pike M. The aetiology of testicular cancer: association with congenital abnormalities, age at puberty, infertility and exercise. *Br Med J* 1994;**308**:1393–1399.

13. Chilvers CED FD, Oliver RTD, Pike MC, Davey G, Coupland CAC, Baker K, Dawson S, *et al.* Social, behavioural and medical factors in the aetiology of testicular cancer – results from the UK study. *Br J Cancer* 1994;**70**(3):513–520.

14. Leahy M, Tonks S, Moses J *et al.* Candidate regions for a testicular cancer susceptibility gene. *Human Mol Gen* 1995;**4**:1551–1555.

15. Fisch H, Goluboff E, Feldshuh J *et al.* Semen analysis in 1283 men from the United States (US) over a 25 year period: no decline in quality. *J Urol* 1996;**155**:(abstract 528).

16. Fisch H, Hendricks J, Klein L, Goluboff E, Andrews H, Olson J. Sperm counts and birth rates: do variations correlate? *J Urol* 1996;**155**:(abstract 664).

17. Lane DP. p53, guardian of the genome. *Nature* 1992;**358**(6381):15–16.

18. Socher S, Yin Y, Dewolf W, Morgentaler A. Heat-induced testicular regression is associated with altered expression of the cell-cycle regulator p53. *J Urol* 1996;**155**:(abstract 531).

19. Fan S, El-Deiry W, Bae I *et al.* p53 Gene mutations are associated with decreased sensitivity of human lymphoma cells to DNA damaging agents. *Cancer Res* 1994;**54**:5824–5830.

20. Huddart RA, Titley J, Robertson D, Williams GT, Horwich A, Cooper CS. Programmed cell death in response to chemotherapeutic agents in human germ cell tumor lines. *Eur J Cancer* 1995;**31A**(5):739–746.

21. Schwartz D, Goldfinger N, Rotter V. Expression of p53 protein in spermatogenesis is confined to the tetraploid pachytene primary spermatocytes. *Oncogene* 1993;**8**(6):1487–1494.

22. Mead G, Stenning S. International germ cell cancer collaborative group prognostic factor scoring system. In: 1995:

23. Fossa S, Droz J, Stoter G *et al.* Cisplatin, vincristine and ifosphanide combination chemotherapy of metastatic seminoma: resuts of EORTC trial 30874. *B J Cancer* 1995;**71**:619–624.

24. Peckham MJ, Horwich A, Blackmore C. Etoposide and cisplatin with or without bleomycin as first line chemotherapy in patients with small volume metastasis of testicular nonseminoma. *Cancer Treatment Report* 1985;**69**:483–488.

25. Mencel PJ, Motzer RJ, Mazumdar M. Advanced seminoma: treatment results, survival and prognostic factors in 142 patients. *J Clin Oncol* 1994;**12**:120–126.

26. Horwich A, Peckham M. Etoposide and cisplatin for small volume non-seminoma. *Br J Cancer* 1985;**49**:135–137.

27. Oliver RTD, Dhaliwal HS, Hope-Stone HF, Blandy JP. Short course etoposide, bleomycin and cisplatin in the treatment of metastatic germ cell tumors. Appraisal of its potential as adjuvant chemotherapy for stage 1 testis tumors. *Br J Urol* 1988;**61**:53–58.

28. Chisholm RA, Dixon AK, Williams MV, Oliver RTD. Bleomycin lung: the effect of different chemotherapeutic regimens. *Cancer Chemother Pharmacol* 1992;**30**:158–160.

29. Williams SD, Birch R, Einhorn LH, Irwin L, Greco F, Loehrer PJ. Treatment of disseminated germ-cell tumors with Cisplatin, Bleomycin, and either Vinblastine or Etoposide. *New Engl J Med* 1987;**316**(23):1435–1440.

30. Dalgleish A, Woods R, Levi J. Bleomycin pulmonary toxicity: its relationship to renal dysfunction. *Medi Paediatric Oncol* 1984;**12**:313–317.

31. Oliver RTD, Love S, Ong J. Alternatives to radiotherapy in management of seminoma. *Br J Urol* 1990;**65**:61–67.

32. Higby D, Wallace H, Albert D, Holland JF. Diaminodichloroplatinum: a phase I study showing responses in testicular and other tumors. *Cancer* 1974;**33**:1219–1255.

33. Samuels M, Logothetis C, Trindade A. Sequential weekly pulse-dose cisplatinum for far-advanced seminoma. *ASCO* 1980;**21**:C-415 (abstract).

34. Logothetis CJ, Samuels ML, Ogden SL. Cyclophosphamide and sequential cisplatin for advanced seminoma: long term follow up 52 patients. *J Urol* 1987;**138**:789–794.

35. Oliver RTD, Hope-Stone HF, Blandy JP. Possible new approaches to the management of seminoma of the testis. *Br J Urol* 1984;**56**:729–733.

36. Oliver RTD. Limitations to the use of surveillance as an option in the management of stage I seminoma. *Int J Androl* 1987;**10**:263–268.

37. Horwich A, Dearnaley D, A'Hern R *et al.* The activity of single-agent carboplatin in advanced seminoma. *Eur J Cancer* 1992;**28A**(89):1307–1310.

38. Schmoll HJ, Harstrick A, Bokemeyer C *et al.* Single-agent carboplatinum for advanced seminoma – a phase-II study. *Cancer* 1993;**72**:237–243.

39. Horwich A, Sleijfer D. Carboplatin-based chemotherapy in good prognosis metastatic non seminoma of the testis (NSGCT): an interim report of an MRC/EORTC randomised trial. *Eur J Cancer Proc ECCO 7* 1993;**29A**:1350 (abstract).

40. Oliver R, Edmonds P, Ong J, Ostrowski M, Jackson A. Pilot studies of 2 and 1 course Carboplatin as adjuvant for Stage I seminoma: should it be tested in a randomized trial against radiotherapy? *Int J Radiation Oncol Biol, Phys* 1994;**29**(1):3–8.

41. Oliver R, Ong J, Gallagher C. Weekly M-BOP as a second line and VIP plus high dose as third line salvage for germ cell cancer. *Eur J Cancer* 1995;**31A**:916.

42. Osterlind A, Berthelsen JG, Abildgaard N. Risk of bilateral testicular germ cell cancer in Denmark; 1960–1984. *J Natl Cancer Inst* 1991;**83**:1391–1395.

43. Boshoff CH, Rustin G, Begent R *et al.* Treatment of good risk, stage II, non-seminomatous testis cancer. *Lancet* 1994;**344**:1085–1086.

44. Oliver R, Ong J, Blandy J, Altman D. Testis conservation studies in germ cell cancer justified by improved primary chemotherapy

response and reduced delay 1978–1994. *B J Urol* 1996;**78**:119–124.

45. Sobeh M, Jenkins B, Paris A, Oliver R. Partial orchidectomy for secondary testis tumors. *Euro J Surgical Onc* 1994;**20**(5):585–586.

46. Duchesne GM, Stenning SP, Aass N, Mead GM, Fossa SD, Olivr RT, Horwich A, Read G, Roberts IT, Rustin G, Cullen MH, Kaye SB, Harland SJ, Cook PA. Radiotherapy after chemotherapy for metastatic seminoma - a diminishing role. MRC Testicular Tumour Working Party. *Eur J Cancer.* 1997;**33**:829–35.

40 Non-germ cell testicular tumors

C E Bermejo and J W Basler

Incidence, etiology and epidemiology

Non-germ cell tumors of the testicle are uncommon accounting for approximately 5% of all primary testicular neoplasms. Leydig and Sertoli cell tumors are the primary non-germ cell tumors of the testis, constituting 1–3% of all testicular tumors[1,2]. Both can occur at any age but the majority have been recognized between the ages of 20 and 60 years[2]. Leydig and Sertoli cell tumors are rare before puberty accounting for about 5–7% and less than 1% respectively of testis tumors[2–5].

The etiology of Leydig and Sertoli cell tumors is unknown[2]. Occurrence in cryptorchid testis has been reported for both tumors. Michalec et al.[6] documents the appearance of Leydig cell tumor in a 71-year-old man with unilateral cryptorchidism. He also states that there have been very few cases reported as coming from undescended testis. Dounis et al. also documents the appearance of a Leydig cell tumor in a cryptorchid man.[7] There is no strong evidence that Sertoli cell and Leydig cell tumors are prone to develop in undescended testis.

Clinical presentation, diagnosis and staging

Clinical presentation

Leydig cell tumors commonly present as a palpable mass in the testicle (most common presenting feature) and less often with precocious puberty, infertility, gynecomastia, decreased libido and impotence[2,5,9–13]. True Sertoli cell mesenchymal tumors are rare in humans. While generally present as palpable testis mass[2], up to one-third of patients have been documented to have gynecomastia, feminization and precocious puberty[2,14–16]. Signs of

precocious puberty include: 1) a growth spurt with an advanced bone age; 2) increased skeletal musculature; 3) increased penile size; 4) increased pigmentation of the penis and scrotal skin; 5) premature pubarche; 6) asymmetry of testicular size; 7) presence of facial hair and acne, and 8) aggressive behavior[5]. Sertoli cell tumors have been associated with Peutz-Jeghers syndrome[17,18], pituitary adenomas[19], adrenocortical hyperplasia[19] and cardiac myxoma[20]. Sertoli cell tumors constitute one of the conditions of Carney's complex. This complex includes unusual testicular tumors, cardiac and cutaneous myxomas, myxoid mammary fibroadenomas, pigmented skin lesions, primary pigmented nodular adrenocortical disease and pituitary adenoma. It is important to recognize this complex, as cardiac myxomas can be lethal. Family members should be screened carefully because of familial occurrence[20]. Virilization may occur in pre-pubertal cases in both Leydig and Sertoli cell tumors[2]. Differential diagnosis for both of these tumors would be feminizing testicular disorders, feminizing adrenocortical disorders and Klinefelter's syndrome. The endocrinologic manifestations may precede the palpable testis mass[2].

Diagnosis

A good history and physical examination are very important in diagnosing Leydig and Sertoli cell tumors. Gynecomastia, feminization, and precocious puberty associated with a palpable testicular mass should orient the physician toward the diagnosis of non-germ cell tumors[3,7,9,21,22]. Scrotal ultrasound is helpful in determining the presence of a testicular tumor but may not be able to differentiate germ cell from non-germ cell tumors. If suspicion is high, MRI may help detect a small non-palpable Leydig or Sertoli cell tumor not seen by ultrasound. Alpha-fetoprotein (AFP) and beta-human chorionic gonadotropin (hCG) are not secreted by these tumors but may be helpful in working through the differential diagnosis[2].

Leydig cell tumors can be differentiated from congenital adrenal hyperplasia by non-suppressible elevations of plasma and urinary 17-ketosteroid[2]. Elevation of urinary and plasma estrogens has been reported with Leydig cell tumors but it remains uncertain whether Sertoli cell tumors produce estrogen[2]. In children, elevated serum testosterone levels, suppressed FSH and LH levels and the accumulation of testosterone metabolites in urine are diagnostic of Leydig cell tumors[5]. When a Leydig cell tumor is suspected but unconfirmed by either physical examination or ultrasound, a selective measurement of testosterone in serum samples obtained from the testicular veins may be helpful[5].

Staging

Due to their rarity, no standard staging system has been developed for Leydig cell and Sertoli cell tumors. The TNM system of staging testes tumors has most relevance to seminoma and non-seminomatous germ cell tumors but can be applied to these tumors as well. Staging of these tumors relies on a physical examination and, because of the approximately 10% malignant potential and inability reliably to distinguish them from the germ cell tumors, the pathologic evaluation after a radical orchiectomy.

Although Leydig cell and Sertoli cell tumors are usually benign, 10% of cases are malignant[2,5,12,22,23]. Detection of metastasis is the only reliable criterion of malignancy. Histologic features are unreliable. Since non-germ cell tumors have been reported to spread to the lung, liver, bone, retroperitoneal and supradiaphragmatic lymph nodes, a metastatic evaluation is usually indicated[2,5,22–26] Radiographic assessment (CT) of the chest, abdomen and pelvis are usually obtained and bone scanning may be clinically indicated in selected patients[2,5].

Pathology

Leydig cell tumors are usually small solid, well-circumscribed masses. They are yellow to brown and rarely will have foci of hemorrhage and necrosis. Microscopically the neoplastic Leydig cells are uniform, polyhedral, have eosinophilic granular cytoplasm with lipoid vacuoles. Brownish pigmentation and Reinke's crystals are characteristic but found only in one-third of cases[2,5].

Sertoli cell tumors usually are gray-white to creamy yellow. They generally are circumscribed and can have foci of hemorrhage. The cells are polygonal with finely vacuolated amphophilic cytoplasm. Call-Exner-like bodies are occasionally seen within the tubules. Charcott-Bottcher crystals are characteristic of Sertoli cell tumors but usually are only seen with electron microscopy[2,17,18]. Three types of Sertoli cell tumor have been described in the literature. These include general Sertoli cell, large cell calcifying Sertoli cell and sclerosing Sertoli cell tumor in order of occurrence[8,13,23,27–29]. Most Leydig and Sertoli cell tumors are immunoreactive with antiinhibin. Immunohistochemistry using this antibody can help in confirming the diagnosis for both tumors and in differentiating these neoplasms from others that may mimic them.[30]

Treatment

Radical orchiectomy is the procedure of choice for any solid testicular mass. This procedure is curative in 90% of cases of Leydig and Sertoli cell tumors[2]. The other 10% of these cases that present with metastasis to the retroperitoneal lymph nodes have been found to benefit from a retroperitoneal lymph node dissection (RPLND). There has not been a uniform treatment regimen with good results. Anecdotal reports suggest that a combination of RPLND, chemotherapy and radiation therapy offer the best results[2,4,15,21,24–26,28].

Cis-platinum, vinblastine, bleomycin, doxorubicin, cyclophosphamide and vincristine have been used in various combination regimens without convincing evidence of efficacy[2]. The data available for the use of chemotherapy and radiotherapy is discouraging[2,4,15,21,24–26,28]. Prognosis for malignant Sertoli and Leydig cell tumors is poor with average survival time after surgery approximately 3 years[2].

Tumor enucleation has been suggested for benign Sertoli and Leydig cell tumors, but data is sparse. Local recurrence after tumor enucleation has been reported[31]. This approach could be considered in bilateral synchronous or metachronous testicular tumors. Frozen section examination in these cases might enable an organ-sparing approach in benign testis tumors thereby benefiting the patient psychologically while maintaining endogenous testosterone and fertility. Conservative surgery might be considered under certain circumstances: 1) a well defined, organ confined tumor without infiltration of the rete testis; 2) no evidence of metastasis; 3) multiple negative biopsies of the tumor bed and peripheral parenchyma at time of resection; 4) and a reliable patient capable of adhering to a close follow up protocol[5,15,23,26,29,32–35].

Since these tumors may recur years after orchiectomy, extended follow up is required[15,21]. In some centers follow up serum hormone levels, abdominal ultrasound and physical examination are taken at 1–4 month intervals during the first 2–3 years post-operatively. Although hormone production is a potential marker for follow up in patients with apparently malignant tumors, clinical evidence of efficacy is again lacking[2,5,21,27,32].

References

1. Mostofi FK. Testicular tumors: Epidemiologic, etiologic and pathologic features. *Cancer* 1973;**32**:1186.

2. Richie JP. Neoplasms of the testis. In: *Campbell's urology* (7th edn) Walsh PC, Retik AB, Vaughan ED, Jr. and Wein AJ, (eds). W.B. Saunders Co., Philadelphia vol. 3, (eds) pp. 2411–2452, 1998.

3. Kaplan GW, Cromie WJ, Kelalis PP *et al.* Prepubertal yolk sac testicular tumors; report of the Testicular Tumor Registry: part 2. *J Urol* 1988;**140**:1109.

4. Rosvoll RV, Woodard JR. Malignant Sertoli cell tumor of the testis. *Cancer*, 1968;**22**:8.

5. Dittrich K, Gyorke Z, Sulyok E *et al.* Picture of the month. *Arch Pediatrics Adolescent Med* 1996;**150**(11):1215–1216.

6. Michalec J, Jardanowski R, Pykalo. Leydigioma – rare testicular tumor diagnosed in an adult male with undescended intraabdominal testis. *Wiadomosci Lekarskie* 1997;**50**(4–6):128–131.

7. Dounis A, Papacharalampous A. Clinically occult Leydig cell tumor in a cryptorchid man. Report of a case presenting with unilateral gynecomastia and impotence. *Eur Urol* 1997;**32**(3):368–370.

8. Zukerberg LR, Young RH, Scully RE. Sclerosing Sertoli cell tumor of the testis. *Am J Surg Path* 1991;**15**(9):829–834.

9. Catala Bauset M, Girbes Borras J, Carmena-Ramon R *et al.* Gynecomastia and Leydig cell tumor. *Anales de Medicina Interna* 1997;**14**(3):131–134.

10. Kondoh N, Koh E, Nakamura M *et al.* Bilateral Leydig cell tumors and male infertility: case report. *Urol Internat* 1991;**46**(1):104–106.

11. Tetu B, Ro JY, Ayala AG. Large cell calcifying Sertoli cell tumor of the testis. A clinicopathological, immunohistochemical, and ultrastructural study of two cases. *Am J Clin Path* 1991;**96**(6):717–722.

12. Fernandez Gomez JM, Fresno M, Martin Benito JL *et al.* Leydig tumor in the adult. *Actas Urologicas Espanolas* 1996;**20**(2):175–180.

13. Cuervo Pinna C, Rodriguez Rincon JP, Abengozar Garcia-Moreno A *et al.* Leydig cell tumor. *Archivos Espanoles de Urologia* 1998;**51**(5):480–482.

14. Blix GW, Levine LA, Goldberg R *et al.* Large cell calcifying Sertoli cell tumor of the testis. *Scand J Urol Nephrol* 1992;**26**(1):73–75.

15. Bruce J, Gough DC. Long term follow-up of children with testicular tumors: surgical issues. *Br J Urol* 1991;**67**(4):429–433.

16. Radhi JM, Garston RG. Large cell, calcifying, Sertoli cell tumor: a case report. *Can J Surg* 1994;**37**(6):500–502.

17. Young S, Gooneratne S, Straus FH II *et al.* Feminizing Sertoli cell tumors in boys with Peutz-Jeghers syndrome. *Am J Surg Path* 1995;**19**(1):50–58.

18. Niewenhuis JC, Wolf MC, Kass EJ. Bilateral asynchronous Sertoli cell tumor in a boy with the Peutz-Jeghers syndrome. *J Urol* 1994;**152**:1246.

19. Young RH, Scully. *Testicular tumors.* American Society of Clinical Pathologists Press, Chicago, 1990; 42.

20. Noszian IM, Balon R, Eitelberger FG *et al.* Bilateral testicular large-cell calcifying Sertoli cell tumor and recurrent cardiac myxoma in a patient with complex Carney's complex. *Ped Radiol* 1995;**25**(suppl 1):S236–7.

21. Kolon TF, Hochman HI. Malignant Sertoli cell tumor in a prebuscent boy. *J Urol* 1997;**158**(2):608–609.

22. Young RH, Koelliker DD, Scully RE. Sertoli cell tumors of the testis, not otherwise specified: a clinicopathologic analysis of 60 cases. *Am J Surg Path* 1998;**22**(6):709–721.

23. Sugimura J, Suzuki Y, Tamura G *et al.* Metachronous development of malignant Leydig cell tumor. *Hum Pathol* 1997;**28**(11):1318–1320.

24. Bertram KA, Bratloff B, Hodges GF *et al.* Treatment of malignant Leydig cell tumor. *Cancer* 1991;**68**(10):2324–2329.

25. Mene MP, Finkelstein LH, Manfrey SJ *et al.* Metastatic Sertoli cell carcinoma of the testis. *J Am Osteo Ass* 1996;**96**(10):612–614.

26. Unluer E, Ozcan D, Altin S. Malignant Leydig cell tumor of the testis: a case report and review of the literature. *Internat Urol Nephrol* 1990;**22**(5):455–460.

27. Anderson GA. Sclerosing Sertoli cell tumor of the testis: a distinct histological subtype. *J Urol* 1995;**154**(5):1756–1758.

28. Nogales FF, Andujar M, Zuluaga A *et al.* Malignant large cell calcifying Sertoli cell tumor of the testis. *J Urol* 1995;**153**(6):1935–1937.

29. White MD, Loughlin MW, Kallakury BVS *et al.* Bilateral large cell calcifying Sertoli cell tumor of the testis in a 7-year-old boy. *J Urol* 1997;**158**(4):1547–1548.

30. McCluggage WG, Shanks JH, Whitside C *et al.* Immunohistochemical study of testicular cord-stromal tumors, including staining with anti-inhibin antibody. *Am J Surg Pathol* 1998;**22**(5):615–619.

31. Wegner HEH, Herbst H, Andresen R *et al.* Leydig cell tumor recurrence after enucleation. *J Urol* 1996;**156**(4):1443–1444.

32. Heidenreich A, Bonfig R, Derschum W *et al.* A conservative approach to bilateral testicular germ cell tumors. *J Urol* 1995;**153**(1):10–13.

33. Heidenreich A, Moul JW, Srivastava S *et al.* Synchronous bilateral testicular tumor: nonseminomatous germ cell tumors and contralateral benign tumors. *Scand J Urol Nephrol* 1997;**31**(4):389–392.

34. Ornstein DK, Dierks SM, Colberg JW. Metachronous presentation of bilateral Leydig cell tumors. *J Urol* 1996;**155**(5):170.

35. Pobil Moreno JL, Martinez Rodriguez J, Maestro Duran JL *et al.* Approximation to conservative surgery of Leydig cell tumor. *Archivos Espanoles de Urologia* 1996;**49**(7):700–705.

PART FIVE
Spermatic cord and scrotal cancer

Chapter 41
Tumors of the spermatic cord

41.1 Epidemiology and etiology

41.2 Presentation, staging and diagnosis

41.3 Pathology of malignant tumors of the spermatic cord

41.4 Paratesticular sarcomas

41.5 Radiotherapy

41.6 Systemic chemotherapy

Chapter 42
Tumors of the Scrotum

42.1 Epidemiology and etiology

42.2 Presentation, diagnosis & staging of squamous cell carcinoma

42.3 Pathology of malignant tumors of the scrotum

42.4 Surgical management of scrotal carcinoma

42.5 Radiotherapy for scrotal carcinoma

42.6 Chemotherapy for scrotal carcinoma

41 Tumors of the spermatic cord

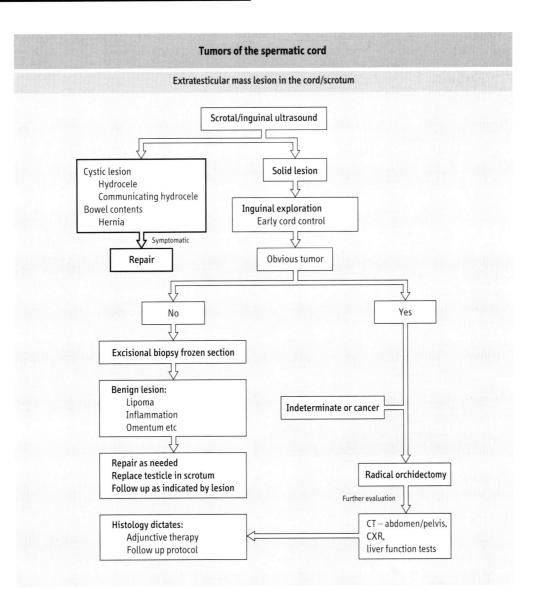

Tumors of the spermatic cord

Extratesticular mass lesion in the cord/scrotum

Scrotal/inguinal ultrasound

Cystic lesion
    Hydrocele
    Communicating hydrocele
Bowel contents
    Hernia

Solid lesion

Inguinal exploration
Early cord control

Symptomatic

Repair

Obvious tumor

No

Yes

Excisional biopsy frozen section

Benign lesion:
    Lipoma
    Inflammation
    Omentum etc

Indeterminate or cancer

Repair as needed
Replace testicle in scrotum
Follow up as indicated by lesion

Radical orchidectomy

Further evaluation

Histology dictates:
    Adjunctive therapy
    Follow up protocol

CT – abdomen/pelvis,
CXR,
liver function tests

41.1 Epidemiology and etiology

J Petros and P D LaFontaine

Malignant tumors of the spermatic chord are rare and account for less than 0.1% of all male genital cancers[1]. From 1973 to 1987 only 93 spermatic cord sarcomas were reported in the SEER tumor registry. The majority of these tumors are soft tissue sarcomas arising from mesenchymal elements and include, in order of frequency, liposarcoma, fibrosarcoma, leiomyosarcoma and rhabdomyosarcoma[1]. Other rare spermatic cord and paratesticular tumors include malignant fibrous histiocytoma, primary osteosarcoma and non-Hodgkins lymphoma. It should be noted that the majority of spermatic cord and paratesticular masses in adults are benign lesions[2]. There is a bimodal age distribution of these tumors, with peaks from 16 to 19 and over age 50[2]. Almost all of the patients under 30 had rhabdomyosarcoma, and rhabdomyosarcoma occurred only rarely over age 40. The etiology of paratesticular sarcomas is unclear, though a number of conditions, such as previous radiation therapy, exposure to Thorotrast radiologic contrast medium, neurofibromatosis and Gardner's syndrome have been associated with the development of soft tissue sarcomas elsewhere in the body[3].

References

1. Gilliland FD, Key CR. Male genital cancers. *Cancer* 1995;**75**:295–315.
2. In: Vogelzang NJ, Scardino PT, Shipley WU, Coffey DS, eds. *Comprehensive textbook of genitourinary oncology*. Williams & Wilkins, Baltimore, MD: 1996, pp. 1131–1133
3. Shiu MH, Brennan MF. *Surgical management of soft tissue sarcoma*. Lea & Febiger, Philadelphia, 1989.

41.2 Presentation, staging and diagnosis

J Petros and P D LaFontaine

Presentation

Paratesticular sarcoma is a rare tumor with only 93 cases reported to the SEER database over a 15 year period[1]. Given the rarity of this tumor and the difficulty in distinguishing it clinically from the more common benign lesions of the cord, the correct pre-operative diagnosis is rarely made. In a series of 22 patients from MSKCC the correct pre-operative diagnosis was not made in a single tumor[2]. These tumors usually present as a slow growing painless mass in the scrotum or groin which may rarely be accompanied by a hydrocele. The average size in one series was 7.8 cm[3], and there is no left or right predilection. Eighty per cent of paratesticular sarcomas present as an intrascrotal mass while 20% present as an inguinal mass[3]. The age at diagnosis and the percentage with metastatic disease at initial presentation depends on the histology of the sarcoma. Rhabdomyosarcoma is most common in the third decade while the other paratesticular sarcomas are more common in the sixth and seventh decades[4]. In one series all patients with rhabdomyosarcoma had metastatic disease at initial presentation[3].

Diagnosis

Correct diagnosis of these uncommon tumors depends on an appropriate clinical suspicion. In addition to paratesticular sarcomas, other benign entities to consider in the differential diagnosis include incarcerated hernia, hydrocele, spermatocele, lipoma, TB or syphilis. Though benign lesions of the chord and scrotum are more common, 20–30% of solid inguinal and scrotal lesions will be malignant[5]. In patients with an enlarging scrotal or inguinal mass an ultrasound is often the first diagnostic test. This will help differentiate solid from cystic lesions and determine the need for further evaluation. For solid lesions of the chord or scrotum we recommend surgical exploration through an inguinal incision. If diagnosis of malignancy is straightforward radical inguinal orchiectomy with high ligation of the chord and en bloc resection is indicated. If the diagnosis is in doubt, incisional biopsy with frozen section analysis and radical orchiectomy if indicated is appropriate. Excisional biopsy will also provide tissue for pathologic examination but risks tumor spillage and inadequate local control. Transscrotal exploration or biopsy of scrotal masses is to be avoided.

Staging

There is no uniformly accepted staging system for paratesticular sarcomas. Some investigators feel that genitourinary sarcomas share prognostic characteristics with sarcomas arising from other sites[3]. At MSKCC Russo *et al.* applied their staging system for soft tissue sarcomas to genitourinary sarcomas[3]. They staged genitourinary sarcomas, including paratesticular, bladder, prostate and renal sarcomas, according to tumor grade, size, depth of invasion and evidence of metastatic disease (Table 41.2.1). They found that patients with tumors less than 5 cm, those with low-grade sarcomas, those who were able to have a complete resection of tumor with negative margins and

Table 41.2.1 MSKCC staging system for soft-tissue sarcoma

Stage	Grade	Size (cm)	Depth
0	Low	<5	Superficial
1	Low	<5	Deep
2	Low	>5	Deep
	High	<5	Deep
3	High	>5	Deep
4	Evidence of metastatic disease		

Adapted from Hajdu SI: *Pathology of soft tissue tumors.* Philadelphia. Lea & Febiger, 1979.

those patients with bladder and paratesticular sarcomas had an improved survival.

Paratesticular sarcomas may arise from the spermatic chord, the epididymis, the tunics of the testicle or the testicular appendages. Metastatic spread may be via hematogenous routes, local extension or via the lymphatics. The lymphatic drainage of these structures is similar to that of the testicle. Appropriate evaluation of the retroperitoneal lymph nodes depends upon tumor histology. Liposarcoma has a very low incidence of spread to the retroperitoneal lymph nodes and thus wide local excision is all that is needed. Rhabdomyosarcoma, leiomyosarcoma and fibrosarcoma should be staged with a CT of the abdomen and pelvis to assess for retroperitoneal adenopathy. The need for retroperitoneal lymph node dissection depends on the findings on CT and the tumor histology. Additional studies should include chest X-ray, CBC and SMA-19.

References

1. Gilliland FD, Key CR. Male genital cancers. *Cancer* 1995;75:295–315.
2. Shiu MH, Brennan MF. Surgical management of soft tissue sarcoma. Lea & Febiger, Philadelphia, 1989.
3. Russo P, Brady MS, Conlon K *et al.* Adult urological sarcoma. *J Urol* 1992;147:1032–1037.
4. Takahashi S, Tsukamoto T, Lieber MM. Genitourinary sarcomas in adults. In: Vogelzang NJ, Scardino PT, Shipley WU, Coffey DS (eds) *Comprehensive textbook of genitourinary oncology.* Williams & Wilkins, Baltimore, Md, 1996; pp. 1131–1133.
5. Lioe TF, Biggart JD. Tumors of the spermatic cord and paratesticular tissue. A clinicopathological study. *Br J Urol* 1993;**71**:600–606.

41.3 Pathology of malignant tumors of the spermatic cord

P A Humphrey

Malignant neoplasms of the paratesticular region, in contrast to the scrotum, are usually sarcomas (Table 41.3)[1–4]. Of the paratesticular sarcomas, rhabdomyosarcoma is the most common type, with over 200 reported cases[1–2,4–7]. In order,

the next most common types are leiomyosarcoma, liposarcoma and malignant fibrous histiocytoma[1–11]. Rare types of paratesticular sarcoma include fibrosarcoma, angiosarcoma, neurofibrosarcoma, chondrosarcoma, malignant ectomesenchyma, malignant mesenchymoma and osteosarcoma[1–4,12]. Malignant mesothelial (mesothelioma)[13] and epithelial malignancies (carcinomas) are uncommon while other types of paratesticular malignancies such as ovarian type epithelial tumors, melanotic neuroectodenual tumor of infancy, malignant lymphoma, plasmacytoma, neuroblastoma, Wilm's tumor, germ cell tumors, desmoplastic small round cell tumor, and malignant rhabdoid tumor are rare[1–4,14,14a]. Also rare are neoplasms that are not uniformly malignant, but which harbor malignant potential, such as ovarian-type epithelial tumors, melanotic neuroectodermal tumor of infancy, hemangiopericytoma and pheochromocyoma (paraganglioma). Metastatic spread to the paratesticular region is rare and such deposits usually emanate from the prostate, kidney and stomach[3].

Paratesticular rhabdomyosarcoma is a childhood/adolescent mesenchymal neoplasm with skeletal muscle differentiation. Macroscopically, the tumors are solitary and tend to be located adjacent to the upper pole of the testis, with involvement of spermatic cord, epididymis and testicular tunics. The gross presentation is of an unencapsulated white to gray or brown mass with focal hemorrhage or cystic change. Size ranges from 1.5 to 20 cm, with a median of 5 cm[15]. Microscopically, there are three distinct subtypes: embryonal, alveolar and pleomorphic. Embryonal rhabdomyosarcoma constitutes the vast majority of cases[1,15] and is heterogeneous in cellular density and appearance of individual tumor cells. Cytologically, the tumor cells vary from small and round to spindled (Figure 41.3.1), to larger cells with abundant acidophilic cytoplasm. In well differentiated tumors, evidence of skeletal muscle features may be discerned in the form of 'strap' cells and cross-striations. For poorly differentiated tumors, special techniques such as immunohistochemical stains (for desmin and muscle-specific actin) and electron microscopy (to demonstrate myofilaments) may be necessary to establish the diagnosis. Diagnostic distinction of the three subtypes of rhabdomyosarcoma is usually on the basis of light microscopic examination. A genetic abnormality that is specific for one of the subtypes – alveolar rhabdomyosarcoma – is a 2;13 translocation which results in fusion of the PAX3 gene on chromosome 2 with the ALV gene on chromosome 13[16,17]. This fusion product, which can be of diagnostic aid in selected cases, may be detected by fluorescence in situ hybridization or reverse transcription polymerase chain reaction[18]. The histologic differential diagnosis of rhabdomyosarcoma includes other pediatric small blue round cell tumors, including lymphoma, Ewing's sarcoma/PNET, Wilm's tumor, and neuroblastoma[19]. The latter three tumors are rare in the

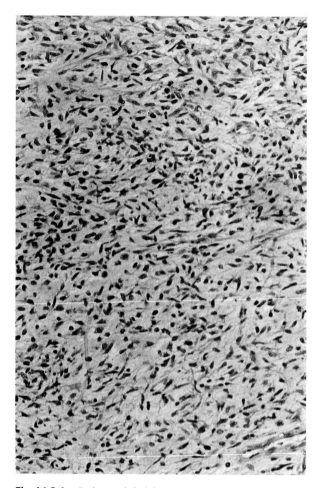

Fig. 41.3.1 Embryonal rhabdomyosarcoma of the paratesticular region,

paratesticular region. Diagnostic separation of these entities is typically accomplished by use of standard H&E sections and a panel of immunohistochemical markers.[4,19]

The essential pathologic prognostic indicators for paratesticular rhabdomyosarcoma are histologic type and stage. The spindle cell variant of embryonal rhabdomyosarcoma (Figure 41.3.1) has the best prognosis while alveolar and pleomorphic rhabdomyosarcoma are more aggressive[20–22]. Staging according to the Intergroup Rhabdomyosarcoma Study guidelines[15,23]. is based on clinical and pathologic assessment of extent of local disease, resection status, presence of gross residual tumor after resection, and metastases. Paratesticular rhabdomyosarcoma has a significant (28–40%) incidence of retroperitoneal or paraaortic lymph node involvement[22,24]. DNA content (ploidy) in tumor cell nuclei does not appear to be a useful prognosticator[25]. Nuclear morphometric analysis has potential in predictive prognostic capacity[26], but currently this is a labor-intensive, experimental tool.

Leiomyosarcoma of the paratesticular area, in contrast to rhabdomyosarcoma, is a tumor mainly of adults. It represents the most common paratesticular sarcoma in adults and overall is the second most common sarcoma of this region (Table 41.3.1). This malignant mesenchymal neoplasm displays smooth muscle differentiation. Grossly, the site of origin is usually spermatic cord and, less often, the epididymis[1,3]. The tumors are often solid, gray-tan masses, with focal necrosis, and an average size of about 6 cm[1,4]. Microscopically, spindled tumor cells are arranged in fascicles (Figure 41.3.2) or a storiform (pinwheel) pattern. Better differentiated neoplasms may be cytologically bland with few mitoses. The differential diagnosis here is with a leiomyoma. Nuclear pleomorphism, necrosis and more than 1 to 2 mitotic figures per ten high-power fields favor a leiomyosarcoma. High-grade leiomyosarcomas may be difficult to distinguish from other high-grade sarcomas and diagnostic work-up may require immunohistochemistry to prove smooth muscle differentiation. Due to the low number of reported cases of paratesticular leiomyosarcoma, it has not been possible to assess for relationships between morphologic features and prognosis.

Liposarcoma of the paratesticular region is overall the third most common sarcoma and should be distinguished from lipoma, which is the most common neoplasm of this region. Grossly, the tumors may be mistaken for lipoma due to the lobulated, yellow appearance of the mass. There are four histologic subtypes of liposarcoma – well-differentiated, myxoid, round cell and pleomorphic – and the low-grade well-differentiated and myxoid subtypes predominate in the paratesticular region. Microscopically, the well-differentiated liposarcomas may simulate the mature adipose tissue of

Table 41.3.1 Histologic types of malignant paratesticular tumors

Histologic type	Number of reported cases[3,4]
Sarcoma	
Rhabdomyosarcoma	200
Leiomyosarcoma	100
Liposarcoma	50
Malignant fibrous histiocytoma	17
Fibrosarcoma	rare
Angiosarcoma	rare
Neurofibrosarcoma	rare
Chondrosarcoma	rare
Osteosarcoma	rare
Malignant ectomesenchymoma	rare
Malignant mesenchymoma	rare
Malignant mesothelioma	60
Epididymal carcinoma	30
Papillary serous carcinoma	6
Malignant lymphoma	rare
Metastatic tumor	rare

Numbers represent minimum estimates.

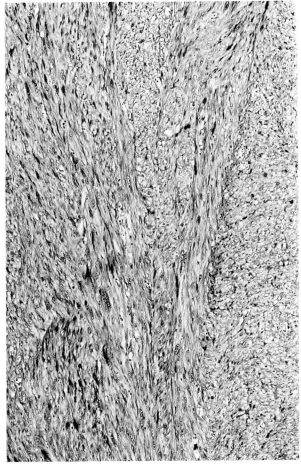

Fig. 41.3.2 Paratesticular spermatic cord leiomyosarcoma, with a fascicular growth of spindled cells.

a lipoma and a thorough search to find lipoblasts (indicative of liposarcoma) may be necessary. The myxoid liposarcoma has a distinctive network of vessels and also a characteristic translocation [t (12;16)(q13;p11)] which may be of diagnostic aid in selected, difficult cases[27,28]. Morphologic prognostic indicators for paratesticular liposarcoma are histologic subtype and stage. The prognosis for patients with well-differentiated and myxoid liposarcoma is good after treatment while pleomorphic, high-grade liposarcomas tend to recur locally and may metastasize[9,29].

Malignant mesotheliomas in the paratesticular region are rare tumors and like the more common peritoneal and pleural mesotheliomas, there is a linkage to asbestos exposure[13,30]. Most arise from the tunica vaginalis and typically present grossly as multiple nodules studding a hydrocele sac[1,13,30]. There may be macroscopic invasion of the tunica albuginea, testis, epididymis and spermatic cord. Microscopically, there is a variable epithelial, spin-

dle cell or biphasic appearance. The epithelial pattern usually has a tubular and/or tubulopapillary architecture and needs to be distinguished from carcinomas, especially those of the rete testis or epididymis. Immunophenotypic analysis may be necessary to confirm the diagnosis of mesothelioma[30]. The differential diagnosis also includes adenomatoid tumor, a benign non-papillary mesothelioma, which is the most common tumor of the epididymis, and second only to lipoma as the most common paratesticular tumor[1]. Paratesticular malignant mesotheliomas have an aggressive natural history, with common local and distant spread[13]. Local spread is into skin of scrotum/penis, epididymis, testis and spermatic cord while metastatic dissemination is to inguinal and retroperitoneal lymph nodes, abdominal peritoneum and lungs.

References

1. Srigley JR, Hartwick RWJ. Tumors and cysts of the paratesticular region. *Pathol Ann* 1990;**25**:51–108.
2. Petersen RO. Testicular adenexa. In: *Urologic pathology* (2nd edn). JB Lippincott Co., Philadelphia, 1992, pp. 526–574.
3. Bostwick DG. Spermatic cord and testicular adenexa. In: Bostwick DG, Eble JN (eds) *Urologic surgical pathology*. Mosby, St Louis, 1997, pp. 663–666.
4. Gaudin PB, Epstein JI. Diseases of the spermatic cord and paratesticular tissue. In: Murphy WM (ed). *Urological pathology* (2nd edn). WB Saunders Co., Philadelphia, 1997, pp. 242–276.
4A. Folpe AL, Weiss SW. Paratesticular soft tissue neoplasms. *Semin Diagn Pathol* 2000;**17**: 307–318.
5. Petersen RO. Scrotum. In: *Urologic pathology* (2nd edn). JB Lippincott Co., Philadelphia, 1992, pp. 710–725.
6. Enzinger FM, Weiss SW. Rhabdomyosarcoma. In: *Soft tissue tumors*. CV Mosby, St Louis: 1995, p. 542.
7. Berkmen F, Celebioglu FS. Adult genitourinary sarcomas – a report of seventeen cases and review of the literature. *J Exp Clin Cancer Res* 1997;**16**:45–58.
8. Stein A, Kaplan A, Sova Y et al. Leiomyosarcoma of the spermatic cord: report of two cases and review of the literature. *World J Urol* 1996;**14**:59–61.
9. Henricks WH, Chu YC, Goldblum JR, Weiss SW. Dedifferentiated liposarcoma – a clinicopathological analysis of 155 cases with a proposal for an expanded definition of dedifferentiation. *Am J Surg Pathol* 1997;**21**:271–281.
10. Ikinger U, Westrich M, Dietz B, Mechtersheimer G, Schmidt C. Combined myxoid liposarcoma and angiolipoma of the spermatic cord. *Urology* 1997;**44**:635–637.
11. Eltorky MA, O'Brien TF, Walzer Y. Primary paratesticular malignant fibrous histiocytoma: Case report and review of the literature. *J Urol Pathol* 1993;**1**:425–430.
12. Beiswanger JC, Woodruff JD, Savage PD, Assimos DG. Primary osteosarcoma of the spermatic cord with synchronous bilateral renal cell carcinoma. *Urology* 1997;**49**:957–959.
13. Jones MA, Young RH, Scully RE. Malignant mesothelioma of the tunica vaginalis. A clinicopathologic analysis of 11 cases with review of the literature. *Am J Surg Pathol* 1995;**19**:815–825.
14. Ferry JA, Young RH. Malignant lymphoma of the genitourinary tract. *Curr Diagn Pathol* 1997;**4**:145–169.
14A. Herley JD, Ferry J, Ulbright TM. Miscellaneous rare paratesticular tumors. *Semin Diagn Pathol* 2000;**17**: 319–339.
15. Raney RB, Tefft M, Lawrence W Jr et al. Paratesticular sarcoma in childhood and adolescence. A report from the Intergroup Rhabdomyosarcoma Studies I and II, 1973–1983. *Cancer* 1987;**60**:2337–2343.

16. Trent J, Casper J, Meltzer P et al. Nonrandom chromosome alterations in rhabdomyosarcoma. *Cancer Genet Cytogenet* 1985;**16**:189–197.

17. Parham DM, Shapiro DN, Downing JR et al. Solid alveolar rhabdomyosarcoma with the t(2;13). Report of two cases with diagnostic implications. *Am J Surg Pathol* 1994;**18**:474–478.

18. Edwards RH, Chatten J, Xiong QG, Barr FG. Detection of gene fusions in rhabdomyosarcoma by reverse-transcriptase-polymerase chain reaction assay of archival samples. *Diagn Mol Pathol* 1998;**6**:91–97.

19. O'Shea PA. Myogenic tumors of soft tissue. In Coffin CM, Dehner LP, O'Shea PA (eds) *Pediatric soft tissue tumors.* Williams and Wilkins, Baltimore, 1997, pp. 222–238.

20. Cavazzana AO, Schmidt D, Ninfo V et al. Spindle cell rhabdomyosarcoma. A prognostically favorable variant of rhabdomyosarcoma. *Am J Surg Pathol* 1992;**16**:229–235.

21. Kodet R, Newton WA Jr, Hamoudi AB et al. Childhood rhabdomyosarcoma with anaplastic (pleomorphic) features. A report of the Intergroup Rhabdomyosarcoma Study. *Am J Surg Pathol* 1993;**17**:443–453.

22. Leuschner I, Newton WA, Schmidt D et al. Spindle cell variants of embryonal rhabdomyosarcoma in the paratesticular region. A report of the Intergroup Rhabdomyosarcoma Study. *Am J Surg Pathol* 1993;**17**:221–230.

23. Crist WM, Garnsey L, Beltangady M et al. Prognosis in children with rhabdomyosarcoma. A report of the Intergroup Rhabdomyosarcoma Studies I and II. *J Clin Oncol* 1990;**8**:443–452.

24. Raney RB Jr, Hays DM, Lawrence W Jr et al. Paratesticular rhabdomyosarcoma in childhood. Cancer 1978;42:729–736.

25. Kilpatrick SE, Teot LA, Geisinger KR et al. Relationship of DNA ploidy to histology and prognosis in rhabdomyosarcoma. Comparison of flow cytometry and image analysis. Cancer 1994;**76**:3227–3233.

26. Leonard MP, Partin AW, Epstein JI, Jeffs RD, Gearhart JP. Nuclear morphometry as a prognostic indicator for genitourinary rhabdomyosarcoma: a preliminary investigation. *J Urol* 1990;**144**:1222–1226.

27. Fletcher CD, Akerman M, Dal Cin P et al. Correlation between clinicopathological features and karyotype in lipomatous tumors. A report of 178 cases from the Chromosomes and Morphology (CHAMP) Collaborative Study Group. *Am J Pathol* 1996;**148**:623–630.

28. Aman P, Ron D, Mandahl N et al. Rearrangement of the transcription factor gene CHOP in myxoid liposarcoma with t(12;16)(q13;p11). *Genes Chromosomes Cancer* 1992;**5**:278–285.

29. Vorstman B, Block NL, Politano VA. The management of spermatic cord liposarcoma. *J Urol* 1984;**131**:66–69.

30. Perez-Ordonez B, Sprigley JR. Mesothelial lesions of the Paratesticular region. *Semin Diagn Pathol* 2000; **17**:294–306.

31. Enzinger FM, Weiss SW. Mesothelioma. In: *Soft tissue tumors.* Mosby, St Louis, 1995, pp. 787–819.

41.4 Paratesticular sarcomas

J Petros and P D LaFontaine

Recommendations on the correct surgical therapy for paratesticular sarcomas are complicated by the rarity of these tumors and the lack of a uniform staging system, making comparison of different treatment modalities difficult. The one universally agreed upon recommendation for treatment of these rare tumors is radical orchiectomy with wide local excision if needed. We recommend an inguinal incision with delivery of the tumor and testis into the wound by division of the gubernaculum. If the pre-operative diagnosis is not in doubt, we recommend radical orchiectomy with high ligation of the spermatic cord and wide local excision for grossly positive margins. A tag should be left on the spermatic cord stump for easy identification should RPLND be indicated later. If the pre-operative diagnosis is in doubt we recommend incisional biopsy with orchiectomy if indicated. Excisional biopsy will provide tissue for diagnosis but has an increased risk of tumor spillage and inadequate local control. If it is necessary to leave a drain post biopsy it should exit through the initial incision to lessen the chance of tumor seeding a separate tract. If wide local excision is needed for adequate local control, surgical defects can be covered with standard rotation flaps, myocutaneous pedicle grafts or prosthetic materials[1].

Paratesticular tumors have the capacity to metastasize through lymphatic or vascular channels as well as by direct local extension. These paratesticular sarcomas share lymphatic drainage with the testicle and have the capacity to spread to the retroperitoneal lymph nodes. The question of whether or not to perform a retroperitoneal lymph node dissection has been debated and depends on several factors, including tumor histology, stage and grade. Though some authors have recommended routine RPLND for paratesticular sarcomas, it does not appear that this is warranted for most histologic subtypes[2]. Currently RPLND is recommended for patients with rhabdomyosarcoma with no evidence of hematogenous spread or for patients with rhabdomyosarcoma who have responded to combined chemotherapy and radiation therapy[3,4]. There is also some evidence that patients with intermediate or high-grade malignant fibrous histiocytoma or liposarcoma may benefit from RPLND[4,5] though the value of RPLND in the management of both of these sarcomas has been questioned[6–8]. There does not appear to be any benefit to RPLND in the management of leiomyosarcoma.

References

1. Stone CA, Payne SR. Perineally-based scrotal skin flap to cover the inguino-scrotal defect resulting from radical removal of scrotal mesothelioma. *Br J Urol* 1993;**71**:621–622.

2. Banowsky LH, Shultz GN. Sarcoma of the spermatic cord and tunics: review of the literature, case report and discussion of the role of retroperitoneal lymph node dissection. *J Urol* 1970;**103**:628–631.

3. Russo P, Brady MS, Conlon K et al. Adult urological sarcoma. *J Urol* 1992;**147**:1032–1037.

4. Catton CN, Cummings BJ, Fornasier V, O'Sullivan B, Quirt I, Warr D. Adult paratesticular sarcomas: a review of 21 cases. *J Urol* 1991;**146**:342–345.

5. Sclama AO, Berger BW, Cherry JM, Young JD, Jr. Malignant fibrous histiocytoma of the spermatic cord: the role of retroperitoneal lymphadenectomy in management. *J Urol* 1983;**130**:577–579.

6. Schwartz SL, Swierzewski SJ III, Sondak VK, Grossman HB. Liposarcoma of the spermatic cord: report of 6 cases and review of the literature. *J Urol* 1995;**153**:154–157.

7. Glazier DB, Vates TS, Cummings KB, Pickens RL. Malignant fibrous histiocytoma of the spermatic cord. *J Urol* 1996;**155**:955–957.

8. Donohue JP. Editorial Comment. *J Urol* 1991;**146**:345.

41.5   Radiotherapy

J Michalski

Soft tissue sarcoma

Radiation therapy is an important adjunctive treatment in the management of soft tissue sarcomas. Following wide local excision, local recurrence rates range from 30% to 60%[1]. With conservative surgery aimed at achieving pathologically negative margins while maintaining reasonable function, postoperative radiation therapy has reduced local failure rates to less than 10%[2–5]. Occasionally patients with small tumors measuring less than 5 cm of low grade may have adequate local control with wide local excision alone[6,7]. Soft tissue sarcomas of the scrotum and spermatic cord behave similarly to those presenting in other sites. Following surgery the risk of local recurrence has been reported to be 33% to 50%[8–11]. The benefits of post-operative radiation therapy in spermatic cord sarcoma has been reported by a retrospective series from the Massachusetts General Hospital. Fagundes *et al.* described 18 patients with soft tissue sarcomas of the spermatic cord who had undergone radical orchiectomy or wide local excision. Five of the nine patients treated with surgery alone developed a local failure, compared with 100% local control in patients receiving adjuvant radiation. This improvement in local control was accompanied by a significant increase in disease-free survival of 100% in irradiated patients compared with only 56% in non-irradiated patients ($P < 0.01$)[12]. Similarly, Catton *et al.* describes a lower risk of local relapse in patients receiving adjuvant irradiation[9].

Adjuvant radiation therapy can be administered in either a pre-operative or post-operative setting with similar rates of local control. Post-operative radiation therapy is generally associated with a lower risk of wound complications following surgery. Post-operative radiation therapy should be given after maximally-debulking surgery. The goal of surgery should be to achieve pathologically negative margins. The radiation therapy treatment volume should encompass the region of the primary tumor with at least a 5 cm margin when possible. In patients who have undergone hemiscrotectomy, extension of the radiation therapy field to the remaining scrotum may be warranted if the tumor was adherent or invading through the fascial coverings of the spermatic cord. Transposition of the contralateral testicle to the pelvis or contralateral thigh should be considered to minimize the risks of infertility or hypogonadism. Proximally the radiation therapy field should cover the entire surgical bed to the internal inguinal ring. A more proximal extension may be necessary if surgical margins

are close to the inguinal ring or if tumor extended retroperitoneally toward the pelvis. Radio-opaque clips placed in the tumor bed at the time of resection may facilitate the radiation therapy treatment planning and field shaping. Tumors that extend proximally to the inguinal ring may need the radiation therapy treatment volume to cover the ipsilateral pelvic region. Elective nodal irradiation of the pelvic or periaortic lymph nodes is generally not required because of the low risk of lymph node metastases in patients with non-rhabdomyosarcoma soft tissue sarcomas. Fractionated external beam irradiation with doses of 50 of 55 Gy generally will control microscopic or subclinical disease. Patients with microscopically positive margins may require slightly higher doses.

Pediatric rhabdomyosarcoma deserves a special consideration. Its natural history and response to treatment is distinctly different from non-rhabdomyosarcoma soft tissue sarcomas. These tumors, despite an increased tendency to metastasize, have a relatively good prognosis because of their high response rate to both chemotherapy and radiation therapy. These tumors have a high risk of micrometastases to the retroperitoneal lymph nodes. If children less than 10 years of age have normal-appearing lymph nodes on fine cut, double contrast CT scans, the risk of relapse in the retroperitoneum after vincristine and actinomycin D chemotherapy is uncommon. Older children require diagnostic retroperitoneal lymph node dissection. Adjuvant radiation therapy remains an important component of the local management of patients with group II (microscopic residual disease or metastatic lymph nodes) or group III (gross residual disease) rhabdomyosarcoma. Children with paratesticular rhabdomyosarcoma who have local tumor spill or wound contamination at the time of radical orchiectomy should be treated as if they have microscopic disease (group II). The radiation therapy volume should be the area of spillage or wound contamination with at least 2 cm margin. Again, if scrotal irradiation is required, temporary transposition of the contralateral testicle to the thigh needs to be carried out to maintain gonadal function.

The radiation dose to control microscopic disease after maximal surgery in paratesticular rhabdomyosarcoma may be as low as 30 Gy[13]. The intergroup rhabdomyosarcoma study is currently testing the adequacy of 36 Gy in a prospective clinical trial. Patients with gross disease require radiation therapy doses of 45 to 50 Gy. Daily fraction sizes of 1.8 Gy are commonly used.

References

1.   McGinn CJ, Lawrence TS. Soft tissue sarcomas. In *Principles and Practice of Radiation Oncology* (3rd edn) 1997;**74**:2051.

2. Huth JF, Eilber FR. Patterns of metastatic spread following resection of extremity soft tissue sarcomas and strategies for treatment. *Sem Surg Oncol* 1988;**4**:20.

3. Potter DA, Glenn J, Kinsella TJ *et al.* Patterns of recurrence in patients with high grade soft tissue sarcomas. *J Clin Oncol* 1985;**4**:353.

4. Suit HD, Mankin HJ, Wood WC *et al.* Treatment of the patient with stage M$_0$ soft tissue sarcoma. *J Clin Oncol* 1988;**6**:854.

5. Williard WC, Hajdu SI, Casper ES *et al.* Comparison of amputation with limb-sparing operations for adults with soft tissue sarcomas of the extremity. *Ann Surg* 1992;**215**:269.

6. Marcus SG, Merino MJ, Glatstein E *et al.* Long term outcome in 87 patients with low grade soft tissue sarcoma. *Arch Surg* 1993;**128**:1336.

7. Pisters WT, Harrison LB, Woodruff JM *et al.* A prospective randomized trial of adjuvant brachytherapy in the management of low grade soft tissue sarcomas of the extremity and superficial trunk. *J Clin Oncol* 1994;**12**:1150.

8. Schwartz SL, Swierzewski III SJ, Sondak VK, Grossman HB. Liposarcoma of the spermatic cord: report of 6 cases and review of the literature. *J Urol* 1995;**153**:154–157.

9. Catton CN, Cummings BJ, Fornasier V, O'Sullivan B, Quirt I, Warr D. Adult paratesticular sarcomas: a review of 21 cases. *J Urol* 1991;**146**:342–345.

10. Russo P, Brady MS, Conlon K *et al.* Adult urologic sarcoma. *J Urol* 1992;**147**:1032–1037.

11. Sogani PC, Grabstald H, Whitmore WF Jr. Spermatic cord sarcoma in adults. *J Urol* 1978;**120**:301–305.

12. Fagundes MA, Zietman AL, Althausen AF, Coen JJ, Shipley WU. The management of spermatic cord sarcoma. *Cancer* 1996;**77**:1873–1876.

13. Mandell L, Ghavimi F, Peretz T. Radiocurability of microscopic disease in childhood rhabdomyosarcoma with radiation doses less than 4000 cGy. *J Clin Oncol* 1990;**8**:1536–1542.

41.6 Systemic chemotherapy

A Tolcher

Systemic chemotherapy for sarcomas of the spermatic cord is generally limited to patients with primary leiomyosarcomas, rhabdomyosarcomas or fibrosarcoma with involved lymph nodes or distant metastases[1–3]. Chemotherapy for soft tissue sarcomas should be viewed as both highly specialized and used as part of a multimodality treatment approach. Furthermore, in light of the rarity of sarcomas of the spermatic cord referral to a center with experience with the treatment of soft tissue sarcomas is encouraged.

References

1. Grey LF, Sorial RF, Shaw WH. Spermatic cord sarcoma. *Urology* 1986;**27**:28–31.

2. Scalama AD, Berger BM, Cherry JM, Young JD. Malignant fibrous histiocytoma of the spermatic cord: role of retroperitoneal lymphadenopathy in management. *J Urology* 1983;**130**:577.

3. Yang JC, Rosenberg SA, Glatstein EJ, Antman KH. Sarcomas of soft tissues. In: Devita VT, Hellman S, Rosenberg SA (eds) *Cancer: principles and practice of oncology* (4th edn), JB Lippincott Company, Philadelphia, 1993, pp. 1436–1488.

42 Tumors of the scrotum

42.1 Epidemiology and etiology

J Petros and P D LaFontaine

Epidemiology

Scrotal malignancies are an uncommon form of genital cancers, accounting for less than 0.1% of invasive male genital cancers[1]. From 1973 to 1987, 149 invasive and 29 in situ scrotal cancers were reported in the SEER study. Of these, 76.5% were carcinomas, 19.5% sarcomas and 3.5% melanomas. Squamous cell carcinoma was the most common histologic subtype and the only one with rates greater than 0.5 per million[1]. It is followed in frequency by basal cell carcinoma, malignant melanoma, extramammary Paget's disease and sarcomas, including leiomyosarcoma, liposarcoma, rhabdomyosarcoma and fibrosarcoma. The average age at diagnosis for carcinomas in whites and blacks was 70 and 58 respectively, and for sarcomas it was 60 and 66.[1] Scrotal carcinoma has been more common in the United Kingdom than in the United States, with an estimated increased incidence of eight to 20 times that in the USA. Social class has also been related to the incidence of scrotal carcinoma. Kennaway and Kennaway examined 1029 cases of scrotal carcinoma in England and, after controlling for occupation, found no cases of scrotal carcinoma in the professional classes and only a single case among white collar workers[2]. There has also been a difference in the incidence between urban and rural populations, most likely related to the fact that rural dwellers have less occupational exposure risks. Finally, race has been a factor in the incidence of scrotal carcinoma. As of 1985 only eight cases of scrotal carcinoma had been reported in American blacks[2].

Etiology

Squamous cell carcinoma has historical significance in that it was the first cancer to be directly associated with a specific occupation. The disease was first described by Bassius in England in 1731 and by Treyling in 1740[3]. However, it was not until 1775 that Sir Percivall Pott linked the lesion with chimney sweepers[4]. Since that time the disease has been associated with other occupations including shale and paraffin workers[3], mule spinners in the cotton industry[5], machine operators in the engineering industry[6], screw makers[6], automatic lathe operators[7] and petroleum wax pressmen[8]. The commonality among these occupations seems to be their exposure to refined mineral oils and heavy lubricating oils. In the 1920s Leitch demonstrated the carcinogenic potential of refined mineral oils in the development of skin cancer in the animal model[9]. Other possible etiologic factors that have been suggested to be important in the development of scrotal cancer include exposure to dust, grease, mechanical irritation, repeated trauma and poor personal hygiene. However, it should be noted that most of the cases now reported in the USA do not have an occupational exposure association[2].

More recently the use of PUVA and psoralens in the treatment of psoriasis has been linked with squamous cell carcinoma of the scrotum. In a recent analysis of almost 900 men treated with PUVA and psoralens, one out of every 89 men developed squamous cell carcinoma of the scrotum[10]. This was found to be a dose dependent relationship with men exposed to high levels of PUVA having a 16-fold increased risk of developing squamous cell carcinoma of the scrotum compared with those with low level exposure and an almost 300-fold increased risk compared with the general population.

Viral factors may also have an etiologic role in the development of scrotal carcinoma. In the recent series of Andrews et al., 45% of the patients had evidence of HPV infection[11]. In this same series they also noted that 22% of the patients had a history of multiple cutaneous epitheliomas located elsewhere on their body.

References

1. Gilliland FD, Key CR. Male genital cancers. *Cancer* 1995;**75**:295–315.
2. Kennaway EL, Kennaway NM. The social distribution of cancer of the scrotum and cancer of the penis. *Cancer Res* 1946;**6**:49–53.

3. Graves RC, Flo S. Carcinoma of the scrotum. *J Urol* 1940;**43**:309–332.
4. Pott P. Cancer scroti. In: Hawes L, Clarke W, Collins R (eds) *Chirurgical works* 1775;**5**:63.
5. Lee WR, McCann JK. Mule spinner's cancer and the wool industry. *Br J Ind Med* 1967;**24**:148–151.
6. Osterling JE, Lowe FC. Squamous cell carcinoma of the scrotum. *AUA Update Series* 1990;**9**:178–183.
7. Avellan L. Breine U, Jacobsson B *et al.* Carcinoma of the scrotum induced by mineral oil. *Scand J Plast Reconstr Surg* 1967;**1**:135–140.
8. Lione JG, Denholm JS. Cancer of the scrotum in wax pressmen. II. Clinical observations. *Arch Ind Health* 1959;**19**:530–539.
9. Leitch A. Mule spinner's cancer and mineral oils. *BMJ* 1924;**2**:941–943.
10. Stern RS, Members of the Photochemotherapy Follow-up Study. Genital tumors among men with psoriasis exposed to psoralens and ultraviolet A radiation (PUVA) and ultraviolet B radiation. *N Engl J Med* 1990;**322**:1093–1097.
11. Andrews PE, Farrow GM, Oesterling JE. Squamous cell carcinoma of the scrotum: long-term followup of 14 patients. *J Urol* 1991;**146**:1299–1304.

42.2   Presentation, diagnosis & staging of squamous cell carcinoma

J Petros and P D LaFontaine

Presentation

Squamous cell carcinoma of the scrotum presents primarily as a solitary lesion[1]. In Ray and Whitmore's series, 90% of the lesions were solitary[1]. The early lesion is usually a slow growing nodule on the anterolateral aspect of the scrotum. These lesions may ulcerate after several months. The base will frequently be indurated with raised edges and a variable amount of seropurulent discharge. The median time from onset of symptoms to presentation was 8 months in one series[1]. Excluding occupational exposure there is no predilection for side[1] The usual age of presentation is in the 6th decade[2]. Between 40% and 50% of men will have palpable inguinal adenopathy at presentation, and of these half will have metastases. Therefore, 25% of men will have metastatic disease at presentation[3].

Diagnosis

As mentioned previously, most men present with an enlarging mass in the scrotum that has been present for several months. Various benign and malignant processes need to be considered in the differential diagnosis. Benign lesions of the scrotum include cutaneous nevus, sebaceous cyst, eczema, psoriasis, folliculitis, manifestations of secondary and tertiary syphillis, tuberculous epidymitis with draining sinus and periurethral abscess. Malignant tumors to be considered include basal cell carcinoma, extra mammary Paget's disease, and various rare tumors such as liposarcoma, leiomyosarcoma, rhabdomyosarcoma, fibrosarcoma, Merkel cell carcinoma, malignant melanoma and peripheral T cell lymphoma.

Staging

The first staging system introduced was by Ray and Whitmore in 1977[1]. This system included all patients who had resectable lymph nodes, both inguinal and pelvic, in the same classification. This staging system was modified by Lowe in 1983 to include all patients who had pelvic lymph node involvement, both resectable and unresectable, in the same staging category since they had similar prognosis. Therefore Lowe included these patients in the same category. This staging system is outlined in Table 42.2.1. Computed tomography has limited use in assessing the ilioinguinal lymph nodes. Although CT has the ability to assess the size of lymph nodes it can not differentiate inflammatory from metastatic adenopathy, nor can it identify micrometastatic disease. CT can be helpful in identifying the extent of pelvic or retroperitoneal lymph node involvement in those patients with bulky inguinal adenopathy, and this may have therapeutic implications.

Pedal lymphangiography has been reported to be between 74% and 95% accurate in differentiating inflammatory from metastatic adenopathy in various pelvic cancers[4]. However, it can not identify micrometastatic disease and therefore contributes little additional information.

References

1. Ray B, Whitmore WF, Jr. Experience with carcinoma of the scrotum. *J Urol* 1977;**117**:741–745.
2. Lowe FC. Squamous cell carcinoma of the scrotum. *Urology* 1985;**25**:63–65.

Table 42.2.1   Staging system for scrotal carcinoma

Stage	Description
A1	Localized to scrotal wall
A2	Locally extensive tumor invading adjacent structures (testis, spermatic cord, penis, pubis, perineum)
B	Metastatic disease involving inguinal lymph nodes only
C	Metastatic disease involving pelvic lymph nodes without evidence of distant spread
D	Metastatic disease beyond the pelvic lymph nodes involving distant organs

Data from Lowe FC: Squamous cell carcinoma of the scrotum. *J Urol* **130**:423, 1983.

3. Osterling JE, Lowe FC. Squamous cell carcinoma of the scrotum. *AUA Update Series* 1990;**9**:178–183.
4. Jing BS, Wallace S, Zornoza J. Metastases to retroperitoneal and pelvic lymph nodes: computed tomography and lymphangiography. *Radiol Clin N Amer* 1982;**20**:511–530.

42.3 Pathology of malignant tumors of the scrotum

P A Humphrey

A number of anatomic structures are the origin of different extratesticular malignancies of the scrotum and its contents. The skin, dartos muscle and fasciae of the scrotum, and paratesticular region, including the testicular tunics (tunica vaginalis and tunica albuginica), the epididymis and spermatic cord may all be the primary sites of development of a malignancy[1–8]. With destructive growth and effacement of normal anatomy, it may be difficult in some cases to determine the precise site of origin of a paratesticular malignancy[1,8].

Malignant neoplasms of the scrotum itself are rare. The most common scrotal malignancy is squamous cell carcinoma[3,4,6,9–24] arising on the scrotal surface in the epidermis. Additional reported malignancies include Paget's disease[3,5,25–33], basal cell carcinoma[3,5,34–36], Merkel cell carcinoma[37], sarcoma[3,5,6,38–47], malignant melanoma[48,49] and malignant lymphoma[50,51] (Table 42.3.1). Metastatic spread to the scrotum is rare and has been reported for gastrointestinal tract[52], lung[53] and prostatic carcinomas[54,55].

Squamous cell carcinoma

This is usually detected as invasive disease but squamous cell carcinoma in situ (Bowen's disease) of the scrotal skin has been reported in rare cases[9,10]. Grossly, scrotal squamous carcinomas initially appear as a solitary nodule or wart-like growth, followed by ulceration and induration.[5] Microscopically, these carcinomas are most often well to moderately differentiated (Figure 42.3.1), with eosinophilic cytoplasm, intercellular bridges and squamous pearls indicative of squamous differentiation. As the carcinomas

Table 42.3.1 Histologic types of primary scrotal cancers

Histologic type	Number of reported cases
Carcinoma	397
Squamous cell carcinoma	347
Basal cell carcinoma	25
Paget's disease	24
Merkel cell carcinoma	1
Malignant melanoma	6
Malignant lymphoma	rare
Sarcoma	rare

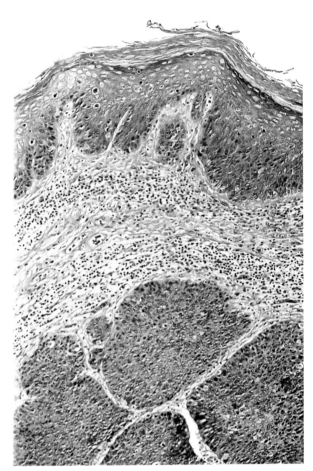

Fig. 42.3.1 Invasive moderately-differentiated squamous cell carcinoma of scrotal skin.

invade, a fibrogenic response is elicited, corresponding to gross induration. A brisk inflammatory cell response is also characteristic. The squamous epithelium adjacent to the carcinoma may display hyperplastic features.

Scrotal squamous cell carcinomas invade locally into the scrotal wall but scrotal contents are usually not involved by direct extension[3,6]. Larger cancers may involve the testis, spermatic cord, penis or perineum[11]. Initial metastatic spread is to regional, ipsilateral inguinal lymph nodes. Important pathologic prognostic factors are tumor size and pathologic stage but not histologic grade[2,5,6,10,11,19]. Tumor size greater than 2 cm seems to portend an increased risk of inguinal lymph node metastasis[2] and pathologic extent of disease, as reflected by staging systems, definitely relates to prognosis. Patients with carcinoma in situ or cancer localized to the scrotum have a favorable prognosis[10,11]. Precise multivariate assessment of these pathologic prognostic indicators has been difficult due to the limited number of patients in a given series. Tumoral genetic abnormalities, including infection with HPV DNA types 16 and 18[23,24], are not currently of practical prognostic value.

Carcinoma in situ

A type of rare carcinoma in situ of the scrotum that merits careful investigation for underlying malignancy is extramammary Paget's disease involving the scrotum. Some patients with scrotal Paget's disease have an underlying carcinoma of the urinary bladder, urethra, prostate or eccrine sweat gland[3,5,25,29]. Grossly, scrotal Paget's disease appears as a red, scaly, eczematous or indurated plaque[3,5,29,31,33]. The lesion may be extensive with involvement of both sides of the scrotum[32], or involvement of skin of the penis, perineum, and inguinal region[3,27,28,33]. Microscopically, scrotal Paget's disease is an intraepithelial malignancy characterized by large pale tumor cells arranged singly or in small groups within the epithelium of the epidermis and sometimes hair shafts. The histological differential diagnosis includes squamous cell carcinoma in situ and malignant melanoma. Histochemical and immunohistochemical stains are valuable in establishment of a definitive diagnosis: the tumor cells in Paget's disease will be mucin positive, carcinoembryonic antigen positive, prostate-specific antigen positive if prostatic in origin, and negative for the melanoma markers HMB-45 and S-100.

Basal cell carcinoma

Basal cell carcinomas of the scrotal skin are as rare as scrotal Paget's disease (Table 42.3.1). Basal cell carcinomas of the scrotum macroscopically appear as a plaque or ulcerated nodule[5]. Microscopically, these carcinomas have the same appearance as the extremely common head and neck basal cell carcinoma, with nests and cords of basaloid tumor cells. Like basal cell carcinomas elsewhere, these tumors are locally aggressive if untreated but there may be a higher propensity for scrotal basal cell carcinomas to exhibit metastatic spread[3,34,35]. Basal cell carcinomas of the scrotum are not as aggressive as scrotal squamous cell carcinomas.

Sarcoma

Sarcomas of the scrotal wall are also rare and should be distinguished from paratesticular, intrascrotal sarcomas, which are sometimes incorrectly designated as 'scrotal sarcomas'. By far the most common type of sarcoma of the scrotal wall is leiomyosarcoma[3,5,6], which likely arises from the dartos muscle[5,38–40]. This spindle cell sarcoma exhibits a well organized fascicular growth pattern. In these cases a sarcomatoid or spindle cell squamous carcinoma should be excluded; an immunohistochemical panel

of antibodies reactive against muscle (actin, desmin) and epithelial (keratin) markers may be of diagnostic value in this context. Additional types of scrotal wall sarcomas have mainly been reported as single cases and include Kaposi's sarcoma[41,42,47], malignant fibrous histiocytoma[43,44], liposarcoma[45] and malignant peripheral nerve sheath tumor (neurofibrosarcoma)[45].

References

1. Srigley JR, Hartwick RWJ. Tumors and cysts of the paratesticular region. *Pathol Ann* 1990;**25**:51–108.
2. Petersen RO. Testicular adenexa. In: *Urologic pathology* (2nd edn). JB Lippincott Co. Philadelphia: 1992, pp. 526–574.
3. Petersen RO. Scrotum. In: *Urologic pathology* (2nd edn) JB Lippincott Co, Philadelphia: 1992, pp. 710–725.
4. Bostwick DG. Spermatic cord and testicular adenexa. In: Bostwick DG, Eble JN (eds) *Urologic surgical pathology*. Mosby, St Louis: 1997, pp. 663–666.
5. Ro JY, Amin MB, Ayala AG. Penis and scrotum. In: Bostwick DG, Eble JN (eds) *Urologic surgical pathology*. Mosby, St Louis: 1997, pp. 712–714.
6. Murphy WM. Diseases of the penis and scrotum. In: Murphy WM (Ed.) *Urological pathology* (2nd edn) WB Saunders Co. Philadelphia: 1997, pp. 401–429.
7. Gaudin PB, Epstein JI. Diseases of the spermatic cord and paratesticular tissue. In: Murphy WM (Ed.) *Urological pathology* (2nd edn) WB Saunders Co, Philadelphia: 1997, pp. 242–276.
8. Richie JP. Neoplasms of the testis. In: Walsh PC, Retik AB, Vaughan ED Jr, Wein AJ (eds) *Campbell's urology* (7th edn) WB Saunders Co, Philadelphia: pp. 2444–2447.
9. Wagner RF Jr, Grande DJ. Solitary pigmented Bowen's disease of the scrotum. *J Dermatol Surg Oncol* 1986;**12**:1114–1115.
10. Andrews PE, Farrow GM, Oesterling JE. Squamous cell carcinoma of the scrotum: long-term follow-up of 14 patients. *J Urol* 1991;**146**:1299–1304.
11. Lowe FC. Squamous cell carcinoma of the scrotum. *J Urol* 1983;**130**:423–429.
12. Rousch GC, Fischer DB, Flannery JT. A population-based study of survival after scrotal carcinoma. *Cancer* 1985;**55**:666–671.
13. Polyak L, Czvalinga I, Frang D. [Primary carcinomas of the scrotum – 5 cases]. [German]. *Urol Nephrol* 1987;**80**:455–458.
14. Saito S, Higa I, Koyama Y, Hatano T, Hayakawa M, Osawa A. [A case of squamous cell carcinoma of the scrotum]. [Japanese]. *Jpn J Urol* 1986;**79**:344–346.
15. McGarry GW, Robertson JR. Scrotal carcinoma following prolonged use of crude coal tar ointment. *Br J Urol* 1989;**63**:211.
16. Gross DJ, Schosser RH. Squamous cell carcinoma of the scrotum. *Cutis* 1991;**47**:402–404.
17. Taniguchi S, Furukawa M, Kutsuna H, Sowa J, Ishii M. Squamous cell carcinoma of the scrotum. *Dermatol* 1996;**193**:253–254.
18. Ray B, Whitmore WF Jr. Experience with carcinoma of the scrotum. *J Urol* 1977;**117**:741–745.
19. McDonald MW. Carcinoma of the scrotum. *Urology* 1982;**19**:269–274.
20. Lowe FC. Squamous cell carcinoma of the scrotum. *Urol Clin North Am* 1992;**19**:397–405.
21. Gerber WL. Scrotal malignancies: the University of Iowa experience and review of the literature. *Urology* 1985;**26**:337–342.
22. Parys BT, Hutton JL. Fifteen-year experience of carcinoma of the scrotum. *Br J Urol* 1991;**68**:414–417.
23. Burmer GC, True LD, Krieger JN. Squamous cell carcinoma of the scrotum associated with human papillomavirus. *J Urol* 1993;**149**:374–377.
24. Orihuela E, Tyring SK, Pow-Sang M *et al.* Development of human papillomavirus type 16 associated squamous cell carcinoma of the scrotum in a patient with Darier's disease treated with systemic isotretinoin. *J Urol* 1995;**153**:1940–1943.
25. Saidi JA, Bose S, Sawczuk I. Eccrine sweat gland carcinoma of the scrotum with associated extramammary Paget's disease. *Urology* 1997;**50**:789–791.

26. Perez MA, LaRossa DD, Tomaszewski JE. Paget's disease primarily involving the scrotum. *Cancer* 1989;**83**:970–975.

27. Weese D, Murphy J, Zimmern PE. ND:YAG laser treatment of extramammary Paget's disease of the penis and scrotum. *J Urologie* 1993;**99**:269–271.

28. Hartley EL, Nambisan RN, Rao U, Karakousis CP. Extramammary Paget disease of the inguinoscrotal area. *NY State J Med* 1988;**88**:546–548.

29. Allan SJR, Mclaren K, Aldridge RD. Paget's disease of the scrotum – a case exhibiting positive prostate-specific antigen staining and associated prostatic adenocarcinoma. *Br J Dermatol* 1998;**138**:689–691.

30. Balducci L, Athar M, Smith GF, Khansur T, MacKenzie D, Crawford ED. Metastatic extramammary Paget's disease: dramatic response to combined modality treatment. *J Surg Oncol* 1988;**38**:38–44.

31. Parikh AR, Aghazarian SG, Orbegoso CM, Schirmer HK. Extramammary Paget's disease of the scrotum: need for early biopsy. *South Med J* 1986;**79**:779–780.

32. Kageyama N, Izumi AK. Bilateral scrotal extramammary Paget's disease in a Chinese man. *Int J Dermatol* 1997;**36**:695–697.

33. Maciejewski W, Brandmann HJ, Schmid MA. [Extramammary Paget's disease]. [German] *Hautarzt* 1979;**30**:271–272.

34. Parys BT. Basal cell carcinoma of the scrotum. A rare clinical entity. *Br J Urol* 1991;**68**:434–435.

35. Nahass GT, Blaurelt A, Leonardi CL *et al.* Basal cell carcinoma of the scrotum. *J Am Acad Dermatol* 1992;**26**:574–578.

36. Schleicher SM, Milstein HJ, Ilowite R. Basal cell carcinoma of the scrotum. *Cutis* 1997;**58**:116.

37. Best TJ, Metcalfe JB, Moore RB, Nguyen GK. Merkel cell carcinoma of the scrotum. *Ann Plast Surg* 1994;**33**:83–85.

38. Flotte FJ, Bell DA, Sidhu GS, Plair CM. Leiomyosarcoma of the dartos muscle. *J Cut Pathol* 1981;**8**:69–74.

39. Collier DS, Pain JA, Hamilton-Dutoit S. Leiomyosarcoma of the scrotum. *J Surg Oncol* 1987;**34**:176–178.

40. Jeddy TA, Vowles RH, Southam JA. Leiomyosarcoma of the dartos muscle. *Br J Urol* 1994;**74**:129–130.

41. Hopkins JA, Hudson PB. Kaposi's sarcoma: penile and scrotal lesions. *Br J Urol* 1953;**25**:233–236.

42. Vyas S, Manabe T, Herman JR *et al.* Kaposi's sarcoma of scrotum. *Urology* 1976;**8**:82–85.

43. Wantanabe K, Ogawa A, Komatsu H *et al.* Malignant fibrous histiocytoma of the scrotal wall. A case report. *J Urol* 1988;**140**:151–152.

44. Konety BR, Campanella SC, Hakam A, Becich MJ. Malignant fibrous histiocytoma of the scrotum. *J Urol Pathol* 1996;**5**:51–56.

45. Bauer JJ, Sesterhenn IA, Costabile RA. Myxoid liposarcoma of the scrotal wall. *J Urol* 1995;**153**:1938–1939.

46. Peters KM, Gonzalez JA. Malignant peripheral nerve sheath tumor of the scrotum: a case report. *J Urol* 1996;**155**:649–650.

47. Vaprek JM, Quivey JM, Carroll PR. Acquired immunodeficiency syndrome-related Kaposi's sarcoma of the male genitalia: management with radiation therapy. *J Urol* 1991;**146**:333–336.

48. Davis NS, Kim CA, Dever DP. Primary malignant melanoma of the scrotum: case report and literature review. *J Urol* 1991;**145**:1056–1057.

49. Konstandoulakis MM, Ricaniadis N, Karakonsis CP. Malignant melanoma of the scrotum: report of two cases. *J Urol* 1994;**151**:161–162.

50. Doll DC, Diaz-Arias AA. Peripheral T-cell lymphoma of the scrotum. *Acta Hematol* 1994;**91**:77–79.

51. Allen DC, Walsh MY. Malignant lymphoma of the scrotum and Wegener's granulomatosis of the penis – genital presentation of systemic disease. *Ulster Med J* 1996;**65**:169–172.

52. Wiesel T, Bohm J, Paul R, Breal J, Hartung R. Rare metastases of signet ring cell carcinomas to the scrotum – report of two cases. *Urology* 1996;**47**:769–771.

53. Ferguson MA, White BA, Johnson DE, Carington PR, Schaefer RF. Carcinoma en cuirasse of the scrotum: an unusual presentation of lung carcinioma metastatic to the scrotum. *J Urol* 1998;**160**: 2154–2155.

54. Doutre MS, Beylot C, Bioulac P, Conte M, De Mascarel A. [Cutaneous metastases of a prostatic cancer. Apropos of a case]. [French]. *Ann Pathol* 1987;**7**:234–236.

55. Fiorelli RL, Finkelstein LH, Fernandes JJ. Metastasis of prostate gland adenocarcinoma to penile and scrotal cutaneous tissues. *J Am Osteopath Assoc* 1989;**89**:349–352.

42.4 Surgical management of scrotal carcinoma

J Petros

Initial therapy for scrotal carcinoma includes wide local excision with a 2 cm margin of normal tissue around the tumor. Excision of scrotal contents is rarely needed and is only indicated if directly invaded by the squamous cell carcinoma. Management of the tissue defect created by wide local excision depends on the extent of the lesion. Small defects may be closed primarily. Larger defects may require the construction of testicular thigh pockets, use of local myocutaneous pedicled flaps or split thickness skin grafting[1]. Local recurrence rates have been reported to be as high as 21%[2]. The management of regional lymph nodes is more controversial. In 1911 Morley elucidated the spread of scrotal carcinoma in the regional lymphatics[3]. He demonstrated that there was free communication between the superficial lymphatic network on both sides of the scrotum and that the median raphe did not act as a barrier. Most importantly, he was not able to identify any case where the lymphatic drainage skipped the inguinal nodes and went directly to the intrapelvic nodes. In addition, there does not appear to be any communication between the superficial lymphatics of the scrotum and those of the testes and chord structures.

One of the controversies in the management of lymph nodes in scrotal carcinoma is the value of primary versus delayed lymph node dissection. Based on the work of Morley[3], early bilateral ilioinguinal node dissection was recommended by several investigators[4,5]. However, these early recommendations for aggressive treatment of regional lymph nodes have since been modified based on our knowledge of the biology of squamous cell carcinoma of the scrotum. Dean was the first to recommend lymphadenectomy only for patients with biopsy proven disease[6]. Since that time it has become clear that only 50% of patients have palpable nodes at presentation, and that only half of these patients will in fact have metastatic disease[1]. Therefore, only 25% of patients will benefit from a lymph node dissection. Patients presenting without clinical lymphadenopathy should have clinical follow up every 2 to 3 months with assessment for the development of regional adenopathy. In patients who present with clinically palpable inguinal nodes a 4 to 6 week course of oral antibiotics should be administered followed by reassessment of inguinal adenopathy. Those patients who continue to have palpable inguinal adenopathy should have a sentinel lymph node biopsy followed by ilioinguinal lymph node dissection if positive. The recommendation for sentinel lymph node biopsy is based on the work of Riveros[7]. Although there has been some controversy on the reliability of sentinel lymph node biopsy in staging squamous cell carcinoma of the penis due to the direct lymphatic drainage of the glans to the deep pelvic nodes[8], Morley has demonstrated that the lymphatic drainage of the scrotal skin goes directly to the inguinal nodes[3]. Daseler added further support to this recommendation by showing that the sentinel lymph node was present in 86% of 450 groin dissections[9].

Another area of controversy in the management of lymph nodes in squamous cell carcinoma of the scrotum is unilateral versus bilateral dissection. Based on Morley's observations that the midline raphe did not act as a barrier to lymphatic dissemination, bilateral ilioinguinal lymph node dissections were recommended by early investigators[3–5]. However, Ray has demonstrated that contralateral nodal involvement with clinically nonpalpable nodes is a rare occurrence, occurring in only 8% of their patients, while in Andrews' series only 14% of patients had contralateral disease with clinically normal nodes[2,10]. To identify this minority of patients who will benefit from contralateral lymph node dissection we recommend contralateral sentinel lymph node biopsy followed by ilioinguinal lymph node dissection if positive.

The last area of controversy in the management of regional lymph nodes in scrotal carcinoma is inguinal versus ilioinguinal lymph node dissection. McDonald has recommended against ilioinguinal node dissection because he believes that these patients 'have such advanced disease that surgery does not seem a reasonable therapeutic solution'. Indeed, in Ray's series none of the five patients with pelvic node involvement survived[2]. However, there have been reports of patients with positive pelvic nodes surviving after ilioinguinal lymph node dissection. Cabanas reported a 20% three year survival rate for patients with penile carcinoma after ilioinguinal lymph node dissection[11]. Since surgery offers the only current cure for these patients, ilioinguinal lymphadenectomy should be performed on patients with biopsy proven inguinal metastasis and minimal or no pelvic lymph node involvement.

Conclusions

We recommend the following treatment plan for squamous cell carcinoma of the scrotum:

1) Wide local excision of the primary tumor with a 2 cm margin.
2) Frequent periodic assessment of regional lymph nodes for patients with clinically normal nodes or those whose palpable nodes normalize after 4 to 6 weeks of antibiotics.
3) Ipsilateral ilioinguinal lymph node dissection with contralateral sentinel lymph node biopsy with completion contralateral ilioinguinal lymph node dissection if sentinel node biopsy positive.

References

1. Osterling JE, Lowe FC. Squamous cell carcinoma of the scrotum. *AUA Update Series* 1990;**9**:178–183.
2. Ray B, Whitmore WF Jr. Experience with carcinoma of the scrotum. *J Urol* 1977;**117**:741–745.
3. Morley J. The lymphatics of the scrotum: in relation to the radical operation for scrotal epithelioma. *Lancet* 1911;**ii**:1545–1547.
4. Graves RC, Flo S. Carcinoma of the scrotum. *J Urol* 1940;**43**:309–332.
5. Kickham CJE, Dufresne M. An assessment of carcinoma of the scrotum. *J Urol* 1967;**98**:108–110.
6. Dean AL. Epithelioma of the scrotum. *J Urol* 1948;**60**:508–518.
7. Riveros M, Garcia R, Cabanas R. Lymphadenography of the dorsal lymphatics of the penis. Techniques and results. *Cancer* 1967;**20**:2026–2031.
8. Perinette E, Crane DB, Catalona WJ. Unreliability of sentinel lymph node biopsy for staging penile carcinoma. *J Urol* 1980;**124**:734–735.
9. Daseler EH, Anson BJ, Reimann AF. Radical excision of the inguinal and iliac lymph glands: study based upon 450 anatomical dissections and upon supportive clinical observations. *Surg Gynecol Obstet* 1948;**87**:679–694.
10. Andrews PE, Farrow GM, Oesterling JE. Squamous cell carcinoma of the scrotum: long term followup of 14 patients. *J Urol* 1991;**146**:1299–1304.
11. Cabanas RM. An approach for the treatment of penile carcinoma. *Cancer* 1977;**39**:456–466.

42.5 Radiotherapy for scrotal carcinoma

J Michalski

Epithelial tumors

Despite the relatively good radiosensitivity of both basal cell and squamous cell cancers of the skin, tumors of the scrotum are uncommonly managed by primary radiation therapy. The radiation therapy dose necessary to gain local control of these tumors ranges from 50 to 65 Gy. This is the dose that almost certainly results in sterility and loss of testosterone production. Radiation therapy is best reserved for patients with unresectable or recurrent lesions, or in patients with positive margins after maximal surgery. Consideration of elective node irradiation for clinical suspicious nodes or pelvic irradiation for patients with positive groin nodes may decrease the risk of regional or nodal relapse[3].

Radiation therapy is useful in the palliative management of AIDS-related or epidemic Kaposi's sarcoma. Superficial X-ray therapy or electron beam treatment to modest doses of 600 to 3000 cGy at 200 to 300 cGy per day will result in a complete response rate of 36% to 70% with durable control[1,2].

References

1. Vapnek JM, Quivey JM, Carroll PR. Acquired immunodeficiency syndrome-related Kaposi's sarcoma of the male genitalia: management with radiation therapy. *J Urol* 1991;**146**:333–336.
2. LeBourgeois JP, Frikha H, Piedbois P, LePechoux C, Martin L, Haddad E. Radiotherapy in the management of epidemic Kaposi's sarcoma of the oral cavity, the eyelid and the genitals. *Radiother Oncol* 1994;**30**:263–266.
3. Homesley HD, Bundy BN, Sedlis A *et al.* Radiation therapy versus pelvic node resection for carcinoma of the vulva with positive groin nodes. *Obstet Gyn* 1986;**68**:733–740.

42.6 Chemotherapy for scrotal carcinoma

J W Basler

The initial treatment of scrotal carcinoma is excision of the lesion and management of the lymph nodes in a manner similar to penile carcinoma. However, in some cases the tumor may be advanced with local extension and/or distant metastases. Radiotherapy may provide local control though it is often complicated by skin breakdown and ulceration. Chemotherapy with methotrexate, bleomycin and cisplatin has shown some efficacy in an isolated case report[1]. In general, the same agents that show activity against penile and other squamous carcinomas may be utilized for scrotal carcinoma[2]. The exception to this statement may be those rare patients with extramammary Paget's disease of the scrotal wall who might gain clinical benefit if not cure from initial topical therapy with 1% 5-fluorouracil cream followed by local excision[3].

References

1. Arai Y, Kinouchi T, Kuroda M, Usami M, Kotake T. A case of scrotal cancer with inguinal lymph node metastasis treated by multidisciplinary modalities including chemotherapy with methotrexate, bleomycin and cisplatin]. *Hinyokika Kiyo* 1997 Sep;**43**(9):683–685.
2. Dexeus FH, Logothetis CJ, Sella A, Amato R, Kilbourn R, Fitz K, Striegel A. Combination chemotherapy with methotrexate, bleomycin and cisplatin for advanced squamous cell carcinoma of the male genital tract. *J Urol* 1991;**146**(5):1284–1287.
3. Haberman HF, Goodall J, Llewellyn M. Extramammary Paget's disease. *Can Med Assoc J* 1978;**118**(2):161–162.

PART SIX
Carcinoma of the penis

Chapter 43
Incidence, etiology and epidemiology

Chapter 44
Presentation, diagnosis and staging

Chapter 45
Pathology of carcinoma of the penis

Chapter 46
Surgical Management

46.1   The role of radiotherapy in the management of squamous carcinoma

46.2   Chemotherapy

43 Incidence, etiology and epidemiology

S D Graham Jr and W H Sanders

Incidence

Squamous cell carcinoma of the penis is a relatively uncommon cancer in the developed world, yet it is a more common disease among developing nations. In the United States, for example, squamous cell carcinoma of the penis accounts for 1% of all malignancies in men, whereas in some regions of India, cancer of the penis accounts for 17% of malignancies in men[1]. The relatively high rate of disease in India may be due to the large Hindu population, which does not practice routine neonatal circumcision. There are between 750 and 1000 cases of carcinoma of the penis in the United States each year (10 cases per million male population) and the incidence has remained stable over the past 25 years. Some regions with a previously high incidence of penile cancer, such as Hong Kong, the Philippines and Puerto Rico, have experienced a significant decline in incidence over the past few decades[2,3]. Migration studies have strengthened the evidence that geographic factors play a role in the differences in incidence rates. The incidence of penile cancer is lower for Chinese living in Hawaii or the continental United States than for Chinese living in Asia. Penile cancer is rare in young men, and the incidence increases with each decade of life without ever reaching a plateau[4].

Etiology

Human papillomavirus (HPV) causes cancer of the penis. DNA from HPV can be detected by the technique of polymerase chain reaction (PCR) in as many as 92% of patients with superficial squamous cell carcinoma of the penis[5]. Remarkably, it is present in only 55% of invasive tumors. Of the HPV positive lesions, 85% have DNA from HPV-16 and 15% have DNA from HPV-18[6]. Other HPV subtypes are rarely associated with cancer of the penis. The HPV gene produces several proteins which bind to the products of tumor suppressor genes, such as the retinoblastoma gene and P53, allowing unregulated cell proliferation[7]. Because a large number of squamous cell carcinomas of the penis do not contain DNA from HPV, there must be a separate and distinct mechanism in the development of this cancer that does not require HPV infection.

HPV infection in men poses an increased risk of cervical cancer in their wives. The risk of cervical cancer in wives of men with cancer of the penis is three times that of wives of men without cancer of the penis[8]. In contrast, the presence of cervical cancer does not increase the risk of penile cancer in men.

Smegma, the accumulated debris of epithelial cells from the glans penis, contains precursors of carcinogens that may play a role in the development of penile carcinoma[9]. While causation remains unproven, the combination of smegma-related carcinogens and phimosis has led to cancer in experimental models[10].

Epidemiology

Three pre-malignant lesions of the penis include 1) Buschke-Lowenstein giant condyloma, 2) balanitis xerotica obliterans (BXO), and 3) leukoplakia. Although metastases are rare, the Buschke-Lowenstein tumor is considered a form of verrucous carcinoma because it is characterized by local invasion and destruction of surrounding tissue. Balanitis xerotica obliterans is a sclerosing inflammation of the glans and prepuce, commonly associated with chronic balanitis and phimosis. The rare but recognized progression of BXO to squamous cell carcinoma of the penis mandates the lifelong follow up of these patients[11]. Leukoplakia is characterized by white plaques involving the meatus, and is often found adjacent to carcinoma. Because of its association with carcinoma, it is important to perform thorough biopsies of all suspected lesions, with close follow up to detect persistent or recurrent disease[12].

Penile cancer is very rare in populations that practice ritual circumcision in infancy. The most striking evidence of the protective effects of circumcision is that of cancer rates in neighboring communities in Uganda with differing circumcision practices. The relative risk of penile cancer in communities that do not practice neonatal circumcision is almost six times the risk of penile cancer in communities that practice ritual circumcision in infancy[13]. The timing of the circumcision and the degree of foreskin excision are also critical to the risk of developing penile cancer. In males undergoing neonatal circumcision, the incidence is very low, while in males undergoing circumcision later in childhood or as adults, circumcision does not appear to have a protective effect. In fact, as many as 11% of patients with penile cancer were circumcised as adults for balanitis and phimosis[14]. While circumcision is protective, other risk factors determine which uncircumcised men develop cancer, because the incidence of penile cancer varies tenfold among uncircumcised communities in Uganda[13]. In addition, the incidence of penile cancer is low in Sweden, a country in which circumcision is not routine[15].

Phimosis is present in 50% of the cases of penile cancer. In contrast, congenital phimosis occurs in 2.4% of the population.[16] Epithelial atypia of the prepuce is present in 35% of men with phimosis, and never present in men without phimosis[17]. Phimosis may prevent adequate hygiene, and allow prolonged exposure to carcinogens associated with smegma[10].

Uncircumcised men are more susceptible to sexually transmitted diseases[17]. While syphilis is no longer considered an independent risk factor for the development of penile cancer, men with history of genital warts have a sixfold increased risk over patients with no history of warts[18,19]. Promiscuity has been suggested as an independent risk factor. There is a direct relation between the number of sexual partners and the risk of becoming infected with papillomavirus[20]. In one study, 28% of patients with penile cancer reported over 30 sexual partners, compared with 10% of matched controls[19].

In a population based case control study, the risk of penile cancer among smokers was three times that of nonsmokers, though the causative agent has not been identified. The tobacco-associated risk is not confined to cigarettes; other forms of tobacco also increase the risk of penile cancer[21]. There has been no association with alcohol intake and the incidence of penile cancer.

It has been difficult to define the role of race as a risk factor. Early studies suggested that penile cancer was less common in African American men than in Caucasians[16].

More recent studies have suggested that cancer of the penis is more common in African Americans[4]. It is unlikely that race is an independent risk factor for the development of penile cancer. Early evidence of socioeconomic factors and occupational hazards as independent risk factors for developing penile cancer has not been supported by subsequent investigations.

Prolonged exposure to certain chemical compounds (insecticides and fertilizers) in combination with poor personal hygiene has been found to be associated with penile SCC[22].

Research has also found that UV radiation exposure can increase the risk of developing penile SCC. The greatest risk is seen in patients undergoing low-dose radiation versus high-dose radiation, for this reason it is believed that more aggressive treatment with higher doses and with rest periods between treatment may be safer[22].

The immunosuppression that accompanies organ transplants is found to increase the risk of developing SCC at all sites by 36-fold. There are reports of penile SCC developing in kidney transplant patients, and in an immunosuppressed HIV-positive man. One study showed 50% of patients with penile SCC had abnormal immunologic responses[22]. These findings point to an immunological risk factor.

References

1. Reddy CRRM, Raghavaiah NV, Mouli KC. Prevalence of carcinoma of the penis with special reference to India. *Internat Surg* 1975;**60**(9):474.
2. Bolamaric J. Malignant tumors in Chinese: a report based on biopsy and autopsy material from Chinese in Hong Kong. *Int J Cancer* 1969;**4**:560.
3. Martinez I: Cancer in Puerto Rico. Estado Libre Asociado de Puerto Rico, Department de Salud, 1977.
4. Hall NEL, Schottenfeld D. Penis. In: Schottenfeld D, Fraumens JF Jr (eds) *Cancer epidemiology and prevention.* WB Saunders, Philadelphia, 1982.
5. Cupp MR, Malek RS, Goellner JR, Smith TF, Espy MJ. The detection of human papillomavirus deoxyribonucleic acid in intraepithelial, in situ, verrucous, and invasive carcinoma of the penis. *J Urol* 1995;**154**(3):104.
6. Wiener JS, Effert PJ, Humphrey PA, Yu L, Liu ET, Walther J. Prevalence of human papillomavirus types 16 and 18 in squamous-cell carcinoma of the penis: a retrospective analysis of primary and metastatic lesions by differential polymerase chain reaction. *Int J Cancer* 1992;**50**(5):694.
7. Munger K, Phelps WC, Bubb V, Howley PM, Schlegel R. The E6 and E7 genes of the human papillomavirus type 16 together are necessary and sufficient for transformation of primary human keratinocytes. *J Virol* 1989;**63**(10):4417.
8. Gajalakshmi CK, Shanta V. Association between cervical and penile cancers in Madras, India. *Acta Oncol* 1993;**32**:617.
9. Pratt-Thomas HR, Heins HC, Latham E. The carcinogenic effect of human smegma: an experimental study. *Cancer* 1956;**9**:671.
10. Shabad AL. The experimental production of penis tumors. *Neoplasm* 1965;**12**:65.
11. Giannakopoulos X, Basioukas K, Dimou S, Agnantis N. Squamous cell carcinoma of the penis arising from balanitis xerotica obliterans. *Int Urol Nephrol* 1996;**28**(2):223.
12. Mikhail GR. Cancers, precancers, and pseudocancers of the male genitalia. A review of clinical appearances, histopathology, and management. *J Dermatol Surg Oncol* 1980;**6**(12):1027.

13. Schmauz R, Jain DF. Geographical variation of carcinoma of the penis in Uganda. *Br J Cancer* 1971;**25**(1):25.

14. Jensen MS. Cancer of the penis in Denmark 1942 to 1962 (511 cases). *Dan Med Bull* 1977;**24**:66.

15. Klauber GT. Circumcision and phallic fallacies or the case against routine circumcision. *Conn Med* 1973;**37**:445.

16. Dean AL. Epithelioma of the penis. *J Urol* 1935;**33**:252.

17. Parker SW, Stewart AJ, Wren MN, Gollow MM, Straton JAY. Circumcision and sexually transmitted disease. *Med J Aust* 1983;**2**:288.

17. Reddy CRRM, Devandrath V, Pratap S. Carcinoma of penis – role of phimosis. *Urology* 1984;**24**(1):85–88.

18. Frisch M, Jorgensen BB, Friis S, Melbye M. Syphilis and the risk of penis cancer. *Sex Transm Dis* 1996;**23**(6):471.

19. Maden C, Sherman KJ, Beckmann AM, Hislop TG, The CZ, Ashley RL, Daling JR. History of circumcision, medical conditions, and sexual activity and risk of penile cancer. *J Natl Cancer Inst* 1993;**85**(1):19.

20. Bosch FX, Castellsague X, Munoz N, de Sanjose S, Ghaffaris AM, Gonzalez LC, Gili M *et al.* Male sexual behavior and human papillomavirus DNA: key risk factors for cervical cancer in Spain. *J Natl Cancer Inst* 1996;**88**(15): 1060.

21. Harish K, Ravi R. The role of tobacco in penile carcinoma. *Br J Urol* 1995;**75**(3):375.

22. Miczli G, Innocenzi D, Nasca MR, Musumeci ML, Ferrau F, Greco M. Squamous cell carcinoma of the penis. *J Am Acad Dermatol* 1996;**35**(3pt1):432–451.

44 Presentation, diagnosis and staging

J Nelson and J W Basler

Signs and symptoms

The first symptoms recognized by the patient are itching and burning under the prepuce or on the shaft of the penis. He may also notice a red or inflamed area that will not recede with usual hygenic measures. If left to progress a node or mass can form. The patient may also present with discharge and a malodorous complaint secondary to a bacterial infection within the lesion. Chronic malaise, fatigue, weight loss and weakness may be seen secondary to this chronic infection[1]. Irritative voiding symptoms and bleeding may also be seen. Pain is typically mild and is usually disproportional to the extensive local destruction, and thus does not cause the patient to seek medical attention.

Presenting symptoms of systemic metastasis are rare due to the far advanced local and regional lymph node disease usually present before distant metastasis. Delayed diagnosis is commonly seen in penile carcinoma from 15–50% of the time. Factors contributing to this are: personal neglect, embarrassment, fear, guilt, ignorance and phimosis obscuring the lesion[1].

The most common sign is the lesion itself. It can occur at any site on the penis, but is most commonly found at the glans, followed by the prepuce, glans and prepuce, coronal sulcus and the shaft[2]. This pattern may be associated with smegma exposure. The lesion can present as papillary and exophytic or flat and ulcerative. The latter lesion, due to it similarity in appearance to inflammation or candidal infection, may be delayed in diagnosis and has a tendency to early nodal metastasis[1]. At presentation 50% of patients will have enlarged inguinal lymph nodes. One half of these are from metastasis and the other half are secondary to bacterial infection of the primary lesion[3]. On physical examination, it is important to characterize the appearance, size, location, involvement of the corporal bodies, secondary superficial locations and lymph node involvement. Adenopathy found in the inguinal lymph nodes is an extremely important finding. Phimosis on physical examination must also be investigated. The base of the penis and scrotum should be viewed in order to rule out extension. Information about perineal body invasion or the presence of a pelvic mass can be obtained from a rectal and bimanual examination[1].

Diagnosis

The diagnosis is made by excisional biopsy for small lesions or incisional biopsy in anticipation of more definitive treatment for large lesions. Common pre-malignant lesions identified in conjunction with evaluation for penile pathology are presented in Table 44.1.

Staging

Typically, laboratory studies reveal no abnormalities. However, in patients with advanced disease, up to one-third may manifest hypercalcemia without obvious osseous metastasis. Hypercalcemia seems to be correlated with the volume of disease due to it increased incidence in node positive cancers. Calcium levels frequently correct after lymph node dissection[4]. Anemia, hypoalbuminemia and leukocytosis may also be findings in patients with a chronic illness or extensive infection[1].

The extent of the primary lesion is usually assessed by physical examination. MRI, ultrasound or CT may be

Table 44.1 Pre-malignant penile lesions

1. Erythroplasia of Queyrat (CIS of mucocutaneous epithelium)
a. Location – glans or prepuce
b. Clinical – single or multiple papules or plaques that may be round or oval. Typically described as a well-marginated lesion appearing red or velvety[6]. May present in the 5th or 6th decade and usually without pain. Very rare in circumcised males.
c. Histology – moderate plaque-like acanthosis with loss of epidermal cell polarity. Atypical epithelial cell may be multinucleated or vacuolated with hyperchromate nuclei and atypical mitosis. Plasma cells can be found in the submucosa and are the dominant component of the inflammatory infiltrate[7].

2. Bowen's disease
a. Location – found in follicle-bearings skin of the genitalia – the shaft of the penis
b. Clinical – a singular, dull-red plaque with areas of oozing and crusting[8]. Rarely painful. The disease may present with or develop visceral malignancies in 70% of patients. Within 5–7 years visceral malignancies can be found in >50% of patients[6].
c. Histology – similar to erythroplasia of Queyrat, Atypical squamous cells with scattered, abnormal multinucleated cells

3. Buschke–Lowenstein giant condyloma
a. Location – glans or prepuce
b. Clinical – typically found in uncircumcised males. These lesions appear as a slow growing, fungating, warty, ulcerating mass that is locally invasive and destructive. Spread tends to be along the proximal corpus urethrae[8,9].
c. Histology – indistinguishable from the benign condyloma with papillary fronds, an undulating keratinized outer layer, and deep margins[10].

4. Balanitis xerotica obliterans
a. Location – glans frenulum, inner prepuce, or urethral meatus. The small multiple lesions may coalesce and therefore extend their area of coverage.
b. Clinical – small erythematous areas that are smooth and shine and may coalesce to form whitish plaques. Often associated with chronic balanitis or phimosis. There are few early symptoms, with late symptoms being obstruction, urethral discharge, and/or pruritus.
c. Histology – hyperkeratosis, atrophy of the malpighian layer with hydropic degeneration of the basal cells, collagen abnormalities in the upper dermis, and mid-dermis inflammatory infiltrates[11].

5. Leukoplakia
a. Location – tends to involve the meatus
b. Clinical – one or more white patches or scaly patches. Associated with chronic irritation or inflammation and with diabetes. Can be found adjacent to or contiguous with SCC
c. Histology – disorderly arrangement of keratinocytes, hyperkeratosis, parakeratosis, irregular acanthosis or malpighian layer atrophy, and possible marked cellular atypia[8].

helpful in this evaluation as well. Chest X-ray, bone scan, and CT scan, MRI or ultrasound of the abdomen and pelvis may be used to evaluate metastasis though only advanced spread of the cancer may be identifiable on radiographic or scanning studies. Metastases are found this way in only 10% at presentation. The effectiveness of lymphangiography alone is not well established due to complications of the study relating to inflammation and metastatic obstruc-

tion. However, in conjunction with fine needle aspiration of suspected nodes it may be very helpful in guiding biopsies.

The rules for classification in the TNM system[5] for clinical staging include examination, endoscopy as indicated to assess urethral involvement and histologic confirmation. Imaging techniques are indicated for metastatic disease detection. For pathologic staging, complete resection of the primary site with appropriate margins is required and where regional lymph node involvement is suspected, assessment of these should be included (Table 44.2).

Table 44.2

Primary tumor (T)

TX	Primary tumor cannot be assessed
T0	No evidence of primary tumor
Tis	Carcinoma in situ
Ta	Non-invasive verrucous carcinoma
T1	Tumor invades subepithelial connective tissue
T2	Tumor invades corpus spongiosum or cavernosum
T3	Tumor invades urethra or prostate
T4	Tumor invades other adjacent structures

Regional lymph nodes (N)

NX	Regional lymph nodes cannot be assessed
N0	No regional lymph node metastasis
N1	Metastasis in a single superficial, inguinal lymph node
N2	Metastasis in multiple or bilateral superficial inguinal lymph nodes
N3	Metastasis in deep inguinal or pelvic lymph node(s) unilateral or bilateral

Distant metastasis (M)

MX	Distant metastasis cannot be assessed
M0	No distant metastasis
M1	Distant metastasis

Stage Grouping

Stage 0	Tis	N0	M0
	Ta	N0	M0
Stage I	T1	N0	M0
Stage II	T1	N1	M0
	T2	N0	M0
	T2	N1	M0
Stage III	T1	N2	M0
	T2	N2	M0
	T3	N0	M0
	T3	N1	M0
	T3	N2	M0
Stage IV	T4	Any N	M0
	Any T	N3	M0
	Any T	Any N	M1

Histopathologic type
Cell types for this staging protocol are limited to carcinomas

Histopathologic grade (G)

GX	Grade cannot be assessed
G1	Well differentiated
G2	Moderately differentiated
G 3–4	Poorly differentiated or undifferentiated

References

1. Walsh PC, Retik AB, Stamey TA, Vaughan ED. Tumors of the penis. In: *Campbell's Urology* (6th edn), Vol. 2, 1992;**31**:1269–1298.
2. Micali G, Innocenzi D, Nasca MR, Musumeci ML, Ferrau F, Greco M. Squamous cell carcinoma of the penis. *J Am Acad Dermat* 1996;**35**:432–451.
3. Stein *et al.* Benign and malignant tumors of the penis, urethra, epididymis, and seminal vesicles. *Clin Urologic Practice* 1991;**34**:1041–1069.
4. Block NL, Rosen P, Whitmore WF. Hemipelvectomy for advanced penile cancer. *J Urol* 1973;**110**:703.
5. Fleming ID, Cooper JS, Henson DE, Hutter RP, Kennedy BJ, Murphy GP, O'Sullivan B *et al. Cancer staging manual* 1997;**33**:215–218.
6. Graham JH, Helwig EB. Erythroplasia of Queyrat: a clinicopathologic and histochemical study. *Cancer* 1973;**32**:1396–1414.
7. Goette DK. Review of erythroplasia of Queyrat and its treatment. *Urology* 1976;**4**:311–315.
8. Mikhail GR. Cancers, precancers, and pseudocancers on the male genitalia: a review of clinical appearances, histopathology, and management. *J Dermatol Surg Oncol* 1980;**6**:1027–1035.
9. Ananthakrishnan N, Ravindran R, Veliath AJ *et al.* Lowenstein–Bushke tumor of the penis – a carcinomimic. *Br J Urol* 1981;**53**:460.
10. Bruns TNC, Lauvetz RJ, Kerr ES *et al.* Buschke-Lowenstein–giant condylomas: Pitfalls in management. *Urology* 1975;**6**:773–776.
11. Rheinschild GW, Olsen BS. Balanitis xerotica obliterans. *J Urol* 1970;**104**:860–863.

45 Pathology of carcinoma of the penis

P A Humphrey

Introduction

The vast majority of malignant neoplasms of the penis are squamous cell carcinomas[1–9,9A], also known as epidermoid carcinomas. Other primary malignancies such as malignant melanoma[10–12], sarcoma[13,14], malignant lymphoma[15], and secondary metastatic cancers[16–18] are rare (Table 45.1). Indeed, it has been estimated that squamous cell carcinomas account for 95% of all penile cancers[19]. These squamous cell carcinomas may be clinically detected as intraepithelial proliferations (carcinoma in situ) or as invasive disease.

Penile intraepithelial squamous cell proliferations span a spectrum from hyperplasia to dysplasia to carcinoma in situ[19–21]. The dysplastic and carcinoma in situ lesions are considered precursors of invasive squamous cell carcinoma and thereby are classified as pre-malignant conditions, but only a minority (5–10%) of patients with atypical penile intraepithelial proliferations progress to invasive carcinoma[22,23]. The diagnostic terminology of these atypical intraepithelial proliferations of the penis has been the source of substantial confusion. Terms such as erythroplasia of Queyrat, Bowen's disease and bowenoid papulosis have been used to classify proliferations with a similar histologic appearance under the light microscope but with different clinical and biologic characteristics. This difference is most marked in the comparison of Bowen's disease/erythroplasia of Queyrat versus bowenoid papulosis. It has been argued that while Bowen's disease and erythroplasia of Queyrat may have different clinical presentations, they are identical or nearly so in clinical course, histopathologic features, and treatment and so should be regarded as one clinicopathologic entity[25].

The unifying designations of penile intraepithelial neoplasia[25] or carcinoma in situ (CIS)[24,26] have been forwarded for Bowen's disease and erythroplasia of Queyrat. In contrast, bowenoid papulosis is an indolent condition of multicentric small papules usually occurring on the shaft of the penis of sexually active, young adults[6,19,20,23,24]. Spontaneous regression is reported as a common occurrence. This diagnosis is a clinicopathologic one. If a biopsy shows carcinoma in situ-like features, with this clinical presentation, bowenoid papulosis should be suspected[24,27].

Grossly, *carcinoma in situ* of the penis may present as a shiny, erythematous, velvety, slightly raised 2–35 mm plaque (54%) or multiple (46%) plaques of the glans or prepuce (erythroplasia of Queyrat)[22–24,26] or as scaly, well demarcated, crusty plaques on the glans or shaft (Bowen's disease)[23,24]. By light microscopy, carcinoma in situ exhibits full-thickness atypia of disordered squamous cells in the epithelium (Figure 45.1). The squamous cells exhibit large, pleomorphic hyperchromatic nuclei, multinucleation, dyskeratosis and mitotic figures, which may be found at any level within the epithelium. Minor histologic differences exist between erythroplasia of Queyrat and Bowen's disease[22,23], but these are mainly the result of differing anatomic locations[23] (with erythroplasia of Queyrat occurring more often in a mucocutaneous location) and again, most believe a separation is usually neither possible nor necessary.

Carcinoma in situ is a frequent finding adjacent to the invasive squamous cell carcinoma, particularly of the superficial spreading and multicentric types[2]. Elegant histologic mapping studies have shown the contiguous carcinoma in situ to be a flat lesion with centrifugal

Table 45.1 Histologic classification of malignant neoplasms of the penis

Histologic type			
I.	Epithelial		
	A.	Squamous cell (epidermoid) carcinoma	
		1.	Superficial spreading
		2.	Vertical growth
		3.	Verruciform
		4.	Multicentric
	B.	Basal cell carcinoma	
	C.	Sarcomatoid (spindle cell) carcinoma	
	D.	Adnexal (sebaceous, eccrine)	
	E.	Adenosquamous carcinoma	
	F.	Basaloid carcinoma	
	G.	Merkel cell carcinoma	
II.	Melanocytic		
	A.	Malignant melanoma	
III.	Mesenchymal		
	A.	Leiomyosarcoma	
	B.	Angiosarcoma	
	C.	Kaposi's sarcoma	
	D.	Rhabdomyosarcoma	
	E.	Malignant fibrous histiocytoma	
	F.	Epithelioid sarcoma	
	G.	Fibrosarcoma	
	H.	Malignant peripheral nerve sheath tumor	
IV.	Hematolymphoid		
	A.	Malignant lymphoma	
V.	Secondary neoplasms		
	A.	Metastatic carcinoma (prostate, bladder, colon, kidney, lung)	

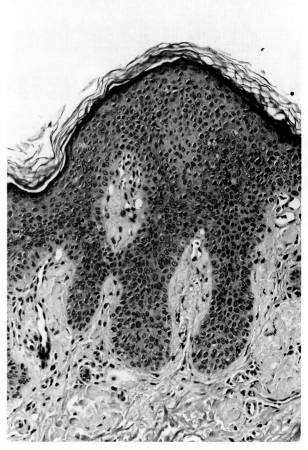

Fig. 45.1 Carcinoma in situ of the penis displaying full-thickness epithelial cell atypia.

growth that extends well beyond the clinically detected mass, corresponding to invasive carcinoma[2]. Mass formation, large lesion size (>2 cm) and ulceration constitute worrying findings for invasion but microscopic examination is necessary for a definitive diagnosis of invasive disease.

Bowenoid papulosis macroscopically usually presents as 2–10 mm papules which may occasionally coalesce to form plaques. Microscopically, the image is quite similar to carcinoma in situ with diffuse intraepithelial squamous cell atypia. Minor morphologic and morphometric differences between bowenoid papulosis and carcinoma in situ have been noted[23] but, for practical purposes, it is usually not possible accurately to distinguish between the two on histologic grounds alone. Human papilloma virus (HPV) DNA, usually type 16 and (less often type 18) has been demonstrated in carcinoma in situ[25,28–30] and bowenoid papulosis[31] and is not useful in the differential diagnosis.

A rare form of intraepithelial malignancy in the penis is *extramammary Paget's disease*. In these cases histological sections of the biopsy demonstrate infiltration of squamous epithelium by single, pale large neoplastic cells or small nests of such cells. These patients are at high risk for harboring an underlying sweat gland carcinoma or associated urothelial carcinoma[32–35].

Invasive squamous cell carcinoma of the penis

Macroscopy

This is usually located on the glans (48%), with a lower frequency of involvement of the prepuce (21%) or concomitant involvement of glans, prepuce and shaft (14%)[23]. Less common sites are glans/prepuce (9%), coronal sulcus alone (6%) and shaft alone (2%)[23]. Macroscopically, the penile squamous cell carcinoma is usually single indurated mass or plaque, with frequent ulceration[6,19]. A variant known as verrucous carcinoma appears cauliflower-like, or fungating and exophytic. This carcinoma should not be mistaken for a condyloma, nor should this malignancy be termed a giant condyloma of Buschke–Lowenstein, a designation that should be abandoned[37].

Microscopy

Microscopically, squamous cell carcinomas of the penis may present with a variety of architectural growth patterns, including superficial spreading (42%), vertical growth (32%), verruciform (including verrucous, warty or condylomatous, and papillary) (18%) or multicentric (8%)[2,9A]. Preliminary data suggest that these types may be predictive of lymph node metastasis[2] and survival[2,36]. Of these four types, the vertical growth carcinomas were the most aggressive, with 82% of patients having inguinal lymph node metastasis[2,36]. At the other end of the spectrum, verrucous carcinomas are slowly growing

malignancies that are locally destructive, with little to no capacity to metastasize[2,37–40]. Most penile squamous cell carcinomas are lower grade[41] and squamous differentiation is readily identified (Figures 45.2 and 45.3). So, squamous pearls (Figure 45.3) and intercellular bridges, which are hallmarks of squamous cells, are easily seen in these tumors. The neoplastic squamous cells invade into stroma as nests and cords, and this invasion typically elicits a fibrogenic and inflammatory cell response (Figures 45.3 + 45.4)[19]. Verrucous carcinomas invade as broad, club-shaped downgrowths and a deep biopsy is needed to facilitate establishment of the histologic diagnosis. The number of mitotic figures in penile squamous carcinomas is related to histological grade, where well differentiated cancers have rare mitoses and poorly differentiated tumors have numerous mitoses[23]. Increasing tumor cell nuclear atypia is also evident with increasing histologic grade[23].

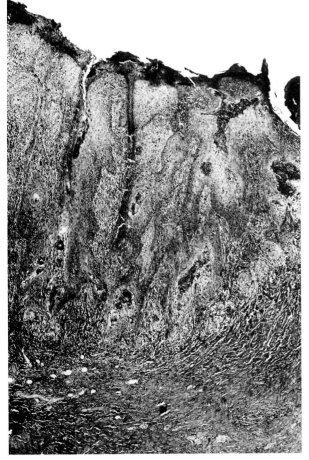

Fig. 45.2 Invasive penile squamous cell carcinoma with irregular lamina propria extension and a prominent inflammatory cell response.

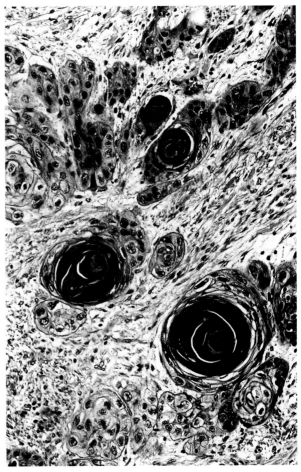

Fig. 45.3 Invasive squamous cell carcinoma with keratin pearl formation.

509

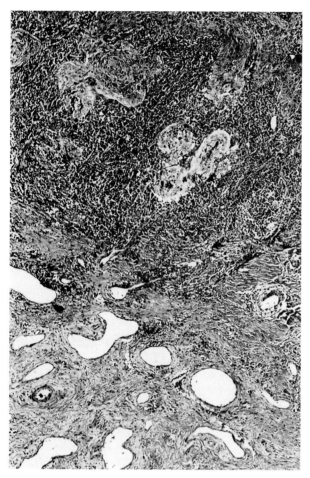

Fig. 45.4   Invasion of penile carcinoma of glans into corpus spongiosum, an indication of pathologic stage T2 disease.

Table 45.2   Penile squamous cell carcinoma histologic grade and incidence of inguinal lymph node metastasis

Study	Grade*	Lymph node metastasis	
Solsona *et al.*[43]	G1	7/36	(19%)
	G2	15/23	(65%)
	G3	6/7	(86%)
Fraley *et al.*[51]	G1	1/19	(5%)
	G2	5/19	(26%)
	G3	16/16	(100%)
Horenblas *et al.*[52]	G1	17/59	(29%)
	G2	13/28	(46%)
	G3	9/11	(82%)
Villavicencio *et al.*[36]	G1	0/3	(0%)
	G2	5/13	(39%)
	G3	8/10	(80%)

* G1 = grade 1 of 3, well differentiated
  G2 = grade 2 of 3, moderately differentiated
  G3 = grade 3 of 3, poorly differentiated

Prognostic factors

The most important pathologic prognostic factors for penile squamous cell carcinoma are pathologic stage and histologic grade, with stage being of primary importance. Size and site of primary tumor, morphologic patterns of growth, histologic subtypes, mitotic rate, and vascular invasion[40A] can also help predict metastasis[9A]. Carcinomas of the coronal sulcus are most aggressive, carcinomas of the glans are intermediate, and carcinomas of the foreskin are in a better prognostic category[9A].

In several series published from 1955 to 1973, a lack of correlation between histologic grade and survival was noted[38]. However, most studies, including more contemporary series, have documented an association between grade and depth of infiltration, inguinal lymph node metastasis and survival[2,35,36,41–53]. Several different grading schemes have been utilized, including three-tiered (well vs. moderately vs. poorly differentiated), four-tiered,[41] and a combined grading staging system[48]. Currently, the

three-tiered one is commonly used. The relationship between three-tiered grade and the likelihood of nodal metastasis is provided in Table 45.2. While there is an increased risk of inguinal lymph node metastasis with increasing grade of the primary tumor, it is essential to recognize that up to 29% of well differentiated (G1) carcinomas spread to inguinal lymph nodes.

Pathologic stage information acquired by assessment of extent of the primary tumor (T stage) and metastatic spread is vital for patient management. Penile squamous cell carcinoma initially invades locally into subepithelial connective tissues (T1 disease), with subsequent contiguous spread into the corpus spongiosum (Figure 45.4) or cavernosum (stage T2 disease). In the glans, there is initial extension into the 2 to 3 mm lamina propria (T1), followed by invasion of the corpus spongiosum (T2). For tumors located on the body or shaft, invasion proceeds in order through the dermis, the dartos (a discontinuous layer of smooth muscle), Buck's fascia, tunica albuginea, and into the corpora cavernosum[54]. Buck's fascia, a fibroelastic membrane that encases the corpora cavernosa and corpus spongiosum[54], provides an initial barrier to invasion of the corpora. In T3 malignancy, tumor invades the urethra or prostate, while in T4 disease, other adjacent structures are invaded[55]. Histologic assessment for the presence and extent of invasion should be made in biopsies taken prior to treatment and in partial and total penectomy specimens. Depth of invasion and grade both have an impact on the likelihood of detection of inguinal lymph node metastasis and the distinction between pathologic stage Tis (carcinoma in situ)/T1 cancer versus T2 or greater disease is important for management of inguinal nodes[42].

Histopathologic assessment of metastasis is also critical for accurate staging. In particular, microscopic examination of sections of inguinal lymph nodes is valuable, since only about 50% of patients with palpable lymphadenopathy have histologic evidence of carcinoma in lymph node tissue[6]. The remaining patients have enlarged lymph nodes on the basis of reactive lymphoid hyperplasia or lymphadenitis. The microscopic evaluation of surgically removed inguinal lymph nodes should entail an accurate count of the number of nodes positive for malignancy, since this is related to patient survival, with an important demarcation between one to two nodes involved versus greater than two nodes positive[42]. It is also important for the surgical pathologist specifically to note whether microscopic extranodal extension by carcinoma into surrounding soft tissue is present, since this is an adverse prognostic finding[56,57]. In more advanced disease, metastases are observed in pelvic lymph nodes. Hematogenous spread with clinically detectable visceral metastatic deposits is distinctly uncommon at the time of initial presentation, with an incidence of less than 2%[23]. Distant metastases to liver, lung, bone and brain have been reported[23,42,58,59].

References

1. Soria JC, Fizazi K, Piron D et al. Squamous cell carcinoma of the penis – multivariate analysis of prognostic factors and natural history in a monocentric study with a conservative policy. Ann Oncol 1997; **8**:1089–1098.
2. Cubilla AL, Barreto J, Caballero C, Ayala G, Riveros M. Pathologic features of epidermoid carcinoma of the penis. A prospective study of 66 cases. Am J Surg Pathol 1993; **17**:753–763.
3. Narayana AS, Olney LE, Loenig SA, Weimar GW, Culp DA. Carcinoma of the penis. Analysis of 217 cases. Cancer 1982; **49**:2185–2191.
4. Merrin CE. Cancer of the penis. Cancer 1980; **45**:1973–1979.
5. Nelson RP, Derrick FC, Allen WR. Epidermoid carcinoma of the penis. Br J Urol 1982; **56**:172–175.
6. Lucia MS, Miller GJ. Histopathology of malignant lesions of the penis. Urol Clin N Am 1992; **19**:227–246.
7. Pow-Sang J, Ojeda J, Ramirez G, Olivares L, Benarente V, Sanchez L. Carcinoma of the penis: analysis of 192 consecutive cases at the Instituto Nacional de Enfermedades Neoplasicas. Int Adv Surg Oncol 1979; **2**:201–221.
8. Hayashi T, Tsuda N, Shimada O et al. A clinicopathologic study of tumors and tumor-like lesions of the penis. Acta Pathol Jpn 1990; **40**:343–351.
9. Heyns CF, Van Vollenhoven P, Steenkamp JW, Allen FJ. Cancer of the penis – a review of 50 patients. S Afr J Surg 1997; **35**:120–124.
9A. Young RN, Srigley JR, Amin MB, Ulbright TM, Cubilla AL. The penis. In: Tumors of the Prostate Gland, Seminal Vesicles, Male Urethra, and penis. Atlas of Tumor Pathology. Armed Forces Institute of Pathology, Washington DC, 2000, pp. 403–488.
10. Khezri AA, Dounis A, Roberts JBM. Primary malignant melanoma of the penis. Two cases and review of the literature. Br J Urol 1979; **51**:147–150.
11. Primus G, Soyer HP, Smolle J, Mertl G, Pummer K, Kerl H. Early 'invasive' malignant melanoma of the glans penis and the male urethra. Eur Urol 1990; **18**:156–159.
12. Rashid A-MM, Williams RM, Horton LW. Malignant melanoma of penis and male urethra. Urology 1993; **41**:470–471.
13. Dehner LP, Smith BH. Soft tissue tumors of the penis. A clinicopathologic study of 46 cases. Cancer 1970; **25**:1431–1447.
14. Blasius S, Brinkschmidt C, Bier B et al. Extraskeletal myxoid chondrosarcoma of the penis. J Urol Pathol 1995; **3**:73–80.
15. Gonzalez-Campora R, Nogales FF, Lerma E, Navarro A, Matilla A. Lymphoma of the penis. J Urol 1981; **126**:270–271.
16. Bosch PC, Forbes KA, Kollin J, Golji H, Miller JB. Secondary carcinoma of the penis. J Urol 1984; **132**:990–991.
17. Belville WD, Cohen JA. Secondary penile malignancies: the spectrum of presentation. J Surg Oncol 1992; **51**: 134–137.
18. Robey EL, Schellhammer PF. Four cases of metastases to the penis and a review of the literature. J Urol 1984; **132**: 992–994.
19. Murphy WM. Diseases of the penis and scrotum. In: Murphy WM (Ed.) Urological pathology. W.B. Saunders Co, Philadelphia, 1997, pp. 401–429.
20. Cubilla AL, Barreto J, Ayala G. The penis. In: Sternberg SS (Ed.) Diagnostic surgical pathology. Raven Press, New York, 1994, pp. 1949–1973.
21. Cubilla AL. In consultation. Carcinoma of the penis. Mod Pathol 1995; **8**: 116–118.
22. Graham JH, Helwing EB. Erythroplasia of Queyrat: a clinicopathologic and histochemical study. Cancer 1973; **32**:1396–1414.
23. Ro JY, Amin MB, Ayala AG. Penis and scrotum. In: Bostwick DG, Eble JN (eds) Urologic surgical pathology. Mosby, St Louis, 1997, pp. 674–722.
24. Gerber GS. Carcinoma in situ of the penis. J Urol 1994; **151**:829–833.
25. Aynaud O, Ionesco M, Barrasso R. Penile intraepithelial neoplasia. Specific clinical features correlate with histologic and virologic findings. Cancer 1994; **74**:1762–1767.
26. Kaye V, Zhang G, Dehner LP, Fraley EE. Carcinoma in situ of penis. Is distinction between erythroplasia of Queyrat and Bowen's disease relevant? Urology 1990; **36**:479–482.
27. Su CK, Shipley WU. Bowenoid papulosis: a benign lesion of the shaft of the penis misdiagnosed as squamous carcinoma. J Urol 1997; **157**:1361–1362.
28. Demeter LM, Stoler MH, Bonnez W et al. Penile intrepithelial neoplasia: clinical presentation and an analysis of the physical state of human papillomavirus DNA. J Infect Dis 1993; **168**:38–46.
29. Cupp MR, Malek RS, Goellner JR, Smith TF, Espy MJ. The detection of human papillomavirus deoxyribonucleic acid in intraepithelial, in situ, verrucous and invasive carcinoma of the penis. J Urol 1995; **154**:1024–1029.
30. Della Torre G, Donghi K, Longoni A et al. HPV DNA in intraepithelial neoplasia and carcinoma of the vulva and penis. Diagn Mol Pathol 1992; **1**:25–30.
31. Obalek S, Jablonska S, Beaudenon S, Walczak L, Orth G. Bowenoid papulosis of the male and female genitalia: risk of cervical neoplasia. J Am Acad Dermatol 1986; **14**:433–444.
32. Smith DJ, Hamdy FC, Evans JWH, Falzon M, Chapple CR. Paget's disease of the glans penis: an unusual urological malignancy. Eur Urol 1994; **25**:316–319.
33. Stevenson JS, Lee RE, Maize JC. Epidermotropic urothelial carcinoma involving the glans penis. Arch Dermatol 1985; **121**:532–534.
34. Kvist E, Osmundsen PE, Sjolin K-E. Primary Paget's disease of the penis. Case report. Scand J Urol Nephrol 1992; **26**:187–190.
35. Mitsudo S, Nakanishi I, Koss LG. Paget's disease of the penis and adjacent skin. Its association with fatal sweat gland carcinoma. Arch Pathol Lab Med 1981; **105**:518–520.
36. Villavicencio H, Rubio-Briones J, Regalada R, Chéchile G, Algaba F, Palou J. Grade, local stage and growth pattern as prognostic factors in carcinoma of the penis. Eur Urol 1997; **32**:442–447.
37. Johnson DE, Lo RK, Srigley J, Ayala AG. Verrucous carcinoma of the penis. J Urol 1985; **133**:216–218.
38. Seixas ALC, Ornellas AA, Marota A, Wisnescky A, Campos F, de Moraes JR. Verrucous carcinoma of the penis: retrospective analysis of 32 cases. J Urol 1994; **152**:1476–1479.
39. Lowe D, McKee PH. Verrucous carcinoma of the penis (Buschke–Lowenstein tumor): a clinicopathological study. Br J Urol 1983; **55**:427–429.
40. McKee PH, Lowe D, Haigh RJ. Penile verrucous carcinoma. Histopathol 1983; **7**:897–906.
40A. Lopes A, Hidalgo GS, Kowalski LP, Torloni H, Rossi BM, Fonseca FP. Prognostic factors in carcinoma of the penis: multivariate analysis of 145 patients treated with amputation and lymphadenectomy. J Urol 1996; **156**:1639–1642.

41. Maiche AG, Pyrhönen S, Karkinen M. Histological grading of squamous cell carcinoma of the penis: A new scoring system. *Br J Urol* 1991; **87**:522–526.

42. Lynch DF Jr, Schellhammer PF. Tumors of the penis. In: Walsh PC, Retik AB, Vaughan ED Jr, Wein AJ (eds) *Campbell's urology.* W.B. Saunders Company, Philadelphia, 1998, pp. 2453–2485.

43. Solsona E, Iborra I, Ricós JV *et al.* Corpus cavernosum invasion and tumor grade in the prediction of lymph node condition in penile carcinoma. *Eur Urol* 1992; **22**:115–118.

44. Horenblas S, van Tinteren H. Squamous cell carcinoma of the penis. IV. Prognostic factors of survival: Analysis of tumor, nodes and metastasis classification system. *J Urol* 1994; **151**:1239–1243.

45. Adeyoju AB, Thornhill J, Corr J, Grainger R, McDermott TED, Butler M. Prognostic factors in squamous cell carcinoma of the penis and implications for management. *Br J Urol* 1997; **80**:937–939.

46. Heyns CF, van Vollenhoven P, Steenkamp JW, Allen FJ, van Velden DJJ. Carcinoma of the penis–appraisal of a modified tumor-staging system. *Br J Urol* 1997; **80**:307–312.

47. Sarin R, Norman AR, Steel GG, Horwich A. Treatment results and prognostic factors in 101 men treated for squamous carcinoma of the penis. *Int J Rad Oncol Biol Phys* 1997; **38**:713–722.

48. Lindegard JC, Nielsen OS, Lundbeck FA, Mamsen A, Studstrup HN, Vondermaase H. A retrospective analysis of 82 cases of cancer of the penis. *Br J Urol* 1996; **77**:883–890.

49. Theodorescu D, Russo P, Zhang ZF, Morash C, Fair WR. Outcomes of initial surveillance of invasive squamous cell carcinoma of the penis and negative nodes. *J Urol* 1996; **155**:1626–1631.

50. Ornellas AA, Seixas ALC, Marota A, Wisnescky A, Campos F, de Moraes JR. Surgical treatment of invasive squamous cell carcinoma of the penis. Retrospective analysis of 350 cases. *J Urol* 1994; **151**:1244–1249.

51. Fraley EE, Zhang G, Manivel C, Niehans GA. The role of ilioinguinal lymphadenectomy and significance of histological differentiation in treatment of carcinoma of the penis. *J Urol* 1989; **142**:1478–1482.

52. Horenblas S, van Tinteren H, Delemarre JFM *et al.* Squamous cell carcinoma of the penis: III. Treatment of regional lymph nodes. *J Urol* 1993; **149**: 492–497.

53. McDougal WS. Carcinoma of the penis: improved survival by early regional lymphadenectomy based on the histological grade and depth of the primary lesion. *J Urol* 1995; **154**:1364–1366.

54. Barreto J, Caballero C, Cubilla A. Penis. In: Sternberg SS (Ed.) *Histology for pathologists* (2nd edn) Lippincott-Raven, Philadelphia, 1997, pp. 1039–1050.

55. Sobin LH, Wittekind Ch (eds) *TNM classification of malignant tumors* (5th edn). John Wiley and Sons, Inc., New York, 1997, pp. 167–169.

56. Ravi R. Correlation between extent of nodal involvement and survival following groin dissection for carcinoma of the penis. *Br J Urol* 1993; **72**:817–819.

57. Svinivas V, Morse MJ, Herr HW *et al.* Penile cancer: relation of extent of nodal metastasis to survival. *J Urol* 1987; **137**:880–882.

58. Wajsman Z, Moore RH, Merrin CE *et al.* Surgical treatment of penile cancer: a follow-up report. *Cancer* 1977; **40**:1697–1701.

59. Johnson DE, Fuerst DE, Ayala AG. Cancer of the penis: experience with 153 cases. *Urology* 1973; **1**:404–408.

46 Surgical management

Algorithm

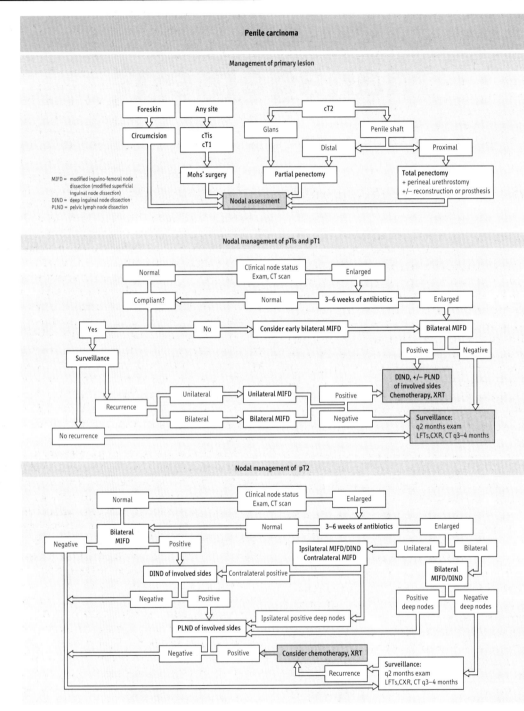

Penile carcinoma

Management of primary lesion

		cT2	

Foreskin — Circumcision

Any site — cTis cT1 — Mohs' surgery

Glans — Partial penectomy

Distal

Penile shaft

Proximal

Total penectomy + perineal urethrostomy +/– reconstruction or prosthesis

MIFD = modified inguino-femoral node dissection (modified superficial inguinal node dissection)
DIND = deep inguinal node dissection
PLND = pelvic lymph node dissection

Nodal assessment

Nodal management of pTis and pT1

Normal — Clinical node status Exam, CT scan — Enlarged

Compliant? — Normal — 3–6 weeks of antibiotics — Enlarged

Yes / No — Consider early bilateral MIFD — Bilateral MIFD

Surveillance

Positive / Negative

DIND, +/– PLND of involved sides Chemotherapy, XRT

Recurrence — Unilateral — Unilateral MIFD — Positive

Bilateral — Bilateral MIFD — Negative

No recurrence

Surveillance: q2 months exam LFTs,CXR, CT q3–4 months

Nodal management of pT2

Normal — Clinical node status Exam, CT scan — Enlarged

Bilateral MIFD — Normal — 3–6 weeks of antibiotics — Enlarged

Negative / Positive

Ipsilateral MIFD/DIND Contralateral MIFD — Unilateral — Bilateral

Bilateral MIFD/DIND

DIND of involved sides — Contralateral positive

Positive deep nodes / Negative deep nodes

Negative / Positive

Ipsilateral positive deep nodes

PLND of involved sides

Negative / Positive — Consider chemotherapy, XRT

Surveillance: q2 months exam LFTs,CXR, CT q3–4 months

Recurrence

46.1 Surgical management

J Petros and P D LaFontaine

Surgical management of carcinoma of the penis remains important in the initial diagnosis, staging, local control and assessment and treatment of regional lymph nodes. Indeed, squamous cell carcinoma of the penis remains one of the few cancers where regional lymphadenectomy may be potentially curative. Until effective systemic therapies exist for patients with advanced disease, timely and appropriate surgical management will remain the mainstay of therapy.

Evaluation and treatment of primary lesion

There are several treatment options available for management of the primary lesion. Which treatment modality is most appropriate depends on tumor stage, location, size and grade. The traditional local approach to squamous cell carcinoma of the penis has included partial or total penectomy. While this may be appropriate therapy for some patients, it is almost uniformly a mutilating procedure and accompanied by severe emotional and psychological trauma. Fortunately for many patients with penile cancer there are now a variety of penile conserving treatments available that may be appropriate for carefully selected patients. It is hoped that with the knowledge that penile conserving therapies are available and efficacious that men will be less reluctant to present for early evaluation of penile lesions.

Circumcision and local excision are the most conservative treatments for the primary lesion. Unfortunately, it is likely only appropriate for patients with small, superficial, non-invasive tumors confined to the prepuce where a 1 to 2 cm tumor-free margin can be obtained. Indeed, local recurrence rates from 18% to 50% have been reported with circumcision and local excision alone[1–4]. The majority of these recurrences occur within 2 years and are easily controlled, though worsening of prognosis and long-term recurrences have been reported[2,4–6]. Therefore, long-term follow up on patients treated with local excision or circumcision is necessary.

Laser therapy has evolved over the past 15 years as a means of conservatively treating benign, pre-malignant and malignant lesions on the penis. Laser therapy using a combination of CO_2, Nd:YAG and KTP lasers has been used to successfully treat small low-stage tumors. Potential advantages of this approach include preservation of normal structure and function while locally eradicating the tumor. Several disadvantages do exist though. It may be difficult to assess the depth of tissue destruction using the laser and there is no histologic confirmation of the depth of tissue invasion or the status of the tumor margin. It is therefore imperative adequately to stage these patients with multiple deep biopsies prior to laser therapy. Nonetheless, lasers have been used successfully on carefully selected patients.

Carcinoma in situ and penile intraepithelial neoplasia (PIN) have been reported to be very responsive to treatment with the Nd:YAG and CO_2 lasers. Cardamakis reports a 96% success rate when the CO_2 laser was combined with topical 5FU in the treatment of PIN III, while several other investigators report a similar success rate using the CO_2 and Nd:YAG laser at a power setting of 15 to 38 Watts treating Tis lesions[7–10]. Lasers have also been used to treat carefully selected T1 lesions. Malloy et al., using a Nd:YAG laser with a focusing handpiece and iced saline, reported on the successful treatment of 6/9 small T1 lesions[9]. The iced saline was used to provide surface cooling, prevent tissue carbonization and allow for a 4 to 6 mm depth of penetration. Several other investigators have used the CO_2 or Nd:YAG laser after first performing circumcision and surgical debulking and have reported success rates from 82–100% treating T1 lesions less than 3.5 cm[2,8,10,11]. The wounds are allowed to heal by secondary intention over a period of 6 to 8 weeks. Other complications are very uncommon. Careful prolonged follow up is important for these patients as recurrence rates up to 50% have been reported in T1 patients, with some patients developing nodal metastasis[5]. Laser therapy is not recommended for T1 lesions larger than 3.5 cm or T2 or greater lesions as the chance of local failure increases substantially[2,5].

The standard approach to squamous cell carcinoma of the penis not amenable to circumcision, local excision or laser therapy, has been total penectomy or partial penectomy with a 2 cm margin of normal tissue. It has been shown that simple wedge excision of tumors on the glans has an unacceptably high local recurrence rate of 40%[4]. This is undoubtedly due to residual carcinoma being left behind at the site of excision. Mohs has shown that skin cancers tend to grow in a contiguous fashion and tend to send out silent extensions, and this correlates with the known poor clinical assessment of tumor margins[12]. However, radical surgery to ensure negative tumor margins requires disfiguring surgery with alterations in sexual function, micturitional capacity and body image. Frederic Mohs introduced microsurgery in 1941. The idea behind microsurgery is to excise the cancerous tissue layer by layer, examining the underside of each layer microscopically to determine the extent of residual cancer. Further resections are then undertaken where residual cancer is present until there is no more cancer at the margin of resection. The benefits of tumor excision under microscopic control are twofold. First, there is maximal assurance that the tumor has been locally eradicated. Secondly, there is maximal preservation of normal tissue and function. The disadvantages of Mohs micrographic technique are that it is time consuming and requires special training to ensure correct performance.

There are two techniques used for Mohs micrographic surgery: the fresh tissue technique and the fixed tissue technique. Historically, the fixed tissue technique was initially used. This is good for lesions that involve the erectile bodies because it cuts down on bleeding by fixing the tissues prior to excision. However, it is painful and time consuming and has been largely replaced by the fresh tissue technique. The fresh tissue technique is an outpatient procedure that starts with obtaining adequate sedation and local anesthesia. The tumor mass is then surgically debulked and a histologic diagnosis obtained if not done previously. A beveled incision is then made circumferentially around the defect created to a depth of 1 to 3 mm. This tissue is then prepared for horizontal frozen section analysis, which allows for review of 100% of the surgical margin, taking great care to maintain the correct orientation of the specimen. Special dyes may be used to mark the edges. The slides are then reviewed and a special map is made of the horizontally oriented frozen sections detailing the area of any remaining cancer. Repeat excision in the appropriate areas is then done using the same frozen section analysis until no more tumor is identified in the specimen. The surgical defect is usually left to heal by secondary intention.

The frozen section technique is also an outpatient procedure that involves surgically debulking the tumor after obtaining adequate anesthesia. A zinc chloride fixative paste is then applied to the surgical defect after dichloroacetic acid has been applied to a 2 mm zone around the tumor, facilitating penetration of the fixative through the epidermis. An occlusive dressing is then applied and the fixative is left in place for 24 hours. The patient then returns for excision similar to that for the fresh tissue technique. Frozen section analysis is then done as in the fresh tissue technique, and the zinc chloride fixative paste is applied to any areas of remaining tumor. The patient returns 24 hours later for excision and this process is continued until tumor is no longer identifiable in the frozen sections. This may require several outpatient visits.

Results of Mohs micrographic surgery for treating the primary lesion of penile cancer have been encouraging to date for carefully selected patients. In Mohs experience a total of 35 patients with primarily Jackson I and II squamous cell carcinoma of the penis were treated with micrographic surgery. They reported a 94% local 5 year control rate and an 86% and 62% overall 5 year cure rate for Jackson stage I and II, respectively[13]. In a similar study Brown evaluated 11 patients with squamous cell carcin-

oma of the penis with clinically negative nodes. He noted a local recurrence in only one of his patients but almost 40% subsequently developed groin nodal metastasis[14]. Partial penectomy remains the gold standard for the treatment of T3, T2 and large T1 (greater than 3.5 cm) penile cancers, as recurrence rates of up to 32% have been reported for large T1 lesions treated with penile conserving therapy[2]. In addition, some investigators do not recommend treating grade 3 lesions with penile conserving therapy[2]. Recurrence rates for partial penectomy with large T1 and T2 lesions run from 0% to 6%[2,3,15]. The goals of partial penectomy are to achieve complete tumor eradication with a 2 cm proximal margin of normal tissue while leaving adequate proximal stump length, usually 3 cm, to allow for micturition in the standing position. We therefore routinely obtain intra-operative frozen sections to assess for adequacy or surgical margins. If we are unable to achieve a 2 cm proximal tumor free margin, if the lesion is located proximally on the shaft of the penis or if micturition in the upright position will not be possible then we perform total penectomy with perineal urethrostomy.

Partial penectomy

We recommend starting the patient on a broad spectrum oral antibiotic 3 to 5 days prior to surgery as these lesions are frequently ulcerated and infected. A cleansing enema is given the night before surgery to prevent post-operative fecal soiling of the perineum. Intravenous broad spectrum antibiotics are administered perioperatively to minimize the chance of wound infection. It is important to discuss with the patient all surgical options, including total penectomy and perineal urethrostomy, prior to surgery.

Total penectomy

If a 2 cm proximal tumor free margin and a 3 cm stump to allow standing micturition can not be achieved then total penectomy is indicated.

Post-operative management and complications

The penrose drains are removed on post-operative day 2 or 3. The urethral catheter is removed on post-operative day 5. Early complications include wound infections and hematomas which may be treated by open drainage and secondary healing. Urinary extravasation is a rare complication unless the urethrostomy is not watertight. This is best treated by re-inserting the urethral catheter for several days. Long-term complications include urethral stenosis which can be managed by self-dilation once it is recognized.

Evaluation and management of regional nodes

The evaluation and management of the regional lymph nodes in patients with squamous cell carcinoma of the penis remains controversial. Currently non-invasive means of assessing lymph nodes are inaccurate. MRI has superior soft tissue visualization and can define the extent of local invasion into the penis. However, both CT and MRI rely on size to evaluate regional lymph nodes and thus suffer the same problems as clinical staging, with high false-positive and false-negative rates. The clinical evaluation of nodal status is also inaccurate, with 30% to 50% of patients presenting with clinically palpable regional adenopathy having inflammatory and not metastatic adenopathy[16–21]. Conversely, 10% to 40% of patients with clinically normal groins will be found to harbor micrometastatic disease[4,16–21]. Some authors currently recommend a 6 week course of oral antibiotics followed by lymph node dissection only if palpable adenopathy persists or if palpable adenopathy develops during surveillance follow up[1,6]. This is obviously advantageous to the majority of patients with clinically normal groins who do not harbor micrometastatic disease as it spares them the significant morbidity of ilioinguinal lymph node dissection. However, numerous studies have shown that there is a correlation between survival and number of positive lymph nodes[5,21]. In addition, several investigators have shown that patients with clinically normal groins who have immediate lymphadenectomy have improved survival rates over those who have delayed lymphadenectomy when nodal disease develops[16,19,22,23]. This indicates that a watch and wait policy in patients with clinically negative groins may not be completely satisfactory because we are missing the opportunity to help the clinically understaged patients who harbor micrometastatic disease and will benefit from immediate lymphadenectomy.

There is however significant morbidity associated with the standard ilioinguinal lymph node dissection, with morbidity rates of 30–50% and mortality rates of up to 3% reported[3,21,24–28]. The controversy thus arises in distinguishing which patients with clinically negative groins will most likely benefit from immediate ilioinguinal lymph node dissection and in which patients this represents needless over treatment with the attendant morbidity and mortality risks.

Recent work has shown a correlation between grade, stage and likelihood of lymph node metastasis. Several investigators have demonstrated a 0% to 5% chance of having or developing regional lymph node disease in patients with T1, G1 primary tumors[20–22,29]. Based on these findings, it would seem safe to assign patients with T1, G1 disease to close clinical follow up and spare them the morbidity of lymph node dissection. Obviously this only applies to patients who can be relied upon to keep their follow up appointments.

Based on the work of Riveros and Cabanas the concept of sentinel lymph node biopsy was developed as a means of determining which patients required standard ilioinguinal lymph node dissection[25,30]. Cabanas describes a technique of sentinel lymph node biopsy where the lymph nodes around the superficial epigastric vein at the saphenous vein junction are removed. In his initial study he found no patient to have lymph node disease whose sentinel lymph node was also not involved, and he reported a 90% 5 year survival rate in patients whose sentinel lymph node was not involved. However, there have since been several reports that have demonstrated the unreliability of sentinel lymph node biopsy as a means of assessing the regional lymph nodes, and its use is no longer recommended[31–33].

In response to the unreliability of sentinel lymph node biopsy in assessing the regional lymph nodes and in light of the significant morbidity and mortality associated with standard ilioinguinal lymph node dissection, Catalona described the modified inguinal lymphadenectomy in 1988[34]. This operation differs from Daseler's classic description of inguinal lymphadenectomy in that the skin incision is reduced, the subcutaneous tissue superficial to Scarpa's fascia is preserved, the dissection does not include the nodal tissue lateral to the femoral artery or inferior to the fossa ovalis, the saphenous vein is preserved and the sartorius muscle is not transposed[34]. Experience with the modified inguinal lymphadenectomy has been encouraging to date. In two separate studies Parra and Colberg et al. report on 21 patients who had a modified bilateral inguinal lymph node dissection. No patient with an initially negative lymph node dissection developed regional nodal disease during follow up[35,36]. All positive nodes have been found in the superomedial quadrant of the dissection. Complications were significantly less than with standard inguinal lymphadenectomy. Prolonged lymph leaks were noted in 10% of patients, all of which resolved spontaneously. No patient developed persistent troubling lymphedema or skin flap necrosis requiring a second procedure. Although we remain optimistic about the utility of modified bilateral inguinal lymphadenectomy, it should be noted that there is at least one report in the literature documenting the inaccuracy of modified bilateral inguinal lymphadenectomy. Lopes reports two patients out of 13 who had retrocrural recurrences following negative modified inguinal lymphadenectomy[37]. Therefore, although we continue to recommend modified bilateral inguinal lymphadenectomy for assessment of regional nodes, more studies will be needed to assess its long-term value. We currently recommend modified bilateral inguinal lymphadenectomy for patients with invasive disease (T2 or greater) and

517

for patients with medium- or high-grade tumors (G2 or 3) who have clinically negative nodes or whose nodes normalize after 6 weeks of antibiotics.

Patients with persistent clinically suspicious nodes after antibiotic therapy have been shown to benefit from immediate ilioinguinal lymph node dissection[30]. We therefore continue to recommend complete ilioinguinal lymphadenectomy for these patients as well as those patients found to have inguinal metastasis during modified dissection.

Post-operative management and complications

Closed suction drains are left post-operatively in the groins and iliac regions until drainage is less than 50 cc per day. The patient is maintained at bed rest for 7 days during which time sequential compression hose are used. Significant morbidity rates of 30% to 50% have been reported as well as up to a 3% mortality rate from the classic inguinal lymphadenectomy[3,21,25,28]. The most common complications are skin flap necrosis, wound infection, lymphocele, chronic lymphedema, deep vein thrombosis and hemorrhage from erosion into the femoral vessels. Skin flap necrosis can be minimized by meticulous attention to handling the skin edges intraoperatively and by taking care not to create skin flaps that are too thin. The management of skin flap necrosis depends on the extent of necrosis. Most can be handled with dressing changes. Rarely a skin or myocutaneous graft may be needed. Wound infections are best drained and allowed to heal secondarily. Lymphoceles should be aspirated initially. If they recur they may require percutaneous drainage. Chronic lymphedema may occur in 30% of patients[25,37]. If severe enough it can be managed with compression stockings, elevation or diuretics. Deep vein thrombosis can be minimized with post-operative compression hose. Some authors recommend post-operative minidose heparin[38]. Major hemorrhage from erosion into the femoral vessels is rare now that the sartorius is transposed over the femoral vessels.

Management of enlarged or ulcerated groin nodes

Squamous cell carcinoma of the penis is characterized by aggressive local invasion and often will present with nodal erosion through the skin in advanced cases. Although the prognosis for patients who present at this stage is poor with few patients surviving more than 1 year, several palliative measures may be employed[16]. When inguinal nodes ulcerate through the skin a standard inguinal lymphadenectomy with excision of the involved skin may be performed. Coverage for the large tissue defects left after such radical excisions may be achieved with a variety of myocutaneous flaps[39-42].

Conclusions

Squamous cell carcinoma of the penis remains a rare disease with surgical management continuing to be the mainstay of therapy. Several options are available for treatment of the primary lesion, including circumcision, local excision, laser therapy, Mohs micrographic surgery and partial and total penectomy. Selection of therapy for the primary lesion depends on the size, stage, location and grade of the primary lesion. Management of regional nodes remains controversial. It is clear that patients with clinically involved groin nodes benefit from ilioinguinal lymph node dissection. Controversy continues to exist for the optimal management of invasive lesions with clinically uninvolved nodes. We currently recommend modified bilateral inguinal lymph node dissection with extended inguinal lymph node dissection and iliac node dissection if nodal metastasis are present. It is hoped that with further experience with this rare malignancy the optimal management protocol will become clear.

References

1. Narayana AS, Olney LE, Loening SA, Weimar GW, Culp DA. Carcinoma of the penis. Analysis of 219 cases. *Cancer* 1982;**49**:2185–2191.
2. Horenblas S, van Tinteren H, Delemare JFM, Boon TA, Moonen LMF, Lustig V. Squamous cell carcinoma of the penis. II. Treatment of the primary tumor. *J Urol* 1992;**147**:1533–1538.
3. McDougal WS, Kirchner FK Jr, Edwards RH, Killion LT. Treatment of carcinoma of the penis: the case for primary lymphadenectomy. *J Urol* 1986;**136**:38–41.
4. Hanash GJ, Furlow WL, Utz DC, Harrison EG Jr. Carcinoma of the penis: a clinicopathologic study. *J Urol* 1970;**104**:291–297.
5. Brkovic D, Kalbe T, Dorsam J *et al*. Surgical treatment of invasive penile cancer – the Heidelberg experience from 1968–1994. *Eur Urol* 1997;**31**:339–342.
6. Lindegaard JC, Nielsen OS, Lundbeck FA, Mamsen A, Studstrup HN, von Der Maase H. A retrospective analysis of 82 cases of cancer of the penis. *Br J Urol* 1996;**77**:883–890.
7. Cardamakis E, Relakis K, Ginopoulos P *et al*. Treatment of penile intraepithelial neoplasia (PIN) with interferon alpha-2a, CO_2 laser (vaporization) and 5-fluorouracil 5% (5-FU). *Eur J Gynaecol Oncol* 1997;**18**:410–413.
8. Windahl T, Hellsten S. Laser treatment of localized squamous cell carcinoma of the penis. *J Urol* 1995;**154**:1020–1023.
9. Malloy TR, Wein AJ, Carpiniello VL. Carcinoma of the penis treated with neodynium YAG laser. *Urology* 1985;**31**:26–29.
10. Malek RS. Laser treatment of premalignant and malignant squamous cell lesions of the penis. *Lasers Surg Med* 1992;**12**:246–253.
11. Hofstetter A. Lasers in urology. *Lasers Surg Med* 1986;**6**:412–414.
12. Mohs FE, Lathrop TE. Modes of spread of cancer of the skin. *Arch Dermatol Syph* 1952;**66**:427–439.

13. Mohs FE, Snow SN, Larson PO. Mohs micrographic surgery for penile tumors. In: Crawford ED, Das S (eds) *Penile, urethral, and scrotal cancer. Urol Clin N Amer* 1992;**19**:291–304.

14. Brown MD, Zachery CB, Grekin RE *et al.* Penile tumors: Their management by Mohs micrographic surgery. *J Dermatol Surg Oncol* 1987;**13**:1163–1167.

15. Frew IDO, Jefferies JD, Swinney J. Carcinoma of the penis. *Br J Urol* 1967;**39**:398–404.

16. Ornellas AA, Seixas ALC, Marota A, Wisnescky A, Campos F, de Moraes JR. Surgical treatment of invasive squamous cell carcinoma of the penis: Retrospective analysis of 350 cases. *J Urol* 1994;**151**:1244–1249.

17. deKernion JB, Tynberg P, Persky L, Fegen JP. Carcinoma of the penis. *Cancer* 1973;**32**:1256–1262.

18. Hardner GJ, Bhanalaph T, Murphy GP, Albert DJ, Moore RH. Carcinoma of the penis: analysis of therapy in 100 consecutive cases. *J Urol* 1972;**108**:428–430.

19. Wajsman Z, Moore RH, Merrin CE, Murphy GP. Surgical treatment of penile cancer. A follow up report. *Cancer* 1977;**40**:1697–1701.

20. Solsona E, Iborra I, Ricos JV *et al.* Corpus cavernosum invasion and tumor grade in the prediction of lymph node condition in penile carcinoma. *Eur Urol* 1992;**22**:115–118.

21. Horenblas S, van Tinteren H, Delemare JFM, Moonen LMF, Lustig V, van Waardenburg EW. Squamous cell carcinoma of the penis. III. Treatment of regional lymph nodes. *J Urol* 1993;**149**:492–497.

22. Fraley EE, Zhang G, Manivel C, Niehans GA. The role of ilioinguinal lymphadenectomy and significance of histological differentiation in treatment of carcinoma of the penis. *J Urol* 1989;**142**:1478–1482.

23. Johnson DE, Lo RK. Management of regional lymph nodes in penile carcinoma. *Urology* 1984;**24**:308–311.

24. Ravi R. Morbidity following groin dissection for penile carcinoma. *Br J Urol* 1993;**72**:941–945.

25. Cabanas RM. An approach for the treatment of penile carcinoma. *Cancer* 1977;**39**:456–466.

26. Whitmore WF, Vagaiwala MR. Technique of ilioinguinal lymph node dissection for carcinoma of the penis. *Surg Gynecol Obstet* 1984;**159**:573–578.

27. Kuruvilla JT, Garlick FH, Mammen KE. Results of surgical treatment of carcinoma of the penis. *Aust N Z J Surg* 1971;**41**:157–159.

28. Theodorescu D, Russo P, Zhang ZF, Morash C, Fair WR. Outcomes of initial surveillance of invasive squamous cell carcinoma of the penis and negative nodes. *J Urol* 1996;**155**:1626–1631.

29. McDougal WS. Carcinoma of the penis: improved survival by early regional lymphadenectomy based on the histological grade and depth of invasion of the primary lesion. *J Urol* 1995;**154**:1364–1366.

30. Riveros M, Garcia R, Cabanas R. Lymphadenography of the dorsal lymphatics of the penis. *Cancer* 1967;**20**:2026–2031.

31. Wespes E, Simon J, Schulman CC. Cabanas approach: Is sentinel node biopsy reliable for staging penile carcinoma? *Urology* 1986;**28**:278–279.

32. Perinetti E, Crane DB, Catalona WJ. Unreliability of sentinel lymph node biopsy for staging penile carcinoma. *J Urol* 1980;**124**:734–735.

33. Pettaway CA, Pisters LL, Dinney CPN, Jularbal FE, Swanson DA, von Eschenbach AC, Ayala A. Sentinel lymph node dissection for penile carcinoma: The M.D. Anderson cancer center experience. *J Urol* 1995;**154**:1999–2003.

34. Catalona WJ. Modified inguinal lymphadenectomy for carcinoma of the penis with preservation of saphenous veins: technique and preliminary results. *J Urol* 1988;**140**:306–310.

35. Colberg JW, Andriole GL, Catalona W. Long term follow-up of men undergoing modified inguinal lymphadenectomy for carcinoma of the penis. *Br J Urol* 1997;**79**:54–57.

36. Parra RO. Accurate staging of carcinoma of the penis in men with nonpalpable inguinal lymph nodes by modified inguinal lymphadenectomy. *J Urol* 1996;**155**:560–563.

37. Lopes A, Rossi BM, Fonseca FP, Morini S. Unreliability of modified inguinal lymphadenectomy for clinical staging of penile carcinoma. *Cancer* 1996;**77**:2099–2102.

38. Crawford ED, Daneshgari F. Management of regional lymphatic drainage in carcinoma of the penis. In: Crawford ED, Das S (eds). *Penile, urethral, and scrotal cancer. Urol Clin N Amer* 1992;**19**:305–318.

39. Hill HL, Nahai F, Vasconez LO. The tensor fascia lata myocutaneous free flap. *Plast Reconstr Surg* 1978;**61**:517–521.

40. Orticochea M. Musculo-cutaneous flap method: Immediate and heroic substitute for the method of delay. *Br J Plast Surg* 1972;**25**:106–110.

41. Taylor GI, Corlett RJ, Boyd JB. The versatile deep epigastric (inferior rectus abdominis) flap. *Br J Plast Surg* 1984;**37**:330–350.

42. Logan SE, Mathes SJ. The use of a rectus abdominis myocutaneous flap to reconstruct a groin defect. *Br J Plast Surg* 1984;**37**:351–353.

46.2 The role of radiotherapy in the management of squamous carcinoma

J T Roberts

Introduction

The management of the primary tumor in patients with penile cancer is controversial. While radical surgery provides best control of the primary tumor, it is mutilating and produces a change of body image, which, with the frequent accompanying loss of sexual function, may result in considerable psychological morbidity. Laser surgery may control limited superficial tumors but for relatively small infiltrating lesions radiotherapy offers the opportunity to control local disease and preserve organ function. Survival after treatment is related to regional nodal disease status. However treatment of the primary tumor effectively prevents distressing local recurrence. Since the risk of local recurrence is related to the depth of invasion and differentiation of the tumor, local recurrence rates vary from series to series according to patient selection. Recurrences after conservative treatment of early lesions can be salvaged surgically, usually by partial penectomy. Salvage rates of 100% may be obtained with T1 tumors but lower rates of salvage are obtained with more advanced lesions[1–3]. Radical surgery should therefore be reserved for cases where an attempt at conservative surgery is not feasible or for relapse after attempted conservative therapy[4].

Radiotherapy techniques

Radiotherapy is the longest established method of conservative therapy for penile cancer. Selection of patients is important; patients with T1 N0 tumors of less than 4 cm are ideal candidates for attempted organ preservation with radiotherapy. Circumcision should be performed if radiotherapy is contemplated. It allows visualization of and access to the tumor and removes the risk of phimosis resulting from post-radiotherapy cicatrization. This is a particular risk following brachytherapy and circumcision is a mandatory precursor of brachytherapy[5].

Radiotherapy may be given either by means of an external beam technique or using brachytherapy. Brachytherapy can be performed with either an external isotope mold or interstitial brachytherapy. A high dose may be delivered to the tumor with an appropriate margin but the inverse square law ensures a rapid fall-off of dose with increasing distance, thus sparing surrounding tissues. An external mould technique involves the use of an inner perspex cylinder, worn over the penis, and an outer cylinder, loaded with iridium-192 wires, which is placed over the inner. A dose of 60 Gy in 6–7 days is given to tumor, while the urethral dose is limited to 50 Gy. The outer cylinder is usually applied and removed by the patient, who can, for example, remove it to pass urine. With treatment times of 8–10 h/day the technique can be used with the patient attending as a day case.

Interstitial brachytherapy involves the implantation of hollow stainless steel needles under general or spinal anesthesia. A urinary catheter is inserted before the implant is performed to prevent the passage of sources through the urethra and to facilitate nursing while the implant is in place. It should move freely at the end of the procedure. A perspex template is used to maintain the spacing and parallelism of the needles. The size and depth of infiltration of the tumor determines the number and position of the needles, which are loaded with iridium-192 wire only when the implant is satisfactory. A typical implant will consist of 4–8 wires of 4 cm in length placed in two parallel planes to give a radiation dose of 50–70 Gy over 5–6 days.

In the case of either a radioactive mold or an implant the patient is nursed in a designated room to provide protection from radiation exposure to staff and others.

For very superficial tumors or carcinoma in situ a low energy (60 to 250 kV) photon beam or an electron beam may be applied directly to the tumor with a 2 cm safety margin beyond the clinical extent of the tumor. External beam irradiation is usually administered using megavoltage photons from a linear accelerator. Doses of the order of 45–60 Gy are given with 15–30 daily fractions over 3–6 weeks. Because megavoltage photons produce a relatively lower dose of radiation at the skin it is usual to encase the penis in a wax block (bolus material) which is worn during each treatment, which is administered with parallel opposed lateral radiation fields.

Results of radiotherapy

The data on the effectiveness of radiotherapy come from small retrospective series spread over the last few decades,

during which there have been major technological advances in radiotherapy. The lack of uniformity of radiation treatment techniques and lack of information about the pathologic staging of the tumors treated hinders analysis of the effectiveness of radiotherapy[6]. The rate of local relapse following radiotherapy depends on tumor stage. Local control rates of up to 91% have been reported for T1 tumors[1] but control rates fall with increasing size and T category: 78–84% for T2, 71–77% for T3 and 50% for T4 lesions[3,8]. In contrast to local recurrences occurring following conservative surgery, which tend to occur within 2 or 3 years, local relapse after radiotherapy may occur after 5 years[5], or, in the case of HPV-related penile cancer, more than 10 years[4]. Patients treated conservatively therefore need long and careful follow up.

Since the rate of development of symptomatic nodal involvement after prophylactic groin irradiation is similar to that seen in the unirradiated patient its routine use cannot be supported. Post-radiation fibrosis makes clinical examination more difficult[6]. The results of radiotherapy are inferior to those of surgery in patients with positive inguinal nodes[2]. However, while there are no randomized series comparing post-operative irradiation with observation in patients with multiple involved inguinal nodes or extracapsular spread, an improvement in 5 year survival has been reported in one series[7].

In two series of patients treated with radioactive iridium-192 wire implants all patients remained sexually active after treatment[1,8].

Treatment-related complications

Minor acute and late complications of radiotherapy for penile cancer are common[9]. Acute reactions such as mucositis (including acute urethritis), edema of the prepuce and local infection may be minimized by prior circumcision and careful attention to hygiene. Minor late complications such as telangiectasia, atrophy and discoloration of the skin have been noted by some in more than 40% of cases[10]. Atrophic skin frequently tears or ulcerates following minor trauma during intercourse. More rarely trauma may precipitate necrosis. Urethral stenosis, which occurs in up to 30% of cases, whichever treatment modality is used, is the commonest late complication. Repeated urethral dilatation usually deals adequately with the problem and surgical correction is only occasionally required[11]. Annular sclerosis of the foreskin will be prevented by circumcision.

Serious late sequelae, such as fibrosis and late necrosis increase in incidence as tumor size and treatment volume increase[3,5,8] and are particularly seen following treatment of tumors >4 cm in diameter or invading the corpora cavernosa. There does not seem to be any relationship between tumor necrosis and dose rate (for brachytherapy[2]) or total dose, either for external beam or brachytherapy[2,3]. Necrosis often occurs after a biopsy has been performed within an irradiated area[4] and is more frequent in patients treated with brachytherapy (15%) than those treated with external beam irradiation (8%). Biopsy should be avoided where possible in these patients.

Conclusions

For early penile cancers radiotherapy to the primary tumor offers the opportunity to remain sexually active with no evidence that local failure of disease control, necessitating salvage surgery impairs survival. For the elderly patient considered unfit for surgical intervention radiotherapy may offer useful palliation or the chance of cure.

References

1. Delannes M, Malavaud B, Douchez J, Donnet J, Daly NJ. Iridium-192 interstitial therapy for squamous cell carcinoma of the penis. *Int J Radiat Oncol Biol Phys* 1992;**24**:479–483.
2. Horenblaas S, van Tinteren H, Delamarre JF et al. Squamous carcinoma of the penis II. Treatment of the primary tumor. *J Urol* 1992;**147**:1533–1538.
3. Rozan R, Albuisson E, Giraud D et al. Interstitial brachytherapy for penile carcinoma: a multicentric survey (259 patients). *Radiother Oncol* 1995;**36**:83–93.
4. Pizzocaro G, Piva L, Bandieramonte G and Tana S. Up-to-date management of carcinoma of the penis. *Eur Urol* 1997;**32**:5–15.
5. Gerbaulet A, Lambin P. Radiotherapy of cancer of the penis. Indications, advantages, pitfalls. *Urol Clin North Am* 1992;**19**:325–332.
6. Jones WG, Elwell CM. Radiation therapy for penile cancer. In: Vogelzang NJ, Scardino PT, Shipley WU, Coffey DS (eds). *Comprehensive textbook of genitourinary oncology.* Williams and Wilkins, Baltimore, 1996.
7. Ekstrom, Edsmyr F. Cancer of the penis; a clinical study of 229 cases. *Acta Chir Scand* 1958;**115**:25–45.
8. Frew IDO, Jeffreys JD, Swinney J. Carcinoma of the penis. *Br J Urol* **39**:398–404.
9. Jones WG, Fossa SD, Harmers H, Van Den Bogaert W. Penis cancer: a review by the Joint Committee of the European Organisation for Research and Treatment of Cancer (EORTC) Genitourinary and Radiotherapy Groups. *J Surg Oncol* 1989, 227–231.
10. Kausal V, Sharma SC. Carcinoma of the penis. *Acta Ocol* 1987;413–417.
11. Mazeron JJ, Langlois D, Lobo PA et al. Interstitial radiation therapy for carcinoma of the penis using iridium 192 wires: the Henri Mondor experience (1970–1979). *Int J Radiat Oncol Biol Phys* 1984;**10**:1891–1895.

46.3 Chemotherapy

A Tolcher

The rarity of metastatic squamous cell carcinoma of the penis limits the experience any one investigator may have with chemotherapy treatment for this disease. However, knowledge of the use of chemotherapy agents in the treatment of other squamous cell carcinomas, notably head and neck car-

cinomas, has led to several small trials of single and multi-agent chemotherapy for this disease. Cisplatin, methotrexate, bleomycin and 5-fluorouracil are the most studied agents to date[1–6]. Antitumor response rates for these agents alone or in combination range from 13–64%, however, complete responses are rare[7–10]. Many series reporting encouraging results included patients who underwent post-chemotherapy surgery to render them disease free[7–10]. Chemotherapy for advanced penile cancer should therefore be used with palliative intent or as an adjunct to further surgery.

Adjuvant chemotherapy for node-positive squamous cell carcinoma

There are insufficient data either to support or refute the use of adjuvant chemotherapy following surgery for lymph node-positive squamous cell carcinoma. Although two small single arm studies suggest adjuvant chemotherapy may reduce the rate of relapse compared with historical controls, these results are subject to considerable bias[11]. Based on the small number of patients who present with this disease, it is unlikely that comparative studies will ever be performed to determine whether adjuvant chemotherapy benefits patients who present with lymph node-positive squamous cell carcinoma versus surgery alone. Individualized discussion with the patient regarding the potential risks and uncertain benefits associated with adjuvant chemotherapy is required.

References

1. Sklaroff RB, Yagoda A. Cis-Diaminedichloride platinum II (DDP) in the treatment of penile carcinoma. *Cancer* 1979;**44**:1563–1565.
2. Gagliano RG, Blumenstein BA, Crawford ED et al. Cis-Diaminedichloroplatinum in the treatment of advanced epidermoid carcinoma of the penis: a Southwest Oncology Group Study. *J Urol* 1989;**141**:66–67.
3. Sklaroff RB, Yagoda A. Methotrexate in the treatment of penile carcinoma. *Cancer* 1980;**45**:214–216.
4. Garnick MB, Skarin AT, Steele GD. Metastatic carcinoma of the penis: complete remission after high-dose methotrexate chemotherapy. *J Urology* 1979;**122**:265.
5. Ichikawa T, Nakano I, Hirokawa I. Bleomycin treatment for tumors of the penis and scrotum. *J Urol* 1969;**102**:699–707.
6. Kyalwazi SK, Bhams D, Harrison NW. Carcinoma of the penis and bleomycin chemotherapy in Uganda. *Br J Urol* 1974;**46**:689–696.
7. Shammas FV, Ous S, Fossa SD. Cisplatin and 5-fluorouracil in advanced cancer of the penis. *J Urol* 1992;**147**:630–632.
8. Hussein AM, Benedetto P, Sridhar KS. Chemotherapy with cisplatin and 5-fluorouracil for penile and urethral squamous cell carcinomas. *Cancer* 1990;**65**:433–438.
9. Sella A, Robinson E, Carrasco H et al. Phase II study of methotrexate, cisplatin and bleomycin combination chemotherapy. *Proc Am Soc Clin Oncol* 1994 (abstract 794).
10. Abratt RP, Barnes RD, Pontin AR. The treatment of clinically fixed inguinal lymph node metastases from carcinoma of the penis by chemotherapy and surgery. *Eur J Surg Oncol* 1989;**15**:285–286.
11. Pizzocaro G, Piva L. Adjuvant and neoadjuvant vincristine, bleomycin, and methotrexate for inguinal metastases from squamous cell carcinoma of the penis. *Acta Oncol* 1988;**27**:823–824.

PART SEVEN
Carcinoma of the urethra

Chapter 47
Carcinoma of the urethra

_____

Chapter 48
Pathology of urethral carcinoma

_____

Chapter 49
Treatment

_____

49.1   Surgery

_____

49.2   Radiotherapy for urethral
       cancer

_____

49.3   Chemotherapy

47 Carcinoma of the urethra

C E Bermejo Jr and J W Basler

Incidence, etiology and epidemiology

Urethral cancer is rare representing less than 1% of all malignancies[1-5]. Most commonly seen between the sixth and seventh decades of life. It is the only genitourinary cancer more common in women than in men (4:1)[1-4]. In men no racial predisposition has been seen[1] but in women urethral cancer is more common in caucasian women[6].

The etiology of male urethral cancer is unknown. Recurrent urinary tract infections and chronic inflammation (venereal disease, prostatitis, urethritis and urethral stricture) have been implicated. Twenty-four to 76% of males with urethral cancer will have urethral strictures at some point. The most common site of this stricture will be in the bulbocavernous urethra, also the most common site of urethral cancer[1-3]. Human papiloma virus (HPV)-16 has been associated with squamous cell carcinoma of the male urethra, especially in the penile urethra[2,7-9]. A few cases of transitional cell carcinoma of the distal urethra associated with HPV-6 have been reported[10-12].

In women the etiology associated with the development of urethral carcinoma is also unknown. Urethral diverticulum[13-18], viral infections (HPV-6)[12], and chronic inflamation secondary to intercourse, infections and caruncles[19-20] have been associated but not proven to be a direct cause.

Classification and histopathology

Epithelial lining of the urethra varies throughout its course for which the histologic type of urethral cancer will also vary depending on where the neoplasm is localized. The most common pathologic types of urethral cancer in males and females in order of frequency are squamous cell carcinoma, transitional cell and adenocarcinoma (Table 47.1)[1-3].

Table 47.1 Histopathology of urethral carcinoma

Type of cancer	Frequency	Observations
Male		
Squamous cell	70–80%	Most commonly seen in bulbomembranous and penile urethral. Most moderate to high grade tumors.
Transitional cell	15–20%	Most commonly seen in prostatic urethra. Should be differentiated from extension of bladder transitional cell carcinoma.
Adenocarcinoma	5–6%	Must be differentiated from extension of adenocarcinoma coming from prostate.
Others	1–2%	Undifferentiated or miscellaneous (i.e. sarcomas, melanomas)
Female		
Squamous cell	70%	Most commonly seen in distal 2/3 of urethra.
Transitional cell	15%	As in men should be differentiated from extension of bladder transitional cell carcinoma.
Adenocarcinoma	10–13%	Two types: clear cell and mucinous/columnar. Patients with tumor generally present at a higher stage. Worse prognosis than squamous cell carcinoma.
Others	1–2%	Undifferentiated or miscellaneous (i.e. sarcoma, melanomas)

Presentation, diagnosis and staging

Presentation

The most common symptom in men with urethral cancer is obstructive voiding symptoms (40–49%) and less common urethral bleeding (40%), urinary retention, irritative voiding symptoms (28%), priapism, penile gangrene, urinary incontinence and perineal pain[1,2,21]. The most common clinical finding in men with urethral cancer is a palpable mass (40%) and less common periurethral abscess and urethrocutaneous fistula[1,2,5,21].

Women with urethral cancer most commonly complain of urethral bleeding or spotting (60–75%) and less commonly of irritative voiding symptoms (20–65%), obstructive voiding symptoms (25–50%) and perineal pain (25–40%)[1,2,5]. The most common physical finding includes a palpable urethral mass (39%) and less often an abscess and urethrocutaneous fistula[1,2,5]. Usually the diagnosis is made 5 months after the appearance of symptoms in both female and male patients[2].

Diagnosis

If there is a high index of suspicion of urethral cancer a careful history and physical examination should be carried out. Special attention should be given to looking for periurethral mass, periurethral or perineal abscess or urethrocutaneous fistula. In men urethral cancer can present as a stricture that bleeds excessively after dilatation and/or has required multiple dilatations for treatment[2].

Cystourethroscopy with transurethral biopsy of the urethral lesion are essential for diagnosis. Special attention should be placed in performing deep biopsies or the tumor may be missed. Cystourethroscopy will help in assessing extent, tumor size and bladder involvement[1–2].

In men retrograde urethrogram can estimate the extent of the tumor. Findings suggesting urethral cancer would be fistulas, irregular strictures, extravasation, and/or urethral intraluminal filling defects[2,22]. Urine cytology can aid in the diagnosis of this tumor[1,2,22]. Nuclear matrix protein 22 (NMP22) in urine has been suggested to be a useful tool for screening of urothelial cancer in patients with microscopic hematuria[24], but data is still lacking.

Benign urethral lesions are more common than urethral cancer. Generally these benign lesions present with similar signs and symptoms of urethral cancer (Table 47.2)[2,3,25]. If any lesion in the urethra is found on a patient who presents with the previously described signs and symptoms urethral cancer should always be a part of the differential diagnosis to avoid delay in the diagnosis of this disease.

Staging

For staging a detailed history and physical examination should be performed. Special attention should be placed to the size, fixation and site of the tumor. A thorough bimanual examination should be carried out to determine the extent of the tumor[1–3]. The inguinal lymph nodes should be palpated; inguinal adenopathy is usually an indication of metastatic disease[1–3,22]. Palpable inguinal lymph nodes occur in approximately 20% of

Table 47.2 Differential diagnosis of urethral cancer

Women	Men
Urethral caruncle	Urethral stricture
Periurethral abscess	Urethrocutaneous fistula
Condylomata acuminata	Perineal abscess
Urethral cyst	Urethral calculus
Urethral diverticulum	Tuberculosis
Urethral prolapse	Foreign body
Hypertrophic mucosa	Metastatic disease (i.e. prostate, bladder, penile
Varicosities	cancer)

cases of male and female patients with urethral cancer; 80% of these patients will have positive lymph nodes at the time of staging. Anterior urethral cancers tend to metastasize to inguinal lymph nodes and posterior urethral cancers metastasize to pelvic lymph nodes[1–3,25]. Cystourethroscopy and retrograde urethrogram can help in determining the site and extent of the urethral neoplasm.

Inguinal and pelvic lymph node involvement can best be assessed with CT scan or MRI[3]. CT scan or MRI can also help in determining the size, extent and extension to adjacent structures of the primary tumor. The most common sites for metastasis of urethral cancer will be in the order of frequency lung, liver and bone. Distant metastasis will occur in 10–14% of patients at time of presentation. The presence of metastasis to bone, lung and liver can be assessed by obtaining a bone scan, chest X-ray and liver function tests, respectively[1–3,26].

In the past most clinicians used the staging systems developed by Ray, Grabstald and associates for staging males and females, respectively, with urethral cancer (Tables 47.3 and 47.4)[3,22]. Recently a staging system based on a TNM classification has been developed for urethral carcinomas (Table 47.5)[27].

Table 47.3 Staging of male urethral carcinoma (Ray and associates staging system)

Stage 0	Confined to mucosa only (in situ)
Stage A	Into but not beyond the lamina propia
Stage B	Into but not beyond the substance of the corpus spongiosum or into but not beyond the prostate
Stage C	Direct extension into tissue beyond the corpus spongiosum (corpora cavernosa, muscle fat, fascia, skin, direct skeletal involvement) or beyond the prostatic capsule
Stage D1	Regional metastasis including inguinal and pelvic lymph nodes (with any primary tumor)
Stage D2	Distant metastasis (with any primary tumor)

Table 47.4 Staging of female urethral carcinoma (Grabstald and associates staging system)

Stage 0	In situ (limited to mucosa)
Stage A	Submucosal (not beyond submucosa)
Stage B	Muscular (infiltrating periurethral muscle)
Stage C	Periurethral
C1	Infiltrating muscular wall of the vagina
C2	Infiltrating muscular wall of the vagina with invasion of vaginal mucosa
C3	Infiltration of other adjacent structures, such as bladder, labia and clitoris
Stage D	Metastasis
D1	Inguinal lymph nodes
D2	Pelvic lymph nodes below the bifurcation of the aorta
D3	Lymph nodes above the bifurcation of the aorta
D4	Distant

Table 47.5 Staging of female and male urethral carcinoma (TNM staging system)

Primary tumor (T) (male and female)

TX	Primary tumor cannot be assessed
T0	No evidence of primary tumor
Ta	Non-invasive papillary, polypoid, or verrucous carcinoma
Tis	Carcinoma in situ
T1	Tumor invades subepithelial connective tissue
T2	Tumor invades any of the following: corpus spongiosum, prostate capsule, anterior vagina, bladder neck
T3	Tumor invades any of the following: corpus cavernosum, beyond prostate capsule, anterior vagina, bladder neck
T4	Tumor invades other adjacent organs

Transitional cell carcinoma of the prostate

Tis pu	Carcinoma in situ, involvement of the prostatic urethra
Tis pd	Carcinoma in situ, involvement of the prostatic ducts
T1	Tumor invades subepithelial connective tissue
T2	Tumor invades any of the following: prostatic stroma, corpus spongiosum, periurethral muscle
T3	Tumor invades any of the following: corpus cavernosum, beyond prostatic capsule, bladder neck (extraprostatic extension)
T4	Tumor invades other adjacent organs (invasion of the bladder)

Regional lymph nodes (N)

NX	Regional lymph nodes cannot be assessed
N0	No regional lymph node metastasis
N1	Metastasis in a single lympph node, 2 cm or less in greatest dimension
N2	Metastasis in a single lymph node, more than 2 cm in greatest dimension, or in multiple lymph nodes

Distant metastasis (M)

MX	Distant metastasis cannot be assessed
M0	No distant metastasis
M1	Distant metastasis

References

1. Herr HW. Surgery of penile and urethral carcinoma. In Walsh PC, Retik AB, Vaughan ED Jr, Wein AJ (eds) *Campbell's urology* (7th edn). W.B. Saunders Company, 1998, pp. 3401–3409.

2. Poore RE, McCullough DL. Urethral carcinoma. In Gillenwater JY, Grayhack JT, Howards SS, Duckett JW (eds) *Adult and pediatric urology* (3rd edn). Mosby, 1996, pp. 1837–1852.

3. Carroll PR. Surgical management of urethral carcinoma. In Crawford ED, Das S (eds) *Current genitourinary cancer surgery* (2nd edn). Williams & Wilkins, 1996, pp. 520–541.

4. Zeidman EJ, Desmond P, Thompson IM Surgical treatment of carcinoma of the male urethra. *Urol Clin North Am* 1992;**19**(2):359–371.

5. Gheiler EL, Tefilli MV, Tiguert R *et al*. Management of primary urethral cancer. *Urology* 1998;**52**(3):487–493.

6. Mostafi FK, Davis CJ, Sesterhenn IA. Carcinoma of the male and female urethra. *Urol Clin North Am* 1992;**19**(2):347–358.

7. Weiner JS, Walther PJ. A high association of oncogenic human papillomavirus with carcinomas of the female urethra: polymerase chain reaction-based analysis of multiple histological types. *J Urol* 1994;**151**(1):49–53.

8. Weiner JS, Walther PJ. The association of oncogenic human papillomavirus with urologic malignancy. The controversies and clinical implications. *Surg Onc Clin North Am* 1995;**4**(2):257–276.

9. Cupp MR, Malek RS, Goellner JR *et al*. Detection of human papillomavirus DNA in primary squamous cell carcinoma of the male urethra. *Urology* 1996;48(4):551–555.

10. Alonso ME, Roma SR, Sanchez MF, Toffoni C. Low-grade papillary transitional-cell carcinoma of the distal urethra with focal squamous differentiation and association with human papillomavirus types 6–11. *Archivos Espanoles de Urologia* 1997;**50**(8):875–878.

11. Shimuzu N, Ichinose Y, Shimo M *et al*. Transitional cell papilloma in the fossa navicularis is positive for human papillomavirus. *Int J Urol* 1998;**5**(3):296–298.

12. Mevorach RA, Cos LR, DiSant'Agnese PA *et al*. Human papillomavirus type 6 in grade I transitional cell carcinoma of the urethra. J *Urol*, 1990;**143**:126.

13. Clayton M, Siani P, Guinan P. Urethral diverticular carcinoma. *Cancer* 1992;**70**:665.

14. Rajan N, Tucci P, Mallouh C *et al*. Carcinoma in female urethral diverticulum: case report and review of management. J *Urol* 1993;**150**:1911.

15. Nakamura Y, Takahashi M, Suga A *et al*. A case of adenocarcinoma arising within a urethral diverticulum diagnosed only by the surgical specimen. *Gynecolog Obstet Invest* 1995;**40**(1):69–70.

16. Kato H, Ogihara S, Kobayashi Y *et al*. Carcinoembryonic antigen positive adenocarcinoma of a female urethral diverticulum: case report and review of the literature. *Int J Urol* 1998;**5**(3):291–293.

17. Seballos RM, Rich RR. Clear cell adenocarcinoma arising from a urethral diverticulum. *J Urol* 1995;**153**(6):1914–1915.

18. Oliva E, Young RH. Clear cell adenocarcinoma of the urethra: a clinicopathologic analysis of 19 cases. *Modern Pathol* 1996;**9**(5): 513–520.

19. Marshall FC, Uson AC, Melicow MM. Neoplasms and caruncles of the female urethra. *Surg Gynecol Obstet* 1960;**110**:723.

20. McCrea LE. Malignancy of the female urethra. *Urol Surv*, 1952;**2**:85.

21. Kaplan GW, Buckley GJ, Grayhack JT. Carcinoma of the male urethra. J *Urol* 1967;**98**:365.

22. Ray B, Canto AR, Whitmore WF Jr. Experience with primary carcinoma of the male urethra. *J Urol* 1977;**117**:591.

23. Grabstald H, Hilaris B, Henschke U *et al*. Cancer of the female urethra. *JAMA*, 1966;**197**:835.

24. Akaza H, Miyanaga N, Tsukamoto T *et al*. Evaluation of urinary NMP22 as a diagnostic marker for urothelial cancer—screening for urothelial cancer in patients with microscopic hematuria. *Japn J Cancer Chemotherapy* 1997;**24**(7):837–842.

25. Sarosdy MF. *Urethral carcinoma*. AUA Update Series, 1987;**6**, lesson 13.

26. Morikawa K, Togashi K, Minami S *et al*. MR and CT appearance of urethral clear cell adenocarcinoma in a woman. *J Computer Assisted Tomography* 1995;**19**(6):1001–1003.

27. Fleming ID, Cooper JS, Henson DE, Hutter RVP, Kennedy BJ, Murphy GP, O'Sullivan B *et al*. (eds) *American Joint Committee on Cancer Cancer Staging Manual* (5th edn) Lippincott-Raven Philadelphia 1997, pp. 247–249.

48 Pathology of urethral carcinoma

P A Humphrey

Primary cancers of the urethra are rare and comprise less than 1% of all urothelial neoplasms[1–17]. Much more common is secondary involvement of the urethra by transitional cell (urothelial) carcinoma of the bladder[18–54]. which occurs in up to 58% of patients with bladder cancer[50].

The most common histologic type of primary malignancy of the urethra is carcinoma and, of the carcinomas, squamous cell carcinoma (Figure 48.1) is the most frequent, followed by transitional cell carcinoma (Figure 48.2) and adenocarcinoma (Figure 48.3) (Table 48.1). Unusual histologic variants of primary urethral carcinoma, which have been mainly reported as single cases, include adenosquamous carcinoma[55], and small cell carcinoma[56,57]. Non-epithelial malignancies of the urethra are exceedingly rare and include malignant melanoma, sarcoma and malignant lymphoma[2–4,58,59]. Carcinomas, usually adenocarcinomas, may arise in the accessory periurethral glands of Cowper, Littre and Skene, and secondarily involve the urethral surface epithelium[3,4]. Other carcinomas that may secondarily involve the urethra include bladder, as mentioned, and carcinomas of uterine cervix, bowel and prostate, which may involve the urethra by direct extension. Metastatic spread to the urethra

Table 48.1 Histologic types of primary urethral malignancies

Histologic type	Percentage
Squamous cell carcinoma	75%
Transitional cell carcinoma	15%
Adenocarcinoma	5%
Adenosquamous carcinoma	Rare
Small cell carcinoma	Rare
Malignant melanoma	Rare
Sarcoma	Rare
Lymphoma	Rare

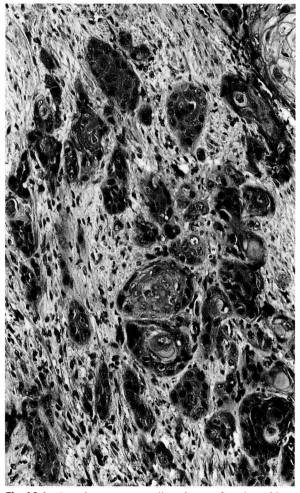

Fig. 48.1 Invasive squamous cell carcinoma of urethra with nests and cords of malignant epithelial cells in fibrous tissue.

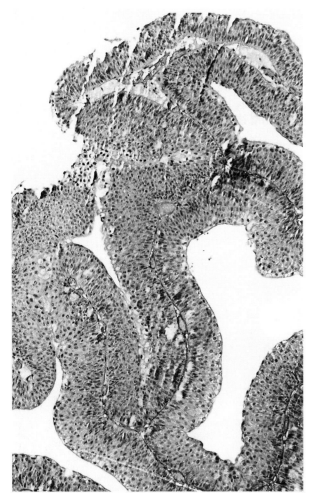

Fig. 48.2 Superficial, low-grade, papillary transitional cell carcinoma of urethra, with fusion of papillary fronds.

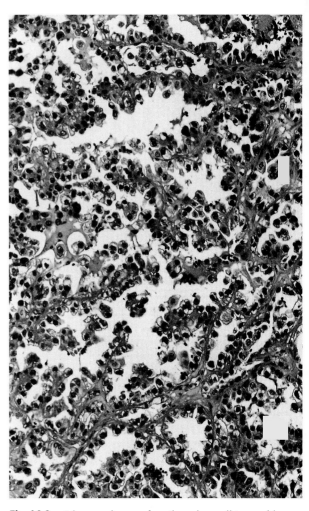

Fig. 48.3 Adenocarcinoma of urethra, clear cell type, with irregular tubules and glandular clefts lined by tumor cells with cleared cytoplasm.

has been reported for lymphoma and for ovarian, lung, prostate, colon, rectum, bladder, kidney, ureter and testis malignancies[2–4].

Primary urethral carcinoma histologic type corresponds to the anatomic site of origin in the urethra. So, in general, proximal neoplasms (prostatic urethra in males, proximal one-third in females) tend to be transitional cell carcinomas while distal tumors (membranous, bulbous or penile in men, distal two-thirds in women) are often squamous cell carcinomas[4]. Adenocarcinomas may arise anywhere along the urethra and may be associated with a diverticulum, or fistula[4]. Often, it is difficult to ascertain the precise site of origin of a urethral carcinoma due to infiltrative growth and normal tissue destruction by tumor.

Grossly, urethral carcinomas assume a variety of morphologic guises including nodular, papillary, ulcerative, cauliflower-like, or an irregular mucosal thickening[1–5].

Urethral carcinoma may be macroscopically misdiagnosed as a caruncle (in women), benign polyp, or benign ulcer. With progression, three main appearances have been described – indurating-ulcerating, annular constricting and fungating[2,64]. The ulcerative variant may occur anywhere along the urethra while the constricting type, which can cause a stricture, favors the proximal urethra and the fungating variety is usually discovered near the external meatus[2,64]. With more advanced disease, abscesses, sinuses and fistulas may form[13]. Gross features of the tumor may not be specific for a histologic type or may correlate with a line of differentiation: squamous cell carcinomas may be grayish-white and scirrhous with necrosis, transitional cell carcinomas or adenocarcinomas may be papillary, and adenocarcinomas may be gelatinous, mucoid, or cystic[1].

Squamous cell carcinoma

Microscopically, *squamous cell carcinomas* of the urethra are typically well to moderately differentiated and deeply invasive, with a fibrogenic response (Figure 48.1). In better differentiated tumors, keratin pearls, intercellular bridges and eosinophilic cytoplasm are indicators of squamous differentiation. Very poorly differentiated, high-grade squamous cell carcinomas may be difficult to impossible to separate histologically from high-grade transitional cell carcinomas. Squamous cell carcinomas of the distal penile urethra frequently invade the corpus cavernosum while more proximal tumors in men may penetrate directly into the urogenital diaphragm, prostate, rectum and bladder neck. Complete excision of these latter neoplasms may be difficult to achieve.

Transitional cell carcinoma

Transitional cell carcinoma in the urethra occurring in the absence of a bladder tumor is much less common than a synchronous or metachronous relationship to bladder neoplasia. This so-called secondary involvement of the urethra by transitional cell carcinoma, occurring in the setting of bladder carcinoma, could represent either direct extension, multifocal disease, or lymphovascular invasion[45]. Secondary involvement has been reported in up to 58% of men[50] and 36% of women[35]. This incidence rate is highly dependent on the degree of urethral sampling, with the highest rates obtained with completely embedded and mapped cystectomy specimens and the lowest rates with limited urethral biopsy. Urethral recurrence after radical cystectomy for transitional cell carcinoma of the bladder has been detected in 4–18% of cases[48,49]. Histopathologically, direct extension of a bladder tumor into the urethra may manifest itself as pagetoid intraurothelial spread of single neoplastic cells or small clusters of neoplastic cells[51–53], pure carcinoma in situ, non-invasive papillary tumors, or invasive carcinoma, with or without a mucosal component. In 70% of cases in men, when carcinoma extends into the prostatic urethra, there is also prostatic involvement (either in situ or stromal invasive disease)[43]. Urethral carcinoma in situ at the 5 and/or 7 o'clock positions of the verumontanum seems to be highly predictive of prostatic involvement[39]. Grossly, secondary urethral involvement by carcinoma may not be visible; papillary tumors are more likely to be visualized than carcinoma in situ[35]. In patients treated with bacillus Calmette-Guérin (BCG), inflammatory changes in the prostatic urethra secondary to BCG may be difficult to distinguish grossly from carcinoma in situ. Important microscopic evaluations in urethral biopsies performed in patients with bladder cancer include assessment for the presence of transitional cell carcinoma and carcinoma in situ. Dysplasia may also be seen in urethral epithelium in patients with bladder cancer[65,66] and tends to be associated with dysplasia/carcinoma in situ in the bladder[65]. When neoplasia is identified, the anatomic structures involved, such as urothelium, submucosa, periurethral glands, prostatic ducts and acini, prostatic stroma and lymphovascular channels, should be specified. Histologic grade of the cancer should be also reported. In bladder cancer cases where cystectomy is performed, and where the urethra is removed, or in delayed urethrectomy cases, tumor histologic type, grade, extent of invasion, tumor size, multicentricity and margin status should be assessed.

Adenocarcinomas

These comprise 10% of all urethral carcinomas in women[6], and are more common in women than men[67–71]. Urethral adenocarcinoma may be broadly classified as clear cell vs. non-clear cell adenocarcinoma. Clear cell adenocarcinoma, known in the past as 'mesonephric' or mesonephroid adenocarcinoma, is rare, with about 50 reported cases[1,72,73] and, unlike other urethral carcinomas, does not exhibit a clinical association with chronic irritation, sexually transmitted disease or stricture[3]. About one-quarter of clear cell adenocarcinomas are found in diverticula[3]. The microscopic patterns of glandular arrangement are tubular, papillary, and tubulocystic (Figure 48.3). The tumor cells display nuclear pleomorphism, with hobnailing, and cytoplasmic clearing. An important entity in the histologic differential diagnosis is nephrogenic adenoma, particularly in small biopsies, but clear cell adenocarcinoma harbors more mitoses and a greater degree of nuclear pleomorphism, and also may demonstrate sheets of clear neoplastic cells with necrosis. The non-clear cell urethral adenocarcinomas may be mucinous, columnar, colloid, signet-ring, or villous[67–71,74]. Clear cell adenocarcinomas of the urethra have a somewhat better prognosis than non-clear cell adenocarcinomas[67].

Prognostic factors

The most significant pathologic prognostic indicators for urethral carcinoma are location of the tumor, tumor size and pathologic stage of the tumor. The more distal tumors have a more favorable prognosis, and for female patients tumor size of greater than 5 cm is associated with poor survival[10]. Many patients with urethral carcinoma present with advanced stage disease[1–5]. Patients often have locally advanced tumor with spread into adjacent structures and 28–50% of patients have lymph node metastases at presentation[10,13,75]. Distant metastases at presentation are uncommon (at 7%)[75]. The most common sites of distant metastases are lung, liver, bone and brain[75].

Genetic abnormalities in urethral carcinoma tissue are currently not of practical clinical prognostic utility. Human papillomavirus DNA of types 16 and 18 have been detected by polymerase chain reaction in squamous cell carcinoma and transitional cell carcinoma[75], but it is not known if this genotype correlates with clinical outcome. DNA content analysis by flow cytometry has been linked to prognosis for male patients with primary squamous cell carcinoma of the urethra[77], but this test has not been widely utilized.

References

1. Amin MB, Young RH. Primary carcinomas of the urethra. *Semin Diagn Pathol* 1997;**14**:147–160.
2. Mostofi FK, Davis CJ Jr, Sesterhenn IA. Carcinoma of the male and female urethra. *Urol Clin N Am* 1992;**19**:347–358.
3. Murphy WM. Diseases of the urinary bladder, urethra, ureters, and renal pelvis. In: Murphy WM (Ed.) *Urological pathology.* WB Saunders Co., Philadelphia, 1997, pp. 119–125.
4. Reuter VE. Urethra. In: Bostwick DG, Eble JN (eds) *Urologic surgical pathology.* Mosby, St Louis, 1997, pp. 434–454.
5. Schellhammer PF. Urethral carcinoma. *Semin Urol* 1983;**1**:82–89.
6. Mandler JI, Pool TL. Primary carcinoma of the male urethra. *J Urol* 1966;**96**:67–72.
7. Kaplan GW, Bulkley GJ, Grayhack JT. Carcinoma of the male urethra. *J Urol* 1967;**98**:365–371.
8. Guinn GA, Ayala AG. Male urethral cancer: report of 15 cases including a primary melanoma. *J Urol* 1970;**103**:176–179.
9. Mullin EM, Anderson EE, Paulson DF. Carcinoma of the male urethra. *J Urol* 1974;**112**:610–613.
10. Bracken RB, Johnson DE, Miller LS, Ayala AG, Gomez JJ, Rutledge F. Primary carcinoma of the female urethra. *J Urol* 1976;**116**:188–192.
11. Bolduan JP, Farah RN. Primary urethral neoplasms. *J Urol* 1981;**125**:198–200.
12. Garden AS, Zagars GK, Delclos L. Primary carcinoma of the female urethra. Results of radiation therapy. *Cancer* 1993;**71**:3102–3108.
13. Ray B, Canto AR, Whitmore WF Jr. Experience with primary carcinoma of the male urethra. *J Urol* 1977;**117**:591–594.
14. Hahn P, Krepart G, Malaker K. Carcinoma of the female urethra. *Urology* 1991;**37**:106–109.
15. Melicow MM, Roberts TW. Pathology and natural history of urethral tumors in males. Review of 142 cases. *Urology* 1978;**11**:83–89.
16. Johnson DE, O'Connell JR. Primary carcinoma of the female urethra. *Urology* 1983;**21**:42–45.
17. Marshall VF. Radical excision of locally extensive carcinoma of the male urethra. *J Urol* 1957;**78**:252–264.
18. Tobisu K, Tanaka Y, Mizutani T *et al.* Transitional cell carcinoma of the urethra in men following cystectomy for bladder cancer: multivariate analysis for risk factors. *J Urol* 1991;**146**:1551–1553.
19. Richie JP, Skinner DG. Carcinoma in situ of the urethra associated with bladder carcinoma: the role of urethrectomy. *J Urol* 1978;**119**:80–81.
20. Hardeman SW, Soloway MS. Urethral recurrence following radical cystectomy. *J Urol* 1990;**144**:666–669.
21. Grabstald H. Tumors of the urethra in men and women. *Cancer* 1973;**32**:1236–1255.
22. Gowing NFC. Urethral carcinoma associated with cancer of the bladder. *Br J Urol* 1960;**32**:428–430.
23. Schellhammer PF, Whitmore WF Jr. Transitional cell carcinoma of the urethra in men having cystectomy for bladder cancer. *J Urol* 1976;**115**:56–60.
24. Melicow MM, Hollowell JW. Intraurothelial cancer: carcinoma in situ. Bowen's disease of the urinary systems. *J Urol* 1952;**68**:763–772.
25. Seemayer TA, Knaack J, Thelmo WL, Wang, NS, Ahmed MN. Further observations on carcinoma in situ of the urinary bladder: silent but extensive intraprostatic involvement. *Cancer* 1975;**36**:514–520.
26. Thelmo WL, Seemayer TA, Madarnas P, Mount BMM, MacKinnon KJ. Carcinoma in situ of the bladder with associated prostatic involvement. *J Urol* 1974;**111**:491–494.
27. Mahadevia PS, Koss LG, Tar IJ. Prostatic involvement in bladder cancer. Prostate mapping in 20 cystoprostatectomy specimens. *Cancer* 1986;**58**:2096–2102.
28. Hillyard RW Jr, Ladaga L, Schellhammer PF. Superficial transitional cell carcinoma of the bladder associated with mucosal involvement of the prostatic urethra: results of treatment with intravesical bacillus Calmette-Guérin. *J Urol* 1988;**139**:290–279.
29. Siref LE, Zincke H. Radical cystectomy for historical and pathological T1, NO, MO (stage A) transitional cell cancer. Need for adjuvant systemic chemotherapy? *Urology* 1988;**31**:309–311.
30. Bretton PR, Herr HW, Whitmore WF Jr *et al.* Intravesical bacillus Calmette-Guérin therapy for in situ transitional cell carcinoma involving the prostatic urethra. *J Urol* 1989;**141**:853–856.
31. Orihuela E, Herr HW, Whitmore WF Jr. Conservative treatment of superficial transitional cell carcinoma of prostatic urethra with intravesical BCG. *Urology* 1989;**34**:231–237.
32. Wood DP Jr, Montie JE, Pontes JE, Medendorp SV, Levin HS. Transitional cell carcinoma of the prostate in cystoprostatectomy specimens removed for bladder cancer. *J Urol* 1989;**141**:346–349.
33. Zincke H, Utz DC, Farrow GM. Review of Mayo Clinic experience with carcinoma in situ. *Oncology* (suppl 4) 1985;**26**:39–46.
34. Malkowicz SB, Nichols P, Lieskovsky G, Boyd SD, Huffman J, Skinner DG. The role of radical cystectomy in the management of high grade superficial bladder cancer (PA, P1, PIS and P2). *J Urol* 1990;**144**:641–645.
35. de Paepe ME, André R, Mahadevia P. Urethral involvement in female patients with bladder cancer. A study of 22 cystectomy specimens. *Cancer* 1990;**65**:1237–1241.
36. Prout GR Jr, Griffin PP, Daly JJ, Heney NM. Carcinoma in situ of the urinary bladder with and without associated vesical neoplasms. *Cancer* 1983;**52**:524–532.
37. Franks LM, Chesterman FC. Intra-epithelial carcinoma of prostatic urethra, periurethral glands and prostatic ducts (Bowen's disease of urinary epithelium). *Br J Cancer* 1956;**10**:223–225.
38. Frazier HA, Robertson JE, Dodge RK, Paulson PF. The value of pathologic factors in predicting cancer-specific survival among patients treated with radical cystectomy for transitional cell carcinoma of the bladder and prostate. *Cancer* 1993;**71**:3993–4001.
39. Sakamoto N, Tsuneyoshi M, Naito S, Kumazawa J. An adequate sampling of the prostate to identify prostatic involvement by urothelial carcinoma in bladder cancer patients. *J Urol* 1993;**149**:318–321.
40. Coloby PJ, Kakizoe T, Tobisu K-I, Sakamoto M-I. Urethral involvement in female bladder cancer patients: mapping of 47 consecutive cysto-urethrectomy specimens. *J Urol* 1994;**152**:1438–1442.
41. Palou J, Xavier B, Laguna P, Montlleo M, Vincente J. In situ transitional cell carcinoma involvement of prostatic urethra: Bacillus Calmette-Guérin therapy without previous transurethral resection of the prostate. *Urology* 1996;**47**:482–484.
42. Erckert M, Stenzl A, Falk M, Bartsch G. Incidence of urethral tumor involvement in 910 men with bladder cancer. *World J Urol* 1996;**14**:3–8.
43. Esrig D, Freeman JA, Elmajian DA *et al.* Transitional cell carcinoma involving the prostate with a proposed staging classification for stromal invasion. *J Urol* 1996;**156**:1071–1076.
44. Tobisu K-i, Kanai Y, Sakamoto M *et al.* Involvement of the anterior urethra in male patients with transitional cell carcinoma of the bladder undergoing radical cystectomy with simultaneous urethrectomy. *Jpn J Clin Oncol* 1997;**27**:406–409.
45. Maralani S, Wood DP Jr, Grignon D, Banerjee M, Sakr W, Pontes JE. Incidence of urethral involvement in female bladder cancer: an anatomic pathologic study. *Urology* 1997;**50**:537–541.

46. Stein JP, Cote RJ, Freeman JA *et al*. Indications for lower urinary tract reconstruction in women after cystectomy for bladder cancer: a pathological review of female cystectomy specimens. *J Urol* 1995;**154**:1329–1333.

47. Chen ME, Pisters LL, Malpica A, Pettaway CA, Dinney CP. Risk of urethral, vaginal and cervical involvement in patients undergoing radical cystectomy for bladder cancer: Results of a contemporary cystectomy series from M.D. Anderson Cancer Center. *J Urol* 1997;**157**:2120–2123.

48. Freeman JA, Esrig D, Stein JP, Skinner DG. Management of the patient with bladder cancer. Urethral recurrence. *Urol Clin North Am* 1994;**21**:645–651.

49. Lebret T, Hervé J-M, Barré P *et al*. Urethral recurrence of transitional cell carcinoma of the bladder. Predictive value of preoperative latero-montanal biopsies and urethral frozen sections during prostatocystectomy. *Eur Urol* 1998;**33**:170–174.

50. Farrow GM, Utz DC, Rife CC. Morphological and clinical observations of patients with early bladder cancer treated with total cystectomy. *Cancer Res* 1976;**36**:2495–2501.

51. Ortega LG, Whitemore WF Jr, Murphy AI. In situ carcinoma of the prostate with intraepithelial extension into the urethra and bladder. A Paget's disease of the urethra and bladder. *Cancer* 1953;**6**:898–923.

52. Tomaszewski JE, Korat OC, LiVolsi VA, Connor AM, Wein A. Paget's disease of the urethral meatus following transitional cell carcinoma of the bladder. *J Urol* 1985;**135**:368–370.

53. Bégin LR, Deschênes J, Mitmaker B. Pagetoid carcinomatous involvement of the penile urethra in association with high-grade transitional cell carcinoma of the urinary bladder. *Arch Pathol Lab Med* 1991;**115**:632–635.

54. Lapham R, Grignon D, Ro JY. Pathologic prognostic parameters in bladder urothelial biopsy, transurethral resection, and cystectomy specimens. *Semin Diagn Pathol* 1997;**14**:109–122.

55. Saito R. An adenosquamous carcinoma of the male urethra with hypercalcemia. *Hum Pathol* 1981;**12**:383–385.

56. Vadmal MS, Steckel J, Teichberg S, Hajdu SI. Primary neuroendocrine carcinoma of the penile urethra. *J Urol* 1997;**159**:956–957.

57. Fukuda T, Kawishima T, Saito T, Itoh S, Suzuki T. Small cell carcinoma arising from the outer urethral orifice – a case report examined by histologic, ultrastructural and immunohistochemical methods. *Pathol Int* 1997;**47**:497–501.

58. Manivel JC, Fraley EE. Malignant melanoma of the penis and male urethra. *J Urol* 1984;**132**:123–125.

59. Hatcher PA, Wilson DD. Primary lymphoma of the male urethra. *Urology* 1997;**49**:142–144.

60. Thomas RB, Maguire B. Adenocarcinomas in a female urethral diverticulum. *Aust NZ J Surg* 1991;**61**:869–871.

61. Patanaphan V, Prempree T, Sewchand W, Hafiz MA, Jaiwatana J. Adenocarcinoma arising in female urethral diverticulum. *Urology* 1983;**22**:259–264.

62. Seballos RM, Rich RR. Clear cell adenocarcinoma arising from a urethral diverticulum. *J Urol* 1995;**153**:1914–1915.

63. Gonzalez MO, Harrison ML, Boileau MA. Carcinoma in diverticulum of female urethra. *Urology* 1985;**26**:328–332.

64. Herbert P. In: *Urological pathology*, vol. 1. Lea and Febiger, Philadelphia, 1952, pp. 20–150.

65. Coutts AG, Grigor KM, Fowler JW. Urethral dysplasia and bladder cancer in cystectomy specimens. *Br J Urol* 1985;**57**:535–541.

66. Bryan RL, Newan J, Suarez V, Kadow C, O'Brien JM. The significance of prostatic urothelial dysplasia. *Histopathology* 1993;**22**:501–503.

67. Meis JM, Ayala AG, Johnson DE. Adenocarcinoma of the urethra. A clinicopathologic study. *Cancer* 1987;**60**:1038–1052.

68. Yachia D, Turani H. Colonic-type adenocarcinoma of male urethra. *Urology* 1991;**37**:568–570.

69. Bostwick DG, Lo R, Stamey TA. Papillary adenocarcinoma of the male urethra. Case report and review of the literature. *Cancer* 1984;**54**:2556–2563.

70. Tran KP, Epstein JI. Mucinous adenocarcinoma of urinary bladder type arising from the prostatic urethra. Distinction from mucinous adenocarcinoma of the prostate. *Am J Surg Pathol* 1996;**20**:1346–1350.

71. Lieber MM, Malek RS, Farrow GM, McMurtry J. Villous adenocarcinoma of the male urethra. *J Urol* 1983;**130**:1191–1193.

72. Oliva E, Young RH. Clear cell adenocarcinoma of the urethra: a clinicopathologic analysis of 19 cases. *Mod Pathol* 1996;**9**:513–520.

73. Drew PA, Murphy WM, Civantos F, Speights VO. The histogenesis of clear cell adenocarcinoma of the lower urinary tract: case series and review of the literature. *Hum Pathol* 1996;**27**:248–252.

74. Loo KT, Chan JKC. Colloid adenocarcinoma of the urethra associated with mucosal in situ carcinoma. *Arch Pathol Lab Med* 1992;**116**:976–977.

75. Grabstald H, Hilaris B, Henschke U *et al*. Cancer of the female urethra. *JAMA* 1966;**197**:835–842.

76. Wiener JS, Walther PJ. A high association of oncogenic human papilloma viruses with carcinomas of the female urethra: polymerase chain reaction-based analysis of multiple histological types. *J Urol* 1994;**151**:49–53.

77. Winkler HZ, Lieber MM. Primary squamous cell carcinoma of the male urethra: Nuclear deoxyribonucleic acid ploidy studied by flow cytometry. *J Urol* 1988;**139**:298–303.

49 Treatment

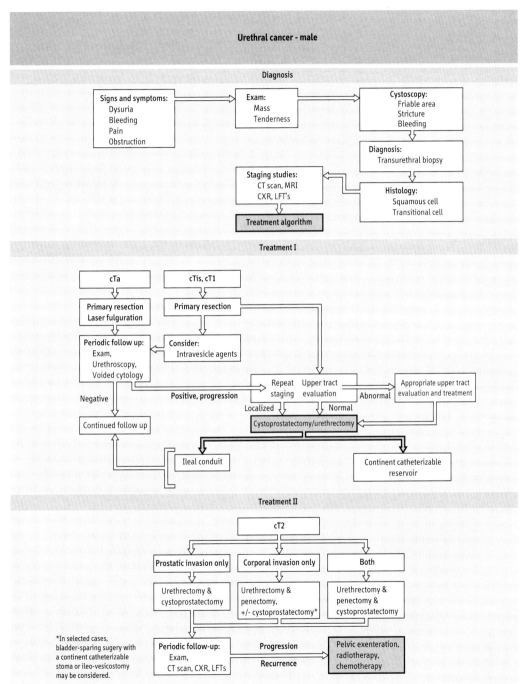

Urethral cancer - male

Diagnosis

Signs and symptoms:
  Dysuria
  Bleeding
  Pain
  Obstruction

Exam:
  Mass
  Tenderness

Cystoscopy:
  Friable area
  Stricture
  Bleeding

Diagnosis:
  Transurethral biopsy

Histology:
  Squamous cell
  Transitional cell

Staging studies:
  CT scan, MRI
  CXR, LFT's

Treatment algorithm

Treatment I

cTa

cTis, cT1

Primary resection
Laser fulguration

Primary resection

Periodic follow up:
  Exam,
  Urethroscopy,
  Voided cytology

Consider:
  Intravesicle agents

Negative

Positive, progression

Repeat staging

Upper tract evaluation

Abnormal

Appropriate upper tract evaluation and treatment

Localized

Normal

Continued follow up

Cystoprostatectomy/urethrectomy

Ileal conduit

Continent catheterizable reservoir

Treatment II

cT2

Prostatic invasion only

Corporal invasion only

Both

Urethrectomy & cystoprostatectomy

Urethrectomy & penectomy, +/- cystoprostatectomy*

Urethrectomy & penectomy & cystoprostatectomy

*In selected cases, bladder-sparing sugery with a continent catheterizable stoma or ileo-vesicostomy may be considered.

Periodic follow-up:
  Exam,
  CT scan, CXR, LFTs

Progression

Recurrence

Pelvic exenteration, radiotherapy, chemotherapy

Algorithm: male

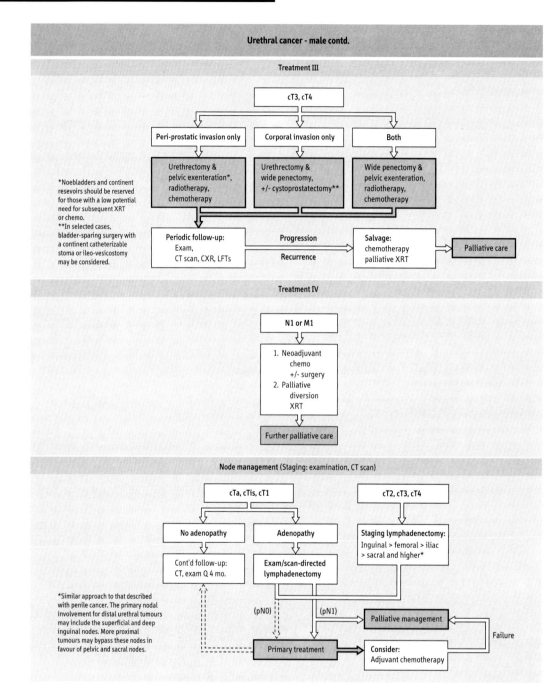

Urethral cancer - male contd.

Treatment III

cT3, cT4

Peri-prostatic invasion only | Corporal invasion only | Both

Urethrectomy & pelvic exenteration*, radiotherapy, chemotherapy | Urethrectomy & wide penectomy, +/- cystoprostatectomy** | Wide penectomy & pelvic exenteration, radiotherapy, chemotherapy

*Noebladders and continent resevoirs should be reserved for those with a low potential need for subsequent XRT or chemo.
**In selected cases, bladder-sparing surgery with a continent catheterizable stoma or ileo-vesicostomy may be considered.

Periodic follow-up: Exam, CT scan, CXR, LFTs → Progression / Recurrence → Salvage: chemotherapy palliative XRT → Palliative care

Treatment IV

N1 or M1

1. Neoadjuvant chemo +/- surgery
2. Palliative diversion XRT

Further palliative care

Node management (Staging: examination, CT scan)

cTa, cTis, cT1 | cT2, cT3, cT4

No adenopathy | Adenopathy | Staging lymphadenectomy: Inguinal > femoral > iliac > sacral and higher*

Cont'd follow-up: CT, exam Q 4 mo. | Exam/scan-directed lymphadenectomy

*Similar approach to that described with penile cancer. The primary nodal involvement for distal urethral tumours may include the superficial and deep inguinal nodes. More proximal tumours may bypass these nodes in favour of pelvic and sacral nodes.

(pN0) | (pN1) → Palliative management

Primary treatment → Consider: Adjuvant chemotherapy → Failure

536

Algorithm: female

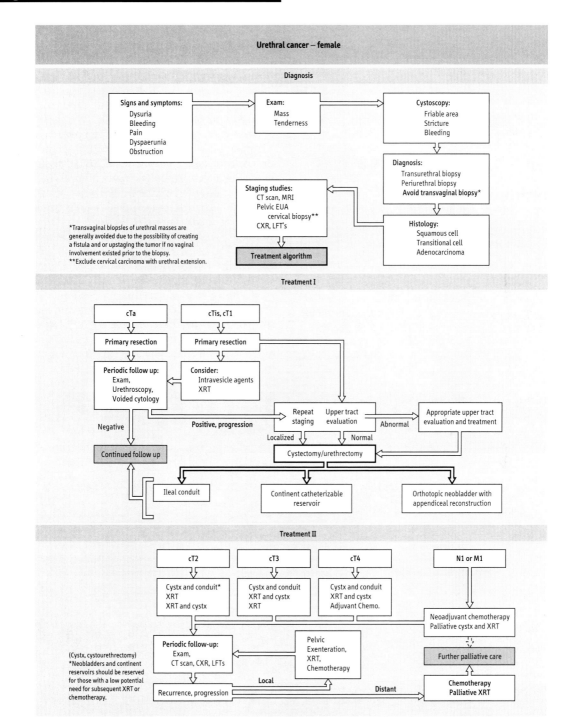

Urethral cancer – female

Diagnosis

Signs and symptoms:
Dysuria
Bleeding
Pain
Dyspaerunia
Obstruction

Exam:
Mass
Tenderness

Cystoscopy:
Friable area
Stricture
Bleeding

Diagnosis:
Transurethral biopsy
Periurethral biopsy
Avoid transvaginal biopsy*

Staging studies:
CT scan, MRI
Pelvic EUA
cervical biopsy**
CXR, LFT's

Treatment algorithm

Histology:
Squamous cell
Transitional cell
Adenocarcinoma

*Transvaginal biopsies of urethral masses are
generally avoided due to the possibility of creating
a fistula and or upstaging the tumor if no vaginal
involvement existed prior to the biopsy.
**Exclude cervical carcinoma with urethral extension.

Treatment I

cTa

cTis, cT1

Primary resection

Primary resection

Periodic follow up:
Exam,
Urethroscopy,
Voided cytology

Consider:
Intravesicle agents
XRT

Repeat
staging

Upper tract
evaluation

Abnormal

Appropriate upper tract
evaluation and treatment

Negative

Positive, progression

Localized

Normal

Continued follow up

Cystectomy/urethrectomy

Ileal conduit

Continent catheterizable
reservoir

Orthotopic neobladder with
appendiceal reconstruction

Treatment II

cT2

cT3

cT4

N1 or M1

Cystx and conduit*
XRT
XRT and cystx

Cystx and conduit
XRT and cystx
XRT

Cystx and conduit
XRT and cystx
Adjuvant Chemo.

Neoadjuvant chemotherapy
Palliative cystx and XRT

Periodic follow-up:
Exam,
CT scan, CXR, LFTs

Pelvic
Exenteration,
XRT,
Chemotherapy

Further palliative care

(Cystx, cystourethrectomy)
*Neobladders and continent
reservoirs should be reserved
for those with a low potential
need for subsequent XRT or
chemotherapy.

Recurrence, progression

Local

Distant

Chemotherapy
Palliative XRT

537

49.1 Surgery

V J Gnanapragasam and H Y Leung

The mainstay of treatment for urethral carcinoma is surgery. Adjunctive management with radiotherapy can however improve prognosis and recurrence rates[1,2]. Surgery can be broadly divided into that for superficial or invasive disease. Invariably the site of disease predicts the stage at presentation, thus surgical management is dependent on the site of disease. Male urethral cancer in particular offers more therapeutic options (Table 49.1.1).

Male urethral carcinoma

Simple

Early stage disease (stage O, stage A) is uncommon and is more likely to be found in the anterior urethra. Though these lesions may be broad based or present as a stricture, TUR may be possible in some cases. There is however a risk of perforation into the cavernosal sinuses. Laser therapy (Nd:Yag) or fulguration may also be performed via the transurethral route. Local excision is also an option with the resection of short segments of urethra and anastomosis. A transcrotal approach is used and the excised urethra is sent for frozen section to check the resection margins[3]. If the defect is too large for primary anastomosis, a pedicle of scrotal skin can be used to fashion a neo-urethra. Adjunctive therapy is rarely used in distal urethral cancers and in stage O and A disease because of the difficulty in precise localization and complications such as strictures.

For more advanced disease (stage B, stage C), and where it is desirous for a one stage remedy, partial or radical penectomy is a safe surgical option. Advanced anterior carcinomas treated via penectomy results in a foreshortened penis or a perineal urethra. Two centimeter margins are mandatory[4] and is associated with a low rate of recurrence. Recurrence if it occurs is relatively easy to detect. Disease of the fossa navicularis has a 5 year survival of 92%, penile urethral carcinoma 34%, and more proximal disease in the order of 16–30%[5–8].

Nash et al. (1996) described a technique using Moh's micrographic surgery combined with distal urethrectomy for reconstruction of the urethra[9]. This technique, although applied to a glanular carcinoma with urethral extension, suggests a way whereby penectomy may be avoided. Bird et al. (1997) have described phallus preservation for urethral carcinoma[10]. Subcutaneous penectomy was used in three men with squamous cell carcinoma of the urethra (proximal bulbous urethra, distal bulb to proximal pendulous urethra and midshaft of urethra). At 22 months, there was no evidence of recurrence in any of these patients.

Posterior or proximal urethral lesions may rarely be treated with TUR or primary resection and anastomosis. More often however the disease is extensive at presentation. In this circumstance, radical resection is required with or without lymphadenectomy. Carcinoma of the prostatic urethra is an aggressive tumor. In a few instances, it may be possible to resect these transurethrally once co-existing bladder tumors have been excluded[11].

Complex

The more proximal the lesions are, the more radical the surgical options become. Advanced anterior urethral

Table 49.1.1 Surgical options for urethral carcinoma

Male urethral carcinoma	
Distal urethra	Transurethral resection (TUR)
	Local excision/fulguration/laser
	Partial amputation (2 cm margins)*
	Radical amputation*
Bulbomembranous urethra	TUR
	Resection and anastamosis
	Radical cystoprostatectomy, pelvic lymphadenectomy, total penectomy* ± resection of pubis and UG diaphragm
Prostatic urethra	TUR
	Cystoprostatectomy, total urethrectomy*
Female urethral carcinoma	
Distal urethra	TUR
	Local excision/fulguration/laser
Proximal urethra	Total urethrectomy (bladder preserving)
	Cystectomy, pelvic node dissection, partial or complete vaginal excision ± resection of pubis and UG diaphragm*

* Inguinal node dissection where appropriate.

carcinomas may be managed with wide radical excision and lymphadenectomy but this is rare. Radical surgery for proximal disease involves cystoprostatectomy, total penectomy, scrotectomy and pelvic lymphadenectomy[4,5,12,13]. Opinion is divided as to whether surgery should include resection of the pubic ramus and urogenital diaphragm. The bulk of the symphysis may be preserved, however, if only the subsymphyseal arch is resected which therefore maintains the integrity of the pelvis. The gap may be filled with omentum and covered with a myocutaneous flap[14]. Adjuvant radiotherapy has been used to debulk these tumors with some success[10,15].

Carcinoma of the prostatic urethra, commonly TCC or adenocarcinoma, is extensive at presentation. These tumors have a high propensity for lymphatic and hematogenous spread. While TUR may be successful in many cases, recurrences occur in up to 50% of patients[16]. Management therefore is usually with cystoprostatectomy and urethrectomy. The role of radiotherapy and chemotherapy is as yet undetermined in this group of patients.

Lymphadenectomy

Of patients with urethral carcinoma 14% to 30% have lymph node involvement at presentation[5,17]. The anterior and posterior urethra drains to the inguinal and pelvic lymph nodes respectively. In both males and females, anterior urethral carcinoma embolize to inguinal nodes that lie superficial to the fascia lata and the lymphatics of the penis, scrotum, vulva and the urethra drain into the medial and central group of these nodes[18]. Subsequent to this, drainage occurs to the deep inguinal nodes or external iliac nodes. Posterior urethral tumors drain into pelvic lymphatic channels[19]. One channel runs alongside the dorsal vein of the penis/clitoris and into the external iliac nodes. Another path is via the lymphatics of the internal pudendal artery and to the obturator lymph nodes. A final pathway is drainage to pre-sacral nodes.

Pelvic and inguinal nodes present different management issues. In anterior disease, inguinal node surgery has not been found to be beneficial unless involved nodes can be demonstrated at presentation. There is a high morbidity associated with inguinal node surgery and traditionally this has been discouraged. Undetected metastasis to lymph nodes may however explain recurrent disease in early treated anterior cancers. Proximal urethral carcinoma has also not been shown to benefit from prophylactic inguinal node dissection. Therapeutic inguinal node surgery is performed during concurrent radical surgery.

Pelvic node dissection is mandatory in surgery for urethral carcinoma involving cystoprostatectomy as metastasis to pelvic lymph nodes is associated with a poor prognosis. If nodes are found to be involved pre-operat-

ively, the 5 year survival in this group is about 18% (work in female urethral cancers)[20].

Female urethral carcinoma

As urethral cancers are commoner in females, surgery in this condition is better defined. Its earlier presentation also allows for less mutilating surgery. Radiotherapy (external beam and brachytherapy) has also been successfully employed for small lesions. Downstaging may also be performed with pre-operative radiotherapy.

Simple

Laser therapy and fulguration can be used to treat early superficial lesions regardless of the site[1]. TUR, as in men, can be performed for early stage O or A lesions and this can be done under local or spinal anesthesia. Local excision is also suitable for low-grade anterior urethral cancers and where good clearance margins are possible. Invasive lesions which have not metastasized can be treated with partial urethrectomy. In some cases total urethrectomy with bladder preservation may be possible for proximal cancers that have only invaded locally or where the whole urethra is involved with superficial disease.

Complex

Proximal urethral cancers tend to be locally advanced at presentation and have invaded extensively by the time of diagnosis[21,22]. The 5 year survival for patients who have surgery is 0% to 57%[1,23,24]. Surgery usually involves cystectomy, urethrectomy, pelvic lymphadenectomy, partial or complete vaginal resection with or without the resection of the pubic symphysis. Even so, local recurrence rates following surgery is about 60%[25] although pre-operative radiotherapy has some marginal benefit in improving these rates[2,21]. Although no prospective trials have been performed, the current recommendation is that bulky proximal lesions should be pre-treated with radiotherapy, this may or may not be helped by adjunctive chemotherapy[12,21].

Lymphadenectomy

Pelvic nodes are resected as part of surgery for proximal cancers. There is no indication for prophylactic inguinal node dissection. As in men, inguinal node surgery should be reserved for patients who present with involved nodes. Modified inguinal dissection techniques however with low morbidity may change this view in the future.

Benign urethral tumors

Benign lesions of the urethra are rare and represent a small part of urological practise (Table 49.1.2). Many have

539

Table 49.1.2   Benign urethral lesions

- Epithelial neoplasms
  - Transitional cell papilloma
  - Inverted papilloma
- Condylomata acuminata
- Fibroepithelial polyp
- Papillary urethritis
- Prostatic urethral polyps
- Villous adenoma

- Metaplastic change
  - Squamous metaplasia
  - Nephrogenic adenoma
- Urethral caruncles

only been reported as case studies. There is no current evidence that papillomas or polyps progress to carcinoma. Metaplastic change however may be a risk factor and is discussed elsewhere in the chapter.

Epithelial neoplasms

Squamous cell papillomas are the most common type of epithelial lesions. These are usually found in the distal urethra but can occur anywhere along the urethra. Histologically, the papilloma is covered with sheets of stratified squamous epithelium. Transitional cell carcinomas tend to occur in the more proximal urethra where bladder epithelium merges into the urethra. In this position, they may rarely cause an obstruction. A further type of papilloma is the rare inverted papilloma.

Condylomata acuminata

The papova virus has been implicated in the genesis of this ubiquitous tumor of the urogenital area. Sexual contact is the main risk factor and urethral involvement, although rare, can be difficult to treat. These can occasionaly become quite large and resemble a branching tree or a cauliflower floret based on a relatively avascular base. Patients may present with urinary obstruction, bleeding, a discharge or the appearance of a tumor/lesion. Treatment is either with topical chemotherapeutics such as 5-flurouracil or Thiotepa, laser fulguration or occasionaly transurethal resection.

Fibroepithelial polyps

These benign lesions are found mainly in men and probably represent congenital malformations. They may cause urinary outflow obstruction which is intermittent in nature as the polyp acts in a ballcock fashion. There may also occasionally be hematuria. Many patients however remain asymptomatic. On histologic sections, the surface of the polyp is covered with normal epithelium and is continuous with the surrounding urethra.

Papillary urethritis

Recurrent inflammation and infection is well known to cause cystic lesions in the bladder. Long-term catheterization in particular is associated with this condition. A similar situation can occur in the urethra and is termed papillary urethritis or polypoid urethritis. It represents an important differential diagnosis of carcinoma. Histologically, there is marked edema and chronic inflammatory cell infiltration.

Urethral caruncles

This condition is almost exclusive to women and probably represents prolapse of the urethra at the urethral meatus. There is considerable inflammation and vascular engorgement and bleeding is a common presentation that accompanies pain and discomfort. It is most common in post-menopausal women and needs to be distinguished from carcinoma in this age group, especially as the lesion may appear quite dysplastic. The covering epithelium is either squamous or transitional but there is always considerable inflammatory infiltration and blood vessels tend to be large and fragile. The surface of large caruncles can ulcerate or become hyperkeratotic.

References

1. Narayan P, Konety B. Surgical treatment of female urethral carcinoma. *Urol Clin N Am* 1992;**19**:373.
2. Johnson DW, Kessler JF, Ferrigni RG, Anderson JD. Low dose combined chemotherapy/radiotherapy in the management of locally advanced urethral squamous cell carcinoma. *J Urol* 1989;**141**:615.
3. Urethra and penis – neoplasms. In: Blandy JP, Fowler C (eds) *Urology* (2nd edn), Blackwell Science Limited London, 1996.
4. Kaplan GW, Buckley GJ, Grayhack JT. Carcinoma of the urethra. *J Urol* 1967;**98**:385.
5. Ray B, Canto AR, Whitmore WF. Experience with primary carcinoma of the urethra. *J Urol* 1977;**117**:591.
6. Urethral tumors In: Vogelzang N, Cardino PTS, Shipley W, Coffey DS, Grigsby PW, Herr HW (eds) *Comprehensive textbook of genitourinary oncology*. William and Wilkins, Baltimore, 1996.
7. Ziedman EJ, Desmond P, Thompson I. Surgical treatment of carcinoma of the male urethra. *Urol Clin N Am* 1992;**19**:3569.
8. Farrer JH, Lupu AN. Carcinoma of the deep male urethra. *Urology* 1984;**24**:527.
9. Nash PA, Bihrle R, Gleason PE, Adams MC, Harke CW. Moh's micrographic surgery and distal urethrectomy with immediate urethral reconstruction for glanular carcinoma in situ with significant urethral extension. *Urology* 1996;**47**:108.
10. Bird E, Coburn M. Phallus preservation for urethral cancer: subcutaneous penectomy. *J Urol* 1997;**158**:2146.
11. Bretton PR, Herr HW. Intravesical BCG therapy for in situ TCC involving the prostatic urethra. *J Urol* 1989;**141**:853.
12. Herr HW. Surgery of the penile and urethra carcinoma. In: Walsh PC, Retik AB, Daracott Vaughn Jr E, Wein AJ (eds) *Campbells urology* (7th edn). WB Saunders, Philadelphia, 1998.
13. Bracken RB, Exenterative surgery for post urethral cancer. *Urology* 1982;**19**:248.
14. Larson DL, Bracken RB. Use of gracilis myocutaneous flap in urologic cancer surgery. *Urology* 1982;**14**:148.
15. Hopkins SC, Nag SK, Soloway MS. Primary carcinoma of the male urethra. *Urology* 1984;**23**:128.
16. Grabstald H. Tumors of the urethra in men and women. *Cancer* 1973;**32**:1236.
17. Anderson KA, McAninch JW. Primary squamous cell carcinoma of the anterior male urethra. *Urology* 1984;**23**:134.

18. McMinn RH (Ed.) *Last's anatomy, regional and applied* (9th edn). Churchill. Livingstone, Edinburgh, 1994.
19. Carroll PR, Dixon CM. Surgical anatomy of the male and female urethra. *Urol Clin N Amer* 1992;**19**:339.
20. Bracken RB, Johnson DE, Miller LS, Ayala AG, Gomez JJ, Rutledge F. Primary carcinoma of the female urethra. *J Urol* 1976;**116**:188.
21. Dalbagni G, Zhang Z, Lacombe L, Herr H. Female urethral carcinoma: an analysis of treatment: outcomes and a plea for a standardized treatment strategy. *J Urol* 1998;**82**:835.
22. Grabstald H, Hilaris B, Henschke U, Whitmore WF Jr. Cancer of the female urethra. *J Am Med Assoc* 1966;**197**:835.
23. Terry PJ, Cookson MS, Sarosdy MF. Carcinoma of the urethra and scrotum. In: Raghavan D, Scher HI, Leibel SA, Lang P (eds) *Principles and practises of genitourinary oncology.* Lippincott-Raven, Philadelphia, 1997.
24. Garden S, Zagars GK, Delclos L. Primary carcinoma of the female urethra: results of radiation treatment. *Cancer* 1993;**71**:3102.
25. Foens CS, Hussey DH, Staples JJ, Doornbos JF, Wen BC, Vigliotti AP. A comparison of the roles of surgery and radiotherapy in the management of carcinoma of the female urethra. *Int J Radiat Oncol Biol Phys* 1991;**21**:961.

49.2 Radiotherapy for urethral cancer

P Grigsby

Introduction

Radiotherapy is employed as curative treatment for some patients with urethral carcinoma. There are many aspects of individual patient management that dictate when radiotherapy alone may be used to treat these patients. Some of the factors to consider are patient gender, size and location of the tumor and the appropriateness of preserving anatomy and organ function.

Carcinoma of the male urethra is very uncommon. Traditionally most men are treated with surgery alone[1]. The role of radiotherapy for men is not well defined. Amputation of part or all of the penis is generally employed for small lesions. If preservation of anatomy and function are of primary consideration then irradiation alone or with chemotherapy may be used[2–4]. For large lesions, en bloc resection is usually performed. There may be consideration of a combined pre-operative irradiation and surgical approach for patients with very large lesions. Irradiation can clearly be employed for prophylactic treatment of the inguinal lymph nodes and for treatment of fixed, unresectable groin lymph nodes.

There is a much larger experience in treating women with urethral carcinoma than there is in men since the disease is much more common in women than in men. This experience has led to a more clearly defined role for irradiation in women than in men. Preservation of the urethra, vagina and bladder are considerations in women. Anatomically, these structures may be preserved when treated with radiotherapy rather than with surgery. Preservation of function of these structures is also possible. Small lesions of the anterior urethra are often treated surgically. However, radiotherapy is an option and should be considered. As lesions become larger, then surgical therapy results in anatomic and functional loss that can be preserved when these patients are treated with irradiation. Radiation techniques may involve brachytherapy or brachytherapy combined with external irradiation[5]. Prophylactic irradiation of inquinal lymph nodes is often performed.

General management

Anterior urethral carcinoma

Surgical management of anterior urethral carcinomas is often performed, most often in stage 0 lesions. For stage I lesions of the anterior urethra, interstitial irradiation (brachytherapy) is an alternative to surgical management. Larger lesions of the anterior urethra (as shown in Figure 49.2.1) require interstitial irradiation combined with external irradiation to the primary site, inguinal lymph nodes and pelvic lymph nodes. The patient in Figure 49.2.1 was found to have a palpable and radiographically demonstrable lymph node in the right groin (Figure 49.2.2). Inguinal lymph node dissection prior to or following groin irradiation may be an option since cure is possible in patients with limited regional lymph node metastasis. Inguinal lymph node dissection is not recommended in patients with clinically negative groins. Prophylactic groin irradiation is the preferred management for patients with invasive disease and clinically negative groins.

Posterior urethral carcinoma

Patients with lesions involving the posterior urethra usually present with large lesions (stages II, III or IV). It is not uncommon for these lesions to involve the entire urethra, to invade the base of the bladder or to metastasize to the inguinal and pelvic lymph nodes. Irradiation alone may be considered in some patients. Other approaches for management of patients with large lesions involving the base of the bladder are pre-operative irradiation or combined irradiation and concurrent chemotherapy[6].

Recurrent urethral carcinoma

The management of non-metastatic, locally recurrent urethral carcinoma is dictated primarily by limitations imposed as a result of the primary therapy. Patients whose initial therapy was surgery alone may be considered for curative therapy with radiotherapy or combined radiotherapy and concurrent chemotherapy for their recurrence. Patients whose initial therapy was radiotherapy are unlikely candidates for additional curative pelvic radiotherapy. Local recurrence after curative radiotherapy may

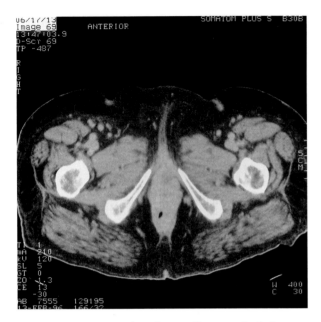

Fig. 49.2.1 Demonstration of a 2 cm diameter spherical urethral carcinoma involving the distal urethra in a 65 year old woman. Biopsy was positive for squamous cell carcinoma.

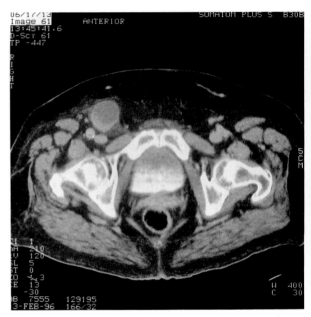

Fig. 49.2.2 Demonstration of a 4 cm diameter lymph node in the right groin of the woman seen in Figure 56.4.1. Fine-needle aspiration cytology was positive for metastatic disease.

be best managed with extensive surgery or neo-adjuvant chemotherapy and surgery.

In the setting of metastatic disease, local recurrences may require palliation for symptoms of pain and bleeding. Palliative radiotherapy should be considered in this situation. Irradiation may be delivered with brachytherapy or external irradiation or a combination of the two types of treatment.

Radiotherapy techniques

Brachytherapy

Brachytherapy for urethral carcinoma can be administered with intracavitary techniques or interstitial techniques. A specific brachytherapy technique for women with urethral cancer has been advocated by Sailer and colleagues[7]. In their technique a special urethral template is attached to a vaginal cylinder. A urinary catheter to drain the bladder exits through the middle of the template. The urinary catheter is surrounded by four implant needles forming a 1 cm diameter circle. An additional 10 implant needles surround the urinary catheter to form a 3 cm diameter circle. A lead shield is placed in the posterior portion of the vaginal cylinder to decrease the irradiation dose to the anterior wall of the rectum.

Grigsby[8] has advocated the use of a circular urethral template through which flexible interstitial needles can be inserted to form a double curved plane implant to encompass the urethral tumor mass. An opening in the urethral template allows for a urinary catheter to be placed.

Garden and colleagues[9] have recommended the use of cystotomy at the time of placement of interstitial needles into urethral lesions. This procedure is advocated to assist with needle placement for women with tumor masses involving the proximal urethra. Direct observation of needle placement for proper spacing of the needles and limiting the size of the implant can be achieved with the aid of a cystotomy. The authors also advocate the instillation of methylene blue into the urinary bladder to determine whether the stainless-steel needles have penetrated the bladder wall.

Gerbaulet and colleagues[10] employ the use of urinary catheters for intraluminal brachytherapy, vaginal mold applicators for intracavitary brachytherapy and hypodermic needles or guide gutters for interstitial brachytherapy. Their system employs IR-192 wires as the radiation source. Therapy for individual patients may include more than one type of implant application.

The current brachytherapy procedure for women with urethral carcinoma treated at the Mallinckrodt Institute of Radiology is demonstrated in Figure 49.2.3. A set of traditional vaginal cylinders for use in the treatment of gynecological malignancies has been modified by drilling holes in the long axis of the cylinder near its surface to allow the

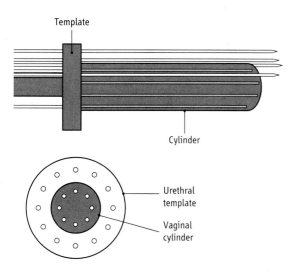

Fig. 49.2.3 Vaginal cylinder with drilled holes near the surface to allow for the placement of flexible interstitial catheters into the long axis of the cylinder and the placement of a single or double plane curved implant into the peri-urethral tissues.

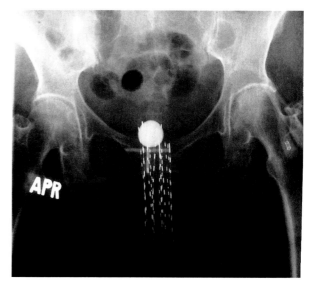

Fig. 49.2.4 AP simulation radiograph demonstrating 'dummy' radioisotope sources present in the vaginal cylinder and the periurethral tissues.

placement of flexible interstitial needles into the cylinder. A complete series of vaginal cylinders with diameters of 2.0, 2.5 and 3.0 cm has been modified. Surrounding the vaginal cylinder is a circular template that allows for the interstitial placement of flexible interstitial needles in the periurethral tissues in a single or double plane configuration dependent upon the size of the tumor mass to be implanted. The use of the vaginal cylinder allows the posterior vaginal mucosa and the anterior rectal wall to be displaced posteriorly to decrease the irradiation dose to those structures. A simulation radiograph demonstrating 'dummy' radiation sources present in the cylinder and the periurethral tissue is shown in Figure 49.2.4. The vaginal cylinder loaded with flexible interstitial needles also permits the expansion of the irradiation isodose curves (Figure 49.2.5) to encompass a larger area of the tumor mass than when interstitial catheters alone are employed. Irradiation dose rates are calculated to be approximately 40 cGy/hour to surround the intended treatment volume. The total irradiation dose from the implant is determined by the initial tumor size and the use of combined treatment with external radiotherapy. One or two interstitial implants may be utilized during the course of treatment.

External irradiation

External radiotherapy may be administered pre-operatively, combined with brachytherapy or delivered post-operatively. The volume to be encompassed with external radiotherapy includes the entire urethra and primary

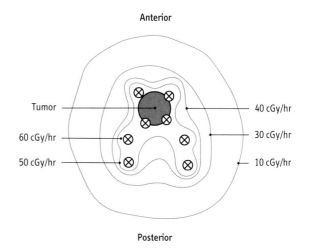

Fig. 49.2.5 Isodose curves from a typical brachytherapy implant utilizing the applicator shown in Figures 56.4.3 and 56.4.4. There is a relative decrease in the dose distribution near the rectum because the interstitial sources are placed anteriorly to encompass the urethral mass.

tumor mass, the inguinal lymph nodes and the pelvic lymph nodes. Figure 49.2.6 demonstrates the external borders of the irradiation ports on the patient's skin and Figure 49.2.7 is a radiotherapy portal radiograph of the same patient. The superior border of the port covers the pelvic lymph nodes to the level of the bifurcation of the common iliac vessels into the external

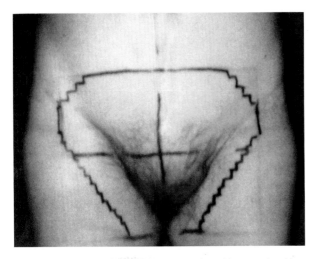

Fig. 49.2.6 External radiotherapy portal markings on the skin of a patient with urethral carcinoma. Volumes encompassed by the port are the entire urethra, the pelvic lymph nodes and the inguinal lymph nodes.

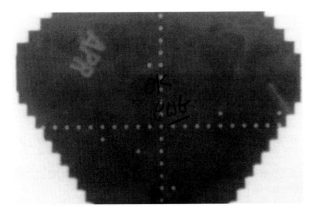

Fig. 49.2.7 AP radiotherapy portal radiograph of the patient seen in Fig. 56.4.6. Volumes encompassed by the port are the pelvic and inguinal lymph nodes and the entire urethra with 'fall-off' of the perineum.

and internal iliacs. Inferiorly, the port covers the entire urethra with 'fall-off' of the perineum. Laterally, the port encompasses the inguinal lymph nodes. The groin region may require the use of bolus depending upon the clinical lymph node status and the patient's anatomy.

Radiation dose

Radiation dose must be individualized. Pre-operative external irradiation is delivered at 180 to 200 cGy per day, five fractions per week, to a total dose of 4500 to 5000 cGy. Similar external irradiation doses are administered in conjunction with brachytherapy when radiotherapy alone is utilized. The radiation dose to the inguinal lymph nodes is 5000 cGy for clinically negative nodes and 6000 to 6600 cGy for palpable lymph nodes. However, large, matted lymph nodes in the groin are best treated with 5000 cGy followed by resection. Brachytherapy may be delivered in one or two procedures to administer a total tumor dose of 7000 to 8500 cGy depending on the size of the tumor. Brachytherapy is usually administered after the completion of external irradiation. When brachytherapy alone is administered to small tumors, a total tumor dose of 5000 to 6500 cGy can be delivered in one or two irradiation implants administered at 40 cGy per hour. Post-operative external irradiation may be delivered for positive lymph nodes or positive resection margins. In this circumstance, 4500 to 5000 cGy is administered as described above. Positive margins receive boost irradiation with either external radiotherapy or brachytherapy to a total dose of 6000 to 6600 cGy. The inguinal regions receive 6000 cGy for resected positive lymph nodes and 6600 if the resected lymph nodes have extracapsular extension.

If the goal of irradiation is palliation, then therapy must be tailored to the individual patient. Treatment may be with brachytherapy alone when the tumor mass is small. One or two brachytherapy procedures may be performed. External irradiation may be delivered with daily treatment over 5 to 6 weeks for a total of 5000 to 6000 cGy. Patients requiring palliation of symptoms and who have a life expectancy of less than 1 year may be treated with external irradiation delivered two times per day (370 cGy, b.i.d.) for 2 days and repeated for two additional courses separated by 2 weeks and delivering a total of 4440 cGy[11].

Results of radiotherapy

Small primary lesions of the urethral meatus and distal urethra may be treated with radiotherapy alone with excellent results. Large lesions of the distal urethra, lesions involving the proximal urethra, and large lesions involving the entire urethra are associated with a high incidence of local failure and a high incidence of lymph node metastasis and are difficult to treat. Proximal urethral lesions and tumors involving the entire urethra may be associated with invasion of the base of the bladder and local recurrences are common.

Bracken and associates[12] treated 81 women with urethral carcinoma with irradiation. The overall 5 and 10 year survival rate was 32% for all patients. Prognosis was correlated to clinical stage of disease. Histologic classification was not a prognostic factor when the results were analyzed by clinical stage.

Johnson and O'Connell[13] reported the use of radiotherapy alone for 12 patients with early stage disease. Local failure occurred in two patients. They recommended the use of pre-operative irradiation and radical surgery for patients with more advanced stage disease.

Prempree and colleagues[14] evaluated the treatment results of 21 women with urethral carcinoma who were treated with radiotherapy alone. Palliative therapy was administered to six patients and one additional patient who did not complete the planned course of therapy. The overall local control was 78% (11/14) in the patients treated with curative intent. The 5 year disease-free survival was 77% for the 14 patients. Prognostic factors were clinical stage and location of the primary lesion. Patients with lesions involving the proximal urethra, base of the bladder and inguinal lymph nodes had a worse outcome. Relief of symptoms occurred in 70% (5/7) of those treated for palliation.

Weghaupt and associates[15] treated 62 women with radiotherapy alone consisting of external irradiation and intracavitary vaginal radium. Patients received 55 to 70 Gy. The posterior urethra was involved in 20 women and the anterior urethra was involved in the remaining 42 women. Inguinal lymph node involvement was present in 31% (19/62). The overall 5 year survival rate was 65% for all patients; it was 71% for those with anterior urethral lesions and 50% for those with posterior urethral lesions.

Radiotherapy alone was employed in the treatment of 28 women with urethral carcinoma at the University of Iowa by Foens and colleagues[16]. Radiotherapy was administered with interstitial therapy alone in seven women, external radiotherapy alone in seven women, and combined external and interstitial therapy in 14 women. Local recurrence occurred in 36% (10/28). The modality of therapy was found to be an important prognostic factor. The 3 year disease-free survivals were 0% for those treated with interstitial therapy alone, 29% for those treated with external radiotherapy alone and 57% for those treated with combined external and interstitial radiotherapy.

Garden and associates[9] reviewed the treatment results for women with urethral carcinoma at the M. D. Anderson Cancer Center. In their summary of 97 women, 86 received radiotherapy alone. The therapeutic modality was combined external and interstitial radiotherapy in 35, brachytherapy alone in 30 and external radiotherapy alone in the remaining 21 women. Total irradiation doses to the tumor ranged from 40 to 106 Gy (median, 65 Gy). The 5 year local control rate was 64% for 84 evaluable patients treated with radiotherapy alone. Involvement of the entire urethra was a predictor of decreased local control. Prognostic factors that were identified for decreased survival were extension of tumor into adjacent structures, involvement of the entire urethra and fixation of the primary lesion.

At the Mallinckrodt Institute of Radiology, Grigsby and Corn[17] reported the results of irradiation alone in 20 women, irradiation and surgery for seven women and surgery only for six women. Their results indicate that either surgery alone or irradiation alone is adequate treatment for patients with lesions less than 2 cm. Lesions 2 to 4 cm may be treated with irradiation alone and lesions larger than 4 cm require combined pre-operative irradiation and surgery.

Sequelae of irradiation

Complications of irradiation for urethral cancers are dependent upon many factors. These include tumor size, invasion of tumor into other structures and total irradiation dose. Acute symptoms during and shortly after completion of irradiation include diarrhea and dysuria. Long-term complications may include dysuria, vaginal stenosis, cystitis, urethral stricture, fistula formation and bowel obstruction[18].

Severe complications occurred in 30% of patients treated with radiotherapy alone in the series reported by Grigsby and Corn[17]. Garden and associates[9] reported that 49% (27/55) of patients treated with radiotherapy alone and who had local control of their tumor developed complications. These complications were urethral stenosis in 11, fistula or necrosis in 10 and cystitis and hemorrhage in six. The complications were mild in five patients, moderate in 14 and severe in eight.

Conclusions

Radiotherapy plays an important role in the management of patients with urethral cancer. Urethral cancer rarely develops in men and the collected experience in treating men with this condition is limited. Therefore, specific recommendations for the use of radiotherapy in men cannot be proposed. Radiotherapy should be considered in the management of individual patients in order to preserve anatomy and organ function.

The experience in treating women with urethral carcinoma is more extensive and general guidelines for management can be proposed. In order to limit the volume of tissue treated with irradiation and therefore decrease the complications of radiotherapy, interstitial irradiation alone should be employed when possible. Small lesions of the anterior urethra may be treated with interstitial radiotherapy alone to total tumor doses of 5000 to 6500 cGy. Large lesions of the anterior urethra and all lesions involving the posterior urethra should be treated with combined external radiotherapy and interstitial or intra-cavitary irradiation to total tumor doses of 7000 to 8500 cGy. The inguinal lymph nodes should be treated in all of these patients. Pre-operative irradiation to doses of 4500 to 5000 cGy should be considered for patients with very large lesions of the urethra. The role of chemotherapy is not defined. Palliative irradiation can be delivered to relieve symptoms in patients who are not considered to be curable.

References

1. Srinivas V, Khan SA. Male urethral cancer. A review. *Int Urol Nephrol* 1988;**20**:61–65.
2. Ravi R, Sastry DV. Innovative treatment of carcinoma of the male urethra. *Urol Int* 1995;**55**:229–231.
3. Baskin LS, Turzan C. Carcinoma of male urethra: management of locally advanced disease with combined chemotherapy, radiotherapy, and penile-preserving surgery. *Urology* 1992;**39**:21–25.
4. Dinney CP, Johnson DE, Swanson DA, Babaian RJ, vonEschenbach AC. Therapy and prognosis for male anterior urethral carcinoma: an update. *Urology* 1994;**43**:506–514.
5. Hahn P, Krepart G, Malaker K. Carcinoma of the female urethra: Manitoba experience, 1958–1987. *Urology* 1991;**37**:106–109.
6. Johnson DW, Kessler JF, Ferrigni RG, Anderson JD. Low dose combined chemotherapy/radiotherapy in the management of locally advanced urethral squamous cell carcinoma. *J Urol* 1989;**141**:615–616.
7. Sailer SL, Shipley WU, Wang CC. Carcinoma of the female urethra: a review of results with radiation therapy. *J Urol* 1988;**140**:1–5.
8. Grigsby PW. Female urethra. In: Perez CA, Brady LW (eds). *Principles and practice of radiation oncology* (2nd edn). J.B. Lippincott Company, Philadelphia, 1992, pp. 1059–1066.
9. Garden AS, Zagars GK, Delclos L. Primary carcinoma of the female urethra. results of radiation therapy. *Cancer* 1993;**71**:3102–3108.
10. Gerbaulet A, Haie-Meder C, Marsiglia H *et al.* Brachytherapy in cancer of the urethra. *Ann Urol* 1994;**28**:312–317.
11. Spanos W, Perez C, Marcus S *et al.* Effect of rest interval on tumor and normal tissue response – a report of phase III study of accelerated split course palliative radiation for advanced pelvic malignancies (RTOG 8502). *Int J Radiat Oncol Biol Phys* 1993;**25**:399–403.
12. Bracken RB, Johnson DE, Miller LS, Ayala AG, Gomez JJ, Rutledge F. Primary carcinoma of the female urethra. *J Urol* 1976;**116**:188–192.
13. Johnson DE, O'Connell JR. Primary carcinoma of female urethra. *Urology* 1983;**21**:42–45.
14. Prempree T, Amornmarn R, Patanaphan V. Radiation therapy in primary carcinoma of the female urethra. *Cancer* 1984;**54**:729–733.
15. Weghaupt K, Gerstner GJ, Kucera H. Radiation therapy for primary carcinoma of the female urethra: a survey over 25 years. *Gynecol Oncol* 1984;**17**:58–63.
16. Foens CS, Hussey JHJ, Staples JJ, Doornbos JF, Wen BC, Vigliotti AP. A comparison of the roles of surgery and radiation therapy in the management of carcinoma of the female urethra. *Int J Radiat Oncol Biol Phys* 1991;**21**:961–968.
17. Grigsby PW, Corn BW. Localized urethral tumors in women: Indications for conservative versus exenterative therapies. *J Urol* 1992;**147**:1516–1520.
18. Marks LB, Carroll PR, Dugan TC, Anscher MS. The response of the urinary bladder, urethra, and ureter to radiation and chemotherapy. *Int J Radiat Oncol Biol Phys* 1995;**31**:1257–1280.

49.3 Chemotherapy

J W Basler

The primary means of treatment for urethral carcinoma involves local excision and/or radiotherapy. However, there will be patients with recurrence or metastatic disease who require systemic therapy despite these local efforts. In general, chemotherapy regimens will be based on the primary histologic type of the urethral tumor: squamous cell, transitional cell or adenocarcinoma. Unfortunately, the number of patients being treated with chemotherapy is low and reports in the literature regarding the use of chemotherapy for urethral carcinoma are sparse. In one report, pre-operative chemo-radiation was found to improve the operative result for a man with locally advanced disease[1]. Other reports from a major cancer center indicated improved survival of patients presenting with metastatic disease after treatment with cis-platinum based regimens[2]. New agents may have some efficacy as well[3]. Due to the rarity of this disease and the lack of specific organized clinical trials, progress in treating advanced stages may be slow at best. Currently there are 12 NCI (US) clinical trials for 'advanced urinary tract cancers' that could accept patients with urethral cancer[4]. Single agents in those trials include pyrazoloacridine, piritrexim and fluorouracil. Multidrug trials include various combinations of paclitaxel, cis-platinum, ifosfamide, methotrexate, vinblastine, interferon-alpha, carboplatin and adriamycin.

References

1. Johnson DW, Kessler JF, Ferrigni RG, Anderson JD. Low dose combined chemotherapy/radiotherapy in the management of locally advanced urethral squamous cell carcinoma. *J Urol* 1989;**141**(3):615–616.
2. Dinney CP, Johnson DE, Swanson DA, Babaian RJ, von Eschenbach AC. Therapy and prognosis for male anterior urethral carcinoma: an update. *Urology* 1994;**43**(4):506–514.
3. Kadan P, Korsh OB, Hiesmayr W. Ukrain in the treatment of urethral recurrent carcinoma (case report). *Drugs Exp Clin Res* 1996; **22**(3–5):271–273.
4. NCI web site reference: http://cancertrials.nci.nih.gov/ NCI_CANCER_TRIALS/zones/TrialInfo/Finding/search: urethral cancer

PART EIGHT
Urological aspects of gynecologic malignancies

Chapter 50
Overview of gynecologic malignancies

50.1   Epithelial ovarian cancer

50.2   Cervical cancer

50.3   Uterine cancer

Chapter 51
The role of exenteration and urinary diversion in gynecological malignancies

Chapter 52
Management of urogynecologic fistulae

50 Overview of gynecologic malignancies

50.1 Epithelial ovarian cancer

K O Easley and D G Mutch

Epithelial ovarian cancer is the leading cause of death from a gynecologic malignancy in the United States. It is the fourth most common cause of cancer death in the USA. There will be an estimated 27 000 cases of ovarian cancer in 1997 with a mortality of greater than 50%[1]. It has been estimated that 1 in 70 women will develop ovarian cancer in her lifetime and one woman in 120 will die of this disease (Figure 50.1.1).

Epidemiology

The age-specific incidence of ovarian cancer increases with age and peaks in the eighth decade. The incidence rates by age are seen in Figure 50.1.1 and are based on the SEER data of the National Cancer Institute[2]. Black women have a slightly lower lifetime risk than whites (1.08% vs. 1.86%)[1]. Overall survival rates for patients with ovarian cancer increased from 36% to 42% in 1991. This is probably due to more accurate staging and the development of new chemotherapeutic protocols.

The cellular events which lead up to the development of ovarian cancer are largely unknown. Numerous studies

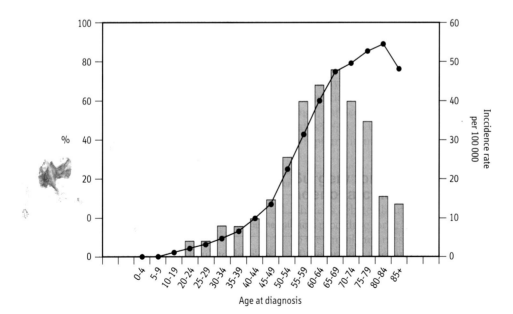

Fig. 50.1.1   Incidence rates of ovarian cancer by age (SEER Data).

have identified some factors which contribute to the risk of developing this disease. These generally include issues related to ovulation. The incidence of ovarian cancer appears to correlate with the number of lifetime ovulations. Multiparity decreases the risk of developing ovarian cancer as does breast feeding and oral contraceptive use[3]. Conversely, the lifetime risk of developing an ovarian neoplasm has been estimated at 4–5% for women with prolonged exposure to fertility medications[4]. These data give credence to the theory that ovulation, with ongoing damage and repair of the epithelium surrounding the ovary, increases the risk of ovarian cancer.

Family history is also an important factor in determining a particular individual's risk of developing ovarian cancer. The risk of a woman developing ovarian cancer in the absence of a positive family history is about 1.6%[5,6]. However, a woman with one first degree relative with ovarian cancer has a risk of 4–5%[6,7]. It should be noted that only about 5% of all ovarian cancers have a familial component[7,8]. Three distinct types of hereditary ovarian cancer have been identified, all of which are autosomal dominant:

1) Breast-ovarian cancer syndrome
2) Site specific ovarian cancer
3) Lynch Type II syndrome: characterized by the inheritance of non-polyposis colorectal cancer, endometrial cancer and ovarian cancer.

Prophylactic oophorectomy may be indicated in patients with a clear family history of ovarian cancer. All patients with a suspected cancer family syndrome should undergo genetic counseling before deciding on any treatment or genetic screening modality.

Pathology

Ovarian tumors may take a wide variety of histologic appearances which are related and described in Table 50.1.1.

Benign common epithelial tumors are almost always serous or mucinous. They are frequently large and microscopically a single cell layer of columnar epithelium lines the cysts.

Tumors of 'borderline malignant potential' are relatively common and carry a relatively good prognosis, yet have distinct histologic features that suggest cancer. Even when these tumors have spread to the abdomen or pelvis about 80% of patients will be alive at 5 years.

The histologic features used to diagnose borderline tumors include:

1) Epithelial papillae
2) Cellular stratification

Table 50.1.1   Histology of ovarian tumors

Serous tumors

Benign
   Cystadenoma and papillary cystadenoma
   Surface papilloma
   Adenofibroma and cystadenofibroma
Borderline malignancy (carcinoma of low malignant potential)
   Cystadenoma and papillary cystadenoma
   Surface papilloma
   Adenofibroma and cystadenofibroma
Malignant
   Adenocarcinoma (papillary adenocarcinoma and papillary cystadenocarcinoma)
   Surface papillary carcinoma
   Malignant adenofibroma and cystadenofibroma
   Mucinous tumors
Benign
   Cystadenoma
   Adenofibroma and cystadenofibroma
Borderline malignancy (carcinoma of low malignant potential)
   Cystadenoma
   Adenofibroma and cystadenofibroma
Malignant
   Adenocarcinoma and cystadenocarcinoma
   Malignant adenofibroma and cystadenofibroma
Endometrioid tumors
Benign
   Adenoma and cystadenoma
   Adenofibroma and cystadenofibroma
Borderline malignancy (carcinoma of low malignant potential).
   Adenoma and cystadenoma
   Adenofibroma and cystadenofibroma
Malignant
   Adenocarcinoma
   Adenoacanthoma
   Adenosquamous carcinoma
   Malignant adenofibroma and cystadenofibroma
     Epithelial-stroma and stromal
   Adenosarcoma
   Stromal sarcoma
Mesodermal (Mullerian) mixed tumors, homologous and heterologous)
   Clear cell tumors
   Benign
   Borderline malignancy (carcinomas of low malignant potential)
   Malignant
   Adenocarcinoma (carcinoma
Transitional cell tumors
   Brenner tumor
   Brenner tumor of borderline malignancy (proliferating)
   Malignant Brenner tumor
   Transitional cell carcinoma (non-Brenner type)
Mixed epithelial tumors
   Benign
   Borderline malignancy
   Malignant
Undifferentiated carcinoma
   Unclassified epithelial tumors

3) Increased mitotic activity
4) Nuclear atypia

Malignant epithelial tumors often present as solid and cystic masses in the pelvis. Most ovarian cancers (70%) present as stage III lesions with peritoneal metastasis. The distinction of pushing, destructive or infiltrative growth is important since it is often the only feature that distinguishes a serous adenocarcinoma from one that is borderline. Other features which may help in distinguishing malignant from non-malignant tumors are:

1) Altered tumor/stromal interface from a broad, uniform front to a focally irregular or ragged border.
2) Change in the normal or edematous stroma to one that is desmoplastic.
3) A chronic inflammatory cell infiltrate.

Staging

Epithelial ovarian cancers are thought to arise from the ovarian surface epithelium. Early in development ovarian cancers are thought to be confined to the ovary but by the time of presentation 75–80% have spread beyond the ovary. Early stage ovarian cancers are relatively uncommon and less than 30% present as stage I or II lesions.

The early spread of this disease is usually occult. A significant number of patients with grossly negative exploration will have microscopic disease present when careful staging is performed (Table 50.1.2).

Since the initial spread of ovarian cancer is occult and many patients have metastatic disease in spite of a grossly negative examination, it is important to be prepared to stage a patient any time removal of an adnexal mass is planned[9]. If no disease can be identified outside of the ovary it is important to biopsy the diaphragm, peritoneal surfaces, sample the pelvic and periaortic nodes, remove the omentum and take washings of the abdominal cavity.

Table 50.1.2   Sites of metastases in ovarian cancer

Site	Number of patients with positive biopsies	Total number of patients	%
Diaphragm	17	223	7.6
Omentum	21	294	7.1
Cytology	13	69	18.8
Peritoneal	6	61	9.8
Pelvic nodes	18	202	8.9
Aortic nodes	35	285	12.3

Reproduced from Rubin and Sutton, *Ovarian cancer*, 1993 McGraw-Hill.

Surgical staging in apparently early ovarian cancer

Vertical incision
Multiple cytologic washings
Intact tumor removal
Complete abdominal exploration
Removal of remaining ovary, uterus and tubes
Omentectomy
Lymph node sampling
Random peritoneal biopsies, including diaphragm

Our understanding of the natural history of ovarian cancer forms the basis of the current staging system. The stage is defined as the extent of the disease at the time of initial laparotomy. It is determined by careful exploration of the abdominal cavity. Separate specimens should be submitted adequately to determine where metastatic disease exists. In a case where frozen section indicates that there is an ovarian cancer, meticulous biopsies should be obtained of all peritoneal surfaces and adhesions should be biopsied and marked. These biopsies should be clearly documented. Table 50.1.3 shows the FIGO staging for ovarian cancer.

Table 50.1.3   Staging for ovarian cancer (FIGO 1986)

Stage I: Growth limited to the ovaries
  IA: Growth limited to one ovary; no ascites; no tumor on the external surfaces, capsule intact.
  IB: Growth limited to both ovaries; no ascites; no tumor on the external surfaces, capsule intact
  IC: Tumor either IA or IB but with tumor on the surface of one or both varies; or with capsule ruptured; or with ascites present, containing malignant cells or with positive peritoneal washings.

Stage II: Growth involving one or both ovaries with pelvic extension
  IIA: Extension and/or metastases to the uterus and or tubes
  IIB: Extension to other pelvic tissues
  IIC: Tumor either IIA or IIB but with tumor on the surface of one or both ovaries; or with capsule(s) ruptured; or with ascites present containing malignant cells or with positive peritoneal washings.

Stage III: Tumor involving one or both ovaries with peritoneal implants outside the pelvis and/or positive retroperitoneal or inguinal nodes; superficial liver metastases; tumor is limited to the true pelvis but with histologically confirmed malignant extension to small bowel or omentum.
  IIIA: Tumor grossly limited to the pelvis with negative nodes but histologically confirmed microscopic seeding of abdominal peritoneal surfaces.
  IIIB: Tumor of one or both ovaries; histologically confirmed implants of abdominal peritoneal surfaces, none exceeding 2 cm in diameter; nodes negative
  IIIC: Abdominal implants greater than 2 cm in greatest diameter and/or positive retroperitoneal or inguinal nodes

Stage IV: Growth involving one or both ovaries with distant metastases; if pleural effusion is present, there must be cytologic test results; presence of parenchymal liver metastases.

551

Prognostic factors

Stage

The long-term survival of patients with ovarian cancer is directly correlated with the stage of the patient at the time of diagnosis. The 5 year survival of patients with stage I disease is as high as 90% in patients who are comprehensively staged[10]. Though stage II disease is uncommon and patients thought to have this stage initially are often upstaged, those who have undergone complete staging may have a survival of 80%. The survival in patients with advanced stage of disease varies with the volume of residual disease but ranges from 5% to 30% over 5 years[11].

Volume of residual disease

The volume of residual disease after primary surgery is directly correlated with survival. Patients are usually described as either optimally debulked (residual tumor less than 1 cm) or suboptimally cytoreduced (residual tumor of greater than 1 cm)[12]. Residual tumor is prognostically related to the size of the largest residual mass and not the number of lesions. Survival in patients who have been optimally cytoreduced is two to three times greater than those patients who have significant residual disease (48 months vs. 21 months).

Histologic subtype and grade

The histologic type is believed to be of less prognostic importance than other clinical factors such as stage, volume of disease and histologic grade. Some series suggest that mucinous tumors have an improved survival over other histologic types but this probably reflects the fact that there are very few poorly differentiated mucinous tumors.

The histologic grade of the tumor has significant prognostic importance particularly in early stage patients. Patients with stage I well or moderately differentiated tumors have a greater than 90% 5 year survival whereas patients with poorly differentiated tumors have a significantly reduced survival[13]. The survival disadvantage for patients with high grade and more advanced stage is less clear than that observed in the early stage patients.

Treatment

Management of tumors of low malignant potential

Patients with tumors of low malignant potential of early stage (I or II) need no further therapy if all gross disease has been removed. Currently there is no demonstrable benefit in treating these tumors.

Approximately 20% of patients with tumors of low malignant potential will present at a late stage. We currently believe that the primary surgical management of this disease should be the same as for invasive cancers. However, the benefit of any type of post-surgical therapy has not been clearly established. Multiple studies have demonstrated conflicting results regarding the benefits of adjuvant therapy[14,15]. The GOG has recently completed accrual on a prospective protocol which follows the natural history of tumors of low malignant potential to determine the efficacy of adjuvant therapy in patients of advanced stage. This study, once the data is mature, should be able to answer definitively the value of adjuvant therapy.

Management of epithelial ovarian cancer

Although only 10–15% of all epithelial ovarian cancer presents as stage I, approximately 30% of all long-term survivors are derived from this group. Most gynecologic oncologists would not treat stage I grade 1 ovarian cancer. However, any stage or grade beyond this requires some adjuvant therapy. Options for treatment include: radiation therapy, intraperitoneal radiocolloid administration and chemotherapy. External radiation therapy has no role in the current management of early stage ovarian cancer.

Currently there is no standard for post-operative treatment of true stage I ovarian cancer of advanced grade. There are several ongoing trials to evaluate the best treatment modality for this situation. GOG Protocol 95 randomized patients to intraperitoneal ^{32}P vs. three cycles of cisplatin and cyclophosphamide. This trial has been closed as it has reached targeted accrual but no data is available. Other studies have randomized patients to three cycles of cisplatin and taxol vs. cisplatin and cytoxan. Over the next few years the important answers about the most effective treatment modality for early stage disease should be available.

Most cases of ovarian cancer are diagnosed in the advanced stages. The standard therapy is cytoreductive surgery followed by chemotherapy. Randomized trials to study the effect of chemotherapy on this disease began in 1978 when Young randomized patients to receive multiagent therapy versus single agent alkylating therapy and showed that multiagent therapy was superior[16]. In the early 1980s platinum based therapy in combination with adriamycin and cyclophosphamide or cyclophosphamide alone became the standard of care. A recently completed trial through the GOG randomizing patients to receive cisplatin and cyclophosphamide vs. cisplatin and paclitaxel demonstrated superior survival in patients treated with the paclitaxel combination. Therefore, at the present time platinum based therapy in combination with paclitaxel is the standard of care for post-operative treatment of advanced stage ovarian cancer[17].

New chemotherapy agents active against ovarian cancer include topotecan, gemcitabine and navelbine. Intraperitoneal therapy as the route of administration is also showing renewed promise. High-dose therapy with stem cell support needs investigation as well as gene therapy. The next decade should bring many advances in the treatment of ovarian cancer.

References

1. Wingo PA, Tong T, Bolden S. Cancer Statistics 1995. *CA Cancer Journal Clin* 1995;**45**:8.
2. Yanik R, Ries LG, Yates JW. Ovarian cancer in the elderly: an analysis of surveillance. *Am J Obstet Gynecol* 1986;**154**:639.
3. Greene MH, Clark JW, Blayney DW. The epidemiology of ovarian cancer. *Semin Oncol* 1984;**1**:209.
4. Whittemore AS, Wu ML, Paffenbarger RS *et al.* Epithelial ovarian cancer and ability to conceive. *Can Res* 1989;**49**:4047.
5. Carlson KJ, Skates SJ, Singer DE. Screening for ovarian cancer. *Ann Int Med* 1994;**121**:124.
6. National Institutes of Health Consensus Development Conference Statement. Ovarian cancer: screening, treatment and follow-up. *Gyn Oncol* 1994;**55**:S4.
7. Schildkraut JM, Thompson WD. Familial ovarian cancer: a population base case-control study. *Am J Epidem* 1988;**128**:456.
8. Whittemore AS. Characteristics relating to ovarian cancer risk: implications for prevention and detection. *Gyn Oncol* 1994;**55**:S15.
9. Piver MS, Barlow JJ, SS L. Incidence of subclinical metastasis in Stage I and II ovarian cancer. *Obstet Gynecol* 1982;**52**:100.
10. Young RC, Walton LA, Ellenberg SS *et al.* Adjuvant therapy in Stage I and II epithelial ovarian cancer: results of two randomized prospective trials. *N Engl J Med* 1990;**322**:1102.
11. Yanik R. Ovarian cancer. Age contrasts in incidence, hisology, disease stage at diagnosis, and mortality. *Cancer* 1993;**71**:517.
12. Hainsworth J, Grosh W, Burnett L *et al.* Advanced ovarian cancer: long term results of treatment with intensive cisplatin based chemotherapy of brief duration. *Ann Int Med* 1988;**108**:165.
13. Rubin SC, Wong GY, Curtin J, Barakat RR, Hakes TB, Hoskins WJ. Platinum-based chemotherapy of high risk stage I epithelial cancer following comprehensive surgical staging. *Obstet Gynecol* 1993;**82**:143.
14. Chambers JT. Borderline ovarian tumors: a review of treatment. *J Biol Med* 1989;**62**:351.
15. Fort MG, Pierce VK, Saigo PE, Hoskins WJ, Lewis JL Jr. Evidence for the efficacy of adjuvant therapy in epithelial ovarian tumors at low malignant potential. *Gyn Oncol* 1989;**32**:269.
16. Young RC, Chabner B, Hubbard S *et al.* Advanced ovarian adenocarcinoma: a prospective randomized trial melphalan vs combination chemotherapy. *N Eng J Med* 1978;**299**:1261.
17. Mcguire WP, Hoskins WJ, Brady MF *et al.* A phase III trial comparing cisplatin/cytoxan and cisplatin/taxol (PI) in advanced ovarian cancer. *Proc ASCO* 1993;**12**:226(abstract 808).

50.2 Cervical cancer

K O Easley and D G Mutch

Pre-invasive disease and epidemiology

Carcinoma of the uterine cervix is the sixth most common female malignancy accounting for approximately 3% of female cancers with 15 800 new cases estimated for 1996 and 4800 estimated cancer deaths[1]. It is one of the most preventable cancers secondary to its generally long pre-invasive state. Numerous epidemiologic studies have shown that the pre-invasive dysplasia is initiated by sexually transmitted carcinogens[2]. While initial studies suggested a link between herpes and genital neoplasia and cancer, convincing evidence is lacking. More recently however numerous studies have implicated the human papillomavirus in the etiology of cervical neoplasia and cancer[3], ulvar neoplasia and cancer[4] as well as penile cancer[5]. Since the introduction of the Papanicolaou smear[6] in the 1940s, an effective cancer-screening method, there has been a significant reduction in mortality from cervical cancer in screened populations[7-9]. In 1988, a workshop sponsored by the National Cancer Institute resulted in new guidelines for reporting the results of cervical and vaginal cytology in an effort further to standardize the reporting of pap smears. Known as the 'Bethesda system' and shown in Table 50.2.1, these guidelines eliminate the usage of the Papanicolaou classification system and instead utilize descriptive terminology including the adequacy of the smear. The Bethesda system also introduced the terms 'low grade and high grade squamous intraepithelial lesions (LGSIL and HGSIL)' but with alcohol. If the cells are allowed to dry before fixation, artifact will result and prevent a reliable interpretation of the smear. An abnormal smear mandates further evaluation and often requires referral for colposcopic examination. Merely repeating the pap smear does not relieve one of the burden to explain by colposcopic examination and biopsy the initial abnormal pap smear. Colposcopy allows 5 × to 40 × magnification of the cervical epithelium and underlying stroma. Usage of a 3% acetic acid solution and a green light filter allows for colposcopic directed biopsies of any abnormal areas. Patients in whom the entire cervical transformation zone is able to be visualized, in whom the entire abnormality is seen and in whom the pap smear, cervical biopsy and colposcopic appearance are in agreement and with no evidence of endocervical involvement, may be treated with conservative means. Cryotherapy or loop electrical excision procedure (LEEP) are commonly used and equally effective. Cryotherapy units use a liquefied gas, usually nitrogen, to cause hypothermia by evaporation of the liquid refrigerant which results in cryonecrosis in a predictable and uniform area. LEEP uses an electrical current applied to a wire loop which is used to excise a cone-shaped portion of the cervix. Both are well tolerated as an office procedure. LEEP also allows a tissue sample to be obtained for pathologic evaluation.

If the colposcopic examination is unsatisfactory due to incomplete visualization, or there is a discordance between the pap smear biopsy or colposcopic appearance, or if there is endocervical involvement, a cold knife conization or

Table 50.2.1   Pap smear classification systems

Bethesda system	Dysplasia/CIN system		Papanicolaou system
Within normal limits	Normal		I
Infection (organism should be specified)	Inflammatory atypia (organism)		I
Reactive and reparative changes			
Squamous cell abnormalities Atypical squamous cells of undetermined significance	Squamous atypia		IIR
Low-grade squamous intraepithelial lesion (LSIL)	HPV atypia Mild dysplasia	CIN 1	
High-grade squamous intraepithelial lesion (HSIL)	Moderate dysplasia	CIN 2	III
Squamous cell carcinoma	Severe dysplasia Carcinoma in situ	CIN 3	IV
	Squamous cell carcinoma		V

CIN = cervical intraepithelial neoplasia
Reproduced from Becker and Hacker, Practical Gynecologic Oncology, 2nd edition, 1994

LEEP procedure is indicated. If there is a suspicion of invasive cancer, a cold knife conization should be performed. While a LEEP procedure has also been used in this situation by some, it is generally not recommended as even very minimal cautery artifact from LEEP may prevent the pathologist from distinguishing a microinvasive lesion from an invasive cancer and consequently may require that the patient undergo a more radical therapy.

Invasive disease

While invasive cervical cancer may be detected by pap smear, false-negative rates for cervical cytology have been reported as 30–40% and may be as high as 50% in the presence of an ulcerated necrotic cancer[12]. Consequently, it is important to remember that the pap smear is only a screening tool, and any suspicious cervical lesion should be biopsied regardless of the pap smear result.

Presenting symptoms vary and may range from completely asymptomatic to uropathy secondary to bilateral ureteral obstruction. More commonly patients will present with complaints of irregular or postcoital bleeding or with an abnormal or malodorous vaginal discharge. Grossly, cervical cancers may present as an obvious exophytic or ulcerated lesion or as an endophytic lesion. The former is easily seen and biopsied while the latter is often not easily seen but may expand the endocervix before detection.

Cervical cancer may spread in several ways including direct extension, lymphatic metastasis, hematogenous metastasis and by intraperitoneal spread. Direct extension into the parametria generally occurs initially. Subsequent migration cephalad into the myometrium and caudad into the vagina also occur. Spread anteriorly and posteriorly into the bladder and rectum also occur, but relatively late because of the vesicouterine and rectouterine spaces. Lymphatic metastasis to lymph nodes generally follows an orderly sequence with initial metastasis to the obturators followed by the external and iliac nodes, the common iliac nodes, the aortics and supraclavicular lymph nodes. Hematogenous spread is a late finding, but when present is commonly to liver, lung and bone. Intraperitoneal spread may also occur, but is rare.

Staging

The current staging system of the International Federation of Gynecology and Obstetrics (FIGO) is shown in Table 50.2.2. The staging of cervical cancer is based upon clinical examination, preferably under anesthesia. Certain additional studies are allowed by FIGO in assessing stage and are listed in Table 50.2.1. Once the stage has been determined, it cannot be changed if at surgery or subsequent treatment additional findings of disease are detected. In general, stage I lesions are confined to the cervix, stage II have spread to the parametria and/or upper vagina, stage III involve the lower third of the vagina, extend to the pelvic side wall or show evidence of ureteral involvement (hydronephrosis or a non-functioning kidney not attributable to other causes) and stage IV indicates extension to the bladder or rectum and with distant spread. The distribution of patients by clinical stage is 38% stage I, 32% stage II, 26% stage III and 4% stage IV[13].

Table 50.2.2   FIGO staging of cervical cancer

TNM[1]	FIGO[2]	Definition
Primary tumor (t)		
TX	——	Primary tumor cannot be assessed
T0	——	No evidence of primary tumor
Tis	0	Carcinoma in situ, intraepithelial tumor
T1	I	Cervical carcinoma confined to cervix (extension to the corpus should be disregarded)
T1a	IA	Invasive carcinoma, diagnosed microscopically only. All gross lesions even with superficial invasion are stage IB cancers. Invasion limited to measured stromal invasion with maximum depth of 5.0 mm and no wider than 7.0 mm
T1a1	IA-1	Minimal microscopically evidence stromal invasion. Measured invasion of stroma no greater than 3.0 mm in depath and no wider than 7.0 mm
T1a2	IA-2	Measured invasion of stroma greater than 3 mm and no greater than 5 mm, and no wider than 7 mm. The depth of invasion should not be more than 5 mm taken from the base of the epithelium, either surface or glandular, from which it originates. Vascular space involvement either venous or lymphatic should not alter the staging
T1b	IB	Clinical lesions confined to the cervix or preclinical lesions greater than stage IA
	IB-1	Clinical lesions no greater than 4.0 cm in size
	IB-2	Clinical lesions greater than 4.0 cm in size
T2	II	Cervical carcinoma invades beyond the uterus, but not to the pelvic wall or to the lower third of the vagina
T2a	IIA	No obvious parametrial invasion
T2b	IIB	Obvious paramtetrial invasion
T3	III	Extends to the pelvic wall and/or involves lower third of the vagina and/or causes hydronephrosis or non-functioning kidney
T3a	IIIA	Tumor involves the lower third of the vagina. no extension to the pelvic wall
T3b	IIIB	Tumor extends to the pelvic wall and/or causes hydronephrosis or non-functioning kidney
T4	IV	The carcinoma has extended beyond the true pelvis or has clinically involved the mucosa of the bladder or rectum. A bullous edema as such does not permit a case to be alloted to stage IV
	IVA	Tumor invades mucosa of the bladder or rectum and/or extends beyond true pelvis
M1	IVB	Distant metastasis

[1] AJCC/UICC, 1992.

[2] Society of Gynecologic Oncologists (1994) *Handbook staging of gynecologic malignancies*, 1st edn. Chicago; Society of Gynecologic Oncologists.

Treatment

Two modalities of therapy are generally available for the primary treatment of cervical cancer: surgery and radiotherapy, with the choice of therapy dependent upon the stage of disease and the general health of the patient. While radiotherapy can be used in all stages of disease,

surgery alone is generally limited to patients with stage I and IIA disease in the United States, while IIb lesions are also occasionally treated by surgery in Europe. The principles of treatment for cervical cancer are to eradicate the primary lesion and treat potential sites of spread. Table 50.2.3 reveals the reported incidence of lymph nodal spread by stage.

Surgical management

Stage I carcinomas are confined to the cervix and can be further classified into stage IA-1 and IA-2, IB-1 and IB-2. Stage IA-1 is a microinvasive carcinoma in which the neoplastic epithelium invades the stroma to a depth of not greater than 3 mm beneath the basement membrane and in which there is no lymphovascular involvement or confluent tongues of tumor. Diagnosis must be based on a cone biopsy of the cervix. The purpose of designating a lesion as microinvasive is to define a group of patients who are not at risk of lymph node metastasis or recurrence and may therefore be treated conservatively by simple hysterectomy or conization if fertility is desired. Stage IA-2a designates a lesion that is identified only microscopically and includes lesions up to 5 mm in depth and 7 mm in width. Stage IB lesions are of greater dimension than IA-2 lesions with stage IA lesions that do not strictly meet microinvasive criteria, as well as stage IB and IIA cervical cancers can be surgically managed by radical procedures. The radical hysterectomy performed most often in the United States is that described by Meigs in 1944[14]. The procedure involves removal of the uterus, upper third of the vagina, the entire uterosacral and uterovesical ligaments, and all of the parametrium bilaterally as well as a meticulous pelvic lymphadenectomy. The operation can be approached through either a midline or transverse incision. These authors prefer to begin the radical surgery by performing the lymphadenectomy first via a retroperitoneal approach. If pelvic or periaortic nodal metastatic disease is found, there is the option of aborting the radical hysterectomy and treating the patient with radiation therapy. Avoidance of entering the peritoneum lessens the likelihood of post-operative adhesion formation which is known to increase the risk of radiation complications. If there is no evidence of metastatic disease, following completion of the lymphadenectomy, the radical hysterectomy is carried out. Upon entering the peritoneum, the peri-

Table 50.2.3   Staging procedures allowed by FIGO

• Colposcopy	• Biopsies
• Endocervical curettage	• Cervical conization
• Chest X-ray	• Intravenous pyelogram
• Barium enema	• Skeletal X-ray
• Hysteroscopy	• Proctoscopy

Table 50.2.4   Incidence of pelvic and para-aortic nodal metastasis by stage

Stage		n	% Positive pelvic nodes	% Positive para-aortic nodes
IA1		23	0	0
IA2	(1–3 mm)	156	0.6	0
	(3–5 mm)	84	4.8	<1
IB		1926	15.9	2.2
IIA		110	24.5	11
IIB		324	31.4	19
III		125	44.8	30
IVA		23	55.0	40

Reproduced from Becker and Hacker, Practical Gynecologic Oncology (2nd edn,) 1994

toneal cavity is explored to exclude metastatic disease with attention directed to the peritoneal surfaces, diaphragm, omentum and liver. The ovaries and fallopian tubes are inspected and if grossly normal are not removed in a patient less than 40–45 years of age, as metastatic disease to the adnexa is extremely rare in cervical cancer. The parametrium are carefully palpated again to ensure no evidence of spread. The bladder should then be carefully dissected from the anterior cervix and vagina with attention to ensure no extension of tumor into the base of the bladder. The uterine artery is isolated and ligated at its origin and gently retracted above the ureter and the ureter is dissected from its peritoneal flap beginning at the uterosacral ligament into the ureteral tunnel and freed from the vesicouterine ligament to the base of the bladder. The peritoneum across the cul-de-sac is incised and the rectovaginal space opened allowing the rectum to be dissected posteriorly and free the uterosacral ligaments. The specimen is then excised by clamping and ligating the uterosacral ligaments midway between uterus and sacrum, paracolpos and upper third of vagina to ensure adequate surgical margins. There are also recent reports of laparoscopic radical hysterectomy as well as combining a radical vaginal hysterectomy with a laparoscopic.

Immediate complications of radical hysterectomy include hemorrhage (800 cc average EBL), infection (<5%) and thromboembolic disease (1–2%). The major reported long-term complications of radical hysterectomy include bladder dysfunction (3%), ureteral fistulae (<1%) and lymphocyst formation. The incidence of each of these complications continues to decrease with the exception of long-term bladder dysfunction.

Immediately after surgery the bladder is hypertonic with a decreased functional bladder capacity, high filling pressure and insensitivity to filling. Difficulty in initiating micturition is common as are reports of overflow incontinence. Over several months, the hypertonia subsides and a picture

of detrusor hypotonia often emerges characterized by urinary retention, overflow incontinence and recurrent infections[15]. A number of theories have been proposed to explain the bladder dysfunction.[16] One theory is that a sympathetic denervation of the bladder during radical surgery results in parasympathetic dominance. A second theory is bladder dysfunction results from associated edema and inflammation to the bladder muscle resulting in an increase in the myogenic tone. Treatment is symptomatic and with time near total recovery occurs in most patients. It is felt that the degree of bladder dysfunction is related to the radicality of the surgery. It has also been reported that adjunctive pelvic radiation is associated with significantly more contracted and unstable bladder[15].

The results of radical surgery in the treatment of cervical cancer is dependent upon several factors. The presence or absence of lymph nodal involvement, lymph vascular space involvement, depth of invasion and tumor size have been found to be the most important prognostic variables. Five year survival rates of 75% to 95% in stages I and IIA with negative prognostic variables can be expected. With metastatic disease, deep invasion, lymph vascular space involvement or large tumors, however, the prognosis significantly worsens.

Post-operative adjuvant radiation therapy should be considered in patients following radical hysterectomy if they are found to have: 1) positive pelvic lymph nodes, 2) microscopic positive margins of resection, 3) deep stromal invasion or 4) lymph-vascular space involvement. It should be prescribed judiciously however, due to the known significant rate of major complications to the intestinal and urinary system that have been reported[17]. In addition, there are no controlled or prospective studies that show improved survival in patients with high-risk factors. Analysis of the retrospective studies available suggest that while post-operative radiotherapy may decrease pelvic recurrences, it has not been shown to change overall survival[18–20]. The only suggestion of a survival benefit with post-operative radiotherapy is in cases of greater than three positive unilateral pelvic nodes or bilateral positive pelvic nodes. The GOG (Gynecology Oncology Group) recently completed a multiinstitutional study looking at patients with poor prognostic factors of deep invasion, large tumor and lymph-vascular space involvement who were randomized to no further treatment versus pelvic radiotherapy. That data is currently being analyzed and hopefully will be soon forthcoming and provide guidance in prescribing post-operative radiotherapy. The usage on neoadjuvant chemotherapy combined with radical hysterectomy or post-operative radiotherapy has also been used, but again, no randomized controlled studies are available. GOG randomized trials are presently underway.

Management with radiation therapy

Radiation therapy is the treatment of choice in patients with advanced stage lesions but can be used for all stages with cure rates of 70% for stage I, 60% for stage II, 45% for stage III and 18% for stage IV[13]. Treatment can be tailored to the particular tumor but generally consists of external radiotherapy to treat the pelvic nodes and intracavitary brachytherapy to boost treatment to the tumor volume. Rectal and bladder tolerance limit the dosages that can be administered. Extended-field radiotherapy to the para-aortic region is also administered in patients with known metastasis to the para-aortic nodes. Elective para-aortic irradiation has been proposed in selected patients without documented para-aortic metastasis based upon a 12% improved survival[21].

Post-treatment surveillance

The majority of recurrences will present within 2 years[22]. The patient should be seen every 3 to 4 months during this period. In addition to a pelvic examination, including a careful rectovaginal examination and pap smear, supraclavicular lymph nodes should also be palpated for evidence of recurrent disease. Some authorities also recommend annual chest X-rays and intravenous pyelogram to screen for evidence of lung or pelvic recurrence, but these may be obtained depending upon the initial stage and extent of disease. CT scan or MRI should also be used if there is a suggestion of recurrence. Any palpable adenopathy or pelvic disease can be further evaluated by FNA cytology as well as an examination under anesthesia with additional biopsies where indicated.

Generally, patients initially treated with surgery will be candidates for radiation therapy, and those treated with radiation therapy may be candidates for surgery. Those patients previously treated with radical hysterectomy and found to have pelvic recurrence are best treated with radiation therapy. Previous studies have commented upon the futility of exenterative procedures with recurrences following radical hysterectomy. Patients previously irradiated and considered for surgical therapy must be carefully selected and limited to only those patients, who after a thorough pre-operative evaluation to rule out metastatic disease, are felt to have only a central pelvic recurrence that is amenable to resection with clear margins. The procedure may include total pelvic exenteration or an anterior or posterior exenteration for isolated anterior or posterior cervical and/or vaginal recurrence. In addition, where total exenteration is indicated and if adequate margins are obtainable, a supralevator exenteration may be possible leaving the rectal stump to allow sigmoid anastomosis and avoid permanent colostomy. Rare reports of radical hysterectomy have also been reported, however complication rates are quite high in advanced stage recurrences and patients considered for less radical treatment must be carefully selected and counseled.

Recurrent cervical cancer not amenable to attempts at curative therapy with radiation or surgery may be considered for palliative chemotherapy. Various studies have shown response rates of 40–50% but complete responses are unusual and long-term survival is unlikely. Cisplatinum has shown the best response rate and presently felt to be as effective as multidrug regimens though further studies are underway.

References

1. 1995 Cancer Statistics. *CA-A Cancer Journal for Clinicians* 1995;45.
2. Rotkin ID. A comparison review of key epidemiologic studies in cervical cancer related to current searches for transmissible agents. *Cancer Res* 1973;**33**:1353.
3. Munoz N, Bosch FX, Shah KV, Meheus A. The epidemiology of HPV and cervical cancer. *International Agency for Research on Cancer* 1992.
4. Park JS, Jownes RW, McLean MR. A possible etiologic heterogeneity of vulvar intraepithelial neoplasia. *Cancer* 1991;**67**:1599.
5. Gross F, Ikenberg H, Gissman L, Hagedorn M. Papillomavirus infection of the anogenital region: correlation between histology, clinical picture and virus type. *J Invest Dermatol* 1985;**85**:146.
6. Papanicolaou G, Traut HF. *The diagnosis of uterine cancer by the vaginal smear.* Commonwealth Fund, New York, 1943.
7. Eddy DM. Appropriateness of cervical cancer screening. *Gynecol Oncol* 1981;**12**:168.
8. Johannesson G, Geitsson G, Day N. The effect of mass screening in Iceland, 1965–1974, on the incidence and mortality of cervical cancer. *Int J Cancer* 1978;**21**:418.
9. Canadian Task Force Report. *Can Med Assoc J* 1976;**114**:1003.
10. Cancer Society. *1991 Facts and Figures.* American Cancer Society, Atlanta 1991.
11. Pearse WH. Consensus report on frequency of Pap smear testing. *ACOG Newsletter* 1988;**32**:3.
12. Hurt GW, Silverberg SG, Fable WJ. Adenocarcinoma of the cervix: Histopathologic and clinical features. *Am J Obstet Gynecol* 1984;**149**:293.
13. Pettersson FE. Annual report on the results of treatment in gynecologic cancer. *Int J Gynecol Obstet* 1991;**36**:1.
14. Miegs J. Radical hysterectomy with bilateral pelvic node dissections: A report of 100 patients operated five or more years ago. *Am J Obstet Gynecol* 1951;**63**:854.
15. Bandy LC, Clarke-Pearson DL, Soper JT, Mutch DG, MacMillan J, Creasman WT. Long-term effects of bladder function following radical hysterectomy with and without postoperative radiation. *Gyn Oncol* 1987;**26**:160.
16. Lee RB, Park RC. Bladder dysfunction following radical abdominal hysterectomy. *Gyn Oncol* 1981;**11**:304.
17. Barter JF, Soong SJ, Shingleton HM. Complications of combined radical hysterectomy: Postoperative radiation therapy in women with early stage cervical cancer. *Gyn Oncol* 1989;**32**:292.
18. Morrow P. Panel report: Is pelvic irradiation beneficial in the postoperative management of stage IB squamous cell carcinoma of the cervix with pelvic node metastases treated by radical hysterectomy and pelvic lymphadenectomy? *Gyn Oncol* 1980;**10**:105.
19. Kinney WK, Alvarez RD, Reid GC. Value of adjuvant whole-pelvic irradiation after Wertheim hysterectomy for early-stage squamous carcinoma of the cervix with pelvic nodal metastasis: a matched-control study. *Gyn Oncol* 1989;**34**:258.

20. Soison AP, Soper JT, Clarke-Pearson DL. Adjuvant radiotherapy following radical hysterectomy for patients with stage IB and IIA cervical cancer. *Gyn Oncol* 1991;**37**:390.

21. Rotman M, Choi K, Pajak T. Prophylactic extended-field irradiation of para-aortic lymph nodes in stages IB, bulky IB and IIA cervical carcinoma: Ten-year treatment results of RTOG 79–20. *JAMA* 1995;**274**:387–393.

22. Shingleton H, Orr J. Posttreatment surveillance. In: Singer A, Jordan J (eds). *Cancer of the cervix*. Churchill Livingstone, New York, 1983:136.

Table 50.3.2   Patients in whom a diagnosis of endometrial cancer should be excluded

- All patients with post-menopausal bleeding
- Post-menopausal women with pyometria
- Asymptomatic post-menopausal women with endometrial cells on a Pap smear
- Perimenopausal patients with intermenstrual bleeding or increasingly heavy periods
- Pre-menopausal patients with abnormal uterine bleeding, particularly if there is a history of anovulation

(Reproduced from Berek and Hacker, *Practical gynecologic oncology* (2nd edn), 1994, Williams and Wilkins)

50.3   Uterine cancer

K O Easley and D G Mutch

In the United States, endometrial cancer is the most common malignancy of the female genital tract. In 1996 an estimated 32 800 new cases are expected with 5900 cancer deaths[1]. The risk of endometrial cancer is felt to correlate with exposure to unopposed estrogens. Consequently nulliparity, amenorrhea, late menopause, obesity, polycystic ovarian disease or unopposed exogenous estrogens place a patient at risk. Factors that decrease exposure to unopposed estrogens or that increase exposure to progesterone will decrease the risk of endometrial cancer, such as oral contraceptives or progesterones[2].

Signs and symptoms

An affluent, obese, low parity, diabetic, hypertensive with abnormal vaginal bleeding is the most common presentation. This may include post-menopausal bleeding or heavy and/or irregular premenopausal vaginal bleeding. As shown in Table 50.3.1, abnormal bleeding may be secondary to a number of causes other than carcinoma, however post-menopausal bleeding or abnormal bleeding warrants further investigation.

Diagnosis

Table 50.3.2 outlines those patients in whom the diagnosis of endometrial carcinoma should be excluded by sampling tissue from the endometrial cavity. An office

Table 50.3.1   Causes of post-menopausal bleeding

• exogenous estrogens	30
• atrophic endometritis	30
• endometrial cancer	15
• endometrial or cervical polyps	10
• endometrial hyperplasia	5
• miscellaneous	10

(Reproduced from Berek and Hacker, *Practical gyncologic oncology* (2nd edn), 1994, Williams and Wilkins)

endometrial biopsy can generally be obtained and is well tolerated by most patients. The usage of a Novaks curette, Pipelle or Vabra aspirator will generally provide an adequate sample to evaluate for evidence of carcinoma, and is reliable approximately 90% of the time. Because of this 10% false-negative rate however, hysteroscopy may be useful to ensure that any abnormal endometrial area has been sampled[3]. While the majority of patients will be able to be adequately evaluated with an office biopsy, some patients may have a stenotic os or be unable to tolerate an office biopsy and require an outpatient dilatation and curettage[4].

The usage of ultrasound has recently been promoted as a screening technique for endometrial cancer. Data suggest that the normal endometrial stripe in a post-menopausal woman, not on estrogen replacement therapy, should be less than 5 mm in thickness[5]. While this modality appears to be used more and more, and may be indicated as a screening technique in asymptomatic high-risk patients, (such as those with a strong family history or with the onset of menopause at a later age), the gold standard for the evaluation of post-menopausal bleeding remains endometrial sampling. On occasion, a pap smear may reveal malignant endometrial cells, however it is not reliable as a screening or a diagnostic technique as only 50% of patients with a known endometrial cancer will have malignant cells on pap smear[6]. If suspicious or frankly malignant cells are present on pap smear in a patient who is found to have endometrial cancer, it is more likely that the patient will have more advanced disease, with higher grade and/or deeper invasion[7]. An asymptomatic patient found to have abnormal endometrial cells on a pap smear however demands endometrial sampling to rule out malignancy as approximately 25% of these will be found to have endometrial cancer. In addition, normal endometrial cells on a pap smear in a post-menopausal patient demands endometrial sampling as well as approximately 5% of these will be found to have endometrial cancer[8].

Endometrial hyperplasia

In the past, it has been felt that endometrial hyperplasia was a precursor to endometrial carcinoma. More recently however, studies have suggested that endometrial hyperplasia and endometrial neoplasia are two distinct diseases[9,10]. Kurman and others found a 1.6% risk of progression of carcinoma in patients with endometrial hyperplasia without cytologic atypia, however in patients with endometrial hyperplasia with cytologic atypia, a 23% risk of progression to carcinoma was found. This suggests that women with endometrial hyperplasia without atypia are not at increased risk for developing carcinoma and may be treated with progestin therapy and follow up. In the presence of hyperplasia with cytologic atypia however, depending on age and childbearing desires, hysterectomy is the recommended treatment. Should a patient with atypical hyperplasia desire uterine conservation, a dilatation and curettage is mandatory to rule out the occasional occult carcinoma. She should then be treated with progestin therapy for at least 10 to 14 days each month and followed every 4 to 6 months with endometrial sampling to assess treatment results.

Pre-operative evaluation in a patient diagnosed with endometrial cancer

Routine pre-operative laboratory evaluations, chest X-ray and EKG should be obtained. In addition a barium enema and mammogram are recommended because of the known association with breast, colon and endometrial cancer[11]. Other studies including cystoscopy, pelvic/abdominal CT scan or MRI may be helpful in cases of suspected advanced disease to help evaluate for the presence of metastatic disease. As an adenocarcinoma can also be primarily of the cervix with endometrial spread, an endocervical curettage should also be carried out pre-operatively to evaluate for endocervical involvement. In the event endocervical stromal involvement is found, it may be difficult to distinguish between a stage IB adenocarcinoma of the cervix and a stage II endometrial carcinoma. These two diseases behave quite differently and are treated very differently, consequently it is important to try to differentiate between these two conditions prior to instituting therapy. Generally an obese, elderly, postmenopausal patient with a bulky uterus is more likely to have an endometrial cancer with cervical extension, whereas a younger patient with a bulky cervix and a normal uterus is more likely to have a cervical cancer with endometrial extension.

Prognostic factors

Prior to 1988 endometrial carcinoma was clinically staged. A number of studies in the literature however demonstrated significant discrepancies in staging compared to patients who were surgically staged[12]. Consequently, the cancer committee of FIGO (International Federation of Gynecologists and Obstetricians) introduced a surgical staging system in 1988 and it is shown in Table 50.3.3.

The majority of endometrial carcinomas are endometrioid adenocarcinomas with an overall survival rate of approximately 90%. A number of less common unfavorable histologic subtypes may also be involved, including papillary serous, clear cell or undifferentiated carcinomas with an overall survival rate of only 33%[13]. An extensive study of more than 1000 stage I and II patients by the Gynecologic Oncology Group (GOG) analyzed histologic grade, depth of myometrial invasion, occult extension to the uterine cervix and lymphovascular space invasion as prognostic factors[14]. Grade and depth of myometrial invasion were found to be particularly related to the risk of extrauterine disease, with depth of invasion found to be the most predictable for risk of nodal metastasis. Lymphovascular space invasion was also felt to be an independent risk factor for nodal spread. The significance of positive peritoneal cytology is unclear and controversial at present[15]. Tumor size has also been reported as an independent prognostic factor with tumors greater than 2 cm in diameter being found to have a fourfold higher incidence of lymph node metastasis compared with tumors less than or equal to 2 cm (15% versus 4%)[16].

Table 50.3.3   1988 FIGO surgical staging for endometrial carcinoma

Stage IA Grade123	Tumor limited to endometrium
Stage IB Grade123	Invasion to less than one-half the myometrium
Stage IC Grade123	Invasion to more than one-half the myometrium
Stage IIA Grade123	Endocervical glandular involvement only
Stage IIB Grade123	Cervical stromal invasion
Stage IIIA Grade123	Tumor invades serosa and/or adnexa, and/or positive peritoneal cytology
Stage IIB Grade123	Vaginal metastases
Stage IIIC Grade123	Metastases to pelvic and/or periaortic lymph nodes
Stage IVA Grade123	Tumor invasion of bladder and/or bowel mucosa
Stage IVB Grade123	Distant metastases including intra-abdominal and/or inguinal lymph nodes

Treatment of endometrial cancer

The mainstay of treatment for endometrial cancer consists of surgical therapy. A midline incision is recommended to allow adequate exploration of the upper abdomen and periaortic lymph node sampling, where indicated. Any ascitic fluid is aspirated or pelvic washings obtained and sent for cytology, followed by exploration of the abdominal cavity and pelvis for evidence of intra-abdominal spread with any suspicious areas biopsied. Surgery consists of a simple hysterectomy with removal of the uterus and cervix. Both fallopian tubes and ovaries should also be removed because of the risk of micrometastasis[14].

While 1988 FIGO surgical staging is based upon pelvic and periaortic lymph nodal sampling, this is not routinely done in early stage well differentiated tumors due to the low risk of metastatic disease[13]. A surgical staging study by the Gynecologic Oncology Group (GOG) has stratified patients into low-risk and high-risk groups for metastatic disease, based upon grade, depth of invasion and histology[14]. Table 50.3.4 outlines those patients in whom surgical staging should be undertaken.

Grade and histology can be determined pre-operatively based upon an endometrial biopsy and can guide the need for lymph node sampling. Grade 2 and 3 tumors and histologic types other than adenocarcinoma or adenosquamous carcinoma are also at high risk for lymph node metastasis and surgical staging is recommended. As previously noted, depth of invasion was found to correlate with risk of lymph node metastasis. Grade 1 tumors found intraoperatively to have myometrial invasion greater than half the depth of the myometrium are also at increased risk for lymph node metastasis and should undergo lymph node sampling. The specimen can be opened in the operating room, and grossly inspected for depth of invasion. It has been shown that gross inspection in grade 1 endometrial carcinomas is accurate greater than 90% of the time in correctly predicting depth of invasion and the need for surgical staging[17].

While the Cancer Committee of FIGO has not detailed the surgical staging requirements for endometrial carcinoma, most authorities recommend lymph node sampling with removal of the fat pad over the vena cava and aorta

Table 50.3.4   Patients on whom surgical staging should be performed

- Patients with grade 2 or 3 lesions
- Patients with non-adeno histology (e.g. clear cell, papillary serous)
- Patients with grade 1 lesions with greater than one-half invasion of the myometrium
- Patients with lower uterine segment involvement or cervical extension
- Patients with large tumors (> 2 cm)

beginning at the bifurcation and extending to the proximity of the renal vessels. In the pelvis, all lymph bearing tissues over the external and common iliac vessels as well as lymph nodal tissue in the obturator fossa above the obturator nerve should be removed.

While an exploratory laparotomy is the recommended approach, in certain situations a vaginal hysterectomy may be considered. A markedly obese or medically compromised patient, in whom abdominal surgery would present an unacceptable high risk, are better served with surgery and post-operative radiation, where indicated, than radiation alone[18]. Patients in whom surgery is medically contraindicated should be treated with radiation therapy. In recent years, laparoscopic assisted vaginal hysterectomy (LAVH) with laparoscopic lymph node sampling has emerged as an additional approach to treatment of the patient with endometrial cancer.

Adjuvant therapy

Following surgical-pathologic staging, any adverse factors can be determined and guide post-operative therapy. Patients at low risk for recurrence are those with a grade 1 or 2 lesion confined to the endometrium and have not been shown to benefit from post-operative radiation therapy[22]. Patients with an intermediate risk for recurrence are those with deep invasion or a high-grade lesion with minimal invasion, lymph vascular space involvement, high-risk histologic subtypes or lower uterine segment involvement and may benefit from intracavitary radiation post-operatively to decrease the incidence of vault recurrence, which carries a very poor prognosis. Intracavitary vaginal radiation has been shown to decrease the incidence of vault recurrence from 14% to 1.7%[19]. High-risk patients include those with metastatic disease to the pelvic and/or periaortic nodes and radiation therapy to these areas has been shown to improve survival in these patients[20].

Data is controversial regarding treatment and benefits in patients found to have positive peritoneal washings or adnexal or peritoneal metastasis and the best mode of therapy is unclear at this time. Total abdominal radiation and intraperitoneal P-32 have been utilized in the past, but results have not been promising.

As previously discussed, it may be difficult to distinguish a stage II endometrial carcinoma with cervical extension from a stage I cervical carcinoma with endometrial extension. Consideration of the clinical history and examination in combination with histopathologic evaluation may help guide therapy. If the diagnosis is felt to be an endometrial cancer, several approaches have been recommended including radical hysterectomy with bilateral salpingo-oophorectomy and lymph node dissection, pre-operative radiation therapy followed by simple hysterectomy and bilateral salpingo-oophorectomy or surgical staging followed by radiation therapy based upon surgical-pathologic findings.

Patients with advanced stage endometrial carcinoma (clinical stage III or IV) are also best served by surgery with removal of all gross tumor[21]. These patients will have a high risk of relapse in the pelvis and upper abdomen as well as distant metastasis and no single combined therapy has been shown to improve survival. Adjuvant chemotherapy has been utilized, but not shown to improve survival over the more traditional therapy of surgery and/or radiation therapy[22].

Recurrence

The majority of recurrences will occur within 3 years with 50% as an isolated vault recurrence, 25% as a distant recurrence and 25% as simultaneous local and distant recurrences[23]. Many patients will be asymptomatic at the time of recurrence with the diagnosis often being made on routine follow-up examinations. If a vaginal recurrence is found, a thorough work-up must be carried out to look for distant disease, including CT or MRI of the chest, abdomen and pelvis and utilization of fine needle aspiration for any suspicious lesions.

An isolated vaginal recurrence in a patient not previously radiated can be treated with a combination of pelvic and intracavitary radiation therapy. Resection of a large vault nodule (>2 cm) prior to radiation may improve local control. If the patient has previously been treated with pelvic radiation, surgical resection with exenteration may be considered provided the recurrence is central and there is no evidence of lymph nodal metastases. There are no large published series on which this is based, however. Treatment in other cases of recurrence must be individualized and may be treated with hormonal therapy or chemotherapy. There is an overall response rate of 15–25% to progestins. Prognostic variables predictive of response include length of disease-free interval, well differentiated tumors and status of estrogen or progesterone receptors. The most active chemotherapeutic agents are adriamycin and cisplatinum with reported responses of 19–38% and 4–42% respectively, but with median responses of only 4–8 months. Most authorities recommend hormonal therapy initially with chemotherapy for failures.

References

1. Boring CC, Squires TS, Tony S. Cancer Statistics. *CA-A Cancer J Clinicians* 1995;**45**:1.
2. Parazzini F, LaBecchia C, Bocciolone L, Franceshi S. The epidemiology of endometrial cancer. *Gyn Oncol* 1991;**41**:1.
3. Stelmachow J. The role of hysteroscopy and gynecologic oncology. *Gyn Oncol* 1982;**14**:392.
4. Koss LG, Schreiber K, Overlander SG. Screening of asymptomatic women for endometrial cancer. *Obstet Gynecol* 1981;**57**:681.
5. Goldstein SR, Nachtigall M, Schneider JR, Nachtigall L. Endometrial assessment by vaginal ultrasonography before endometrial sampling in patients with postmenopausal bleeding. *Am J Obstet Gynecol* 1990;**163**:119.
6. Gusberg SB, Malano C. Detection of endometrial carcinoma and its precursors. *Cancer* 1981;**47**:1173.
7. DuBeshter V, Warshal DB, Angel C. The relevance of cervical cytology. *Obstet Gynecol* 1991;**77**:458.
8. Ing NG, Reagan JW, Hawliczek CT, Wince BW. Significance of endometrial cells and the detection of endometrial carcinoma and its precursors. *Acta Cytol* 1974;**18**:356.
9. Carman RJ, Kaminski BF, Norris HJ. The behaviour of endometrial hyperplasia: A long-term study of "untreated" hyperplasia in 170 patients. *Cancer* 1985;**56**:403.
10. Ferenczy A, Gelfan NE, Tziprasf. The cytodynamics of endometrial hyperplasia in carcinoma: a review. *Ann Pathol* 1983;**3**:189.
11. Lynch HT, Conway T, Lynch J. Hereditary ovarian cancer. In: Sharp N, Mason WP, Leake RE (eds) *Ovarian cancer: biological and therapeutic challenges.* Chapman and Hall Medical, Cambridge 1990, pp. 719.
12. Cowles TA, Magrina JF, Matterson BJ, Capen CD. Comparison of clinical and surgical staging in patients with endometrial carcinoma. *Obstet Gynecol* 1985;**66**:413.
13. Wilson TD, Podratz KC, Gaffy TA. The unfavorable histologic subtypes and endometrial adenocarcinoma. *Am J Obstet Gynecol* 1990;**162**:418.
14. Creasman WT, Morrow CT, Bundy BN, Mesley HD, Graham JW, Heller PB. Surgical pathologic spread patterns of endometrial cancer: a Gynecologic Oncology Group Study. *Cancer* 1987;**60**:2035.
15. Lorraine JR. The significance of positive peritoneal cytology in endometrial cancer. *Gyn Oncol* 1992;**46**:143.
16. Schink JC, Lorraine JR, Wallemark CT, Chmiel JS. Tumor size and endometrial cancer: a prognostic factor for lymph node metastases. *Obstet Gynecol* 1987;**70**:216.
17. Goff BA, Rice LW. The assessment of depth of myometrial invasion and endometrial adenocarcinoma. *Gyn Oncol* 1990;**38**:46.
18. Peters WA, Andersen WA, Thornton Jr. N, Morley GW. The selective use of vaginal hysterectomy in the management of adenocarcinoma of the endometrium. *Am J Obstet Gynecol* 1983;**146**:285.
19. Lotkochi RJ, Copeland LJ, DePetrillo AD, Muirhead W. Stage I endometrial adenocarcinoma: Human results of 835 patients. *Am J Obstet Gynecol* 1983;**146**:141.
20. Piver MS, Yazigi R, Blumenson L, Tsukada Y. A prospective trail comparing hysterectomy, hysterectomy plus vaginal radium, and uterine radium plus hysterectomy in stage I endometrial carcinoma. *Obstet Gynecol.* 197;**54**:85–9.
21. Aalders SJ, Abeler V, Kolstad P. Clinical (Stage III) as compared to subclinical intrapelvic extrauterine tumor spread in endometrial carcinoma: A clinical and histopathological study of 175 patients. *Gyn Oncol* 1984;**17**:64.
22. Mora C, Bundy B, Holmesly H. Doxorubicin as an adjuvant following surgery and radiation therapy in patients with high risk endometrial carcinoma Stage I and II: a Gynecologic Oncology Group Study. 1990, 36.
23. Aalders J, Abeler V, Kolstad P. Recurrent adenocarcinoma of the endometrium: a clinical and histopathological study of 379 patients. *Gyn Oncol* 1984;**17**:85.

51 The role of exenteration and urinary diversion in gynecological malignancies

A R Mundy

Introduction

In this context gynecological malignancy generally refers to carcinoma of the cervix or carcinoma of the body of the uterus and carcinoma of the cervix is much more common. This is generally treated by a combination of surgery and radiotherapy or both. Local recurrence after treatment is generally known as 'central recurrence' and may present for further surgical treatment for one of two reasons: 1) for a possible cure; or 2) to deal with disabling symptoms irrespective of the long-term outcome. A long-term cure with a central recurrence is not commonly achieved but is achieved sufficiently commonly to make it worth trying[1], if there is no evidence of distant spread.

Disabling symptoms generally arise in patients with fistulae or with an infected mass or a combination of the two, in which anaerobic infection causes a profound foul smelling discharge which is disabling both physically and socially. This particular problem is compounded by difficulty in proving whether there is residual or recurrent disease in some patients.

Although gynecological malignancies are the commonest to fall into the category considered in this chapter, other unusual malignancies are seen in which exenteration rather than just radical resection of a single organ may be the treatment of choice. Pelvic sarcomata are typical of this type but vaginal, urethral and other unusual tumors would also fall into this category.

Assessment

Assessment is generally unsatisfactory. It may be possible to obtain a good biopsy but the report commonly reports the presence of just a few cells in amongst a mass of fibrous or inflammatory tissue and this can be unhelpful[2]. MRI and CT imaging are sometimes helpful[3] (Figure 51.1)

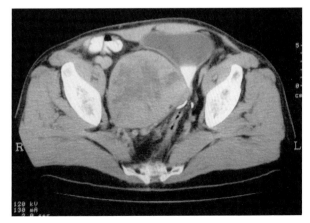

Fig. 51.1 CT scan demonstrating a mass in the pelvis.

but generally only to exclude disease outside the pelvis. It is unusual to obtain image of the local tumor within the pelvis sufficient to allow pre-operative planning with any degree of certainty.

Very often the most useful form of assessment, taken in conjunction with the severity and nature of the symptoms, is an examination under anesthetic together with cystoscopy and proctoscopy, sigmoidoscopy or colonoscopy. If the tumor feels operable on EUA it will usually be so. If it feels inoperable and fixed on EUA then it may not necessarily be so and the decision to proceed to surgery will be based on the severity of the patients' symptoms and whether or not they justify the surgical attempt.

Any patient who has had radiotherapy and suffered complications as a result of it should have a barium meal to look for abnormalities of the sigmoid colon or irradiation disease elsewhere in the bowel.

For the same reason, at the time of EUA it is sensible to biopsy the bladder, vagina and rectum to look for evidence of irradiation damage. Having said that the state of the skin over the sacrum and the presence or absence of pubic hair are good guides to the severity of the reaction. Dense retracted abdominal scars, absence of pubic hair and puffiness of the pubic and sacral skin all indicate severe irradiation damage and the consequent likelihood of per-operative and post-operative irradiation related problems.

The vulval skin and labial skin may also show features of irradiation damage but these features are equally likely to be due to excoriation of the skin because of intractable incontinence.

Having assessed the patient by these various means, it is important to establish exactly what the patient wishes to achieve by surgery particularly if long-term survival is not anticipated. The problems that the patient will most likely want to have dealt with are first to be rid of a foul smelling discharging abscess cavity, secondly to be continent of urine and faeces and thirdly to have a functioning vagina. When the rectum is substantially involved in a pelvic mass, or when the sigmoid colon has suffered severe irradiation damage, or when the anal sphincter mechanism is no longer competent, then it will not be possible to achieve these aims without both urinary and fecal diversion in the majority of cases. Localized rectal problems, for example a small fistula, may be surgically correctable if the bowel is otherwise normal but, very often, if the bowel is involved at all it is extensively involved and not easily salvageable.

If the bowel is intact and has not suffered irradiation damage then it is usually possible to perform an anterior exenteration combined with some form of bladder substitution procedure and some form of vaginoplasty in order to achieve a satisfactory result. An alternative to a bladder substitution would be an ileal conduit urinary diversion

and this should be discussed with the patient as it may suit her better. Equally not all patients want a vaginoplasty particularly if it might prove to be a difficult undertaking.

Total urinary tract reconstruction[4] (Figures 51.2 and 51.3) or an externally draining continent diversion[5] after exenteration are possible but increase the scale and complexity of the surgery and the uretero-sigmoidostomy variant, popularized in Mainz[6], is generally quicker and easier and gives a satisfactory result without the same risk of post-operative complications, and is quite suitable (in my experience) for those with a limited life expectancy. In those with a long-term prognosis a formal Mitrofanoff-type continent diversion or urinary tract reconstruction can be performed at a later stage if indicated.

In patients with a vesico-vaginal fistula and evidence of metastatic disease a conduit urinary diversion is a satisfactory solution to their problem; and in those who are clearly inoperable, urinary or fecal diversion or both may improve the quality of life sufficiently to justify their use in some patients; but surgery is not commonly indicated in such patients for these reasons – one is usually operating either in the hope of a cure or because of an infected or fistulous mass involving the bladder and vagina.

Ureteric obstruction is another common presenting problem and again there is often a problem establishing or refuting the diagnosis of residual or recurrent cancer. The diagnostic difficulty is usually to distinguish between residual or recurrent nodal or retroperitoneal malignancy on the one hand or the effects of radiotherapy or surgery on the other. The next considerations are whether or not any obstruction is progressive and whether or not intervention is necessary. There is a growing tendency to rely on internal stenting for such patients but the requirement for histologic evidence to see if further treatment might be indicated means that the urologist is often asked to intervene.

Ureteric obstruction after radiotherapy alone is rare[7]. It is more common after surgery[8], including internal stenting, but it is most commonly associated with recurrent tumor. Whether or not to treat the obstruction depends on the prognosis of the tumor in relation to rate of deterioration of renal function unless there is a consideration such as pain relief that warrants intervention in its own right, assuming of course that the pain is due to the ureteric obstruction and not to the presence of recurrence per se. Internal stenting may be as uncomfortable as the pain of mild obstruction particularly if the lower end of a stent irritates an already hypersensitive bladder so if treatment of ureteric obstruction is indicated then either percutaneous nephrostomy for temporary relief or open surgical correction will usually be necessary. In general, treating minor or moderate degrees of ureteric obstruction generally creates more problems than

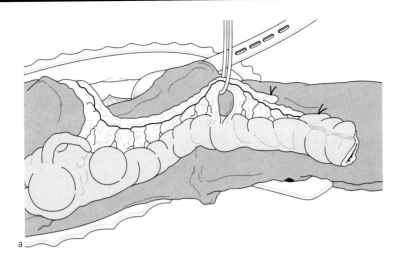

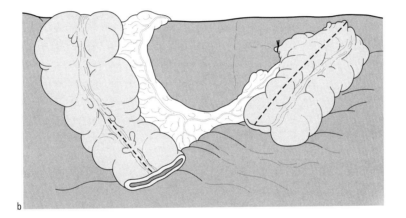

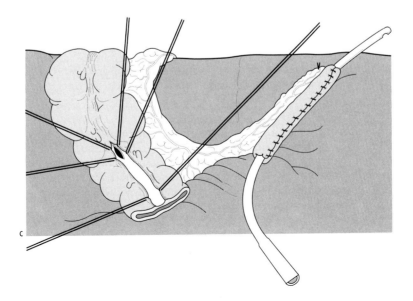

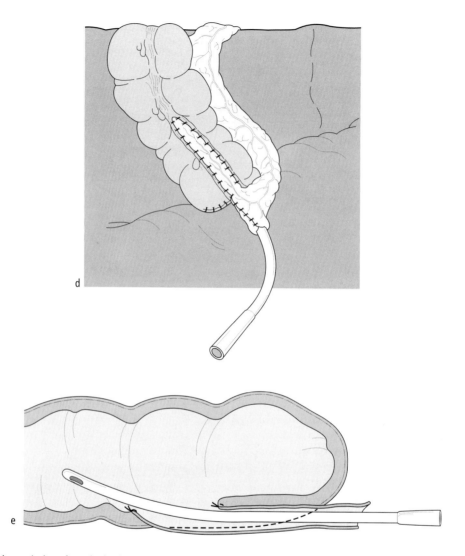

Fig. 51.2   Operative technique for substitution cystourethroplasty: a) isolation of a segment of bowel; b) division of segment to use for bladder and urethra (or vagina); c) tailoring of the segment to form a neo-urethra; d) implantation of urethral tube into neobladder (Mitrofanoff technique); e) demonstration of the valve mechanism.

is solves and when there is a temptation to intervene it should be resisted unless there is a clear advantage to be gained by doing so[9].

Any radiotherapy reaction sufficient to cause ureteric obstruction is likely to be sufficient to make conduit urinary diversion impossible by traditional means and a colon conduit using the transverse colon[10] is usually the best option. If large bowel is unavailable I have on occasions used a gastric conduit with satisfactory results. Surgery in such circumstances requires a great deal of care to avoid damage to the small bowel as this may lead to a fistula, and sometimes multiple fistulae, as a result. Such entero-

enteric, enterocutaneous or enteroconduit fistulae (Figure 51.4) are very often more of a problem then the ureteric obstruction would have been had it been left alone or treated by internal stents and such surgery is therefore not recommended in those who have had multiple previous laparotomies.

Practical aspects of surgery

These patients are often nutritionally and metabolically fragile if not overtly anemic and malnourished. A couple of days of inpatient preparation before surgery are

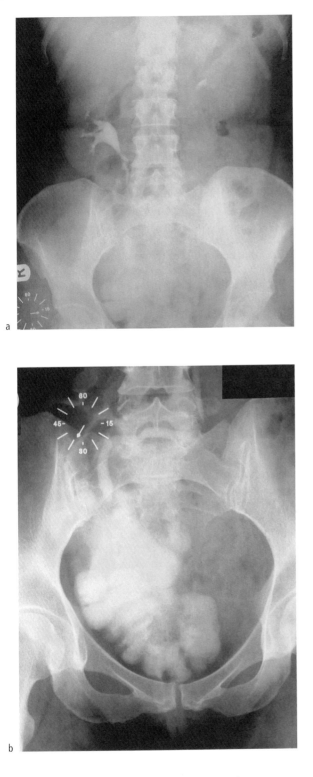

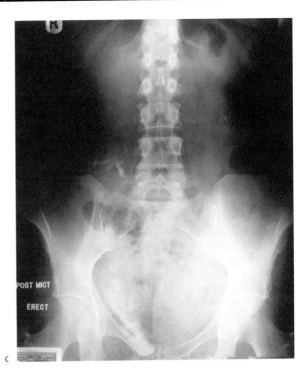

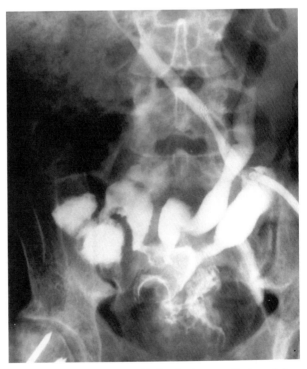

Fig. 51.3 IVU of a patient who has had a substitution cystoplasty: a) at 15 min, b) at 35 min, c) post-micturition.

Fig. 51.4 IVU of a patient with fistulae between ileal conduit, small bowel and rectum.

generally well spent. Most patients bleed more than one might be accustomed to so blood should always be cross-matched and ready, particularly in those who have had previous radiotherapy. Bowel preparation may be desirable but impossible or intolerable in some patients. Antibiotic cover should be provided either with the pre-medication or per-operatively – rarely pre-operatively. Full length stockings, at least, should be used to reduce the risk of deep vein thrombosis.

Finally always remember a last minute chest X-ray – this very often has not been done for some time and it is embarrassing to find metastases on an early post-operative lung film which means that the whole undertaking was pointless (although not always).

The only sensible incision in the vast majority of patients is a long midline abdominal incision to give adequate access to everything. Many patients will require a transperineal approach as well and so the low lithotomy position is best for the patient and for this reason inflatable leggings are a further useful precaution against deep vein thrombosis and compartment syndromes.

In the irradiated patient the risk of damaging the small bowel and causing fistulae is such that the surgeon should resist the urge to divide adhesions any more than is necessary to retract the small bowel out of the pelvis in order to expose the pelvic viscera adequately for the purpose in hand.

This is not the place to describe anterior exenteration but it is worth making one or two points. First, the retropubic space is often obliterated and the best way of identifying the planes of the pelvis is to start at the level of the external iliac vessels and work down into the pelvis from there. Secondly, these adhesions in the retropubic space are such that the bladder has to be carved off the pubis with a scalpel or with diathermy. This does not mean that the patient is necessarily unsalvageable, just that the surgery is likely to be difficult and tedious.

Thirdly, before proceeding too far it is wise to define the anterior aspect of the lateral pedicle from the retropubic space and the posterior aspect of the pedicle antero-lateral to the rectum so that the pedicle can be cross-clamped or pinched or simply cut across and oversewn if bleeding becomes uncontrollable.

Finally in this category of general caveats, if the rectum and colon are undamaged at the start of the procedure, the greatest care should be taken to make sure it stays that way during the course of the surgery.

Diversion and reconstruction

This is not the place to discuss the details of such surgery anymore than it is to discuss the details of exenteration; only the general principles will be outlined.

It is often impossible to decide on the type of surgery until the exenteration has been performed. In a true exenteration there will be nothing left in the pelvis beyond the musculo-skeletal elements. On the other hand a total exenteration is uncommon – an anterior exenteration leaving the colon, rectum and anus intact is much more common. Even in an anterior exenteration the urogenital viscera are not removed in their entirety except when a cure is intended and so enough of these structures may be salvageable, if they do not have to be sacrificed, to serve as building blocks for reconstructive surgery.

The crucial factor in the urinary tract is the outflow and its control mechanism – the urethra and its sphincter. If these can be left behind then all that is required is a substitution cystoplasty and reimplantation of the ureters[4] and this is a straightforward procedure if the bowel has not been irradiated and is otherwise intact. In circumstances in which orthotopic reconstruction is going to be difficult it is likely that continent diversion using an isolated segment of bowel and a surgically created valve mechanism will also be a problem for the same reasons. In addition, a continent diversion of this type, like orthotopic reconstruction in the absence of a urethra or a sphincter mechanism, is a complicated and time-consuming procedure which is also prone to a relatively high incidence of post-operative complications[5]. For all of these reasons they are only indicated when the patient has an assured long-term prognosis.

Continent 'internal' urinary diversion by means of a variant of the uretero-sigmoidostomy technique has considerable advantages. It is relatively simple to perform with few post-operative complications and if the anal sphincter is competent then continence is more or less assured. The problem with ureterosigmoidostomy is twofold. First, if the bowel has been irradiated and the patient has post-irradiation problems then the technique is not suitable and she will be better off with a conduit urinary diversion using a section of bowel such as the transverse colon as alluded to above. In the non-irradiated patient this problem does not usually apply. The second problem with ureterosigmoidostomy is that after the standard procedure in which the bowel is not modified in any way the patient often has frequency and urgency and may be incontinent as a result of these. Fortunately with the Mainz modification[6] this is rarely a problem. In this the lower sigmoid colon is formed into a pouch involving one or two adjacent loops (Figure 51.5) and this seems to reduce the problems of frequency and urgency considerably; the patient can expect to empty the bowel of 'slurry' (the urine–feces mix) five times a day or thereabouts and without suffering problems of peri-anal skin excoriation. There is a further modification of this procedure to include intussusception of the sigmoid at the upper end of the pouch in order to reduce the back flow of urine to the proximal colon[11] but this seems to be more

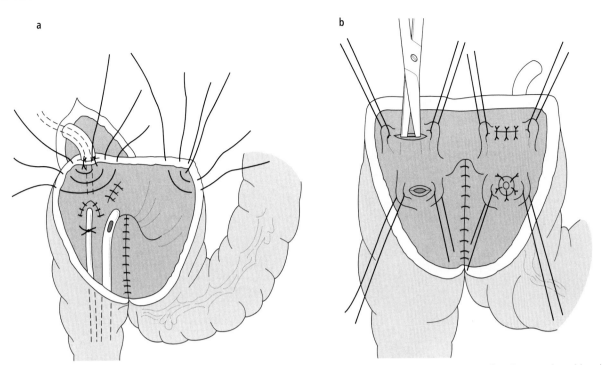

Fig. 51.5   Demonstration of operative technique for Mainz 11 sigma rectum pouch: a) pouch formed by opening the rectosigmoid and forming a pouch; b) ureters tunneled to form an antireflux anastomosis.

of a potential cause of problems than an advantage and is not recommended (Figure 51.6).

Techniques of vaginal reconstruction largely depend on what has been left behind. If the vagina has been excised down to the introitus then extraneous tissue will have to be used to replace it in its entirety. Very often however it is possible to preserve at least a posterior tongue of vaginal wall which not only protects the anorectal junction and anal canal but serves as a substrate for vaginal reconstruction. If a large posterior tongue is preserved this can be rolled down anteriorly to give a shortened but altogether natural vagina. If only a short posterior tongue exists or if there is no vagina at all then a pedicled segment of sigmoid colon can be swung down as a substitution vaginoplasty as described by Goligher[12] (Figure 51.7). The alternative vaginal substitute for the non-irradiated patient is local perineal skin using the technique described by Wee[13], but this produces considerable scarring and is not recommended.

A ureterosigmoidostomy does not need to be covered by a colostomy but it is wise to splint the ureters and bring them out through the anal sphincter as a temporary measure during healing. Whenever possible the omentum should be brought down into the pelvis to wrap round anastomoses and particularly to keep adjacent anastomoses apart. Finally, to prevent the formation of hematomas that might become infected, wound drains should be used liberally.

Post-operative care

The particular problem to anticipate is with wound healing and specifically the patients' ability to heal. It should be expected that these people will have a difficult post-operative course and enteral and parenteral nutrition should be instituted early. It is much easier to stop it if it proves unnecessary than to start it late and to be forced to try and catch up with the situation – often too late.

Post-operative antibiotic cover with a broad spectrum antibiotic and one that will cover anaerobic species is a sensible precaution. Early mobilization is also advisable because these patients are at risk of deep vein thrombosis.

Conclusions

Persistent and recurrent malignancy can be psychologically devastating but the impact of a foul smelling vaginal discharge due to an infected or fistulous mass can be worse leading to isolation at the one time in the patients' life when support is generally most needed. The indications for surgery are therefore based on a consideration of the patients' symptoms rather than just the nature of the disease and its prognosis. Equally the surgeon has to be sensible and realistic about what he can achieve but generally the cause of the patient's symptoms can be removed

569

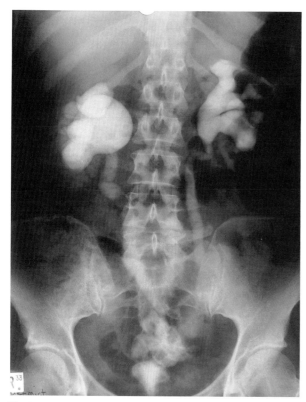

Fig. 51.6 IVU of a patient with a Mainx 11 sigma rectum pouch demonstrating limited reflux into the colon.

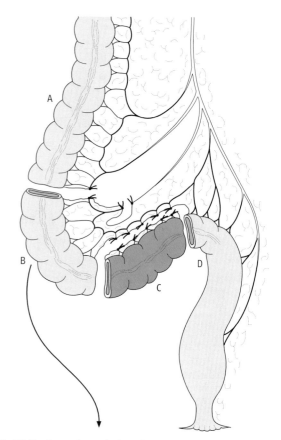

Fig. 51.7 Operative technique for vaginoplasty. B is used to form the vagina, C is discarded. The sigmoid (A) is anastomosed to the rectum (D).

and so the principal aim can be achieved even if the prognosis for the patient is short. Reconstruction or diversion should be kept as simple as possible and this is usually achievable by internal urinary diversion and substitution vaginoplasty in the non-irradiated patient. In the irradiated patient in whom the bowel is compromised a conduit urinary diversion may be a more realistic proposition and vaginoplasty may not be feasible. Alternatives exist for exceptional circumstances.

References

1. Robertson G, Lopes A, Beynon G, Monaghan JM. Pelvic exenteration: a review of the Gateshead experience 1974–1992. *B J Obstet Gynaecol* 1994; **101**:529–531.
2. Jaques PF, Staab E, Richey W, Photopulos G, Swanton M. CT-assisted pelvic and abdominal aspiration biopsies in gynaecological malignancy. *Radiol* 1978; **128**:651–655.
3. Blies JR, Ellis JH, Kopecky KK, Sutton GP, Klatte EC, Stehman FB, Ehrlich CE. Assessment of primary gynaecologic malignanies: comparison of 0.15-T resistive MRI with CT. *AJR* 1984; **143**:1249–1257.
4. Mundy AR. A technique for total substitution of the lower urinary tract without the use of a prosthesis. *BJU* 1988; **62**:334–338.
5. Woodhouse CR, MacNeily AE. The Mitrofanoff principle. *BJU* 1994; **74**(4):447–453.
6. Fisch M, Wammack R, Muller SC, Hohenfellner R. The Mainz 11 (sigma rectum pouch). *J Urol* 1993; **149**:258–263.
7. Kontturi M, Kauppila A. Ureteric complications following treatment of gynaecological cancer. *Ann Chir Gynaecol* 1982; **71**:232–238.
8. Ulmsten U. Obstruction of the upper urinary tract after treatment of carcinoma of the uterine cervix. *Acta Obstet Gynaecol Scand* 1975; **54**:297–301.
9. Hoe JW, Tung KH, Tan EC. Re-evaluation of the indications for percutaneous nephrostomy and interventional uroradiological procedures in pelvic malignancy. *BJU* 1993; **71**:469–472.
10. Ravi R, Dewan AK, Pandey KK. Transverse colon conduit urinary diversion in patients treated with very high dose pelvic irradiation. *BJU* 1994; **73**:51–54.
11. Ghoneim MA, Ashamallah AK, Mahran MR, Kock NG. Further experience with the modified rectal bladder (the augmented and valved rectum) for urine diversion. *J Urol* 1992; **147**:1252–1255.
12. Goligher JC. The use of pedicled transplants of sigmoid or other parts of the intestinal tract for vaginal construction. *Ann R Coll Surg Engl* 1983; **65**:353–355.
13. Wee JT, Joseph VT. A new technique of vaginal reconstruction using neurovascular pudendal-thigh flaps: a preliminary report. *Plast Reconstr Surg* 1989; **83**:701–709.

52 Management of urogynecologic fistulae

L D Kowalski and D G Mutch

Injuries to the urogynecologic tract which result in fistulae occasionally complicate the treatment of patients with gynecologic cancers. Managing genitourinary fistulae in the setting of a pelvic malignancy can be quite challenging, and careful attention to surgical, psychosocial and medicolegal considerations are imperative.

Anatomic considerations

Ureterovaginal and vesicovaginal fistulae account for the vast majority of genitourinary fistulae and will be specifically considered in this treatise. Less commonly, urethrovaginal, vesicocervical or uterovesical fistulae may be encountered (Figure 52.1), and similar principles of management may be applied to these clinical entities. However, reports of rare sites of fistulae, including ureteroiliac[1], enterovesical[2], vesicosacral[3], and vesicoovarian[4] illustrate that fistulae can form anywhere sufficient injury and/or devascularization compromise the integrity of the urogenital tract.

Most ureterovaginal fistulae (UVF) result from surgical injury, while tumor recurrence and radiation fibrosis more commonly present with ureteral obstruction[5]. Seventy-five per cent of all ureteral injuries result from gynecological operations, and 50% of injuries requiring intervention result in fistulae[6]. The incidence of fistulae is highest following radical hysterectomy for carcinoma of the cervix (1%–2%)[7,8], but 0.5%–1% of abdominal hysterectomies and 0.1% of vaginal hysterectomies for benign disease are complicated by ureteral injuries[9]. More recently, ureteral injuries from laparoscopy-assisted vaginal hysterectomy have been reported[10].

In the United States, three-fourths of vesicovaginal fistulae (VVF) occur after total abdominal hysterectomy (TAH) or vaginal hysterectomy for benign disease[11,12]. However, 1–3% of patients treated for invasive cervical cancer either by radical hysterectomy or radiation therapy (RT) develop VVF. The incidence rises fourfold when RT and surgery are combined[13]. Most injuries associated with hysterectomy occur at the bladder base between the anterior vaginal wall and the posterior bladder wall.

Mechanisms of fistula formation

The three primary mechanisms of fistula formation include surgical injury, radiation injury and direct tumor invasion. Tissue necrosis underlies the pathophysiology of fistula formation in all cases, and management decisions primarily rest upon the surgeon's assessment of the vitality of the involved tissues.

Surgical injuries

Ureteral injury complicates 0.1% to 1.5% of all cases of pelvic surgery[9]. Operative trauma may result from crush injury, inadvertent ligation or transection, secondary obstruction by angulation, ischemia due to devascularization, or intentional resection. However, only 30% of ureteral injuries are recognized at the time of operation[14], and the incidence of silent injury may rise to 36–46% after radical hysterectomy[15,16]. The classic experiments of Sampson[17] demonstrated in a canine model the events which lead to ureterovaginal fistula after the extensive ureterolysis attendant to radical hysterectomy. Following destruction of the periurethral arterial plexus, Sampson noted ischemia leading to a localized hemorrhagic infarct.

571

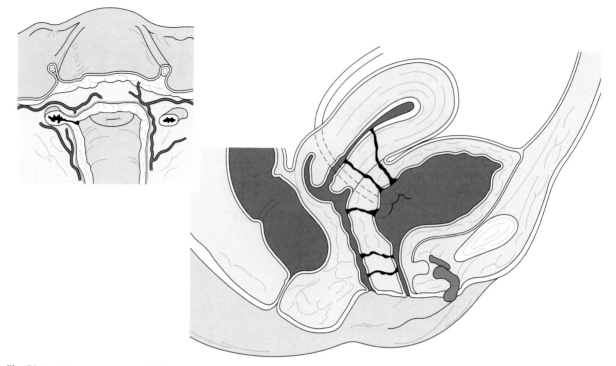

Fig. 52.1 Common urogynecologic fistulae include uterovesical (A), vesicocervical (B), vesicovaginal (C), urethrovesicovaginal (D), urethrovaginal (E) and ureterovaginal (F). The relative proximity of these structures illustrates how localized tissue necrosis may result in fistula. Multiple fistulae may occur simultaneously.

In most cases, necrosis with ureteral wall rupture ensued, with urinoma formation and drainage through the vagina. In the case of inadvertent ureteral ligation, transection, or obstruction, ureteral dilatation leads to an increase in intraluminal pressure and eventual wall necrosis, rupture and urinary extravasation.

Surgical injury to the bladder usually occurs during dissection of the pubovesicocervical fascia during hysterectomy. When mobilization is inadequate, the surgeon may inadvertently suture the bladder base to the vaginal cuff, resulting in tissue necrosis and possible fistula.

Radiation injury

Urogynecologic fistulae resulting from radiation therapy most commonly occur after treatment of invasive cervical cancer. In contrast to surgical injury, isolated ureteral fistulae due to RT are rare, but VVF complicate 1–2% of cases and may occur several years following therapy. Acutely, RT may result in fistulae due to destruction and sloughing of tumor. However, the primary chronic lesion of RT is a progressive, obliterative endarteritis which results in tissue devascularization and necrosis. Van Nagell *et al*. reported that a history of underlying vascular disease was more predictive of fistula formation than radi-

ation dose[18], illustrating the crucial role vascular injury may play in fistula formation.

Direct tumor invasion

While invasion of the ureter by tumor usually leads to ureteral stricture, direct tumor extension into the bladder will often result in a fistula. Replacement of normal tissues by malignancy leads to tissue necrosis, ulceration and fistula formation.

Principles of fistula diagnosis and management

When a patient first presents with urinary incontinence per vagina and fistula is suspected, the initial goals are to determine the fistula location and assure normal kidney function. Impairment of kidney function is usually heralded by hydroureteronephrosis, and excretory urography is the best initial study. One can often delineate bladder vs. ureteral injury by filling the bladder with methylene blue and placing a tampon in the vagina. If the tampon becomes wet from urinary leakage but remains free of blue dye, a ureteral fistula is implicated. In addition, water cystoscopy is usually employed to examine the bladder and to attempt passage of a ureteral catheter on the suspected side. In most cases of ureteral injury, passage of a catheter is difficult due to ureteral stricture and/or edema.

Because the closely juxtaposed pelvic tissues may be equally exposed to a common mechanism of injury, the potential exists for coexistent fistulae in any given patient. Complex ureterovaginal and vesicovaginal fistulae have been reported in 25% and 12% of cases, respectively[19]. Therefore, the evaluation of patients with a newly diagnosed fistula must exclude both tumor recurrence and multiple fistulae.

Once initial evaluation is complete, there are two primary modalities for managing urogynecologic fistulae: drain and repair or divert. Although small fistulae following surgery will spontaneously close 15–20% of the time with drainage alone[20–22], large fistulae or fistulae complicating radiation therapy generally require either primary repair or urinary diversion.

The goals of drainage include improving patient comfort, preserving renal function, and diverting the urinary flow to allow local inflammation and edema to subside. Kidney drainage for ureteral fistulae is usually accomplished by percutaneous nephrostomy with or without concomitant bladder drainage depending on the degree of continued incontinence. For VVF, a large indwelling Foley catheter is usually sufficient.

Fistulae resulting from direct tumor invasion should never be repaired primarily. Depending on the patient's life expectancy and overall functional status, permanent urinary diversion may be considered to improve quality of remaining life. However, for terminal care in the more debilitated patient, percutaneous nephrostomy is often the simplest and safest alternative.

Surgical correction of urogynecologic fistulae

The optimal timing for primary repair has long been debated. Traditionally, repair was delayed 3 to 6 months to allow resolution of all tissue inflammation and edema. However, more recently successes in immediate repair have been reported[22–25]. Persky et al. described six small fistulae which were successfully repaired from 1 to 10 weeks after diagnosis. The largest fistula in the series (3 cm) accounted for their only failure. In the setting of a radiation-induced fistula, the traditional delay of at least 6 months seems prudent to allow establishment of the farthest limits of tissue necrosis prior to repair attempts.

Ureterovaginal fistulae

In the case of a UVF resulting from surgical injury and/or RT, careful surgical technique is imperative. In almost all cases, the repair should be performed via a transperitoneal approach. The ureter must be handled with care while the ureter is mobilized and the site of injury identified. The damaged segment must be excised and the surrounding tissue debrided. Any ureteral anastamosis must be tension-free, and ureteral stenting as well as local drainage are the rule to prevent fibrosis and obstruction postoperatively. Often the specific procedure is chosen intraoperatively, when the scope and location of the injury may be fully evaluated. The surgeon (and the patient) should be prepared for all possible outcomes, including the use of a segment of bowel for a conduit or a cutaneous ostomy. This includes a good mechanical and antibiotic bowel preparation and appropriate informed consent. Greenstein et al.[26] provides a detailed discussion of the principles of successful ureteral surgery.

With the exception of a purely palliative procedure in the face of limited expected survival, the goal should be permanent and definitive repair. The procedure of choice will entirely depend upon the anatomic location of the injury. As depicted in Figure 52.2, injuries to the lower third of the ureter are usually best treated by bladder implantation, utilizing bladder extension or mobilization techniques if necessary to avoid tension on the anastomosis. Ureteroureterostomy is most often the best technique for injuries above the pelvic brim, but interposition of an ileal segment may help bridge a gap when a large segment of ureter must be excised[27]. Transureterostomy is rarely performed due to the chance of injuring the normal reno-ureteral unit, but may be considered when there is loss of a large portion of the lower ureter. Finally, permanent diversion is always an option and will be considered below.

Vesicovaginal fistulae

The gynecologic literature generally supports VVF repair by the transvaginal route while the urologic literature favors the transabdominal/transvesical approach. This discrepancy appears to reflect the innate biases of the specialties, but most cases attempted by gynecologists follow simple hysterectomy and are located on the anterior aspect of the vagina, easily accessible transvaginally. In contrast, fistulae managed by urologists are more often complex or follow a previously failed repair attempt.

For the repair of simple VVF, the transvaginal approach is preferable. The best described transvaginal procedure is the Latzko technique of partial colpecleisis[21], with a reported cure rate of 93–100%. Briefly, the damaged epithelium around the fistula is excised, and the bladder and vaginal wall is then closed in layers. More recently, Leach and Raz[28,29] described advancing a flap of vaginal tissue over the fistula site, thereby separating the bladder and vaginal suture lines.

Complicated fistulae, more commonly encountered in the setting of a gynecologic malignancy, are often larger,

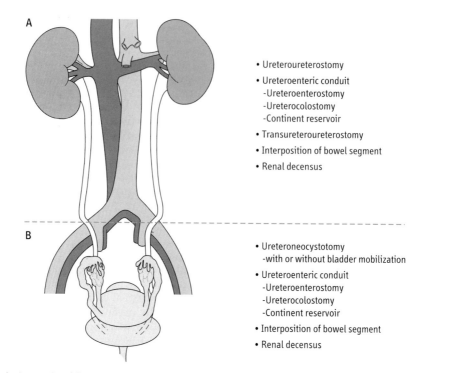

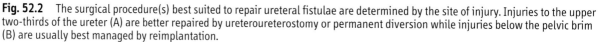

- Ureteroureterostomy
- Ureteroenteric conduit
  - Ureteroenterostomy
  - Ureterocolostomy
  - Continent reservoir
- Transureteroureterostomy
- Interposition of bowel segment
- Renal decensus

- Ureteroneocystotomy
  - with or without bladder mobilization
- Ureteroenteric conduit
  - Ureteroenterostomy
  - Ureterocolostomy
  - Continent reservoir
- Interposition of bowel segment
- Renal decensus

Fig. 52.2 The surgical procedure(s) best suited to repair ureteral fistulae are determined by the site of injury. Injuries to the upper two-thirds of the ureter (A) are better repaired by ureteroureterostomy or permanent diversion while injuries below the pelvic brim (B) are usually best managed by reimplantation.

occur in less accessible locations, and result from global mechanisms of tissue devascularization. The surgical approach to primary repair is usually transabdominal, utilizing the technique best described by O'Connor, Jr[30].

Several techniques for neovascularization or tissue substitution have been described and are advocated in the primary repair of complicated VVF. Transvaginally, the use of bulbocavernosus flaps[31] or bulbocavernosus myocutaneous flaps[32] as well as abductor[33], sartorius[34] and gracilis[33,35] muscle flaps can provide tissue and vascular support. For the transabdominal approach, rectus abdominus muscle flaps[33] and omental interposition[36] have been described. One report recommends routine use of omental grafts for fistula prevention when abdominal hysterectomy is required following radiation therapy for cervical cancer[37].

References

1. Mutch D. Personal communication, 1995.
2. Levenback C, Gershenson D, McGehee R, Eifel P, Morris M, Burke T. Enterovesical fistula following radiotherapy for gynecologic cancer. *Gynecol Oncol* 1994;**52**:296–300.
3. Lentz S, Homesley H. Radiation-induced vesicosacral fistula: treatment with continent urinary diversion. *Gynecol Oncol* 1995;**58**:278–280.
4. Ulstein M, Baydia J, Pradhan U. Fistula between the urinary bladder and an ovarian dermoid tumor. *Acta Obstet Gynecol Scand* 1987;**66**:723–724.
5. McIntyre J, Eifel P, Levenback C, Oswald M. Ureteral stricture as a late complication of radiotherapy for Stage IB carcinoma of the uterine cervix. *Cancer* 1995;**75**:836–843.
6. Higgins C. Ureteral injuries during surgery. *J Am Med Assoc* 1967;**199**:118–124.
7. Hatch K, Parham G, Shingleton H, Orr J Jr, Austin J Jr. Ureteral strictures and fistulae following radical hysterectomy. *Gynecol Oncol* 1984;**19**:17–23.
8. Larson D, Malone J Jr, Copeland L *et al.* Ureteral assessment after radical hysterectomy. *Obstet Gynecol* 1987;**69**:612–616.
9. Thompson J. Operative injuries to the ureter: prevention, recognition, and management. In: *Thompson, J. Rock J.* (eds) *Te Linde's operative gynecology.* J.B. Lippincott, Philadelphia, 1992, pp. 749–783.
10. Woodland M. Ureter injury during laparoscopy-assisted vaginal hysterectomy with the endoscopic linear stapler. *Am J Obstet Gynecol* 1992;**167**:756–757.
11. Miller N, George H. Lower urinary tract fistulas in women. A study based on 292 cases. *Am J Obstet Gynecol* 1954;**68**:436–445.
12. Lee R, Symmonds R, Williams T. Current status of genitourinary fistula. *Obstet Gynecol* 1988;**72**:313–319.
13. Boronow R, Rutledge F. Vesicovaginal fistula, radiation, and gynecologic cancer. *Am J Obstet Gynecol* 1971;**111**:85–90.
14. Mann Q, Arato M, Patsner B *et al.* Ureteral injuries in an obstetrics and gynecology training program: etiology and management. *Obstet Gynecol* 1988;**72**:82–85.
15. Mattsson T. Frequency and management of urological and some other complications following radical surgery for carcinoma of the cervix uteri, stages I and II. *Acta Obstet Gynecol Scand* 1975;**54**:271–280.
16. Ulmsten U. Obstruction of the upper urinary tract after treatment of carcinoma of the uterine cervix. *Acta Obstet Gynecol Scand* 1975;**54**:297–301.

17. Sampson J. Ureteral fistulae as sequelae of pelvic operations. *Surg Gynecol Obstet* 1909;**8**:479–497.

18. Van Nagell J Jr, Parker J Jr, Maruyama Y, Utley J, Luckett P. Bladder or rectal injury following radiation therapy for cervical cancer. *Am J Obstet Gynecol* 1974;**119**:727–732.

19. Goodwin W, Scardino P. Vesicovaginal and ureterovaginal fistulas: a summary of 25 years of experience. *J Urol* 1980;**123**:370–374.

20. Lang E, Lanasa J, Garrett J, Stripling J, Palomar J. The management of urinary fistulas and strictures with percutaneous ureteral stent catheters. *J Urol* 1979;**122**:736–740.

21. Latzko W. Postoperative vesicovaginal fistulas. *Am J Surg* 1942; **58**:211–228.

22. Thompson J. Vesicovaginal fistulas. In: J. Thompson, J. Rock (eds) *Te Linde's operative gynecology*. J.B. Lippincott Company, Philadelphia, 1992, pp. 785–818.

23. Collins C, Pent D, Jones F. Results of early repair of vesicovaginal fistula with preliminary cortisone treatment. *Am J Obstet Gynecol* 1960;**80**:1005–1012.

24. Cruikshank S. Early closure of post-hysterectomy vesicovaginal fistulas. *S Med J* 1988;**81**:1525–1528.

25. Persky L, Herman G, Guerrier K. Nondelay in vesicovaginal fistula repair. *Urology* 1979;**13**:273–275.

26. Greenstein A, Vernon Smith M, Koontz W Jr. Surgery of the ureter. In: Walsh *et al. Campbell's urology*. WB Saunders, Philadelphia, 1992, pp. 2552–2570.

27. Krupp P, Hoffman M, Roeling W. Terminal ileum as ureteral substitute. *Obstet Gynecol* 1970;**35**:416–426.

28. Leach G, Raz S. Vaginal flap technique: a method of transvaginal vesicovaginal fistula repair. In: Raz S. (Ed.) *Female urology*. WB Saunders, Philadelphia 1983, p. 372.

29. Stothers L, Chopra A, Raz S. Vesicovaginal fistula. In: Raz S. (Ed.) *Female urology*. WB Saunders, Philadelphia, 1996, pp. 493–497.

30. O'Connor V Jr. Review of experience with vesicovaginal fistula repair. *Trans Am Assoc Genito-Urinary Surgeons* 1979;**71**:120–122.

31. Martius H. Die operative Wiedeherstellung der volkommen fehlenden Harnrohre und des Schiessmuskels derselben. *Zentralbl Gynakol* 1928;**52**:480.

32. Leuchter R, Lagasse L, Hacker N, Berek J. Management of post-exenteration perineal hernias by myocutaneous axial flaps. *Gynecol Oncol* 1982; **14**:15–22.

33. Ingleman-Sundberg A. Pathogenesis and operative treatment of urinary fistulae in irradiated tissue. In: Youssef A. (Ed.) *Gynecologic urology*. Charles C Thomas, Springfield, 1960, pp. 263–279.

34. Byron R, Ostergard D. Sartorius muscle interposition for the treatment of the radiation-induced vaginal fistula. *Am J Obstet Gynecol* 1969, p. 120.

35. Garlock J. The cure of an intractable vesicovaginal fistula by the use of a pedicled muscle flap: a new concept. *Surg Gynecol Obstet* 1928; **47**:255–260.

36. Bastiaanse NvB. Bastiaanse's method for surgical closure of very large irradiation fistulae of the bladder and rectum. In: Youssef A. (Ed.) *Gynecologic urology*. Charles C Thomas, Springfield, 1960, pp. 280–297.

37. Petty W, Lowy R, Oyama A. Total abdominal hysterectomy after radiation therapy for cervical cancer: use of omental graft for fistula prevention. *Am J Obstet Gynecol* 1986;**154**:1222–1226.

PART NINE
Common pediatric urologic malignancies

Chapter 53
Neuroblastoma

Chapter 54
Wilms' tumor

Chapter 55
Urologic manifestations of pediatric rhabdomyosarcoma

50 Neuroblastoma

D C S Gough and N Wright

Neuroblastoma is a malignant tumor composed predominantly or totally of neuroblasts. These cells are derived from the primitive neural crest in the embryo and are subsequently to be found along the sympathetic chain and in the adrenal gland. These are, therefore, the sites where primary neuroblastoma arises. Two-thirds of all cases present with abdominal disease and nearly two-thirds of these cases probably have their origin in the adrenal gland.

Fifteen per cent of patients present with a thoracic primary tumor and approximately 3% with neck lesions.

The primary site of origin remains unknown in 15% of cases and children frequently present with widespread metastatic disease.

It is the most common solid tumor in childhood occurring outside the brain and accounts for 7% of all the tumors of childhood, yet it is still rare and the case incidence is 9.7 per million children per annum[1].

Presentation

Because of its various primary sites and the high incidence of bony metastases, this tumor can present in many different ways and has even been found antenatally on ultrasound scans, but in the majority of instances the child presents ill with a large abdominal mass.

Pathologic fractures of the humerus and ribs and the appearance of a 'black eye' when orbital bony metastases occur can mimic the features of trauma and hence the need to exclude neuroblastoma in suspected cases of child abuse.

Unusual neurologic manifestations of neuroblastoma include cerebellar encephalopathy, myasthenia gravis or a strange random eye movement termed the 'dancing eye syndrome'. 'Dumb bell' tumors in the abdomen or thorax extend through spinal foramina into the extradural space and can lead to temporary or permanent paralysis with the need to manage a neuropathic bladder in those patients during treatment and as survivors of treatment.

Additional features of this tumor are its relatively high incidence of bone marrow involvement and bony metastases and its universal ability to secrete catecholamines.

Diagnosis

Measurement of the metabolites of catecholamines in the urine is used in both diagnosis and follow up of patients. There are very large numbers of these metabolites which can be present in the urine, but laboratory diagnosis of raised vanillylmandelic acid (VMA) or homovanillic acid (HVA) are relatively inexpensive and measurement of these metabolites in conjunction with 3-methoxy-4-hydroxy phenylethyleneglycol (MHPG) will identify 97% of patients with proven neuroblastoma

The problems with this investigation as a method of diagnosis are the small percentage of patients who do not secrete these commonly measured catecholamine metabolites and the difficulties of 24 hour urine collection and measurements in children. In addition dietary substance, such as fruit, vanilla, coffee and some proprietary and non-proprietary drugs cause elevation of catecholamines in the urine of patients[2].

The clinical effects of these metabolites are infrequently seen in patients with neuroblastoma, but hypertension or diarrhea are both rare manifestations of this catecholamine release.

Tumor behavior and staging

Neuroblastoma is essentially a tumor of very young children and has even been reported in fetal life causing death in utero[3].

Routine post-mortem examination of children under 3 months of age will reveal one in 250 have apparent neuroblastoma in situ in their adrenal glands. The clinical incidence of neuroblastoma is approximately one in 10 000 live born infants, suggesting that there is a spontaneous regression of huge numbers of these in situ lesions which never cause symptoms[4].

Spontaneous regression of malignancy is not unknown, but this particular pattern of behavior is relatively frequent in patients with neuroblastoma and occurs in approximately 1% of all cases[5].

The tumor may also mature to a benign form – ganglioneuroma[6].

For some years it has been appreciated that there is apparently an advanced stage of neuroblastoma which is termed 4S where the patients present with liver, skin and bone marrow involvement, usually within the first year of life, and that there is a very favorable prognosis. Some have suggested that this special stage of neuroblastoma might even require no treatment at all as 10% of the patients in the initial report died of complications of treatment not disease. It would be the experience of most workers, however, that some form of treatment is needed, especially for those with bone marrow involvement as there is also a 10% incidence of progressive disease with death[7].

One of the most important factors in the prognosis of patients with neuroblastoma is their age, with a high incidence of spontaneous cure, regression or response to treatment in patients under 1 year of age. It is almost unknown for a patient over the age of 2 years to show spontaneous regression and there is a high incidence of osseous metastases at presentation in this age group and a poor response to treatment.

Staging

All the historical published data with regard to neuroblastoma and the results of treatment relate to the Evans Staging System which was developed more than 20 years ago.

Stage I   Tumor confined to the organ or structure of origin.

Stage II   Tumor extending beyond the organ or structure of origin, but does not cross the midline and ipsilateral, but contralateral lymph nodes may be involved.

Stage III   Tumor extends in continuity beyond the midline with bilateral nodal involvement.

Stage IV   Metastatic disease.

Stage IVs   Special category. Patients who would otherwise be stage I or II, but who have remote disease confined to the liver, skin or bone marrow and who have no radiologic evidence of bone metastases on complete skeletal survey.

Metastatic disease

Bony metastases to the skull, ribs, spine, pelvis, femur and humerus are found in almost half of patients with neuroblastoma at presentation. There are usually lytic lesions and indicate a poor prognosis, being more frequently seen in children over the age of 2 years.

Bone marrow involvement is common and a histologic confirmation of the diagnosis frequently comes from marrow aspiration and is invariable in stage 4S disease. Marrow involvement can frequently occur without bony lytic lesions and does not carry the same sinister prognosis.

Tumor biology and its effect on prognosis

A number of recent investigations suggest there are prognostic factors related to the cellular biology of the tumor, with particular emphasis on its genetic structure.

The NMYC gene product activates transcription of genes involved in cell proliferation and so amplification, or over-expression of this gene increases proliferative activity[8].

The cellular DNA content of the tumor cells has also been shown to have a prognostic effect with DNA index indicating diploidy giving a poor prognosis[9].

The level of serum lactic dehydrogenase (LDH) has also been implicated in a poor prognosis when the level of this is measured in the serum at >1500 international units per liter.

It has to be appreciated, however, that all these three features are associated with rapid duplication of tumor cells and a high tumor bulk and perhaps they all mean the same thing: a large rapidly dividing cellular tumor.

Some other serum markers that have prognostic significance do not readily lend themselves to this explanation and the serum ferritin has been found to be low in patients with stage III and IV tumors and, therefore, has a direct correlation with poor prognosis[10].

Correlation has been sought between these and other markers of neuroblastoma and there is a feeling that the grade of tumor can be assessed directly from formal histology when features such as calcification of the tumor and its mitotic rate are assessed under direct microscopy. Where there is a high degree of calcification and a low mitotic rate then the prognosis based on histologic criteria alone show 90% of patients with 5 year survival[11].

With so many factors known to be involved in the prognosis of neuroblastoma, such as primary site, stage, age, tumor biology, serum markers and histologic classification, it is difficult to predict in the individual what is likely to happen[12].

In a study of 83 patients, successful surgical treatment and radiotherapy plus single agent chemotherapy gave an overall survival rate at 5 years of 90% in patients with favorable histologic factors, but only 30% in those with unfavorable histology survived[13].

Overall survival has probably changed little over the last 25 years, with a recent study showing survival at 5 years of 65% in stage III cases, where multiple agent chemotherapy has been utilized along with an attempt at resectional surgery[14].

Imaging neuroblastoma

Radiology is used to identify the primary tumor mass, the extent of the disease and the subsequent response to treatment. For tumor staging, there are two distinct areas which require evaluation, each utilizing different imaging modalities; the local extent of the tumor including the pattern of lymph node involvement and the presence of distant metastases.

The evaluation of the primary tumor and local disease

Abdominal radiology is an insensitive technique for the diagnosis of neuroblastoma with calcification being visible in 38–66% of tumors. Ultrasound is frequently the first imaging modality used to investigate an abdominal mass and the diagnosis of neuroblastoma can be made on ultrasound grounds alone[15]. Ultrasound is limited, however, by its inability to assess intrathoracic and some retroperitoneal disease, and intraspinal extension. Computed tomography can detect calcification in up to 85% of tumors, can clearly demonstrate vascular encasement following the use of intravenous contrast and can be used to assess intraspinal extension. Despite this, there is evidence that magnetic resonance imaging is the single most useful imaging modality for the diagnosis and staging of neuroblastoma.[16] Its multiplanar ability and excellent soft tissue contrast mean the extent of the primary tumor can be accurately assessed (Figure 53.1), including involvement of the spinal canal (Figure 53.2), and the presence of bone marrow metastases evaluated. Contrast injection is not required to demonstrate vascular encasement (Figure 53.3), but may improve sensitivity in assessing bone marrow involvement.

The cross-sectional imaging techniques, such as magnetic resonance and computed tomography, are generally used to assess nodal size, with ultrasound being less useful. No currently available imaging modality can confidently distinguish benign from malignant lymphadenopathy.

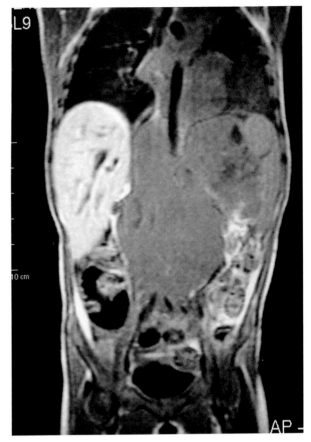

Fig. 53.1

Imaging techniques can also be used to perform guided biopsies of the primary or metastatic lesions when this is felt appropriate.

Distant metastases

Skeletal metastases are common, with the skull and orbit most frequently involved, followed by the ribs, femora, vertebrae, pelvic bones and appendicular skeleton in descending frequency. Both technetium-99m-methylene diphosphonate (MDP) and metaiodobenzylguanidine (MIBG) scintigraphy have been used to identify skeletal metastases as well as the primary tumor.

Both techniques are more sensitive than conventional skeletal surveys. MDP is taken up by cells active in bone metabolism and metastases, therefore, generally show as areas of increased tracer uptake (Figure 53.4). It has a sensitivity of 77%[17]. Metaphyseal involvement may be difficult to assess and may lead to false positives, and conversely lytic lesions can lead to false-negative results. MIBG is an amine precursor treated by the

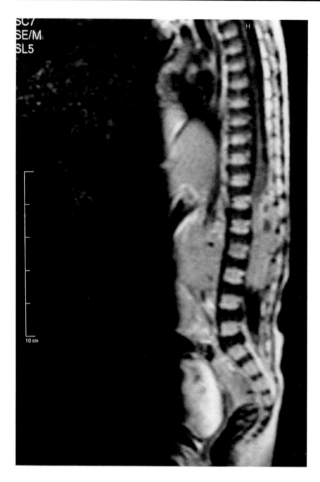

Fig. 53.2

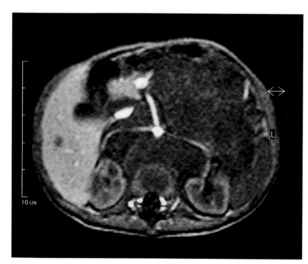

Fig. 53.3

neurosecretory chromaffin granules in neuroblasts in a similar fashion to noradrenaline. More than 90% of neuroblastomas can concentrate MIBG[18]. Four high spots on an MIBG under these circumstances gives a very poor prognosis[19]; yet the results for the detection of metastases with MIBG are conflicting. Both MDP and MIBG may show some metastatic lesions that the other fails to demonstrate.

Some investigators have suggested both MDP and MIBG scans should be performed to detect skeletal metastases. Again metaphyseal assessment may be difficult.

Bone marrow metastases are generally assessed by bone marrow aspiration and/or trephine biopsy, possibly at multiple sites. MRI is also sensitive to bone marrow changes, however, and contrast injection may improve the sensivity. 99m-Tc-labelled monoclonal antibody scanning and MIBG have been used for the detection of bone marrow metastases and have been found to be comparable.

Liver metastases can be detected by ultrasound, computed tomography and magnetic resonance. Evaluation of the liver usually forms part of the initial evaluation when assessing the primary tumor. Liver scintigraphy is not routinely performed.

Pulmonary metastases, although rare at presentation, are best demonstrated by computed tomography, preferably acquired using a helical or spiral technique to improve sensitivity. Contrast is generally not required.

Central nervous involvement is optimally imaged by magnetic resonance imaging and may require the use of contrast to improve sensitivity.

Treatment of neuroblastoma

Surgery is undoubtedly the treatment of choice for localized disease and is important in obtaining tissue for diagnosis in patients with more advanced disease where this is not forthcoming from bone marrow aspiration or biopsy.

The main challenge of surgical treatment in patients with stage III neuroblastoma is where extensive local infiltration and vascular encasement has occurred and this poses a huge technical challenge.

For many years it has not been clear whether extensive surgery of this nature has improved the prognosis, but a recent large study from the European Neuroblastoma Group confirmed an earlier report from the Children's Cancer Study Group and showed an advantage in terms of survival for patients whose surgeon had achieved 100% resection[14,20]. Resections are generally performed after chemical de-bulking with six courses of OPEC (Cisplatinum, Etoposide, Cyclophosphamide and Vincristine).

Screening for neuroblastoma

Poor historical results in the treatment of advanced neuroblastoma and the huge technical challenge posed to

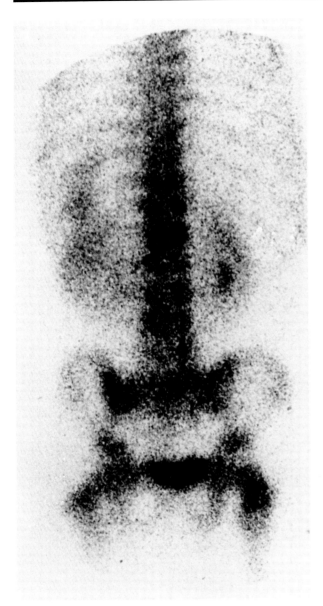

Fig. 53.4a

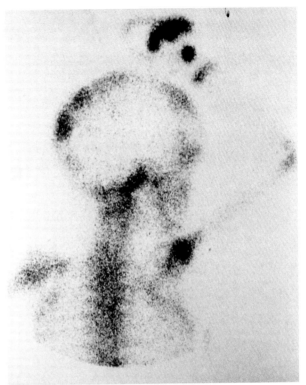

Fig. 53.4b

the surgeon in trying to resect major abdominothoracic disease, coupled with the ability to diagnose this lesion from the urine, led some authors to suggest that screening programs ought to be introduced to make an earlier diagnosis.

In stage III and IV disease the prognosis for survival overall is 25% at 5 years and as almost half the patients present at this stage, it is understandable that the impetus for screening has developed.

Screening children's urine for catecholamines started in Japan in 1972 and became nationwide in that country in 1985. Asymptomatic disease is identified in the first year of life and 97% of patients are alive, and only three children of 342 identified cases had died of the disease[21].

Results such as these suggest there is a way forward with neuroblastoma, but when attempted in the United Kingdom there was a high incidence of false-positive results during screening programs. Factors still to be evaluated are the lead time bias where cases diagnosed earlier seem to be living longer and length bias, whereby slower growing tumors are detected earlier and, therefore, appear in early studies and give a favorable prognosis. As yet no national screening program is evolving in the United Kingdom and neuroblastoma remains a challenge to the pathologist, the oncologist and the surgeon and currently defies a breakthrough in its treatment.

References

1. Gurney JG, Severson RK, Davies S, Robison LL. Incidence of cancer in children in the United States. *Cancer* 1995;**75**:2186–2195.
2. Gitlow SE, Bertani, LM, Rausen A *et al.* Diagnosis of neuroblastoma by quantitative determination of catecholamine metabolites in urine. *Cancer* 1970;**25**:1377–1383.
3. Potter E, Parish RR. Neuroblastoma, ganglioneuroma and fibroneuroma in a stillborn fetus. *Am J Pathol* 1942;**18**:141–151.

4. Beckwith JB, Perrin E. In situ neuroblastomas; a contribution to the natural history of neurocrest tumors. *Am J Pathol* 1963;**43**:1089–1104.

5. Pochedly C. *Neuroblastoma*. Mass. Publishing Sciences Group Acton 1976, p. 278.

6. Griffin ME, Bolande RP. Familial neuroblastoma with regression and maturation into ganglioneurofibroma. *Paediatrics* 1969;**43**:377–382.

7. D'Angio GJ, Evans A, Koop CE. Special patterns of widespread neuroblastoma with a favourable prognosis. *Lancet* 1971;**i**:1046–1049.

8. Seeger RC, Brodeur GM, Sather H *et al.* Association of multiple copies of N-myc with rapid progression of neuroblastoma. *N Engl J Med* 1985;**313**:1111–1116.

9. Look TA, Hayes FA, Nitschke R *et al.* Cellular DNA content as a predictor of response to chemotherapy in infants with unresectable neuroblastoma. *N Engl J Med* 1984;**311**:231–235.

10. Han HWL, Evans AE, Siegel SE *et al.* Prognostic importance of serum ferritin in patients with stages III and IV neuroblastoma. The Children's Cancer Study Group Experience. *Cancer Res* 1985;**45**:1843–1848.

11. Joshi V, Cantor AB, Broduer GM *et al.* Correlation between morphologic and other prognostic markers of neuroblastoma. *Cancer* 1993;**71**:3173–3181.

12. Shimada H, Chatten J, Newton WA *et al.* Histopathologic prognostic factors in neuroblastic tumors. Definition of subtypes of ganglioneuroblastoma and an age-linked classification of neuroblastomas. *J Nat Cancer Inst* 1984;**73**:405–416.

13. O'Neil JA, Littman P, Blizter P *et al.* The role of surgery in localised neuroblastoma. *J Pediatr Surg* 1985;**20**:708–712.

14. Powiss MR, Immison JG, Holmes SKJ. The effect of complete excision on stage III neuroblastoma: a report of the European Neuroblastoma Study Group. *J Pediatr Surg* 1996;**31**:516–519.

15. Bousvaros A, Kirks DR, Grossman H. Imaging of neuroblastoma: an overview. *Pediat Radiol* 1986;**16**:89–106.

16. Dietrich RB, Kangarloo H, Lenarsky C, Feig SA. Neuroblastoma: the role of MR imaging. *Am J Roentgenol* 1987;**48**:937–942.

17. Stark DD, Moss AA, Brasch RC, de Lorimier AA, Albin AR, London DA *et al.* Neuroblastoma: diagnosis imaging and staging. *Radiology* 1983;**148**:101–105.

18. Voute PA, Hoefnagel CA, de Kraker J. 131-I-meta-iodobenzylguanidine in diagnosis and treatment of neuroblastoma. *Bulletin du Cancer (Paris)* 1988;**75**:107–111.

19. Suc A, Lumbroso J, Rubie H *et al.* Metastatic neuroblastoma in children older than 1 year. *Cancer* 1996;**77**:805–811.

20. Haase GM, Atkinson JB, Stram DO et al. Surgical management and outcome of locoregional neuroblastoma. Comparison of the Children's Cancer Study Group and the International Staging system. *J Pediatr* 1995;**30**:289–295.

21. Huddart SN, Mann JR. Screening for neuroblastoma. *Arch Dis Childhood* 1991;**66**:1272–1274.

54 Wilms' tumor

H M Landa

Introduction

When advances in the treatment of cancer are discussed, Wilms' tumor is frequently brought forth as a paradigm of the success of multimodal cancer therapy. Seventy years ago, when nephrectomy was the only real therapeutic modality, the cure rate was below 20%. Currently, a combination of better diagnosis and radiologic staging, improved surgical technique, and subsequent chemo- and radiation therapy, provide a cure rate that exceeds 90%. The incredible success story of Wilms' tumor really begins in 1969, with the founding of the National Wilms' Tumor Study (NWTS) group. There have been four randomized, prospective studies to date, and the fifth study began in late 1995.

NWTS 1, 2, and 3 made many contributions to the therapy of Wilms' tumor. These studies showed that routine radiation to the flank is unnecessary in all stage 1 and favorable histology (FH) stage 2 Wilms' tumors. They demonstrated that cyclophosphamide did not improve the prognosis of stage 4 FH Wilms', and that stage 3 FH tumors are best treated with dactinomycin, vincristine, and 2000 cGy of radiation; or dactinomycin, vincristine, doxorubicin and 1000 cGy of radiation. NWTS-4 demonstrated that 'pulse intensive' regimens produced less hematological toxicity that standard protocols at a lower cost per patient, without sacrificing curability.

The fifth National Wilms' Tumor Study[1] is an ambitious project that endeavors to continue to improve the survival of children with renal tumors while reducing the morbidity of treatment. It will evaluate new protocols for unfavorable histology Wilms' tumor and clear cell sarcoma of the kidney utilizing etoposide and cyclophosphamide, and evaluate the treatment of rhabdoid tumor of the kidney with an aggressive combination of carboplatin, etoposide and cyclophosphamide. NWTS-5 will also explore the impact of recently identified chromosomal markers on the prognosis and therapy of Wilms' tumor, and evaluate treatment options for children with bilateral tumors. The NWTS group has made such significant contributions, it is my belief that any child who is eligible for the NWTS should be offered enrolment.

Epidemiology

Wilms' tumor is the most common solid malignancy of childhood and accounts for approximately 5% of all childhood cancers[2]. Its incidence is approximately eight cases per million children. It is more common in blacks than in caucasians, and more common in caucasians than in asians. The mean age of diagnosis is 3.5–4 years age for unilateral tumors and 2.5–3 years for bilateral tumors. Wilms' accounts for over 90% of childhood renal tumors.

There are many congenital anomalies that are associated with an increased incidence of Wilms' tumor[3]. These include: Beckwith-Weideman Syndrome (BWS); Denys-Drash Syndrome (DDS); and the combination of Wilms' tumor, Aniridia, Genitourinary anomalies and mental Retardation (WAGR) (Table 54.1). There have also been suggestions that environment exposures (e.g. lead, pesticide and hydrocarbons) may play a role, but these remain controversial and, as yet, unproven.[4]

There are other renal tumors that occur in childhood that are much less frequent than classic Wilms' tumor. Clear cell sarcoma of the kidney (CCSK), also known as bone metastasizing tumor of childhood, accounts for about 3% of all renal tumors of children, and rhabdoid tumor of the kidney (RTK) accounts for about 2%. Both CCSK and RTK tend to be more aggressive than Wilms' tumor and are associated with a worse prognosis, despite aggressive chemo- and radiotherapy. Congenital mesoblastic nephroma (CMN) is a rare renal tumor, usually presenting in much younger children (mean age 3.5 months). CMN is a tumor which rarely metastasizes but it can be locally invasive and mandates thorough resection. In very rare cases renal cell carcinoma may also present in childhood.

Genetics

The genetics of Wilms' tumor is undergoing its own very rapid and confusing evolution[5]. Chromosome 11p has been strongly implicated in the genesis of Wilms' tumor. The WT1 gene is believed to reside at 11p13, and is a tumor suppressor gene. It is involved in only a limited number of Wilms' tumors and is thought to act by the conventional two hit theory of oncogenesis. The first hit can be either a pre-zygotic (germline) or post-zygotic (somatic) mutation. In the first case, a germline mutation would cause a heritable condition as well as predispose to multiple tumors. The second hit would occur later, to the contralateral allele, and would result in the loss of expression of WT1. The loss of WT1 binding can result in Wilms' tumor formation. WT1 is expressed in the kidneys, gonads, uterus and spleen. Its expression is higher in the fetal kidney than in more mature renal tissue. WT1 also plays a role in gonadal development as might be expected from the study of WAGR and DDS patients.

Heritable Wilms' needs to be differentiated from familial Wilms' tumor. Familial Wilms' accounts for about 2% of all Wilms' tumors and is autosomal dominant with incomplete penetrance. Data suggest that an additional locus, as yet unidentified, is responsible for familial Wilms' tumor.

The second Wilms' tumor suppressor gene (WT2) is thought to reside at the 11p15 position. Patients with BWS are thought to have two copies of an abnormal gene located at 11p15, both of paternal origin without associated maternal genetic material. This situation (two chromosomal segments from one parent) is termed 'genomic imprinting.' It is unclear at this time if WT2 and the BWS gene are one in the same or are merely adjacent at 11p15. Chromosome 16q has also been identified as a possible tumor locus and is currently under investigation.

Presentation and evaluation

Wilms tumor may present with abdominal pain, hematuria or fever, but a palpable abdominal mass is the most common manifestation[3]. It may be difficult to differentiate a large renal mass from either hepatic or splenic enlargement by physical examination. There may also be a varicocele present. This can be caused by direct pressure on the venous system by the tumor mass, or by a renal vein or vena caval thrombus. In addition, the patient needs to be evaluated for other anomalies associated with Wilms' tumors (Table 54.1).

Laboratory studies for these patients include complete blood count with differential and platelet count, liver and renal function tests, serum calcium and a urinalysis[1]. The first radiologic evaluation of any child with a suspected renal mass should be an ultrasound. Palpable abdominal masses of renal origin that are not malignant (e.g. hydronephrosis, multicystic dysplasia, etc.) are still much more common than Wilms' tumor, and are best evaluated by ultrasound. When a renal mass with solid components is identified, however, abdominal computed tomography (CT) is indicated[1,6]. Although there is some controversy over whether a CT scan is required in the face of a diagnostic ultrasound, most clinicians obtain one prior to exploration.

Knowledge of the status of the renal vein and vena cava, as well as that of the contralateral kidney, is very important before proceeding with surgery. Renal vein involvement has been demonstrated in 11.3% of patients with Wilms, tumor and vena caval involvement has been seen in 4%[7,8]. Ultrasound and/or CT scans generally provide enough information to assess these vascular structures, but occasionally magnetic resonance imaging (MRI) or contrast studies of the vena cava are required.

Chest radiographs are required for staging but the role of chest CT remains controversial. It is unusual to see metastatic lesions on a chest CT that are missed on an

Table 54.1   Table of associated anomalies

Strong association
Denys-Drash syndrome
Renal mesangial sclerosis
Male pseudohermaphroditism
WAGR
Aniridia
Genital abnormalities
Mental retardation
Risk of Wilms' tumor 40%
Beckwith-Weideman syndrome
Visceromegaly
Aniridia
Hemihypertrophy
Macroglossia
85% sporadic, 15% inherited
Risk of Wilms' tumor 10–20%
Hemihypertrophy
Risk of Wilms' tumor 3–5%
Aniridia
Familial or sporadic
Almost all Wilms' tumors occur in sporadic cases
Risk of Wilms' tumor 1%
Minimal association
Horseshoe kidney
Hypospadias
Cryptorchidism

adequate posterior/anterior and lateral chest radiograph[9]. Bone scans are indicated only in children with CCSK and an MRI of the brain is indicated in children with CCSK or RTK.[1]

Staging

The National Wilms' Tumor Study staging system is predominately a pathologic staging system (Table 54.2). The local stage is easily determined intra-operatively, but distant metastases are troublesome. Lesions identified on chest X-rays are felt to be metastatic but if lesions are noted only on chest CT scans, the recommendation is to biopsy these before considering the patient as stage four.

The adaption of this pathologic staging system to a clinical one is relevant in two clinical situations: bilateral Wilms' tumors (or tumor in a solitary kidney), and advanced local disease making resection difficult or impossible. The second category includes patient with vena caval thrombi and/or disease locally invasive into vital organs. These cases may be best handled with preoperative cyto-reductive therapy[10,11].

Pathology

The gross appearance of Wilms' tumor is that of a soft tan or grey mass that is sometimes gelatinous. There may be areas of the mass which are necrotic, hemorrhagic, or cystic, and the renal parenchyma adjacent to the mass is compressed and forms a pseudo-capsule. Wilms' tumor develops from the immature kidney and, histologically, it can consist of any one or all of three classic components. These are primitive blastemal cells, stromal cells (muscle, cartilage, fat, etc.), and epithelial cells. Wilms' tumors with classic histology have all three components and distinctive patterns of blastemal cell proliferation. In favorable histology (FH) tumors, these cells have modest nuclear enlargement and mitotic figures are very rare. Unfavorable histology (UFH) Wilms' tumors have anaplastic cells with greatly enlarged hyperchromatic nuclei and frequent mitotic figures. These anaplastic changes can be focal or diffuse, the latter carrying a much worse prognosis.

Nephrogenic rests are lesions which histologically are easily mistaken for Wilms' tumors and predispose to the development of Wilms' tumors[12]. They are present in approximately one-third of all cases of Wilms' tumor. Nephroblastomatosis is the term used for multiple collections of these rests. These lesions can be perilobar in location or intralobar. These rests commonly regress and sclerose over time, but some may degenerate into Wilms, tumors. Their gross shape is probably the single most important factor in differentiating these rests from FH tumors (Figure 54.1)[13]. The presence of nephrogenic rests in one kidney implies their contralateral presence, so a patient with a Wilms' tumor and rests within the parenchyma of the resected kidney has a higher likelihood of contralateral synchronous or metachronous Wilms' tumors.

Treatment

The treatment of Wilms' tumor has improved dramatically over the last few decades, predominately by the work of the NWTS and its investigators. The standard treatment for a child with a solitary, resectable renal mass, begins with a thorough transperitoneal abdominal exploration, including visualization and examination of the contralateral kidney. This is important because small renal tumors and flat areas of nephroblastomatosis may be missed on pre-operative imaging studies. If the contralateral kidney is found to be uninvolved, a radical nephrectomy is performed and the ipsilateral adrenal gland is excised if it is adherent to the kidney, or if the upper pole of the kidney is involved with the tumor. Resection of any grossly enlarged para-aortic lymph nodes should be performed and lymph node sampling should be undertaken if the nodes are grossly normal. Patients are generally entered in the National Wilms' Tumor Study after nephrectomy and tumor staging and grading. The NWTS-4 treatment protocols are summarized[1] in Table 54.3 for children who have resectable disease. Subsequent to nephrectomy, the NWTS guidelines for follow up are listed in Table 54.4[1]. The overall cure

Table 54.2   Staging

Stage 1
   Tumor is confined to the kidney and completely resected. The renal capsule is intact.

Stage 2
   Tumor extends beyond the kidney but is completely resected...or...
   tumor is stage 1 but was previously biopsied (except fine needle aspirate)
   ...or...
   tumor spillage occurred but was confined to the flank.
   In all cases, the tumor is completely resected.

Stage 3
   Residual non-hematogenous tumor left behind...or...
   positive lymph nodal disease...or...
   tumor penetrated or present, on the peritoneal surface...or...
   tumor spillage occurred not limited to the flank.

Stage 4
   Hematogenous metastasis present (lung, liver, bone, brain, etc.)

Stage 5
   Bilateral renal disease

587

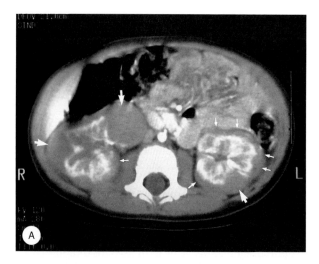

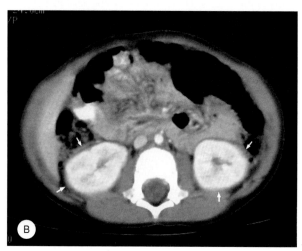

Fig. 54.1 Abdominal CTs of a 2-year-old male with Beckwith-Weideman Syndrome. (A) Development of bilateral spheroidal renal masses which are felt to be Wilms' tumors (indicated by large arrows) within a mantle of nephroblastomatosis (small arrows). (B) Same child after 3 months of chemotherapy (no resection performed). Note the resolution of the tumors and decrease in thickness of the mantle of nephroblastomatosis (small arrows).

Table 54.3 NWTS treatment protocols, S/P radical nephrectomy

Age	Stage	Histology	Chemo	Flank XRT	Other XRT
<2 years	1, tumor < 550 g	Favorable	None	No	No
>= 2 years	1	FH, focal or diffuse anaplasia	EE-4A	No	No
Any age	1	Focal anaplasia	EE-4A	No	No
Any age	2	Favorable	EE-4A	No	No
Any age	2	Focal anaplasia	DD-4A	Yes	No
Any age	3	FH or focal anaplasia	DD-4A	Yes	No
Any age	4	Favorable	DD-4A	Yes	2
Any age	2–4	Diffuse anaplasia	Reg I	Yes	2
Any age	1–4	CCSK	Reg I	Yes	2
Any age	1–4	RTK	Reg RTK	1, 2	2

EE-4A: Dactinomycin, Vincristine.
DD-4A: Dactinomycin, Vincristine, Doxorubicin.
Regimen I: Vincristine, Doxorubicin, Cyclophosphamide, Mesna, Etoposide, Granulocyte colony stimulating factor,
Regimen RTK: Carboplatin, Cyclophosphamide, Mesna, Etoposide, Granulocyte colony stimulating factor,

[1] No XRT for stage 1 and 2. No flank XRT for stage 4 if renal tumor is stage 1 or 2.
[2] Chest XRT if CXR positive or biopsy proven pulmonary metastasis. CT scan only disease is at discretion of investigator, biopsy recommended.
    For infants < 18 months. can hold off chest XRT for 4 weeks to determine if there has been a response to chemotherapy.
    Metastasis to brain, bone, liver, etc. are also treated with XRT.

the biopsy specimen. Patients should be evaluated after 5 weeks and an exploration is suggested with local excisions if feasible.

Patients with inoperable local disease (particularly vena caval thrombi above the hepatic veins) should be treated in a similar fashion with either DD-4A for FH or Regimen I for UFH.

Relapse

Relapse can occur locally in the flank or abdomen, in the contralateral kidney, or at distant sites (lung, brain, bone, etc.). The recurrence rate is approximately 10% for stage 1 and 2 FH tumors and 22% for stage 3 and 4 FH tumors. The rate for UFH tumors increases to 36% for stages 1, 2 and 3, and to 46% for stage 4 tumors[14]. The treatment of a patient who has suffered a relapse has not been standardized previously, but a protocol has been established in NWTS-5[1].

Late effects

A great deal of work is ongoing to evaluate the late effects of the treatment of Wilms' tumor. This is particularly important as now the great majority of children are cured

rate (based on NWTS-4) of Wilms' tumor stage for stage is described in Table 54.5[14].

Children with bilateral disease (stage 5) are usually treated with renal biopsy and chemotherapy, followed by a renal parenchymal sparing operation. The NWTS protocol (Table 54.3) used to treat these patient is regimen EE-4A if each kidney appears to be stage 1 or 2 and has favorable histology. Regimen DD-4A is recommended if either kidney demonstrates a local stage 3 or 4 and favorable histology, and Regimen I if there is any anaplasia in

Table 54.4   NWTS follow up protocols after nephrectomy

Age	Stage	Histology	0	3	6	9	12	15	18	21	24	27
< 2 years	1, tumor < 550 g	Favorable	1	1	1	1	1	1	1	1		
≥2 years	1	FH, focal or diffuse anaplasia	2	3	2	3	3	2	3	2		
Any age	1	Focal anaplasia	2	3	2	3	3	2	3	2		
Any age	2	Favorable	2	3	2	3	3	2	3	2		
Any age	2	Focal anaplasia	2,5,6	3	3	2	3	3	3	2	3	2
Any age	3	FH or focal anaplasia	2,5,6	3	3	2	3	3	3	2	3	2
Any age	4	Favorable	2,5,6	3	3	2	3	3	3	2	3	2
Any age	2–4	Diffuse anaplasia	8	4	4	2	4	4	4	2,6	4	8
Any age	1–4	CCSK	8,9	4	4	2	4	4	4	2,6	4	8
Any age	1–4	RTK	7	4	4	2	4	4	4	2	4	6

CBC with differential every week while on chemotherapy
[1]Chest X-ray and abdominal U/S.
[2]Liver/renal function tests, UA, chest X-ray, chest CT (if positive previously), and abdominal U/S.
[3]Liver function tests.
[4]Liver/renal function tests, UA.
[5]Abd. CT.
[6]Muga scan, echocardiogram.
[7]Liver/renal function tests, UA, Chest X-ray, Chest CT, abdominal U/S, MRI of brain.
[8]Liver/renal function tests, UA, Chest X-ray, chest and abdominal CT, abdominal U/S, Muga scan, echocardiogram.
[9]MRI of brain, skeletal survey, bone scan, bone marrow aspirate and biopsy.

Table 54.5   Wilm's tumor survival by stage

Stage	Four year survival	Four year recurrence-free survival
1	96%	89%
2	91%	87%
3	91%	82%
4	81%	79%

of their primary disease, and face a lifetime of risks due to the late effects of their curative therapy. An NWTS late effects study exists for children who are alive 5 years after completion of therapy. The late effects are what would be expected from chemo- and irradiation therapy in childhood. Infertility and hormonal dysfunction are common in both sexes and those women who do become pregnant have a higher incidence of complications[15]. Truncal growth abnormalities are still a problem in those children who have received abdominal irradiation[16] and all treated patients are at risk for the development of secondary malignancies[17], especially within radiated fields. Congestive heart failure is a well recognized complication of treatment with doxorubicin and chest radiotherapy worsens this effect[18]. Renal insufficiency is a rare late complication, presumably due to a combination of hyperfiltration from decreased renal mass and the nephrotoxicity of the cancer treatment. This has led to the suggestion by some[19] that renal sparing surgery (with pre-operative chemotherapy when necessary) be considered even in patients with unilateral disease. Currently, the incidence of renal failure in patients with unilateral disease and no associated anomalies is less than 0.2%[20].

Conclusion

The outlook for patients with Wilms' tumor has improved dramatically over the past few decades. Long-term follow up of previously treated patients and support of the NWTS group will continue to improve the curability of Wilms' tumor, while reducing the morbidity of its treatment.

References

1. National Wilms Tumor Study Group Committee. National Wilms Tumor Study-5: Therapeutic Trial and Biology Study. National Wilms Tumor Study Group.
2. Breslow N, Olshan A, Beckwith JB, Green DM. Epidemiology of Wilms tumor. *Med Pediatr Oncol* 1993;**21**(3):172–181.
3. Ritchey ML, Andrassy RJ, Kelalis PP. Pediatric urologic oncology. In: Gillenwater JY, Grayhac JT, Howard SS, Duckett JW (eds) *Adult and pediatric urology*. United States: Mosby. 1996, pp. 2675–2719.
4. Olshan AF, Breslow NE, Falletta JM et al. Risk factors for Wilms tumor. Report from the National Wilms Tumor Study. *Cancer* 1993;**72**(3):938–944.
5. Coppes MJ, Williams BRG. The molecular genetics of Wilms tumor. *Cancer Invest* 1994;**12**(1):57–65.
6. Green DM, D'Angio GJ, Beckwith JB, Breslow NE, Grundy PE, Ritchey ML, Thomas PRM. Wilms tumor. *CA Cancer J Clin* 1996;**46**:46–63.
7. Ritchey ML, Othersen HB Jr, de-Lorimier AA, Kramer SA, Benson C, Kelalis PP. Renal vein involvement with nephroblastoma: a report of the National Wilms Tumor Study-3. *Eur Urol* 1990;**17**(2):139–144.

8. Ritchey ML, Kelalis PP, Haase GM, Shochat SJ, Green DM, D'Angio G. Preoperative therapy for intracaval and atrial extension of Wilms tumor. *Cancer* 1993;**71**(12):4104–4110.

9. Wilimas JA, Douglass EC, Magill HL, Fitch S, Hustu HO. Significance of pulmonary computed tomography at diagnosis in Wilms tumor. *J Clin Oncol* 1988;**6**(7):1144–1146.

10. Beagler M, Landa HM. Preoperative chemotherapy in the treatment of high stage Wilms tumor. Presented at the annual meeting of the American Urological Association, 1994.

11. Greenberg M, Burnweit C, Filler R *et al.* Preoperative chemotherapy for children with Wilms' tumor. *J Pediatr Surg* 1991;**26**(8):949–953; discussion 953–956.

12. Beckwith JB. Precursor lesions of Wilms tumor: clinical and biological implications. *Med Pediatr Oncol* 1993;**21**(3):158–168.

13. Beckwith JB. Personal communication, 1995.

14. D'Angio GJ, Breslow N, Beckwith JB *et al.* Treatment of Wilms' tumor. Results of the Third National Wilms' Tumor Study. *Cancer* 1989;**64**(2):349–360.

15. Li FP, Gimbrere K, Gelber RD, Sallan SE, Flamant F, Green DM, Heyn RM. Outcome of pregnancy in survivors of Wilms tumor. *JAMA* 1987;**257**(2):216–219.

16. Wallace WH, Shalet SM, Morris-Jones PH, Swindell R, Gattamaneni HR. Effect of abdominal irradiation on growth in boys treated for a Wilms tumor. *Med Pediatr Oncol* 1990;**18**:441–446.

17. Breslow NE, Norkool PA, Olshan A, Evans A, D'Angio GJ. Second malignant neoplasms in survivors of Wilms' tumor: a report from the National Wilms' Tumor Study. *J Natl Cancer Inst* 1988;**80**(8):592–595.

18. Sorensen K, Levitt G, Sebag-Montefiore D, Bull C, Sullivan I. Cardiac function in Wilms' tumor survivors. *J Clin Oncol* 1995;**13**(7):1546–1556.

19. McLorie GA, McKenna PH, Greenberg M. Reduction in tumor burden allowing partial nephrectomy following preoperative chemotherapy in biopsy proved Wilms tumor [see comments]. *J Urol* 1991;**146**(2 (2)):509–513.

20. Ritchey ML, Green DM, Thomas PR *et al.* Renal failure in Wilms' tumor patients: a report from the National Wilms Tumor Study Group. *Med Pediatr Oncol* 1996;**26**(2):75–80.

55 Urologic manifestations of pediatric rhabdomyosarcoma

O Lesani, E Espinosa and J W Basler

Incidence

Rhabdomyosarcoma (RMS) is the most common soft tissue sarcoma in infants and children, accounting for greater than 50% of pediatric soft tissue sarcomas. It accounts for 15% of all pediatric solid tumors. 15–20% of all rhabdomyosarcomas in children arise in the genitourinary system[1]. The ratio of males to females is 1. 4 : 1, demonstrating a slight male predominance in genitourinary (GU) rhabdomyosarcoma[2]. RMS typically grows from embryonal mesenchymal tissue and morphologically resembles developing fetal skeletal muscle[3].

Pediatric RMS is characterized by a different anatomic distribution to that of adults. The most common primary sites for pediatric RMS are head, neck, and genitourinary organs, whereas the majority of soft tissue sarcomas in adults arise from extremities[1]. Genitourinary tumors, in order of occurrence, are prostate, bladder, vagina, and paratesticular RMS. Other pelvic tumors carry a worse prognosis than the aforementioned genitourinary sites[4]. This is possibly due to the fact that pelvic tumors must grow to a large size before presenting with symptoms of obstruction. Lawrence and colleagues have demonstrated that the anatomical site of the primary directly affects patient survival rates. Bladder and prostate RMS cases are considered a less favorable group of anatomical sites compared with paratesticular and vaginal tumors. Three year survival was estimated to be only 60–70% for bladder and prostate compared with 94% survival in other genitourinary tumors[5].

Many researchers have suggested possible genetic causes of rhabdomyosarcoma. In 1969, Li and Fraumeni[6] proposed familial aggregation of rhabdomyosarcoma with other sarcomas and types of cancers including breast. This predisposition to a family cancer syndrome was attributed to the susceptibility gene p53. Mutations in p53 have been identified in sporadic rhabdomyosarcomas[7]. McKeen et al (1978) have suggested an increased incidence of RMS in association with neurofibromatosis[8]. Genetic studies have pointed to chromosome 11p as the locus of embryonal rhabdomyosarcoma[9]. Other molecular characteristics of RMS, such as persistent expression of MyoD gene family, may be used as possible diagnostic markers in the future[10].

Clinical staging

Two different staging systems for RMS exist. The Intergroup Rhabdomyosarcoma Study Group (IRSG) has devised a Pretreatment Staging System (Table 55.1) using data from their second study. This system classifies RMS based on physical examination, imaging studies and laboratory findings. Tumor location, size, and involvement of regional nodes were found to be most predictive of survival[5]. The traditional TNM system differs from the IRSG system in that it does not incorporate anatomical location in its classification and has no basis on survival data. As new treatment staging technologies emerge, the IRSG Pretreatment Staging Systems must be modified to readjust our ability to predict patient outcome[11].

Table 55.1 Intergroup Rhabdomyosarcoma Study Group (IRSG) Pretreatment Staging System

Stage	Sites	T	Tumor size	N	M
I	Orbit	T1 or T2	a or b	N0 or N1 or N2	M0
	Head and neck (excluding parameningeal)				
	GU-nonbladder/nonprostate				
II	Bladder/prostate	T1 or T2	a	N0 or Nx	M0
	Extremity				
	Head and neck parameningeal				
	Other (including trunk, retroperitoneum, etc.)				
III	Bladder/prostate	T1 or T2	a	N1	M0
	Extremity		b	N0 or N1 or Nx	
	Head and neck parameningeal				
	Other (including trunk, retroperitoneum, etc.)				
IV	All	T1 or T2	a or b	N0 or N1	M1

T1 = confined to anatomic site of origin, T2 = extension and/or fixation to surrounding tissue, a = <5 cm in diameter, b = >5 cm in diameter, N0 = regional lymph nodes not clinically involved, N1 = regional lymph nodes clinically involved by neoplasm, Nx = clinical status of regional lymph nodes unknown (especially with sites that preclude lymph node evaluation), M0 = no distant metastases, M1 = metastases present

Pathology

WHO and the IRSG committee recognize three primary histologic subtypes: embryonal, alveolar and pleomorphic. The embryonal subtype is the most prevalent, making up 50–60% of rhabdomyosarcomas in children[2]. It can present in a solid form and sarcoma botryoides, a polypoid variety. The solid form is seen more commonly in the trunk and extremities, whereas the sarcoma botryoides is found more frequently in hollow organs such as bladder and vagina. The alveolar subtype, the second most common subtype, is found more frequently in the extremities than the GU system. Its higher rate of dissemination and local recurrence gives alveolar tumors a worse prognosis. Any scattered alveolar component in a tumor is now considered to be adequate for designation of the tumor as alveolar[12]. The third subtype, pleomorphic, exhibits features of both embryonal and alveolar subtypes. IRSG-I and IRSG-II committees found only five pure cases of this subtype in their study of 1600 tumors. A controversy exists as to whether pleomorphic tumors deserve a part in the classification[12]. Recent discoveries of chromosomal abnormalities and translocation in these tumors may possibly prove to be beneficial in both classification and assignment of prognosis.

RMS has a natural course of rapid growth and local invasion. These tumors disseminate through both lymphatic channels and bloodstream with a predilection for metastasis to the lungs. Risk of widespread metastasis warrants a complete metastatic evaluation including CT scan of pelvis, chest, bone scan and bone marrow biopsy for accurate staging.

Paratesticular

Paratesticular rhabdomyosarcoma is the primary tumor in 10% of all rhabdomyosarcomas. While it can present from infancy to early adulthood, the incidence peaks between 2 and 5 years of age. It originates from embryonal mesenchyme of the tunics surrounding the spermatic cord[13]. It commonly presents as a unilateral painless intrascrotal mass, distinct from the testes. With enlargement, the lesion can compress the testes. Ultrasound will reveal its solid nature.

This lesion is best treated by multimodal management that combines surgery, chemotherapy and radiation. The surgical option is radical inguinal orchiectomy unless the scrotal skin integrity is compromised; in which case a hemiscrotectomy is warranted. Diagnosis requires evaluation of nodal and distant metastasis by chest and retroperitoneal CT. Weiner and colleagues have noted that among 121 IRS-III patients, CT evaluation failed to confirm pathologic presence of nodal metastasis in 14% of these patients[14]. Limited unilateral para-aortic and iliac lymph node biopsy should therefore be considered adequately to evaluate nodes not identified on CT scan even in the absence of gross metastatic disease[3]. Radiation therapy is recommended for those with evidence of nodal involvement or gross metastasis. Recommended chemotherapy is vincristine-dactinomyosin-cyclophosphamide. The 5 year survival rate using multimodal therapy is 72% as projected by IRSG-III[15].

Bladder and prostate

Bladder and prostate RMS commonly present with symptoms of urinary obstruction. Frequency, urinary retention, stranguria and hematuria have all been mentioned. The tumor mass or distended bladder present as an abdominal mass on the physical examination. Contrast studies will reveal a filling defect in tumors involving the bladder. Prostatic primary tumors can displace the bladder, which is also apparent in excretory urogram. Cystoscopy with transurethral biopsy confirms the diagnosis. Bladder tumors are mostly botryoid subtype arising from the trigone, in contrast to solid embryonal tumors, arising from the prostate[16].

Partial cystectomy has been employed in vesicular rhabdomyosarcomas that is confined to vesicular wall and bladder dome successfully[17]. Problems have been encountered in utilizing partial cystectomy with RMS that initially arises in the prostate or trigone. Chemotherapy can be used to shrink tumors in these locations. If successful reduction in tumor size in these locations occurs, partial cystectomy may be adequate therapy. Current conservative management of bladder cancer includes bladder salvage in case of bladder wall tumors (with or without initial chemotherapy) and routine administration of radiation. Partial resection of the bladder wall has demonstrated overall survival of 80%, allowing the majority of patients to be free of bladder malfunction[18].

The early treatment for prostatic RMS was an anterior exenteration, which achieved excellent results, but with unacceptable morbidity for these long-term survivors[19]. Attempts were made in IRSG I and II to fashion a therapy that integrated early, high-dose chemotherapy followed by radiotherapy, and conservative surgery if necessary[16]. The resulting cure rates (57%) were less than expected, leading to the search for new therapeutic approaches. The IRSG-III protocol 37-B is much more impressive, with cure rates of 82% and a bladder salvage rate of 64%[20]. The earlier utilization of radiotherapy is believed to have played a role in this success, as well as the addition of other chemotherapeutics. Most important is the finding that chemotherapy and radiotherapy, not surgery, are the best initial treatments for prostatic RMS. This can be followed by conservative surgery in select cases[21].

Vaginal, vulvar and uterine

Initial presentations for rhabdomyosarcomas are often in the first few years of life, with a protruding vaginal mass at introitus or vaginal bleeding/discharge. Vulvar tumors can be palpated as a firm nodule within the labial fold or around the clitoris[22]. Vaginal rhabdomyosarcoma originates mainly from the anterior vaginal wall in the area of the embryonic urogenital sinus. Uterine tumors may involve the cervix or the uterine body. Tumors arising from the cervix may present with a vaginal mass or bleeding while those arising from the uterus may present with an abdominal mass. Diagnosis is made by biopsy of the lesion. Full metastatic evaluation with pelvic and chest CT, bone scan and aspiration, vaginoscopy and cystoscopy should accompany biopsy.

Andrassy and colleagues (1995)[22] report success with chemotherapy (VAC plus adriamycin and cisplatin) and recommend it as the primary treatment modality for vaginal and vulvar rhabdomyosarcoma. Whenever indicated, conservative surgery and adjunctive radiotherapy in addition to the above mentioned chemotherapy can effectively halt local recurrence and distant metastases. Primary chemotherapy and delayed resection may also be a workable approach to treating uterine rhabdomyosarcoma as well as preserving pelvic organs[23]. IRSG-III and IRSG-IV pilot study of patients with primary uterine tumors revealed survival rates ranging from 1.5–6 years. However, chemotherapy resulted in chemotoxicity-associated mortality independent of the mortality caused by the tumor. The outcome of the study points to the need for modifications in combination therapy necessary further to maximize the cure rate, while minimizing treatment associated morbidity and mortality.

The Third Intergroup Rhabdomyosarcoma Study reports that the cure rate for rhabdomyosarcoma has improved dramatically in the past 25 years, from an estimated 25% in 1971 to 70% in 1991[24]. Triple agent therapy, VAC (vincristine, actinomycin-D and cyclophosphamide) have been traditionally used for treatment of RMS. Arndt and colleagues have reported an overall 3 year survival of 91% in patients with intermediate RMS treated with newer chemotherapies including doxorubicin, etoposide and ifosfamide[25]. Multimodality therapy with surgery, chemotherapy and radiation is the current recommended management for RMS. Clinical use of molecular markers, modification of chemotherapy regimen, and hematopoietic growth factors are yet to be explored and assessed for their effect in increasing survival rates[20].

References

1. Maurer HM, Beltangady M, Gehan EA *et al.* The Intergroup Rhabdomyosarcoma Study – I. A final report. *Cancer* 1988;**61**:209.

2. Maurer HM, Moon T, Donaldson M, Fernandez C, Gehan EA, Hammond D, Hays DM *et al.* The Intergroup Rhabdomyosarcoma Study: a preliminary report. *Cancer* 1977;**40**:2015–2026.

3. Skoog SJ. Benign and malignant pediatric scrotal masses. *Ped Urol* 1997;**44**(5):1229–1250.

4. Crist WM, Raney RB, Tefft M, Heyn R, Hays DM, Newton W, Beltangady M, Maurer HM: Soft tissue sarcomas arising in the peritoneal space in children: A report from the Intergroup Rhabdomyosarcoma Study (IRS) Committee. *Cancer* 1985;**56**:2125–2132.

5. Lawrence W Jr, Gehan EA, Hays DM, Beltangady M, Maurer HM. Prognostic significance of staging factors of the U.I.C.C. staging system in childhood rhabdomyosarcomas. A report from the Intergroup Rhabdomyosarcoma Study (IRS II). *J Clin Oncol* 1987;**5**:46–54.

6. Li FP, Fraumeni JF Jr. Soft tissue sarcomas, breast cancer and other neoplasms. A familial syndrome? *Ann Intern Med* 1969;**71**:747–752.

7. Malkin D, Li FP, Strong LC, Fraumeni JF, Nelson CE *et al.* Germline p53 mutations in a familial syndrome, breast cancer, and other neoplasms. *Science* 1990;**250**:1233–1238.

8. McKeen EA, Bodurtha J, Meadows AT *et al.* Rhabdomyosarcomas complicating multiple neurofibromatosis. *J Pediatr* 1978;**93**:992–993.

9. Douglass EC, Valentine M, Etcubanas E. A specific chromosomal abnormality in rhabdomyosarcoma. *Cytogenet Cell Genet* 1987;**45**:148–155.

10. Scrable H, Witte D, Shimada H, Seemayer T, Sheng WW, Soukup S, Koufos A *et al.* Molecular differential pathology in rhabdomyosarcoma. *Genes Chromosom Cancer* 1989;**1**:23–35.

11. Lawrence W, Anderson J, Gehan E, Maurer H. Pretreatment TNM staging of childhood rhabdomyosarcoma: A report of the Intergroup Rhabdomyosarcoma Study Group. *Cancer* 1997;**80**:1165–1170.

12. Pappo AS, Shapiro DN, Crist WM, Maurer HM. Biology and therapy of pediatric rhabdomyosarcoma. *J Clin Oncol* 1995;**13**:2123–2139.

13. Ritchey ML, Andrassy RJ, Kelalis PP. Pediatric urologic oncology. In Gillenwater JY, Grayhack JT, Howards SS (eds). *Adult and pediatric urology* (3rd edn). Mosby Year Book, St Louis, 1996, pp. 2706.

14. Wiener ES, Lawrence W, Hays D, Lobe TE, Andrassy R, Donaldson S, Crist W *et al.* Retroperitoneal node biopsy in paratesticular rhabdomyosarcoma. *J Pediatr Surg* 1994;**29**:171.

15. Donaldson SS, Anderson J. Factors that influence treatment decisions in childhood rhabdomyosarcoma. *Radiology* 1997;**203**:17–22.

16. Hays DM, Raney RB Jr, Lawrence W Jr, Tefft M, Soule EH, Crist WM, Foulkes M, Maurer HM. Primary chemotherapy in the treatment of children with bladder-prostate tumors in the Intergroup Rhabdomyosarcoma Study (IRS-II). *J Pediatr Surg* 1982;**17**:812–819.

17. Hays DM, Lawrence W Jr, Crist WM, Wiener E, Raney RB Jr, Ragab A, Tefft M *et al.* Partial cystectomy in the management of rhabdomyosarcoma of the bladder: a report from the Intergroup from the Intergroup Rhabdomyosarcoma Study (IRS). *J Pediatr Surg* 1990;**25**:719.

18. Hays DM: Bladder/prostate rhabdomyosarcoma. Results of the multi-institutional trials of the Intergroup Rhabdomyosarcoma Study. *Sem Surg Oncol* 1993;**9**:520–523.

19. Grosfeld JL *et al.* Rhabdomyosarcoma in childhood: analysis of survival in 98 cases. *J Pediatr Surg* 1983;**18**:141–146.

20. Crist WM, Gehan EA, Ragab AH, Dickman PS, Donaldson SS, Fryer C, Hammond D *et al.* The Third Intergroup Rhabdomyosarcoma Study. *J Clin Oncol* 1995;**13**:610–630.

21. Lobe TE, Andrassy RJ, Crist WM *et al.* The argument for conservative delayed surgery in the management of prostatic rhabdomyosarcoma. *J Pediatr Surg* 1996;**31**:1084–1087.

22. Andrassy RJ, Hays DM, Raney RB, Wiener ES, Lawrence W, Lobe TE, Corpron CA *et al.* Conservative surgical management of vaginal and vulvar pediatric rhabdomyosarcoma: a report from the Intergroup Rhabdomyosarcoma Study III. *J Pediat Surg* 1995;**30**:1034–1036.

23. Corporan CA, Andrassy RJ, Hays DM, Raney RB, Weiner ES, Lawrence W, Lobe TE, Maurer HM. Conservative management of uterine pediatric rhabdomyosarcoma: a report from the Intergroup Study III and IV pilot. *J Pediatr Surg* 1995;**30**:942–944.

24. Crist WM, Kun LE. Common solid tumors of childhood. *N Engl J Med* 1991;**324**:461–471.

25. Arndt CA, Nascimento AG, Schroeder G, Schomberg PJ, Neglia JP, Sencer SF, Silberman TL *et al.* Treatment of intermediate risk rhabdomyosarcoma and undifferentiated sarcoma with alternating cycles of vincristine/doxorubicin/cyclophosphamide and etoposide/ifosfamide. *Eur J Cancer* 1998;**34**(8):1224–1229.

PART TEN
Patient support and palliative care

Chapter 56
Palliative care

56 Palliative care

P McNamara and C Regnard

Introduction

Although palliative care is the right of every patient and is the duty of every clinician[1], it is a sad reality that severe pain remains unrelieved in over half of cancer patients[2]. At the core of effective palliative care is the creation of a 'Safe place to suffer'[3]. This has nothing to do with a building, but with a relationship where the patient feels safe to express their distress. Adequate symptom control is implicit in this care (no-one will tell you what frightens them while they are vomiting). Also central to the care is the willingness for the clinician to listen to what a patient says about their feelings (no-one will tell you how they feel if you are showing you are not listening). Finally, this care acknowledges that you cannot fix everything; patients will still feel distress at their situation. The key is that expressing that distress is therapeutic in itself, and they will do this if they feel safe to do so.

Palliative care services

The traditional (medieval) model of hospice was as a resting place for travelers, usually a religious institution. In the UK, Trinity Hospice is the oldest hospice (1894) with St Joseph's, Hackney (1905). Places like Conrad House, Newcastle, opened in 1957 by Marie Curie Cancer Care, were able to provide high quality nursing to terminally ill patients. The UK is the place where the modern hospice originated a generation ago, St Christopher's in Sydenham, London. When it opened its doors in 1967, it was in response to a perceived inadequacy in the way terminally ill patients were cared for on general hospital wards. In the 30 or so years since then, there has been an explosion of palliative care services in the UK. There are now over 200 independent hospices in the UK and somewhat less than 30 NHS Units, with as many units again worldwide. In the last 15 years or so, the emergence of specialist and non-specialist palliative care services has begun and there are numerous hospital palliative care support teams, day hospices and community based services. There is now a considerable body of literature and information about palliative care principles and approaches[4–7].

At the end of 1987, palliative medicine was adopted as a medical specialty by the Royal College of Physicians, London. This recognized that palliative medicine was a clinical area with its own set of specialist knowledge and skills, and there are now over 100 specialist registrars in palliative medicine in the UK. There are now national definitions of what constitutes a specialist palliative care service or hospice[1]. Non-specialist palliative care services are expected to have had training and education in palliative care, with regular updating, but need not have accredited staff or have palliative care as their central work, e.g. Marie Curie sitting and home nursing service, palliative care designated beds in a nursing home, etc. Specialist services are provided by staff accredited in the specialty and whose core function is palliative care. In the case of inpatient units, there will be one or more consultants in palliative medicine on staff. Additionally, there will be the full interdisciplinary team, including physiotherapy, social worker, occupational therapy, psychosocial resources, chaplaincy, etc. This is to fulfil the object of holistic care for the patient, physical, psychological, social and spiritual. There is also support offered to the family and carers (with involvement of the patient and their family in decisions about their care), as well as bereavement support.

Following the Calman-Hine Report into cancer services in England and Wales[9], one of the requirements for accreditation of cancer centers and units, was the regular sessional input of consultants in palliative medicine. This is often by way of support and advice to a hospital palliative care/support team, a specialist team to resource the hospital, clinically and educationally. The nurses on the team will be specialist palliative care nurses, with their equivalents in the community often called Macmillan nurses. Macmillan nurses are community clinical nurse specialists in palliative care, whose initial funding was pump-primed by Macmillan Cancer Relief. Macmillan and

Marie Curie are the UK's two major national cancer charities.

Palliative care may be applicable to anyone with advancing life threatening illness, not just cancer. Other 'traditional' diagnoses seen in palliative care are motor neurone disease (MND) and acquired immune deficiency syndrome (AIDS). However, it is being increasingly recognized that multiple sclerosis and other neurodegenerative diseases, end stage heart and respiratory disease and a host of other diagnoses have palliative care needs. The percentage of people with advancing life threatening illnesses who need palliative care probably approaches 100%. But the percentage of this group with specialist palliative care needs is probably 10–25%.

As with the Calman-Hine Report's concern to reduce the inequality in services available, geographically, so the next step is to reduce the inequality of palliative care in primary health care. Macmillan nurses are usually community based and there to assist the primary health care teams with palliative care difficulties. Recently, Macmillan GP Facilitators have been commissioned: practicing GPs with a remit to help their peers review and improve their palliative care knowledge and skills. An important part of the role of specialist palliative care is to act as a resource to educate and update those providing non-specialist palliative care. The range of palliative care services, specialist and non-specialist, is listed below. The extent of the services will probably vary a little from area to area in the UK:

Specialist
- Consultants in palliative medicine
- Community or hospital specialist nurses (may be called Macmillan Nurses)
- Specialist palliative care inpatient units or specialist hospices with their full interdisciplinary team
- Specialist Day Hospice
- Specialist Day Treatment[8]
- Specialist outpatient clinics: medical, lymphedema, breathlessness etc.
- Specialist hospital palliative care teams
- Specialist community palliative care teams

Non-specialist
- Non-specialist hospices
- Nursing homes with designated 'palliative care' beds
- Community hospitals with palliative care facilities
- Community sitting and nursing services, e.g. Marie Curie nurses, local 'hospice at home' services, etc.

Palliative care services specifically for children are developed in a limited number of places and being planned more widely. Children's hospices deal less with terminally ill children with cancer (for which services are well developed) and more with children with advancing life threatening ill-

nesses. Diagnoses such as the neurodegenerative diseases, cystic fibrosis, etc. are often the main focus of these hospices, where short respite for the family are often the most urgent need, in a facility with fully trained children's nurses and medical back up. A full compendium of palliative care services, updated annually, is available from St Christopher's Hospice Information Service[9] (Tel. No. 020 8778 9252).

Breaking bad news

Having to break bad news is always uncomfortable. One effect can be that doctors tell the relative or partner first, forgetting the burden they now place upon the relative. You cannot make bad news less bad, but it is possible to break bad news in a way that makes acceptance and understanding easier.

People react to bad news in different ways, whether they are a patient, a relative or a partner. Many people adapt to bad news because they have had time to prepare or a previous experience has made them aware of the reality. Sometimes a person may be relieved that there is an explanation for the problems they have been experiencing, although they may still react emotionally later. Denial is less common than acceptance, but many people cope with denial to some extent. A few people react with strong denial and will refuse absolutely to believe the news given. Many of these people will describe themselves as 'fighters' and may ask for second opinions from other specialists. Other people are ambivalent and fluctuate between appearing to accept the bad news and then denying there is a problem. Those who are in denial or who are ambivalent can have unrealistic expectations leading to demands for inappropriate treatment which can cause considerable difficulties. This may result in a relative asking for drips to be put up or for tubes to be put down. Overwhelming distress is unusual, but can happen if the news is broken abruptly without warning. This distress may then prevent any further information being taken in. Collusion is usually the result of one person trying to protect another from the truth. The person colluding will argue clearly that they know the patient or their partner better than anyone in the health care team, and that they know the individual could not take the bad news. There will be considerable pressure for the information to be kept hidden. If the patient asks that others are not told of their diagnosis, this is their legal right, although it can cause problems for the health professionals. If, however, the relative or partner asks that the patient is not told, this causes bigger problems since the patient has a legal right to know their own diagnosis and its prognosis if they wish.

To break bad news effectively a patient must be physically capable of understanding information. If this is prevented by a reversible cause this needs to be treated. In other situations the cause is severe and irreversible (e.g. coma due to end stage disease) or it is inappropriate to

Breaking bad news

Breaking bad news is never easy but can be given in a positive way that the individual can both accept and understand. Remember this also applies to relatives and partners.

Table 56.1   Clinical decisions in breaking bad news in advanced cancer[5]. The initial approach

Key decision	Management
Is patient physically unable to understand?	● If this is irreversible: unless patient has previously objected, inform relative or partner using this clinical decision table to do so. ● If reversible: treat cause.
Is relative or partner withholding information from patient?	Collusion by relative or partner: ● Accept that carer *does* know patient better than any professional. ● Explore reasons for collusion (the carer is doing what they think is best at the time). ● Ask permission to speak to the patient to find out what they themselves are making of the situation. ● Check the cost of the collusion on the relationship with the relative.

● If possible, find somewhere that is confidential, quiet, comfortable and free of interruptions.
● Explore what the person already knows and check understanding.
e.g. 'What do you make of what's happening to you' or 'How do you see things going from here?'

Does the person already know?	● No further information requested:
	   – *for patient*: go to Table 56.2.
	   – *for relative*: if patient agrees inform relative or partner or patient's level of knowledge. Use this table.
	 ● If more information is requested, but this is not bad news:
	   – supply the required information (ideally with written or taped backup), and go to Table 56.2

● WARN (e.g. 'We have the result, and I'm afraid they're more serious than we thought.')
● PAUSE to allow person to respond.

| ● CHECK
 Has the person responded to the warning shot? | e.g. 'What do you mean, more serious?' 'Are you saying it's cancer?'
 ● Answer invitation for more information, giving first part of news. (e.g. 'I'm afraid we found some abnormal cells.')
 ● Ensure person understands information.
 ● Keep giving information as long as person is responding positively to questions (e.g. 'What do you mean, abnormal?') |

treat the cause (e.g. obstructive renal failure due to advanced retroperitoneal tumor). What to do will depend on previous commitments or the family's views. If the relative or partner are colluding (e.g. 'You won't tell him, will you?') it must be acknowledged by the professional that this is usually an act of love and that the relative or partner knows the patient much better than anyone in the health care team. It is possible to give a promise that bad news will not be blurted out, but will only be confirmed if the patient is obviously ready to know. The aim is to bring them together so they can talk through any mutual problems.

The place where bad news is broken should be somewhere that cannot be overheard by others, and if possible should also be quiet, comfortable and free of interruptions. It is not acceptable to break bad news in the middle of a busy corridor. The person may also want a friend or relative to be present for support, and may also agree to another professional carer being in attendance.

The key role for the professional in breaking bad news is not deciding how much the person should know, but asking the person how much they want to know. This is usually easier than it seems. The first step is to find out what they already know (never assume). Their clarity or otherwise will already given an indication of how aware they are. Asking how much they want to know can be done safely by direct questions (e.g. 'Do you want me to explain the result of your test?') or more open questions (e.g. 'Are you the sort of person who prefers to know what's going on?'). Most people's response is clear, but when it is ambiguous this simply reflects that they are ambivalent themselves about knowing. Ambivalence is not a problem if it is acknowledged and the professional leaves open the possibility of further discussion. These initial questions act as a 'warning shot' since this will give some indication to the person that they need to come to grips with something that could be unpleasant. The questions should now be at the person's pace (not the professional's), pausing to

Table 56.2   Clinical decisions in breaking bad news in advanced cancer[5]. Handling the effects of bad news

Key decision	Management
• Pause to check person's reaction • Acknowledge any distress.	
Is the person accepting the bad news?	• Acknowledge and explore any feelings and concerns. • Monitor regularly for anger, withdrawal, feelings of defeat and spiritual anguish.
Is the person overwhelmingly distressed?	• Acknowledge distress. • Explore the individual concerns to work out why the reaction has been so disturbing.
Is the person denying or holding unrealistic expectations?	• Acknowledge denial or unrealistic expectations (e.g. 'I can see how you're feeling about this.'). • Check for a window on the denial (e.g. 'Are there any times, even for a second, when you're less sure that everything is alright?'). • Challenge any inconsistencies (e.g. 'You say everything is fine, but you're still continuing to lose weight.') • Do not be defensive about unrealistic expectations (e.g. Patient: 'You doctors have got it all wrong.') **NB. If they are coping well,** *do not persist in challenging* **denial or unrealistic expectations (remember, these people** *are* **coping!).**
Is the person ambivalent?	Denial will fluctuate, therefore keep to reality. • *When in acceptance*: offer any requested information. • *When in denial*: confront the ambivalence (e.g. 'Yesterday you seemed to accept that your situation was quite serious, but today you say you're going to get better. I wonder which of these you want me to work with?') • *If person is responding with uncertainty* (e.g. Person: 'I'm not sure.' or 'I need to think about that.') Acknowledge uncertainty (e.g. 'I can see you're not sure about this.') and offer time or help (e.g. 'Do you want more time or any help.')
Is patient colluding?	• Recognize that this is often a need to protect the partner out of love. • Accept that the patient *does* know the relative or partner better than any professional. • Explore the reasons for the collusion (the patient is doing what they think best at the time). • Negotiate permission to speak to the relative or carer to find out what they are making of the situation. • Check the cost of the collusion with both patient and relative or partner.

allow the person to respond to what has been said. This allows the person to stop the flow of bad news at any point. This stage can vary from a few minutes to at least several days. When the person is asking for more information a common mistake is too much information is given at once. If they have just been told they have a carcinoma of the bladder any details on treatment will be forgotten while they assimilate the news of the cancer. Time is needed for the person to absorb what has happened. It is then vital for the health professional to ask how the person is feeling, even if it will be another professional who picks up the pieces. The 'Warn, Pause, Check' approach is shown in more detail in Table 56.1. How to handle the effects of bad news is shown in Table 56.2, but it is important to understand that the health professional who breaks the news does not have to be the one who later supports or

counsels the patient – we all have legitimate limits to our skills! Consequently, having an additional professional colleague present can be supportive and will help interprofessional communication if that colleague is from a different discipline. It is also essential that a summary of the interview, including the information given, is recorded and included in any correspondence.

Pain is a complex experience and relief is only possible if the four cornerstones to management are applied to each pain: assessment, planning, treatment and reassessment.

Assessment

Assessment is the keystone. Pain severity is often difficult to assess and is of little value in choosing treatment. In

Pain

Pain can be complex in advanced cancer, but the principles of management are no different from managing the simplest pain.

Table 56.3 Clinical decisions in diagnosing and treating pain[5]

Key decision	Management

● Is the pain worsened or precipitated by movement?	● On the slightest passive movement:
	  −*fracture*: −immobilize + regional anesthesia + strong opioid.
	    −arrange for X-ray ± orthopedic surgery.
	    −if malignant arrange for radiotherapy
	  −*acute nerve compression*: see nerve compression below
	  −*soft tissue tumor infiltration*: commence opioid; consider dexamethasone or radiotherapy.
	  −*acute infection*: treat appropriately.
	● Only on straining a bone on examination:
	  −*pain over bone* suggests a bone metastasis: commence opioid + arrange DXT. NSAIDs help in a small proportion of patients (beware adverse effects).
	    If skeletal instability consider orthopedic surgery ± radiotherapy.
	  −*pain in the distribution of a nerve or nerve root* suggests nerve compression: commence opioid and consider dexamethasone 12 mg PO daily, reducing to maintenance of 4–6 mg daily.
	● Mainly on active movement suggests skeletal muscle pain. A trigger point (tender area in muscle, often with underlying tight band) suggests a myofascial pain – a common type of skeletal pain treated by injection of 0.25% bupivacaine into trigger point in muscle; a TENS (with the electrodes over the trigger point) may also help.
	● Only on inspiration: look for pathology involving pleura, ribs, muscle or skin and treat appropriately.
	● Consider other movement related pains (arthritis, organ distention, local infection) and treat appropriately.

Is the pain periodic?	● *Colic*: source is usually indicated by the site of pain.
	● *Bowel*: exclude constipation, obstruction or bowel irritation due to drugs or infection. Use hyoscine butylbromide SC 10–20 mg.
	● *Bladder*: exclude infection, outflow obstruction, unstable bladder. For persistent bladder irritation consider instillation of 20 ml 0.25% bupivacaine 8–12 hourly.
	● *Ureter*: exclude infection.
	  Give 10–20 mg hyoscine butylbromide for immediate relief.
	  Diclofenac 75 mg IM can be used for longer lasting relief.
	  For low obstruction consider stent, otherwise try dexamethasone 12 mg daily, reducing to maintenance of 4–6 mg daily.

Is the pain related to a procedure?	● Change the technique (e.g. different dressings, topical anesthetic cream) ● Try: − Entonox if available and patient can comply − 4- hourly dose of usual analgesic given PO or SC ● Consider sedation with midazolam 1–5 mg titrated IV.
Is the pain related to eating?	● Consider problems in the mouth, esophagus or stomach and treat according to cause.
Is there skin damage?	● Consider trauma, tumor, infection, irritation and treat according to cause.
Are there unpleasant sensory changes at rest?	Suggests neuropathic pain (often associated with increased sensitivity or pain on light touch): ● Amitriptyline 10–50 mg at night. Consider gabapentin 300–900 mg bd. twice daily. If pain persists, contact local pain specialist for further advice and consideration of regional analgesia.

Is the pain in an area supplied by a nerve or nerve root?	● *Nerve compression*:
	  − start an opioid and titrate.
	  − exclude skeletal instability as a cause
	  − for compression by tumor consider dexamethasone ± radiotherapy.

Is the pain persisting?	● Consider:
	  − unresolved anger, fear or depression
	  −poor compliance because of fear, misunderstanding of instructions or an unacceptable form of medication.
	  −onset of a new pain: go through previous 9 clinical decisions.

contrast, diagnosing the cause of the pain is the essential first step.

Pain related to movement

Pain that is precipitated or worsened by movement suggests a limited range of possibilities (see Table 56.3):

Fracture: The immediate priority in a fracture is to relieve distress at rest. If immobilization is insufficient a strong opioid may help, or even titrated sedation (e.g. midazolam by subcutaneous infusion[10]). Spinal analgesia can be invaluable[11,12], and allows time to plan elective orthopedic surgery.

Bone metastases: Pain from skeletal instability will respond poorly to strong opioids or to nonsteroidal anti-in-flammatory drugs (NSAIDs). The instability must be treated by surgery, by treating the metastasis (usually with radiotherapy) or by encouraging bone healing (e.g. bis-phosphonates in breast carcinoma)[13]. Rest pain from bone metastases can be helped with a strong opioid. A small proportion of such patients may also be helped by NSAIDs, but their adverse effects make these second line. If the pain radiates along the distribution of a discrete nerve, this suggests accompanying nerve compression which may require regional anesthesia, or high-dose dexamethasone.

Myofascial pains are common and a discretely tender spot, often with an underlying band of muscle in spasm, is typical of a myofascial trigger point. Such pains have typical sites and radiations depending on the muscle involved[14], and respond to injection of the trigger point with local anesthesia, or transcutaneous electrical nerve stimulation (TENS)[15].

Other movement-related pains may arise from joints, organ distension (e.g. hepatomegaly) or local inflammation, and the management will depend on the cause.

Periodic pain

Regular, sharp episodes of pain, suggest smooth muscle spasm (colic), with the site and radiation depending on the source. Treatment involves either removing the source of irritation (e.g. drugs irritating the bowel), instillations of topical local anesthesia (in bladder irritation due to tumor), or the use of an antispasmodic (e.g. hyoscine butyl-bromide).

Neuropathic pain

This type of pain does not involve pain receptors and can be due to continuing nerve damage (neuropathy), or can persist after the damage has occurred (de-afferentation pain, sympathetically maintained pain). It can follow nerve damage within 1–3 months, occasionally in hours. A dermatomal or peripheral nerve distribution is usual, but a vascular distribution suggests altered sympathetic activity, usually accompanied by localized sympathetic hyper-

activity or hypoactivity. Patients describe sensations such as burning, shooting, pins and needles, sandpaper, scalding or freezing. Hyperesthesia (increased sensitivity to stroking) or allodynia (pain which is provoked by a normally non-painful stimulus such as stroking) are strongly suggestive of neuropathic pain. Although neuropathic pain is usually partly or totally unresponsive to opioids, in cancer it is often part of a mixed pain and it is worth starting a trial with morphine since other components of the pain may respond[16]. Otherwise, low doses of tricyclic antidepressants, or anticonvulsants in standard doses, can be effective singly or in combination. Other drugs and techniques can be useful, and the advice of a pain or palliative care specialist is essential if the first line treatments are ineffective.

Explanation and planning

Explanation follows assessment. It is often a relief to patients that a likely cause is now known. Realistic goals then need to be set. These goals need to be negotiated with the patient, for example, expecting freedom from pain on walking in the presence of skeletal instability will result in disappointment for patient and carers alike. Patient goals that seem distant should not be dismissed (after all, they may be achieved), but additional, closer goals should be negotiated. For patients with goals that seem too close, their fears should be explored and longer-term goals negotiated. With appropriate goals it is then possible to plan pain relief over the next 4 hours, 24 hours and in the future.

Treatment

The analgesic ladder was devised by the World Health Organization to guide world-wide analgesic prescribing in malignancy (Figure 56.1)[17]. This applies where pain is continuous, dull and unremitting. As the pain is continuous, analgesia must be continuous, aiming at full pain relief. Strong opioids are a logical progression from weak opioids and not 'reserved for the end'. Morphine is the strong opioid of choice, and should be started when weak opioids are found to be no longer fully effective. The initial dose is 10 mg morphine 4 hourly (or 30 mg controlled release morphine b.d – half this dose in the elderly or in renal failure). Adverse effects on first starting morphine are nausea, drowsiness and constipation. These effects disappear after a few days, except the constipation, hence prescribe an antiemetic, e.g. low-dose haloperidol 1.5 mg nocte, and a laxative, e.g. senna/docusate nocte, when prescribing morphine, and warn about the drowsiness. Where analgesia is good with morphine, but side effects are intolerable, a change of strong opioid may reduce the adverse effects, e.g. to hydromorphone. Not all cancer pains

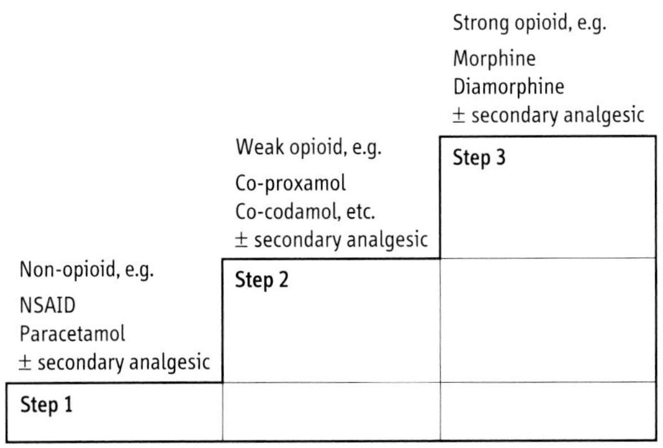

Fig. 56.1   The analgesis ladder.

respond to morphine (although about 70% do) and 'secondary analgesics' may be required, e.g.

dexamethasone can reduce peritumor edema, so is helpful in nerve compression (incl. cord compression), raised intracranial pressure, 'raised intrapelvic pressure';

amitriptyline ± gabapentin can help in neuropathic pains;
baclofen can settle painful skeletal muscle spasms;
hyoscine butylbromide can settle smooth muscle colic;

antibiotics can reduce painful inflammation when this is due to infection.

These 'secondary' approaches may need the guidance of an experienced local pain relief resource, e.g. palliative medicine consultant, or anesthetist specialist in pain. Where the urologic malignancy has given risen to predominantly intrapelvic disease, the pain may be very difficult to control, often giving rise to lower body severe pain. A spinal line may be effective with an infusion of bupivacaine and morphine. Experience with intrathecal spinal lines has demonstrated good efficacy and low morbidity, the caveat being that the team caring for the line must be suitably trained[11,12]. Where the pain is in unilateral site, e.g. affecting one limb, a nerve block is worth considering[11]. A lumbar sympathectomy can be effective for tenesmoid pain and a celiac plexus block for upper abdominal pain.

Reassessment

Regular assessment is essential. Relying on pain severity assessments can be used but it is better to rely on a patient's ability to perform daily functions. If the pain is still present it is worth considering unresolved psychosocial issues, poor compliance with medication, or inappropriate analgesic dose or timing. Since new pains can arise

Constipation

Constipation is common in cancer – prevention is the key.

Table 56.4   Clinical decisions in managing constipation[5,18]

Key decision	Management
Is obstruction present?	• If stool is an unlikely cause then see Table 54.5 on bowel obstruction.

Have feces been easy and comfortable to pass?	• Exclude constipation by rectal, abdominal and, if necessary, X-ray examination.
	• If constipation is a risk:
	  – *constipating drugs* (e.g. opioids): docusate 100mg ± senna 1 tab daily
	  – *immobility*: docusate 100 mg daily
	• Titrate laxative to maintain passage of comfortable stool.
	• Reassess daily.

Is the rectum full?	• If the feces are hard: encourage fluids and use glycerin suppositories. If this fails try a docusate enema to soften stool. • If this fails consider manual evacuation (always under sedative cover). • If the feces are soft: commence senna or bisacodyl PO. • If no success: manual evacuation under sedative cover (e.g. midazolam titrated IV).
Is the colon full?	• If colic is a problem: use docusate 100 mg daily and titrate dose or split up any stimulant laxative into divided doses. Consider a high arachis oil enema. • If colic is absent: commence docusate + senna
Is privacy lacking?	• Offer privacy by helping patient to the toilet. Avoid commodes or bed pans.

in the site of the original pain, persistent pain should prompt reassessment.

Constipation

Constipation here is defined as the difficult or uncomfortable passage of feces. Frequency of stool is unhelpful in advanced cancer since it is invariably reduced. Symptoms include pain, anorexia and diarrhea. Signs include 'overflow diarrhea' (small amounts of fecal fluid in the presence of an empty rectum), abdominal masses or distention. Prevention is the key. Stimulant laxatives such as senna, danthron and bisacodyl, act mainly on the large bowel. Danthron (in co-danthrusate) occasionally colors the urine red, and can occasionally cause a perianal rash. Docusate is a weak contact stimulant, but with surface wetting properties which is useful when softening stool is a priority. Lactulose is an osmotic laxative and can cause postural hypotension, even in well hydrated patients. Therefore no laxative is ideal, but combinations of docusate and senna or lactulose and senna often produce a comfortable stool. Laxatives should be taken on a regular basis with the dose adjusted every 3–5 days using stool consistency as the guide, not frequency. Enemas are not often required. If a manual evacuation is necessary it should always be carried out under sedative cover such as diazepam or midazolam intravenously – it is simply unkind to do otherwise.

Nausea and vomiting

Nausea and vomiting are the final common pathway of a variety of stimuli. The vomiting centers in the medulla can be activated by vagal stimulation (gastric distention, bowel distention, liver capsule stretch, irritation of gastrointestinal mucosa by drugs, infection or radiotherapy, unpleasant genitourinary stimulation, or mediastinal disease); direct stimulation (raised intracranial pressure, radiotherapy to the head and neck, or brain stem metastases); stimulation from the chemoreceptor trigger zone in the floor of the fourth ventricle (drugs, bacterial toxins and biochemical disturbances); stimulation from the inner or middle ear (infection, movement, ototoxic drugs or local tumor); or stimulation from higher central nervous system centers such as anxiety, fear, or revulsion.

In assessing the cause it is helpful to know the extent of tumor spread, previous treatment, current drugs, biochemistry and clinical examination. Most causes of nausea and vomiting produce a non-specific pattern. Gastric related causes are the exception since they produce vomiting with brief nausea or no nausea (see Table 56.5).

Choice of antiemetics is limited initially to three types. Cyclizine is effective in vagally mediated emesis, haloperidol for chemically mediated causes, and metoclopramide (or domperidone) for most gastric related causes. These can be taken singly or in combination if it is felt several causes are present. If these first line antiemetics fail, low-dose levomepromazine can be helpful. In contrast to their effectiveness in chemotherapy-induced vomiting, odansetron and granisetron seem of no value in the emesis of advanced disease. Although this scheme is based on the distribution of dopamine and histamine receptors in the ferret, it has been shown to be effective in 93% of patients with advanced disease[19,20]. Parenteral hydration may be needed until the oral route can be tolerated. The intravenous route is commonly used but the subcutaneous route into sites in the upper, lateral back is effective, can be delivered at home and hyaluronidase is unnecessary[21].

Bowel obstruction

The commonly used terms 'acute' and 'sub-acute' are unhelpful in assessing bowel obstruction. Obstruction is either complete or partial, and is either continuous or intermittent. Using these terms gives a much clearer picture of events. It is important at the outset to exclude constipation and a medically treatable ileus. Diagnosis is sometimes difficult but is helped by the history (e.g. altered bowel habit, absent flatus, vomiting, pain), observation (e.g. distention, visible peristalsis), examination (e.g. resonant percussion, succussion splash), and investigation (radiology). In obstructions of the distal ileum and colon, vomiting is less frequent and develops later, while high obstructions cause frequent vomiting at an early stage, but with little or no abdominal distention. The more complete and continuous the obstruction, the more obvious and severe the symptoms.

The first step is to eliminate nausea, the second to reduce vomiting to 1–3 times a day. Occasional vomiting may continue, but patients find this is preferable to constant nausea. An antihistaminic antiemetic (e.g. cyclizine) is the first line, adding a dopamine antagonist (e.g. haloperidol) if the nausea persists. Alternatives are to replace the cyclizine with low-dose levomepromazine (5–10 mg once at night), or to consider the use of octreotide[23,24].

It is always right to consider surgery especially as bowel obstructions in cancer are due to a benign cause or to an unrelated second primary tumor in up to 38% of patients[22]. There are indicators of a good prognosis in patients suggesting surgery is worthwhile (see Table 56.6), but some patients are too ill, their tumor is too extensive or they do not wish further intervention. These patients can still be successfully palliated.

Hydration is used automatically in hospital at the first suggestion of an obstruction. While this is good pre-operative practice, it is not always necessary with inoperable obstruction. Distal obstructions (rectum, colon, ileum) still leave enough area for fluid absorption to prevent symptomatic dehydration. More proximal obstructions may cause mild symptoms such as a dry mouth which can be treated by frequent mouth care. In many patients, slowly developing dehydration in the last days of their lives is not perceived by them as distressing. A few patients will feel thirsty, especially in more proximal obstructions, and it is appropriate for these to be parenterally hydrated, subcutaneously if necessary (see notes on nausea and vomiting). Nasogastric suction fails to control symptoms of obstruction in at least 86% of patients[25]. It therefore has a limited place in palliative care (see notes). Patients with partial obstructions may manage small frequent snacks of low-fibre foods. Patients with complete obstructions should still be allowed to enjoy snacks as often as they wish. As a patient deteriorates the aim of feeding is for pleasure, not survival. Families and staff need to understand this as much as the patient.

Patients palliated in this way have been shown to survive for a mean of 3.7 months, with some surviving for more than 10 months, a result comparable to survival after surgery for malignant obstruction[22]. In addition, this approach allows patients with obstruction to be managed at home. If it is clear the obstruction is inoperable it is no longer necessary to admit them to hospital for care, or they can be discharged back home if that is their wish.

Nausea and vomiting

The key is to target antiemetics at specific causes.

Table 56.5   Clinical decisions in managing nausea and vomiting[5]

Key decision	Management

Is patient mainly vomiting with little or no nausea?	• Large volume vomiting (may also have hiccups, early satiation, heartburn, fullness)
	  If dehydrating rapidly: consider gastric outflow obstruction and start parenteral hydration. Consider surgery.
	  Little or no dehydration: this is probably gastric stasis due to drugs or partial outflow obstruction (e.g. hepatomegaly, ascites).
	  Start metoclopramide 30–90 mg SC infusion per 24 hours or domperidone 30–60 mg PR 8 hourly).
	  Consider erythromycin 250–500 mg 8 hourly or percutaneous gastrostomy.
	• Small volume vomiting:
	  −*if stomach not distended*: 'squashed stomach syndrome' due to hepatomegaly or ascites: treat as for gastric stasis.
	  −*if stomach distended*: 'floppy stomach syndrome' (gastric atony): brief nasogastric suction until stomach empty of air and fluid.
	  −*If regurgitation*: exclude oesophageal causes.
	  −*if raised intracranial pressure*: see below.

Could chemicals be stimulating the CTZ?	e.g. drugs (morphine, metronidazole), uremia, bacterial toxins. • haloperidol 1.5–3 mg PO or SC once daily at bedtime.
Could vagal afferents be involved?	e.g. pharyngeal irritation by candida, hepatomegaly, bowel obstruction • Cyclizine 25–50 mg PO 8 hourly or 75–150 mg SC infusion per 24 hours.
Is the bowel obstructed?	See Table 56.6 on bowel obstruction.
Is intracranial pressure raised	• Cyclizine 25–50 mg PO 8 hourly or 75–150 mg SC infusion per 24 hours. • If due to cerebral tumor: start high-dose dexamethasone and refer to clinical oncologist for cranial irradiation.
Is gastritis present?	Epigastric pain is usually a feature • If on NSAIDs stop drug or add omeprazole (*not* an H_2 blocker) • Start sucralfate suspension 10 ml PO 6 hourly • Metoclopramide or domperidone as above.

• If nausea and vomiting still present:
  −exclude fear or anxiety and manage if present.
  −consider levomepromazine 5–15 mg PO or SC once at night.

Bowel obstruction

When bowel obstruction is inoperable, symptoms can be palliated and patients kept at home if they wish.

Table 56.6   Clinical decisions in managing bowel obstruction in advanced cancer[5]

Key decision	Management
Is there any doubt that this is bowel obstruction?	History, observation, clinical examination, radiology. • Consider other causes of nausea and vomiting, abdominal distention, colic (e.g. laxatives), or altered bowel habit (e.g. constipation).
Is constipation the sole cause?	• Clear rectum and commence laxative.
Is a physical blockage absent?	Peristaltic failure (absent bowel sounds, distention, little vomiting): • Exclude peritonitis / septicemia / recent cord compression • Stop antiperistaltic drugs (e.g. anticholinergics, loperamide) and osmotic laxatives. • Start mild stimulant laxative, e.g. docusate 100 mg 8 hourly • Consider metoclopramide SC infusion 30–90 mg per 24 hours.
Is troublesome thirst present?	• Parenterally hydrate (usually IV, but up to 2 liters can be infused into upper, lateral back subcutaneously in 24 hours).
Is this an operable obstruction and is patient fit for surgery?	*Indicators of a good prognosis*: no ascites or abdominal masses, no previous radiotherapy, large bowel blockage, single blockage, single blockage, good nutritional and medical condition. • Consider surgical exploration if patient agrees.
Is nausea and/or vomiting present?	• Cyclizine 50 mg PO 8 hourly or 150 mg per day by continuous subcutaneous infusion (reduce these doses by 50% if >70 years age). • If nausea is still present and colon is distended: *add* haloperidol 5 mg PO or SC once at night. • If no improvement, consider replacing above with —levomepromazine 5–15 PO or mg SC once at night. or —octreotide 300–600 μg/24 hours SC infusion. • If vomiting persistent, feculant or fecal, consider nasogastric tube.
Is obstruction complete and continuous?	• Stop all laxatives. Treat dry mouth. • Treat colic if present with hyoscine butylbromide 30 mg per day by continuous subcutaneous infusion (up to 180 mg). • Continue to hydrate and feed orally in occasional snacks. • Consider high-dose dexamethasone (see text).
Is obstruction incomplete or partial?	• Stop osmotic and strong contact laxatives. Treat dry mouth. • Start docusate 100 mg 8 hourly and titrate dose. • Intermittent colic: hyoscine hydrobromide 300 μg sublingually (max. 1200 μg in 24 hours). • Treat other pain: see Table 56.3 on pain. • Hydration and feeding orally in small frequent snacks.

Diarrhea

Causes of *intermittent diarrhea* should be considered. Constipation or partial bowel obstruction can both cause episodes of diarrhea. Gastrointestinal infection can cause diarrhea, but repeated episodes suggest persistent infection – this can become chronic in immunocompromised patients such as those with AIDS.

Color changes: Dark or black stools suggest bleeding from the upper gastrointestinal tract. Steatorrhea causes diarrhea, usually with pale stools that float and have an offensive odor. *Previous surgery* can cause diarrhea. Examples are gastrectomy (dumping syndrome); ileal resection (bile irritation of colon); blind loops (bacterial overgrowth); and anterior resection (mucous discharge).

Clear fluid in low volume may be mucus from colon (total bowel obstruction), rectum (surgically formed rectal stump) or from a mucus secreting tumor involving bowel. A larger volume may be urine from a vesicocolic or

Diarrhea

A loose or frequent stool is an added insult to the patient with advanced disease, especially if accompanied by perianal soreness, fecal incontinence, dehydration or abdominal pain.

Table 56.7   Clinical decisions in managing diarrhea in advanced cancer[5]

Key decision	Management
Is patient dehydrated?	• Hydrate orally or subcutaneously. IV hydration is not usually needed in advanced disease.
Is the diarrhea intermittent?	• Exclude: constipation with spurious diarrhea, or partial bowel obstruction. • Exclude infection: culture stool if diarrhea persists for more than 5 days or contacts are affected. • High osmotic load: NG feeding – dilute feeds / increase length of feeding time. Gastric dumping – small, frequent snacks (no large meals).
Are stools darker than usual?	• Upper gastrointestinal blood loss – consider surgery or embolisation if appropriate/ sucralfate suspension 10 ml 4- hourly if stomach is the source.
Are stools paler than usual?	Steatorrhea: • Pancreatic insufficiency: pancreatin +H_2 blocker + dietary supplement. • Obstructive jaundice: H_2 blocker (consider corticosteroids, surgery or stent). • Intestinal surgery – see below.
Has there been previous surgery?	• Post-gastrectomy (dumping syndrome) – small, frequent snacks. • Ileal resection (causing bile salt irritation of colon) – cholestyramine 12–16G • Extensive intestinal resection (causing steatorrhea) – as for ileal resection. • Blind loop – tetracycline or metronidazole for 2 weeks. • Blind rectum with ostomy (causing mucous rectal discharge) – see below.
Is the stool mixed with blood or discharge?	• Fungating tumor involving rectum – topical corticosteroids ± metronidazole. • Infection (e.g. shigella or salmonella) – identify and treat. • Inflammatory (NSAIDs / radiotherapy) – stop drug.

Is there clear fluid in the stool?	• If the volume is less than 1 l/24 hours consider:
	  –urine (vesicocolic or vesicorectal fistula)– if surgery is not possible, pass a urethral catheter or give nasal desmopressin at night.
	  –mucus (total bowel obstruction / blind rectum / rectal or colonic tumor secreting mucus) – try hyoscine hydrobromide (orally / SC/ topically) in rectal tumor.
	• If the volume is greater than 1 l/24 hours, this may be a secretory diarrhea due to infection: if severe consider octreotide (100–600) μg per 24 hours as subcutaneous infusion) ± rectal tube.

Exclude
• Drugs (e.g. excess laxatives / antibiotics / NSAIDs / β-blockers / diuretics / magnesium antacids)
• Infection (bacterial / protozoal / viral, including HIV-related). Note that to diagnose AIDS-related diarrhoea, up to six stool specimens may be required ± rectal biopsy.
• Gastrocolic fistula – consider colostomy
• Irritable colon
• Recent radiotherapy
• Anxiety, fear

• Treat symptomatically:
–loperamide 2–4 mg with each loose stool (up to 16 mg / day) (see caution in notes)
–barrier agent (e.g. dimethicone cream) or protective covering (e.g. hydrocolloid such as Granuflex).
–consider octreotide (100–600 μg per 24 hours as subcutaneous infusion).

vesicorectal fistula – this can be confirmed by the instillation of methylene blue into the bladder. Volumes greater than 1 l/24 hours, however, are usually secretory and the commonest cause of this type is infection.

Blood or offensive discharge in the stool suggests a carcinoma involving the bowel wall, infection (especially shigella or salmonella), or mucosal inflammation of rectum or colon (non-steroidal anti-inflammatory drugs, radiotherapy).

Causes which are easily missed include drugs (e.g. laxatives, magnesium antacids, antibiotics, β-blockers, diuretics); a gastrocolic fistula; an irritable colon; recent radiotherapy to the lower spine or pelvis; and anxiety or fear.

Treatment of diarrhea

Fluid replacement: Some water loss is inevitable with diarrhea, but symptomatic dehydration is unusual in diarrhea related to advanced cancer. Oral rehydration is therefore often sufficient for most patients. In addition, water absorption can be increased by slowing peristalsis with loperamide. The exception to this approach is infection which may cause fluid loss requiring parenteral replacement. It is also important to avoid slowing peristalsis in infection, since this would increase the absorption of bacterial toxins.

Drug approaches: The diarrhoea due to steatorrhea can be helped with loperamide. It is also helpful to increase duodenal pH to encourage lipid micelle formation by starting an H_2 blocker. Magnesium antacids should not be used since they can cause diarrhea and also reduce lipid absorption, problems not shared by aluminium antacids. Pancreatic insufficiency may require enzyme replacement using pancreatin tablets or capsules. Where obstructive jaundice is due to bile duct obstruction, high-dose corticosteroids may reduce peritumor edema and inflammation, with relief of the obstruction. Intestinal resection diminishes the release of gastrin inhibiting hormones resulting in increased gastrin – this increases gastric acid output which further reduces lipid micelle formation by making the duodenal content too acid. An H_2 blocker should therefore be added. If bile salt irritation is the problem, the salts can be sequestrated using cholestyramine. Loperamide can be used in doses up to 16 mg or more daily and is preferable to atropine or opioids with central actions such as morphine. Octreotide has been used in AIDS to reduce motility and bowel secretion and can be helpful in persistent diarrhea in doses of 100–300 mg/24 hours.

Fistulae pose special problems. Urine from a fistula may be helped by a urethral catheter. Urine formation can be stopped at night with nasal desmopressin – this at least allows for night-time continence[26]. The discharge from a bowel fistula can be reduced with octreotide[27], and will reduce the diarrhea from an enterocolic fistula.

Bleeding from rectal tumors can be reduced with topical 1% alum solution[28], or sucralfate[29].

Offensive discharge may be reduced with systemic or topical metronidazole, or topical corticosteroids. Radiotherapy may help both bleeding and discharge.

The skin around the anus or a fistula needs to be protected from the excoriating effects of fecal fluid. Barrier agents such as dimethicone cream help, but if the skin is severely damaged, protective coverings such as hydrocolloid dressings (e.g. Granuflex) provide additional protection. In severe, persistent diarrhea, fecal collecting devices may help and are obtainable from the stoma specialist.

Leg edema

Causes: Leg edema Lymphedema is the commonest form of edema in patients with urological malignancies, although the low protein edemas are sometimes seen (e.g. water accumulation such as cardiac ventricular failure, reduced venous return such as venous thrombosis or protein loss such as hypoalbuminemia due to poor nutrition, liver disease or protein losing nephropathy). In addition, any condition which severely limits limb mobility (e.g. paraparesis due to lumbosacral plexopathy) may result in a mixed picture due to venous and lymphatic stasis. There are four cornerstones to treatment: skin care, support, massage and movement. Units that see lymphedema regularly should have a keyworker trained in lymphedema management, and all units should have access to a specialist lymphedema clinic. Lymphedema clinics are often run by, or linked to, specialist palliative care teams.

Skin care: If the onset of the edema has been rapid and acute, the skin is thin and vulnerable to trauma. In contrast, the skin in chronic lymphedema is usually thickened and dry, and may progress to warty changes and hyperkeratosis. Overnight moisturizing cream ensures that any dry skin stays supple. Any individual skin breaks must be dressed aseptically. Cellulitis is an extremely common complication of lymphedema and if suspected this should be treated promptly with antibiotics (penicillin V since *Streptococcus* is the commonest cause). Compression hosiery should not be applied to traumatized skin, but bandages can be used until the skin condition improves.

Support and compression is achieved with elastic hosiery or compression bandages. Compression is used when a reduction in edema is expected or desired, while support is used when a reduction in edema is not anticipated or desired. The contraindications to hosiery and bandaging are shown in Table 56.8. Massage is based on the principles of manual lymph drainage[30], with the aim of moving fluid from a congested, edematous area of the body to

Leg edema

Lymphedema in pelvic malignancy is common and treatable.

Table 56.8   Clinical decisions in managing edema in advanced cancer[5]

Key decision	Management
Is arterial insufficiency present?	• Measure Doppler ankle/brachial arterial pressure: —if ratio < 0.75: do not apply bandage, hosiery or garment and ask for advice from vascular specialist.

Is infection present?	Affected area redder or warmer than normal limb (signs may be subtle)
	• Acute cellulitis: start penicillin V 500 mg 6 hourly.
	  —treat any obvious focus of infection (e.g. antifungal for tinea pedis, potassium permanganate soaks for infected eczematous reactions).
	  —if no improvement after 3 days, add flucloxacillin 250 mg 6 hourly.
	  —for patients allergic to penicillin use erythromycin 500 mg 6 hourly.
	• Recurrent cellulitis: treat as above then continue penicillin or erythromycin 250 mg twice daily for 3 months.

Is venous obstruction present?	• Peripheral thrombosis: anticoagulate and wait 8 weeks before applying compression. • Central thrombosis or obstruction (e.g. affecting inferior vena cava, or pelvic veins): support bandaging or hosiery can be used but avoid compression pump.
Is this a low protein edema?	e.g. ventricular failure, hypoalbuminemia. *If skin is in good condition*: • Fit class 1 or class 2 hosiery. • Treat primary cause if possible.
Is prognosis too short to allow limb reduction?	i.e. patient deteriorating week by week. • Use massage and support bandaging or hosiery. • Active or passive movements for stiff joints. • If advanced local tumor, consider high-dose dexamethasone and diuretics.

Is edema limited to trunk or genitalia?	• Massage the trunk at least three times daily.
	  —*abdomen*: support garment (e.g. Tubipad lumbar) if genitals free of edema.
	  —*genitals and perineum*: use made measure compression pants, tights or scrotal support.

Is support bandaging indicated?	e.g. limb too large or painful for hosiery, irregular shape or hosiery unsuccessful. • Refer to lymphedema clinic for compression bandaging, massage, exercises and skin care. **Do not use bandages if** in severe ventricular failure, within 8 weeks of peripheral venous thrombosis or Doppler ankle/brachial index below 0.75. **Use with caution if** sensation is absent.

- Fit compression hosiery: see notes for aims and types.
- Exercise limb regularly.
- Moisturize skin regularly.
- Review regularly: if maintained on hosiery, return to beginning.
- **Do not use hosiery if**: skin is damaged, limb is too large, abnormally shaped or painful to fit hosiery, patient is in severe ventricular failure, within 8 weeks of peripheral venous thrombosis, Doppler ankle/brachial index below 0.75, sensation is absent.

one where lymph drainage is normal. The essential principle is to clear the way ahead, so that massage always begins in a healthy quadrant of the trunk, before moving gradually to the swollen side[30,31]. Patients should be encouraged to use their limbs as normally as possible. Some gentle exercise whilst wearing compression seems to be particularly beneficial. Elevation is not a treatment for lymphedema since it discourages mobility.

Intermittent pneumatic compression pumps (e.g. Flowtron) are of limited value. They work mainly by pushing water back into the capillaries and are therefore only helpful in low protein oedemas or in the intensive treatment phase of lymphedema. In lymphedema, they should always be used in conjunction with truncal massage and pressures should not exceed 60 mmHg. Contraindications to using a pump are shown in Table 56.8. Progress can be

Urinary problems

Most urinary problems in advanced cancer can be managed by standard protocols, but some benefit from a different approach.

Table 56.9   Clinical decisions in managing urinary problems in advanced cancer[5]

Key decision	Management

Is the urine cloudy, but a normal colour?	• Test for nitrites, leukocyte esterase and protein: a positive result suggests infection.
	• In the absence of UTI symptoms: if protein present exclude a protein losing nephropathy.
	• In the presence of UTI symptoms:
	  –if urine dipstick is negative: consider candida.
	  –if GU tract is normal: give trimethoprim 200 mg 12 hourly for 3 days.
	• If infection persists: culture and give 7 day course of a cephalosporin (6 weeks for pyelonephritis).
	  –exclude unusual microbial organisms (eg. candida, mycobacterium).
	  –enterovesical fistula (mixed enterococci): treat only if urinary symptoms troublesome, since eradication of infection is impossible.

Has the urine changed colour?	• If positive for blood on testing:
	  –*if bleeding is severe*, see Table 56.10 on managing bleeding.
	  –culture urine to exclude UTI
	  –*if clots are causing retention*: insert 24F gauge catheter and irrigate with 0.9% saline;
	  –consider instilling 1% alum solution 50 ml for 30 min or as continuous infusion 5 ml/hour for 24–72 hours.
	  –start ethamyslate PO 500 mg 6 hourly.
	• If this is not blood: reassure patient and consider other causes of colour change (e.g. drugs, food).

Is pain present?	• **In the midline:**
	  In penis or urethra:
	  –*mucosal irritation*: instil 20 ml bupivacaine 0.25% for 15 minutes.
	  –*trigone irritation due to* – catheter: reduce balloon volume or intermittent catheterization.
	  –tumor: instil bupivacaine as above and consider radiotherapy.
	
	  In midline abdomen, suggests bladder irritability or spasm
	  –*catheter*: reduce balloon volume, consider intermittent catheterization.
	  –*urinary retention*: see below
	  –*tumor*: instil bupivacaine, consider radiotherapy.
	  –*unstable bladder*: imipramine ± hyoscine butylbromide.
	  –*anxiety*: support, relaxation.
	
	• **Unilateral pain:**
	  In groin suggests ureteric colic: diclofenac 75 mg IM (hyoscine butylbromide 10–20 mg can be given IV for rapid relief). Consider relieving obstruction (high-dose dexamethasone, stent).
	
	  In loin or abdomen suggests renal capsule distention or irritation:
	  –*tumor*: opioids ± NSAIDs or corticosteroid or radiotherapy.
	  –*hemorrhage*: parenteral strong opioid. Consider nerve block.
	  –*infection*: exclude TB and treat appropriately.

Urinary incontinence?	• If fistula present (e.g. vesicovaginal, vesicorectal): try pads, regular voiding and intermittent catheterization. Desmopressin nasal spray 10–30 µg at bedtime will at least provide night-time dryness and a better sleep. • If confusion present: see Table 56.11 on managing confusion. • For other causes of incontinence, manage according to standard urologic protocols. If incontinence persists, consider bedtime desmopressin as for urinary fistulae. • Manage the consequences of incontinence, especially skin care, personal hygiene and altered body image.

(continued)

Table 56.9 (continued)

Has urine output changed?	<ul><li>Increased:
	  −*diuretics*: consider if previous dose is still necessary.
	  −*endocrine*: exclude hypercalcemia, diabetes mellitus, diabetes insipidus.
	  −*cardiac failure with nocturia*: diuretics or ACE inhibitor.
	  −*renal failure*: unless obstructive, usually no action is appropriate.</li><li>Decreased:
	  −*dehydration*: only occasionally requires IV fluids (see notes on nausea and vomiting)
	  −*obstruction of*:
	    −*ureters by tumor*: high dose corticosteroids or stent.
	    −*urethra (tumor/prostate)*: catheter. Consider radiotherapy.
	    (*fecal impaction*): see Table 56.4 on constipation.
	  −*neuropathic bladder*: intermittent catheterization.
	  −*endocrine (inappropriate ADH)*: demeclocycline.</li></ul>

Has urinary frequency changed?	<ul><li>Increased:
	  −*bladder irritability* (e.g. small capacity bladder, unstable bladder, anxiety, obstruction with overflow): manage according to standard urologic protocols.
	  −*causes of increased urine output*: see above.</li><li>Decreased:
	  −*increased sphincter tone due to anticholinergic drugs.*
	  −*Poorly relaxed sphincter (detrusor-sphincter dyssynergia)*: intermittent catheterization plus imipramine.
	  −*causes of reduced urinary output*: see above.</li></ul>

most easily monitored with three circumferential measurements at the hand or foot, mid forearm or calf, and at a fixed point in the mid upper arm or thigh. Volume measurements can be made by taking multiple circumferential measurements[32].

Urinary Problems

Most patients with a urologic malignancy who develop symptoms and signs of a urinary tract infection will need their urine cultured and started on an appropriate antibiotic until symptoms resolve. Antibiotics are appropriate for all patients who can take oral medication – there are no ethical issues to consider as there is no evidence they prolong life unnecessarily and they are the most appropriate treatment. Perhaps the only exception is the patient with an entero-vesical fistula in whom eradication of microbes is impossible and treatment is aimed at the symptoms (e.g. using bupivacaine bladder instillations for comfort). Microscopic hematuria does not need further action, once infection has been excluded. Heavy bleeding producing clots or anemia should be treated with a 1% solution of alum[33], following which oral ethamsylate should be started (avoid tranaxamic acid as this may produce hard clots which are difficult to remove). Patients with persistent bleeding can be considered for palliative radiotherapy. Arterial embolization may also be helpful.

Pain in urologic malignancies often need approaches with secondary analgesics, rather than morphine. For example, mucosal pain from the bladder, trigone or urethra can be effectively relieved by instilling bupivacaine, while bladder or ureteric colic are rapidly eased by hyoscine butylbromide. This can be given by a continuous subcutaneous infusion of 30–180 mg in 24 hours with few central effects, but with an inhibiting action on bowel motility. Pain due to obstructions can be relieved with ureteric stents inserted at cystoscopy, while obstructions due to peritumor edema may be eased by high-dose corticosteroids (18–24 mg dexamethasone starting dose). A percutaneous nephrostomy (ideally done under ultrasound control) can be helpful as a temporary measure if more radical tumor control is planned, but other patients do not find it offers any advantage. Pain due to tumor expansion or pressure will usually require strong opioids with the addition of a non-steroidal anti-inflammatory drug. Radiotherapy can palliate a painful renal tumor, if there is a functioning kidney on the other side.

Urinary fistulae are easily missed, but can be readily identified by instilling methylene blue into the bladder through a temporary catheter. Pads, frequent voiding and continuous catheterization may help, and for a vesicovaginal fistula a vaginal prosthesis can be made of silicone which incorporates a catheter using the technique suggested by Green and Phillips[34]. Urinary diversion is not usually appropriate. Other causes of incontinence are managed according to standard urologic protocols, but these may be inappropriate for some patients. Intermittent catheterization can be very helpful in these patients, particularly in a neuropathic bladder, since it gives them control over emptying their bladder. Knowing their bladder is

611

empty frees them to go out when previously they may have felt trapped. Even though intermittent catheterization is safe and the treatment of choice in a neuropathic bladder it remains an infrequently used technique[35]. If all else fails, dry nights can be provided using nasal desmopressin[26,36].

Bleeding

There are many potential sources of bleeding with several potential causes, but treatment is limited to radiotherapeutic, pharmacologic or physical approaches.

Radiotherapy can help a superficial bleeding tumor but sites such as vulva and perineum tolerate treatment less well, causing troublesome skin reactions in a debilitated patient. Radiotherapy to urological tumors is also limited by the sensitivity of the remaining gastrointestinal tract and surrounding tissues. Single treatments are possible in frail patients and some situations are amenable to brachytherapy, where the radioactive source is placed close to the tumor.

Pharmacological approaches involve modifying the coagulation mechanism. Tranaxamic acid is contraindicated in urinary tract bleeding and, in addition, causes a number of troublesome adverse effects, including nausea. Ethamsylate is thought to enhance platelet adhesion, most is excreted unchanged in the urine and adverse effects are less troublesome. Tranexamic acid has been used topically in bleeding rectal carcinoma[38]. Sucralfate is a useful and rapid topical coagulant which enhances protection against further injury as well as making the protective layer a thick gel[39,40]. A 1% solution of alum has been used to treat severe bladder hemorrhage – published evidence describes 24–72 hours of constant irrigation at a rate of 5 ml/hour[33], but less severe bleeding can be managed with 30 minute instillations from 1–5 times daily. Vasoconstrictors such as adrenaline are of little use since rebleeding often recurs within 10 minutes. Sclerosing agents such as phenol, silver nitrate and formalin should be avoided because they cause tissue damage with pain and impaired healing. Homeostatic dressings (e.g. calcium alginate dressing such as Kaltostat) act as a matrix for coagulation.

Accessible bleeding lesions can be debulked using laser, but diathermy may make hematuria worse[41]. Embolization is occasionally used for renal malignancy and can also be helpful in hematuria arising from the bladder[42]. Pain and pyrexia for a few days after embolization are the usual adverse effects.

Coping with massive hemorrhage: if the blood loss is a terminal event, sheets and dark towels can be placed in the bed temporarily to soak up the loss. The hypotension will make the patient feel cold and will be helped by warm blankets or heat pads. In any type of massive hemorrhage patients will feel frightened. Whilst some will

be eased by gentle support, others will need pharmacological help. Intravenous diazepam is the most rapid and effective method. Alternatives are diazepam injection solution rectally or midazolam into deltoid muscle. Usually both will be absorbed and act within 5–15 minutes. Both family and staff will need support after such an experience.

Confusional states

Assessment is complicated because effective two-way communication is limited by the patient's fear about what is happening and their difficulty in clarifying incoming information, together with the carer's difficulty in seeing a clear way forward. Clarity for both is more likely if the carer follows the few clinical decisions in Table 56.11.

Recent memory failure is common in confusional states and is due to a failure to take in information. This type of memory failure is reversible, while persistent memory failure suggests a neurological problem. This second type of memory failure is due to the inability to retain information and is usually caused by the dementias. Both types can exist together and early dementia can be unmasked by the stress of serious illness. A much less common cause of persistent memory failure are cerebral metastases, but other cognitive functioning is usually intact. Management of memory failure requires frequent re-orientation in time and place, in a light, quiet environment with the minimum of staff changes. The symptoms of cerebral tumors may be helped by corticosteroids[43] or cranial radiotherapy in sensitive tumors.

Alertness in altered in confusional states and is usually reduced but can be increased. There are a number of possible causes. Drugs are a common cause and opioids are often blamed for reduced alertness, but while these may certainly cause confusion, they are an unlikely cause in a patient on long-term opioids whose renal function is unaltered. Overlooked pharmacological causes of confusion are non-steroidal anti-inflammatory drugs, antidepressants, corticosteroids and commonly forgotten, drug withdrawal (night sedation, alcohol). Infection is a common cause of confusion in the elderly in whom the infection may produce few signs and symptoms, and any confused patient should have their chest and urine examined. Hypercalcemia occurs in 5–7% of solid tumors, producing many symptoms (sedation, confusion, nausea, vomiting, constipation, thirst, polyuria). Since there are no specific signs and the symptoms may occur singly or be masked by other concurrent problems[44], checking serum calcium and albumin. Previous cardiac disease may be unsuspected and produce ventricular failure and previous or new respiratory disease may produce hypoxia without warning.

Bleeding

The risk of major, external hemorrhage is often exaggerated amongst staff. Bleeding is the cause of death in only 6% of patients[37], and in most of these patients internal, unseen bleeding is more common.

Table 56.10   Clinical decisions in managing bleeding in advanced cancer[5]

Key decision	Management
Is there a risk of bleeding?	• If on warfarin: keep INR to between 1.5 and 3. • Coagulation disorder: correct if appropriate and possible. • Erosive tumor: keep dark green or dark blue towel and sedation to hand. Consider radiotherapy or embolization.
Is the patient hypotensive?	• If resuscitation is appropriate: obtain IV access —start rapid infusion of 0.9% saline and cross match. —start blood transfusion Then: find bleeding source: visual / endoscopy / radiology. • If resuscitation inappropriate: —if patient is distressed give sedation: e.g. diazepam 5–30 mg titrated IV (if no IV access give diazepam PR or midazolam 5–15 mg IM into deltoid). —external bleeding: use green or blue towel to make appearance of the blood less frightening. Place warm blankets over patient. Do not leave patient
Is there a coagulation disorder?	e.g. low or abnormal platelets, reduced warfarin metabolism or displaced warfarin, disseminated intravascular coagulopathy, severe hepatic impairment. • Treatment can be difficult – the advice of a hematologist is essential.
Is the bleeding source external?	If vessel can be identified: apply pressure to stop flow. • Promote clotting: apply sucralfate paste or calcium alginate dressing. • Prevent rebleeding: —start ethamsylate PO 500 mg 6 hourly or tranexamic acid 1G 8 hourly. —apply sucralfate paste under totally non-adherent dressing (e.g. Mepitel). The dressing can be left for up to 7 days, although rebleeding may require up to daily • Consider diathermy, radiotherapy or embolization.
Is the urinary tract the source?	• Culture urine to exclude UTI • See Table 56.9 on urinary problems.
Is the source the rectum or vagina?	• If minor (streaking only): observe. Consider pads. • If troublesome (clots, frequent bleeds, anemia): ethamsylate PO 500 mg 6 hourly or tranexamic acid 1G 8 hourly. Consider radiotherapy / topical sucralfate paste / topical tranexamic acid.
Hemoptysis only?	• If minor (streaked sputum): —exclude pulmonary embolus and infection —ethamsylate PO 500 mg 6 hourly or tranexamic acid 1 G 8 hourly. • If troublesome (clots, anemia or frequent bleeds): —radiotherapy, laser or embolization.
Hematemesis only?	• Stop gastric irritants, e.g. NSAIDs • If minor (altered blood in vomit or positive fecal occult blood): —2G sucralfate on waking and at night. • If troublesome (fresh blood, malena or anemia): —2G sucralfate 4 hourly plus ranitidine 300 mg 12 hourly or omeprazole 20 mg daily. —if source is non-malignant, consider referral for endoscopy.
Is bleeding coming from multiple sites?	• Exclude: trauma / coagulation disorder / vitamin C deficiency / altered warfarin handling / bone marrow suppression (due to tumor invasion, chemotherapy): treat appropriately if possible.

Confusional states

Despite the many potential causes of confusion, and the difficulty of accessing a confused patient, it is possible to assess, manage and treat a confused patient in a logical way. Contrary to popular belief, cerebral metastases are an unusual cause of confusion.

Table 56.11   Clinical decisions in managing confusional states in advanced cancer[5]

Key decision	Management
Is there a failure of memory?	• Exclude dementia (no localizing signs, static from day to day, symptoms of deficit, no change in alertness).
Has alertness changed?	NB. Alertness may decrease *or* increase in confusion. • Drugs: suspect all recently started (and stopped) drugs. • Infection: check urine and chest. • Biochemical: hypercalcemia is the commonest and is diagnosed by suspicion (50% present with drowsiness as the sole symptom). • Cardiac: check for ventricular failure (common in the elderly). • Respiratory: check for causes of hypoxia (infection, pleural effusion, pulmonary metastases). See elsewhere for treatment of dyspnea. • Trauma: exclude long bone fracture or subdural hematoma.
Is concentration impaired?	• In the presence of anxiety: consider communication problems, ignorance about diagnosis, social problems. • Consider distraction due to pain, depression or uncommonly, a psychiatric illness.
Is patient having abnormal experiences?	*If seeing or hearing things*: • Ensure environment is light, quiet and consistent. • *Misperception* (due to altered alertness or reduced concentration): see above. • *Hallucinations*: —exclude drugs or alcohol withdrawal. —control with haloperidol or levomepromazine (see doses below). —consider psychotic illness and refer as appropriate.
Has behavior altered?	*If wandering, paranoia, euphoria, mania or depression are present (one or more)*: • Exclude memory failure (see above). • Consider drugs as cause (especially corticosteroids). • Consider psychiatric illness and refer or manage as appropriate.
Are specific neurologic deficits present?	e.g. hemiparesis, visual field defects, gait abnormalities. • Exclude a cerebral metastasis. • Consider radiotherapy or dexamethasone.
Is control of disturbance urgent?	Emergency treatment while awaiting the effects of specific treatments or further assessment. • Ensure light, quiet, consistent environment. • *In absence of abnormal experience or behavior*: —with minimal sedation: lorazepam 0.5–1 mg PO or sublingually. —if sedation required: midazolam 2–10 mg SC, IM or PR (or SC infusion 20–120 mg per 24 hours). • *In presence of abnormal experience or behavior*: —with minimal sedation: haloperidol 2.5–10 mg PO or SC (3–20 mg per 24 hours) —if sedation required: levomepromazine 12.5–100 mg PO or SC (25–200 mg per 24 hours).

• Explain cause of confusion, possible treatment, and management to patient, family, staff.
• Reassess frequently.

Concentration can be impaired regardless of any change in alertness. Anxiety, severe physical symptoms, can affect concentration. Anxiety can be severe enough to block awareness – so-called 'frozen terror'[45].

Confused patients may describe seeing or hearing things and it is important to decide whether these abnormal experiences are misperceptions or hallucinations[46]. Misperceptions are prompted by an external stimulus which is misinterpreted, especially in the presence of reduced alertness or concentration. In contrast hallucinations have no outside stimulus, being generated internally as a consequence of drugs, alcohol withdrawal or a psychotic illness. With morphine, for example, reduced alertness is temporary and may cause a misinterpretation, but a slower titration will allow tolerance to the sedative effect to occur. In contrast a true hallucination due to morphine will not wear off and the dose must be reduced or an alternative means of pain control used.

Behavior may alter with aimless wandering, paranoid behavior, paranoid thoughts, euphoria or mania, or depression[47,48]. It is important to exclude causes of memory failure (see above), and then to consider other causes such as drugs (e.g. corticosteroids) or psychiatric illness.

Drugs should only be considered as a last resort and after the initial assessment is complete. Confusion is frightening and it is hardly surprising that some patients become very disturbed at what is happening to them. Even very agitated patients, however, will respond to a light, quiet, comforting environment, in which a care giver spends time gently exploring what is distressing to the patient. What reassures patients most is a feeling that their caregiver wants to understand what is the matter, and knows what to do. There are occasions when the disturbance is so severe that access is impossible, or patients are at risk of injuring themselves or others. If there is no altered behavior or abnormal experiences midazolam is a useful short acting anxiety suppressant[10]. Lorazepam is an alternative oral preparation with less sedation, but diazepam should be avoided because of its very long half-life (7–10 days in older patients). If altered behavior or abnormal experiences are present an antipsychotic is needed with a choice of haloperidol for minimal sedation, or thioridazine or levomepromazine if sedation is felt to be necessary.

Explanation is an essential component in managing the confused patient. Patients usually understand what is being said to them and explanations of the likely cause of confusion to a patient can lessen their anxiety and make it easier gently to explore their worries. It is equally important to provide the family with an explanation since they too will be frightened by the change and need to understand the reasons for the patient's distress and that the confusion is invariably manageable even if it is irreversible.

References

1. National Council for Hospice & Specialist Palliative Care Services. *Specialist palliative care. A statement of definitions.* Occasional Paper, 8 October 1995.
2. Addington-Hall J, McCarthy M. Dying from cancer: results of a national population based investigation. *Palliative Medicine* 1995;9:295–305.
3. Stedeford A. A safe place to suffer. *Palliative Medicine.*
4. Twycross R, *Introducing Palliative Care.* Radcliffe Medical Press, Oxford, 1995.
5. Regnard CFB and Tempest S. *A guide to symptom relief in advanced disease* (4th edn). Hochland & Hochland, Manchester, 1998.
6. Doyle D, MacDonald N, Hanks G (eds) *Oxford textbook of palliative medicine* (2nd edn). Oxford University Press, 1997.
7. Twycross R, Wilcock A, Thorpe S. *Palliative care formulary.* Radcliffe Medical Press, Oxford, 1999.
8. Clarke K. Personal communication. St. Oswald's Hospice Day Treatment Unit.
9. St. Christopher's Hospice Information Service. *Directory of Hospice & Palliative Care Services in the UK and Republic of Ireland.*
10. McNamara P, Minton M, Twycross RG. Use of midazolam in palliative care. *Palliative Medicine* 1991;5:244–249.
11. Swarm RA, Cousins MJ. Anaesthetic techniques for pain control. In: Doyle D, Hanks G, MacDonald N (eds) *Oxford textbook of medicine.* Oxford University Press, Oxford, 1993, pp. 204–221.
12. Sjoberg M, Appelgren S, Einarsson S et al. Long-term intrathecal morphine and bupivacaine in 'refractory' cancer pain. I. Results from the first series of 52 patients. *Palliative Medicine* 1991;35:30–43.
13. Ernst DS, MacDonald RN, Paterson AHG et al. A double blind, cross-over trial of intravenous clodronate in metastatic bone pain. *J Pain Symp Manag* 1992;7:4–11.
14. Simons DG, Travell JG. Myofascial pain syndromes, In: Wall PD, Melzack R (eds) *Textbook of pain* (3rd edn). Churchill Livingstone, Edinburgh, 1994.
15. Thompson JW, Filshie J. TENS and acupuncture. In: Doyle D, Hanks G, MacDonald N (eds) *Oxford textbook of palliative medicine.* Oxford University Press, Oxford, 1993, pp. 229–224.
16. Hanks GW, Portenoy RK, MacDonald N, O'Neill W. Difficult pain problems. In: Doyle D, Hanks G, MacDonald N (eds) *Oxford textbook of palliative medicine.* Oxford University Press, Oxford, 1993, pp. 187–203.
17. *Cancer Pain Relief* (2nd edn) Geneva: WHO, 1996.
18. Regnard C. Constipation. In: *Flow diagrams in advanced cancer and other diseases.* Edward Arnold, London, 1995, pp. 11–13.
19. Lichter I. Results of antiemetic management in terminal illness. *J Pall Care* 1993;9:19–21.
20. Peroutka SJ, Snyder SH. Antiemetics: neurotransmitter receptor binding predicts therapeutic actions. *Lancet* 1982;i:658–659.
21. Constans T, Dutertre J, Froge E. Hypodermoclysis in dehydrated elderly patients: local effects with and without hyaluronidase. *J Pall Care* 1991;7:10–12.
22. Baines M. The pathophysiology and management of malignant intestinal obstruction. In: Doyle D, Hanks G, MacDonald N (eds) *Oxford textbook of palliative medicine.* Oxford University Press, Oxford, 1993, pp. 311–316.
23. Riley, Fallon MT. Octreotide in terminal malignant obstruction of the gastrointestinal tract. *Eur J Pall Care* 1994;1:23–25.
24. Mercadante S, Maddaloni S. Octreotide in the management of inoperable gastrointestinal obstruction in terminal cancer patients. *J Pain Symp Manag* 1992;7:496–498.
25. Bizer LS, Liebling RW, Delany HM, Gliedman ML. Small bowel obstruction. *Surgery* 1981;89:407–413.
26. Meadow SR, Evans JHC. Desmopressin for enuresis. *Br Med J* 1989;298:1596–1597.
27. Nubiola P, Badia JM, Martinez-Rodenas F et al. Treatment of 27 postoperative enterocutaneous fistulas with the long half life somatostatin analogue SMS 201–995. *Ann Surg* 1989;210:56–58.
28. Paes TRF, Marsh GDJ, Morecroft JA, Hale JE. Alum solution in the control of intractable haemorrhage from advanced carcinoma. *Br J Surg* 1986;73:192.
29. Regnard CFB. Control of bleeding in advanced cancer. *Lancet* 1991;337:974.
30. Badger C. External compression and support in the management of chronic oedema. In: *The Royal Marsden Hospital manual of clinical nursing procedures* (3rd edn). Blackwell Scientific Publications, Oxford, 1992.
31. Földi E, Földi M, Clodius L. The lymphoedema chaos: a lancet. *Ann Plas Surg* 1989;22:505–515.
32. Regnard C, Badger C, Mortimer P. *Lymphoedema: advice on treatment* (2nd edn). Beaconsfield Publishers, Beaconsfield, 1990.

33. Goel AK, Rao MS, Bhagwat AG *et al.* Intravesical irrigation with alum for the control of massive bladder haemorrhage. *J Urol* 1985;**133**:956–957.

34. Green DE, Phillips GL. Vaginal prosthesis for control of vesicovaginal fistula. *Gynaecol Oncol* 1986;**23**:119–123.

35. Anonymous. Underused: intermittent self catheterisation. *Drug Ther Bull* 1991;**29**:37–39.

36. Rittig S, Knusden B, Sorensen S *et al.* Longterm double-blind crossover study of desmopressin intranasal spray in the management of nocturnal enuresis. In: Medow SR (Ed.) *Desmopressin in nocturnal enuresis.* Horus Medical, Sutton Coldfield, 1989, pp. 43–55.

37. Carter RL. Some pathological aspects of advanced malignant disease. In: Saunders C (Ed.) *The management of terminal malignant disease* (3rd edn). Edward Arnold, London, 1993.

38. McElligot E, Quigley C, Hanks GW. Tranexamic acid and rectal bleeding. *Lancet* 1991;**337**:431.

39. Hollander D, Tarnawski A. The protective and therapeutic mechanisms of sucralfate. *Scand J Gastroenterol* 1990;**25**(suppl 173):1–5.

40. Regnard CFB. Control of bleeding in advanced cancer. *Lancet* 1991;**337**:974.

41. Bullock N, Whitaker RH. Massive bladder haemorrhage. *Br Med J* 1985;**291**:1522–1523.

42. Lang EK, Deutsch JS, Goodman JR *et al.* Transcatheter embolization of hypogastric branch arteries in the management of intractable bladder haemorrhage. *J Urol* 1979;**121**:30–36.

43. Kirkham SR. The palliation of cerebral tumours with high dose dexamethasone: a review. *Palliative Medicine* 1988;**2**:27–33.

44. Heath DA. Hypercalcaemia of malignancy. *Palliative Medicine* 1989;**3**:1–11.

45. Brittlebank A, Regnard C. Terror or depression? A case report. *Palliative Medicine* 1990;**4**:317–319.

46. Stedeford A. Confusion. In: *Facing death: patients, families and professionals* (2nd edn). Sobell Publications, Oxford, 1994, pp. 149–163.

47. Stedeford A. Depression. In: *Facing death: patients, families and professionals* (2nd edn). Sobell Publications, Oxford, 1994, pp. 136–139.

48. Stedeford A. Paranoid reactions and other problems. In: *Facing death: patients, families and professionals* (2nd edn). Sobell Publications, Oxford, 1994, pp. 165–175.

Index

Page numbers in *italic* indicate figures and tables.

A

Acrivastine, *340*
Adenocarcinoma
  of adrenal cortex, 392–3, 407–8
  of bladder, 95–100
  of prostate *see* Prostate cancer
Adenoma
  adrenal cortex, 392, *407*
  metanephric, 280
  nephrogenic, 42
  papillary, 279–80
  renal, 385
Adrenal gland, 390
Adrenal tumors
  adrenal cortex
    adenocarcinoma, 392–3, 407–8
    adenoma, 392, *407*
    myelolipoma, 408
    neuroblastic tumors, *408*, *409*
  incidental adrenal masses, *390*, *391*, 392
  pathology, 407–9
  pheochromocytoma, 393–4, *395*, 409
  treatment algorithm, *389*
Adriamycin
  invasive transitional cell carcinoma, 91
  renal cell carcinoma, *239*, *240*
Age
  and bladder adenocarcinoma incidence, 95
  and testicular cancer incidence, 415–16
Alkylating agents, *339*
Amphotericin B, *340*
Amsacrine, *339*
Androgen withdrawal, 135, 180–6, 212–16
  antiandrogens, 215–16
  clinical trials, 181–4
    clinically organ confined prostate cancer, 183, *184*
    locally advanced prostate cancer, 181, *182*, *183*
  complications, 230–1
  experimental basis, 180, *181*

immediate versus delayed, 226–32
  Medical Research Council study, *227–31*
  Veterans Administration studies, 226
intermittent, 220–1
and irradiation, 200–1, 205
medical castration, 212–15, *214*
sequential, 221–2
superiority to castration, 218–19
surgical castration, 213
timing of, 219–20
Androgens
  biological effects, 212
  mechanism of action, 210–12, *211*
  and prostate gland, 210
  renal cell carcinoma, *338*
Angiomyolipoma, 280, 383–4
Anthracycline, 255
Antiandrogens, *214*, 215–16
  side effects, *266*
Antiestrogens, *338*
Antimetabolites, *339*
Antitumor antibiotics, *339*
Autolymphocyte therapy, 332–3

B

Bacillus Calmette-Guérin *see* BCG
BCG
  carcinoma in situ, 59–61, *60*
  potential toxicity, 49–50
  transitional cell carcinoma, 47, 380–1
  trials versus chemotherapy, 47–8, *47*
Benign prostatic hyperplasia, 43–4, 113
Bicalutamide, *214*, 215
  side effects, *266*
Bilharziasis, and squamous cell carcinoma of bladder, 102–3
Biopsy
  bladder cancer, 53
  carcinoma in situ, *58*
  prostate cancer, 127–8

after androgen deprivation therapy, 135
after cryosurgery, 136
after radiation therapy, 135, 196–7
TRUS-guided, *142*
Bisantrene, *339*
Bisphosphonates in prostate cancer, 244–5, 244–7
  clinical studies, 245–6
  morbidity, 245
  pathophysiology, 244–5
  rationale for, 244
Bladder
  microanatomy, 17–18, *17*
  perforation, 44
  TNM staging, *25*, *40*
Bladder cancer
  adenocarcinoma, 32, *33*, 95–100
    age and sex distribution, 95
    etiology and pathogenesis, 95–6
    grading and staging, 97
    incidence, 95
    mestastatic secondary, 98
    pathology, 31, *32*, 96
    presentation and investigation, 96–7
    prognosis, 99
    treatment, 97–8
  algorithm, *37*
  diagnosis, 38
  epidemiology, 3–4
  etiology, 3–4
  follow-up, 52–5
    alternative diagnostic tests, 54–5
    flexible versus rigid cystoscopy, 53
    frequency of, 52–3
    imaging, 54
    random mucosal biopsies, 53
    urine cytology, 54
  genetics, 4–7
    genetic markers, 7
    proto-oncogenes, 4–5
    schistosomiasis-associated bladder cancer, 7

Bladder cancer (*cont.*)
    tumor suppressor genes, 5–6
    histological classification, 18
    incidence of, 3
    interpretation of test results, *38, 39, 40*
    management of urethra, 72–3
    muscle invasive disease, *14*
    natural history, 12–13
    pathology, 17–36
        glandular epithelial tumors, 31, *32*
        histological classification, 18
        hyperplasia, 28–30
    presentation, 38
    primary adenocarcinoma, 31, *32*
    prognosis, 12–13
    radiotherapy, 105–7
    rhabdomyocarcoma, 592–3
    schistosomiasis-associated, 3, 4
    squamous carcinoma, 101–7
        adjuvant pre-operative radiation, 103, *104*
        bilharzial bladder, 102–3
            clinicopathological features, 102
            treatment, 102–3
        chemotherapy, 104
        non-bilharzial bladder, 101–2
        pathology, *30, 31*
        radiotherapy, 105–7
    staging, 11, 24, *25, 26, 27,* 39, 40, *43*
        detrusor muscle invasion, 26
        lamina propria invasion, *25*
        muscularis mucosae invasion, *25, 26*
        prostatic involvement, *26, 27*
        vascular invasion, 27
    superficial tumors
        carcinoma in situ, 13–14
        grade, *13*
        T1 disease, 13
        Ta disease, 13
    tumor grade, 11–12
    urothelial abnormalities, 12
    see also Carcinoma in situ; Transitional cell carcinoma
Bladder conservation, 90–1
Bladder neck contracture, 173
Bladder outlet obstruction, 263–4
Bladder preservation, 85–8
    follow-up and risk of recurrence, 87
    radiotherapy, 86
    systemic chemotherapy, 87
    transurethral resection and partial cystectomy, 86
Bladder reconstruction, 80–1
    see also Urinary diversion
Bladder washing, *59*
Bone fractures, pathologic, 262
Bone metastases
    prostate cancer, 236–9

external local irradiation, *236, 237*
hemibody irradiation, 237, *238*
phosphorus-32, *239*
rhenium-186, 239
strontium[89], 238, *239,* 242–4
yttrium[90] hypophysectomy, 239
renal cell carcinoma, 325–6
Bone pain, 261–2
Bone scan, 155
Brachytherapy
    interstitial, 176–7
        implant procedure, 177
        treatment planning, 177
    urethral carcinoma, 542, *543*
Brain metastases, 239–40
Bropirimine
    carcinoma in situ, 59, 61
    transitional cell carcinoma, 50, 381
BTA dipstick test, 54
Buserelin acetate, *214*

C

Calcium losses, 78–9
[111]In-Capromab pendetide, 250–2
Carboplatin, *339,* 454
Carcinoma in situ, 12, 13–14, *42*
    bladder washing, *59*
    concomitant, 14
    cytology, 58
    diagnostic assessment, 58
    imaging, 59
    primary, 14
    prostatic urethra, *27,* 65
    scrotum, 492
    secondary, 14
    selected site biopsies, *58*
    staging, *59*
    testis *see* Intratubular germ cell neoplasia
    treatment, 57–64
        algorithm, *57*
        BCG, 59–61, *60*
        bropirimine, 61
        chemotherapy, 59, *61*
        cystectomy, 62
        interferon, 61
        photodynamic therapy, 62
        prostatic urethral involvement, 61
        transurethral resection, 59
    urothelial, 28–30, *29*
Cellular therapy, 332–3
Cepharanthine, *340*
Cervical cancer
    invasive disease, 554
    post-treatment surveillance, 557
    pre-invasive disease and epidemiology, 553, *554*
    radiotherapy, 557

staging, 554, *555*
surgical management, 555, *556*
treatment, *555*
Chemotherapy
    adjuvant, 89–90
    bladder adenocarcinoma, 98
    carcinoma in situ, 59, *61*
    muscle invasive bladder cancer, 87
    neoadjuvant, 89–90
    non-seminomatous germ-cell tumors, 452–9
        chemo-sensitivity, 457
        choice of, 454, *455*
        clinical trials, *454,* 455
        late events, 455–6
        patient selection, 453–4
        practical issues, 453
        primary management, 452, *453*
        seminoma, *457*
        stage 1 and 2 disease, *456*
        testis conservation, 456–7
    penile carcinoma, 521
    prostate cancer, 253–7, *254*
    renal cell carcinoma, 338–41
    scrotal tumors, 495
    spermatic cord tumors, 488
    toxicity, 49
    transitional cell carcinoma, *45, 46,* 87, 88–91
        bladder conservation, 90–1
        choice of agent, *48*
        locally advanced bladder cancer, 89–90
        metastatic disease, 89
        single dose, 46, *47*
        upper urinary tract, 379–82
    urethral carcinoma, 546
    see also individual chemotherapeutic agents
Chlorambucil, *339*
Chromophobe renal carcinoma, 278, *279*
CIS *see* Carcinoma in situ
Cisplatin
    germ cell tumors, 437
    invasive transitional cell carcinoma, 91
    testicular cancer, *454,* 472
Clear cell renal carcinoma, 277, *278*
Clear cell renal sarcoma, 282–3
Clodronate, 245–6
Collecting duct carcinoma, 279
Colon cancer, secondary adenocarcinoma, 98
Comedonecrosis, *27*
Computed tomography
    prostate cancer, 140, *141*
    renal cell carcinoma, 286, *287*
Condylomata acuminata, 540
Continence mechanism in bladder replacement, 81

Cryosurgery, 136
Cryotherapy, 316
Cryptorchidism, and testicular cancer, 417
Cyclophosphamide, *341*
Cyclosporin, *340*
Cyproterone acetate, *214*, 216
 side effects, *266*
Cystectomy
 bladder adenocarcinoma, 97, 98
 carcinoma in situ, 62
 complications, 74
 partial, 44, 86
 radical, 45, 68–72
  abdominal exploration, 69
  anterior apical dissection in male
   patients, 71–2
  anterior dissection in female patients,
   72
  bladder squamous cell carcinoma,
   103
  bowel mobilization, 69–70
  definition, 72
  incision, 69
  ligation of lateral vascular pedicle to
   bladder, 70–1
  ligation of posterior vascular pedicle
   to bladder, 74–5
  patient positioning, 69
  pelvic lymphadenectomy, 70
  post-operative care, 74
  pre-operative evaluation, 68
  pre-operative preparation, 69
  pre-operative radiation therapy, 72–3
  ureteral dissection, 70
 salvage, 73–4
Cystic nephroma, 282
Cystic partially differentiated
 nephroblastoma, 282
Cystitis cystica, 42
Cystitis glandularis, 42
Cystoscopy
 flexible versus rigid, 53
 follow-up of superficial bladder cancer,
  52–3
Cytology
 bladder cancer, 54
 carcinoma in situ, 58–9

D

Deep venous thrombosis, 170
Denonvilliers' space, 70
Detrusor muscle, 18
 invasion of, 26
Dexamethasone suppression test, *391*
Dexverapamil, *340*
Diaziquone, *339*
Dietary fat, as risk factor for prostate
 cancer, 112

Digital rectal examination, 140, 153
Dipyridamole, *340*
Disseminated intravascular coagulation,
 264–5
DNA-flow cytometry, 436
Docetaxel, 91
Doxorubicin
 bladder adenocarcinoma, 98
 dose, *47*
 patient response, *45*
 prophylaxis, *46*
 renal cell carcinoma, *241*, *339*
 toxicity, 49

E

Electrolyte disturbances, 78–9
 gastric reservoirs, 78
 hyperammonemia, 79
 hyperchloremic acidosis, 78
 jejunal conduits, 78
 magnesium and calcium, 78–9
Elliptinium, *339*
Endocrine therapy
 prostate cancer, 203–5, 210–26
  androgen withdrawal, 135, 180–6,
   212–16
   antiandrogens, 215–16
   clinical trials, 181–4, *182*, *183*, *184*
   early versus delayed, 204–5
   experimental basis, 180, *181*
   immediate versus delayed, 226–32
   intermittent, 220–1
    sequential, 221–2
   and irradiation, 200–1, 205
   medical castration, 212–15, *214*
   superiority to castration, 218–19
   surgical castration, 213
   timing of, 219–20
  controversies surrounding, 217–22
  hormonal manipulation, *203*, 204
  and irradiation, 200–1, 205
  treatment of emergency conditions,
   222
  treatment of hot flushes, 222
 renal cell carcinoma, 337, *338*
Endometrial cancer *see* Uterine cancer
Endometrial hyperplasia, 559
Epirubicin
 patient response, *45*
 prophylaxis, *46*
 renal cell carcinoma, *339*, *341*
 toxicity, 49
Epodyl
 dose, *47*
 patient response, *45*
 prophylaxis, *46*
Estramustine, 254–5
Estrogens, 213, *214*

side effects, *266*
Ethnic differences
 prostate cancer, 112
 testicular cancer, 416
Etidronate, 245
External beam irradiation, 176, 190, *191–4*
 prognostic factors, 191–2, *193*
 survival, 191, *192*

F

Fibroepithelial polyps, 363, *364*, 540
Fistulae *see* Urogynecologic fistulae
Flow cytometry, 54
Fludarabine, *339*
5-Fluorouracil
 adenocarcinoma of bladder, 98
 renal cell carcinoma, *339*, *341*
Flutamide, *214*, 215
 side effects, *266*
Focused ultrasound ablation, 311–16
 application to kidney, 313, *314*
 clinical application, 312–13
 malignant tumors, 311, *312*
 technical principle, 311

G

Gastric reservoirs, 78
Gemcitabine, 91, *339*
Gene therapy, 333–4
Genetics
 bladder cancer, 7
 renal cell carcinoma, 274–5
 testicular cancer, 418–20
 transitional cell carcinoma, 351–2
 urologic malignancy, 4, *5*
 Wilms' tumor, 586
Glandular epithelial tumors, 30, *31*
Goserelin acetate, *214*
 side effects, *266*
Grading of tumors, 11–12, *13*
 alternative grading systems, 22–3
 bladder cancer, 11–12, *13*, 97
 and prognosis, 22
 prostate cancer, 131–3, *132*, 153
 reproducibility of, 22
 transitional cell carcinoma, 20–2
Granulomatous orchitis, 427
Granulomatous seminoma, 427
Gynecologic malignancies
 cervical cancer
  invasive disease, 554
  post-treatment surveillance, 557
  pre-invasive disease and
   epidemiology, 553, *554*
  radiotherapy, 557

Gynecologic malignancies (*cont.*)
    staging, 554, *555*
    surgical management, 555, *556*
    treatment, *555*
  exenteration and urinary diversion,
    563–70
    assessment, 563–4, *565, 566, 567*
    diversion and reconstruction, 568,
    569, 570
    post-operative care, 569
    surgery, 566, 568
  ovarian cancer, 549–53
    epidemiology, 549–50
    incidence, *549*
    management, 552–3
    pathology, *550–1*
    prognostic factors, 552
    staging, *551*
    treatment, 552
  uterine cancer
    adjuvant therapy, 560–1
    diagnosis, *558*
    endometrial hyperplasia, 559
    incidence, 558
    pre-operative evaluation, 559
    prognostic factors, *559*
    recurrence, 561
    signs and symptoms, *558*
    staging, *559*
    treatment, *560*

H

Histological classification, 18
Hormone status
  and prostate cancer, 113
  and testicular cancer, 417
Hormone therapy
  prostate cancer, *203, 204*–5
    see also Androgen withdrawal
  renal cell carcinoma, 337, *338*
Hyperammonemia, 79
Hyperchloremic acidosis, 78

I

Idarubicin, *339*
Ifosfamide, 91, *339, 341*
Ileo-cecal pouch, 82
Imaging
  carcinoma in situ, 59
  prostate cancer, 140–2
  superficial bladder cancer, 54
  see also Computed tomography;
    Magnetic resonance imaging
Immunotherapy, 329–37
  cellular therapy, 332–3
  combination therapy, 331, *332*
  gene therapy, 333–4

interferons, *330*
interleukin-2, 330, *331*
surgery, 334
transitional cell carcinoma, *380*–1
Impotence, post-prostatectomy, 172–3
Incontinence, post-prostatectomy, 172
Infertility, and testicular cancer, 417
Inguinal hernia, and testicular cancer, 417
Interferon
  carcinoma in situ, 61
  combined with chemotherapy, *341*
  immunotherapy, *330*
  transitional cell carcinoma, 50
Interleukin-2, 330, *331*
Interstitial brachytherapy, 176–7
  implant procedure, 177
  treatment planning, 177
Intratubular germ cell neoplasia, *424,*
  435–8
  characteristics and origin, *435*
  definition, 435
  diagnosis, *436*
  management, 437
  prevalence, 435
  screening, 435–6
  versus degenerate germ cells, 426–7
  versus intratubular spread of neoplasia,
    427
  versus spermatogenic arrest at
    spermatogonia stage, 427
Intravenous urography, 286
Invasive transitional cell carcinoma
  bladder preserving treatment, 85–8
    follow-up and risk of recurrence, 87
    radiotherapy, 86
    systemic chemotherapy, 87
    transurethral resection and partial
      cystectomy, 86
  chemotherapy, 88–91
    in bladder conserving strategy, 90–1
    future developments, 91
    locally advanced cancer, 89–90
    metastatic disease, 89
  radical cystectomy, 67–76
    abdominal exploration, 69
    anterior apical dissection in male
      patients, 71–2
    anterior dissection in female patients,
      72
    bowel mobilization, 69–70
    definition, 68
    incision, 69
    ligation of lateral vascular pedicle to
      bladder, 70
    ligation of posterior pedicle to bladder,
      70–1
    patient positioning, 69
    pelvic lymphadenectomy, 70
    post-operative care, 74

    pre-operative evaluation, 68, 73
    pre-operative radiation therapy,
      68–9
    ureteral dissection, 70
  salvage cystectomy, 73–4
  treatment algorithms, 66, 67
  urethrectomy
    in female patients, 72–3
    in male patients, 73
  urinary diversion and bladder
    replacement, 76–84
    conduit diversion, *80*
    continent diversion and bladder
      reconstruction, 80–1
      continence mechanism in bladder
        replacement, 81
      continence mechanism in continent
        diversion, 81
      features of reservoir, 80–1
      Mitrofanoff principle, 81
      nipple valve, 81
      tapered efferent loop, 81
    electrolyte disturbances, 78–9
      gastric reservoirs, 78
      hyperammonemia, 79
      hyperchloremic acidosis, 78
      jejunal conduits, 78
      magnesium and calcium, 78–9
    emptying of reservoir and
      reconstructed bladder, 82
    functional results and urinary
      continence, 83
    ileo-cecal pouches, 82
    Kock pouch, 82
    metabolic and bowel problems, 79
    pre-operative assessment and
      counselling, 77
    sigmoid neo-bladder, 82–3
    Ulm bladder, 82
    uretero-intestinal anastomosis, 76–7
    uretero-sigmoidostomy, 83
  see also Transitional cell carcinoma
Inverted transitional cell papilloma, *18, 19*
ITGCN *see* Intratubular germ cell
  neoplasia

J

Jejunal conduits, 78
Juxtaglomerular cell tumor, 280, 384–5

K

Ketoconazole, *214*
Keyhole limpet hemocyanin
  carcinoma in situ, 59
  transitional cell carcinoma, 50
Kidney tumors *see* Renal cell carcinoma
Kock pouch, 82

L

LAK cells, 332–3
Lamina propria invasion, 25–6, *25*
Laparoscopic surgery
  partial radical nephrectomy, 318
  prostatectomy, 169
  radical nephrectomy, 318–20
  renal cell carcinoma, 316–21
  transitional cell carcinoma, 376
Laser fulguration, 48
Leiomyosarcoma, 18, *411*
  paratesticular, *484*, *485*
Leukovorin, *241*
Leuprolide acetate, *214*
  side effects, *266*
LHRH agonists, 213–15, *214*
  side effects, *266*
Liposarcoma, *410*, 411
Lomustine, *339*, *340*
Lymph node metastases
  prostate cancer, 187
  renal cell carcinoma, 326
Lymphadenectomy, 539

M

Magnesium losses, 78–9
Magnetic resonance imaging
  prostate cancer, 140, *141*, 154
  renal cell carcinoma, *287*, 288
Malignant fibrous histiocytoma, 411
Malignant rhabdoid tumor of kidney, 282
Malignant teratoma
  differentiated, 425–6
    versus epidermal cyst, 428
  intermediate, 426
  trophoblastic, 426, 427
  undifferentiated, *425*
Marital status, as risk factor for prostate
  cancer, 113
Medical castration, 213–15
  estrogens, 213, *214*
  LHRH agonists, 213–15, *214*
Megestrol acetate, *214*
Melphalan, *339*
Mesoblastic nephroma, 282
Metanephric adenoma, 280
Metastatic disease
  invasive transitional cell carcinoma, 89
  neuroblastoma, 581–2, *583*
  prostate cancer, 236–9
  renal cell carcinoma, 323–9
Methotrexate, 91
Metyrapone stimulation test, *391*
Microwave therapy, 316
Mitoguazone, *339*
Mitomycin

adenocarcinoma of bladder, 98
  dose, *47*
  patient response, *45*
  prophylaxis, *46*
  renal cell carcinoma, *341*
  toxicity, 49
  transitional cell carcinoma, 380
Mitoxantrone, *339*
Mitrofanoff procedure, 81
Monoclonal antibody imaging in prostate
  cancer, 247–53
  ^{111}In-capromab pendetide studies,
    250–2
  anti-PSA and anti-PAP antibodies, 248,
    250
  imaging technique, 248, *250*
  monoclonal antibody 7E11-C5.3,
    250
  radioimmunoconjugates, 248, *249*
MTD *see* Malignant teratoma,
  differentiated
Mucosal biopsy, 53
Muscle invasive bladder cancer, *14*
  bladder preserving treatment, 85–8
Muscularis mucosae invasion, *26*
Myelolipoma, 408

N

Nationality, as risk factor for prostate
  cancer, 112
Navelbine, *339*
Nephrectomy
  adjunctive, for unresectable metastases,
    328
  initial, 327–8
  palliative, 327
  partial radical, 304–6
    indications, 304
    intraoperative sonography, 304
    laparoscopic, 318
    operative technique, 304, *305*, *306*
    pre-operative evaluation, 304
  radical, 296–300
    indications, *296*
    intra-operative complications, 298–9
    laparoscopic, 318–20
    operative approach, 296, *297*
    operative procedure, 297, *298*, *299*
    results, 299–300
  and spontaneous regression of
    metastases, 328–9
Nephro-ureterectomy, 368–70
  incision, *369*
  rationale, *368*, 369
  renal dissection, 369–70
Nephroblastoma *see* Wilms' tumor
Nephrogenic adenoma, 42
Nephrogenic rests, 281–2

Nests of von Brunn, 17
Neuroblastic tumors, *408*, *409*
Neuroblastoma, 579–84
  diagnosis, 579
  distant metastases, 581–2, *583*
  evaluation of primary tumor, *581*, *582*
  imaging, 581
  presentation, 579
  screening for, 582–3
  treatment, 582
  tumor behavior and staging, 579–80
  tumor biology and prognosis, 580–1
Nifedipine, *340*
Nilutamide, *214*, 215
  side effects, *266*
Nipple valves, 81
NMP 22 urinary immunoassay, 54
Non-seminomatous germ-cell tumors,
  433–59
  adjuvant chemotherapy, 442–4
    management preferences, 443–4
    Medical Research Council study, 442,
      443
  algorithms, *439*, *440*
  chemotherapy, 452–9
    chemo-sensitivity, 457
    choice of, 454, *455*
    clinical trials, 454, 455
    late events, 455–6
    patient selection, 453–4
    practical issues, 453
    primary management, 452, *453*
    seminoma, *457*
    stage 1 and 2 disease, *456*
    testis conservation, 456–7
  surgical treatment
    radical orchiectomy, 445
    retroperitoneal lymph node dissection,
      445–6, *447–51*
  surveillance, 440–2
    drawbacks of, 442
    Medical Research Council studies,
      441, *442*
    stage I, 441

O

Obturator nerve injury, 170
Occupation
  and prostate cancer, 113
  and testicular cancer, 113
Oncocytoma, *279*, 384
Oncogenes, 419
Orchiectomy *see* Surgical castration
Ovarian cancer, 549–53
  epidemiology, 549–50
  incidence, *549*
  management, 552–3
  pathology, *550–1*

Ovarian cancer (*cont.*)
  prognostic factors, 552
  secondary adenocarcinoma, 98
  staging, *551*
  treatment, 552

P

Paclitaxel, 91
Palliative care, 597–616
  assessment of pain, 600, *601*, 602
    neuropathic pain, 602
    pain related to movement, 602
    periodic pain, 602
  bleeding, 612, *613*
  bowel obstruction, 604–5, *606*
  breaking bad news, 598, *599*, *600*, *601*
  care services, 597–8
  confusional states, 612, *614*, 615
  constipation, *603*, 604
  diarrhea, 606, *607*, 608
  explanation and planning, 602
  leg edema, 608, *609*, 611
  nausea and vomiting, 604, *605*
  reassessment, 603–4
  treatment of pain, 602, *603*
  urinary problems, *610*, 611–12
Pamidronate, 246
Papillary adenoma, 279–80
Papillary carcinoma, *362*
Papillary renal carcinoma, *278*
Papillary urethritis, 540
Paratesticular sarcoma, 486
Partial radical nephrectomy *see*
    Nephrectomy
Pathology
  adrenal tumors, 407–9
  bladder cancer, 17–36, 96
  dysplasia, 28–30, *28*
  indifferentiated carcinoma, 33, *34*
  inverted transitional cell papilloma, *18*, *19*
  penile carcinoma, 507, *508–10*, 511–12
  prostate cancer, 127–38
  reactive atypia, 28–30
  renal cell carcinoma, 277–83
  retroperitoneal tumors, 409, *410*, 411
  scrotal tumors, *491–3*
  spermatic cord tumors, 483, *484*, *485*
  testicular cancer, 423–9
  transitional cell carcinoma, 19–23, 361
    additional prognostic factors, 23
    alternative grading systems, 22–3
    grading, 20–2, *20*, *21*
    prognostic factors, 22
    reproducibility of grading, 22
    tumor growth and macroscopic
      appearances, 19–20
    variants of, 23, *24*
  transitional cell papilloma, 18

  inverted, *18*, *19*
  urethral carcinoma, *529*, *530*, 531–2
  urothelial carcinoma in situ, 28–30, *29*
Pediatric urologic malignancies
  neuroblastoma, 579–84
    diagnosis, 579
    distant metastases, 581–2, *583*
    evaluation of primary tumor, *581*, *582*
    imaging, 581
    presentation, 579
    screening for, 582–3
    treatment, 582
    tumor behavior and staging, 579–80
    tumor biology and prognosis, 580–1
  rhabdomyosarcoma, 591–4
    bladder and prostate, 592–3
    clinical staging, 591, *592*
    incidence, 591
    paratesticular, 592
    pathology, 592
    vaginal, vulvar and uterine, 593
  Wilms' tumor, 280, *281*, 585–90
    epidemiology, 585, *586*
    genetics, 586
    late effects, 588, *589*
    pathology, 587
    presentation and evaluation, 586–7
    relapse, 588
    staging, *587*
    survival, *589*
    treatment, 587, *588*
Pelvic exenteration, 563–70
  assessment, *563–4*, *565*, *566*, *567*
  diversion and reconstruction, 568, *569*,
    570
  post-operative care, 569
  surgery, 566, 568
  see also Urinary diversion
Pelvic lymph node dissection, 155–6
Pelvic lymphadenectomy, 74
Penile carcinoma
  chemotherapy, 521
  diagnosis, 503
  epidemiology, 499–500
  etiology, 499
  incidence, 499
  pathology, 507, *508–10*, 511–12
    histologic classification, *508*
    macroscopy, *508–9*
    microscopy, *509*, *510*
    prognostic factors, *510–11*
  radiotherapy, 519–21
    results, 520
    techniques, 519–20
    treatment-related complications,
      520–1
  signs and symptoms, 503
  staging, 503, *504*
  surgical management

  algorithm, *514*
  evaluation and management of
    regional nodes, 517–18
  evaluation and treatment of primary
    lesion, 515–16
  management of enlarged/ulcerated
    groin nodes, 518
  partial penectomy, 516
  post-operative management and
    complications, 516, 518
  total penectomy, 516
Pheochromocytoma, 393–4, *395*, 409
Phosphorus[32], *239*
Photodynamic therapy, 62
Plant alkaloids, *339*
Progestins, *338*
Prognosis, 12–13
Prostascint scan, 155
Prostate cancer
  biopsy, 127–8
    after androgen deprivation therapy,
      135
    after cryosurgery, 136
    after radiation therapy, 135, 196–7
  chemotherapy, 253–7, *254*
    anthracycline, 255
    estramustine, 254–5
    suramin, 255
  complications, 261–5
    bladder outlet obstruction, 263–4
    bony destruction and bone pain,
      261–2
    disseminated intravascular
      coagulation, 264–5
    pathologic fractures, 262
    spinal cord compression, 262–3
    ureteral obstruction, 264
  definition, 117
  delayed treatment, 117–21
    localized disease, 118
    locally symptomatic cancer, 121, *122*
    mortality, 121
    overview analysis, 118, *119*
    registry-based studies, 119–21, *120*
    requirements for informative studies,
      117–18
    single institution series, *118*
  diagnostic markers, 136
  digital rectal examination, 140
  early diagnosis and prognostic markers,
    121, 123
    PSA detection, 121, *123*
  early versus late therapy, 117
  endocrine therapy, 203–5, 210–26
    androgen withdrawal, 135, 180–6,
      212–16
      antiandrogens, 215–16
      clinical trials, 181, 181–4, *182*, *183*,
        184

early versus delayed, 204–5
experimental basis, 180, *181*
immediate versus delayed,
226–32
intermittent, 220–1
sequential, 221–2
and irradiation, 200–1, 205
medical castration, 212–15, *214*
prognostic markers, 216–17
quality of life, 220–2, *221*
superiority to castration, 218–19
surgical castration, 213
timing of, 219–20
controversies surrounding,
217–22
hormonal manipulation, *203*, 204
and irradiation, 200–1, 205
side effects, 265, *266*
treatment of emergency conditions,
222
treatment of hot flushes, 222
epidemiology and etiology, 111–16
extraprostatic extension, 133–5
adipose tissue, 133, *134*
anterior muscle, 135
perineural spaces of neurovascular
bundles, 134–5
grading, 131–3, *132*, 153
histological variants of, *133*
imaging studies, 140–2
computed tomography, 140, *141*
magnetic resonance imaging, 140,
141
TRUS, *141*
TRUS-guided sextant biopsy, *142*
incidence, 111
intraepithelial neoplasia, 128–30, *128*,
129
laboratory studies, 142–5
age-specific reference ranges for
PSA, *143*, *144*
molecular PSA, 145
prostate-specific antigen, 142, *143*
PSA density, *144*
PSA velocity, 144, *145*
management of sequelae, algorithm,
260
metastases, 194–5, *196*
androgen withdrawal therapy, 217
bone, 236–9, 244–5
brain, 239–40
liver, 240
palliative radiation therapy, *236–8*,
239–40
treatment algorithms, *207–9*
molecular biology, 136, *137*
monoclonal antibody imaging, 247–53
anti-PSA and anti-PAP antibodies,
248, 250

In-capromab pendetide studies,
250–2
imaging technique, 248, *250*
monoclonal antibody 7E11-C5.3,
250
radioimmunoconjugates, 248, *249*
mortality, *112*
natural history, 117–25
outcome of treatment, 123
pathologic diagnosis, 130–1, *130*
pathology, 127–38
patient history, 149
prevalence, 111–12
prognostic markers, 123, 136
prostatectomy *see* Prostatectomy
radiotherapy, 135, 176–7, 190–203,
233–42
external beam irradiation, 176, 190,
191, *192*
failure of, 192–5
distant metastases, 194, *195*
pelvic, 192, *193*, *194*
interstitial brachytherapy, 176
locally recurrent carcinoma, 233–6,
234, *235*
morbidity, 197, *198*
palliative
bone metastases, *236–8*, 239
brain metastases, 239–40
pelvic recurrence, 235–6
positive biopsy after, 196, *197*
pre-treatment PSA and results of,
195, *196*
results, 177
side effects, 266–7
three-dimensional treatment planning,
198, *199*
rhabdomyocarcoma, 592–3
risk factors
benign prostatic hyperplasia, 113
dietary fat, 112
family history, 114
hormone status, 113
occupation, 113
race and nationality, 112
sexual activity and marital status, 113
vasectomy, 113
viral, 113–14
vitamins, 113
screening, 145–7
effectiveness of, 146, *147*
optimal use of diagnostic tools, 145,
146
secondary adenocarcinoma, 98
side effects of cancer management,
265–8
hormone manipulation, 265, *266*
radiotherapy, 266–7
surgery, 267–8

spinal cord compression, 240–1
staging, 151–7, 186–7
digital rectal examination, 153
evaluation of distant spread, 155–6
evaluation of local mass, 152–5, *154*
influence of high-grade disease on
prognosis, 187
lymph node metastases, 187
magnetic resonance imaging,
154
over/understaging, 186–7
prostate-specific angigen, 153,
154
RTPCR, 155
TNM system, *152*
transrectal ultrasound, 153–4
volume, 154–5
Whitmore/Jewett system, 151, *152*
surgery *see* Prostatectomy
survival, *120*, 188
treatment
algorithms, *160*, *161*, 179
patient factors, 162, *163*
radiotherapy, 176–7
tumor factors, 162
watchful waiting, 164–7
Prostate gland, androgen effects on,
210
Prostate-specific antigen, 121, *123*, 142,
143
age-specific reference ranges for, *143*,
144
and androgen withdrawal therapy,
216–17
density, *144*
molecular, 145
molecular forms, *143*
in monitoring of prostate cancer, 231
post-prostatectomy elevation, 233
pre-treatment levels and therapy results,
195–6, *197*
role in staging, 153, *154*
velocity, 144, *145*
Prostatectomy, 133, 167–74
biochemical progression, 189
cancer-specific survival, 188
candidates for, *168*
clinical progression, 188, *189*
complications, 169, *170*, *171–2*, 189,
267–8
intraoperative, 170
post-operative, 170–3
bladder neck contracture, 173
impotence, 172–3
incontinence, 172
lymphocele, 171–2
post-operative pain, *171*
thromboembolic events, 170–1
laparoscopic, 169

Prostatectomy (*cont.*)
    local recurrence, 188, *189*
    management of margin positive disease, 173–4
    outcomes, *173*
        clinically locally advanced disease, 187, *188*, *189*
        overall survival, 187, *188*
        perineal versus radical retropubic, 168–9
        pre-operative preparation, 168
        rationale for, 186–90
        side effects, 267–8
Prostatic intraepithelial neoplasia, 128–30, *128*, *129*
    molecular biology, 136, *137*
    see also Prostate cancer
Prostatic urethral CIS, *27*, 61
Proto-oncogenes, 4–5
PSA *see* Prostate-specific antigen
Pulmonary embolism, 170

Q

Quinidine, *340*

R

Race *see* Ethnic differences
Radical cystectomy *see* Cystectomy
Radical nephrectomy *see* Nephrectomy
Radical prostatectomy *see* Prostatectomy
Radioimmunoconjugates, 248
Radiotherapy
    bladder adenocarcinoma, 98
    bladder cancer, 105–7
    bladder squamous cell carcinoma, 103, *104*
    cervical cancer, 556
    muscle invasive bladder cancer, 86
    penile carcinoma, 519–21
    pre-operative
        invasive transitional cell carcinoma, 68–9
        radical cystectomy, 72–3
    prostate cancer, 135, 176–7, 190–203, 233–42
        external beam irradiation, 176, 190, *191*, *192*
        failure of, 192–5
            distant metastases, 194, *195*
            pelvic, 192, *193*, *194*
        interstitial brachytherapy, 176, 176–7
        locally recurrent carcinoma, 233–6, *234*, *235*
        morbidity, 197, *198*
        palliative
            bone metastases, *236–8*, 239
            brain metastases, 239–40
        pelvic recurrence, 235–6

positive biopsy after, 196, *197*
    pre-treatment PSA and results of, 195, *196*
    results, 177
    side effects, 266–7
    three-dimensional treatment planning, 198, *199*
scrotal tumors, 494–5
seminoma, 464–5
    bulky seminomas, 464–5
    dose, 464
    and response to chemotherapy, *471*
    stage 1 disease, 464
    stage 2 disease, 464
    supra-diaphragmatic irradiation, 464
    toxicity, 465
spermatic cord tumors, 487–8
urethral carcinoma, 541, *542–4*, 545–6
Renal adenoma, 385
Renal cell carcinoma
    benign adult tumors
        angiomyolipoma, 280
        juxtaglomerular cell tumor, 280
        metanephric adenoma, 280
        oncocytoma, *279*
        papillary adenoma, 279–80
    chemotherapy, 338, *339*, *340*
        biological therapy combined with, 339–40, *341*
    cryotherapy, 316
    diagnosis, 286–90
        cystic renal masses, *290*, 291
        radiologic imaging, *286*, *287*, 288
        solid renal masses, *288*, *299*
    epidemiology, 274
    etiology, 273–4
    focused ultrasound ablation, 311–16
        application to kidney, *313*, *314*
        clinical application, 312–13
        malignant tumors, 311, *312*
        technical principle, 311
    genetics/molecular biology, 274–5
    hormonal therapy, 337, *338*
    immunotherapy, 329–37
        cellular therapy, 332–3
        combination therapy, 331, *332*
        gene therapy, 333–4
        interferons, *330*
        interleukin-2, 330, *331*
        surgery, 335
    incidence, 273
    laparoscopic surgery, 316–21
        background, 317
        current status, 317
        diagnosis, 317
        partial nephrectomy, 318
        radical nephrectomy, 318–20
        wedge excision, 318

localized symptoms from primary tumor mass, 285
malignant adult tumors, *277*
    chromophobe renal carcinoma, 278, *279*
    clear cell carcinoma, 277, *278*
    collecting duct carcinoma, 279
    papillary renal carcinoma, *278*
metastases
    lymph node resection, 326
    non-regional, 326–7
    spontaneous regression, 328–9
    treatment algorithm, *323*, *324*
    tumor embolization, 325–6
    unresectable, 327, 328
microwave therapy, 316
pathology, 277–83
pediatric tumors
    clear cell sarcoma, 282–3
    cystic nephroma and cystic partially differentiated nephroblastoma, 282
    malignant rhabdoid tumor of kidney, 282
    mesoblastic nephroma, 282
    nephroblastoma, 280, *281*
    nephrogenic rests, 281–2
presentation, 285
staging, 290–2
    prognosis based on, 291, *292*
    radiologic imaging, 290–1
    staging systems, *291*
surgery
    algorithm, *295*
    neoplastic involvement of renal vein and inferior vena cava, 300–3
        operative technique, *301*, *302*, *303*
        pre-operative evaluation and management, 301
    partial radical nephrectomy, 304–6, 318
        indications, 304
        intraoperative sonography, 304
        operative technique, 304, *305*, *306*
        pre-operative evaluation, 304
    radical nephrectomy, 296–300, 318–20
        indications, *296*
        intra-operative complications, 298–9
        operative approach, 296, *297*
        operative procedure, 297, *298*, *299*
        results, 299–300
    wedge excision, 318
Renal leiomyoma, 385
Renal medullary carcinoma, 383
Renal pelvis
    percutaneous tumor resection, *373*, 374–5

transitional cell carcinoma, 355–9,
  373–4
Renal sarcoma, 385–6
Retinoic acid, *341*
Retrograde pyelography, 43–4
Retroperitoneal fibrosis, 403, *404*
Retroperitoneal lymph node dissection
  high-stage testicular cancer, 446
  low-stage testicular cancer, 445–6
  morbidity, 451
  results, *451*
  technique
    basics, 446, *447*, *448*
    high-stage modifications, 449, *450*,
      451
    low-stage modifications, *448*, 449
Retroperitoneal tumors
  algorithm, *397*, *398*
  clinical presentation, 402
  diagnostic imaging, 402
  leiomyosarcoma, *411*
  liposarcoma, *410*, 411
  lymphoma, 401
  malignant fibrous histiocytoma, 411
  metastatic disease, *401*
  pathology, 409, *410*, 411
  primary, *399*, 400
  retroperitoneal fibrosis, 403, *404*
  sarcoma, *400*, 401, 410
  treatment and prognosis, 403
  types of, 401–2
  ureteral obstruction, 402
Reverse transcription of prostate cell
    mRNA, 155
Rhabdomyosarcoma, 18
  paratesticular, *484*, 592
  pediatric, 591–4
    bladder and prostate, 592–3
    clinical staging, 591, *592*
    incidence, 591
    paratesticular, 592
    pathology, 592
    vaginal, vulvar and uterine, 593
Rhenium-186, 239
Rhizoxin, *339*
Risk of recurrence, *12*

S

Salvage cystectomy, 73–4
Sarcoma
  clear cell of kidney, 282–3
  paratesticular, 486
  renal, 385–6
  retroperitoneal, *400*, 401, *410*
  scrotum, 492
Schistosomiasis-associated bladder
    cancer, 3, 4
  genetic alterations in, 7

Screening
  intratubular germ cell neoplasia, 435–6
  prostate cancer, 145–7
  Von Hippel-Lindau disease, *308*
Scrotal tumors
  chemotherapy, 495
  diagnosis, 490
  epidemiology, 489
  etiology, 489
  pathology, *491–3*
    basal cell carcinoma, 492
    carcinoma in situ, 492
    sarcoma, 492
    squamous cell carcinoma, *491–2*
  presentation, 490
  radiotherapy, 494–5
  staging, *490*
  surgical management, 493–4
Seminal fluid analyses, *436*
Seminoma, *424*, *425*, 461–74
  algorithm, *461*
  chemotherapy, 457, 467–74
    lymph node metastases, 470, *471*
    prognosis and response to, 469, *470*
    results, 472
    small volume metastatic seminoma,
      471, 472
    superiority to radiation, *467*, *468*, 469
  extra-gonadal, 465
  granulomatous, 427
  mortality, *468*
  post-surgery treatment, 463
  preservation of fertility, 463
  prognostic indicators, 428
  radiotherapy, 464–5
    bulky seminomas, 464–5
    dose, 464
    and response to chemotherapy, *471*
    stage 1 disease, 464
    stage 2 disease, 464
    supra-diaphragmatic irradiation, 464
    toxicity, 465
  serum tumor markers, 463
  spermatocytic, 425
  staging, *461*
  surgery, 463
  therapeutic options, 462
  treatment, 462
  versus malignant teratoma trophoblastic,
    427
  versus Sertoli cell tumor, 427–8
  versus undifferentiated teratoma, 427
  versus yolk sac tumor, 427
Sertoli cell tumor, 427–8
Sexual activity, as risk factor for prostate
    cancer, 113
Sigmoid neo-bladder, 82–3
Small cell carcinoma, 32, *33*
Smoking, and bladder cancer, 3

Spermatic cord tumors
  algorithm, *481*
  diagnosis, 482
  epidemiology, 482
  etiology, 482
  paratesticular sarcoma, 486
  pathology, 483, *484*, *485*
  presentation, 482
  radiotherapy, 487–8
  staging, 482, *483*
  systemic chemotherapy, 488
Spinal cord compression, 240–1,
    262–3
Squamous cell carcinoma, 29, 30, 363
Squamous metaplasia, 42
Staging *see* Tumor staging
Stone disease, 47
Stricture disease, 43
Strontium[89], *238*, *239*, 242–4
  administration, 243
  cost, 243
  efficacy, 243
  physiology, *242*, 243
  radiation protection, 243
  re-treatment, 243
  toxicity, 243
Superficial tumors
  carcinoma in situ, 13–14
  grade, *13*
  T1 disease, 13
  Ta disease, 13
Suramin, 255, *339*
Surgical castration, 213
  germ cell tumors, 445, 462
  side effects, *266*

T

Taxol, *339*
Taxotere, *339*
Telomerase, 54
Teniposide, *340*
Testicular cancer
  algorithm, *431*
  carcinoma in situ *see* Intratubular germ
    cell neoplasia
  classification, *423*, 424
  diagnosis, 424–6, 432
  differential diagnosis, 426, *427–8*
  etiology, 417–18
    cryptorchidism, 417
    hormones, 417–18
    infectious diseases, 418
    infertility, 417
    inguinal hernia, 417
    prenatal/perinatal risk factors, 418
    trauma, 418
    vasectomy, 417
  genetics, 418–20

Testicular cancer (*cont.*)
cytogenetic studies, 418–19
oncogenes, 419
tumor suppressor genes, 419–20
germ cell tumors
intratubular *see* Intratubular germ cell
neoplasia
non-seminomatous *see* Non-
seminomatous germ-cell tumors
seminomatous *see* Seminoma
incidence, 415–17
age, 415–16
frequency, histology, laterality and
bilaterality, 416–17
occupation, 416
racial differences, 416
malignant teratoma
differentiated, 425–6
intermediate, 426
trophoblastic, 426
undifferentiated, *425*
non-germ cell tumors, 475–7
clinical presentation, 475
diagnosis, 475–6
incidence, etiology and epidemiology,
475
pathology, 476
staging, 476
treatment, 476
non-seminomatous germ-cell tumors
see Non-seminomatous germ-cell
tumors
pathology, 423–9
presentation, 432
prognostic indicators, 428–9
spermatocytic seminoma, 425
staging, 432, *433, 434*
yolk sac tumor, 426
Thiotepa
dose, *47*
patient response, *45*
prophylaxis, *46*
toxicity, 49
transitional cell carcinoma, 380
TNM staging, *11*
bladder, *25, 40*
prostate cancer, *152*
urethra, *26*
Topotecan, *339*
Transitional cell carcinoma, 18, 19–23
additional prognostic factors, 23
chemotherapy, 49, *50*
bropirime, 55
choice of agent and course of
therapy, 52–3, *52*
doxorubicin, 53
epirubicin, 54
mitomycin, 53–4
single dose, 50, *51*

thiotepa, 53
grading, 20–2, *20, 21*
alternative systems, 22–3
and prognosis, 22
reproducibility of, 22
incidence, 3
invasive *see* Invasive transitional cell
carcinoma
macroscopic appearance, 19–20
pathology, 19–23, 361
additional prognostic factors, 23
grade and prognosis, 22
grading, reproducibility of, 22
tumor growth and macroscopic
appearances, 19–20
pattern of tumor growth, 19–20
prognosis, 22
prostatic involvement, *26, 27*
proto-oncogenes, 4–5
risk factors, 3
surgery
complications, 44
laser fulguration, 44
partial cystectomy, 44
total cystectomy, 45
transurethral resection, 42–4
treatment, 41–55
algorithm, 41
BCG, *51, 52*
definition of failure, 48–9
interferon, 54–5
intravesicular, 49–57
keyhole limpet hemocyanin, 50
systemic, 88–94
bladder conservation, 90–1
locally advanced cancer, 89–90
metastatic disease, 89
tumor suppressor genes, 5–7, *5*
upper urinary tract, 349–53
benign conditions simulating
fibroepithelial polyp, 363, *364*
urothelial metaplasia, 363,
364
benign tumors, 361
chemotherapy, 379–82
diagnosis, 355–7, *356*
etiology, 349–51
genetics, 351–2
incidence and epidemiology, 349
invasive carcinoma, 362, *363*
inverted papilloma, 361–2
laparoscopic resection, 376
papillary carcinoma, *362*
pathology, 361
presentation, 355
squamous cell carcinoma, 363
staging, *357, 358*
surgical treatment
algorithm, *367*

biolateral disease or solitary
kidneys, 371
conservative open surgery, 372–3
follow up, *370, 371*
nephro-ureterectomy, *368, 369,*
370
patient and operation selection, 370
percutaneous treatment of renal
pelvic tumors, *373, 374*–5
prognosis, 371
ureterectomy, 370
ureteroscopic management, *375, 376*
see also Renal cell carcinoma
urethra, 531
variants of, 23, *24*
Transitional cell papilloma, 18
inverted, *18, 19*
Transrectal ultrasound, *141,* 153–4
sextant biopsy, *142*
Transurethral resection
adenocarcinoma of bladder, 97
carcinoma in situ, 59
complications, 44
concurrent urologic problems
BPH, 43–4
retrograde pyelography, 43
stone disease, 43
stricture disease, 43
invasive transitional cell carcinoma, 86
of prostate (TURP), 192
special situations, 43
transitional cell carcinoma, 42–3
Trauma, and testicular cancer, 418
Trimetrexate, *339*
Triptorelin, *214*
TRUS *see* Transrectal ultrasound
Tumor embolization, 325–6
Tumor grade *see* Grading of tumors
Tumor infiltrating lymphocytes, 332–3
Tumor size, *12*
Tumor staging
bladder cancer, 11, 24, *25, 26, 27, 43*
adenocarcinoma, 97
detrusor muscle invasion, 26
lamina propria invasion, 25–6, *25*
muscularis mucosae invasion, 26
prostatic involvement, *26, 27*
vascular invasion, 27–8
carcinoma in situ, 63
cervical cancer, 554, *555*
neuroblastoma, 579–80
non-germ cell tumors, 476
ovarian cancer, *551*
penile carcinoma, 503, *504*
prostate cancer, 151–7, 186–7
digital rectal examination, 153
evaluation of distant spread, 155–6
evaluation of local mass, 152–5, *154*
grade, 153

influence of high-grade disease on
  prognosis, 187
lymph node metastases, 187
magnetic resonance imaging, 154
over/understaging, 186–7
prostate-specific antigen, 153, *154*
RTPCR, 155
TNM system, *152*
transrectal ultrasound, 153–4
volume, 154–5
Whitmore/Jewett system, 151, *152*
renal cell carcinoma, 290–2
  prognosis based on stage, 291, *292*
  radiologic imaging, 290, *291*
  staging, *291*
scrotal tumors, *490*
seminoma, *461*
spermatic cord tumors, 482–3
testicular cancer, 432, *433, 434*
TNM system, *11*
transitional cell carcinoma, *357*, 358
urethral carcinoma, *526, 527*
uterine cancer, *559*
Wilms' tumor, *587*
Tumor suppressor genes, *5–7*, 419–20

U

Ulm bladder, 82
Ultrasonography, renal, 287
Umbrella cells, 17, 18
Upper urinary tract, transitional cell
    carcinoma *see* Transitional cell
    carcinoma
Ureter
  dissection of, 70
  injury during prostatectomy, 170
  obstruction, 264
  transitional cell carcinoma, 355–9
Ureterectomy, 370
Uretero-intestinal anastomosis, 76–7
Uretero-sigmoidostomy, 83
Ureterovaginal fistulae, 573, *574*
Urethra
  benign tumors of, 539, *540*
    condylomata acuminata, 540
    epithelial neoplasms, 540
    fibroepithelial polyps, 540
    papillary urethritis, 540
    urethral caruncles, 540
  involvement in carcinoma in situ, 61
  management in bladder cancer, 72–3
  TNM staging, *26*
Urethral carcinoma
  chemotherapy, 546
  classification and histopathology, *525*
  diagnosis, 526
  epidemiology, 525
  etiology, 525

incidence, 525
pathology, *529, 530*, 531–2
  adenocarcinoma, 531
  prognostic factors, 531–2
  squamous cell carcinoma, 531
  transitional cell carcinoma, 531
presentation, 525–6
radiotherapy, 541–6
  anterior urethral carcinoma, 541, *542*
  brachytherapy, 542, *543*
  external irradiation, 543, *544*
  posterior urethral carcinoma, 541
  radiation dose, 544
  recurrent urethral carcinoma,
    541–2
  results, 544–5
  sequelae, 545
staging, *526, 527*
surgery, *538–41*
  benign urethral tumors, 539, *540*
  female urethral carcinoma, 539
  male urethral carcinoma, 538–9
treatment algorithms, *535, 536, 537*
Urethral caruncles, 540
Urethrectomy
  female patients, 72–3
  male patients, 73
Urinary diversion, 76–84
  conduit diversion, *80*
    continence mechanism, 81
    continent diversion and bladder
      reconstruction, 80–1
    Mitrofanoff principle, 81
    nipple valve, 81
    patient follow-up, *80*
    reservoir features, 80–1
    tapered efferent loop, 81
  electrolyte disturbances, 78–9
    gastric reservoirs, 78
    hyperammonemia, 79
    hyperchloremic acidosis, 78
    jejunal conduits, 78
    magnesium and calcium, 78–9
  emptying of reservoir and reconstructed
      bladder, 82
  functional results and urinary
      continence, 83
  ileo-cecal pouches, 82
  Kock pouch, 82
  metabolic and bowel problems, 79
  pre-operative assessment and
      counselling, 77
  risk of tumor formation, 79
  sigmoid neo-bladder, 82–3
  Ulm bladder, 82
  uretero-intestinal anastomosis, 76–7
  utero-sigmoidostomy, 83
  see also Pelvic exenteration
Urine cytology, 54

Urogynecologic fistulae, 571–5
  anatomic considerations, 571, *572*
  diagnosis and management, 572–3
  mechanisms of formation
    direct tumor invasion, 572
    radiation injury, 572
    surgical injuries, 571–2
  surgical correction, 573–4
    ureterovaginal fistulae, 573, *574*
    vesicovaginal fistulae, 573–4
Urothelial carcinoma *see* Transitional cell
    carcinoma
Urothelial carcinoma in situ, 28–30, *29*
Urothelial dysplasia, 27–9, *28*
Urothelial hyperplasia, 27–9
Urothelial metaplasia, 363, *364*
Uterine cancer
  adjuvant therapy, 560–1
  diagnosis, *558*
  endometrial hyperplasia, 559
  incidence, 558
  pre-operative evaluation, 559
  prognostic factors, *559*
  recurrence, 561
  rhabdomyosarcoma, 593
  signs and symptoms, *558*
  staging, *559*
  treatment, *560*

V

Vaginal rhabdomyosarcoma, 593
Vasectomy
  and prostate cancer, 113
  and testicular cancer, 417
Verapamil, *340*
Verrucous carcinoma, 31
Vesicovaginal fistulae, 573–4
Vinblastine
  invasive transitional cell carcinoma,
    91
  renal cell carcinoma, *240, 339, 341*
Vindesine, *339*
Vitamins, as risk factor for prostate cancer,
    113
Von Hippel-Lindau disease, 306–10
  ascertainment and screening, *308*
  clinical features and natural history, 306,
    307, 308
  management of renal lesions, 308–9
Vulval rhabdomyosarcoma, 593

W

Watchful waiting in prostate cancer,
    164–7
  benefits and risks of, 165
  management by, 164–5
  outcomes of, 165–6

Whitmore/Jewett staging system, 151, *152*
Wilms' tumor, 280, *281*, 585–90
  epidemiology, 585, *586*
  genetics, 586
  late effects, 588, *589*
  pathology, 587
  presentation and evaluation, 586–7
  relapse, 588

staging, *587*
survival, *589*
treatment, 587, *588*

Y

Yolk sac tumor, 426, 427
Yttrium-90, 239